Practical Pharmacology in Rehabilitation

Effect of Medication on Therapy

Lynette L. Carl, PharmD, BCPS
University of Florida
South University

Joseph A. Gallo, DSc
Salem State University

Peter R. Johnson, PhD
Select Medical Rehabilitation Services

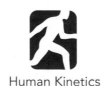

Human Kinetics

Library of Congress Cataloging-in-Publication Data

Carl, Lynette L.
  Practical pharmacology in rehabilitation : effect of medication on therapy / Lynette L. Carl, Joseph A. Gallo, Peter R. Johnson.
    p. ; cm.
  Includes bibliographical references and index.
  I. Gallo, Joseph A., 1968- II. Johnson, Peter R. (Peter Roy), 1942- III. Title.
  [DNLM: 1. Pharmacological Phenomena. 2. Drug Therapy--adverse effects. 3. Recovery of Function--drug effects. 4. Rehabilitation. QV 37]

  615.1--dc23

                           2012041414

ISBN-10: 0-7360-9604-3 (print)
ISBN-13: 978-0-7360-9604-1 (print)

The authors have made every effort to ensure the accuracy of the information herein, particularly with regard to drug selection and dose. However, appropriate information sources should be consulted, especially for new or unfamiliar drugs or procedures. It is the responsibility of every practitioner to evaluate the appropriateness of a particular opinion in the context of actual clinical situations and with due consideration to new developments.

The web addresses cited in this text were current as of March 2013, unless otherwise noted.

Acquisitions Editors: Loarn D. Robertson, PhD, and Amy N. Tocco; **Developmental Editor:** Amanda S. Ewing; **Assistant Editor:** Casey A. Gentis; **Copyeditor:** Amanda M. Eastin-Allen; **Indexer:** Susan Danzi Hernandez; **Permissions Manager:** Dalene Reeder; **Graphic Designer:** Nancy Rasmus; **Graphic Artist:** Dawn Sills; **Cover Designer:** Susan Rothermel Allen; **Photo Production Manager:** Jason Allen; **Printer:** Sheridan Books

Printed in the United States of America   10 9 8 7 6 5 4 3 2 1

The paper in this book is certified under a sustainable forestry program.

Human Kinetics
Website: www.HumanKinetics.com

United States: Human Kinetics
P.O. Box 5076
Champaign, IL 61825-5076
800-747-4457
e-mail: humank@hkusa.com

Canada: Human Kinetics
475 Devonshire Road Unit 100
Windsor, ON N8Y 2L5
800-465-7301 (in Canada only)
e-mail: info@hkcanada.com

Europe: Human Kinetics
107 Bradford Road
Stanningley
Leeds LS28 6AT, United Kingdom
+44 (0) 113 255 5665
e-mail: hk@hkeurope.com

Australia: Human Kinetics
57A Price Avenue
Lower Mitcham, South Australia 5062
08 8372 0999
e-mail: info@hkaustralia.com

New Zealand: Human Kinetics
P.O. Box 80
Torrens Park, South Australia 5062
0800 222 062
e-mail: info@hknewzealand.com

E5204

This book is dedicated to our spouses: Randy Sturgeon, Gina Gallo, and Joanne Johnson. Without their love, support, and encouragement this book would not have been written.

CONTENTS

PART VI Medications Used to Treat Chronic Disease

PREFACE

Clinicians and teachers are often left with questions when using currently available pharmacology textbooks written for those who care for patients undergoing rehabilitation. These textbooks tend to discuss pharmacology as a separate entity and fail to integrate pharmacology into clinical practice in a practical manner that helps the rehabilitation therapist or specialist design a patient-specific therapy plan based on each patient's coexisting disease states and medication therapies.

Practical Pharmacology in Rehabilitation grew out of awareness that a need exists for a textbook for students and a reference book for practicing rehabilitation professionals that takes an interdisciplinary approach to discussing medications and integrates medication use with nonpharmacologic therapies in the rehabilitation patient. *Practical Pharmacology in Rehabilitation*, written by a team that includes a clinical pharmacist, a speech–language pathologist, and a physical therapist and athletic trainer, provides a practical text for rehabilitation practitioners.

Practical Pharmacology in Rehabilitation is a working guide for optimizing rehabilitation sessions through appropriately timing medication administration. It also discusses medication-associated issues that affect the patient's rehabilitation progress and provides examples of appropriate interventions the rehabilitation therapist can make regarding medication use in patients. The text summarizes the pathophysiology associated with specific conditions, the medications used to treat these conditions, methods for optimizing dosing, the most commonly encountered adverse effects, and rehabilitation implications associated with both medication use and the disease state. Each chapter includes patient cases that highlight how medications, drug interactions, and drug intolerances affect speech and language, cognition, activities of daily living, and motor functioning. These patient cases provide a detailed and clear picture of how medications can positively or negatively affect the rehabilitation process.

Organization

The text comprises six parts that are grouped by category of clinical disease. Each chapter provides an overview of the pathophysiology of the diseases discussed, pharmacology of medications used to treat the diseases (i.e., mechanism of action, dosing, monitoring for effects, side effects, effects on rehabilitation, pertinent drug-drug and food-drug interactions), and the roles of the different rehabilitation specialists in providing safe and effective rehabilitation. Almost every chapter includes patient cases that will help the clinician understand and apply the presented concepts.

Part I of the text consists of three introductory chapters that provide the foundational concepts for understanding the clinical disease states and the effect on rehabilitation of the medications used to treat each of these disease states. Chapter 1 explains why the rehabilitation therapist should be familiar with the effects of medications that patients take. It provides an overview of terms used when discussing medications and discusses how medications provide therapeutic effects as well as undesired side effects and how drug interactions can alter the effects of other medications. Every rehabilitation specialist providing patient care should understand these concepts and be able to share them with patients.

Chapter 2 explains how medications can alter the function of the different parts of the nervous system, and in turn, how these medications can affect voluntary and involuntary muscle function. Chapter 2 also provides an introduction to cognition and memory

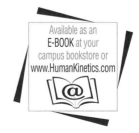

and explains how different medications can affect patients' cognitive function and learning in the rehabilitation process.

Chapter 3 describes the effect of nutrition on rehabilitation and discusses how the different components of a patient's diet may need to be altered in different disease states to provide adequate nutrition and avoid toxicity associated with nutritional imbalances. This chapter also outlines how these disease states and the medications used to treat the clinical conditions can affect nutritional status and immune status and provide effective healing. The section on medication-induced dysphagia discusses how medications can alter the patient's ability to eat and swallow and how they can affect the patient's nutritional status.

Parts II through VI comprise chapters on important disease states that are often encountered in providing rehabilitation therapy. Each part consists of several chapters that cover related disease states grouped together for ease of use. Each chapter begins with an introduction to the condition or special population that is the focus of the chapter. The introduction includes a definition of the condition and a discussion of the incidence, etiology, pathophysiology, and clinical manifestations of the disorder. The next section of each chapter discusses the specific classes or classifications of medications used to treat the patient population being discussed. Topics in the medication section include indications, physiologic action of the medication, contraindications, in-depth information on initiating and titrating the dose to minimize adverse effects, the most commonly encountered side effects, and important drug interactions. The text includes patient cases, generated from the authors' own clinical experience, that make the discussion of the medications more relevant to the reader. Each chapter then discusses rehabilitation considerations, including the effects of medications on speech, language, cognition (including sensory memory, working memory, the declarative memory system, and the nondeclarative memory system), activities of daily living, and motor functioning as well as how the condition affects the patient's performance in rehabilitation and activities of daily living. Each chapter

ends with a short summary of the important aspects covered in the chapter.

The tables in each chapter present material in a format that is easy to access. Each chapter strongly emphasizes how the medications being discussed affect the patient during the rehabilitation process and during activities of daily living. More comprehensive tables, available in the text's web resource, provide additional detail, including dosing information for each medication and more detailed information on drug interactions and considerations. An icon in the book next to each abbreviated table directs the reader to the web resource. (See the "Web Resource" section that follows for more information.)

Practical Pharmacology in Rehabilitation emphasizes the use of a proactive approach in educating the patient and caregiver and monitoring the patient for side effects. The rehabilitation specialist will be able to prevent adverse occurrences such as falls and other medical complications by using the provided information to implement proactive approaches, and initiate important dialogue with the patient's prescriber and pharmacist. The case studies engage the reader in the process of recognizing the adverse responses associated with both the patient's condition and the medications used to treat the condition and determining possible solutions to the scenarios provided.

Part II of this text discusses psychiatric and cognitive disorders commonly seen in rehabilitation practice. Although patients may not be referred to rehabilitation for these clinical conditions, these conditions and the medications used to treat them will affect rehabilitation and therefore need to be considered when developing a patient-specific treatment plan.

Chapter 4 discusses the clinical disease states of depression and bipolar (manic–depressive) disease as well as the medications used to treat these disorders. Chapter 5 reviews the psychiatric diseases of psychosis and schizophrenia, describes how these disorders can affect rehabilitation, and discusses the therapeutic effects, side effects, and drug interactions of medications used to treat these disorders. The rehabilitation therapist should consider these effects when developing therapy sessions and monitoring the patient in order to maintain a safe rehabilitation environment. Chapter 6 provides an overview of cognitive disorders such as delirium and the dementias, including Alzheimer's disease, and discusses the effect of medication use on these disorders and the rehabilitation progress. Chapter 7 differentiates general symptoms of anxiety that we all experience in everyday living from the clinical disease states that comprise anxiety disorders. A discussion is provided regarding pathophysiology and treatments for insomnia. Finally, this chapter provides information on pharmacologic and nonpharmacologic treatments of these disorders and explains how these disorders can affect rehabilitation progress, while providing guidance on how to adjust therapy sessions for patients with these disorders to optimize progress while maintaining a safe environment.

The chapters in part III deal with neurologic and movement disorders, including Parkinson's disease, stroke, seizure disorders, skeletal muscle disorders, and some of the demyelinating neuromuscular diseases. Chapter 8 discusses seizure disorders, and chapter 9 reviews the treatment of spasticity and of muscle spasm. Chapter 10 reviews Parkinson's disease and related treatments of the motor symptoms of the disease. Chapter 11 discusses amyotrophic lateral sclerosis, multiple sclerosis, and myasthenia gravis and the associated therapies used to treat these disorders. Chapter 12 reviews clinical conditions that result in movement disorders as well as medication-induced movement disorders. Each chapter discusses medication use and methods for optimizing therapy sessions and patient outcomes.

Part IV deals with the treatment of pain and provides an overview of commonly encountered substance-abuse disorders. Although pain management may not be the primary reason a patient is referred to rehabilitation therapy, pain can significantly affect the patient's rehabilitative progress. Chapter 13 reviews common conditions associated with acute pain, discusses the impact of failure to control pain on rehabilitation success, and provides an overview of pharmacologic and nonpharmacologic treatments commonly used to manage acute pain. Chapter 14 reviews

common syndromes associated with chronic pain and explains how therapy for managing chronic pain differs from treatment of acute pain associated with injury. Chapter 15 reviews substance-use disorders, including abuse of prescription drugs, alcohol, and illicit drugs and the effect of these disorders on rehabilitation. This chapter also provides an overview of medications commonly used to treat substance-use disorders, methods for monitoring patients with substance-use disorders, and methods for appropriately altering rehabilitation sessions. The rehabilitation therapist should understand the symptoms associated with substance-use disorders as well as symptoms of withdrawal in order to effectively monitor the patient and ensure that rehabilitation sessions are safe and effective.

Part V provides information on disorders that affect the immune system, including infections, rheumatic disease, and cancer. All chapters summarize the clinical disease state and discuss the impact of these disease states, medication therapies, and other therapies on the patient's rehabilitation. Chapter 16 provides an overview of the infections most commonly encountered in the patient undergoing rehabilitation as well as the medications and other treatments used to treat them. It also discusses concepts of infection control that the rehabilitation therapist must use to prevent the spread of infections to other patients and caregivers. Chapter 17 reviews osteoarthritis, gout, and rheumatoid arthritis disorders and the associated treatments. Chapter 18 introduces the treatment of different types of cancer and supportive therapies that are commonly used in these patients, such as methods for managing radiation- or chemotherapy-associated nausea and vomiting, anemia, neutropenia, and mucositis. A section also discusses cancer-associated fatigue.

The chapters in part VI summarize chronic diseases commonly encountered in rehabilitation, including diabetes, cardiac disease, thyroid and parathyroid disease, respiratory disease, and gastrointestinal disease, as well as dysphagia associated with these diseases. Patients may not be referred to rehabilitation for these diseases. However, because these diseases and the associated medication therapies can affect rehabilitation, the rehabilitation therapist must consider them when developing an effective rehabilitative treatment plan. All chapters summarize the clinical disease states and discuss the impact of these diseases, and the medications and other types of therapies used to treat them, on rehabilitation. Chapter 19 summarizes the cardiac diseases of hypertension, congestive heart failure, and cardiac arrhythmias. Chapter 20 reviews disease states associated with atherosclerosis, including peripheral artery disease, stroke, and coronary heart disease. Chapter 21 provides an overview of diabetes and some of the complications associated with diabetes, such as peripheral neuropathy and diabetic foot infections, that can affect the rehabilitation plan. Chapter 22 discusses common respiratory diseases such as chronic obstructive pulmonary disease, which includes chronic bronchitis, emphysema, and asthma. This chapter discusses medications and other therapies used to treat these conditions as well as methods for adjusting patient therapy sessions appropriately. Chapter 23 reviews thyroid disease, parathyroid disease, and osteoporosis and discusses current treatments of these disease states and methods for preventing osteoporosis. Chapter 24 reviews commonly seen gastrointestinal disorders and medication-induced dysphagia, as well as methods of identifying, preventing, and treating dysphagia.

The appendix provides information on administering medications using iontophoresis and phonophoresis. A glossary of terms is provided at the end of the book; glossary terms are in bold font in the text. Two indexes follow the glossary. The first index lists all medications discussed in the text, and the second index lists important terms. The authors look forward to and welcome feedback from the reader, which will help improve future editions of this text.

Web Resource

The web resource includes 48 tables that provide more than 200 pages of information. These tables include medication names, indications, dosing recommendations, side effects, and, often, other side effects or considerations. Because the tables are delivered in PDF format, searching for specific medications is easy.

Throughout the chapters, this wording points readers to these full tables:

@ See table 4.1 in the web resource for a full list of medication-specific indications, dosing recommendations, and side effects.

The tables can be accessed at www.Human Kinetics.com/PracticalPharmacologyIn Rehabilitation.

This text serves as both a textbook for students in the rehabilitation field and related health care fields and a go-to reference for practicing clinicians who want to access practical, evidence-based information quickly and efficiently during clinical practice.

ACKNOWLEDGMENTS

We would like to thank Joseph Murphy for authoring the appendix on medication delivery using iontophoresis and phonophoresis; Lori Eskridge and Michele Fox for providing valuable feedback and guidance as reviewers of this textbook; Loarn Robertson, PhD for serving as our acquisitions editor at Human Kinetics prior to his retirement; Amy Tocco, senior acquisitions editor, for all of her efforts and assistance with this project; and Amanda Ewing, our developmental editor at Human Kinetics, for all of her insight and support.

REVIEWERS AND CONTRIBUTORS

Reviewers

Lori Eskridge, PharmD, BCPS
Clinical manager at Pharmacy Solutions
Town and Country Hospital
Tampa, FL

Michele Fox, PT, DPT, CSCS
Associate director of clinical education, lecturer
Doctor of physical therapy program
University of Massachusetts at Lowell
Lowell, MA

Contributor

Joseph Murphy, PhD, ATC
Assistant professor
Athletic training program clinical education
coordinator
Salem State University
Salem, MA

Foundations

Part I consists of three introductory chapters that provide the foundational concepts for understanding clinical disease states and the effects of the medications used to treat common disease states encountered in patients undergoing rehabilitation.

Chapter 1 explains why the rehabilitation therapist should be familiar with the effects of medications that patients take. It provides an overview of terms used when discussing medications and discusses how medications provide therapeutic effects as well as undesired side effects and how drug interactions can alter the effects of other medications. Every therapist providing patient care should understand these concepts and be able to share them with patients.

Chapter 2 reviews the role of the nervous system in controlling muscle function and cognition. It introduces the parts of the nervous system, including the central nervous system, peripheral nervous system, and enteric nervous system. This chapter also details the role of chemical messengers, called neurotransmitters, in communicating between different nerves and between the nerves and muscles in the body and how this communication affects cognition, learning, and muscle function. The chapter reviews the neurotransmitters most often involved in cognition, motor function, and behavior in the central nervous system, resulting in central nervous system stimulation or depression. The chapter also delineates which neurotransmitters are involved in the coordination of sensory and motor function and how they can affect voluntary and involuntary muscle function. Finally, the chapter explains how medications can affect the levels and effects of these neurotransmitters and alter neurotransmission and function of the different parts of the neuromuscular system.

Chapter 3 describes the effect of nutrition on rehabilitation and discusses how the different components of a patient's diet may need to be altered in different disease states (e.g., cardiac disease, diabetes, respiratory disease, kidney disease, liver disease, pancreatitis, and cancer) to provide adequate nutrition and avoid toxicity associated with nutritional imbalances. This chapter also outlines how these disease states and the medications used to treat the clinical conditions can affect nutritional status and immune status and provide effective healing. The section on medication-induced dysphagia discusses how medications can alter the patient's ability to eat and swallow.

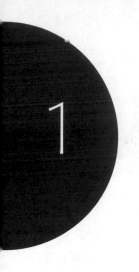

Introduction to Medication Monitoring by the Rehabilitation Therapist

Data released by the U.S. Department of Health and Human Services indicate that at least one half of all Americans take at least one prescription drug and that one in six Americans takes three or more medications. Use of prescription drugs is increasing among all age groups. Five out of six people aged 65 yr or older take at least one medication, and almost one half of seniors take three or more prescription medications. Patients on multiple medications are subject to drug interactions. This is especially true for older patients, who frequently have more than one disease state and may be taking several medications to control these conditions. In addition, many patients take nonprescription medications and herbal therapies on a routine basis; these can alter the effects of prescription medications. Medications can significantly affect a patient's progress in rehabilitation. The individualized therapy plan should involve a review of the medications that a patient is taking, and during this review the rehabilitation therapist should always ask patients about their use of nonprescription medications, herbal therapies, and other alternative medication such as homeopathic therapies (Niles, 2001; Ross & Kenakin, 2001; Wilkinson, 2001).

A rehabilitation therapist should be knowledgeable about medications for several reasons. First, therapists must know the usual effects of a medication in order to anticipate how it might affect the ability of the patient to participate in rehabilitation therapy. For instance, certain medications may cause fatigue and sedation that interferes with cognition, impairs motor function, and increases the patient's risk of falling during prescribed exercise. Second, a clinician should understand the timing of medication effects in relation to medication administration and schedule rehabilitation sessions for times when medication effects are optimal in order to enhance patient participation and benefit. For example, a clinician could schedule a patient with Parkinson's disease for physical therapy when optimal control of tremors is obtained after taking a medication dose. Another example would be to schedule administration of a short-acting pain medication 1 h before an exercise session in order to enhance patient participation in therapy. Third, a therapist should be able to anticipate the effects of interventions used in rehabilitation therapy on patients taking certain medications and be able to adjust the session to prevent adverse events caused by medications. For example, whirlpool treatments may cause peripheral **vasodilation** in a patient undergoing vasodilator therapy for blood pressure control, and such treatments may result in an acute drop in blood pressure, which could result in a patient fall. In order to achieve these objectives, the rehabilitation therapist should carefully review the medications a patient is taking upon admission to their service and should question the patient before each rehabilitation session about any changes in their medication regimen (Ciccone, 2002; Gadson, 2006; Malone, 1989).

Although medications are prescribed to achieve certain therapeutic effects, their use also can cause undesired effects, called side effects or adverse drug reactions. The therapist must be alert in monitoring for any adverse drug reaction or side effect that a patient may be experiencing, especially with the addition of a new medication or after a dosing change. If such a side effect is identified and interferes with the patient's ability to participate in rehabilitation, the therapist should be proactive in communicating this information to the patient's physician, who may need to adjust the patient's medication dose or therapy.

The therapist also needs to be cognizant of the potential for drug interactions in their patients. A drug interaction occurs when the use of one medication changes the effects of a second medication, resulting in an increase or decrease in the effects of one or both medications. The potential for drug interactions is increased in patients taking multiple medications, in patients with liver or kidney disease, and in the elderly population. For instance, combining the antidepressant fluoxetine (Prozac) with an antipsychotic medication such as haloperidol (Haldol) can lead to increased **extrapyramidal** symptoms such as involuntary movements that may impair motor function and the ability to ambulate. Another example would be adding a medication, such as prochlorperazine for nausea, to the medication regimen of a patient with Parkinson's disease who is being treated with Sinemet with the adverse outcome of reduced control of tremor. Drug interactions can significantly influence rehabilitation. The clinician should be alert to the possibility that new symptoms affecting a patient may be related to a drug interaction or side effect caused by a change in medication or dose (Carl & Johnson, 2006).

This chapter discusses the principles of pharmacotherapy, pharmacokinetics, and pharmacodynamics and explains how medications provide therapeutic effects, why medications are dosed in a certain way, how medications can cause undesired side effects, and how medications can alter the effects of other medications. All of these factors can influence the way a patient responds to medications and can affect patient rehabilitation.

Principles of Pharmacotherapy

Pharmacotherapy is the study of the use of medications to prevent, diagnose, and cure disease. Pharmacotherapy integrates principles of anatomy and physiology, pathophysiology, and pharmacology. Pharmacotherapy may be further divided into two domains: pharmacokinetics and pharmacodynamics.

Pharmacokinetics

Pharmacokinetics is the study of how medications are absorbed, distributed, metabolized, and eliminated in the body based on an individual patient's characteristics. Pharmacokinetics is useful in predicting the drug level achieved in an individual patient after administration of a specified dose. It also helps one predict how long it will take for the medication to have the desired effect, how long those effects will continue, and when it will become necessary to redose the medication. The pharmacokinetic characteristics of a medication help one determine an effective dosing regimen in order to achieve and maintain therapeutic effects (Bauer, 2002; Blumenthal & Garrison, 2011; Buxton & Benet, 2011).

Absorption (Route) of Medications

Absorption of medications can occur through many different routes. Most popular is the oral route, in which a capsule, tablet, or liquid is swallowed, absorbed into the gastrointestinal tract, and distributed to other parts of the body through the circulatory system (bloodstream). Oral absorption usually takes between 30 and 60 min; however, this can vary based on the dosage form of the medication (extended release versus immediate release), the motility of the gastrointestinal tract, the extent that the different parts of the gastrointestinal system break down the medication, and the extent that the liver breaks down the medication before passing it into the circulatory system.

Diabetic gastroparesis is an example of a patient condition that can significantly affect the motility of the gastrointestinal tract. Gastroparesis results in decreased gastric emptying and delayed absorption, thus delaying the effects of the medication (Buxton & Benet, 2011; Carl & Johnson, 2006; Niles, 2001; Ross & Kenakin, 2001; Wilkinson, 2001).

Enteric-coated medications are formulated with a protective coating that minimizes acid breakdown of the medication and allows the medication to pass intact from the stomach into the small bowel, where it is absorbed. The enteric-coated dosage form also protects the patient from stomach damage from such products as aspirin. The Institute of Safe Medical Practices website (www.ismp.org/tools/donotcrush.pdf) includes a list of medications that are specially formulated for optimal absorption and that should not be crushed before administration (Buxton & Benet, 2011).

The absorption of medications through the sublingual, buccal, and rectal routes of administration is more rapid than absorption through the oral route because the medications are absorbed by mucous membrane and directly enter the bloodstream, thus avoiding the delay of transit through the gastrointestinal tract. In sublingual administration, medications are placed under the tongue and provide effects within 5 min. For example, nitroglycerin may be sublingually administered to a patient who has chest pain. In buccal administration, the medication is sucked and is delivered directly through the mucosal layer in the cheek portion of the mouth. For example, Actiq buccal lollipops, which contain fentanyl, provide rapid pain relief in patients with severe breakthrough pain (Buxton & Benet, 2011). In rectal administration of medications, drug absorption is more variable than with oral administration. However, the onset of effects is rapid and usually occurs within 5 min. Patients who are not able to swallow, such as patients in hospice care, often receive medications via this route. This route is also helpful in patients with nausea and vomiting and is an alternative route for medication administration that the patient or a family member can use (Buxton & Benet, 2011).

The inhalation route is a very effective way of administering medications directly to the respiratory tract for treatment of patients with respiratory disease. Examples of inhaled medications include nebulized medications or medications given through an inhaler for patients with asthma or chronic obstructive pulmonary disease. Because inhaled medications bypass the gastrointestinal tract and are absorbed directly into the respiratory tract, onset of action is very rapid. Administering medications by the inhalation route also minimizes side effects because the dosage requirement is much lower than that of medications administered in an oral or injectable dosage form (Buxton & Benet, 2011).

The transdermal route is another route of medication administration that bypasses the gastrointestinal tract. In transdermal administration, the medication, which can be an ointment or cream or can be embedded in a patch, is absorbed through the skin. Examples of medications that are administered by this route include nitroglycerin ointment or patches used in patients with angina, scopolamine (Transderm Scop) patches used in motion sickness, and fentanyl (Duragesic) patches used in the patient with chronic pain. Transdermal medication should always be placed in an area where circulation and adipose tissue are adequate to assist with medication absorption. Transdermal patches administer medication through a slow-release mechanism and need to be replaced every 1 to 7 days, depending on the medication. Local irritation can occur at the site where the transdermal medication is placed, so one should rotate the site of placement. To avoid unintentional overdose of the medication, one must take care to remove the old patch when placing a new patch (Bauer, 2002; Buxton & Benet, 2011; Carl & Johnson, 2006; Niles, 2001; Ross & Kenakin, 2001; Vogel et al., 2000; Wilkinson, 2001).

Medications are administered via the **parenteral** (injectable) route when other forms of administration are not possible. Parenteral medications are administered through an intravenous (IV) catheter or via subcutaneous or intramuscular injection. Examples of parenteral medications include insulin administered subcutaneously, iron administered intramuscularly, and **antibiotics** such as vancomycin administered through IV infusion (diluted medications given slowly over longer time periods). Administration of medication via subcutaneous or intramuscular injection can be painful, and administration via the parenteral route is associated with increased complications of infection and local reactions at the injection site. With IV administration, absorption into the bloodstream is very rapid and usually occurs within 15 min. Subcutaneous or intramuscular administration also provides very good blood levels, but absorption into the bloodstream is more delayed (15-30 min for subcutaneous administration and 30-60 min for intramuscular injections). If medications are repeatedly administered via the subcutaneous or intramuscular route, the site of injection must be rotated with each administration and the injection sites should be monitored for any localized irritation from the medication (Bauer, 2002; Buxton & Benet, 2011; Niles, 2001; Ross & Kenakin, 2001; Wilkinson, 2001).

Provision of certain medications may require a special IV catheter called a central line, which is surgically inserted into a central vein. Central veins rapidly transport large volumes of blood from other areas of the body to the heart for delivery to the lungs and oxygenation before recirculation. Medications that are administered through the central catheters are rapidly diluted, thus reducing medication-associated irritation to the vein. Central lines are used to administer medications that are irritating to the veins and that can cause **phlebitis** (inflammation of a vein) or are used for long-term therapy, such as chemotherapy or total parenteral nutrition, that include IV medications. Examples of central lines include subclavian catheters, surgically inserted ports, peripherally inserted central catheters, Hickman catheters, and Broviac catheters. IV catheters provide a portal for administering medications directly into the bloodstream, but they also provide a portal of entry for bacteria and can be associated with IV catheter-associated infections and bloodstream infections. When providing catheter care, one must frequently inspect the IV catheter site and meticulously use appropriate infection-control techniques (Bauer, 2002;

Buxton & Benet, 2011; Niles, 2001; Ross & Kenakin, 2001; Wilkinson, 2001).

The activity level and temperature of the patient and the effectiveness of heart function and blood flow can also affect the extent of absorption of medications. The absorption of medications via the oral route is also affected by the effectiveness of gastrointestinal lubrication, the level of acidity in the stomach, and the rate of motility of medications moving through the gastrointestinal system. The medications that a patient is taking can alter these factors dramatically. For example, anticholinergic agents such as diphenhydramine (Benadryl) can slow gastrointestinal transport of another medication through the gastrointestinal tract and delay its absorption and onset of action (Carl & Johnson, 2006).

Distribution of Medications in the Body

Drug distribution occurs after the medication is absorbed. In drug distribution, the medication is taken to different parts of the body via the circulatory system (bloodstream) and eventually to its target site. Medication may be distributed to different parts of the body, including **interstitial** and intracellular fluids and extravascular tissue such as the different organs. Where a medication eventually collects in the body after the bloodstream delivers it to the tissues is its **drug compartment**. The size of the drug compartment of each medication is its volume of distribution. The volume of distribution is unique for each medication and can vary with the characteristics of the patient receiving the medication. For example, patients who are fluid overloaded will have a larger drug compartment for water-soluble medications, and patients who are obese will have a larger drug compartment for fat-soluble medications. The size of the drug compartment determines the size of the dose that is needed to obtain effective medication concentrations. Using a pool as an example, more chlorine is required to chlorinate an Olympic-size pool (large drug compartment) than to chlorinate a hot tub (small drug compartment) (Bauer, 2002; Buxton & Benet, 2011; Carl & Johnson, 2006; Niles, 2001; Ross & Kenakin, 2001; Wilkinson, 2001).

The drug compartment is also determined by the chemical structure of the medication, which can be charged or uncharged. Charged medications have more difficulty passing through cell membranes. The chemical structure of the medication also determines whether the medication tends to accumulate in fat or water tissues. Water-soluble medications tend to attain higher levels in the bloodstream, are more easily removed by the kidneys, and have a shorter duration of action, whereas lipid-soluble medications tend to accumulate in tissue compartments, remain in the body longer, and have more prolonged effects. The concentration of medication achieved in a particular part of the body depends on a variety of factors, including the perfusion (extent of circulation of blood) of the particular part of the body and the chemical characteristics of the medication, such as the size of its chemical structure (molecular weight), whether it is water or lipid soluble, and how extensively it is bound by circulating proteins such as albumin and globulin in the blood (Buxton & Benet, 2011).

Medications that are extensively bound by proteins in the blood are prevented from easily crossing from the bloodstream into the tissues and to the drug target area, called the **drug receptor**. Plasma proteins normally found in the blood that can bind medications include albumin and alpha-1 glycoprotein. Albumin binds many medications that are acidic. Many basic drugs bind to the plasma protein alpha-1 glycoprotein. The nutritional status of the patient can determine the amount of plasma proteins that are available in the bloodstream. Malnourished patients with liver disease tend to have less protein available for binding to medications and, as a result, more unbound (free) medication is available to cross into the tissues and act at the drug receptor. Because of this, malnourished patients are more susceptible to higher drug levels and more toxicity with the same dose of medication than are those who are well nourished. Higher medication levels can increase the patient's response to the medication, increase side effects associated with the medication, and interfere with the patient's ability to participate in rehabilitation. Provision of adequate nutrition should always be part of a patient's rehabilitation plan (Blumenthal & Garrison, 2011; Buxton & Benet, 2011; Carl & Johnson, 2006; Ciccone, 2002; Gadson, 2006; Malone, 1989).

When a medication enters the bloodstream, the blood flow of the circulatory system determines the initial distribution of the medication. The brain, heart, liver, and kidneys are all highly perfused organs; therefore, medications are delivered to these organs very soon after entry into the bloodstream. Distribution to other compartments, such as muscle, skin, and fat, takes longer, and medications that are distributed to these tissues may not reach their normal area of distribution, or their drug compartment, for several hours after administration. The amount of time it takes for a medication to reach its final drug compartment and receptor site can determine how quickly it works, which is termed its **onset of action** (Blumenthal & Garrison, 2011; Buxton & Benet, 2011).

Some medications undergo a **first-pass effect**. After oral administration, these medications undergo extensive metabolism in the liver before entering the bloodstream or circulatory system. As a result, when given orally, the levels of these medications are significantly reduced before distribution. Therefore, significantly larger oral doses of these medications are required in order to achieve therapeutic levels. This is important when converting medications from oral to injectable doses because injectable doses do not undergo a first-pass effect and doses are substantially lower to avoid unintentional overdose. For example, the oral dose of propranolol (Inderal) is 40-80 mg and the equivalent injectable dose is 1 mg (Buxton & Benet, 2011).

Agents that are very lipid soluble tend to accumulate in fat tissue and then slowly diffuse into the rest of the body compartments. Medications such as anesthetic agents and sedatives are frequently lipid soluble and tend to accumulate and stay in the fat (lipid) compartment of the body. These medications tend to reenter the bloodstream slowly, resulting in prolonged effects of sedation. This explains the hangover effect that a patient may experience after administration of sedatives or anesthesia. The hangover effect is also influenced by the length of time a patient is under sedation or anesthesia as well the depth of the anesthesia. For example, patients undergoing open-heart surgery are under deep anesthesia for a prolonged period of time. As a result, it is not uncommon for such patients to experience cognitive decline after surgery that affects the patient's response to rehabilitation. Short-term memory loss and difficulty finding words are frequently reported sequelae of surgery. Modern anesthesiology seeks to attain the proper depth of anesthesia to prevent awareness without encumbering the patient with drugs that are not vital to the surgical procedure (Buxton & Benet, 2011; Carl & Johnson, 2006; Ciccone, 2002; Gadson, 2006; Malone, 1989).

Two mechanisms that are important in protecting patients from medication toxicity are the blood–brain barrier and the placenta. The **blood–brain barrier** prevents medications from entering the central nervous system from the circulatory system. The blood–brain barrier comprises a series of tight junctions at the area where the capillaries provide blood flow into the central nervous system. Medications must be transported across the blood–brain barrier by carrier proteins, which protect the brain from the toxic effects of many medications. The placenta has a low rate of blood flow, reducing the rate and extent of medication diffusion from maternal blood to the fetus and thereby helping protect the unborn child from exposure to the high levels of medications found in the mother's blood (Carl & Johnson, 2006; Ciccone, 2002; Gadson, 2006; Malone, 1989).

Elimination of Medications

How the body eliminates a medication is determined by the chemical characteristics of the medication. Elimination of medications from the body occurs by two main mechanisms: metabolism by the liver and elimination by the kidney. A medication can also be eliminated by both the liver and kidneys. Medications that are ionized with an acid or base charge, those that are water soluble, and those that are of small molecular size are more easily

removed by the kidneys. Medications that are lipid soluble and are of larger molecular size are more often prepared for elimination by the process of **metabolism**. Metabolism converts medications into metabolites that are more water soluble in order to assist in their elimination. Medications that are metabolized by the liver can be eliminated through the feces or kidneys. In most cases, metabolism changes a medication from an active form to an inactive form, but some medications are metabolized to another active form. These are called active **metabolites**. Other routes of drug elimination include breast milk, saliva, respiration, tears, and sweat (Buxton & Benet, 2011; Niles, 2001; Ross & Kenakin, 2001; Wilkinson, 2001).

The two major types of metabolism are phase 1 and phase 2. Phase 1 metabolism changes the chemical structure of the medication by **oxidation**, **reduction**, or **hydrolysis**. Most of these chemical reactions are mediated by the cytochrome P450 enzymes. Several hundred forms of these enzymes exist. These enzymes are found primarily in the liver; however, they are also found in smaller quantities in the lungs, kidneys, and gastrointestinal tract. A specific group of cytochrome P450 enzymes is involved in the metabolism of each medication. Phase 2 metabolism involves the **conjugation** (chemical combining) of the medication with more water-soluble groups such as glucuronic acid, glutathione, acetate, or sulfate. This reduces the lipid solubility of the medication, making it easier for the body to eliminate the medication (Bauer, 2002; Buxton & Benet, 2011; Carl & Johnson, 2006; Niles, 2001; Ross & Kenakin, 2001; Wilkinson, 2001).

The age of the patient can also affect the extent of absorption, rate of metabolism, and rate of renal elimination. In pediatric patients, the processes of metabolism and elimination undergo major changes during the transition from neonate to infant and then throughout childhood and adolescence. Special attention to adjustment of dosing is required as children get older. Metabolism and renal elimination of medications become less efficient in the adult patient with each decade of age. Because of this, the senior adult may require a lower dose of medication than a younger adult to maintain the desired medication levels. Failure to decrease dose in the older patient may result in increased side effects and toxicity, can affect medication adherence (taking the medication as prescribed), and may impair progress in rehabilitation (Blumenthal & Garrison, 2011; Carl & Johnson, 2006).

Drug Interactions and Altered Metabolism

The specific pathway through which a medication is metabolized can help a clinician predict drug interactions between one or more medications. A drug interaction occurs when one medication influences the action of another medication. Several types of drug interactions can occur. Antagonism occurs when one medication reduces the action of another medication. One example of this is enzymatic induction, in which the metabolism of one medication is sped up (or induced) by a second medication. This results in decreased action of the first medication and may require an increase in dose of the first medication to maintain the desired therapeutic effect. **Potentiation** occurs when the one medication potentiates, or makes stronger, the action of the second medication. An example is enzymatic inhibition, in which the metabolism of one medication is reduced by a second medication. This drug interaction can result in higher levels of the first medication and can increase the risk of drug toxicity associated with the first medication. Drug interactions involving altered metabolism (enzymatic induction or inhibition) frequently occur when the two involved medications are both metabolized by the same type of cytochrome P450 enzymes in the liver (Blumenthal & Garrison, 2011).

Some medications can actually increase their own metabolism; this is termed **metabolic autoinduction**. An increase in dosage may be required in order to maintain therapeutic levels and effects over time. A requirement for increased dose over time is termed drug tolerance. Tolerance frequently occurs with the use of narcotic pain medications and **anticonvulsants** such as carbamazepine (Tegretol) (Blumenthal & Garrison, 2011).

In addition, patients may have different metabolic rates due to heredity and genetic makeup; some are termed fast metabolizers and others are termed slow metabolizers. Such differences can change the effects of medications and dosage required to maintain therapeutic concentrations as well as the likelihood of encountering side effects with the use of certain medications (Blumenthal & Garrison, 2011).

Drug Interactions and Absorption

Drug interactions in which one medication affects the absorption of another medication in the gastrointestinal tract can occur when one medication binds to another medication (**chelation**), thus preventing its absorption. For example, when the antibiotic tetracycline is given at the same time as medications containing aluminum, magnesium, or calcium, the absorption and effects of the tetracycline are decreased. This form of drug interaction can be avoided by adequately spacing the times of administration of the two medications. On the other hand, absorption of some medications can be altered by medications that change the acidity (pH) of the stomach. **Antacids** can decrease stomach acidity and thus affect the absorption of other medications that require stomach acid for chemical degradation and absorption. Antacids can cause enteric-coated medications to be absorbed in the stomach rather than in the small intestine. Administration of an acidic medication such as vitamin C with certain medications such as dextroamphetamine can cause the dextroamphetamine to become chemically charged (**ionized**), thus reducing its absorption and therapeutic effects (Buxton & Benet, 2011; Carl & Johnson, 2006; Ciccone, 2002; Gadson, 2006; Malone, 1989).

Pharmacodynamics

Whereas pharmacokinetic principles study how the body processes medications, the field of pharmacodynamics determines how and where in the body a medication elicits its actions (Bauer, 2002; Blumenthal & Garrison, 2011; Buxton & Benet, 2011). Pharmacodynamics helps to describe the mechanism of action of the medication at the cellular and organ-system levels. Pharmacodynamic studies identify the sites in the body with which medications interact (target drug receptors) to achieve their desired therapeutic effects as well other drug receptors with which medications interact that cause their undesired side effects.

Target Receptors for Medication Action

Medications work by binding to target areas in the body, called **receptors**, to elicit the desired pharmacologic (therapeutic) response. These target areas include intracellular receptors, ion channels, transport molecules, and enzymes that catalyze chemical reactions. Intracellular receptors such as the deoxyribonucleic acid-coupled receptors and kinase-linked receptors mediate protein synthesis and transcription of genes. Examples of intracellular receptors include receptors for hormones such as estrogen, cortisol, and insulin (Blumenthal & Garrison, 2011; Carl & Johnson, 2006).

In order to reach these receptors from the bloodstream medications must be able to pass through cell membranes to the target receptor. Cell membranes comprise a fat-soluble layer and a water-soluble layer. Most medications can cross the cell membrane in three ways. The first is passive diffusion through the lipid membrane. This is the primary method by which medications cross cell membranes. Medications that are fat soluble are able to diffuse readily across cell membranes to their target site. The second is diffusion through the water-filled ion channels located throughout the cell membrane. Ion receptors are proteins arranged around a central aqueous channel or pore. These channels or pores open in response to a medication binding to the site and allow transport of ions across a tissue membrane. Examples of such receptors include sodium and calcium channels. When these receptors are activated, the result is **depolarization** of nerve tissue and resultant nerve transmission. Small ionized or water-soluble medications, such as sodium, potassium, or lithium, also pass through these ion channels (Blumenthal & Garrison, 2011; Carl & Johnson, 2006). The third is facilitated diffusion or active transport using carrier proteins, which bind to the drug and facilitate transport across the membrane. Carrier-mediated processes involve movement of drugs across the blood–brain barrier, the gastrointestinal tract, and the renal tubules in

the kidneys. Energy is required when a drug requires transport across the concentration gradient; this is termed active transport. Guanosine protein (G-protein)-linked receptors assist in transporting medications across the cell membrane and mediate enzymatic activity, muscle contraction, ion channel transport, and cytokine production. G-protein receptors include **muscarinic** acetylcholine receptors, dopamine receptors, norepinephrine receptors, and hormone receptors. A less common method of transport across the cell membrane is pinocytosis, in which the cell membrane engulfs, and subsequently absorbs, a very large molecule (Blumenthal & Garrison, 2011).

Medications that act on only one type of receptor are termed receptor specific. Receptors may have several subtypes. Medications that act on only one of these subtypes are termed selective. Receptor selectivity is often concentration dependent; that is, the medication acts at only one subtype of receptor at low concentrations but may affect more than one subtype at higher concentrations. Medications that are highly selective for a specific receptor provide more targeted action and minimize undesired side effects caused by binding to receptors other than the target receptors (Blumenthal & Garrison, 2011).

Medication binding to a receptor can elicit several different responses. When a medication binds to a target receptor and triggers a desired response, the medication is termed an **agonist**. When a medication binds to a receptor without producing the desired response but prevents a second medication from acting at that receptor, the first medication is termed an **antagonist**. Competitive antagonism occurs when the first medication can be displaced from the receptor by increasing the levels of the second medication (Bauer, 2002; Carl & Johnson, 2006; Niles, 2001; Ross & Kenakin, 2001; Wilkinson, 2001).

Therapeutic Response of Medications

Medication is administered to a patient to achieve a desired therapeutic response. The magnitude of the response tends to increase when higher doses of medication are administered and higher concentrations are achieved at the receptor. Each medication has an associated

therapeutic index, which establishes the desired levels of medication concentration to maintain the desired therapeutic effect while avoiding toxicity (Blumenthal & Garrison, 2011).

Onset of action, or how quickly this therapeutic drug level is achieved, depends on several factors. The route of administration determines the rate of absorption and distribution of the medication to the receptor site. However, reaching a therapeutic drug level and achieving the desired response may take more than one dose. The optimal frequency of dosing is determined by the duration of action of the medication, which depends on the rate of elimination of the medication. *Half-life*, a term used to describe the rate of elimination of a medication, is defined as the time it takes for half of the drug concentration in the body to be eliminated. Half-life is very specific for each medication and for each patient. **Steady-state** levels are usually required to determine whether a dose of medication will achieve therapeutic concentrations and avoid toxic levels. Steady-state levels are achieved once the medication concentrations achieve steady levels in the body and occur when the dose being given each day is equal to the total amount being eliminated each day. Steady-state concentrations are usually achieved after continued dosing for a period equivalent to five times the medication's half-life in that particular patient. How quickly a steady state is reached is highly specific to the medication and the patient and depends on the patient's rate of medication elimination. Some medications must be used for an extended period of treatment even after therapeutic levels are obtained in order to realize the full therapeutic effects. For example, with medications used to treat depression, the full effects of the medication dose may not be seen for several weeks after initiation (Blumenthal & Garrison, 2011; Carl & Johnson, 2006; Ciccone, 2002; Gadson, 2006; Malone, 1989).

Generic Medications

Medications have three names: a chemical name, a generic name, and a trade name.

The trade name is used by the manufacturer when advertising the medication to the prescriber and consumer. The U.S. Food and Drug Administration (FDA) regulates the manufacture of generic products, and the majority of generic drugs are as effective as the brand-name products. Once the patent expires on a medication, other pharmaceutical companies can manufacture the medication. Once the new manufacturer proves to the FDA that the efficacy and safety of its generic product is equivalent to that of the trade-name product, the FDA approves the generic product and the medication is offered to the public under the generic name. Once the drug is offered in a generic form, competition usually drives down the cost of the drug to the consumer. A limited number of medications are manufactured with a specialized delivery system or have special characteristics that make generic products less effective. A pharmacist cannot substitute these products with a generic product without specific authorization from the prescriber. The list of these medications, termed the Negative Formulary, varies from state to state (Carl & Johnson, 2006; Niles, 2001; Rivera & Gilman, 2011; Ross & Kenakin, 2001; Wilkinson, 2001).

Side Effects of Medications

Undesired effects associated with medication use are called **side effects**. The patient information provided by the pharmacist at the time of dispensing includes a list of the most common side effects seen with a particular medication. Patients and family should be aware of the side effects that are expected with initiation of any new medication and should know that these side effects may recur with each change in dose of the medication. The severity of a side effect is often related to the size of the initial dose. Dose-related side effects can be minimized by initiating medications in lower doses and slowly titrating the dose to the desired effects. This is particularly true if the patient is taking more than one medication that has similar side effects. Examples of dose-related side effects include sedation and nausea. Tolerance to dose-related side effects generally occurs within the first 5 to 7 days of medication initiation. If side effects do not resolve after this time period, the patient should contact the prescriber because a decrease in dose may be indicated. In addition, patients and families should be educated to consult with a pharmacist before self-medicating with a non-prescription medication or herbal product. The pharmacist can assist the patient and family by ensuring that the medication is safe to use and that the symptoms they are self-treating are not related to a medication the patient is taking (Blumenthal & Garrison, 2011; Carl & Johnson, 2006).

The occurrence of some side effects, such as allergic or hypersensitivity reactions, is not predictable. These side effects are termed idiosyncratic. **Anaphylactic** reactions, which involve the skin and the pulmonary and cardiovascular systems, are the most severe allergic reactions. Signs and symptoms associated with anaphylaxis include skin or mucous membrane reactions such as flushing, **erythema**, **pruritus**, swelling, or **maculopapular rash**, cardiac symptoms such as hypotension, tachycardia, or other changes in heart rate, and breathing difficulties such as **bronchospasm**, laryngeal **edema**, **stridor**, or respiratory arrest. Once a patient has had an anaphylactic reaction to medication, the medication should be added to the patient's allergy list in the medical record and should not be readministered. When documenting or obtaining drug allergy information, it is important to ask what symptoms accompanied the allergic reaction. Patients often refer to a side effect such as nausea as an allergy, which may inappropriately prevent related medications from being used (Carl & Johnson, 2006; Ciccone, 2002; Gadson, 2006; Malone, 1989).

Medications that cause sedation should not be combined with alcohol, which can potentiate this side effect. Patients started on medications associated with sedation should not drive or operate machinery until these effects subside. Gastrointestinal upset such as nausea often may be minimized by taking the medication with food or milk. Side effects are also possible with long-term use of a medication. For example, chronic use of benzodiazepines can result in significant pharyngeal **dysphagia**,

including **aspiration** (Carl & Johnson, 2006; Ciccone, 2002; Gadson, 2006; Malone, 1989).

Special Populations and Medication Risk

Patient caregivers should be aware that side effects can occur as a result of drug interactions, particularly when the patient is taking more than four medications. Adverse drug reactions are more common in patients who are older and in patients with cardiac, respiratory, liver, or kidney disease. In addition, certain patients are at risk due to genetic factors associated with metabolism and receptor binding. A published list of medications, called the Beer's List (www. americangeriatrics.org), details medications that are not recommended for use in the elderly. Patients and caregivers should especially monitor for adverse drug reactions with the initiation of any new medication, and timely communication with the prescriber is indicated if an adverse drug reaction is suspected (Campbell-Taylor, 2001; Carl & Johnson, 2006; Ciccone, 2002; Gadson, 2006; Malone, 1989).

Patient Education and Medication Use

The role of the rehabilitation specialist in ensuring that patients understand how to correctly take their medications and in facilitating medication adherence cannot be underestimated. The rehabilitation specialist can monitor patients for medication effects and can assist in educating the patient and family about safe and effective medication use (Carl & Johnson, 2006).

The rehabilitation specialist should instruct patients to ask these questions when getting a new medication (Carl & Johnson, 2006):

- What is the name of the medicine?
- What is it supposed to do?
- How and when do I take this medication and for how long?
- Should I avoid certain foods, caffeine, alcohol, other medicines, or certain activities such as driving?

- Will It work well with the other medicines I am taking?
- Are there side effects? What do I do if they occur?
- Will it affect my sleep or activity level?
- What should I do if I miss a dose?
- Is written material about the medicine available?

In addition to the information provided by the pharmacist, information on medications can be obtained on the Internet. Manufacturer websites often provide information about their medications in a format written for patients. The website www.healthline.com/druginteractions is a patient friendly and useful resource that can be used for identifying potential drug interactions. Another site that provides useful information in layman's terms on medications, food–drug interactions, and drug interactions is www.drugs.com/drug_interactions.html. In addition, sites such as the Mayo Clinic website provide information on medications used to treat different disease states in language that is appropriate for the non-health professional (Carl & Johnson, 2006; Malone, 1989).

In addition to instructing patients to ask the aforementioned questions when they are started on a new medication, the rehabilitation therapist should instruct patients to do the following (Malone, 1989):

- Keep a list of your current medications, the names of your physicians, and any medication allergies in your purse or wallet at all times.
- Use adequate light to read labels carefully before taking doses.
- Ask the doctor or pharmacist before crushing or splitting tablets; some can only be swallowed whole.
- Contact the doctor or pharmacist if new or unexpected symptoms occur after taking a medication.
- Never stop taking medicine the doctor has told you to finish just because the symptoms disappear.

- Ask your family physician and pharmacist to periodically reevaluate whether you still need all of your long-term medications.
- Talk to your pharmacist or doctor before using an over-the-counter (nonprescription) or herbal medicine.
- Carefully read labels of over-the-counter medicines for ingredients, proper uses, directions, warnings, and expiration dates.
- Discard outdated medicine.
- Never take someone else's medication.
- Keep medications away from heat, light, and moisture. Never store medications in the bathroom medicine cabinet.

Medications cannot work if they are not taken. Helping the rehabilitation patient take their medications requires the help of each member of the health care team. The therapist can assist with medication adherence by doing the following (Malone, 1989):

- Determine the proper vials to use for people with poor vision, decreased fine-motor control, or arthritis.
- Determine the proper memory aid to increase a patient's adherence in taking their medications.
- Educate the caregiver or family of those with memory impairments or other challenges and identify the most useful tools and strategies to prevent errors.
- Recommend special aids and devices that can assist with medication use. These special aids and devices include
  ○ medication containers or watches that beep when it is time for the next dose,
  ○ pill boxes by the day or the week,
  ○ computerized drug organizers or dispensers, and
  ○ special caps that count the openings of a prescription vial so the patient can tell whether he has taken the day's dose.

Safe and Effective Use of Medications

Approximately 7% of hospital admissions are due to serious adverse drug reactions (ADRs). It is estimated that the percent of hospital admissions that are caused by ADRs in patients older than 65 yr of age increases to about 20%. The Institute for Safe Medication Practices (2011) estimates that adverse drug reactions are between the fourth and sixth leading cause of death in U.S. hospitals.

Patients and health professionals caring for these older patients must understand how to take medications correctly and safely. Elderly patients tend to take more medications and have more cognitive deficits and frequently have difficulty understanding and remembering how to safely take their medications. The importance of ensuring that patients understand how to correctly take their medications and facilitating medication adherence cannot be underestimated. Weekly or monthly medication organizers that assist in setting up medications ahead of time for daily administration are useful tools, especially in the older patient or the patient with cognitive impairment (Carl & Johnson, 2006; Ciccone, 2002; Gadson, 2006; Malone, 1989).

Invaluable interventions in optimizing rehabilitation progress include educating patients about medication use, monitoring for therapeutic effects and side effects of medications during therapy, making appropriate adjustments to a patient's therapy sessions, and contacting a patient's prescriber when one suspects that medications may be affecting rehabilitative progress (Carl & Johnson, 2006; Ciccone, 2002; Gadson, 2006; Malone, 1989).

Summary

This chapter discusses the principles of medication use. Pharmacotherapy combines the disciplines of pharmacokinetics and pharmacodynamics to optimize medication use in individual patients. Pharmacokinetics describes how medications are absorbed, distributed, metabolized, and eliminated from the body and helps clinicians decide the best dosing regimen for a patient. Pharmacodynamics describes how and where medications act at a cellular level to elicit therapeutic effects and undesired side effects. Pharmacodynamics and pharmacokinetic concepts help clinicians predict and identify drug interactions that alter medication effects. Being aware of expected therapeutic effects, side effects, and drug interactions associated with a patient's medication regimen can help the therapist design the safest and most effective therapy session for the patient.

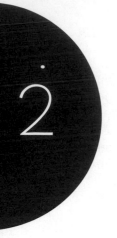

2

Medication's Effects on the Nervous System, Muscle Function, and Cognition

The nervous system controls the function of all muscle, including both voluntary muscle, such as the leg muscles used in walking, and involuntary muscle, such as that which controls the movement of food through the lower gastrointestinal tract. Medications can affect the function of nerves and, subsequently, the function of muscles.

The nervous system also controls cognition and learning. The term *cognition*, from Latin, means "to know." Cognition is further defined as the ability of an individual to process information and apply knowledge. Cognition usually refers to the processes of perceiving, conceiving, judging, recognizing, and reasoning, all of which are important in learning and training in the rehabilitative session. **Metacognition** is the patient's ability to understand their own cognition and cognitive difficulties and understand strategies for improving their cognition. The rehabilitation therapist often needs to develop individualized strategies to improve a patient's cognition and to help the patient learn new skills such as eating, walking, and communication as they undergo rehabilitation.

Rehabilitation requires working with neuromuscular function, cognition function, and memory. Patients with neurogenic disorders such as Alzheimer's disease (AD), Parkinson's disease (PD), and traumatic brain injury (TBI) can exhibit changes in neuromuscular function, cognition, and memory. In addition, patients receiving rehabilitation may take medications for chronic diseases other than

the disease state requiring rehabilitation. Medications for these chronic diseases also can alter neuromuscular, cognitive, memory, and muscle function. Understanding the effect of medications on processes used in the rehabilitation session and being able to appropriately alter the planned session can greatly affect the patient's ability to participate in therapy.

This chapter reviews the major parts of the nervous system—the central nervous system and the peripheral nervous system—and outlines how different parts of the nervous system affect muscle and endocrine functions. This chapter also explains how medications can change the function of these systems.

Central Nervous System

The central nervous system (CNS) comprises the brain and spinal cord. The CNS contains both sensory (afferent) and motor (efferent) pathways. The CNS is divided into three major levels of function. First, the spinal cord level includes sensory signals that are transmitted through the spinal nerves into each segment of the spinal cord; these signals trigger automatic and instantaneous localized motor responses called reflexes. Second, the lower brain controls most unconscious activities such as respiration, feeding reflexes, and blood pressure as well as emotional patterns such as anger. Third, the cortical level involves storage of information and patterns of motor responses that are consciously controlled (Carl & Johnson, 2006).

Brain, Cognition, and Rehabilitation

Rehabilitation teaches the patient how to regain function using new processes such as walking using a prosthetic device, safely eating with a swallowing disorder, or regaining muscle function of an affected limb after a stroke. The patient's ability to understand and apply new concepts and to safely incorporate new processes into daily life requires cognitive function. Many patients have impaired cognition due to a disease state that may or may not be the reason for their referral for rehabilitation. For example, patients with chronic cardiac disease, respiratory disease, or psychiatric disease may have decreased cognitive function that interferes with their therapy for stroke rehabilitation. Knowing what type of cognitive impairment is associated with different disease states and the best approach for teaching these patients can be useful when designing a rehabilitative regimen for the patient. Medications that a patient is taking can also affect cognitive function. Most of the chapters in this book review the effect of specific disease states on cognitive and motor function and outline how medications used to treat these disease states affect cognition, memory, and motor function. This chapter introduces the neurophysiology associated with cognition, memory, and motor function in the rehabilitation patient.

Temporal Lobe

No one area of the brain controls the entire process of memory; all areas of the brain play a part. This is particularly evident with damage to the **temporal lobe**. The temporal lobe is responsible for functions relating to auditory and visual attention, auditory and visual perception, organizing verbal information, comprehending language, long-term memory, personality, and affective behavior (Berube, 2002; Vogel et al., 2000; Zemlin, 1998).

The hippocampus, which is in the medial temporal lobe and is part of the limbic system, plays an important role in spatial navigation and long-term memory. The medial temporal lobe and hippocampus are involved in the storage of episodic information. In neurode-generative diseases such as AD, the hippocampus is one of the first areas of the brain to suffer damage. As a result, the patient becomes disoriented and experiences difficulty with memory, particularly episodic memory. Extensive damage to the hippocampus, frontal lobe, and medial temporal lobe can result in amnesia (Berube, 2002; Emilien et al., 2004; Vogel et al., 2000; Zemlin, 1998).

The hippocampal region of the brain plays a part in episodic memory, semantic memory, recall memory, and recognition memory (Emilien et al., 2004). Individuals have a right and left hippocampus. The right hippocampus is responsible for recall of visual information, whereas the left hippocampus is responsible for recall of verbal information. Subsequently, removal of the right hippocampus results in impaired visual memory and little problem with recall of verbal information. Left-sided removal results in the reverse (Parente & Herrmann, 2003).

The **amygdala**, also part of the limbic system, is involved in emotional memory. Emotional arousal can strengthen episodic memory and can slow forgetting after learning (Emilien et al., 2004).

PATIENT CASE 1

M.J. is a 40-yr-old right-handed woman who was recently hospitalized secondary to multiple (50-100) seizures on a daily basis. Medications are not controlling the seizures. The surgeon suggests removing the right hippocampus. The patient is quite concerned that the surgery will affect her cognition.

Question

What information can the rehabilitation therapist give M.J. regarding the expected effects of this surgery on her memory?

Answer

The surgeon suggested removing the hippocampus because it is damaged and is generating her seizures. The hippocampus functions primarily in working memory and short-term memory conditions. Sensory memory and, in particular, attention are critical for the working memory. In fact, another term for working memory is *working attention*. The right hippocampus governs visual memory, whereas the left hippocampus governs verbal memory. The therapist can explain to M.J. that she may experience postoperative difficulties with short-term visual memory.

Frontal Lobe

The **frontal lobe** is the emotion and personality center. The frontal lobe is responsible for social and impulse control, memory, problem solving, and motor function. Upper-body fine-motor movement and strength (Kuypers, 1981), motor chaining (Leonard et al., 1988), facial expression (Kolb & Milner, 1981), and expressive language (Brown, 1972) are associated with frontal lobe function. The left frontal lobe is involved with language, whereas the right frontal lobe is involved with nonverbal activities. Frontal lobe damage may result in difficulty organizing, sequencing, and setting time markers that identify the past and the present. The frontal lobe is involved when a patient experiences retrograde or **anterograde amnesia**. The patient with frontal lobe damage may also exhibit proactive interference in which the learning of new information is impaired due to confusion with older information (Parente & Herrmann, 2003). Also common with damage to the frontal lobe are problems interpreting environmental feedback, perseveration (repeated speech patterns) (Milner, 1964), risk taking and noncompliance with rules (Miller, 1985), and reduced associated learning (Drewe, 1975). Semmes and colleagues (1963) also report that the frontal lobe plays some role in spatial orientation. The frontal lobe also influences memory retention. Long-term episodic memory learning and working memory are usually associated with activation of the frontal lobe. Executive planning, including monitoring behavior, evaluating outcomes, formulating plans, and initiating action, is also usually associated with activities of the frontal lobe (Emilien et al., 2004).

Parietal Lobe

Damage to the **parietal lobe** affects memory retention and retrieval. Memory difficulties differ according to the location of the damage to the parietal lobe. Damage to the juncture of the occipital and parietal lobes results in short-term memory loss. The patient will be unable to recall digits presented visually but will be able to recall digits presented with auditory stimuli. When the juncture of the temporal and parietal lobes is damaged, the patient can recall digits visually but not auditorily. Damage to the posterior parietal lobe affects the patient's memory for the location of objects. Damage to the left parietal–temporal area affects short-term retention of verbal information, and damage to the right parietal–occipital area affects short-term retention of nonverbal information (Parente & Herrmann, 2003).

PATIENT CASE 2

P.L., a 75-yr-old male, approaches his therapist in rehabilitation and says that he is very concerned about his memory—in particular, his short-term memory. He states that he tends to rely on rituals and routines more than he has in the past because of his problems with short-term memory. He is concerned that he may be developing AD.

Question
How should the rehabilitation therapist advise P.L.?

Answer
The rehabilitation therapist should advise the patient to see his physician and ask for a referral to see a neurologist. The neurologist should review P.L.'s list of medications to rule out medication-induced problems with his memory. In addition, neuropsychological testing may be warranted to differentiate between age-associated memory loss and mild cognitive impairment. Rehabilitation may help provide therapeutic interventions that assist with the cognitive decline and initiate programs to prevent complications such as falls.

Processes of Memory   The processes involved in memory include **encoding**, **storage**, and **retrieval**. Encoding is the processing of material to be learned. The success of encoding determines how efficiently material is stored and retrieved in the future. A number of variables, such as sensory memory deficits, attention or concentration deficits, hearing and vision deficits, and frontal lobe deficits, can negatively affect encoding. The mechanics of encoding can range from simple repetitive rehearsal to complex organization of the information to be retained. The most effective way to encode new information is generally to associate that information with previously learned information. The role of the therapist is to establish a strong encoding message in the patient to ensure storage and retrieval (Sander et al., 2007).

Storage refers to the manner in which information is retained in memory for future use. Encoding and storage are interactive in nature. Short-term retention and storage, or working memory, involves a number of variables that are discussed in the next section. Long-term retention or storage is generally considered to be permanent memory (Sander et al., 2007). Retrieval, or recall, is thought to be the action of obtaining information from long-term storage. This is usually referred to as delayed recall on tests of memory. Retrieval is usually assisted by recognition, as evidenced by multiple-choice or true–false examinations. Although recognition is important, recall is critical for memory. Retrieval, storage, and encoding are interactive. For example, an individual is more likely to recall information that is important and is organized in a logical manner (Sander et al., 2007).

PATIENT CASE 3

T.J. is a patient with AD. The rehabilitation therapist spends several sessions developing a memory book for the patient. A few days later the therapist discovers that T.J. has placed the memory book in a bedside drawer and has not opened the book.

Question

Should the rehabilitation therapist stop trying to get the patient to use the memory book?

Answer

No. Patients may be instructed in the use of compensatory strategies, such as memory books, but may not use the strategies if they do not appreciate that they have memory difficulties. T.J.'s metacognition (ability to detect one's cognitive impairment) may be impaired. The rehabilitation therapist needs to help T.J. realize her difficulty with memory tasks and instruct her to begin using compensatory strategies such as memory books.

System Models of Memory   Each of the four system models of memory—sensory, working, declarative, and nondeclarative—depends on the integrity of different neuroanatomical structures (Mahendra & Apple, 2007). The rehabilitation therapist must have a strong understanding of the various memory systems in order to select the most appropriate therapeutic intervention for each patient.

Sensory memory is considered the lowest form of memory. Sensory memory involves two functions: attention and processing. Use of sensory memory requires sustained shifting or selective attention abilities and the ability to process presented stimuli at an adequate speed (Wiig at al., 2008). A good sensory memory allows the patient to quickly process and attend to information being presented in a timely manner. A good example of a patient with poor sensory memory is the patient with TBI (Levin, 1990), who may be comatose or have poor concentration or attention skills that greatly impair the input of data. This is comparable with a computer that is not plugged into the wall or that has a defective plug that allows electricity to pass through only intermittently (Mahendra & Apple, 2007).

Working memory, also called working attention, involves information manipulation. The model for working memory involves a central executive officer that acts as a supervisor and coordinates all other aspects of working memory. The central executive officer allows recently acquired information to be recirculated (task maintenance) and focuses attention on tasks, thus reducing information that may be competing in nature. For example, an author might become lost in his writing to the point where outside distractions are not relevant. Working memory makes possible the organization and planning of memory to facilitate the encoding and retrieval of information (Emilien et al., 2004).

The model for working memory is divided into several components: the visual–spatial sketchpad, the auditory–phonological loop, and the episodic buffer. The visual–spatial sketchpad, governed by the right hemisphere, is responsible for the retention of visual information (Emilien et al., 2004). An example of the sketchpad is a student recalling via a picture in the mind's eye the exact location in their class notes of the answer to a question.

The auditory–phonological loop, which is associated with the left hemisphere, contains the subvocalization rehearsal process. This is the process of retaining information by saying it over and over in your head subvocally. This is frequently used to retain new information. It maintains subvocal material, to be later retrieved and translated into verbal material, in primary memory through short-term storage (Emilien et al., 2004). A student may use the auditory–phonological loop when learning lines for a play.

The episodic buffer, which holds episodes of information (Emilien et al., 2004), is controlled by the central executive and serves as a temporary, limited-capacity storage system for combined visual and verbal information and for data that exceed the limits of the sketchpad or loop. Use of the episodic buffer can be seen in patients with long-term memory problems who still exhibit normal performances on tasks of immediate recall that typically exceed their visual or verbal memory span. The episodic buffer depends on frontal lobe integrity. This ability to recall begins to decline after age 40 (Sander et al., 2007). Individuals can generally hold up to seven recognizable pieces of data and can manipulate that data for approxi-

mately 20 s without rehearsal (Cone, 2008).

Working memory depends on a functional frontal lobe. The prefrontal regions are connected with the sensory-processing systems that form the basis for emotion. The visual–spatial sketchpad depends on an intact occipital–parietal cortex, which mediates spatial and visual components. The auditory–phonological loop depends on Broca's area as well as the inferior temporal and parietal cortexes (Bayles & Tomoeda, 2007).

Many disorders involve difficulty with working memory; this difficulty is caused by dysfunction of the frontal lobe (Bayles & Tomeada, 2007). For example, AD patients may exhibit a decline in working memory. Executive function decreases, resulting in reduced ability to create ideas and deal with multiple units of information. As a result, verbal output is reduced. Attention span also declines in the AD patient, resulting in a reduced ability to maintain information in consciousness for a length of time (Casper, 2007). Impairment of the frontal lobe can affect executive function in a variety of ways. The patient with frontal lobe dysfunction may have difficulty with inhibition, judgment, insight, problem-solving skills, processing speed, attention and concentration, abstract reasoning, mental flexibility, or initiating or persisting in an activity (Cone, 2008). The patient's disinhibition can result in highly distractible, emotionally liable behavior. The patient may have difficulty maintaining their premorbid level of social behavior. In addition, the patient may be unable to function independently due to poor problem-solving skills (Cone, 2008).

Long-term memory is divided into **declarative** and **nondeclarative memory**. Declarative memory is a process that can assimilate new facts and events. Declarative memory is divided into semantic memory, episodic memory, and lexical memory. Declarative memory depends on the integrity of the medial temporal lobe and hippocampus (Emilien et al., 2004).

Semantic memory is the knowledge of facts learned over time, such as multiplication tables, vocabulary, and spelling (Sander et al., 2007). Semantic memory is also defined as general knowledge of the world in the absence of contextual cues for retrieval (Emilien et al., 2004). Damage to the temporal lobe can result in disorders such as frontotemporal dementia. Semantic deficits result in word-retrieval problems (Cone, 2008). The general fund of information in semantic memory does not depend on contextual cues for word retrieval. Semantic memory generally does not decline with age; however, access to semantic memory may decline after age 40 due to an age-related decrease in temporal lobe functioning (Cone, 2005, 2008). Semantic memory is also helpful in activating associated concepts. For example, the concept *July 4th* can activate concepts such as fireworks, family reunions, and hotdogs.

Episodic memory involves conscious recall of specific episodes. Episodic memory is identified with consciousness that allows recollection of past situations in which the subject was present. Episodic memory also allows the individual to view the future where he is present (Gardiner, 2001). Normal aging plays a significant role in the reduction of episodic memory ability. Disorders such as AD demonstrate reductions in episodic memory. Semantic memory and episodic memory interact. For example, learning the navigational rules of sailing involves semantic memory. Remembering where one learned how to sail involves episodic memory.

In patients with certain forms of early dementia, access to information previously stored in semantic memory is preserved. In the later stages of dementia, even semantic memory is impaired (Sander et al., 2007). The decline of semantic memory in AD patients is characterized by diminished auditory comprehension, bizarre content of speech, and empty language. The decline of episodic memory in AD patients is characterized by reduced topic maintenance, diminished auditory comprehension, and sentence fragments. The AD patient usually exhibits spared procedural memory, resulting in retention of some social verbal phrases, adequate pronunciation, and preserved grammar (Casper, 2007).

Lexical memory, the final declarative memory system, is a store of word knowledge (Mahendra & Apple, 2007). Lexical memory,

episodic memory, and semantic memory interact. Difficulty with lexical memory in the AD patient can result in **anomia**, poor vocabulary, and **paraphasia** (Casper, 2007). Because of the prominence of difficulties with episodic memory and problems with semantic memory in the AD patient, the clinician may overlook difficulties with lexical memory.

PATIENT CASE 4

R.P. is a 79-yr-old male with a history of academic achievement. The patient, a tenured professor, recently went in for unilateral knee replacement. Postoperatively, the professor had a premorbid difficulty with word finding (anomia). When asked when he published his last book he had to ask his wife for the answer. His wife stated that he had published the book 1 yr ago. When asked the name of his book he asked his wife, who stated the title.

Question
What types of memory difficulties does this patient exhibit?

Answer
This patient exhibits decline in semantic memory. He is unable to recall factual information, such as when he published his book or the title of his book.

Nondeclarative memory is divided into procedural memory, priming, conditioned responses, and habits. **Procedural memory** facilitates learning motor tasks and developing cognitive skills (e.g., solving a Sudoku puzzle) by repetition (Mahendra & Apple, 2007). Procedural memory may also be called motor memory, skilled memory, or implicit memory. It involves connections among the cerebellum, neocortex, and basal ganglia. The **neostriatum** mediates this type of learning. Damage to these connections results in subcortical dementia such as Huntington's disease (Sander et al., 2007). Procedural memory typically does not require consciousness and usually does not decline with age. Subsequently, the procedural memory abilities of AD patients (cortical dementia) are routinely spared. As a result, rehabilitative treatment for AD patients revolves around stimulating procedural memory to replace lost episodic or semantic memory (Cone, 2005, 2008).

Priming is an unconscious ability to detect, identify, or respond to a stimulus after recent or repeated exposure to it (Mahendra & Apple, 2007). Priming can be perceptual or conceptual. An example of perceptual priming is producing a word after seeing the same word or a similar word. An example of conceptual priming is producing a concept after hearing a word (Bayles & Tomoeda, 2007). In contrast to declarative (semantic, episodic, and lexical) memory, which relies on the medial temporal lobe, priming is mediated by the posterior neocortex (visual cortex). Priming is also assisted by some subcortical structures, particularly the basal ganglia. Generally, the nature of the stimulus determines which areas of the cortex are activated. A visual stimulus involves the inferior temporal lobe, and an auditory stimulus involves both the right and left auditory cortexes. The left auditory cortex processes phonologic information, and the right auditory cortex processes information about the voice of the speaker (Bayles & Tomoeda, 2007). The difference between declarative and nondeclarative memory is evident in patients with amnesia, who demonstrates preserved learning (e.g., playing the piano) even though they are unable to recall the learning event (e.g., learning how to play the piano). This is called implicit learning.

Conditioned responses are behaviors that one automatically produces in response to a stimulus (Bayles & Tomoeda, 2007). Motor conditioning is affected by the integrity of the cerebellum. Subsequently, patients with impairment of the cerebellum may have difficulty acquiring conditioned responses (Bayles & Tomoeda, 2007).

PATIENT CASE 5

X.P. is an 80-yr-old male diagnosed with AD. The patient has episodic memory decline, short-term memory difficulties, and sensory memory problems in the areas of attention span and processing speed. The rehabilitation therapist wants to initiate functional goals for getting out of a wheelchair safely.

Question
What memory systems would the rehabilitation therapist use to teach the patient how to safely get out of a wheelchair?

Answer
The rehabilitation therapist would use spaced retrieval techniques to teach the patient safety procedures. Spaced retrieval uses nondeclarative memory systems such as procedural memory, priming, and conditioned responses to elicit the proper response from the patient. The spaced aspect of spaced retrieval requires that the patient retain the message for longer and longer periods. The spaced retrieval techniques would incorporate shaping and errorless learning techniques to encode proper techniques in the patient.

Habits are behavioral routines that are almost unconscious (Mahendra & Apple, 2007). These routines, which are mediated by the **striatum**, act as a chain in which one behavior tends to facilitate subsequent behaviors (Bayles & Tomoeda, 2007).

Neurotransmission and Effects of Medication on Neuromuscular Function

The nervous system comprises specialized cells called **neurons** that are able to send and receive messages through an electrochemical process. Chemical messengers called **neurotransmitters** facilitate all communication among the nerves by transmitting nerve signals. Neurotransmitters are released by one nerve cell into the gap between the cells, called the **synapse**, and carry the message that stimulates the next nerve cell. Changing the amount of neurotransmitter in the synapse at the site of their action can decrease or increase the efficiency of the nerve transmission (Carl & Johnson, 2006).

Neurotransmitters that function in the CNS to enhance excitability and propagation of neuronal activity include **glutamate**, aspartate, acetylcholine, dopamine, norepinephrine, purines, peptides, cytokines, and steroid hormones. In contrast, **gamma amino butyric acid** (GABA) and glycine inhibit transmission and reduce neural activity. Medications can affect CNS transmission by increasing or decreasing the action of these neurotransmitters in the CNS or by binding to the receptors in the brain that these neurotransmitters normally act on. For example, many medications that are used to promote sleep or to control seizures work by binding to the receptors usually acted on by the sedating neurotransmitter GABA. This action reduces neural excitability and activity, thus promoting sleep or preventing seizure activity (Emilien et al., 2004; Iversen et al., 2009).

Medications can affect neurotransmission by changing the rates of destruction of the different neurotransmitters, by inhibiting or increasing release of neurotransmitter into the synapse, or by enhancing **reuptake** of neurotransmitter into the cell itself, leaving less neurotransmitter in the synapse to elicit neurotransmission. Medications that increase the amount of neurotransmitter in the synapse potentiate (increase) the effects of the neurotransmitter and elicit a stronger response. For example, the increase in norepinephrine levels associated with the use of antidepressant medications increases neurotransmission and improves mood. Medications that reduce neurotransmitter levels antagonize (decrease) the effects of the neurotransmitter, leading to decreased neurotransmission and decreased response. For example, medications used to treat schizophrenia reduce the effects of dopamine, resulting in reduced neurotransmission and reduced agitation (Carl & Johnson, 2006).

Dopamine, norepinephrine, epinephrine, serotonin, acetylcholine, **histamine**, and amino acids are the most common neurotransmitters in the body. Neurotransmitters can be thought of as the software for the body; they are instrumental in synaptic activity. One must appreciate neurotransmitter activity in order to understand how medications can affect nervous system function and impact cognition, emotion, learning, and motor processes involved in rehabilitation.

Dopamine

Catecholamines are neurotransmitters derived from the amino acid tyrosine. These catecholamines include epinephrine, norepinephrine, and dopamine. The neurotransmitter dopamine composes one half of the catecholamines found in the brain. Dopamine is particularly important in the regulation of movement, cognition, and emotional response. It is the main transmitter of the extrapyramidal system and several mesocortical and mesolimbic pathways. Dopamine is involved in the pathophysiology of depression, PD, and schizophrenia (Carl & Johnson, 2006). Dopamine levels are reduced in patients with PD and administration of dopamine reduces symptoms in these patients. In contrast, excessive central dopamine activity occurs in schizophrenia and antipsychotic medications that block dopamine reduce symptoms of agitation and hallucinations in these patients. Dopamine blocking also contributes to the improved mood associated with the use of the antidepressant amoxapine (Asendin) (Carl & Johnson, 2006; Iversen et al., 2009).

Norepinephrine

Norepinephrine, the main neurotransmitter for sympathetic postganglionic fibers, is also found in all parts of the brain; large amounts are found in the hypothalamus (which controls body temperature, hunger, and thirst) and in the limbic system (which controls emotion, behavior, smell, and long-term memory). This neurotransmitter affects mood and many of the **antidepressant** medications act by increasing levels of norepinephrine in the central nervous system (Carl & Johnson, 2006).

Epinephrine

Epinephrine is found in the medullar reticular formation, but associated physiological properties of this catecholamine in this region have not yet been identified. In the peripheral nervous system epinephrine is the primary neurotransmitter in mediating sympathetic nervous system response, also known as the fight or flight response (Carl & Johnson, 2006).

Serotonin

Serotonin is found in regions of the CNS that are associated with mood and anxiety. Serotonin mediates functions of sleep, cognition, sensory perception, temperature regulation, motor activity, sexual behavior, hormone secretion, and appetite. Serotonin stimulates smooth-muscle activity in the **autonomic nervous system**, which stimulates gastrointestinal motility. The serotonin-1A receptor is highly concentrated in the hippocampus, which has been demonstrated to play a critical role in sensory memory and working memory. Reduced serotonin levels have been shown in age-related cognitive disorders and in AD. Medications that increase serotonin levels and neurotransmission include many antidepressants; use of these medications can affect appetite, sleep, cognition, and sexual function. Triptans, which are used to treat migraine headache, are another group of medications that increase serotonin levels and activity. **Serotonin receptor antagonists** such as ondansetron (Zofran) are effective in the treatment of nausea and vomiting (Carl & Johnson, 2006; Emilien et al., 2004).

Acetylcholine

The existence of acetylcholine has been known since the 19th century; its role as a neurotransmitter was identified in the 1920s. Acetylcholine affects neuronal activity through nicotinic and muscarinic types of **cholinergic** receptors. Cholinergic neurons, which are found in both the CNS and the peripheral nervous system, are associated with cognition, stimulus processing, sleep, arousal, motivation, and reward. Nicotinic cholinergic receptors are important in regulating cognitive functions such as attention and in regulating release of other neurotransmitters. In the peripheral nervous system, acetylcholine is the most important neurotransmitter in the promotion of gastrointestinal function and in processes mediated by the parasympathetic nervous system (Emilien et al., 2004; Iversen et al., 2009).

Altered acetylcholine activity in the hippocampus and neocortex is associated with AD. The cholinergic neurons in the pons provide cholinergic transmission to the striatum and thalamus. The cholinergic neurons in the medulla provide transmission to the brainstem and midbrain. One of the most important aspects of brain neural degeneration and impaired cognition in AD patients is the loss of the basal forebrain cholinergic system. Medications used to treat AD increase the level and activity of acetylcholine in the brain (Carl & Johnson, 2006; Emilien et al., 2004).

Histamine

Histamine was discovered as a neurotransmitter in the early part of the 20th century. Histamine, which is a central neurotransmitter, originates in the hypothalamus and regulates body temperature, arousal, and vascular dynamics. Histamine receptors are identified as histamine-1 (H1), histamine-2 (H2), and histamine-3 (H3) receptors. H1 receptors are involved in smooth-muscle contraction, hormone release, and capillary permeability in response to exposure to allergens. **Antihistamines**, used to treat allergy, block H1 receptors. H2 receptors are involved in a number of functions, including smooth-muscle contraction, inhibitory effects on the immune system, and secretion of gastric acid. H2 receptor blockers such as cimetidine (Tagamet) are used to reduce gastric acid production in the treatment of peptic ulcer disease. H3 receptors act as autoreceptors and regulate presynaptic release of histamine, dopamine, gamma aminobutyric acid, acetylcholine, norepinephrine, and serotonin (Carl & Johnson, 2006; Iversen et al., 2009).

Amino Acids

Amino acids that act as central neurotransmitters include GABA, aspartate, glutamate, and glycine. The amino acid transmitters that inhibit neurotransmission and reduce the excitatory response in the brain are GABA and glycine. GABA, which mediates presynaptic function in the brain and spinal cord, is the major inhibitory neurotransmitter in the brain. As such, many medications promote GABA activity by acting on GABA receptors. The GABA receptors mediate sedative, anticonvulsant, **anxiolytic**, amnesic, and muscle-relaxant activities and are targeted by many medications that treat anxiety, insomnia, and seizures (Carl & Johnson, 2006; Iversen et al., 2009).

Aspartate and glutamine, which are excitatory neurotransmitters, are located in every part of the CNS. These two neurotransmitters exercise very powerful stimulatory effects. They play a role in the synthesis of peptides and proteins and in the detoxification of ammonia in the brain. These amino acids act as precursors and are used as building blocks in the formation of the neurotransmitter GABA. Memantine (Namenda) is a newer medication used to treat AD and targets activity at glutamate receptors within the CNS (Carl & Johnson, 2006; Iversen et al., 2009).

Peripheral Nervous System

The peripheral nervous system is divided into two sections: the sensory–somatic nervous system, which controls voluntary muscle function, and the autonomic nervous system, which controls involuntary function, including endocrine function (Carl & Johnson, 2006).

Autonomic Pathways Affecting Glands and Organ Function

The autonomic (involuntary) nervous system, which is activated in centers located in the spinal cord, brainstem, and hypothalamus, regulates visceral function and functions that occur without conscious control. This system helps control gastrointestinal motility, salivation, and secretions that assist in digestion. The endocrine system and the nervous system are so closely associated that they are sometimes referred to as the neuroendocrine system. Neural control centers in the brain control the endocrine glands, helping regulate and maintain various body functions by making and releasing hormones. These glands include the pituitary, pineal, hypothalamus, thyroid, parathyroid, thymus, and adrenal glands, reproductive organs, and pancreas. The autonomic nervous system is further divided into three systems: the sympathetic, parasympathetic, and enteric nervous systems (Carl & Johnson, 2006).

The **sympathetic nervous system** prepares the body for action ("fight or flight") during times of perceived emergency. Activation of this system results in dilated pupils, inhibition of saliva flow, acceleration of heart rate, dilation of the bronchi, inhibition of peristalsis and secretions, conversion of glycogen to glucose, secretion of adrenalin and noradrenalin, and inhibition of bladder function. Most of the postganglionic nerve endings in the sympathetic system secrete norepinephrine. Norepinephrine is found in all parts of the brain, particularly the hypothalamus and limbic system. The hypothalamus is responsible for functions such as body temperature, thirst, and hunger. The limbic system is associated with emotion, behavior, smell, and long-term memory. Patients with depression have lower levels of norepinephrine; many medications used to treat depression optimize activity of norepinephrine in the CNS (Carl & Johnson, 2006; Grimsley, 1998).

The **parasympathetic nervous system**, on the other hand, stimulates activities associated with relaxation and restorative functions such as digestion, rest, micturition, and defecation. The parasympathetic system communicates with the CNS via the cranial nerves, sacral nerves, and vagus nerve. Parasympathetic nerves are called cholinergic nerves, as they are regulated by the neurotransmitter acetylcholine. Activation of the parasympathetic nervous system results in stimulation of saliva flow, slower heart rate, decreased respiratory rate, stimulation of peristalsis, increased gastrointestinal secretions, stimulation of bile release, contraction of the bladder, and effective defecation. In addition, the parasympathetic nerves interact with and assist in regulation of the enteric nervous system (Carl & Johnson, 2006).

The **enteric** nervous system innervates the gallbladder, pancreas, and gastrointestinal tract. Much of its function is mediated by acetylcholine and serotonin. Many disease states can result in impaired gastrointestinal function; medications can also affect levels and activity of neurotransmitters and can inadvertently cause difficulties with eating and swallowing, GI motility, and production of gastrointestinal secretions needed in the digestive process. Eating and swallowing require a coordinated effort between muscles and the nervous system mediated by neurotransmitters.

Medications can alter neurotransmitter levels and affect neurotransmission in the central and autonomic nervous systems. In addition, unintended side effects from medications can result in an altered cognition, sedation, nausea and vomiting, constipation, xerostomia, and esophageal injury that can contribute to nutritional compromise and impaired ability to participate in rehabilitation (Carl & Johnson, 2006).

Sensory–Somatic Nervous System

The sensory–somatic nervous system controls voluntary muscles via the neurotransmitter acetylcholine. The **somatic** system contains sensory fibers that send information from sensory organs to the CNS and motor fibers that control voluntary movements of skeletal muscle. The **somatic nervous system** controls the function of the skeletal (voluntary, striated) muscles. Somatic nerves are unique in that their cell bodies are all located in the ventral horn of the spinal cord and their synapses are all housed in the cerebrospinal column. An **axon** divides into many branches, and each of these branches innervates a single muscle fiber. The nerves are **myelinated** and connect to the muscle fibers via the motor end plate. The motor end plate contains acetylcholine receptors. When acetylcholine stimulates these receptors, the end plate is depolarized, resulting in muscle contraction. Paralysis and, eventually, muscle atrophy occur when the transmission of the spinal nerves controlling the muscle is interrupted. Medications can alter neurotransmission associated with the sensory somatic nervous system and can result in impaired motor function and movement disorders (Carl & Johnson, 2006).

Medication-Induced Movement Disorders

Movement disorders affect the speed, fluency, quality, and ease of movement. Abnormal fluency or speed of movement (dyskinesia) may involve excessive or involuntary movement (e.g., essential tremor, tics) or slowed or absent voluntary movement (hypokinesia). Movement disorders can cause ataxia (lack of coordination, often producing jerky movements) and dystonia (involuntary movement and prolonged muscle contraction) (Emilien et al., 2004; Mendez & Cummings, 2003).

Many medications can cause or worsen movement disorders. Medications that change the level of the neurotransmitter dopamine can affect motor function. In most cases of drug-induced movement disorders, the medication induces an acute imbalance in the levels of dopamine in the neostriatum portion of the extra-pyramidal system. Medications that are most frequently associated with altered dopamine levels and potential for inducing movement disorders include antipsychotic medications, antidepressant medications, lithium, and medications used to treat PD. Antipsychotic medications can also induce a life-threatening disorder called **neuroleptic malignant syndrome**, which is characterized by muscle rigidity, fever, autonomic instability, and cognitive changes such as delirium and is associated with elevated creatine phosphokinase, a byproduct of muscle breakdown (Carl & Johnson, 2006).

High levels of serotonin can cause a movement disorder called **serotonin syndrome**. Serotonin syndrome is potentially life threatening and usually occurs as a result of a drug interaction. Symptoms can include agitation, hallucinations, loss of coordination, overactive reflexes, elevated heart rate and blood pressure, nausea, and vomiting. Table 2.1 lists common drug combinations that can lead to serotonin syndrome (Grimsley et al., 2006) as well as medications that can induce or worsen tremor. Most drug-induced movement disorders are dose related, and many occur as the result of additive effects of other agents or drug interactions that increase levels and effects of the medication. Movement disorders significantly affect the patient's ability to participate in rehabilitation sessions. Table 2.1 summarizes medications that commonly cause movement disorders (Carl & Johnson, 2006; Emilien et al., 2004; Mendez & Cummings, 2003).

Table 2.1 Medications That Can Cause Movement Disorders

Movement disorder	Medications	Corrective actions
Extrapyramidal symptoms	Antipsychotics: haloperidol (Haldol), trifluoperazine (Stelazine), thioridazine (Mellaril), chlorpromazine (Thorazine), quetiapine (Seroquel), ziprasidone (Geodon), aripiprazole (Abilify), risperidone (Risperdal), asenapine (Saphris) Benzamides: metoclopramide (Reglan) Antihypertensives: reserpine, methyldopa (Aldomet) Calcium channel blockers: diltiazem (Cardizem), nifedipine (Procardia), verapamil (Calan, Isoptin, Verelan) Mood stabilizer: lithium (Eskalith) Benzodiazepine: high-dose diazepam (Valium) Chemotherapy: cytosine arabinoside (Ara-C) Anticonvulsant: long-term use of valproic acid (Depakene)	• Reduce dose or discontinue medication. • Add an anticholinergic in the short term to antipsychotic therapy and adjust therapy or dose.
Akathisia	Antidepressants: tricyclic antidepressants such as amitriptyline (Elavil), imipramine (Tofranil), doxepin, (Sinequan), or trazodone (Desyrel); mirtazapine (Remeron); selective serotonin reuptake inhibitors such as citalopram (Celexa), fluoxetine (Prozac), fluvoxamine (Luvox), or paroxetine (Paxil); monoamine oxidase inhibitors such as isocarboxazid (Marplan), phenelzine (Nardil), selegiline (Eldepryl), or tranylcypromine (Parnate) Antipsychotics: haloperidol (Haldol), trifluoperazine (Stelazine), thioridazine (Mellaril), chlorpromazine (Thorazine), quetiapine (Seroquel), ziprasidone (Geodon), aripiprazole (Abilify), risperidone (Risperdal), asenapine (Saphris) Calcium channel blockers: diltiazem (Cardizem), nifedipine (Procardia), verapamil (Calan, Isoptin, Verelan)	• Reduce dose of the offending medication. • Administer propranolol (Inderal) or a benzodiazepine such as lorazepam (Ativan). • Do not treat with anticholinergic medications such as benztropine (Cogentin) or trihexyphenidyl (Artane).
Dystonia	Antipsychotics: haloperidol (Haldol), trifluoperazine (Stelazine), thioridazine (Mellaril), chlorpromazine (Thorazine), quetiapine (Seroquel), ziprasidone (Geodon), aripiprazole (Abilify), risperidone (Risperdal), asenapine (Saphris) Abrupt withdrawal of anticholinergic therapy such as benztropine (Cogentin) or trihexyphenidyl (Artane)	• Discontinue antipsychotic or reduce dose. • Administer parenteral anticholinergic medications such as benztropine (Cogentin) or diphenhydramine (Benadryl).
Serotonin syndrome	*Any of this group of agents:* Selective serotonin reuptake inhibitor antidepressants: citalopram (Celexa), fluoxetine (Prozac), fluvoxamine (Luvox), paroxetine (Paxil) Monoamine oxidase inhibitors: isocarboxazid (Marplan), phenelzine (Nardil), selegiline (Eldepryl), tranylcypromine (Parnate), linezolid (Zyvox) Serotonin and norepinephrine reuptake inhibitor antidepressants: duloxetine (Cymbalta), venlafaxine (Effexor) *Combined with any of these medications that increase serotonin levels:* Tricyclic antidepressants: amitriptyline (Elavil), imipramine (Tofranil), doxepin, (Sinequan) Atypical antidepressants: trazodone (Desyrel), mirtazapine (Remeron) Migraine therapy: ergot alkaloids	• Discontinue the offending medications. • Relieve behavioral symptoms with lorazepam (Ativan), autonomic symptoms with cyproheptadine (Periactin), cardiac ischemia with nitroglycerin, and hypertension and tachycardia with propranolol (Inderal).

› continued

Table 2.1 › *continued*

Movement disorder	Medications	Corrective actions
Serotonin syndrome *(continued)*	Triptans: sumatriptan (Imitrex), almotriptan (Axert), eletriptan (Relpax), frovatriptan (Frova), naratriptan (Amerge), rizatriptan (Maxalt)	
	Pain medications or muscle relaxants: morphine, tramadol (Ultram), meperidine (Demerol), fentanyl (Duragesic), methadone, cyclobenzaprine (Flexeril)	
	Antiemetics: ondansetron (Zofran)	
	Anticonvulsants: valproic acid (Depakote), dextromethorphan (a cough suppressant used in over-the-counter cough syrups; Robitussin DM)	
	Others: buspirone (Buspar), cocaine, lithium, amphetamines	
	Foods, supplements, or herbals: L-tryptophan, tyramine-rich foods (aged cheeses, wines, meats), St. John's wort	
Neuroleptic malignant syndrome	Antipsychotics: haloperidol (Haldol), trifluoperazine (Stelazine), thioridazine (Mellaril), chlorpromazine (Thorazine), quetiapine (Seroquel), ziprasidone (Geodon), aripiprazole (Abilify), risperidone (Risperdal), asenapine (Saphris)	• Discontinue the antipsychotic. • Treat with bromocriptine 30 mg/day or dantrolene 400 mg/day.
Tremor	Alcohol: chronic use	• Discontinue the offending medication or reduce dose.
	Antiarrhythmics: amiodarone (Cordarone), mexiletine (Mexitil), procainamide (Pronestyl)	
	Anticonvulsants: carbamazepine (Tegretol), phenytoin (Dilantin), valproic acid (Depakene)	
	Selective serotonin reuptake inhibitor antidepressants: citalopram (Celexa), fluoxetine (Prozac), fluvoxamine (Luvox), paroxetine (Paxil)	
	Tricyclic antidepressants: amitriptyline (Elavil), imipramine (Tofranil), doxepin, (Sinequan)	
	Antipsychotic: haloperidol (Haldol)	
	Bronchodilators: albuterol (Ventolin), salmeterol (Serevent, Advair)	
	Corticosteroids: prednisone, methylprednisolone (Medrol), cyclosporine (Neoral, Sandimmune)	
	Heavy metals: arsenic, manganese, lead, mercury	
	Lithium (Eskalith) combined with antidepressants	
	Metoclopramide (Reglan)	
	Methylxanthines: caffeine, theophylline (Theodor)	
	Nicotine	
	Reserpine	
	Sympathomimetics: amphetamines, cocaine, ephedrine, methylphenidate (Ritalin), pseudoephedrine (Sudafed), weight-reduction preparations such as phentermine (Ionamin)	
	Thyroid supplements	

Summary

The clinician must be familiar with how the neurotransmitters in the central and peripheral nervous systems affect voluntary and involuntary muscle function, cognition and learning, enteric processes, and endocrine function. This chapter reviews neuroanatomy and summarizes the functions of important neurotransmitters in both the central and peripheral nervous systems. This chapter also introduces concepts of how medications can affect neurotransmission, motor function, and cognition.

The rehabilitation therapist should be aware of the normal processes of cognition and memory and how these affect the rehabilitative process. This chapter introduces the forms of memory and learning and relates them to the portions of the brain involved in these processes. The rehabilitation therapist who works with a patient with cognitive disabilities should attempt to assess the memory function of the patient. Memory assessment can help the rehabilitation therapist develop or implement the goals for treatment and can provide the baseline for comparing improvements as a result of treatment. Memory assessment can also help the rehabilitation therapist develop compensatory strategies for the patient and can be useful when discussing these strategies with caregivers and families. When caring for patients with impaired cognition, one must identify which forms of memory are preserved and target those processes to facilitate the effective learning needed for individualized treatment of each patient. The clinician should be able to identify existing cognitive deficits and neuromuscular disease before looking at the additional effect that medications can have on motor function, cognitive function, and learning (Sander et al., 2007).

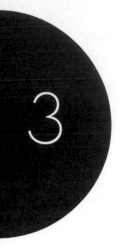

3

Nutrition in the Rehabilitation Patient

This chapter summarizes the role of nutrition in the healing process of the rehabilitation patient. The rehabilitation therapist should assess the patient's nutritional status and nutritional needs with the initial evaluation and facilitate the development of a nutritional plan for patients in rehabilitation. Carefully monitoring the weight, nutritional intake, and fluid and electrolyte status of the patient ensures that the patient's nutritional needs are being met and that complications are avoided during rehabilitation. The rehabilitation therapist should understand how different disease states affect a patient's nutritional requirements and the patient's ability to process different components of nutritional therapy. This chapter discusses how to assess the nutritional and fluid requirements of patients, introduces components of nutrition, and explains how different disease states can change the patient's ability to process nutrition and can change nutritional needs. The chapter also covers important considerations in developing a nutrition plan based on the patient's concurrent disease states and summarizes important parameters for monitoring and assessing the adequacy of nutrition provided and for detecting any toxicity associated with the nutrition.

Physiology of Nutrition

Energy is essential for all biochemical and physiologic functions in the body. Dietary protein provides amino acids for the synthesis of body muscle, organs, nerve cells, neurotransmitters, and hormones. Micronutrients are essential cofactors in transport of nutrients and enzymatic processes of metabolism and utilization of provided nutrition.

The appearance, taste, and smell of food are integrated and can affect palatability, which can affect appetite. The sense of smell is mediated by olfactory receptor cells derived from the central nervous system. Secondary olfactory tracts pass through the hypothalamus, thalamus, hippocampus, and brainstem nuclei to stimulate automatic feeding activities as well as emotional response. The smell of food initiates an impulse from the nose to the vagal, glossopharyngeal, and salivary nucleus of the brainstem. Parasympathetic nerves stimulate the secretion of digestive juices before food even enters the mouth. Taste signals are transmitted through the 5th, 7th, 9th, and 10th cranial nerves to the smell centers in the hypothalamus and to the salivary centers in the maxillary and parotid glands to control salivary secretions. Lubrication of the nasal passages enhances the sense of smell, and adequate presence of saliva is important in the sensation of taste. Medications may cause changes in cognition, taste, smell, and appetite, resulting in decreased oral intake. Medications can also change gastrointestinal tract motility and alter production of saliva, further contributing to a decline in intake. Certain medications, such as anticholinergic medications (e.g., antihistamines), can reduce both saliva production and the lubrication of the nasal passages, affecting taste and smell. Ensuring adequate fluid intake and moisturizing the mouth and nasal passages can minimize some of these effects. Anticholinergic medications can also impair movement of food through the digestive tract and contribute to impaired nutrition (Alvi, 1999; Campbell-Taylor, 1996, 2001; Carl & Johnson, 2006, 2010; Huckabee & Pelletier, 1999; Willoughby, 1983).

Malnutrition occurs when nutritional intake is insufficient to supply the energy the body needs to maintain growth and cellular function. Malnutrition affects the function of all organ systems and contributes to overall functional decline, muscle breakdown and weakness, osteoporosis, decreased immune function, and anemia associated with decreased tissue oxygenation. Malnutrition can reduce cognitive status and can result in skin breakdown and poor wound healing. Malnutrition can be classified as marasmus, kwashiorkor, or a combination of these. Marasmus malnutrition is seen when intake of both protein and calories is inadequate. This type of malnutrition causes catabolism; the body breaks down its own tissues to produce needed calories and amino acids. Kwashiorkor malnutrition is seen when intake of protein is inadequate but intake of calories is sufficient and is associated with decreased protein components in the blood, resulting in fluid imbalances and edema (Harohalli et al., 2010; Scheinfeld & Mokashi, 2010).

Incidence, Etiology, and Pathophysiology of Malnutrition

Children and the elderly are at a higher risk for malnutrition than the general population. Malnutrition, which is the most important risk factor for illness and death, contributes to more than half of deaths in children worldwide. Malnutrition in children less than 5 yr of age causes an estimated 50% of the 10 million annual deaths in developing countries. Risk factors for malnutrition in children include dependence on others for food, increased protein and energy requirements, and an immature immune system that makes the child susceptible to infection with exposure to contaminated food and water sources. Common and significant micronutrient deficiencies, which occur in up to 2 billion children, include deficiencies of iron, iodine, zinc, and vitamin A (Harohalli et al., 2010; Rabinowitz et al., 2010; Scheinfeld & Mokashi, 2010).

Institutionalized patients are also at higher risk for malnutrition. In a survey conducted in a large children's hospital, more than one half of patients experienced acute or chronic protein-energy malnutrition (Rabinowitz et al., 2010). Up to 55% of elderly persons who are hospitalized are malnourished, and up to 85% of elderly persons in extended-care facilities are malnourished (Scheinfeld & Mokashi, 2010). Studies have shown that the vitamin and mineral intake of up to 50% of elderly institutionalized patients is less than the recommended dietary allowance and that the levels of vitamins and minerals in up to 30% of elderly persons are below normal (Harohalli et al., 2010; Kayser-Jones, 2000; Morley & Kraenzle, 1994; Scheinfeld & Mokashi, 2010).

In developed countries, conditions in children such as prematurity, food allergies, cystic fibrosis, chronic renal failure, childhood malignancies, congenital heart disease, and neuromuscular diseases contribute to malnutrition. During adolescence, self-imposed dietary restrictions such as fad diets, inappropriate management of food allergies, and psychiatric diseases such as **anorexia nervosa** can also lead to severe protein-energy malnutrition. Malnutrition can lead to fatty degeneration of the liver and heart, atrophy of the small bowel, and dehydration, leading to increased **aldosterone** levels and fluid retention (Harohalli et al., 2010; Rabinowitz et al., 2010; Scheinfeld & Mokashi, 2010).

Risk factors for malnutrition in the elderly include decreased appetite, decreased sensation of thirst, impaired cognition, isolation, depression, dietary changes affected by limited income, monotony of diet, poor dentition, and dysphagia. In this population, dehydration can increase the risk of renal failure, infection, falls, and confusion (Huckabee & Pelletier, 1999; Kayser-Jones et al., 1999). This is particularly true when the patient depends on others to provide hydration or nutrition (Winchester et al., 2001).

Initial signs and symptoms of dehydration include thirst, fatigue, weakness, confusion, muscle cramps, postural dizziness, and syncope. Monitoring for dehydration includes monitoring for rapid changes in weight, monitoring for decreases in blood pressure when sitting or standing compared with when lying, and monitoring for diminished skin turgor and dryness of mucous membranes. High levels of sodium and chloride and a high blood urea nitrogen to creatinine ratio help confirm the presence of dehydration. Normal laboratory values for these laboratory tests vary by laboratory. Normal sodium levels are between 135 and 145 mEq/L, normal chloride levels are between 95 and 107 mEq/L, normal creatinine levels are between 0.6 and 1.5 mg/dl, normal blood urea nitrogen levels are between 7 and 18 mg/dl, and normal blood urea nitrogen to creatinine ratios are less than 20:1. Severe dehydration can cause decreased perfusion of organs and result in elevated liver enzymes, cardiac arrhythmia, syncope, renal failure, and coma. Dehydration can also result in elevated levels of lactic acid and other metabolic acids, resulting in metabolic acidosis. Frequent causes of dehydration include diarrhea, vomiting, blood loss, fluid losses from drains or fistulas, decreased fluid intake, and overuse of **diuretics** (Carey et al., 1998; Fischbach, 2002).

Certain disease states (e.g., cancer, diabetes) and organ dysfunction (e.g., cardiac, renal, or respiratory failure) can also increase the risk of malnutrition and require special consideration when providing hydration and nutrition in order to avoid toxicity and avoid worsening the patient's condition. Thyroid disease can cause changes in appetite and result in significant changes in body weight. Other disease states such as cancer, depression, pulmonary disease, and Parkinson's disease can also be associated with decreased appetite and weight loss. Dietary deficiencies can cause changes in taste or smell. For instance, magnesium deficiency decreases salt perception, and zinc deficiency can cause loss of taste. Parkinson's disease and Alzheimer's disease can both cause loss of smell. Medications can also contribute to altered taste, smell, and appetite (Carl & John-

son, 2006; Carson & Gormican, 1976; Griffin, 1992; Henkin, 1994; Willoughby, 1983).

Nutritional Screening, Assessment, and Monitoring

The rehabilitation therapist should screen patients at the time of admission to identify those with nutrition risk that may require diet therapy, and these patients should be routinely reassessed for nutritional adequacy. Patients at risk for malnutrition include those with chronic debilitating disease, alcoholics, cancer patients, the elderly, those with confusion or mental illness, those with poor wound healing, those with skin breakdown, and those with infection. When the rehabilitation therapist finds risk for malnutrition, the therapist should refer the patient to a clinical dietitian for a comprehensive nutrition assessment and development of a diet plan that includes appropriate education for the patient and family. The assistance of a speech–language pathologist and a dietitian in the development of a nutrition plan can be invaluable in patients with identified swallowing, chewing, and nutrition disorders (Frankenfield et al., 2005; Mifflin et al., 1990).

The diet or specialized nutrition therapy plan for the patient includes **macronutrients** that provide the amount of protein as well as nonprotein calories provided by fat and carbohydrate as determined by the nutritional assessment. The proportion of protein, fat, and calories in a diet is customized to include consideration of the patient's concurrent disease states, any organ dysfunction, and any specific fluid or electrolyte requirements or restrictions. Consideration of fluid and electrolyte requirements should always take into account the effects of the patient's medications (Frankenfield et al., 2005; Mifflin et al., 1990).

Methods of assessing calorie and protein needs depend on patient height, weight, age, sex, activity factors, and stress factors and take into account chronic and acute states of illness. Skeletal muscle loss is assessed by measuring body weight, arm muscle circumference, and creatinine height index. Visceral protein loss is assessed by measuring serum albumin, transferrin, and prealbumin levels. Immune function is assessed by measuring total lymphocyte count, and immunosuppression is verified by **antigen** skin testing. Resting energy expenditure can be measured using indirect **calorimetry**, and initial needs can be estimated using the Harris Benedict equations; the Mifflin-St. Jeor equations; the Owen equation; and the World Health Organization, Food and Agriculture Organization, and United Nations University (WHO/FAO/UNU) equations. The clinician determines nutritional needs using body composition analysis, clinical examination, and biochemical assessment. **Adipose** tissue loss can be assessed using skinfold measurements and body mass index (Langley, 2007; Frankenfield et al., 2005; Mifflin et al., 1990).

When patients who are malnourished are provided with oral or **enteral** nutrition therapy, they often exhibit feeding intolerance in the form of diarrhea. Nutrition therapy should be initiated gradually and with caution in malnourished patients because it can also result in refeeding syndrome. Refeeding syndrome, which can be life threatening, occurs when patients who are chronically malnourished are reintroduced to nutrition. Chronic malnutrition may result in depletion of total body stores of thiamine, potassium, magnesium, and phosphorus. Reintroduction of nutrition in a patient at risk for refeeding syndrome requires repletion of these components before initiation of nutrition. Nutrition should be carefully introduced; fluids should be restricted to less than 800 ml/day and sodium restricted to 20 mEq/day. Carbohydrate should be initiated cautiously (100-150 g/day) in order to avoid **hyperglycemia**. Potassium, magnesium, and phosphorus levels should be reassessed and aggressively repleted as nutrition is slowly advanced because adequate levels are required to facilitate intracellular delivery of the nutrition provided. Complications associated with refeeding syndrome can include renal retention of sodium and fluids and resultant fluid overload; pulmonary edema; respiratory failure; **lysis** of red blood cells, platelets, and white blood cells; seizures; gastrointestinal dysmotility; cardiac decompensation; and even sudden cardiac death (Langley, 2007; Brooks & Melnik, 1995).

Routine monitoring of weight is important; however, increases in weight associated with fluid retention may mask nutritional losses. Monitoring intake of fluids and of the meals provided and monitoring urine output and other fluids lost through ostomy or fistula drainage is important in assessing and maintaining fluid and electrolyte balance. Sodium levels may actually decrease in patients with fluid overload due to a dilutional effect, and rapid gains in weight are more often a reflection of fluid overload than of improved nutritional status. Monitoring of daily weights can identify rapid weight gain associated with excessive salt or fluid intake or acute changes in renal function. Monitoring serum electrolytes such as sodium, potassium, magnesium, and phosphorus can help ensure that adequate electrolytes are available to transport the provided nutrition into the cells via the cellular transport pumps (Langley, 2007; Beck & Rosenthal, 2002; Frankenfield et al., 2005; Mifflin et al., 1990).

Improvement in protein status is reflected by increases in albumin and prealbumin levels and has been shown to correlate with positive patient outcomes. Albumin is a traditional marker of protein stores; however, levels can be altered with changes in fluids. Increases in albumin that reflect improved nutritional status are not evident until weeks after initiation of nutrition therapy (Beck & Rosenthal, 2002). The normal range for albumin in adults is 3.8 to 5.0 g/dl but can vary from laboratory to laboratory (Fischbach, 2002).

Prealbumin, which is a more useful marker for assessment of protein status, has a short half-life of 2 days and increases within 2 days of provision of adequate protein. Unlike albumin, it is not dependent on fluid status, and it provides a more accurate and timely assessment of whether the patient is able to process the provided nutrition and use it to build body cells and tissue. The normal range for prealbumin in adults is 14.0 to 42 mg/dl (2.5-7.6 μmol/L) but may vary depending on the laboratory. Normal levels in patients over 60 yr of age are 20% lower, and normal levels in premenopausal females are lower than in males (Fischbach, 2002). In high-risk patients, measuring prealbumin levels twice weekly can alert the clinician to declining nutrition status (Beck & Rosenthal, 2002).

Prealbumin that fails to increase by at least 4 mg/dl after 8 days of nutrition therapy indicates poor utilization of provided nutrition and the need for adjustment of the provided nutritional components. Confounding factors that can reduce prealbumin levels include concurrent steroid therapy (increases levels), zinc deficiency (lowers levels), and acute stress associated with sepsis or critical illness (can lower levels). Con-current increases in levels of C-reactive protein can indicate acute stress, which may make prealbumin levels less useful as an nutritional assessment tool. Table 3.1 provides recommendations for providing initial protein and calorie requirements in adults based on specific disease states and lists additional monitoring considerations associated with providing and monitoring nutrition therapy in these patients (Langley, 2007; Beck & Rosenthal, 2002; Frankenfield et al., 2005; Gottschlich, 2007; Mifflin et al., 1990).

Table 3.1 Initial Estimation of Nutritional Needs in the Adult Based on Patient Disease State

Disease state	Protein needs	Kilocalorie needs	Kilocalories as carbohydrate	Kilocalories as fat	Comments
Promotion of weight loss	0.8 g/kg/day	20-25 kcal/kg/day	50%-60%	20%-30%	These are needs in patients who are not metabolically stressed.
Weight maintenance	0.8-1.0 g/kg/day	25-30 kcal/kg/day	50%-60%	20%-30%	
Promotion of weight gain	1 g/kg/day	30-40 kcal/kg/day	50%-60%	20%-30%	
Age >65 yr	1 g/kg/day	25-35 kcal/kg/day	50%-60%	20%-30%	
NPO after elective surgery	1-1.5 g/kg/day	35 kcal/kg/day	50%-60%	20%-30%	Monitor for acute decreases in K, Mg, and phosphate.
Bariatric surgery	First 2 mo after surgery: 40-60 g/day Long term: 80-100 g/day	First 6 mo: 1000 kcal/day Long term: 1200-1600 kcal/day	50%-60%	20%-30%	
Respiratory disease: chronic obstructive pulmonary disease	1.2-1.5 g/kg/day	Repletion in malnourished: 35-45 kcal/day Maintenance: 25-35 kcal/day (1.3 × the basal energy requirement)	Start at 150 g/day and titrate as tolerated; maximum of 4 mg/kg/min	30%-40%	Check phosphate, Mg, K, and calcium and replete; all contribute to respiratory muscle dysfunction. 50% of patients with chronic obstructive pulmonary disease have low phosphate levels; excess glucose increases CO_2 retention and can worsen respiratory function.
Respiratory disease: ventilated	1.5-2.5 g/kg/day	30-35 kcal/day	Start at 150 g/day and titrate as tolerated; maximum of 4 mg/kg/min	30%-40%	Propofol provides 1.1 kcal/ml of fat; reduce fat in TPN for any daily propofol intake. Excess glucose increases CO_2 retention and can worsen respiratory function and failure to wean off ventilator.

Disease state	Protein needs	Kilocalorie needs	Kilocalories as carbohydrate	Kilocalories as fat	Comments
Renal disease: acute renal failure	1 g/kg/day Keep BUN:Cr ratio <30	25-35 kcal/kg/day	40%-50% Start at 150 g/day and titrate as tolerated; maximum of 4 mg/kg/min	30%-40%; keep TG <200	Restrict Na (<2 g) and fluids (<2 L). Consider dialysis for provision of needed nutrition. Monitor closely for acute decreases in K, Mg, and phosphate. Use bolus replacements.
Renal disease: chronic renal failure, no dialysis	0.5-0.8 g/kg/day Keep BUN:Cr ratio <30	25-35 kcal/kg/day	40%-50% Start at 150 g/day and titrate as tolerated; maximum of 4 mg/kg/ min	30%-40%; keep TG <200	Restrict Na (<2 g), fluids (<2 L), K, and Mg. Use phosphate binder and activated vitamin D.
Renal disease: chronic renal failure, hemodialysis	1-1.2 g/kg/day Keep BUN:Cr ratio <30	35-50 kcal/kg/day	40%-50% Start at 150 g/day and titrate as tolerated; maximum of 4 mg/kg/ min	30%-40%; keep TG <200	Restrict Na (<2 g), fluids (<2 L), K, and Mg. Use acetate rather than chloride salts, folic acid, ascorbic acid, and pyridoxine. Use phosphate binder and activated vitamin D.
Renal disease: chronic renal failure, continuous arteriovenous hemodialysis	1.6-1.8 g/kg/day Keep BUN:Cr ratio <30	Reduce glucose by 600-800 kcal/day	40%-50%	30%-40%; keep TG <200	Fluid and other electrolytes are less restricted due to losses from dialysis.
Renal disease: chronic renal failure, peritoneal dialysis	1-1.5 g/kg/day Keep BUN:Cr ratio <30	Reduce glucose by 500 kcal/day	40%-50%	30%-40%; keep TG <200	Restrict Na (<2 g), fluids (<2 L), K, and Mg. Use phosphate binder and activated vitamin D.
Diabetes	1.2-1.5 g/kg/day	25-35 kcal/kg/day	Start at 100-150 g/day and titrate to maximum of 4 mg/kg/min	30%	For TPN in critical care initiate insulin drip and adjust following insulin protocols. In more stable patients, add two thirds of previous day's insulin coverage in TPN and continue to titrate based on glucose testing. Monitor Na, K, Mg, and phosphate levels. Monitor for refeeding syndrome. For oral enteral diet: High fiber, low fat, avoid processed sugars.
Refeeding syndrome	1.2-1.5 g/kg/day	Start at 20 kcal/kg/day; increase after 3.5 days to goal by 10-14 days	Start at <150 g/day and titrate as tolerated; maximum of 4 mg/kg/ min	30%-40%	Initiate fluids <800 ml/day. Restrict Na to 20 mEq/day. Monitor and replete K, Mg, and phosphate via bolus per protocol.

› continued

Table 3.1 › *continued*

Disease state	Protein needs	Kilocalorie needs	Kilocalories as carbohydrate	Kilocalories as fat	Comments
Cancer	Repletion: 1.5-2.0 g/kg/day Maintenance: 1-1.5 g/kg/day	Repletion: 35-50 kcal/kg/day Maintenance: 25-35 kcal/kg/day	Start at 100-150 g/day and titrate as tolerated; maximum of 4 mg/kg/min	20%-40%	Na with fluid status (syndrome of inappropriate antidiuretic hormone). Monitor for refeeding syndrome and tumor lysis syndrome with high dose chemotherapy administration in patients with high tumor loads.
Critical illness	1.5-2.0 g/kg/day (adjusted body weight); up to 3 g/kg/d BCAA products are preferred Obese patients: Use ideal body weight	15 kcal/kg/day using enteral nutrition during initial week of admission in intensive care unit; slowly titrate to 30-35 kcal/kg/day. Avoid hyperglycemia and excessive carbohydrate loads while providing adequate protein.	Glucose intolerance: Start at 100-150 g/day and titrate as tolerated. Maximum of 4 mg/kg/min. Preferential use of free fatty acids and branched-chain amino acids in patients who are in a stressed state.	30%-40%	Initiate trickle or trophic feeds (10-30 ml/h) with enteral nutrition even in the absence of bowel sounds within 24-48 h of critical care admission. TPN is not recommended for initial 7 days of stay in intensive care unit; enteral nutrition is preferred. Permissive underfeeding is recommended for patients with BMI >30: provide 2-2.5 g/kg of protein but only 11-14 kcal/kg of total body weight or 22%-25% of ideal body weight to avoid hyperglycemic complications. TPN indicated only in patients undergoing surgery who are malnourished. In these patients, 7 preoperative days of TPN is recommended prior to the surgery. Transition TPN to enteral therapy as soon as possible.
Pressure ulcers, stage I	1.25-1.5 g/kg/day	30-35 kcal/kg/day	Depends on stage of ulcer	20%-40%	Multivitamin with mineral, vitamin C, vitamin A, and zinc supplementation is helpful.
Pressure ulcers, stage II	1.25-1.5 g/kg/day	30-35 kcal/kg/day			
Pressure ulcers, stage III	1.25-1.5 g/kg/day	30 kcal/kg/day			
Pressure ulcers, stage IV	1.5-2.0 g/kg/day	35-40 kcal/kg/day			
Hepatic failure	0.8 g/kg/day initially and 1.2-1.5 g/kg/day for positive nitrogen balance. Patients with cirrhosis: 1.5 g/kg/day; do not restrict protein. BCAA for >grade 2 encephalopathy, which may indicate protein intolerance.	25-35 kcal/kg/day Acute hepatitis requires more kilocalories than does stable cirrhosis to facilitate liver regeneration.	Glucose intolerance: Use higher percentage of lipids. Start at 100-150 g/day and titrate as tolerated. Maximum of 4 mg/kg/min.	20%-40%	Restrict fluids and Na. Monitor for refeeding syndrome, hepatic encephalopathy, and ascites. Monitor liver function tests including AST, ALT, bilirubin, alkaline phosphatase, and prothrombin time.

Disease state	Protein needs	Kilocalorie needs	Kilocalories as carbohydrate	Kilocalories as fat	Comments
Acute pancreatitis	1.5-2.5 g/kg/day	Increase to 1.7-1.9 times basal energy requirement (40-50 kcal/kg/day)	Glucose intolerance: Start at 100-150 g/day and titrate as tolerated; maximum of 4 mg/kg/min	Limit fats to <20% of kilocalories to prevent worsening of acute pancreatitis symptoms of belly pain and prevent further increases in TG.	Monitor amylase, lipase, TG, abdominal pain, and white blood cells. Concurrent intravenous hydration and NPO or J-tube enteral feedings are required.
Inflammatory bowel disease	1-1.5 g/kg/day	30-40 kcal/kg/day	50%-60%	<20% by fat; monitor for fat intolerance with associated increases in belly pain and TG levels	Supplement with iron, zinc, copper, selenium, manganese, folic acid, and vitamins B$_{12}$, A, D, E, and K. Monitor electrolytes, fluid status, and stool output daily. Monitor for refeeding syndrome.
Bowel resection and short bowel syndrome	Acute: 1-1.5 g/kg/day Maintenance: 1.2-2.5 g/kg/day to compensate for malabsorption (20%-30% of diet)	Acute TPN: 30-35 kcal/kg/day Oral maintenance: 30-40 kcal/kg/day; increase by 200%-400% to compensate for malabsorption	Intact colon: 50%-60% Jejunostomy/ileostomy: 20%-30%	Intact colon: 20%-30% Jejunostomy/ileostomy: 50%-60%	Administer small, frequent meals and liquids between meals to minimize dumping. Supplement with pancreatic enzymes. For patients with oxalate stones, provide a low-oxalate, low-fat diet with high fluid intake.
Fistulas	High output: 1.5-2.5 g/kg/day Low output: 1-1.5 g/kg/day	25-35 kcal/kg/day	Glucose intolerance: Start at 100-150 g/day and titrate as tolerated; maximum of 4 mg/kg/min	30%-50%	Monitor fluids and electrolyte loss via fistula drainage and replace in TPN. Monitor for refeeding syndrome.
Human immunodeficiency virus and acquired immune deficiency syndrome	1-2 g/kg of adjusted body weight/day	Repletion: 35-45 kcal/kg/day Maintenance: 30-35 kcal/kg/day	Start at 100-150 g/day and titrate as tolerated; maximum of 4 mg/kg/min	20%-40%	Monitor glucose tolerance and lipid profile; human immunodeficiency virus antiviral medications may alter these.

AST = aspartate aminotransferase; ALT = alanine aminotransferase; BCAA = branched chain amino acids; BUN= blood urea nitrogen; Cr = creatinine; K = potassium; Mg = magnesium; Na = sodium; NPO = nothing by mouth; TG = triglyceride, TPN = total parenteral nutrition.

Rehabilitation Considerations

Many clinical conditions that contribute to malnutrition in the patient undergoing rehabilitation may require the rehabilitation team to revise the patient's nutritional plan.

Previous hospitalization or critical illness can contribute to malnutrition when the patient is admitted to rehabilitation services. Malnutrition risk is especially high in the elderly and in patients with dysphagia. Cancer and gastrointestinal disease such as pancreatitis, inflammatory bowel disease, or short bowel syndrome resulting from surgery can significantly increase nutritional risk. A therapist may also encounter pediatric patients with failure to thrive and associated malnutrition. Other common diseases that require the therapy team to adjust the nutritional plan include respiratory disease, diabetes, kidney disease, and liver disease. Recommended medication and nonmedication therapies for these diseases are discussed in later chapters.

Nutrition in the Hospitalized Patient

To provide both short-term and long-term nutritional plans that are appropriate for the patient, members of the rehabilitation therapy team, particularly the clinical dietitian, must take a careful diet history and pay close attention to likes and dislikes, food allergies, and identified barriers of oral intake. In patients who cannot or should not use the gastrointestinal tract due to their clinical disease, short-term nutrition can take the form of total parenteral nutrition (TPN) administered via a central catheter, or peripheral nutrition support, administered via a peripheral catheter. However, parenteral nutrition should not be considered a long-term option unless the gut cannot or should not be used. Oral and enteral nutrition are safer alternatives to parenteral nutrition and should be used in any patient with a functional gut unless contraindicated by concurrent disease. Whenever possible, use of the gastrointestinal tract is recommended as it is important to maintaining gut integrity and avoiding complications. When the gastrointestinal tract is not used, the epithelial lining of the gastrointestinal tract breaks down and the villi associated with nutrient absorption shorten. Complications associated with loss of gut integrity can include sepsis associated with bacterial translocation across the impaired gastrointestinal tract and immunosuppression associated with decreased production of hormones by the gastrointestinal tract (Harohalli et al., 2010; Scheinfeld & Mokashi, 2010).

Complications associated with parenteral nutrition include increased catheter-related infections and catheter sepsis, deficiencies of vitamins and trace elements, diarrhea and intolerance to enteral intake, and liver toxicity associated with long-term parenteral nutrition. Specialized nutrition support may be needed. This nutrition may be provided by an oral diet plus oral supplements or by enteral nutrition via a nasogastric tube or percutaneous gastric tube. A percutaneous gastric tube (PEG), which is a catheter placed directly into the stomach through the skin, reduces discomfort associated with having a feeding tube down the nasal or oral passageway and restores the protective function of the epiglottis. In patients with continued aspiration associated with gastric feeding tubes, a feeding tube can be surgically placed directly into the jejunum and be used to provide long-term enteral nutrition using elemental enteral formulas (Harohalli et al., 2010; Kumpf & Gervasi, 2007; Scheinfeld & Mokashi, 2010).

Hospitalized patients and, in particular, elderly patients who are institutionalized are at high risk for malnutrition because many medical conditions, surgical treatments, and medications can cause fluid and nutrient losses. Nutrient and fluid loss can be associated with malabsorption associated with diarrhea, abscess drainage, ostomy losses, fistulas, and nothing by mouth (NPO) status for procedures and tests. In addition, diseases such as pneumonia or respiratory failure that require mechanical ventilation can interfere with intake in the critically ill. Renal failure that requires hemodialysis can result in significant protein loss associated with the procedure. Nutritional deficiencies accompanied by immobility can contribute to skin breakdown and formation of pressure sores (Harohalli et al., 2010; Scheinfeld & Mokashi, 2010).

The nutritional needs of critically ill patients are often increased, but their stress response to critical illness often prevents them from effectively using the nutrition provided. Providing nutritional support can lead to hyperglycemia and associated increases in complications that can increase hospital length of stay and patient mortality. Alterations in the metabolism of critically ill patients are mediated through interactions of the neuroendocrine, cardiovascular, toxic, and starvation responses. These responses mobilize nutritional substrates to maintain vital organ function and immune defenses (Mirtallo, 2007).

Neuroendocrine responses include stress responses mediated by the sympathetic nervous system. Increased catecholamines, epinephrine, and cortisol stimulate glucagon release, which increases gluconeogenesis, glycogenolysis, and hyperglycemia. Growth hormone increases and stimulation of the renin–angiotensin–aldosterone system can result in hyponatremia, **oliguria**, and volume overload. Cardiovascular responses include shock, cellular dysfunction, poor wound healing, fluid imbalance, and poor tissue perfusion that leads to tissue destruction. Toxic response is associated with infection and is mediated by increases in interleukin-1 and tissue necrosis factor. Interleukin-1 causes fever and increased gluconeogenesis by the liver as well as increased production of the stress hormones cortisol and catecholamines. Tissue necrosis factor antagonizes lipoprotein lipase, resulting in hypertriglyceridemia. Results include increased metabolic rate, increased energy expenditure accompanied by catabolism of lean body mass, and increased excretion of urinary nitrogen. Critical illness also results in a starvation response that differs from changes associated with the normal starvation response seen with long term starvation (Mirtallo, 2007).

With critical illness, the normal starvation response that spares protein breakdown is altered. Interleukin-1 and tissue necrosis factor cause muscle breakdown and increased production of gluconeogenesis and ammonia, and fat stores are mobilized to produce FFA for energy. Nutritional requirements in critically ill patients include up to 3 g/kg/day of protein. Protein is often provided as branched-chain amino acids (BCAAs) to minimize breakdown of skeletal muscle.

Critically ill patients exhibit glucose intolerance and insulin resistance, and providing calories using carbohydrate can lead to hyperglycemia in this population. High carbohydrate loads can also lead to CO_2 retention and subsequent respiratory failure. Fats are a more concentrated source of nonprotein calories, assist with fluid restriction in critically ill patients,

and are better tolerated in glucose-intolerant patients; therefore, they are used to provide a larger proportion (20%-40%) of the patient's total nonprotein calories. Because of the glucose intolerance that normally accompanies critical illness, patients who are not malnourished receive permissive underfeeding with enteral nutrition for the first 4 to 7 days in the critical care unit to minimize hyperglycemic complications. Permissive underfeeding provides adequate protein but only half of the estimated caloric requirements recommended. TPN, which contains high amounts of concentrated glucose, is avoided to improve surgical outcome in all but malnourished patients with critical illness or in critically ill patients being nutritionally repleted for at least 7 days before planned surgery (McClave et al., 2009).

During critical illness the body loses large amounts of phosphate, potassium, and urea.

Daily monitoring of electrolyte and fluid status by measuring fluid intake and urine output is critical. The critical care clinicians must monitor for sodium and fluid overload and associated dilutional hyponatremia in these patients. Such fluid overload can lead to congestive heart failure (CHF), pulmonary edema, and elevation of intracranial pressure. Conversely, severe fluid restriction can result in dehydration, hypernatremia, and hyperosmolality. Depletion of intravascular volume can result in decreased renal perfusion, resulting in shock and acute renal failure. Critical care clinicians should also monitor patients for refeeding syndrome when initiating nutritional therapy in patients with critical illness.

Nutrition in the Elderly Patient With Dysphagia

Providing adequate nutrition in the elderly patient with dysphagia presents special challenges (Scheinfeld & Mokashi, 2010). Patients who are elderly often have several disease states and require multiple medications that may cause side effects and drug interactions that contribute to changes in cognition, taste, smell, and appetite and result in decreased intake. Medications can also change gastrointestinal tract motility and alter production of saliva, further contributing to dysphagia. Certain medications, such as anticholinergic medications (e.g., antihistamines), can reduce both saliva production and the lubrication of the nasal passages, affecting taste and smell. Ensuring adequate fluid intake and moisturizing the mouth and nasal passages can minimize some of these effects. Table 3.2 summarizes some medications that commonly affect appetite, nutritional intake, and weight. Chapter 24 provides additional information on medication-induced dysphagia. The rehabilitation specialist should investigate medication use when detecting symptoms of dehydration or changes in a patient's weight (Carl & Johnson, 2006, 2010; Harohalli et al., 2010; Scheinfeld & Mokashi, 2010).

PATIENT CASE 1

Y.P. is an 81-yr-old female who was recently discharged after a prolonged hospitalization for a stroke. During her hospitalization she developed aspiration pneumonia secondary to dysphagia and lost 15 lb (6.8 kg). She has residual hemiplegia and suffers from dysphagia.

Table 3.2   Medications That Can Affect Nutrition

Mechanism affecting nutrition	Medication classes with associated examples
Medications that affect smell	Anticholinergics (Phenergan), anti-infectives (amoxicillin), cardiac medications (Procardia), cholesterol-lowering agents (Lopid), inhaled products (intranasal), nasal decongestant sprays (Afrin), anti-inflammatory agents (prednisone), gastrointestinal agents (Tagamet), medications that affect thyroid function (Tapazole), medications for Parkinson's disease (levodopa, Sinemet)
Medications that affect taste	Agents that prevent alcohol abuse (Antabuse; metallic taste); antidepressants (Prozac; unpleasant taste); anti-infectives (ampicillin; taste loss); anticonvulsants (Dilantin; taste loss); antihypertensive, antiarrhythmic, or cardiac medications (Procardia; unpleasant taste); antianxiety or insomnia medications (Xanax; taste loss); antispasmodic agents (baclofen; taste loss); antipsychotic agents (Risperdal; bitter taste); chemotherapy and immunosuppressant medications (Imuran; taste loss); gastrointestinal medications (Pepcid; unpleasant taste); hormonal or endocrine agents (insulin; taste loss); inhaled medications (Albuterol; unpleasant taste); medications for Parkinson's disease (Permax; unpleasant taste); medications for hyperlipidemia (Pravastatin; unpleasant taste)
Medications that promote weight loss	Medications that increase levels of the neurotransmitter norepinephrine can decrease appetite and promote weight loss. Many of these products are found in diet aids, decongestants used in cough and cold products, and herbals used in weight reduction. Some medications used for weight reduction increase central levels of serotonin, resulting in decreased food intake, and prolong the time between meals. Selective serotonin reuptake inhibitors, antidepressants, and the herbal product St. John's wort also can increase serotonin and promote weight loss.
Medications associated with weight gain	Corticosteroid use can be associated with significant increases in appetite, changes in fat distribution, and significant increases in fluid accumulation and weight gain. Lithium, tricyclic antidepressants, and the phenothiazine class of antipsychotic medications have all been associated with significant unintentional weight gain. Medications used specifically to promote weight gain include anabolic steroids such as oxandrolone (Oxandrin), progestins such as megestrol (Megace), the antihistamine cyproheptadine (Periactin), and the antidepressant mirtazapine (Remeron), which promote weight gain by blocking histamine receptors. Use of these agents is recommended only once treatable causes of weight loss are sought and addressed. Dronabinol (Marinol) is used to stimulate appetite and prevent weight loss in patients with human immune deficiency virus and acquired immune deficiency syndrome.

The medications listed in parenthesis are examples only and not the only such medications.

Question
What are some risk factors for malnutrition in Y.P.?

Answer
Identified risk factors in Y.P. include her age, prolonged hospitalization, and the hemiplegia and dysphagia associated with her stroke.

Dietary modification is one component of dysphagia treatment. A patient's protein and calorie intake may be enhanced with thickening agents, prethickened beverages, oral liquid supplements, and modular components. An altered diet of pureed or mechanical soft foods may be recommended for patients who have difficulties with the oral preparatory phase of swallowing, who pocket food, or who have significant pharyngeal retention of foods. The speech–language pathologist may also recommend thickened liquids such as nectar and honey. A uniform and viscous bolus of food or beverage may enable a patient with a delayed swallow reflex to control mastication and transport. It may also allow the individual to swallow with less risk of aspirating residue material (Moses, 2010; Scheinfeld & Mokashi, 2010). The dysphagia diet is classified by the severity level of the dysphagia, and the associated recommended diet varies by viscosity and ease of chewing and swallowing to minimize aspiration risk (see table 3.3). Liquids may need to be thickened with thickening agents to minimize aspiration risk. The degree to which they are thickened is described by four classifications: thin liquids (regular fluids), nectar thick liquids (thickened but still may be sipped through a straw), honey thick (too thick to be sipped through a straw), and pudding thick (holds its shape in a spoon) (Harohalli et al., 2010).

Nutrition in the Pediatric Failure-to-Thrive Patient

Pediatric patients with unexplained weight loss may be diagnosed with failure to thrive. Evaluation of the family's psychosocial situation by an interdisciplinary team of specialists in pediatric rehabilitation, mental health, and social services is necessary to determine what support is needed. Support may include a psychologist

Table 3.3 Levels in the Dysphagia Diet

Severity level of dysphagia	Consequence of the dysphagia with recommended diet alterations and recommendations for medication administration. As swallowing function improves, the diet may be advanced to the next level of soft and semisolid foods of regular consistencies.
Level I: Severe dysphagia	The patient is unable to safely swallow chewable foods and is unable to safely drink thin liquids. The patient requires thick, homogenous, semiliquid textures. No coarse textures, raw fruits or vegetables, or nuts. Medications cannot be swallowed whole and must be crushed and mixed with food. The patient may require foods with a puréed consistency (e.g., pudding, mashed potatoes) and thickened liquids.
Level II: Moderate dysphagia	The patient can tolerate minimal foods that are easily chewed. The patient may not safely tolerate thin liquids and may require thickened liquids. The patient may be unable to tolerate coarse textures such as raw fruits and vegetables and nuts. Medications may need to be crushed and mixed with food. The patient may require minced foods.
Level III: Difficulty chewing	The patient may have difficulty manipulating and chewing foods. Mechanically soft foods are provided for this level of dysphagia. Patients should not consume nuts or raw foods. Liquids may require thickening and are given as tolerated. Medications may need to be crushed and mixed with food.
Level IV: Mild dysphagia	The patient chews soft textures and swallows liquids safely. Provided foods are finely chopped or provided as textured foods that do not require grinding or chopping. No nuts, raw fruits, vegetables, or deep-fried or crisp foods are permitted. Whole medications and unthickened liquids are cautiously reintroduced and given as tolerated.

and may require referral to child protective services if neglect is suspected. Home visits can help determine any underlying reason for the child's failure to thrive and can help support the caregiver.

If outpatient care is unsuccessful, hospitalization may be necessary to determine physical reasons for weight loss. The clinician should initially observe the interaction between the caregiver and the child during feeding. During hospitalization the caregiver should provide feedings under close observation. If weight loss continues, hospital staff should perform feedings. If feedings are unsuccessful, the clinician should implement a trial of nasogastric tube feeding to determine whether the gastrointestinal tract can absorb adequate nutrition. Malabsorption can be treated with predigested enteral nutrition or even short-term parenteral nutrition. Speech–language pathologists specially trained in pediatric feeding can perform an assessment to determine any oral, pharyngeal, or esophageal dysphagia and, in collaboration with the dietitian, can develop a feeding plan that involves training the family to provide adequate intake for growth. High-calorie products (e.g., protein powders, rice cereals, nonfat dry milk powders, concentrated infant formulas, and coconut, safflower, and corn oils) can be incorporated in the diet to increase nutrition intake (Rabinowitz et al., 2010).

Nutrition in the Patient With Cancer

Malnutrition in patients with cancer often results from either the progression of the tumor itself or cancer treatment. Cancer cachexia is caused by increased tumor necrosis factor and results in weight loss, muscle wasting, anorexia, decreased nutrient intake and absorption, and inability to appropriately utilize provided nutrients. The average survival of cancer patients with weight loss is reduced by 30%, and these patients show a reduced response to chemotherapy treatment. Weight loss is seen in 85% of patients with gastric or pancreatic cancer, 55% of patients with colorectal, prostate, or lung cancer, and 35% of patients with breast cancer, **sarcoma**, or non-Hodgkin's lymphoma. Cancer-associated weight loss occurs late in the disease and progresses rapidly (Douglass, 1984; Finley & LaCivitia, 1992; Grunwald, 2003; Roberts & Mattox, 2007).

Cancer cachexia is associated with glucose intolerance, gluconeogenesis, increased mobilization of free fatty acids, and muscle wasting. Muscle wasting is associated with preferential breakdown of skeletal muscle (branched-chain amino acid) and protein and preferential utilization of fat in place of carbohydrate. Each 1 kg (2.2 lb) of tumor consumes 140 g of carbohydrate/day. Metabolism of glucose by cancer cells is **anaerobic**. Glucose is converted to **pyruvate** and large amounts of lactic acid are dumped into the circulating blood, resulting in metabolic acidosis. Protein-calorie malnutrition results in decreased synthesis of deoxyribonucleic acid (DNA) and ribonucleic acid (RNA), diminished total mass in organs with the highest cellular turnover, and increased risk of infection due to reduced neutrophil production and reduced phagocytosis of bacterial pathogens. Effects of malnutrition include decreased ability to replicate cells and repair intestinal tissues. This can cause shortening of the gastrointestinal villi, reduced intestinal enzymes, reduced immune hormone production, reduced brush border activity, and decreased intestinal absorption. Intestinal atrophy can result in diarrhea and intolerance of nutrition provided in oral or enteral form. Other complications include pancreatic atrophy, fatty liver, osteoporosis, and muscle atrophy (and associated impairment of respiratory and cardiac function) due to **catabolism** (Douglass, 1984; Finley & LaCivitia, 1992; Grunwald, 2003; Roberts & Mattox, 2007).

Mucositis often accompanies chemotherapy, especially when combined with radiation therapy. In high-dose chemotherapy patients, oral intake of food and liquids may be reduced by more than 50% for 7 to 14 days after each treatment. The median survival of patients who receive radiation and chemotherapy is 40 wk, whereas the median survival of patients receiving chemotherapy alone is 75 wk. The combination of chemotherapy and radiation results in severe nausea and vomiting in two thirds of these patients. Autopsy revealed that most of these deaths were due to **inanition** rather than progression of cancer (Carl & Johnson, 2006; Douglass, 1984; Finley & LaCivitia, 1992; Grunwald, 2003; Roberts & Mattox, 2007).

PATIENT CASE 2

E.K. is a 65-yr-old man with small-cell lung cancer. He has had surgical resection of the tumor and now is undergoing chemotherapy and radiation therapy. He has lost 24 lb (10.9 kg) in the past 6 wk. His physician has diagnosed him with cancer cachexia and referred him for cancer rehabilitation to deal with his weight loss and progressive muscle weakness. E.K. is complaining about mouth pain that is preventing him from eating many foods.

Question:
What are some factors contributing to malnutrition in E.K.?

Answer:
His cancer cachexia and his nausea and vomiting associated with chemotherapy can be contributing to his weight loss. It is also highly likely that he has mucositis associated with his chemotherapy and radiation treatments.

Nutrition support as an adjuvant to cancer chemotherapy, surgical resection, or radiation helps the patient survive the metabolic insult and reduces morbidity and mortality associated with cancer. However, its use is controversial and benefits associated with nutritional support vary with the type of cancer. Nutritional support does reduce the time spent in the hospital for surgical treatment in cancer patients. The enteral route should be used when a functional gut exists, but patients with weight loss of greater than 20% require resuscitation with parenteral nutrition. In well-nourished patients with solid tumors receiving standard chemotherapy, parenteral nutrition may not be warranted and may actually be harmful. Studies have shown that patients receiving chemotherapy benefit from nutrition support, but some studies demonstrate that **stomatitis**, myelosuppression, diarrhea, and infections increased when parenteral nutrition was used. Parenteral nutrition is beneficial in patients undergoing bone marrow transplant. Parenteral nutrition also reduces incidence of **anastomosis** leakage after bowel resection in patients with gastrointestinal cancer (Ignoffo, 1992).

In cancer patients, protein requirements are 1 to 1.5 g/kg/day for maintenance and 1.5 to 2.0 g/kg/day for repletion of protein stores lost while receiving chemotherapy, radiation, or surgical intervention. Caloric requirements are 25 to 35 kcal/kg/day for maintenance and 35 to 50 kcal/kg/day for repletion. The recommended percentage of calories provided by fat is usually 20% to 40% of the calories, depending on the degree of glucose intolerance.

Fluid and electrolyte imbalances are common in the cancer patient. One of the most serious complications of chemotherapy is tumor lysis syndrome. It is caused by tumor cell death and lysis, which leads to release of intracellular potassium, phosphate, and uric acid. This can lead to **hyperkalemia**, hyperphosphatemia, hypocalcemia, hyperuricemia, uric acid nephropathy, and acute renal failure (Krishnan, 2012). Cancer patients who are malnourished are at high risk for refeeding syndrome. In addition, hyponatremia and fluid retention are commonly seen in the cancer patient due to syndrome of inappropriate **antidiuretic hormone** caused by the tumor or the chemotherapy medications (Douglass, 1984; Finley & LaCivitia, 1992; Grunwald, 2003; McDonald & Dubose, 1993; Roberts & Mattox, 2007).

Nutrition in the Patient With Respiratory Disease

The most common type of chronic respiratory disease is **chronic obstructive pulmonary disease** (COPD), which includes both chronic bronchitis and emphysema. Failure to take into account the specialized needs of the COPD patient can worsen respiratory function and interfere with the patient's participation in rehabilitation.

About 50% of hospitalized patients with COPD suffer from protein and calorie malnutrition. The total energy expenditure associated with breathing in the normal patient is 2% to 5% of total daily needs, but in patients with respiratory disease the calories needed for breathing can increase to 10% to 20% of total daily needs. Providing calories 1.7 times the resting energy expenditure is recommended. The metabolism of carbohydrate in the diet is associated with production of CO_2. Patients with respiratory disease tend to retain CO_2, and hypercapnea (high CO_2 levels) associated with excessive carbohydrate intake can worsen respiratory function. For patients with respiratory disease, 30% to 40% of nonprotein calories should be provided by fat, which carries a lower respiratory quotient and produces less CO_2 (Btaiche & Khalidi, 2004a; Cochran et al., 1989; Frankenfield et al., 2005; Hoffer, 2003; Ireton-Jones et al., 1993; Lemoyne & Jeejeebhoy, 1986).

Weakening of the respiratory or intercostal muscles due to protein and electrolyte deficiencies can also worsen breathing difficulty. Patients with chronic respiratory disease require at least 1.7 g/kg of protein/day to replete and preserve the muscle protein utilized in breathing (Btaiche & Khalidi, 2004b; Cochran et al., 1989; Frankenfield et al., 2005; Hoffer, 2003; Ireton-Jones et al., 1993; Lemoyne & Jeejeebhoy, 1986).

Patients with respiratory disease must take in adequate micronutrients to ensure that they are able to properly utilize the nutrition provided. Fifty percent of patients with COPD have low phosphate levels due to the increased energy associated with breathing. Phosphate, which is required for muscle function and energy utilization, is the most important electrolyte associated with pulmonary function and is found in many protein sources. Hypophosphatemia can exacerbate respiratory failure and result in neuromuscular dysfunction. Phosphate is also required for the synthesis of adenosine triphosphate (ATP) which is part of the ATP cellular pump that transports energy into muscle cells. Inadequate ATP production can lead to respiratory muscle weakness. Other important electrolytes include magnesium, calcium, and potassium. These also affect cell transport of nutrients into the muscle cell, and depletion of these electrolytes can result in respiratory muscle dysfunction. Medications such as diuretics and steroids may contribute to the loss of these electrolytes, and renal dysfunction can cause retention of potassium, magnesium, and phosphate. The clinician should always consider drug interactions and the effects of other disease states when designing a nutritional plan (Btaiche & Khalidi, 2004b; Cochran et al., 1989; Frankenfield et al., 2005; Hoffer, 2003; Ireton-Jones et al., 1993; Lemoyne & Jeejeebhoy, 1986).

The onset of weight loss in a patient with chronic respiratory disease is an indicator of a poor prognosis. Progressive weight loss can occur with inadequate dietary intake. Nutrition counseling and meals that address the needs of the pulmonary patient are essential to the success of pulmonary rehabilitation. Obesity may also be detrimental to respiratory function because the work of the compromised respiratory system is increased. Weight loss should be part of the rehabilitation plan in obese patients (Btaiche & Khalidi, 2004a; Cochran et al., 1989; Frankenfield et al., 2005; Hoffer, 2003; Ireton-Jones et al., 1993; Lemoyne & Jeejeebhoy, 1986).

PATIENT CASE 3

W.P. is a 75-yr-old man with severe COPD and a history of smoking 60 packs/yr. He quit smoking 5 yr ago and has found it increasingly difficult to continue his daily routine due to increased shortness of breath and progressive weakness in his extremities. His doctor refers him for pulmonary rehabilitation. After taking the initial history, the rehabilitation therapist determines that W.P. has lost 25 pounds in the past year. The therapist refers W.P. to a clinical dietitian, who formulates a new diet plan. W.P. complains that the diet restricts many of the carbohydrate foods he usually eats and requires too much meat. He asks how important this diet is and states that he cannot afford the grocery bill associated with this new diet.

Question
What can the therapist tell W.P. about his dietary requirements and how they affect his respiratory function?

Answer
The dietitian has adjusted W.P.'s diet to provide more protein, less carbohydrate, and more fat for calories. W.P. requires more protein to maintain the muscles needed for breathing. Carbohydrate increases CO_2 production, which can worsen his breathing and even cause respiratory failure, whereas fats provide a more concentrated source of calories that do not cause CO_2 accumulation.

Nutrition in the Patient With Diabetes

Diabetes is a disorder of metabolism that results from insulin deficiency or peripheral tissue resistance to the effects of insulin that results in hyperglycemia, metabolic derangement, and toxicity resulting in complications at the microvascular and macrovascular levels. Diabetes affects the metabolism of all fuels (carbohydrate, fat, protein, and ketones). Insulin is a hormone produced by beta cells of the pancreas. Insulin-dependent diabetes is associated with a deficiency in insulin levels due to pancreatic damage, whereas non-insulin-dependent diabetes is associated with a relative deficiency of insulin with resistance at target receptors at the cellular level to the effects of insulin that prevents cells from absorbing and utilizing glucose. In the diabetic patient, the regulatory function of insulin is impaired and intake of excessive amounts of carbohydrate or fat can result in high glucose levels. Severe stress associated with injury or infection or the administration of medications such as steroids can increase levels of glucagon, cortisol, and catecholamines and can induce or worsen hyperglycemia with insulin resistance. New-onset hyperglycemia in the diabetic who was previously well controlled may be the first warning sign of infection (DeHart & Worthington, 2005; McDonnell & Aprovian, 2007; McMahon et al., 1989).

Diet management includes education about the timing, size, frequency, and composition of meals to avoid hypoglycemia or postprandial hyperglycemia. All patients should receive a comprehensive diet plan that includes a prescription for daily caloric intake; recommendations for amounts of dietary carbohydrate, fat, and protein; and instructions for dividing calories among meals and snacks. Distributing calorie intake throughout the day is important for diabetics. They should consume 20% of daily calories at breakfast, 35% at lunch, 30% at dinner, and 15% as a late-evening snack. Some patients with insulin-dependent diabetes may also need midmorning and midafternoon snacks in order to avoid hypoglycemia. Protein requirements range from 1 to 1.5 g/kg/day; protein intake should be reduced in patients with diabetic nephropathy (Lamb, 2010; McDonnell & Aprovian, 2007; Sherman & Echeverry, 2010; Votey & Peters, 2010).

The diabetic diet is a healthy-eating plan that is naturally rich in fiber and nutrients and low in fat and calories and that emphasizes fruits, vegetables, and whole grains. Patients should be encouraged to increase intake of the healthiest sources of carbohydrate such as fruits, vegetables, whole grains, legumes (e.g., beans, peas, lentils), and low-fat dairy products. Increased intake of dietary fiber decreases the risk of heart disease and helps control blood sugar levels. Foods high in fiber include vegetables, fruits, nuts, legumes (e.g., beans, peas, lentils), whole-wheat flour, and wheat bran. Patients should eat heart-healthy fish (e.g., cod, tuna, halibut) at least 2 times/wk. Fish such as salmon, mackerel, and herring are rich in omega-3 fatty acids, which reduce triglycerides (Mayo Clinic, 2010).

Because diabetics are at increased risk for high cholesterol and associated heart disease and stroke, the amount of fat and sodium in the diet should be limited. Patients should avoid added table salt and salty foods and limit sodium intake to less than 2000 mg/day. Clinicians should teach patients to limit intake of high-fat dairy products and animal proteins containing high amounts of saturated fats (e.g., bacon, hotdogs, sausage) to less than 7% of daily caloric intake. They should also teach patients to read the labels of food products for sodium and fat contents per serving. Trans fat is found in processed snacks, baked goods, shortening, and stick margarines and should be avoided completely. Patients should limit cholesterol intake to no more than 200 mg/day. Foods high in cholesterol include high-fat dairy products, high-fat animal proteins, egg yolks, shellfish, liver, and other organ meats (Mayo Clinic, 2010).

Weight loss can be important in managing glucose levels in the non-insulin-dependent diabetic who is overweight, and exercise is an important aspect of diabetes management. Clinicians should encourage patients to exercise regularly and should educate patients about the effects of exercise on blood glucose level, especially if the patient is taking insulin. If patients participate in rigorous exercise for more than 30 min, they may develop hypoglycemia. To prevent hypoglycemia, they can have an extra snack prior to exercise. These patients must stay hydrated during exercise (Lamb, 2010; McDonnell & Aprovian, 2007; Sherman & Echeverry, 2010; Votey & Peters, 2010).

Nutrition in the Patient With Renal Failure

Two types of renal failure exist: acute and chronic. Acute renal failure (ARF) can result from acute reduction in renal perfusion seen with sudden hypotension associated with hemorrhage, anaphylaxis, low cardiac output, or sepsis. In ARF, the kidneys lose the ability to regulate fluid balance, maintain electrolyte and acid–base balance, and eliminate toxic waste products. ARF patients have increased metabolic rates due to increased concentrations of endogenous stress hormones such as glucagon, catecholamines, glucocorticoids, growth hormone, aldosterone, and antidiuretic hormone. Stress hormones result in increased gluconeogenesis and increased catabolism of muscle protein, which lead to increased accumulation of **urea** and **creatinine**. Fifty percent of patients with acute renal failure will be glucose intolerant and will have high insulin levels due to impaired insulin excretion. Insulin resistance also results in high levels of

circulating triglycerides. Forty-two percent of patients who develop acute renal failure are severely malnourished. The clinician should restrict protein intake in ARF patients in order to prevent worsened uremic symptoms. If the patient is dialyzed, the clinician can increase protein intake because protein losses occur with dialysis. Providing 29 kcal/kg usually achieves positive nitrogen balance in stressed patients with ARF who require hemodialysis. Because of glucose intolerance, a higher percentage (20%-40%) of nonprotein calories are provided as fat. Fat intake should be adjusted to keep triglyceride levels less than 200 mg/dl (Awdishu & Mehta, 2007; Chima et al., 1993; Feinstein, 1988; Harm, 1990; Horton & Godley, 1988; Krenitsky, 2004; Mirtallo et al., 1984; Wolk, et al., 2007).

PATIENT CASE 4

U.B. is a 56-yr-old female who has chronic kidney disease and peripheral neuropathy in her feet that is affecting her ability to ambulate. Both are complications associated with her diabetes. She is 5 ft 6 in. (1.7 m) tall and weighs 250 lb (113.4 kg), and her glycosylated hemoglobin (A1C) is high at 8.5 (desired levels are less than 7.0) which reflects long term uncontrolled glucose levels. She is referred to the rehabilitation specialist for exercise training and education about diet therapy.

Question
What are dietary considerations in the diabetic with chronic kidney disease?

Answer
U.B. should carefully follow her prescribed diet plan, which includes avoiding fast foods and foods with high sugar and fat content. Her diet plan encourages the intake of whole grains, fresh fruits, and vegetables, with limited amounts of healthy protein sources (white meat) in scheduled and appropriately proportioned meals and snacks that meet her assessed caloric needs. U.B.'s diet plan should also include restriction of fluids, electrolytes (sodium, potassium, phosphate, and magnesium),

and protein to maintain stable fluid and electrolyte balance in light of her poor renal function. Daily weights are an excellent way to ensure that her fluid status remains stable and that her kidney function does not worsen.

In contrast to ARF, chronic renal failure does not involve alterations of fat, carbohydrate, or glycogen metabolism. It does require restricting sodium to less than 2000 mg/day, restricting fluid to 2000 ml/day, and restricting protein to 0.5 to 0.8 g/kg/day in patients not receiving dialysis. Maintaining a blood urea nitrogen:creatinine ratio of less than 30:1 is recommended in order to avoid worsening renal function and prevent the development of ARF. Maintaining such a ratio is accomplished by restricting protein and maintaining euvolemia. Monitoring daily weight is an excellent tool for assessing whether a patient is retaining or losing fluids. When practical, monitoring intake and output of fluids can also be helpful in the acute care setting. Patients with renal failure tend to accumulate potassium, phosphate, and magnesium because they are eliminated by the kidney; therefore, these electrolytes should be carefully restricted in the diet. During exercise patients should avoid sport drinks, which contain high amounts of sugar and these electrolytes, and instead rehydrate with water.

Hyponatremia is usually dilutional and associated with fluid overload. **Hypocalcemia** is common in the patient with renal failure because the kidney fails to activate vitamin D (vitamin D supplementation with ergocalciferol is recommended) or hypocalcemia can result from uncontrolled hyperphosphatemia. When interpreting calcium level results to determine whether a patient requires calcium replacement, the level should always be adjusted using a correction factor and concurrent albumin levels (termed a corrected calcium). Excretion of fat-soluble vitamins is impaired in patients with kidney disease and these patients should be advised not take supplements of vitamins A, D, E, or K without a physician's prescription. On the other hand, because water-soluble vitamins can be lost in dialysis, dialysis patients should take supplemental B vitamins and vitamin C (Awdishu & Mehta, 2007; Chima et al., 1993; Feinstein, 1988; Harm, 1990; Horton & Godley, 1988; Krenitsky, 2004; Mirtallo et al., 1984; Wolk et al., 2007).

When chronic kidney disease worsens to the point that dialysis is needed, the frequency and type of dialysis will alter nutritional requirements. Dialysis can improve insulin resistance, correct fluid overload and hyperkalemia, and remove protein waste and acidic waste products. Patients on long-term hemodialysis also may develop protein-energy malnutrition that is associated with increased morbidity and mortality. Hemodialysis can result in glucose losses of 20 to 50 g per dialysis session; therefore, it is recommended to provide up to 50 kcal/kg/day in these patients to provide positive nitrogen balance, and liberalization of protein intake to 1 to 1.2 g/kg/day is recommended. Peritoneal dialysis results in significant absorption of glucose from the dialysate; therefore, reduction of calories by 500 kcal/day in these patients is recommended. Peritoneal dialysis also removes 40 to 60 g of amino acids/day; therefore, liberalization of protein to 1 to 1.5 g/kg/day in these patients is also recommended (Awdishu & Mehta, 2007; Chima et al., 1993; Feinstein, 1988; Harm, 1990; Horton & Godley, 1988; Krenitsky, 2004; Mirtallo et al., 1984; Wolk et al., 2007).

Nutrition in the Patient With Liver Disease

The liver is the main organ involved in the digestion, synthesis, metabolism, and storage of nutrients. The liver synthesizes glucose, plasma proteins, blood-clotting factors, and bile; metabolizes proteins, carbohydrate, and fat; stores vitamins and minerals; converts ammonia produced from deamination of amino acids to urea; converts fatty acids to ketones; and degrades and eliminates drugs and hormones. The liver produces secretory proteins (albumin, fibrinogen, prothrombin, and blood-clotting factors V, VII, IX, and X) that are released into the bloodstream. It also synthesizes amino acids through transamination and deamination. Deamination removes amino groups from amino acids and converts them to ketoacids and ammonia. Ammonia is converted to urea in the liver and excreted by the kidneys. In carbohydrate metabolism, the liver stores excess glucose as glycogen and releases glucose into circulation when blood glucose levels decrease. The liver synthesizes glucose from glycerol, amino acids, and lactic acid during times of fasting or increased needs. It also converts excess carbohydrate to triglycerides, which are stored in adipose tissue (Delich et al., 2007).

In liver disease, protein production and urea synthesis are impaired. Blood ammonia accumulates, which can result in altered mental status (encephalopathy). Liver disease also results in decreased production of clotting factors, which can increase bleeding risk. Liver disease can impair carbohydrate metabolism through impaired gluconeogenesis and impaired uptake of excess glucose levels by glycogen via glycogenesis. Liver disease also affects fat metabolism. The liver functions in lipid metabolism to derive energy as triglycerides are split into glycerol and fatty acids. The liver also converts excess carbohydrate and protein into triglycerides and fatty acids, which can be stored as adipose tissue. Beta oxidation converts fatty acids into acetyl coenzyme A. Acetyl coenzyme A goes through the citric acid cycle to produce ATP and is used to synthesize cholesterol, which is needed for the synthesis and repair of cell membranes, and bile acids, which are needed for the absorption of fats and synthesis of cholesterol. These normal functions are impaired with liver disease (Barber & Teasley, 1984; Delich et al., 2007).

The liver is the major organ that eliminates toxins from the body. Hepatic detoxification and metabolism of drugs and chemicals involve phase 1 and phase 2 reactions. Phase 1 reactions involve oxidation, reduction, and hydroxylation of drugs and chemicals. Many medications are oxidized by the liver's cytochrome P450 (CYP 450) enzyme system. Phase 2 reactions involve converting lipid-soluble products to water-soluble products via conjugation and glutathione; this enables the kidney to eliminate these products. The liver inactivates insulin and glucagon, metabolizes thyroxine and tri-iodothyronine, and inactivates steroids via phase 1 and phase 2 reactions (Barber & Teasley, 1984; Buchman, 2006; DeHart & Worthington, 2005; Hamaoui, 1986).

Hepatic disease can be acute, or chronic, or both. Symptoms include low serum albumin, elevated prothrombin time, elevated liver enzyme levels, fatigue, pruritus, jaundice, palma erythema, spider angioma, **gynecomastia**, ascites, edema, anorexia, and weight loss. Acute hepatic failure can result from a sudden decrease in hepatic blood flow, trauma, surgery, sepsis, **hepatotoxic** drugs (acetaminophen overdose, herbals, environmental toxins), or viral infection (DeHart & Worthington, 2005).

Chronic liver failure is caused by long-term alcohol abuse, hepatitis B and C, or hemochromatosis and can lead to cirrhosis. Cirrhosis results from destruction of the hepatocytes by fibrotic changes and is associated with portal hypertension, varices (alternative blood flow around the liver), and hepatic encephalopathy. Bleeding risk from esophageal varices is due to tension on the variceal wall from cirrhosis and portal vein pressure. Hemorrhage occurs in 25% to 40% of patients. Beta blockers or nitrates are used to reduce portal hypertension, and octreotide can be used to reduce splanchnic blood flow in acute bleeding episodes. Bleeding is treated with intravenous fluids and albumin and transfusion of red blood cells, platelets, and fresh frozen plasma. Sclerotherapy can be used to stop bleeding. Surgical shunts are also used to reduce pressure from the accumulation of fluid in the peritoneal cavity (ascites). Hepatic encephalopathy occurs in 50% to 80% of patients with cirrhosis and is caused by the accumulation of nitrogenous substances (elevated ammonia and aromatic amino acids) in the central nervous system. Hepatic encephalopathy is classified from grade 0 (normal) to grade 4 (coma, decerebrate posture, electroencephalograph abnormalities). Symptoms of hepatic encephalopathy include altered sleep, confusion, agitation, tremors, asterixis, ataxia, muscle rigidity, and disorientation. Hepatic encephalopathy is treated with protein restriction, and lactulose or neomycin are administered to promote ammonia clearance in the stool (Barber & Teasley, 1984;

Buchman, 2006; DeHart & Worthington, 2005; Delich et al., 2007; Hamaoui, 1986).

Eighty percent of patients with alcoholic liver disease are malnourished. These patients exhibit intolerance of fats, proteins, and glucose. In cirrhosis, energy metabolism shifts from carbohydrate to fat oxidation and breakdown of skeletal muscle is accelerated. In carbohydrate-intolerant patients with cirrhosis, 25% to 40% of calories may have to be provided as fat. Patients with liver disease require 35 to 45 kcal/kg/day. Protein should be initiated in low doses to prevent hepatic encephalopathy and advanced to 1.5 g/kg/day as tolerated. Interventions that can help the patient maintain an adequate oral diet include eating frequent, smaller meals and an evening snack, using liquid supplements, and optimizing gastric emptying by avoiding excess fiber and medications that slow gastric emptying (Barber & Teasley, 1984; Buchman, 2006; DeHart & Worthington, 2005; Delich et al., 2007; Hamaoui, 1986).

PATIENT CASE 5

T.K. is a 75-yr-old man with alcoholic cirrhosis and ascites. He was recently discharged from the hospital after surviving a massive bleeding episode associated with esophageal varices. His clinician referred him to Alcoholics Anonymous and to rehabilitation for reconditioning and dietary education. He is not hungry most of the time and has difficulty eating enough to prevent losing weight. He also has symptoms of shortness of breath associated with his ascites.

Question
What would help T.K. increase his nutritional intake?

Answer
Ascites can limit nutritional intake and contribute to a feeling of fullness. Limiting fluid and sodium intake can help prevent fluid accumulation and worsening of his ascites. Other interventions that can help T.K. maintain an adequate oral diet include eating frequent, smaller meals that contain protein and an evening snack and using liquid supplements. T.K. should avoid drinking fluids during meals in order to avoid overloading the stomach and to allow him to eat more of the meal. T.K. can check and record his weight every day to ensure that his fluid status is stable. He should optimize gastric emptying by avoiding excess fiber and medications that slow gastric emptying (e.g., antihistamines).

Enteral therapy containing branched-chain amino acids can be useful in patients exhibiting protein intolerance denoted by encephalopathy of grade 2 or greater. The clinician can initiate branched-chain amino acids at 0.5 to 0.75 g/kg/day and increase them by 0.25 to 0.5 g/kg/day until the daily protein goal of 1.5 g/kg/day is met. In patients with worsening ascites, restricting fluids to 1 to 1.5 ml/kg/day and sodium to no more than 30 mEq/day is recommended. When initiating nutrition, the clinician should monitor for the development of refeeding syndrome with careful monitoring of potassium, phosphate, and magnesium levels. Any drops in these levels should be treated with aggressive replacement therapy. Sodium and fluid intake should be restricted to avoid acute fluid overload associated with refeeding syndrome. In addition, supplementation with a multiple-vitamin formula and additional vitamin B_{12}, folate, thiamine, and zinc is recommended. Liver-function tests that should be monitored include prothrombin, liver enzymes, bilirubin, and alkaline phosphatase. Bilirubin levels greater than 3.6 have been associated with 100% mortality within 10 mo (Barber & Teasley, 1984; Buchman, 2006; DeHart & Worthington, 2005; Delich et al., 2007; Hamaoui, 1986).

Nutrition in the Patient With Pancreatitis

Pancreatitis, which is defined as inflammation of the pancreas, starts with pancreatic ischemia, pancreatic duct obstruction, or premature zymogen activation, which results in activation of pancreatic enzymes in the pancreas instead of in the small intestine. The resulting activated pancreatic enzymes cause autodigestion of the pancreas and surrounding tissue and increased inflammation as a result of activation of the complement system. Pancreatitis results in dysfunction of both the exocrine and the endocrine functions of the pancreas. Exocrine functions affected include secretion of proteolytic enzymes (trypsinogen, chymotrypsinogen, procarboxypeptidase, proaminopeptidase, amylase, and ribonuclease) and lipolytic enzymes (lipase, prophospholipase A2, and carboxylesterase lipase). Endocrine functions affected include insulin production, glucagon production, and somatostatin production.

Primary causes of pancreatitis include gallstones and alcohol abuse (60%-80% of cases). Other causes include biliary tract disease, infections caused by cytomegalovirus (CMV) and cryptosporidiosis, trauma, gastrointestinal surgery, hyperlipidemia, hypocalcemia, endoscopic retrograde cholangiopancreatography, pregnancy, and use of medications such as furosemide, didanosine, estrogens, sulfonamides, **tetracyclines**, hydrochlorothiazide, pentamidine, chemotherapy agents, and **corticosteroids** (Sitzman et al., 1989).

Metabolic responses to pancreatitis include increased energy expenditure, increased gluconeogenesis along with decreased insulin responsiveness, and increased protein degradation. Energy requirements of patients with pancreatitis are 1.7 to 1.9 times basal energy requirements, protein needs are 1.5 to 2.5 g/kg/day, and the optimal ratio for provided nitrogen grams to nonprotein calories is 100:1. Signs and symptoms of pancreatitis include hyperglycemia with glucose intolerance, abdominal pain, nausea and vomiting, tachycardia, increased amylase and lipase levels, and increased triglycerides levels in the blood. Complications include fluid collection, development of pseudo cysts, pancreatic **necrosis**, abdominal infections, and catheter sepsis. Treatment includes pancreatic rest, nothing by mouth (NPO) status, nasogastric suctioning, intravenous administration of fluids, reduction of gastric acid with proton

pump inhibitors or histamine-2 blockers, and pain management. Additional interventions may include antibiotic therapy and surgery to remove gallstones, drain pseudo cysts, or remove the necrotic, infected, and inflamed tissue (phlegmon). Fistulas can form from the pancreas to adjacent areas and can result in fluid and electrolyte disorders (Gardner & Berk, 2010; Tiu & McClave, 2007).

Support with enteral nutrition via a jejunostomy tube should start early. If initiated within 72 h, the complication rate is 24% and mortality rate 13%; if initiated later than 72 h, the complication rate is 96% and mortality increases to 38%. Mortality increases tenfold when positive nitrogen balance through aggressive nutritional support is not achieved. Mortality is increased in patients with persistent hypertriglyceridemia, hypoalbuminemia, and higher insulin requirements. TPN is indicated in patients who are unable to tolerate enteral nutrition. The use of lipids is controversial, and using lipids to provide more than 20% of needed calories is not recommended; most clinicians avoid lipids when pancreatitis is caused by hyperlipidemia. Lipids may be used in patients with elevated triglyceride levels but should be reduced if triglyceride levels increase or if abdominal pain worsens with lipid administration (Gossum et al., 1998; Tiu & McClave, 2007; Pisters & Ranson, 1992).

Nutrition in the Patient With Inflammatory Bowel Disease

Two types of inflammatory bowel disease exist: ulcerative colitis and Crohn's disease. Ulcerative colitis is a mucosal inflammatory disease of the colon and rectum, whereas Crohn's disease is characterized by transmural inflammation of any part of the gastrointestinal tract, from the mouth to the anus. Triggers of inflammatory bowel disease exacerbation include increased refined sugars, chemical food additives, reduced fiber intake in the diet, smoking, and use of nonsteroidal anti-inflammatory drugs. Inflammation can cause bowel scarring and thickening of the intestinal walls, frequently leading to obstruction, fistula, perforations, and strictures of the gastrointestinal tract. Abdominal masses and tenderness and perianal fissure may also be present. The goal of treatment is to resolve acute inflammation; alleviate systemic symptoms of fever, malaise, abdominal pain, weight loss, arthritis, and diarrhea; and maintain remission. Surgery for palliation or cure is used in some patients. Malnutrition results from malabsorption and the catabolic effects of the disease. Caloric needs are 30 to 40 kcal/kg/day (<20% provided by fat), and protein needs are 1 to 1.5 g/kg/day. Additional supplementation of iron, zinc, copper, selenium, manganese, folic acid, and vitamins B_{12}, A, D, E, and K is needed. Electrolyte and fluid losses in the stool can be significant, and serum electrolytes, fluid status, and stool production should be carefully monitored. Intravenous replacement of electrolytes and fluids should be initiated as needed (Dombrowski & Mirtallo, 1984; Farthing, 1983; Tiu & McClave, 2007).

Fistulas are tunnels connecting two tissues that are not normally connected. Gastrointestinal fistulas connect as a result of surgery, infection, or inflammation and are believed to evolve from a bowel perforation that connects to an adjacent tissue. Fistulas are classified as low or high output; high-output fistulas drain more than 500 ml/day. Vesicoenteric fistulas connect bowel to bladder, and colovesicular fistulas, which connect the colon to the bladder, are commonly associated with diverticulitis. Fifty-three percent of patients with gastrointestinal fistulas are malnourished and require nutrition support. Adequate nutrition leads to an 89% closure rate and a 12% mortality rate. In patients who do not receive adequate nutrition support, the closure rate is 37% and the mortality rate is 55%. Primary causes of death in patients with gastrointestinal fistulas include malnutrition, electrolyte imbalances, and sepsis (Dombrowski & Mirtallo, 1984).

Treatment of fistulas includes NPO status and treatment with parenteral nutrition support providing 25 to 35 kcal/kg/day and 1 to 1.5 g/kg/day of protein (for low output fistulas) or 1.5 to 2.5 g/kg/day of protein (for high-output fistulas). Providing 30% to 50% of calories via lipids is recommended due to insulin resistance and glucose intolerance in these patients. The type of electrolytes that are lost in fistula drainage vary depending on the location of the fistula in the gastrointestinal tract. Method and content of repletion of fluid and electrolytes is determined by the electrolyte content of the drainage and the amount of fluid lost. Ten percent of patients with fistulas develop refeeding syndrome; therefore, nutrition should be initiated slowly. Carbohydrate should be restricted to less than 150 g/day, sodium to less than 20 mEq/day, and fluid to 800 to 1000 ml/day. The clinician should closely monitor and replace serum potassium, magnesium, phosphorus, and fluids (Dombrowski & Mirtallo, 1984; Farthing, 1983; Tiu & McClave, 2007).

Nutrition in the Patient With Short-Bowel Syndrome

Normal small bowel size is 600 cm and most nutrients are absorbed in the first 100 to 150 cm of the small bowel. Short-bowel syndrome (SBS) is associated with extensive small bowel resection with a subsequent decrease in the functional surface area of the intestine and rapid transit of abdominal contents through the lower intestinal tract leading to nutrient, fluid, and weight loss. SBS occurs when 70% to 75% of the bowel is resected or from bowel surgery that leaves less than 200 cm of jejunum and ileum. Common causes of these extensive bowel resections include enterocutaneous fistulas, radiation enteritis, or severe inflammatory bowel disease. Removal of the duodenum results in poor tolerance of lactose and concentrated sugars and malabsorption of folic acid, iron, and calcium (Parrish et al., 2007; Sundaram et al., 2002).

The jejunum is 200 to 300 cm long and absorbs proteins, carbohydrate, fats, vitamins, and minerals. The jejunum also secretes peptides that limit gastrin production. Loss of the jejunum results in fluid losses of 3 L/day and 90 mEq/L of sodium, increased acidity from gastric sections, and inactivation of pancreatic enzymes, which results in decreased digestion of lipids and protein. This excess in gastric acid also damages bowel mucosa and increases peristalsis. Proton pump inhibitors or histamine-2 blocker medications are used to reduce acid production (Parrish et al., 2007).

The **ileum** is 300 to 400 cm long and slows peristalsis (Sundaram et al., 2002). Loss of the ileum results in loss of bile acids, fat malabsorption, and deficiencies of calcium and vitamins A, D, E, and K. The ileum can perform the functions of the jejunum, but the jejunum cannot perform the functions of the ileum. The colon absorbs 1 L/day of water and sodium and excretes bicarbonate and potassium. The colon ferments 60 to 80 g/day of unabsorbed carbohydrate into short-chain fatty acids, which provide a source of calories. Preserving at least half of the colon reduces fecal loss of nutrients and slows intestinal transit. Diarrhea is treated with loperamide or codeine, and lactase supplements assist with bloating and diarrhea associated with lactose intolerance (Charney, 1995; Parrish et al., 2007; Sundaram et al., 2002).

Malabsorption of carbohydrate, lactose, and protein occurs after extensive bowel surgery that results in short bowel syndrome. The remaining bowel begins to adapt 12 to 24 h postoperation, and changes continue for up to 2 yr. High-volume fluid losses of up to 3 L/day can occur immediately postoperation and can last for 1 to 3 wk. With each liter lost, a sodium loss of 90 mEq/L, a potassium loss of 15 mEq/L, and a chloride loss of 60 to 140 mEq/L occur. Magnesium and calcium are lost also and need to be repleted. Zinc, vitamin B_{12}, iron, fat-soluble vitamins, and selenium should be supplemented. Complications of fluid and electrolyte loss associated with SBS include metabolic acidosis, cholesterol bile stones, renal oxalate stones, dehydration, diarrhea, weight loss, and transient hyperbilirubinemia (Charney, 1995; Parrish et al., 2007; Sundaram et al., 2002).

The acute phase of SBS lasts for 1 to 3 mo and is marked by poor absorption of water, electrolytes, protein, fat, vitamins, carbohydrate, trace elements, and vitamins; transient hyperbilirubinemia; and large losses of fluid. Aggressive fluid and electrolyte replacement is needed and oral antibiotics (neomycin and metronidazole) are given to prevent bacterial translocation through the gut. Early initiation of nutrition support with TPN at 30 to 35 kcal/kg/day (20%-30% of kilocalories as fat) and with 1 to 1.5 g/kg/day of protein is recommended. When fluid and electrolytes stabilize and diarrhea is less than 2 L/day, an elemental diet may be initiated. Providing early, high-viscosity enteral feedings tends to reduce the length of TPN therapy. Elemental diets are efficiently absorbed within the first 100 cm of the jejunum. Polymeric diets are often used in place of elemental supplements because they are more palatable, cause less diarrhea, and are less expensive (Charney, 1995; Parrish et al., 2007; Sundaram et al., 2002).

The adaptive phase begins 24 to 48 h after surgery and lasts for 1 to 2 yr. An additional 5% to 10% improvement in bowel adaptation is possible during this phase. Fluid and electrolyte levels stabilize and mucosal surface areas increase as intestinal dilatation and lengthening occur. In this phase the colon salvages calories by converting unabsorbed carbohydrate into absorbable short-chain fatty acids (Charney, 1995; Parrish et al., 2007; Sundaram et al., 2002).

During the final phase, the maintenance phase, nutrition continues with initiation of small meals and continued supplementation with vitamins and minerals. Patients with SBS absorb less of their diet and so must increase caloric intake between 200%-400% to compensate, and the diet should be high in calories and protein to facilitate recovery. Energy requirements are 30 to 40 kcal/kg/day, and the oral diet should provide at least 2.5 times the basal energy requirement. Patients should not take liquids with meals in order to minimize the volume load and minimize dumping. A low-oxalate, low-fat diet and high fluid intake are recommended for patients with oxalate stones. Pancreatic enzymes are administered to facilitate digestion of protein and fat. Most patients require home cyclic TPN or enteral feedings. Patients with less than 30 cm of small bowel and a competent ileocecal valve, less than 60 cm and no ileocecal valve, or less than 50 cm of jejunum require lifetime TPN to supplement their oral intake. Other patients have a good chance of transitioning to a normal diet as the remaining bowel adapts during this maintenance phase (Charney, 1995; Parrish et al., 2007; Sundaram et al., 2002).

Summary

This chapter summarizes factors such as disease states and medications that increase risk for malnutrition. It includes specialized considerations for providing nutrition to patients with organ dysfunction and disease states such as renal failure, liver failure, and respiratory failure and provides guidance for managing the patient with dysphagia. This chapter also provides methods for assessing and monitoring a patient's nutritional needs and fluid requirements. Finally, the chapter summarizes medications that can affect nutritional status.

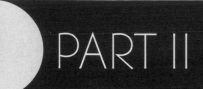

Medications Used to Treat Psychiatric and Cognitive Disorders

Part II of this text discusses psychiatric and cognitive disorders commonly seen in rehabilitation practice. Although patients may not be referred to rehabilitation for these clinical conditions, these conditions and the medications used to treat them affect rehabilitation and therefore need to be considered when developing a patient-specific treatment plan.

Chapter 4 discusses the clinical disease states of depression and bipolar (manic–depressive) disease as well as the medications used to treat these disorders. It provides insight into how these disorders can affect cognition, communication, and behavior, all of which significantly affect rehabilitation. This chapter also explains therapeutic effects of these medications and how they can enhance rehabilitation as well as important side effects and drug interactions associated with the use of these agents that should be considered when monitoring these

patients and in developing an individualized rehabilitation plan.

Chapter 5 reviews the psychiatric diseases of psychosis and schizophrenia, the most common type of psychosis. The chapter also differentiates between the symptoms associated with agitation and those seen with the clinical disease states of psychosis and outlines differences in recommended treatments. It discusses how these disorders can affect cognition, communication, motor function, and behavior, all of which significantly impact rehabilitation. It also discusses the therapeutic effects, side effects, and drug interactions of medications used to treat these disorders. The rehabilitation therapist should consider these effects when developing therapy sessions and monitoring the patient in order to maintain a safe rehabilitation environment. The chapter discusses the differences between first- and second-generation antipsychotics and their associated efficacy in treatment of positive and negative symptoms of psychosis as well as their effects on cognition and nonpsychiatric symptoms. It also presents side effects and toxicities associated with first-generation antipsychotics (e.g., parkinsonism, tardive dyskinesia) and contrasts them with those associated with second-generation antipsychotics (e.g., metabolic syndrome, weight gain).

Chapter 6 provides an overview of cognitive disorders such as delirium, dementia, and Alzheimer's disease and discusses the effect of medication use on these disorders and rehabilitation progress. Delirium is a reversible disorder that is associated with medication use or other clinical conditions. This chapter provides information on medications and conditions commonly associated with delirium and appropriated interventions for treating delirium. The dementias, which include Alzheimer's disease, are irreversible cognitive impairments. This chapter reviews methods for assessing cognition and categorizing dementias. Because appropriate treatment (i.e., medications, behavioral therapies, altered environment, and strategies that focus on the use of areas of preserved cognition) varies by type of dementia, accurately diagnosing the cognitive disorder is vital in developing a plan for rehabilitation.

Chapter 7 reviews the differences between the symptoms of anxiety that all people experience as part of everyday life and the clinical disease states of anxiety disorders and insomnia. This chapter provides information on pharmacologic and nonpharmacologic treatments of these disorders and explains how these disorders can affect rehabilitation progress. Methods of altering the rehabilitation plan for patients with different types of anxiety disorders to provide maximum benefit to the patient while maintaining a safe environment are also discussed in this chapter. The chapter also includes a universally applicable review of interventions associated with good sleep hygiene.

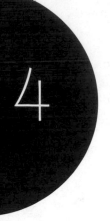

4

Medications Used to Treat Depression and Bipolar Disorder

The rehabilitation therapist will care for patients who use medications to treat mood disorders (i.e., depression and bipolar illness) as well as patients who are being treated with antidepressants for **neuropathic pain**. Therapy for mood disorders involves a combination of cognitive restructuring, behavioral therapies, psychosocial intervention, and pharmacotherapy. A significant percentage of patients referred to a rehabilitation therapist have underlying depression that can affect their rehabilitation progress. This chapter introduces mood disorders and their therapies and outlines important considerations that the rehabilitation specialist should incorporate into the individual patient's rehabilitation plan.

Depression

Depression (major depressive disorder) is a psychiatric illness that occurs in both adults and children. Symptoms associated with depression include sadness, despair, loss of ability to experience pleasure, apathy, social withdrawal, guilt, sleep and appetite disturbances, fatigue, decreased sex drive, psychomotor retardation, and impaired cognition (Dopheide, 2006; Tom-Revson & Lee, 2006).

Children with depression also exhibit symptoms of irritability and hostility. In children between 3 and 5 yr of age, interest in play is diminished and suicidal and self-destructive themes are persistent in play. Children between 6 and 8 yr of age exhibit outbursts of crying, shouting, and irritability that are accompanied by somatic complaints. Children between 9 and 12 yr exhibit low self-esteem, hopelessness, and fear of death, and commonly run away from home. Adolescents aged 12-18 yr exhibit impulsivity, irritability, reckless behavior, poor school performance, appetite and sleep disturbance, and suicide attempts. The depression rate in female adolescents doubles after puberty. Additional risk factors for depression include substance abuse, anxiety disorders, genetic predisposition, and psychosocial stressors (e.g., maternal mental illness, physical or sexual abuse, parental loss or absence). Childhood depression can interfere with the developmental process, result in difficulty with concentration and motivation, affect academic performance, impair social functioning, reduce self-esteem, and increase suicide risk. Suicidal thoughts occur in 19% of nondepressed youths, whereas 35% to 50% of youths with depression attempt suicide. Of those patients, 2% to 8% are successful in committing suicide. Behavioral disorders found in adolescents who are treated with antidepressants or mood stabilizers include major depressive disorder, eating disorders such as anorexia nervosa or bulimia nervosa, and bipolar disorder (Dopheide, 2006; Tom-Revson & Lee, 2006).

Incidence

Depression is a significant public health problem worldwide and is the fourth leading cause of disease burden. Depression is the largest nonfatal burden and accounts for approximately 12% of all years lived with disability

(Uston et al., 2004). Depression affects about 15 million people in the United States each year. Major depression is the leading cause of disability in adults between 15 and 44 yr of age and is the leading cause of suicide in children and adults. Depression occurs in 0.3% of pre-schoolers, 2% of children in elementary school, and 5% to 10% of adolescents. Among adolescents, depression occurs in 29% of American Indians, 22% of Hispanics, 18% of Caucasians, 17% of Asian-Americans, and 15% of African Americans. Untreated depressive episodes can last for up to 9 mo and recur in 50% of depressed patients within 5 yr (Tom-Revson & Lee, 2006).

Etiology and Pathophysiology

Depression is associated with an imbalance in the levels and activity of the neurotransmitters serotonin, norepinephrine, and dopamine. Serotonin is found in regions of the central nervous system that are associated with mood and anxiety. Serotonin also affects functions of sleep, cognition, sensory perception, memory, temperature regulation, motor activity, sexual behavior, hormone secretion, and appetite. Norepinephrine is found in all parts of the brain and large amounts are found in the hypo-thalamus, which regulates body temperature, hunger, and thirst; and in the limbic system, which governs emotion, behavior, smell, and long-term memory. Norepinephrine, the "fight or flight" neurotransmitter, is the main neu-rotransmitter for sympathetic–postganglionic fibers. Norepinephrine is also associated with mood and is one of the neurotransmitters that antidepressants target. Dopamine is particu-larly important in the regulation of movement, cognition, and emotional response. Antide-pressant medications reestablish a balance in the levels and activities of one or more of these neurotransmitters (Bostwick & Diez, 2008; Carl & Johnson, 2006; DeSimone et al., 2006; Dopheide, 2006; Dunlay et al., 2008).

Effects of Depression on Cognition

A number of studies have reported difficulties with cognition and memory in the depressed population. Geriatric depression is associated with a loss of executive functioning. Depres-sion has been shown to contribute to func-tional impairment by altering cognition and impairing communication. Depressed patients are more likely to have difficulty with instru-mental activities of daily living (ADL), such as handling one's finances. The elderly depressed patient is at risk for falls and malnutrition because the depressed patient may not main-tain their health by eating healthy meals (Hazif et al., 2009; Kindermann et al., 2000).

The hippocampus plays a very important part in memory and learning. Stress associated with major depression can cause the hippo-campus to shrink, thus impairing new learn-ing, episodic memory, and semantic memory (Sapolsky, 2001). Depressed patients also exhibit impaired recall (Hart et al., 1987) and difficulty updating of the contents of working memory, which results in problems with short-term memory (Nebes et al., 2000). The length of time that the patient has been depressed seems to influence the severity of impairment of updating skills. Impaired memory is asso-ciated more with recurrent depression than with initial episodes of depression (Basso & Bornstein, 1999). Depressed patients have difficulty with verbal-fluency tasks and story recall (Bate et al., 1993; Dunlay et al., 2008; Fossati, 2002; Fossati et al., 2004; Hill et al., 1993; Schuck et al., 2003; Suslow, 2009). The depressed patient can also have difficulty with effortful processing (i.e., learning or storing information that requires attention and effort). Effortful processing is the opposite of implicit learning, or learning without really thinking about the learning process. An example of effortful processing is memorizing informa-tion for an examination or rehearsing lines for a play. The depressed population tends to retain more automatic learning (Suslow, 2009). Depression can also affect processing speed (Fahlander et al., 1999; Kizibash et al., 2002; Nebes et al., 2000).

The depressed patient can experience dif-ficulty with set shifting and inhibition deficits, resulting in the inability to shift from one stimulus to another in a timely and appropriate fashion. This may explain why the depressed patient might stay on one subject. This inability to shift stimuli reduces the ability of the patient to benefit from instruction given by a rehabilitation therapist and can potentially increase the risk of falls (Brooks, 2011; Burt et al., 2000; Butters et al., 2000; Harvey et al., 2004).

Effects of Depression on Communication

Depression affects patterns of verbal and nonverbal communication. Depressed patients tend to show reduced **prosody** (i.e., rhythm, stress, and intonation) during speech (Alpert, 2001). Studies have shown that patients with depression speak at a reduced rate (Teasdale et al., 1980) and may have a significantly lengthened time of vocal onset (Flint et al., 1993). The length of time that the patient with depression pauses between utterances also appears to be longer (Darby et al., 1984; Greden & Carroll, 1980). In depressed patients, the process of speaking is often laborious, slow, and fixated on one subject. Body posture is described as limp and bent, and limbs tend to be tense (Eligring, 1989). Other studies show that language processing is different between depressed and normal elderly subjects (Emery & Breslau, 1989) and that depressed patients tend to use more negatively valenced words and use the word *I* more often than do patients without depression (Rude et al., 2004).

Rehabilitation Considerations

The use of regular aerobic exercise and resistance-training programs is advocated in the treatment of depression. In a study by Blumenthal and colleagues (1999), 30 min of aerobic exercise at 75% to 85% of heart rate reserve a minimum of 3 times/wk for 16 wk resulted in a clinically significant reduction in depression. The mode and intensity of exercise need to be adapted to the patient's level of fitness and other health conditions. Several mechanisms may be related to the positive effects: the production of endorphins that is associated with aerobic exercise, a reduction of anxiety, and the social benefits of group exercise. Improvements in concentration, cognition, and information processing have also been shown with bouts of submaximal aerobic exercise (Tomporowski, 2003).

Antidepressant medications can improve depressive symptoms but may be associated with side effects and drug interactions that can alter cognition and communication. Antidepressant medications can impair motor function by effects on the central and peripheral nervous system. This motor impairment may affect the progress of rehabilitation in depressed patients. During sessions, the rehabilitation therapist should monitor the patient for abnormal changes in heart rate (most notably tachycardia), symptoms of dizziness or orthostasis, or difficulty breathing and should question the patient about the presence of any medication side effects. The therapist should also monitor the patient for excessive drowsiness that interferes with learning and concentration during the treatment session. Sedation is especially problematic during the first and second weeks of therapy and immediately after a change in dosage, but the patient generally develops a tolerance to sedation. If sedation persists for more than 2 wk, the patient's physician should lower the dose or review the patient's regimen to identify a possible drug interaction that may be causing prolonged sedation (Jackson, 2002; Kando et al., 2002; Watanabe, 2007).

Because medication-related side effects can alter the patient's ability to participate in a rehabilitation session, the rehabilitation therapist should question the patient at the beginning of each session about any changes in medications or doses; most side effects are dose related and appear each time a dose is increased. The therapist should encourage the patient to adhere to the medication and should ensure that the patient has been adequately educated about their antidepressant medications. The patient should understand the purpose of the medication, the delayed onset of effects, pertinent side effects and drug interactions, and how long to continue therapy. The rehabilitation therapist can also help educate the patient and family about medication use and help monitor for side effects that affect rehabilitation. The value of acting as a patient advocate by communicating with the prescriber when necessary and facilitating medication adherence through patient and family education cannot be overstated (Fitz & Teri, 1994).

Medication Therapy

Antidepressant therapies are used in the treatment of depression and numerous anxiety disorders, such as obsessive–compulsive disorder (OCD), posttraumatic stress syndrome (PTSD), and other panic disorders. Antidepressant therapies are also used in the management of neuropathic pain syndromes (Kirkwood et al., 2011).

All antidepressant agents work by increasing the binding of one or more of the central neurotransmitters (norepinephrine, serotonin, and dopamine) to their target receptors, which can occur in several different ways. Antidepressants may enhance the action of these neurotransmitters by decreasing the metabolism of the neurotransmitter and increasing neurotransmitter levels; by decreasing the cellular reuptake of the neurotransmitter, thus leaving higher amounts to exert action at the receptor site in the synapse; or by acting as a substitute neurotransmitter and actively binding to these receptors, thus enhancing activity. They differ in selectivity and the extent to which they affect each of these neurotransmitters, which affects both their therapeutic actions and their side effects (Bloom, 2001; Carl & Johnson, 2006).

Generally, when choosing an antidepressant, the prescribing physician considers the patient's concurrent drug therapy and disease states in an effort to minimize adverse drug reactions (side effects) and drug interactions. An antidepressant that has worked for the patient or the patient's family member in the past often will have good antidepressant effects. Concurrent disease states that should be considered include neuropathic pain, **enuresis**, migraine headache, OCD, PTSD, generalized anxiety disorder, anorexia, bulimia, insomnia, seizure disorders, and cardiovascular disease (Baldessarini, 2001; Jackson, 2002; Kando et al., 2002; Kirkwood et al., 2011; Meyer, 2011; O'Donnell & Shelton, 2011).

The onset of antidepressant action is delayed, and a minimum of 4 wk is needed to assess antidepressant response. The physician should explain this to the patient so that failure to see immediate results does not result in discouragement and discontinuation of therapy during the initial titration phase. Antidepressant therapy should be initiated at low doses and titrated every 1 to 3 days until a usually effective dose is achieved; this dose should be maintained for at least 4 wk in order to assess the therapeutic effect of the medication. This minimizes the time that the patient experiences dose-related side effects, which occur during the titration period (Baldessarini, 2001; Jackson, 2002; Kando et al., 2002; Meyer, 2011; O'Donnell & Shelton, 2011).

Most antidepressants have long half-lives—typically 12 to 36 h. Therefore, they are often administered only once daily. A few antidepressants have a short half-life and are dosed more often than once daily. These include trazodone (Desyrel), nefazodone (Serzone), and venlafaxine (Effexor); these products are also available in slow-release formulations. Several agents have active metabolites that can double or even triple the length of the effects. These include amitriptyline (Elavil), clomipramine (Anafranil), doxepin (Sinequan), imipramine (Tofranil), trimipramine (Surmontil), amoxapine (Asendin), fluoxetine (Prozac), sertraline (Zoloft), and venlafaxine (Effexor). Fluoxetine (Prozac) has a half-life of 50 h and an active metabolite that extends action to 240 h. It comes in a delayed-release formulation that allows once-weekly dosing (Baldessarini, 2001; Chapman et al., 2003; Jackson, 2002; Kando et al., 2002; Meyer, 2011; O'Donnell & Shelton, 2011; Teter et al., 2011).

Patients taking antidepressants for at least 6 wk should not abruptly discontinue the medication but rather should taper the dose before discontinuance. At least 20% of patients who abruptly discontinue antidepressant therapy develop discontinuation syndrome. Symptoms of discontinuation syndrome include flu-like symptoms, insomnia, nausea, imbalance, sensory disturbances, hyperarousal, agitation, crying spells, and irritability. More serious cases can involve development of psychosis, catatonia, or severe cognitive impairment. Discontinuation syndrome is most often associated with long-term use or with use of shorter-acting antidepressants such as bupropion (Wellbutrin; half-life of 12-30 h), duloxetine (Cymbalta;

half-life of 8-17 h), and venlafaxine (Effexor; half-life of 3-13 h). Symptoms associated with discontinuation syndrome usually resolve in 7 to 10 days (Guthrie, 2007).

Antidepressants are classified into four categories based on mechanism of action: tricyclic antidepressants (TCA), **monoamine oxidase inhibitors** (MAOI), selective serotonin reuptake inhibitors (SSRI), and selective serotonin and norepinephrine reuptake inhibitors (SSNRI). SSRI and SSNRI have become preferred over the older TCA and MAOI because their side effect and drug interaction profiles are improved (Baldessarini, 2001; Jackson, 2002; Kando et al., 2002; Meyer, 2011; O'Donnell & Shelton, 2011).

- *TCAs.* Tricyclic agents (TCAs), which have been available since the 1960s, include amitriptyline (Elavil), clomipramine (Anafranil), doxepin (Sinequan), imipramine (Tofranil), trimipramine (Surmontil), amoxapine (Asendin), desipramine (Norpramin), maprotiline (Ludiomil), nortriptyline (Pamelor), and protriptyline (Vivactil). TCAs block serotonin and norepinephrine reuptake, thus enhancing the availability of these neurotransmitters at the synapse. TCAs are structurally related to the phenothiazine antipsychotic agents. In fact, the significant dopamine-blocking action of amoxapine (Asendin) causes neuroleptic effects and side effects in addition to antidepressant effects. Although TCAs are effective, most have a delayed onset of 2 to 3 wk and require slow upward titration due to their side effects, which include anticholinergic side effects, sedation, and orthostatic hypotension. Once they have been titrated over several weeks to the maximum effects, most TCA can be administered as a single bedtime dose. Some TCAs with strong sedative properties are used at bedtime to assist with depression-associated insomnia. Once the agents of choice, TCAs use as antidepressants has declined because their associated side effects of seizures and cardiac arrhythmias are difficult to treat and can be deadly in the case of an overdose. In addition, because many TCAs have strong anticholinergic effects that can increase sedation, altered cognition, and the risk of falls, their use is discouraged in the elderly. TCAs can cause weight gain, and the side effects of unpleasant

taste, altered taste, and xerostomia can affect medication adherence (Baldessarini, 2001; Jackson, 2002; Kando et al., 2002; Meyer, 2011; O'Donnell & Shelton, 2011; Tom-Revson & Lee, 2006).

- *MAOIs. Monoamines* is another name for the catecholamines, which include the neurotransmitters norepinephrine, epinephrine, and dopamine. The enzyme **monoamine oxidase** (MAO) metabolizes catecholamines to inactive products. MAO inhibitors (MAOIs) block this metabolism, leaving more active neurotransmitters available to act at the receptors, thus enhancing neurotransmitter effects. MAOIs are antidepressants which first became available in the 1960s and include phenelzine (Nardil), tranylcypromine (Parnate), and isocarboxazid (Marplan). Use of MAOIs in the treatment of depression is limited by serious toxicity associated with interactions with certain medications and foods. MAOIs are generally not considered first-line agents for treating depression due to these interactions and the necessary medication and dietary restrictions. A transdermal form of selegiline (Emsam) was recently introduced for the treatment of major depression. In low doses, selegiline is selective for monoamine oxidase-B and does not pose the risk of many of the food and drug interactions that occur with the monoamine oxidase-A inhibitors. However, because this selectivity is lost in high doses, many of the food and drug interactions exist when the transdermal form (Emsam) is used (Baldessarini, 2001; Jackson, 2002; Jacobson et al., 2007; Kando et al., 2002; Meyer, 2011; O'Donnell & Shelton, 2011).

- *SSRIs.* Selective serotonin reuptake inhibitors (SSRIs) selectively block the reuptake of serotonin by the cell, thus providing more serotonin at the site of the receptor in the synapse and enhanced effects of serotonin. Their blocking effects on norepinephrine and dopamine neuronal uptake are weak. SSRIs are the agents most often used in the treatment of depression. They are also useful in treating OCD, generalized anxiety disorder, anorexia, bulimia, panic disorder, and PTSD. Compared with TCAs, SSRIs have fewer cardiac side effects and pose less chance of precipitating seizures. However, they do have significant drug interactions that can precipitate a serious condition called serotonin syndrome. Although akathisia is normally associated with anti-psychotics, SSRIs can also produce akathisia (Jacobson et al., 2007; Kirkwood, 2011; Tom-Revson & Lee, 2006).

• **SSNRIs.** Selective serotonin and norepinephrine reuptake inhibitors (SSNRIs) block reuptake of serotonin and norepinephrine and weakly block reuptake of dopamine, resulting in increased levels and effects of these neurotransmitters. SSNRIs include bupropion (Wellbutrin, Zyban), duloxetine (Cymbalta), mirtazapine (Remeron), nefazodone (Serzone), and trazodone (Desyrel). The brand name nefazodone is no longer available due to concerns regarding its hepatotoxicity, but the generic product is still made. Zyban is used to help with smoking cessation, Cymbalta is used to treat neuropathic pain, and Remeron is frequently used to improve appetite and insomnia associated with depression (Baldessarini, 2001; Jackson, 2002; Kando et al., 2002; Meyer, 2011; O'Donnell & Shelton, 2011).

Table 4.1 lists the antidepressants and provides information on dosing and important side effects that can affect rehabilitation. The risk and type of drug interactions vary widely depending on the class of antidepressant used.

 See table 4.1 in the web resource for a full list of medication-specific indications, dosing recommendations, and side effects.

Table 4.1 Medications Used to Treat Depression

Medication	Side effects affecting rehab	Other side effects or considerations
Tricyclic antidepressants: Enhance norepinephrine or serotonin; used to treat depression; additional indications also listed.		
Amitriptyline (Elavil)	Cog ++++ S ++++ A 0 Motor ++ D ++++ Com ++++ F ++++	Weight gain +++ Seizure +++ Cardiac +++ Sexual ++ Treats depression and neuropathic pain and PTSD. Not recommended in elderly due to high sedative and anticholinergic effects that increase fall risk.
Amoxapine (Asendin)	Cog + S + A 0 Motor +++ D 0/+ Com + F +	Weight gain + Seizure ++ Cardiac ++ Sexual ++ Treats depression.
Clomipramine (Anafranil)	Cog ++++ S ++++ A 0 Motor ++ D ++ Com ++++ F ++	Weight gain ++ Seizure ++++ Cardiac +++ Sexual + Treats depression and OCD. Relatively selective for serotonin.
Desipramine (Norpramin)	Cog ++ S ++ A + Motor ++ D ++ Com ++ F ++	Weight gain + Seizure ++ Cardiac ++ Sexual ++ Treats depression and neuropathic pain. Prolongs QT interval.
Doxepin (Sinequan)	Cog ++++ S ++++ A 0 Motor ++ D +++ Com ++++ F ++	Weight gain ++ Seizure +++ Cardiac ++ Sexual ++ Treats depression and neuropathic pain.
Imipramine (Tofranil) nocturnal enuresis	Cog +++ S +++ A + Motor ++ D +++ Com +++ F ++++	Weight gain ++ Seizure +++ Cardiac +++ Sexual ++ Treats depression, neuropathic pain, and PTSD.

› continued

Table 4.1 › *continued*

Medication	Side effects affecting rehab							Other side effects or considerations
Maprotiline (Ludiomil)	Cog ++	S ++	A +	Motor ++	D ++	Com ++	F ++	Weight gain + Seizure ++ Cardiac ++ Sexual ++ Treats depression.
Nortriptyline (Pamelor)	Cog +++	S ++	A 0	Motor ++	D ++	Com ++	F +	Weight gain + Seizure ++ Cardiac ++ Sexual ++ Treats depression and neuropathic pain. Preferred tricyclic antidepressant in elderly due to low anticholinergic and sedative effects.
Protriptyline (Vivactil)	Cog +	S +	A ++	Motor ++	D +	Com +	F ++	Weight gain + Seizure ++ Cardiac +++ Sexual ++ Treats depression. Avoid doses >20 mg in elderly due to cardiac effects.
Trimipramine (Surmontil)	Cog +++	S +++	A 0	Motor ++	D ++	Com ++	F +++	Weight gain ++ Seizure ++ Cardiac +++ Sexual ++ Treats depression.
Selective serotonin reuptake inhibitors: Enhance effects of serotonin.								
Citalopram (Celexa)	Cog 0	S +	A 0/+	Motor 0	D +++	Com 0	F 0	Weight gain 0 Seizure ++ Cardiac 0 Sexual +++ Used to treat depression, PTSD, OCD, and panic disorder. 20% incidence of dry mouth and nausea; take with food.
Escitalopram (Lexapro)	Cog 0	S 0/+	A 0/+	Motor 0	D +	Com 0	F 0	Weight gain 0 Seizure 0 Cardiac 0 Sexual +++ Used to treat depression, PTSD, OCD, and panic disorder. S-isomer of citalopram causes less dry mouth and nausea than citalopram.
Fluoxetine (Prozac)	Cog 0/+	S 0/+	A +	Motor 0	D 0/+	Com 0/+	F 0	Weight gain 0/+ Seizure ++ Cardiac 0/+ Sexual +++ Used to treat depression, PTSD, OCD, and panic disorder. 20% incidence of nausea; take with food. 20% incidence of insomnia; take in the morning.
Fluvoxamine (Luvox, Luvox CR sustained release)	Cog 0/+	S 0/+	A +	Motor +	D 0/+	Com 0/+	F 0	Weight gain 0 Seizure ++ Cardiac 0 Sexual +++ Used to treat depression, PTSD, OCD, and panic disorder. 40% incidence of nausea, 20% incidence of dry mouth, 20% incidence of somnolence, and 20% incidence of insomnia; take with food. May be associated with tremor and hyperkinesis.

Medication	Side effects affecting rehab							Other side effects or considerations			
Sertraline (Zoloft)	Cog	S	A	Motor	D	Com	F	Weight gain	Seizure	Cardiac	Sexual
	+	+	+	0	+	+	+	0	++	0	+++
	Used to treat depression, PTSD, OCD, and panic disorder.										
Paroxetine (Paxil)	Cog	S	A	Motor	D	Com	F	Weight gain	Seizure	Cardiac	Sexual
	0/+	+	+	0	+	+++	0/+	0	0	0	+++
	Used to treat depression, PTSD, OCD, and panic disorder.										
Vilazodone (Viibryd)	Cog	S	A	Motor	D	Com	F	Weight gain	Seizure	Cardiac	Sexual
	0/+	0/+	+	0	+++	+	0	0	++	0	0
	Used to treat depression.										

Selective serotonin and norepinephrine reuptake inhibitors: Enhance effects of norepinephrine and serotonin.

Medication	Side effects affecting rehab							Other side effects or considerations			
Venlafaxine (Effexor, Effexor XR)	Cog	S	A	Motor	D	Com	F	Weight gain	Seizure	Cardiac	Sexual
	+	+	0/+	0	+	+	+	0	++	+	+++
	Used to treat depression and neuropathic pain.										
Desvenlafaxine (Pristiq)	Cog	S	A	Motor	D	Com	F	Weight gain	Seizure	Cardiac	Sexual
	+	+	0/+	0	+	+	+	0	++	+	+++
	Used to treat depression. Major metabolite of venlafaxine.										
Bupropion (Wellbutrin SR and XR, Zyban)	Cog	S	A	Motor	D	Com	F	Weight gain	Seizure	Cardiac	Sexual
	0	++	++	0	++	0	0	0	++++	0	0
	Used to treat depression and for smoking cessation. Contraindicated in seizure disorder. 23% incidence of gastrointestinal upset, 28% incidence of dry mouth, 28% incidence of anorexia, 22% incidence of insomnia, 22% incidence of agitation, and 20% incidence of tremor and sedation; take with food.										
Duloxetine (Cymbalta)	Cog	S	A	Motor	D	Com	F	Weight gain	Seizure	Cardiac	Sexual
	+	0	+	0	++	0	+	0/+	0	0	+
	Used to treat depression and neuropathic pain. Metabolized by CYP1A2 and CYP2D6. Should not be used in hepatic disease or in patients with creatinine clearance <30 ml/min.										
Mirtazapine (Remeron)	Cog	S	A	Motor	D	Com	F	Weight gain	Seizure	Cardiac	Sexual
	++	++	0	0	0/+	++	+	++	0	+	0
	Used to treat depression and enhance appetite. Useful in patient with weight loss associated with depression. Take at bedtime to minimize effects of sedation.										

› continued

Table 4.1   › *continued*

Medication	Side effects affecting rehab							Other side effects or considerations			
Nefazodone (Serzone)*	Cog +++	S +++	A 0	Motor ++	D ++	Com +++	F +++	Weight gain 0/+	Seizure ++	Cardiac +	Sexual 0/+
								Used to treat depression.			
Trazodone (Desyrel)	Cog ++++	S ++++	A 0	Motor ++	D ++	Com +++	F +++	Weight gain +	Seizure ++	Cardiac +	Sexual +
								Used to treat depression.			
Monoamine oxidase inhibitors: Enhance effects of norepinephrine, dopamine, and serotonin; used to treat depression not responsive to other classes of antidepressants and PTSD. Tyramine-rich foods and beverages should be avoided starting on day 1 and for 2 wk after discontinuance (see table 4.4). See table 4.3 for monoamine oxidase inhibitor drug interactions.											
Phenelzine (Nardil)	Cog ++	S ++	A 0/+	Motor 0	D +	Com ++	F +	Weight gain +	Seizure +	Cardiac +	Sexual +++
Tranylcypromine (Parnate)	Cog +	S +	A ++	Motor 0	D +	Com +	F ++	Weight gain +	Seizure +	Cardiac +	Sexual ++
Isocarboxazid (Marplan)	Cog +	S +	A ++	Motor 0	D +	Com +	F ++	Weight gain +	Seizure +	Cardiac +	Sexual ++
Selegiline (Emsam) transdermal patch	Cog +	S +	A ++	Motor +++	D 0	Com +	F ++	Weight gain 0	Seizure 0	Cardiac 0	Sexual +

*Brand not made due to hepatotoxicity concerns; generic still available.

Cog = cognition; S = sedation; A = agitation or mania; Motor = discoordination; D = dysphagia; Com = communication; F = falls; OCD = obsessive–compulsive disorder; PTSD = posttraumatic stress disorder; XR = extended release.

Sexual is associated with gynecomastia and other sexual dysfunction.

The likelihood rating scale for encountering the side effects is as follows: 0 = Almost no probability of encountering side effects. 0/+ = Slight probability of encountering side effects with use of higher doses. + = Little likelihood of encountering side effects. +/++ = Low probability of encountering side effects; however, probability increases with increased dosage. ++ = Medium likelihood of encountering side effects. +++ = High likelihood of encountering side effects, particularly with high doses. ++++ = Highest likelihood of encountering side effects; best to avoid in at-risk patients.

Antidepressant Use in Pain Management

Pain and depression frequently occur together and are linked in the central and peripheral nervous systems. In fact, depression is often an outcome of unrelieved chronic pain. Eighty percent of depressed patients report painful somatic symptoms. Chronic neuropathic pain is often associated with diabetes, immune disorders, cancer, and ischemic disorders and is one of the most difficult types of pain to relieve. Neuropathic pain can also originate from injury to the brain or spinal cord (e.g., stroke, multiple sclerosis) and peripheral injury (e.g., neuropathies, herpes zoster, injury amputations, trigeminal neuralgia). Neuropathic pain is characterized by decreased afferent sensory function accompanied by painful hypersensitivities such as **hyperalgesia** and **allodynia**. Nociceptive pain and neuropathic pain originate in the primary sensory neurons and terminate in the dorsal horn of the spinal cord. Neural pathways from the dorsal horn activate the brain through ascending pathways via the autonomic, perceptual, and cognitive systems, resulting in the pain response. Descending pain is transmitted through serotonin pathways in the dorsal raphe nucleus and norepinephrine pathways in the locus coeruleus. In depressed patients the dysregulation of serotonin and norepinephrine can affect these pathways and may result in nonspecific pain symptoms in depressed patients. TCAs and the SSNRIs duloxetine and venlafaxine alleviate chronic pain and treat depression. SSRIs affect only the serotonin receptors and are effective in only 33% of patients with chronic pain, whereas TCAs and SSNRIs, which affect levels of both serotonin and norepinephrine, are effective in 80% of patients. TCAs carry the disadvantage of being associated with motor coordination problems that are not seen with use of the SSNRIs (Jann & Slade, 2007).

Suicide Risk

In February of 2004, a report at a hearing of the U.S. Food and Drug Administration (FDA) indicated that suicide was the third leading cause of death in adolescents aged 15 to 19 yr. This report led to an investigation into whether these suicides were related to use of antidepressants and, as a result of this investigation, an FDA warning was added to all antidepressants. The warning states that risk of suicidal thinking and behavior increases during the first few months of antidepressant treatment in children and adolescents and recommends weighing the risks and balances before prescribing the medication and educating family and caregivers about the risk and need for close supervision during this period. In 2007, this FDA warning was extended to include adults aged 18 to 24 yr. In 2008, the FDA added to 23 anticonvulsant agents a warning about increased suicidal thoughts and behaviors. Risk of suicide is highest in the first months of therapy or when dosage is increased or decreased. Risk of suicide increases when children or adults exhibit increased anxiety, agitation, irritability, hostility, impulsivity, restlessness, hypomania, or mania while receiving antidepressant therapy. If symptoms of hypomania or mania occur, the prescriber should be notified immediately (Dopheide, 2006; McCain, 2009; Tom-Revson & Lee, 2006).

Antidepressant Use in Children

In younger children and in pediatric patients with mild depression, cognitive restructuring and behavioral therapy are first line-therapies. The addition of antidepressants is indicated in youths with moderate or severe depression. Studies have documented a 33% decrease in risk of suicide in adult and pediatric patients who were treated with antidepressants com-

pared with those who were not treated (Gibbons et al., 2005). SSRIs are safe and effective in treating depression in children or adolescents. Fluoxetine (Prozac), the only antidepressant approved for treating depression in children aged 8 yr or older, is the agent of choice because its efficacy is clearly established and it poses low risk of suicidal behaviors. In 2009, escitalopram (Lexapro) was approved for treating depression in adolescents aged 12-17 yr. SSNRIs have been used successfully in pediatric and adolescent patients with conduct disorders, substance abuse issues, and attention deficit–hyperactivity disorder and in pediatric patients who have failed SSRI therapy. TCAs and MAOIs are not recommended for treating depression in pediatric patients (Dopheide, 2006; Tom-Revson & Lee, 2006).

Antidepressant Use in Pregnancy

Antidepressant use in the pregnant patient is a challenge because none of the antidepressants are categorized as safe to use in pregnancy. Paroxetine (Paxil) should be avoided in all three trimesters because its use has been associated with a twofold increase in major malformations and a threefold increase in cardiac malformations. When SSRI are given in the first trimester, toxicity to the embryo includes tremor, feeding difficulties, irritability, agitation, rigidity, and respiratory distress. Other symptoms that occur in the neonate include seizures, excessive crying, hyperreflexia, and sleep disturbances that resolve in 1 to 2 wk. These symptoms are likely attributable to serotonin withdrawal. Anticholinergic side effects limit the use of TCAs in pregnancy. Nortriptyline (Pamelor) and desipramine (Norpramin) are the safest to use in pregnancy. When TCAs are used during the third trimester, neonates exhibit symptoms of diarrhea, jitteriness, and muscle weakness attributed to rebound cholinergic hyperactivity. The safety of SSNRI use during pregnancy is not yet established (Baylor & Patterson, 2009).

Side Effects of Antidepressants

The alteration of norepinephrine, serotonin, and dopamine levels determines the therapeutic actions of an antidepressant, and how it binds to other receptors helps shape its side effect profile. Antidepressants can alter central neurotransmission of acetylcholine, histamine, norepinephrine, serotonin, dopamine, and gamma amino butyric acid (GABA), resulting in altered cognition, sedation, agitation, seizures, and sleep disturbances. In the peripheral nervous system, antidepressants can alter effects of acetylcholine and norepinephrine at the peripheral receptors and alter sodium or potassium in cellular transport, resulting in symptoms of orthostatic hypotension and arrhythmia, problems with balance and dizziness, and gastrointestinal effects of nausea, vomiting, and xerostomia that can contribute to dysphagia and impair nutritional intake (Carl & Johnson, 2006).

Medication Adherence

Medication therapy is a mainstay in the treatment of mood disorders such as depression and bipolar disorder. However, medication adherence can be a significant issue. Medications cannot work if a patient does not take them. Factors that affect adherence include the cognitive deficits associated with the disease, social stigma associated with the disease, lack of family or social support systems, and lack of understanding about the role of medication therapy in managing the illness. Many patients have misconceptions about psychotropic medications. Twenty-three percent of Americans believe that psychotropic medications are harmful to the body. Also, many patients do not understand the importance of taking their medications or the expected side effects of their medications. Nearly 30% of patients who start an antidepressant stop taking the medication within the first month (Svarstad et al., 2004).

Effects of Medication on Cognition

Cognitive impairment, already a symptom of depression, can worsen when the antidepressant therapy causes the binding and subsequent blocking of acetylcholine and histamine at their receptor sites. These cognitive difficulties put the patient at risk for falls and can greatly influence the success of rehabilitation. The prevalence of antidepressant-induced cognitive impairment varies from agent to agent and depends on the extent of binding

and inhibition at the muscarinic acetylcholine receptors and histamine-1 receptors. Table 4.1 shows the propensity of each agent to be associated with impaired cognition; this side effect is listed as *Cog*. Sedation associated with binding of the antidepressant to muscarinic acetylcholine receptors or histamine-1 receptors can have a marked effect on rehabilitation; this side effect is listed in table 4.1 as *S*. Medication-induced sedation can exacerbate existing depression-induced cognitive difficulties affecting ADL and instrumental ADL functioning. Sedation associated with the use of antidepressants can impair mental or physical abilities, affect the patient's ability to communicate, and decrease appetite and attention to eating, especially upon initiation of therapy or after a change in dosage. Table 4.1 lists the risk for decreased communication ability associated with each agent; this side effect is listed as *Com*. Sedation also increases risk for falls and aspiration. Because sedation can be dose related, beginning with a low dose and titrating slowly may help minimize the impact of this side effect. The patient may develop tolerance to the effects of sedation, but onset of tolerance may be delayed. Once an effective dose of antidepressant is reached, sedation may be minimized by administering the medication as a single daily dose at bedtime (Alvi, 1999; Campbell-Taylor, 1996, 2001; Feinberg, 1997; Rooney & Johnson, 2000).

Agitation, mania, and insomnia can also be associated with the use of antidepressants; this side effect is listed as *A* in table 4.1. Antidepressants increase norepinephrine, a "flight or fight" neurotransmitter. This increases the **sympathomimetic** response and decreases the effects of GABA, resulting in increased anxiety, agitation, and insomnia. Insomnia is particularly debilitating in the beginning of treatment as the antidepressant takes effect. Antidepressants have been known to induce mania in patients who have bipolar disorder. If mania occurs, the antidepressant medication should be tapered off and a mood stabilizer such as lithium or an anticonvulsant should be introduced. Antidepressants that are less likely to induce mania include those with fewer effects on norepinephrine and more effects on serotonin, such as venlafaxine (Effexor), bupropion (Wellbutrin), and the SSRIs. Mania can be a complicating factor in rehabilitation (Jacobson et al., 2007). Symptoms such as impulsiveness, decreased attention, excessive talkativeness, and inability to focus on rehabilitation tasks can lead to noncompliance and jeopardize the patient's safety during a therapy session. Patients may also overestimate their abilities due to a sense of euphoria. The rehabilitation therapist must be alert to the onset of manic symptoms.

Antidepressants can also cause delirium in the elderly. This is associated with the anticholinergic effects of these medications and is particularly evident with the use of TCAs. Delirium may be preceded by nightmares and restlessness. As delirium becomes more fully developed, the patient may develop central anticholinergic syndrome, which includes symptoms such as myoclonus (muscle twitching) and choreoathetoid (jerky muscle) movements. These movements can directly affect rehabilitation (Jacobson et al., 2007). The rehabilitation therapist may be the first to observe these signs and symptoms and should report these motor-system abnormalities to the patient's prescriber or pharmacist to determine whether a change in dosage or type of medication may be indicated. The rehabilitation therapist should monitor the patient for related changes in balance, posture, and frequency and severity of involuntary movements. These involuntary movements can impede the patients' psychomotor performance in therapy and may negatively influence neuromuscular control during transfers and gait, thus putting the patient at risk for falls. The fine motor coordination necessary for many ADL such as dressing, grooming, and personal hygiene may also be negatively influenced.

Medication Effects on Motor Function

Motor discoordination, which is associated with blockage of dopamine by the antidepressant medication, can occur. This side effect is listed in table 4.1 as *Motor*. Resting tremors have been reported with the use of SSRI and TCA. Some studies have shown that SSRI use has resulted in extrapyramidal symptoms

(pseudoparkinsonism), particularly in the medically complex or elderly patient. Concurrent therapy using both SSRI and antipsychotics can produce extrapyramidal symptoms in the patient. Motor dysfunction can negatively affect rehabilitation. The health care practitioner needs to be particularly diligent in looking for motor dysfunction among patients who are taking multiple medications or who are elderly. Motor dysfunction can put the patient at risk for dysphagia as well as falls (Jacobson et al., 2007).

Effects of Anticholinergic Medications on Rehabilitation

Peripheral anticholinergic side effects include xerostomia (dry mouth), constipation, urinary retention, and vision problems. Urinary retention can increase the patient's risk for urinary tract infection. If the patient presents with even moderate urinary retention symptoms, the prescriber should be notified and the medication should be discontinued or reduced. The anticholinergic medication may also result in blurred vision, which can have a major effect on the patient's safety and independent functioning. A physician may prescribe 1% pilocarpine eye drops for patients who experience blurred vision. TCAs and other anticholinergic medications are contraindicated in patients with narrow-angle glaucoma (Jacobson et al., 2007).

Dysphagia

Dysphagia is commonly seen in patients taking antidepressant agents. The most commonly seen adverse drug reactions (side effects) associated with the use of antidepressants that can contribute to dysphagia include sedation, anticholinergic effects, and gastrointestinal symptoms of nausea, vomiting, diarrhea, and abdominal pain. Anticholinergic effects that contribute to dysphagia include anticholinergic-induced dry mouth (xerostomia) that results in difficulty forming a food bolus and initiating a swallow, reduced peristalsis due to anticholinergic effects on smooth visceral muscle, and effects on the esophageal striated or smooth muscle that result in deglutitive inhibition (Carl & Johnson, 2006).

Cardiac Side Effects and Fall Risk

Antidepressants can contribute to both cardiac arrhythmia and changes in blood pressure, which can affect balance and fall risk and significantly affect rehabilitation success. Orthostatic hypotension is a reduction in systolic blood pressure when changing positions or bending. Orthostatic hypotension can occur with the use of TCA. Antidepressant binding at the alpha-1 adrenergic binding can result in orthostatic hypotension. Hypertension and hypertensive crisis can result from excessive catecholamine levels that occur with MAOI or SSRI drug interactions (Baldessari, 2001; Glassman et al., 1993; Lichtman et al., 2008).

Impaired cognition and increased sedation can also increase fall risk. Table 4.1 lists the tendency of each agent to be associated with fall risk; this side effect is listed as *F*. The rehabilitation therapist can help reduce falls by encouraging the patient to perform active contractions of the ankle and knee muscles before standing. Activities such as ankle pumps (active dorsiflexion and plantar flexion), seated knee extensions, and seated marching can help increase venous return and circulation and help the patient slowly go from a sitting position to a standing position. The therapist should also encourage the patient to dorsiflex the feet before standing. Elastic stockings and abdominal binders may assist the patient. Geriatric patients tend to exhibit reduced orthostatic hypotension with strength training (Jacobson et al., 2007).

Elevated blood pressure, which can increase the risk of stroke, is associated with medications with the increased effects of norepinephrine. Diastolic or systolic blood pressure or both may be elevated, and the elevation may be related to the antidepressant dose. The physical therapist working with a patient using antidepressants should be aware that the patient's blood pressure may be elevated even when the patient is reclining (Jacobson et al., 2007).

The rehabilitation therapist must be aware that altered blood pressure can be a side effect of antidepressant medications. The therapist should measure the patient's blood pressure while the patient is in supine, sitting, and standing positions and should notify the patient's physician once hypertension is identified. Hypertensive crisis can also occur if a patient uses MAOI concurrently with certain medications and foods. Refer to tables 4.2 through 4.7 later in this chapter for additional information on food and drug interactions associated with antidepressants (Jacobson et al., 2007).

Antidepressants can also affect sodium and potassium transport and prolong cardiac contraction by prolonging the QT interval, resulting in arrhythmias such as torsades de pointes, which can be life threatening (Zemrak & Kenna, 2008). Table 4.1 lists the tendency of each agent to be associated with cardiac arrhythmia. This side effect is listed as *Cardiac*, and a severity rating of 0 to 4 is used (0 = little risk; ++++ = highest risk). Physicians should consider this toxicity when choosing an antidepressant in a patient with underlying heart disease, bradycardia, heart failure, or ischemic heart disease. QT prolongation has been most often associated with the use of SSRIs but can also occur with the use of TCAs and SSNRIs. The SSRI effects of slowed entry of sodium and potassium into cardiac muscle is believed to be the mechanism of slowed contraction and QT prolongation, which most often causes bradycardia. The SSNRI trazodone (Desyrel) also causes QT prolongation by inhibiting entry of potassium into the cardiac cell. The TCA imipramine (Tofranil) and amitriptyline (Elavil), are also associated with QT prolongation and slow entry of calcium and potassium into the cardiac cells. The risk of QT prolongation increases when antidepressants are combined with other medications that cause QT prolongation, such as antipsychotics, many cardiac medications used to treat arrhythmia, quinolone antibiotics, and macrolide antibiotics. Tables 4.2 through 4.5 provide additional detail regarding these drug interactions (Baldessarini, 2001; Jackson, 2002; Kando et al., 2002; Meyer, 2011; O'Donnell & Shelton, 2011; Zemrak & Kenna, 2008).

Seizure Risk

All antidepressants can potentially lower the seizure threshold, but bupropion (Wellbutrin, Zyban) and the TCAs carry the highest risk for this side effect. Table 4.1 lists the seizure risk associated with each agent. This side effect is listed as *Seizure*, and a severity rating of 0 to 4 is used (0 = little risk; ++++ = highest risk) (Baldessarini, 2001; Jackson, 2002; Kando et al., 2002; Meyer, 2011; O'Donnell & Shelton, 2011). All rehabilitation patients taking these medications should be closely monitored for seizure activity, and additional caution should be taken with those who have a history of seizure. Various factors may trigger a seizure, including stress, poor nutrition, flickering lights, illness, fever, allergies, lack of sleep, negative emotions, and heat and humidity (Goodman et al., 2003). The rehabilitation therapist should be mindful of potential triggers and minimize the patient's exposure to triggers during therapy.

When a seizure does occur during a therapy session, the therapist should take special care to prevent serious injury to the patient by ensuring that the immediate area is clear of harmful objects and that the patient is laying on a surface that will prevent a fall. Resting the patient's head on something soft to prevent the head from repeatedly striking the floor is recommended, but the therapist should not restrain the patient in any way. Rolling the patient onto the side may help keep the airway clear. Most seizures are not life threatening; however, a type of seizure known as **status epilepticus** can cause permanent brain damage due to **hypoxia**. In this instance the patient may need emergency intubation to establish an airway. It is not unusual for the victim to be unresponsive or confused for a short time after a seizure. The rehabilitation specialist should document how long the seizure lasted and other characteristics of the seizure that may be helpful to the patient's physician, who may need to change the dosage or type of antidepressant medication in order to prevent further medication-related seizures.

Weight Gain

Weight gain is common with antidepressant use. Weight gain is most common with use of the TCAs and mirtazapine (Remeron) and is less common with the use of the SSRIs and bupropion (Wellbutrin, Zyban). Table 4.1 lists the risk of weight gain associated with each agent. This side effect is listed as *Weight gain*, and a severity rating of 0 to 4 is used (0 = little risk; ++++ = highest risk) (Baldessarini, 2001; Jackson, 2002; Kando et al., 2002; Meyer, 2011; O'Donnell & Shelton, 2011).

Sexual Dysfunction

Sexual dysfunction is common with the use of SSRIs and TCAs and is less common with use of the SSNRIs bupropion (Wellbutrin), nefazodone (Serzone), and mirtazapine (Remeron). Table 4.1 lists the risk of sexual dysfunction associated with each agent. This side effect is listed as *Sexual*, and a severity rating of 0 to 4 is used (0 = little risk; ++++ = highest risk) (Baldessarini, 2001; Jackson, 2002; Kando et al., 2002; Meyer, 2011; O'Donnell & Shelton, 2011).

PATIENT CASE 1

S.S. is a 40-yr-old male accountant who has been in a romantic relationship for the past 7 yr. Recently, his girlfriend left him for another man. Because S.S. was not aware that his girlfriend was seeing another individual, he was not prepared for the breakup. After the breakup, S.S. began having difficulty at work. He found it hard to concentrate on his job and was written up by his boss for numerous accounting errors, lack of productivity, missed project deadlines, and difficulty getting along with his coworkers. S.S. was in danger of losing his job. S.S. is also behind in paying his bills because he has had difficulty concentrating on writing checks. Subsequently, several bills have gone to a collection agency. In addition, S.S. has had difficulty sleeping since the breakup and has lost 15 lb (6.8 kg) over the past 2 mo. He states that he is not actively trying to lose weight but merely has no appetite. S.S. complains that he has no interest in anything at this time, is fatigued, and finds it impossible to enjoy life. He recently suffered a fall and has undergone surgery for a fractured hip. When S.S. sees his physician in the hospital for the fractured hip, the physician diagnoses him with clinical depression.

Question

What signs and symptoms does S.S. exhibit that are consistent with the diagnosis of depression?

Answer

S.S. exhibits many of the communication, behavioral, and cognitive signs of depression. For instance, S.S. is speaking slower than normal. The duration of pauses in an utterance was also longer than normal for this patient. Behaviorally, S.S. is having difficulty with instrumental ADL; his difficulty concentrating on paying bills reflects a marked change in his behavior and is not consistent with his occupation as an accountant. S.S.'s loss of appetite and subsequent reduction in weight is also a behavioral change that can be attributed to his clinical depression, as can his difficulty sleeping and subsequent daytime fatigue. S.S. also demonstrates several cognitive changes that may indicate clinical depression. S.S. missed several project deadlines due to difficulty concentrating on a task. His clinical depression has affected his sensory memory and, in particular, his concentration and speed of processing. In addition, the depression has affected his short-term and working memory abilities. His physician considers prescribing the antidepressant mirtazapine (Remeron) at a dose of 30 mg twice/day because one of the reported side effects of Remeron is weight gain, which would help S.S. at this time. In a team meeting, the surgical resident speaks with the rehabilitation specialist about the choice of antidepressant.

Question

What factors should the rehabilitation team consider when selecting this antidepressant for S.S.?

Answer

The rehabilitation therapist assesses the other effects of Remeron and points out that it has a high incidence of sedation, which could significantly affect rehabilitation. Drowsiness, dizziness, and confusion are other frequent side effects; these effects could impair S.S.'s ability to work effectively in his job. One role of the rehabilitation team is to report to the team's physician and pharmacist any communication, behavior, and cognitive changes observed in the patient. The pharmacist suggests that the physician consider adjusting the mirtazapine (Remeron) dosage to 15 mg at bedtime. This dosage would reduce the amount of sedation present in the patient and follows the adage that the key to managing side effects and improving adherence is to start low and go slow. The pharmacist agrees that Remeron would help decrease S.S.'s depression and increase his appetite.

Drug Interactions With Antidepressants

The rehabilitation therapist should be aware of the most common and more serious side effects that can be associated with antidepressant medications. For example, serotonin syndrome, a serious side effect that may become evident during rehabilitation, can be life threatening if not identified and treated promptly. At the beginning of any rehabilitation session, the therapist should carefully review the patient's medication regimen and any identified changes or new symptoms in order to implement appropriate cautions or alter the planned session as needed. The therapist should question the patient about use of any new over-the-counter medications, nutraceuticals, herbal products, and prescription medications because any of these has the potential to interact with antidepressant medications (Jacobson et al., 2007; Meyer, 2011; O'Donnell & Shelton, 2011).

Drug Interactions With TCA

TCA agents can potentiate the effects of anesthetics, sedatives, analgesics, antihistamines, cold remedies, and alcohol, resulting in excessive sedation, respiratory depression, and potentiation of anticholinergic effects. TCA have anticholinergic effects that can cause confusion and delirium, particularly when combined with other anticholinergics such as antipsychotic or antiparkinson agents. Amoxapine (Asendin) causes mild dopamine blockage and therefore can antagonize the effects of dopamine agonists and levodopa (L-dopa, Sinemet) used in patients with Parkinson's disease (Baldessarini, 2001; Carl & Johnson, 2006; Jackson, 2002; Kando et al., 2002; Meyer, 2011; O'Donnell & Shelton, 2011).

Antidepressant agents are metabolized by the liver via the cytochrome P450 enzymes and by glucuronide conjugation. TCAs, SSRIs, and some SSNRIs have significant metabolic pathways that involve the cytochrome P450 enzyme systems of the liver. Because more than 80% of medications currently on the market are metabolized via the cytochrome P450 enzyme systems classified as CYP2D6 and CYP3A4, adding an antidepressant that affects these systems introduces the potential for numerous drug interactions. Refer to tables 4.2 and 4.5 (later in this chapter) for additional details. Venlafaxine (Effexor), bupropion (Wellbutrin), and mirtazapine (Remeron) have only minor effects via the cytochrome P450 enzyme systems; use of these antidepressants prevents many potential drug interactions. Combining any of the SSRIs with the pain medication tramadol (Ultram) is contraindicated because this drug interaction increases tramadol (Ultram) levels and can increase risk of seizures. Drug interactions can increase or decrease therapeutic effects or can potentiate adverse effects. Table 4.2 summarizes the drug interactions commonly associated with TCAs (Baldessarini, 2001; Jackson, 2002; Kando et al., 2002; Mascarenas, 2012; Meyer, 2011; O'Donnell & Shelton, 2011; Teter et al., 2011).

Table 4.2   Drug Interactions With Tricyclic Antidepressants

Interacting medication	Resulting effect
Alcohol, other sedatives	Increased central nervous system depression (sedation)
Amphetamines, stimulant diet pills	Enhanced amphetamine effects and toxicity
Anticonvulsants: carbamazepine (Tegretol), phenobarbital, phenytoin (Dilantin)	Decreased antidepressant effects, increased seizures
Antihypertensives: clonidine (Catapres), guanethidine (Ismelin), methyldopa (Aldomet)	Decreased control of blood pressure
Antipsychotics: haloperidol (Haldol), phenothiazines	Increased levels of tricyclic antidepressants
Cardiac medications: amiodarone (Cordarone), quinidine, procainamide, disopyramide (Norpace), sotalol (Betapace), ibutilide (Corvert), diltiazem (Cardizem), labetalol (Normodyne), quinidine, verapamil (Calan, Isoptin, Covera, Verelan)	Increased risk of QT prolongation and arrhythmias when combined with tricyclic antidepressants, increased levels of tricyclic antidepressants
Cimetidine (Tagamet)	Increased levels of tricyclic antidepressants
Disulfiram (Antabuse)	Acute organic brain syndrome
Estrogens, oral contraceptives	Change in antidepressant effects and toxicity
Insulin, oral hypoglycemics	Increased lowering of blood sugar
Levodopa (Sinemet, L-dopa)	Decreased effects of levodopa
Lithium	Increased risk of seizure
Monoamine oxidase inhibitors	Hypertensive crisis, delirium, seizures, serotonin syndrome
Selective serotonin reuptake inhibitor antidepressants	Increased levels and effects of tricyclic antidepressants
Thyroid hormones	Increased effects and toxicity of both drugs
Warfarin (Coumadin)	Increased INR and risk of bleeding

INR = international normalized ratio.

Drug Interactions With MAOIs

Very significant drug interactions are associated with the use of MAOIs. MAOIs should not be used with medications that increase catecholamine (monoamine) levels in the body. Contraindicated medications include certain over-the-counter **decongestants** containing pseudoephedrine or phenylephrine and over-the-counter diet aids containing ephedra, ma huang, or phenylpropanolamine. Contraindicated prescription medications include epinephrine (adrenalin), norepinephrine (Levophed), methylphenidate (Ritalin), **amphetamines**, or TCA. When transitioning a patient from an SSRI or atypical antidepressant to an MAOI antidepressant, the prescriber should allow at minimum a 2 wk washout (drug-free) period to prevent the occurrence of serotonin syndrome. The prescriber should extend this washout period to 5 wk if the patient has been on fluoxetine (Prozac) due to its prolonged elimination time. Table 4.3 summarizes important drug interactions associated with the use of MAOIs. Patients taking MAOIs should avoid the medications listed in table 4.3 in order to prevent life-threatening hypertensive crisis due to excess catecholamine levels.

Food Interactions With MAOIs

Because tyramine is a precursor of the catecholamines, MAOIs significantly interact with foods containing high amounts of **tyramine**. Patients who take an MAOI and eat foods containing high amounts of tyramine or other **vasopressor** agents may experience a life-threatening hypertensive crisis (Baldessarini, 2001; Carl & Johnson, 2006; Jackson, 2002; Kando et al., 2002; Meyer, 2011; O'Donnell & Shelton, 2011). Table 4.4 summarizes common food–drug interactions associated with MAOIs.

Drug Interactions With SSRI and Atypical Antidepressants

The SSRIs fluoxetine (Prozac), fluvoxamine (Luvox), paroxetine (Paxil), sertraline (Zoloft), citalopram (Celexa), and the SSNRIs mirtazapine (Remeron), nefazodone (Serzone), and venlafaxine (Effexor) are extensively metabolized in the liver by cytochrome P450 enzyme

Table 4.3   Medications to Avoid in Patients Using Monoamine Oxidase Inhibitors

Amphetamines
Appetite suppressants: ma huang, phenylpropanolamine, Dexatrim, ephedra
Asthma inhalants with ephedrine, albuterol, or isoproterenol (Isuprel)
Buspirone (Buspar)
Carbamazepine (Tegretol)
Cocaine
Cyclobenzaprine (Flexeril)
Decongestants (topical and systemic): phenylephrine (Neo-Synephrine), pseudoephedrine (Sudafed, Actifed)
Dextromethorphan (Robitussin DM)
Dopamine
Ephedrine
Epinephrine (including local anesthetics with epinephrine)
Guanethidine (Ismelin)
Levodopa (Sinemet)
Meperidine (Demerol)
Methyldopa (Aldomet)
Reserpine
Tryptophan

oxidation. These agents can change the levels and effects of other agents metabolized via the same cytochrome P450 enzyme pathway; these changes may be clinically significant (Mascarenas, 2012).

Because SSRIs and SSNRIs increase effective levels of serotonin, these agents interact with other medications that affect serotonin levels. One of the most serious adverse reactions seen with the use of these agents is serotonin syndrome, which is characterized by an excess amount of serotonin in the periphery. Associated symptoms include gastrointestinal symptoms of abdominal cramping, bloating, and diarrhea and neurological symptoms of tremor, myoclonus (muscle twitching), dysarthria, hyperreflexia, manic symptoms, mental confusion, agitation, hypertension, hypothermia, sweating, and visual and tactile hallucinations. Serotonin syndrome has been associated with combining SSRI with one of the following: MAOI, TCA, a second SSRI, linezolid (Zyvox), trazodone (Desyrel), nefazodone (Serzone), ondansetron (Zofran), sumatriptan (Imitrex), and St. John's wort. Table 4.5 lists other medications that should be avoided in patients taking SSRI or SSNRI (Baldessarini, 2001; Brown, 2008; Carl & Johnson, 2006; Jackson, 2002; Kando et al., 2002; Mascarenas, 2012; Meyer, 2011; O'Donnell & Shelton, 2011).

Table 4.4   Dietary Guidelines for Patients Treated With Monoamine Oxidase Inhibitors

Foods to avoid	
Alcoholic beverages: imported beers, red wine (particularly Chianti), sherry, vermouth, cognac, Drambuie, Chartreuse	**Fruits and vegetables:** bean curd, dried fruits, overripe fruits (e.g., avocados, bananas, figs), raspberries, sauerkraut, soy sauce, yeast extracts (e.g., marmite)
Cheese and dairy products: American, blue, Boursault, brie, Camembert, cheddar, Emmental, gruyere, mozzarella, parmesan, Romano, Roquefort, and Swiss cheeses; sour cream; yogurt	**Foods containing vasopressors:** broad beans (e.g., fava), ginseng
Meat and fish: anchovies, beef or chicken liver, caviar, fermented meats or sausages, dried fish, game meat, meat extracts, smoked or pickled herring, shrimp paste, protein supplements found in health-food stores or diet programs	

Foods that are safe
Beverages containing caffeine (e.g., coffee, tea, cola), chocolate, fresh figs, raisins, yeast breads, meat tenderizers, cream cheese, cottage cheese

Table 4.5   Drug Interactions With Selective Serotonin Reuptake Inhibitors (SSRIs), and Selective Serotonin and Norepinephrine Reuptake Inhibitors (SSNRIs)

Interacting medication	Effects of drug interaction
Antianxiety medications	
Alprazolam (Xanax)	Increased sedation when used with nefazodone (Serzone), fluoxetine (Prozac), or fluvoxamine (Luvox)
Buspirone (Buspar)	Decreased effects when used with fluoxetine (Prozac)
Diazepam (Valium)	Increased sedation when used with fluvoxamine (Luvox)
Triazolam (Halcion)	Increased sedation when used with nefazodone (Serzone)
Antiasthmatic: theophylline	Increased levels when used with fluvoxamine (Luvox)
Antibiotic: ciprofloxacin (Cipro)	Increased (2-3 times) levels of the antidepressants fluvoxamine (Luvox) and duloxetine (Cymbalta); increased toxicity such as hypertensive crisis, orthostasis, syncope, and serotonin syndrome
Anticoagulant: warfarin (Coumadin)	Increased anticoagulant effect (bleeding risk) when used with fluoxetine (Prozac), fluvoxamine (Luvox), paroxetine (Paxil), or sertraline (Zoloft); decreased anticoagulant effect when used with trazodone (Desyrel)
Anticonvulsants: carbamazepine (Tegretol), phenytoin (Dilantin)	Tegretol increases the antidepressant levels when used with fluoxetine (Prozac), fluvoxamine (Luvox), or sertraline (Zoloft); phenytoin increases antidepressant levels when used with trazodone (Desyrel) or fluoxetine (Prozac)
Antipsychotic agent: haloperidol (Haldol)	Increased levels when used with nefazodone (Serzone), fluoxetine (Prozac), or fluvoxamine (Luvox)
Antacid: cimetidine (Tagamet)	Increased levels of citalopram (Celexa) and paroxetine (Paxil), decreased levels of venlafaxine (Effexor)

› continued

Table 4.5 › *continued*

Interacting medication	Effects of drug interaction
Antidepressants and antimania medications	
Lithium	Increased neurotoxicity and seizures when used with fluoxetine (Prozac) or fluvoxamine (Luvox)
Monoamine oxidase inhibitors	Serotonin syndrome, seizures, delirium, hypertensive crisis
St. John's wort	Induced CYP34A enzymes; decreased levels of fluoxetine (Prozac), sertraline (Zoloft), fluvoxamine (Luvox), citalopram (Celexa), and nefazodone (Serzone); increased risk of serotonin syndrome when combined with other antidepressants
Fluoxetine (Prozac)	Increased levels of trazodone (Desyrel), haloperidol (Haldol), fluphenazine (Prolixin), risperidone (Risperdal), and clozapine (Clozaril); increased EPS; increased levels and toxicity of diazepam (Valium), alprazolam (Xanax), phenytoin (Dilantin), warfarin (Coumadin), propranolol (Inderal), nifedipine (Procardia), and verapamil (Calan, Verelan)
Fluvoxamine (Luvox)	Increased (3-4 times) levels of imipramine (Tofranil), amitriptyline (Elavil), clomipramine (Anafranil), and mirtazapine (Remeron); increased (2-4 times) levels of haloperidol (Haldol); increased (5-10 times) levels of clozapine (Clozaril); increased (2 times) levels of olanzapine (Zyprexa); increased levels of diazepam (Valium) and alprazolam (Xanax); increased (5 times) levels and toxicity of theophylline, warfarin (Coumadin), and propranolol (Inderal); increased (30%-50%) levels of methadone
Paroxetine (Paxil)	Increased (3-4 times) levels of desipramine (Norpramin); increased (2-13 times) levels of perphenazine (Trilafon) along with sedation and extrapyramidal side effects; increased (3-9 times) levels of risperidone (Risperdal) along with extrapyramidal side effects; moderately increased levels of clozapine (Clozaril)
Sertraline (Zoloft)	Moderately increased levels of tricyclic antidepressants
Citalopram (Celexa)	No known drug interactions; safest selective serotonin reuptake inhibitor
Mirtazapine (Remeron)	No significant drug interactions; safe selective serotonin reuptake inhibitor
Nefazodone (Serzone)	Increased levels of cyclosporine (Sandimmune, Neoral) or tacrolimus (Prograf) along with nephrotoxicity and neurotoxicity; increased (2 times) levels of triazolam (Halcion); increased (3 times) levels of alprazolam; increased levels of simvastatin (Zocor) along with myositis and rhabdomyolysis. Contraindicated with cisapride (Propulsid) and loratadine (Claritin) due to fatal ventricular arrhythmias and QT prolongation
Tricyclic antidepressants	Increased levels and toxicities of tricyclic antidepressants
Cardiac agents	
Digoxin (Lanoxin)	Decreased heart rate when used with nefazodone (Serzone) or trazodone (Desyrel)
Calcium channel blocker: diltiazem (Cardizem)	Bradycardia and hypotension occur due to enhanced effects of diltiazem when combined with CYP34A inhibitors felodipine (Plendil), fluvoxamine (Luvox), nisoldipine (Sular), fluoxetine (Prozac), sertraline (Zoloft), citalopram (Celexa), or nefazodone (Serzone)
Beta blockers: propranolol (Inderal), metoprolol (Lopressor)	Hypotension and bradycardia when used with fluoxetine (Prozac), fluvoxamine (Luvox), or paroxetine (Paxil); decreased effects of Inderal when used with nefazodone (Serzone); increased (5 times) levels, hypotension, and bradycardia when used with fluvoxamine (Luvox)
Pain medications	
Codeine, opioids, tramadol (Ultram)	Decreased pain control with codeine when used with fluoxetine (Prozac) or paroxetine (Paxil); increased opioid levels when used with fluoxetine (Prozac) or paroxetine (Paxil). Avoid using Ultram with fluoxetine (Prozac) or paroxetine (Paxil)—increased risk of seizures and serotonin syndrome.

Bipolar Disorder

Bipolar disorder (formerly called manic–depressive illness), which occurs in about 1.5% of the population of the United States, can be serious and debilitating. Bipolar disorder is genetically linked and is characterized by multiple recurring cycles of mania or hypomania alternating with cycles of depression. Mania is characterized by insomnia, rapid speech, flight of ideas, grandiosity, increased impulsivity, delusions, and even psychotic symptoms such as hallucinations or catatonia. With hypomania, the patient experiences the symptoms of mania but with less intensity and is able to function socially or occupationally. Major depressive symptoms are listed earlier in this chapter.

Incidence

Worldwide, bipolar disease accounts for more disability adjusted life years than all neurologic conditions and cancer combined. This is attributable to the early onset and chronic nature of the disease. Depressive episodes tend to be more severe than manic episodes. In addition, 75% of patients with bipolar disorder report at least one other disorder. Generally, this disorder is undertreated in low-income countries; less than 25% of patients report access to treatment (Merikangas et al., 2011). In patients with a family history, the incidence of bipolar disorder can range up to 14.5% and the incidence of unipolar depression (depression without mania) can be up to 24.5%. No differences in risk that are associated with ethnicity, race, or sex have been identified. The diagnosis of bipolar disease requires the presence of elevated mood (expansive or irritable) for a period of at least 1 wk along with three or four of the following: inflated self-esteem, decreased need for sleep, racing thoughts or flight of ideas, pressure speech, distractibility, increased psychomotor activity, or increased involvement in pleasurable activities that have a high risk of negative consequences. Four types of mood disorders are associated with bipolar disease: manic, major depressive, hypomanic, or mixed. Patients are termed rapid cyclers if they have four or more mood episodes in 1 yr (Baldessarini, 2001; Jackson, 2002; Kemrak & Kenna, 2008; Kando et al., 2002; Meyer, 2011; Miller & Miller, 2012; O'Donnell & Shelton, 2011; Teter et al., 2011; Tom-Revson & Lee, 2006).

Patients with mania and especially hypomania seldom seek help because most enjoy this phase of the illness or fail to identify a problem with their behavior. Because patients with bipolar disease will present more often with symptoms of depression, the physician must take a careful history of the patient's previous mood alterations in order to avoid missing the diagnosis of bipolar illness. The use of traditional antidepressant therapies in the treatment of bipolar illness can actually worsen symptoms and trigger an episode of mania. Pediatric bipolar disorder can result in impaired family and peer relationships, poor academic performance, higher levels of substance abuse, and increased risk of suicide completions and attempts. Children and adolescents with bipolar disorder frequently present with symptoms of severe mood swings, disruptive behaviors, shortened sleep, intrusiveness, and hypersexuality. They are also more prone to violent behavior. A careful medication history to rule out the use of antidepressants, stimulants, or steroids should be done to rule out medication-induced behavior(Baldessarini, 2001; Drayton, 2011; Jackson, 2002; Kando et al., 2002; Meyer, 2011; O'Donnell & Shelton, 2011; Teter et al., 2011; Tom-Revson & Lee, 2006).

Etiology and Pathophysiology

Bipolar disease is thought to be caused by excessive levels of norepinephrine and a depletion of dopamine and serotonin. Treatment of bipolar disease should include a combination of cognitive restructuring and behavioral therapies, psychosocial intervention, and medication therapy. Medications used in the treatment of bipolar disease treat acute symptoms, balance the levels and actions of the neurotransmitters, and reduce the frequency of the mood cycles (cycling) the patient experiences. Hypothyroidism occurs in a large percentage of patients with bipolar disorder, especially those who are rapid cyclers or who are resistant to therapy. Patients diagnosed with bipolar disease should always have their thyroid function evaluated because thyroid supplementation can help to stabilize this mood disorder (Bostick & Diez, 2008; Drayton, 2011; Watanabe, 2007).

Rehabilitation Considerations

Manic patients typically exhibit poor judgment and a lack of resistance to inhibit manic episodes. They may exhibit rapid speech that may be difficult to understand. Sentences may be incomplete along with labile pitch. The manic patient may also have what is described as "flights of ideas," during which they continuously switch topics. The patient with mania typically exhibits deficits in sustained attention and difficulties with verbal learning; these difficulties should be the focus of therapeutic interventions. Other difficulties include impairment of working memory, set shifting, and planning ability (Sigfried et al., 2010); the impact of these difficulties on rehabilitation is minor. To address patient difficulties with sustained attention and verbal learning, the clinician can use procedural learning methods that emphasize repeatedly performing step-by-step tasks until the tasks become automatic. The clinician should then progress the procedural learning methods to the point of introducing new variables to the task or environment so that the patient is able to execute the task under more than one set of constraints. The therapist should also initially focus on eliminating distractions in the treatment area and establishing the patient's attention before the initiation of the task. The use of eye contact, tactile cues, and verbal cues has been found to help focus patients' attention on a specific psychomotor task (Clark et al., 2001; Martinez-Aran et al., 2004; Rubinsztein et al., 2001; Vogel et al., 2000).

Medication Therapy

Medication therapy is a mainstay in treating the patient with bipolar disorder. The medications used depend on the symptoms associated with the cycle the patient is experiencing. Medications used to manage an acute cycle of mania may differ from those used to treat acute depression, and other agents may be used to stabilize mood or prevent further relapses. Several weeks of continuous therapy may be required before the full therapeutic effects of medications used to stabilize mood in bipolar disorder become evident. The therapist should counsel patients about this delay of onset and encourage patients to continue taking their medications in order to achieve successful use of medication therapy (Baldessarini, 2001; Carl & Johnson, 2006; Drayton, 2011; Jackson, 2002; Kando et al., 2002; Meyer, 2011; Miller & Miller, 2012; Watanabe, 2007).

The goal of using medication therapy in acute treatment of an episode of mania is to control the symptoms and return the patient to normal levels of psychosocial function. This is done with a combination of short-acting agents that initially stabilize symptoms and a mood-stabilizing agent. Short-acting agents can include **antianxiety agents** used to treat agitation or anxiety or antipsychotic agents used to control initial symptoms of agitation or psychosis. Mood stabilization is accomplished with higher doses of lithium with or without an anticonvulsant such as **valproic acid** (Depakene), carbamazepine (Tegretol), or lamotrigine (Lamictal). Other options include the use of olanzapine–fluoxetine (Symbyax) or quetiapine (Seroquel) (Drayton, 2011). Table 4.6 lists the medications used to treat bipolar disorder (Miller & Miller, 2012).

Acute depressive episodes can be treated with higher doses of lithium to achieve desired serum levels of 1.0 to 1.2 mEq/L. Antidepressants should be used with caution because they can switch the episode of depression to an episode of mania, especially when used as monotherapy. Use of antidepressants can also cause rapid cycling of mania and depression. To reduce this risk, prescribers use a mood stabilizer as adjunctive therapy with the antidepressant. SSRIs or SSNRI antidepressants such as trazodone (Desyrel), nefazodone (Serzone), mirtazapine (Remeron), or venlafaxine (Effexor) have been used with success in combination with a mood stabilizer such as lithium or one of the anticonvulsants. TCAs are associated with a high risk of triggering mania and rapid cycling and should not be used in patients with bipolar disorder (Baldessarini,

See table 4.6 in the web resource for a full list of medication-specific indications, dosing recommendations, side effects, and other considerations.

Table 4.6 Medications Used to Treat Bipolar (Manic–Depressive) Disorder

Medication	Side effects affecting rehab							Other side effects or considerations
Lithium: High dose for acute mania or depression—target level is 1.0 to 1.2 mEq/L. Low dose for maintenance therapy to prevent recurrence—target level is 0.6 to 1.0 mEq/L. Toxicity with levels >1.5 mEq/L: lethargy, severe diarrhea, and incoordination can occur. Levels of 2.5 to 3.0 mEq/L: myoclonic twitches, dysarthria, coarse tremors, confusion, dyskinesia, choreoathetoid movements, and urinary and fecal incontinence can occur. Levels >3.0 mEq/L: seizures, cardiogenic shock, peripheral vascular collapse, coma, and death can occur.								
Lithium (Eskalith)	Cog ++	S ++	A +	Motor +++	D +++	Com ++	F ++	Gastrointestinal disturbance, xerostomia, tremors, dysphagia, neuromuscular weakness, ataxia, sedation, polyuria, polydipsia, edema, weight gain, leukocytosis, delirium, cardiac arrhythmias, hypotension, tinnitus, oral or facial tremor, slurred speech
Anticonvulsants: For acute mania/mixed therapy. Valproic acid can also be used for maintenance therapy. Lamotrigine is used for acute depression only.								
Carbamaze-pine (Tegretol)	Cog ++	S ++	A +	Motor ++	D ++	Com ++	F +++	Ataxia, blurred vision, drowsiness, agitation, disequilibrium, dizziness, benign leukopenia, cardiac arrhythmias, congestive heart failure, hepatic failure (rare), syndrome of inappropriate antidiuretic hormone (rare), aplastic anemia (rare). Therapeutic levels are 8-12 mg/dl. Autoinduction of its own metabolism occurs after 30 days; may need to adjust dose to maintain levels.
Valproic acid (Depakote)	Cog ++	S ++	A ++	Motor ++	D ++	Com ++	F ++	Weight gain, hepatotoxicity, dyspepsia, pancreatitis that can be life threatening, alopecia, tremor, thrombocytopenia, platelet dysfunction, rash, hair loss
Lamotrigine (Lamictal)	Cog ++	S 0	A +	Motor ++	D 0	Com ++	F ++	Insomnia, rash that can progress to Stevens-Johnson syndrome. If used with valproic acid, decrease dose by 50% to minimize rash (Stevens-Johnson syndrome).
Antipsychotic medications: Used to treat acute mania and mixed episodes. Quetiapine, ziprasidone, aripiprazole, paliperidone, and asenapine are also used to treat bipolar depression.								
Aripiprazole (Abilify)	Cog +	S +	A +	Motor +	D +	Com +	F +	Weight gain + · Seizure 0 · Cardiac + · Sexual +
Asenapine (Saphris)	Cog +	S +	A +	Motor ++	D +	Com +	F ++	Weight gain + · Seizure 0 · Cardiac + · Sexual +
Olanzapine (Zyprexa)	Cog ++	S ++	A +	Motor ++	D ++	Com ++	F ++	Weight gain ++++ · Seizure + · Cardiac + · Sexual + · High risk of metabolic effects and weight gain.
Quetiapine (Seroquel)	Cog ++	S ++	A +	Motor +	D +	Com ++	F ++	Weight gain ++ · Seizure 0 · Cardiac ++ · Sexual +
Risperidone (Risperdal)	Cog +	S +	A +	Motor ++	D +	Com +	F ++	Weight gain ++ · Seizure 0 · Cardiac ++ · Sexual ++++

› continued

Table 4.6 › continued

Medication	Side effects affecting rehab							Other side effects or considerations
Ziprasidone (Geodon)	Cog ++	S +	A +	Motor ++	D +	Com ++	F +	Weight gain Seizure Cardiac Sexual + 0 +++ + High risk of QT prolongation and torsades de pointes with higher doses and injectable form.
Antianxiety medications: Used short term only until anxiety symptoms resolve.								
Clonazepam (Klonopin)	Cog +	S +	A 0	Motor ++	D ++	Com ++	F +	Drowsiness, headache, fatigue, nausea, ataxia, sedation, dependence
Lorazepam (Ativan)	Cog +++	S +++	A 0	Motor ++	D ++	Com ++	F +++	Ataxia, sedation, headache, nausea, fatigue, dependence; higher risk of withdrawal symptoms

Selective serotonin and norepinephrine reuptake inhibitor antidepressants and selective serotonin reuptake inhibitor antidepressants are used in combination with a mood stabilizer in acute management of depression. Tricyclic antidepressants are contraindicated; do not use in bipolar disease.

Cog = cognition; S = sedation; A = agitation or mania; Motor = discoordination; D = dysphagia; Com = communication; F = falls. Sexual is associated with gynecomastia and other sexual dysfunction.

The likelihood rating scale for encountering the side effects is as follows: 0 = Almost no probability of encountering side effects. 0/+ = Slight probability of encountering side effects with use of higher doses. + = Little likelihood of encountering side effects. +/++ = Low probability of encountering side effects; however, probability increases with increased dosage. ++ = Medium likelihood of encountering side effects. +++ = High likelihood of encountering side effects, particularly with high doses. ++++ = Highest likelihood of encountering side effects; best to avoid in at-risk patients.

2001; Drayton, 2011; Jackson, 2002; Kando et al., 2002; Meyer, 2011; Watanabe, 2007).

Chronic medication therapy includes lower maintenance doses of lithium to achieve serum levels of 0.8 to 1.0 mEq/L or an anticonvulsant, valproic acid (Depakene), carbamazepine (Tegretol), lamotrigine (Lamictal), or the antipsychotic quetiapine (Seroquel). Some newer anticonvulsants that show promise in preliminary studies include lamotrigine (Lamictal) and gabapentin (Neurontin). Episodes of stress often trigger the cycles; therefore, anticonvulsant medications are useful in treating patients with rapid cycling (frequently occurring episodes of mania alternating with depression) because they reduce the threshold of neurological activity (kindling effect) in a manner that is similar to their action in suppressing seizures (Baldessarini, 2001; Jackson, 2002; Kando et al., 2002; Meyer, 2011; O'Donnell & Shelton, 2011).

Lithium

Lithium, an alkali salt, is chemically related to sodium and potassium. Its usefulness in treating mood disorders was recognized in patients using the agent as a salt substitute. Lithium acts as a substitute for sodium, magnesium, potassium, and calcium at receptors which cause blocking of dopamine action and enhanced activity of the neurotransmitters acetylcholine, serotonin, and GABA. Lithium also decreases levels of cyclic adenylcycline monophosphate, which is required in intracellular transport of energy required for neurotransmission. Lithium achieves an overall response rate of 78% in patients when used to manage symptoms of acute mania; in these cases, onset of full effects requires up to 2 wk of continuous therapy. The use of lithium as monotherapy for managing acute symptoms of depression is associated with a response rate of 60% to 80%; in these cases, onset of full effects requires 6 to 8 wk of continuous therapy. Adjunctive treatment with an antidepressant or a second mood stabilizer and psychotherapy may shorten onset of response (Baldessarini, 2001; Drayton, 2011; Jackson, 2002; Kando et al., 2002; Meyer, 2011; Watanabe, 2007).

Lithium dosing is initiated at 300 mg 2 or 3 times/day and increased to 1200 mg/day as needed to achieve desired serum drug levels (1.0-1.2 mEq/L). Serum drug levels are taken after 5 to 7 days, when levels are at a steady state, and levels are drawn 12 h after a dose. Lithium has a narrow therapeutic range and requires close monitoring to prevent dose-related toxicity. Higher doses are needed when treating episodes of acute mania and acute depression. Use of lithium as maintenance therapy reduces suicide risk eight- to tenfold. When the drug is used in maintenance therapy to prevent recurrence of depressive or manic episodes, lower dosing is recommended (target levels of 0.6-1.0 mEq/L) to postpone the occurrence of long-term toxicity to the kidney and thyroid caused by drug accumulation in these organs (Baldessarini, 2001; Drayton, 2011; Jackson, 2002; Kando et al., 2002; Meyer, 2011; Watanabe, 2007).

Patients receiving lithium in therapeutic doses can develop side effects of gastrointestinal disturbance, xerostomia, dysphagia, tremors, neuromuscular weakness, ataxia, and sedation. Lithium use can be associated with dysphagia that results from dry mouth (xerostomia), deglutitive inhibition on the esophageal striated or smooth muscle, or abnormal peristalsis on the smooth visceral muscle. In addition, sedation can impair mental abilities and result in decreased appetite, impaired motor coordination, and inattention to eating. Lithium side effects of sedation, ataxia, dizziness, and discoordination can interfere with the communication, learning, and motor activities required in rehabilitation sessions (Carl & Johnson, 2006; Ciccone, 2002). Additional side effects of lithium include **polyuria**, **polydipsia**, edema, weight gain, and **leukocytosis** (increased white blood cell count). Table 4.6 summarizes side effects and dosing associated with lithium (Baldessarini, 2001; Ciccone, 2002; Drayton, 2011; Jackson, 2002; Kando et al., 2002; Meyer, 2011).

Symptoms of toxicity occur when serum lithium levels exceed 1.5 mEq/L and can include lethargy, severe diarrhea, incoordination, delirium, ataxia, cardiac arrhythmias, hypotension, **tinnitus**, oral or facial tremor, and slurred speech. At serum levels of 2.5 to 3.0 mEq/L, myoclonic twitches, dysarthria, coarse tremors, confusion, dyskinesia, choreoathetoid movements, and urinary and fecal incontinence can occur. Seizures, cardiogenic shock, peripheral vascular collapse, coma, and death

can occur at serum lithium levels greater than 3.0 mEq/L (Baldessarini, 2001; Ciccone, 2002; Drayton, 2011; Jackson, 2002). The rehabilitation therapist should be aware of these side effects and how they affect the patient's ability to participate in rehabilitation sessions. Upon identifying side effects associated with toxic levels of lithium, the therapist should immediately notify the prescriber and the patient's lithium blood levels should be checked. The therapist should question the patient about any changes in use of over-the-counter medications, changes in use or dose of prescription medications, and any changes in diet or herbal therapy in order to identify possible causes of these side effects and to alter the rehabilitation regimen to maximize patient safety and participation (Carl & Johnson, 2006).

PATIENT CASE 2

M.O. is a 45-yr-old female with a 20 yr history of depression, hypothyroidism, and hypertension. She was not well controlled with previous trials of antidepressants, including amitriptyline (Elavil), fluoxetine (Prozac), paroxetine (Paxil), and mirtazapine (Remeron). Her current medications include Lithium-SR/300 mg/day, Synthroid 0.1 mg/day, Hydrodiuril (hydrochlorothiazide) 50 mg/day, Cardizem-SR (diltiazem) 300 mg/day, and Seroquel (quetiapine) 100 mg twice/day. Seroquel and lithium were added and use of Paxil (paroxetine) was discontinued after a recent hospital admission for extreme agitation, combativeness, and hallucinations. During this admission she was diagnosed with bipolar disorder. She complains of difficulty swallowing and is referred to the speech-language pathologist (SLP) for evaluation.

Question
What risk factors for dysphagia does M.O. have?

Answer
Seroquel (quetiapine) and lithium both carry risk of dysphagia. Seroquel carries the risk of sedation, xerostomia, and extrapyramidal side effects such as dystonia that can affect

the motor functions involved in swallowing. Lithium can also cause sedation, xerostomia, ataxia, and neuromuscular weakness. The side effects associated with both of these medications are more prominent when the medications are initiated or when dosage is adjusted. With the use of lithium, dietary changes and medications that increase loss of salt and water can contribute to lithium toxicity. The diuretic (water pill) hydrochlorothiazide removes both water and salt. This loss causes an increase in lithium levels, which increases risk for developing associated side effects and toxicity. M.O.'s physician should check her lithium blood levels periodically to ensure that her lithium levels stay in the therapeutic range.

Medication Use in Pregnancy

Lithium is associated with a slight increase in fetal malformations when administered during the first trimester. Anticonvulsants used include valproic acid (Depakote).This has a risk of neural tube defects when administered in the first trimester, and fetal valproate syndrome is associated with fetal growth restriction, limb and heart defects, and facial changes. Carbamazepine (Tegretol) is also used and can cause fetal carbamazepine syndrome, which includes fetal dimorphisms and fingernail hypoplasia, in neonates. Use of carbamazepine also increases the risk for spina bifida. Lamotrigine (Lamictal) is not associated with increased risk of fetal malformation when given in the first trimester (Baylor & Patterson, 2009).

Drug Interaction With Lithium

Drug interactions with lithium involve medications and foods that alter sodium levels. Reduction of sodium results in compensatory retention of lithium by the kidney, leading to lithium accumulation and toxicity. Conversely, increases in sodium intake are associated with excretion of lithium by the kidney and resultant decreases in levels and effects. Table 4.7 summarizes lithium drug interactions.

Anticonvulsant Therapy

In 1995, valproic acid was approved for first-line use in the treatment of acute mania in doses of 750 to 3000 mg/day in 2 to 3 divided doses; dosing targets blood levels of 50 to 125 μg/ml. Valproic acid is also used as a third-line agent in combination with another agent for treating acute depression. Some studies show that valproic acid is as effective as lithium when used as maintenance therapy. Carbamazepine (Tegretol) is used as a first-line agent in treating acute mania or as a third-line agent in combination with another agent for treating acute depression. Dosing is 200 to 1600 mg/day in 2 divided doses. Carbamazepine is not helpful as a maintenance therapy. Lamotrigine (Lamictal) is used as a third-line agent in combination with another agent for treating acute mania and as monotherapy or in combination with another agent as a first line-agent in treating acute depression. Dosing is 50 to 1400 mg/day in divided doses that are slowly titrated up. Lamotrigine is effective when used as maintenance therapy. If given with valproic acid, the dose should be reduced by

Table 4.7   Food and Medication Interactions With Lithium

Medications	Examples	Effects
Nonsteroidal anti-inflammatory drugs	Ibuprofen (Motrin), naproxen (Aleve)	Sodium and fluid retention, decreased lithium accumulation and effects
Thiazide diuretics	Hydrochlorothiazide (Diuril)	Decreased sodium and fluid retention, increased lithium accumulation and effects
Angiotensin-converting enzyme inhibitors	Captopril (Capoten), lisinopril, enalapril (Vasotec)	Decreased sodium and fluid retention, increased lithium accumulation and effects
Salt substitutes	Potassium chloride salt (low salt, no salt)	Decreased sodium and fluid retention, increased lithium accumulation and effects

50% to avoid a serious dose-related rash called **Stevens-Johnson syndrome**. If rash occurs, the medication should be discontinued and not restarted. Females taking valproic acid (Depakene) should avoid becoming pregnant because this medication is **teratogenic**. In addition, females taking carbamazepine (Tegretol) or oxcarbazepine (Trileptal) should understand that these agents can reduce the effectiveness of oral contraceptives (Tom-Revson & Lee, 2006; Watanabe, 2007).

Second-Generation Antipsychotic Therapy

Second-generation antipsychotic agents are used as first-line treatment of acute mania as monotherapy or in combination with other agents. Quetiapine (Seroquel) and olanzapine–fluoxetine (Symbyax) are also used as second-line agents for treating acute depression. Other agents may be used as third-line agents for treating depression unless concurrent psychotic symptoms are present. In one study, the use of 300 mg or 600 mg doses of quetiapine (Seroquel) was associated with dry mouth (44%), sedation, somnolence (30%), and dizziness (17%) but was also associated with a minimal weight gain of 1 to 1.6 kg and improved quality of life in patients (Endicott et al., 2007). The efficacy of olanzapine (Zyprexa) is comparable with that of lithium or valproic acid when used as maintenance therapy but is associated with increased risk of weight gain and associated metabolic syndrome that can result in increased cardiac risk. Aripiprazole (Abilify) is also effective when used as maintenance therapy (Endicott et al., 2007; Miller & Miller, 2012; Thase et al., 2006; Watanabe, 2007).

Summary

This chapter reviews depression and bipolar disorder and summarizes how these mood disorders can alter cognition, impair communication and learning, and result in impaired motor coordination in rehabilitation sessions. This chapter also provides information about the medications used to treat these disorders and how they may also contribute to cognitive and motor impairment, particularly when initiating therapy or altering dose. The rehabilitation therapist should monitor the patient for impaired cognition and learning and for changes in balance, posture, and the frequency and severity of involuntary movements. Involuntary movements can impede the patient's psychomotor performance in therapy and may negatively influence neuromuscular control during transfers and gait, thereby putting the patient at risk for falls. These movements may also negatively affect the fine motor coordination necessary for many ADL such as dressing, grooming, and personal hygiene. In addition, such side effects may indicate drug toxicity that necessitates a dosage adjustment. The rehabilitation therapist should alter the therapy plan to address any impairment in learning or attention and incorporate appropriate interventions such as verbal cueing.

Serotonin syndrome and lithium toxicity are toxic effects that may become evident during rehabilitation and can become life threatening if not identified and treated promptly. Tables 4.1 and 4.6 list common side effects associated with medications used to treat mood disorders that affect rehabilitation. Food and drug interactions can increase or decrease therapeutic effects or potentiate adverse effects. The rehabilitation therapist should be aware of important drug and food interactions associated with these agents; these interactions are summarized in tables 4.2 through 4.7. At the beginning of each rehabilitation session, the therapist should carefully review the patient's medication regimen and identify any changes or new symptoms and should alter the patient's planned session if necessary. The therapist should also question the patient about use of new over-the-counter medications, herbal products, and prescription medications because any of these can potentially interact with antidepressant medications. Communication with the patient's prescriber in a timely manner about any identified medication-related issues can greatly affect patient progress and quality of life.

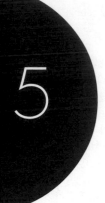

5

Medications Used to Treat Psychosis and Schizophrenia

In clinical practice, the rehabilitation therapist will encounter patients who are taking antipsychotic medications. Antipsychotic medications are used to treat symptoms of agitation or psychosis. Agitation is defined as excessive motor or verbal activity and can include hyperactivity, assaultiveness, verbal abuse, threatening gestures and language, physical destructiveness, vocal outbursts, and excessive verbalizations of distress. Psychosis is a psychiatric disease that is characterized by a disturbance of thinking and personality. This chapter reviews the pathophysiology associated with agitation and psychotic disorders and provides a summary of effective treatments.

Psychosis

The most common type of psychosis is schizophrenia. Psychotic symptoms can also occur in patients with other psychiatric disorders such as bipolar disorder, major depression, cognitive disorders such as the dementias and Alzheimer's disease, and Parkinson's disease. Antipsychotic medications are increasingly used to treat psychotic symptoms in these other diseases and in refractory major depression. In pediatric patients, behavioral disorders (e.g., autism, oppositional defiant disorder, and conduct disorder) that have components of psychotic behaviors may also be treated with **antipsychotic** medications (Crismon et al., 2011).

Incidence

Approximately 1% of the U.S. population is affected by schizophrenia, which is usually triggered by an environmental stressor. Genetic predisposition to the disease is strong. In the United States, patients being treated for schizophrenia occupy 20% of all hospital bed days and 50% of all psychiatric bed days. Schizophrenia costs the U.S. economy $35 billion annually. Onset typically occurs between 16 and 25 yr of age (5 to 7 yr earlier in males than in females) and persists throughout the patient's life. Substance abuse is common in patients with schizophrenia. More than 75% of patients with schizophrenia are addicted to nicotine, 30% to 50% are addicted to alcohol, 15% to 25% are addicted to cannabis, and 5% to 10% are addicted to cocaine or amphetamines (Maguire, 2002; Masand, 2007; Patel & Hlavinka, 2007).

Etiology and Pathophysiology

Psychosis is caused by an imbalance of neurotransmitters in the central nervous system and is primarily associated with excessive levels and activity of dopamine in the brain. This excessive activity makes the brain hypersensitive to stimuli and results in distorted perceptions. Symptoms of psychosis are categorized as positive, negative, cognitive, or mood.

Positive symptoms associated with schizophrenia include extra symptoms that are not usually seen in patients without psychosis.

These symptoms, which include disorganized speech or behavior, delusions, and hallucinations, are believed to be caused by hyperactive transmission of dopamine in the mesolimbic pathway. A flooding of sensations, described as increased awareness of environmental noises and increased perception of color and detail, occurs (Vogel et al., 2000). As a result, the patient may be unable to select, attend to, and focus on a stimulus. Stimulus distractions may affect the patient's cognitive speed (Sommer et al., 2008).

Delusions are fixed false beliefs. They occur when a patient misinterprets an experience and lead to erroneous beliefs that are associated with paranoia or persecution. Delusions may be grandiose, persecutory, or religious. **Hallucinations**, which can be auditory, visual, olfactory, tactile, or gustatory, involve disruption of perception and processing of sensory information. Auditory hallucinations, which occur more often than visual hallucinations, are generally associated with increased neurotransmission and activity in the right inferior frontal section of the brain (Eon & Durham, 2009; Masand, 2007; Patel & Hlavinka, 2007; Woodruff et al., 1997). Positive symptoms generally respond well to both first- and second-generation antipsychotic medications (Guthrie, 2002a; Iversen et al., 2009; Maguire, 2002; Masand, 2007; Patel & Hlavinka, 2007).

Negative symptoms is a term used to describe normal symptoms that are lacking in schizophrenics and include decreases or absence of normal expression, affective flattening (reduction in emotional expression), alogia (poverty of speech or lack of spontaneous conversation), **anhedonia** (emotional or social withdrawal), and avolition (lack of desire to pursue goals). Negative symptoms are thought to be due to decreased dopamine transmission in the mesocortical pathways of the brain and deficient dopamine in the medial prefrontal, anterior cingulated, and orbitofrontal cortexes (Eon & Durham, 2009; Maguire, 2002; Masand, 2007; Patel & Hlavinka, 2007).

Cognitive symptoms in schizophrenia are one of the major difficulties in this population. Most cognitive symptoms are associated with prefrontal deficits of dopamine transmission (Iversen et al., 2009). Cognitive symptoms can include short-term memory loss and impaired attention, executive function, working memory, and semantic memory. The patient can have language deficiencies in comprehension, generation of complex sentences, and verbal fluency. Affective reactivity of speech (communication disturbances exacerbated by stress) is also seen in some patients with schizophrenia. Alogia (poverty of speech content and increasing latency of response) is exacerbated by disorganization of semantic memory. Manipulating a patient's working memory load can assist with language difficulties (Gawel, 1981; Harvey & Serper, 1990; Melinder & Barch, 2003). Other common language disorders include **perseveration**, bizarre content with **neologisms**, **dysprosody**, **echolalia**, concreteness, derailment (inability to stay on track), blocking (abrupt interruptions), clang associations (using words that have no logical association), unintelligible speech (incoherent mixture of words), inappropriate nonverbal communication, and **mutism** (Eon & Durham, 2009; Gawel, 1981; Harvey & Serper, 1990; Maguire, 2002; Masand, 2007; Patel & Hlavinka, 2007; Salome et al., 2000; Sumiyoshi, 2001; Sumiyoshi et al., 2005; Tahir, 2007; Vogel et al., 2000).

Mood symptoms that are common in schizophrenia include anxiety, hostility, depression, and excitement. Identifying and appropriately treating these symptoms can reduce suicidal actions and decline in quality of life (Eon & Durham, 2009; Maguire, 2002; Masand, 2007; Patel & Hlavinka, 2007).

Rehabilitation Considerations

The rehabilitation therapist is confronted with a number of problems when working with the psychotic patient. The psychotic patient presents a cadre of symptoms affecting prognosis. In addition, the patient may have drug- and alcohol-related difficulties further complicating the remediation process. The side effect profile of the antipsychotic medications themselves may present additional challenges. The rehabilitation therapist needs to be fully versed in the medicines used to treat this population.

Medication Therapy

Antipsychotics are among the most widely used **psychotropic** (psychiatric) medications. Antipsychotic agents (formerly called major tranquilizers) are used to treat positive, negative, cognitive, and mood symptoms associated with psychosis or schizophrenia. Positive symptoms usually respond to medication treatment, whereas negative, mood, and cognitive symptoms are more difficult to reverse with medication therapy. All antipsychotic agents work by blocking the central neurotransmitter dopamine and other neurotransmitters in the brain's basal ganglia, hypothalamus, limbic system, brainstem, and medulla. All antipsychotic agents are effective in treating positive symptoms associated with psychosis, but they differ in selectivity of binding to the central dopamine and serotonin neuroreceptors. This selectiveness and extent of binding to these different receptors determines the antipsychotic actions of a medication (Miller & Holliday, 2012).

Typical or first-generation antipsychotics block the dopamine type-2 receptor in the mesolimbic pathway, resulting in decreasing positive symptoms, and block dopamine receptors in the mesocortical, tuberoinfundibular, and nigrostriatal pathways. Blocking dopamine in the nigrostriatal pathways results in worsened negative symptoms and cognition, and causes a particular set of motor symptoms termed extrapyramidal side effects (EPS). Atypical or second-generation antipsychotics reduce the effects of both serotonin and dopamine neurotransmission. They target and bind to serotonin 2A receptors to a much greater extent than the typical antipsychotics and bind less to dopamine 2A receptors than the older agents, resulting in improved negative symptoms with fewer EPS (Goldberg & Weinberger, 1995; Miller & Holliday, 2012).

The side effect profile of each antipsychotic medication depends on which receptors the medication binds to. In the autonomic nervous system, binding to the alpha-1 and alpha-2 adrenergic receptors can result in **orthostatic hypotension** and **cardiac arrhythmias**; binding to the histamine-1 receptors can increase level of sedation and decrease cognition and communication; and binding to the muscarinic acetylcholine receptors can increase sedation and cause autonomic dysfunction (e.g., balance disorders or dysphagia associated with decreased saliva production and impaired gastrointestinal motility). Table 5.1 lists the side effects associated with antipsychotic agents (Eon & Durham, 2009; Lee

 See table 5.1 in the web resource for a full list of medication-specific indications, dosing recommendations, and side effects.

Table 5.1   Medications Used to Treat Psychosis

Medication	Side effects affecting rehab					Other side effects or considerations			
First-generation (typical) agents: Used to treat psychosis in nonadherent patients or patients not responsive to single or dual atypical agent therapy. Haloperidol is also used to treat acute agitation.									
Chlorpromazine (Thorazine)	Cog ++++	Motor +++	D +++	Com +++	F +++	Weight gain ++++	Seizure +++	Cardiac ++	Sexual +++
Chlorprothixene (Taractan)	Cog +++	Motor ++	D ++	Com +++	F +++	Weight gain ++	Seizure ++	Cardiac +	Sexual ++
Fluphenazine (Prolixin)	Cog +	Motor ++++	D +	Com +	F +	Weight gain +	Seizure 0	Cardiac 0	Sexual ++++
Haloperidol (Haldol)	Cog +	Motor ++++	D +++	Com +	F ++	Weight gain +	Seizure 0	Cardiac 0	Sexual ++++

Medication	Side effects affecting rehab					Other side effects or considerations			
Loxapine (Loxitane)	Cog ++	Motor +++	D ++	Com ++	F ++	Weight gain +	Seizure +	Cardiac +	Sexual ++
Mesoridazine (Serentil)	Cog +++	Motor +	D +++	Com +++	F +++	Weight gain ++	Seizure +++	Cardiac ++	Sexual ++
Molindone (Moban)	Cog +	Motor +++	D ++	Com +	F ++	Weight gain +	Seizure +	Cardiac +	Sexual ++
Pimozide (Orap)	Cog +	Motor +++	D ++	Com +	F ++	Weight gain +	Seizure 0	Cardiac ++	Sexual ++
Perphenazine (Trilafon)	Cog ++	Motor ++++	D ++	Com ++	F ++++	Weight gain ++	Seizure +	Cardiac +	Sexual ++++
Thioridazine (Mellaril)	Cog ++++	Motor +++	D +++	Com ++++	F ++++	Weight gain +	Seizure +++	Cardiac ++	Sexual +++
						Agent with highest risk for anticholinergic side effects, orthostasis, sedation, and cardiac arrhythmia.			
Thiothixene (Navane)	Cog +	Motor ++++	D +	Com +	F ++	Weight gain +	Seizure +++	Cardiac 0	Sexual ++++
Trifluoperazine (Stelazine)	Cog +	Motor +++	D +++	Com +	F ++	Weight gain +	Seizure 0	Cardiac 0	Sexual ++++
						High risk for extrapyramidal side effects.			

Second-generation agents: Used in treatment of acute agitation or in initial treatment of psychosis.

Medication	Side effects affecting rehab					Other side effects or considerations			
Iloperidone (Fanapt)	Cog +	Motor +	D ++	Com +	F +++	Weight gain ++	Seizure 0	Cardiac ++	Sexual +
						High risk of orthostasis; titrate slowly. Prolongs QT interval.			
Risperidone (Risperdal)	Cog +	Motor ++	D +	Com +	F ++	Weight gain ++	Seizure 0	Cardiac ++	Sexual ++++
						Prolongs QT interval.			
Ziprasidone (Geodon)	Cog ++	Motor ++	D +	Com ++	F +	Weight gain +	Seizure 0	Cardiac +++	Sexual +
						High risk of QT prolongation and torsades de pointes with higher doses and injectable form.			

Second-generation (atypical) agents: Used as initial therapy in treatment of psychosis and in patients with bipolar disorder and as an adjunct to antidepressants in patients with depression not responsive to antidepressant therapy alone.

Medication	Side effects affecting rehab					Other side effects or considerations			
Aripiprazole (Abilify)	Cog +	Motor +	D +	Com +	F +	Weight gain +	Seizure 0	Cardiac +	Sexual +
Asenapine (Saphris)	Cog +	Motor ++	D +	Com +	F ++	Weight gain +	Seizure 0	Cardiac +	Sexual +
Lurasidone (Latuda)	Cog +	Motor +	D +	Com +	F +	Weight gain +	Seizure 0	Cardiac +	Sexual +
						Prolongs QT interval.			

› continued

Table 5.1 › *continued*

Medication	Side effects affecting rehab					Other side effects or considerations			
Olanzapine (Zyprexa)	Cog ++	Motor ++	D ++	Com ++	F ++	Weight gain ++++	Seizure +	Cardiac +	Sexual +
						High risk of metabolic effects and weight gain.			
Quetiapine IR (Seroquel IR; Seroquel XR)	Cog ++	Motor ++	D +	Com ++	F +++	Weight gain ++	Seizure 0	Cardiac ++	Sexual +
						High risk for orthostasis and falls.			
Paliperidone (Invega ER)	Cog +	Motor ++	D +	Com +	F ++	Weight gain ++	Seizure 0	Cardiac +++	Sexual ++++
						Active metabolite of risperidone. Avoid in patients with creatinine clearance <50 ml/min. Prolongs QT interval.			

Fourth-line agent: Added with failure of triple therapy for treatment of psychosis. Clozapine has the worst side effect profile (i.e., risk of seizures, anticholinergic effects, hypersalivation, myocarditis, agranulocytosis) and requires pharmacist and prescriber registration with the manufacturer's Clozaril National Registry, a dispensing and monitoring program that requires white blood counts to be done weekly for the first 6 mo of therapy and then continuously throughout.

Medication	Side effects affecting rehab					Other side effects or considerations			
Clozapine (Clozaril)	Cog ++++	Motor +	D ++++	Com ++++	F ++++	Weight gain ++++	Seizure ++++	Cardiac +++	Sexual +

Long-acting depot formulations: Used to treat psychosis in patients with adherence problems.

Medication	Side effects affecting rehab					Other side effects or considerations			
Fluphenazine decanoate IM (Prolixin Decanoate)	Cog +	Motor ++++	D +	Com +	F +	Weight gain +	Seizure 0/+	Cardiac 0	Sexual ++++
Haloperidol decanoate IM (Haldol Decanoate)	Cog +	Motor ++++	D +++	Com +	F ++	Weight gain +	Seizure 0	Cardiac 0	Sexual ++++
						Prolongs QT interval.			
Risperidone IM (Risperdal Consta)	Cog +	Motor ++	D +	Com +	F ++	Weight gain ++	Seizure 0	Cardiac ++	Sexual ++++
						Prolongs QT interval.			
Paliperidone (Oral: Invega extended release; IM: Invega Sustenna)	Cog +	Motor ++	D +	Com +	F ++	Weight gain ++	Seizure 0	Cardiac +++	Sexual ++++
						Active metabolite of risperidone. Not recommended in patients with renal creatinine clearance <50 ml/min. Prolongs QT interval.			

Cog = cognition; Motor = discoordination; D = dysphagia; Com = communication; F = falls; IM = intramuscular.

Weight gain is associated with metabolic effects such as increased risk for diabetes, coronary heart disease, myocardial infarction, and stroke. Seizure indicates risk for worsening or new onset of seizures. Cardiac side effects include arrhythmia and orthostatic hypotension. Sexual is associated with gynecomastia and other sexual side effects.

The likelihood rating scale for encountering side effects is as follows: 0 = Almost no probability of encountering side effects. 0/+ = Slight probability of encountering side effects with higher doses. + = Little likelihood of encountering side effects. +/++ = Low probability of encountering side effects; however, probability increases with increased dosage. ++ = Medium likelihood of encountering side effects. +++ = High likelihood of encountering side effects, particularly with high doses. ++++ = Highest likelihood of encountering side effects; best to avoid in at-risk patients.

et al., 2004; Masand, 2007; Miller & Holliday, 2012; Preston & Johnson, 2009; Schatzberg et al., 2007; Wang et al., 2005).

First-generation antipsychotics, also referred to as typical antipsychotics, act primarily by binding to dopamine-2 receptors in the brain. The introduction of first-generation antipsychotics in the 1960s provided the first effective treatment of psychosis and allowed many institutionalized patients to transition to outpatient care. The effects and side effects of these medications are related to the size of the dose, which determines what percentage of dopamine receptors these medications bind. Desired antipsychotic effects are seen when the medication binds at least 65% of the dopamine receptors in the brain. The extent of binding to the dopamine receptors also increases the risk of EPS and **tardive dyskinesia** (TD) seen with these agents. EPS side effects occur when the medication blocks at least 78% of the dopamine receptors. This leaves a narrow range for dosing that achieves the desired percentage bound and avoids EPS side effects (Masand, 2007).

First-generation agents are classified by their chemical structure. Phenothiazines include chlorpromazine (Thorazine), mesoridazine (Serentil), thioridazine (Mellaril), fluphenazine (Prolixin), perphenazine (Trilafon), and trifluoperazine (Stelazine). Thiothixanthines include chlorprothixene (Taractan) and thiothixene (Navane). Diphenylbutylpiperidines include haloperidol (Haldol) and pimozide (Orap). Haloperidol is classified as a butyrophenone. Molindone (Moban) is classified as a dihydroindolone, and loxapine (Loxitane) is classified as a dibenzoxazepine (Carl & Johnson, 2006).

First-generation antipsychotics are also divided into two classes based on their potency. Low potency agents are associated with more sedation and include chlorpromazine (Thorazine) and thioridazine (Mellaril). Medium potency agents include mesoridazine (Serentil), chlorprothixene (Taractan), molindone (Moban), and loxapine (Loxitane). High potency agents include fluphenazine (Prolixin), trifluoperazine (Stelazine), and haloperidol (Haldol) and have less sedative effects.

They are helpful in increasing activity levels in patients with negative symptoms but are more frequently associated with the development of extrapyramidal side effects (EPS) (Carl & Johnson, 2006; Eon & Durham, 2009).

Second-generation antipsychotics, also called atypical antipsychotics, were introduced in the 1990s. Clinicians prefer to initiate these agents in newly diagnosed patients. Atypical agents can be beneficial in the treatment of negative, mood, and cognitive symptoms, which usually do not respond to first-generation antipsychotics. These agents bind to norepinephrine and serotonin receptors as well as dopamine receptors. Because these agents bind less to dopamine receptors in the extrapyramidal portions of the brain, the occurrence of EPS is reduced. Their effects on negative, mood, and cognitive symptoms are attributable to their action on serotonin-2A and norepinephrine receptors (Green, 2002; Masand, 2007; Patel & Hlavinka, 2007; Sumiyoshi et al., 2005; Terri, 2008).

The clinician must consider the patient's current medications and concurrent disease states when choosing the patient's initial antipsychotic medication. Although symptoms of insomnia and agitation may begin to improve within the first 24 to 48 h of therapy, a minimum of 2 wk is needed to observe the onset of response to antipsychotic medications. A medication trial of 6 to 8 wk is appropriate to determine whether the patient will respond to therapy. Because it takes about 1 wk to see the full effects of a change in dosage, the clinician should change the maintenance dosage no more frequently than every 7 days and should always use the lowest effective dose. If the patient reports no improvement in symptoms after 2 to 4 wk, the clinician should increase the dose. Lack of response after 6 to 8 wk requires trial of an alternative agent (Eon & Durham, 2009; Petersen et al., 2005; Zemrak & Kenna, 2008).

PATIENT CASE 1

B.J. is a 72-yr-old male with a history of schizophrenia characterized by disturbed thinking, loss of interest in life, and strong emotions. B.J. has been seeing a speech–language pathologist because he has difficulty swallowing. His doctor prescribed 5 mg of Zyprexa, an atypical antipsychotic medication. Shortly after initiating the medication, B.J. began to complain that he was excessively tired, had a very dry mouth, and had begun to gain weight. B.J.'s blood sugar levels on his laboratory tests were higher than they had been in the past and he had begun to fall when getting up from a chair.

Question

What should the speech–language pathologist do after observing these behaviors during the evaluation?

Answer

The rehabilitation therapist is often the first to notice changes in a patient's behavior after the patient begins taking a new medication. The rehabilitation therapist should immediately notify the prescribing physician of any changes in a patient's behavior. In B.J.'s case, Zyprexa is noted to increase sedation in patients. In addition, this medication frequently causes anticholinergic effects such as xerostomia (dry mouth), which can have a negative effect on the patient's ability to masticate food. A lack of saliva can influence bolus formation and bolus transfer. Xerostomia can also put the patient at risk because it leads to undiluted oral bacteria in the mouth. Use of this medication can also result in weight gain and can increase the probability of hyperglycemia. Orthostatic hypotension can also occur, increasing the risk of falls. B.J.'s physician may consider changing the medication to one that is less sedating and has fewer anticholinergic side effects, such as Geodon or Abilify.

Antipsychotic therapy is usually initiated with an atypical antipsychotic. If antipsychotic side effects result in patient nonadherence or if no therapeutic response occurs, the clinician should try combination therapy with two agents: either a different atypical agent with a conventional agent or two atypical agents with different side effect profiles. If the patient does not show an adequate response with a regimen involving two antipsychotics, the clinician should add a third agent: a typical agent in the noncompliant patient or an atypical agent in the compliant patient with inadequate response. A trial with three agents that does not result in therapeutic success is usually followed by a trial with clozapine (Clozaril) with or without other antipsychotic agents (Wick & Zanni, 2006; Zemrak & Kenna, 2008).

Once the patient attains a good clinical response, antipsychotic medications are continued indefinitely. If side effects necessitate switching to another antipsychotic, the old agent should be gradually tapered while the new agent is slowly increased (cross-tapering) in order to avoid discontinuation reactions. Discontinuation reactions include restlessness, insomnia, anxiety, confusion, nausea, muscle aches, and pains associated with cholinergic rebound (Wick & Zanni, 2006; Zemrak & Kenna, 2008).

Antipsychotics have long half-lives, typically 1 to 2 days, and many have active metabolites that can further prolong effects. Therefore, most antipsychotics can be administered once daily. Agents with active metabolites include chlorpromazine (Thorazine), mesoridazine (Serentil), and risperidone (Risperdal). In addition, many of these agents are available in a long-acting depot injection form that helps patients adhere to the medication regimen (Wick & Zanni, 2006; Zemrak & Kenna, 2008).

Agitation

Agitation, which is defined as excessive motor or verbal activity, includes hyperactivity, assaultiveness, verbal abuse, threatening gestures and language, physical destructiveness, vocal outbursts, and excessive verbalizations of distress. It is an acute symptom of psychosis but may occur in patients without psychosis. Medication therapy is used to rapidly control symptoms in order to protect the patient and others from harm while identifying and treating the cause of the symptom.

Incidence

Agitation is seen in a number of disorders from psychosis to traumatic brain injury to dementia. The incidence of agitation has ranged from 15% to more than 50%. This range indicates that there is a lack of reliability among observers about what constitutes agitation (Zasler, Katz, & Zafonte, 2006).

Etiology

The causes of agitation are multiple. Agitation can be seen in patients suffering from organic illnesses such as dehydration, diabetes, cardiovascular disease, and neurologic diseases. Agitation is also present in anxiety and depressive illnesses. The consequences can range from falls, dehydration, decrease in alimentary intake, and noncompliance in medication to changes in daily life activities (Leger et al., 2000).

Pathophysiology

Agitation is a nonspecific group of unrelated behaviors seen in a variety of conditions. The pathophysiology of agitation involves dysregulations of serotonergic, noradrenergic, dopaminergic, and GABAergic systems (Lindenmayer, 2000).

Rehabilitation Considerations

Agitation presents a challenge to the rehabilitation clinician. Agitation can decrease the amount of rehabilitation that can be given successfully, as this behavior sharply decreases attention span and focus for rehabilitative efforts. In addition, agitation can be harmful to both the patient as well as the rehabilitation clinician. Each rehabilitation clinician needs to develop an approach to the agitated patient for training as well as safety. The first order of approach is usually the initiation of medications to control the agitation. The medications need to be initiated and titrated carefully so that the patient does not go from agitation to stupor. Identification of the underlying cause of agitation and treatment of the cause is critical (e.g., dehydration, infection, hypoglycemia).

Medication Therapy

Medications used to treat acute agitation should resolve the symptoms. The initial dose should be administered by injection until acute symptoms are controlled and then treatment should be transitioned to oral therapy as soon as possible. Traditional treatment for acute agitation includes intramuscular injections of haloperidol (Haldol) 5 mg and lorazepam (Ativan) 2 mg, which are readministered as needed. Injected medications resolve symptoms more rapidly and may provide higher concentrations of medication in the blood than oral formulations. Research shows that haloperidol 2.5 to 10 mg given intramuscularly initially and then repeated every 4 h to a maximum daily dose of 40 mg is an effective regimen. An updated method of treatment involves the use of newer antipsychotics, such as olanzapine (Zyprexa) or ziprasidone (Geodon), which are also available in an injectable form and effectively treat acute agitation. Olanzapine (Zyprexa) is dosed 2.5 to 10 mg initially and is repeated after 2 h and again after 1 to 2 h to a maximum of 3 doses in 24 h. Olanzapine (Zyprexa) achieves maximum concentrations in the blood in only 15 min. Ziprasidone (Geodon) is dosed intramuscularly at 5 to 20 mg every 4 to 6 h to a maximum daily dose of 80 mg; it is followed with oral doses of 40 to 200 mg/day. Ziprasidone (Geodon) achieves maximum concentrations in 30 to 40 min. Side effects associated with injected antipsychotics include acute **dystonia**, most commonly seen with haloperidol (Haldol), and cardiac arrhythmias associated with prolongation of the QT interval, most commonly with ziprasidone (Geodon) (Bellnier, 2002).

Side Effects Associated With Antipsychotic Agents

The most common side effects associated with antipsychotic medications that can affect the patient's rehabilitative progress include EPS, anticholinergic effects, neurocognitive effects and sedation, cardiac effects, and dysphagia. Antipsychotic therapy can also cause metabolic effects that can significantly affect long-term morbidity and mortality. This section discusses these effects as well as the effects of antipsychotic agents in pregnant women. The rehabilitation therapist must be aware of the potential side effects of antipsychotic medications and should incorporate methods for minimizing the impact of these effects into the patient's plan of care.

EPS

First-generation (typical) antipsychotic agents have been associated with a high incidence of extrapyramidal symptoms (EPS) and tardive dyskinesia (TD), which has limited their use. Because the newer second-generation (atypical) antipsychotic agents pose a much lower risk of EPS and TD, they are preferred over the older typical agents when initiating therapy. EPS can include muscle rigidity, resting and intentional tremor, pill rolling, **cogwheel rigidity**, shuffling gait, difficulty initiating motor plans, **masked facies**, dysphagia, dysarthria, akathisia, restlessness, and dystonia (Laporta et al., 1990). EPS may be acutely treated with administration of anticholinergic agents such as benztropine (Cogentin) or diphenhydramine (Benadryl) (Carl & Johnson, 2006).

EPS usually occur within days of initiating **neuroleptic** medications, whereas the onset of TD is insidious. TD occurs in about 14% of patients treated with an antipsychotic. The risk of developing TD is related to the cumulative dose of the antipsychotic. TD is a syndrome of involuntary dyskinetic movements that are potentially irreversible. An early symptom of TD is fine, **vermicular** tongue movements. The rehabilitation therapist should monitor for this initial symptom. If it appears, the patient must immediately discontinue the therapy in order to prevent the TD from worsening. As TD progresses, involuntary movement of the eyelids, lips, jaw, tongue, neck, and fingers, lip smacking, repetitive tongue protrusions, and repetitive chewing motions can occur and can interfere with speech and even respiratory function (Garrett et al., 1984; Goldberg et al., 2000). Because no effective treatment of TD is known, the patient should stop using the antipsychotic medication as soon as TD is detected.

If antipsychotic therapy needs to be restarted, the lowest possible dose of an atypical agent should be used (Carl & Johnson, 2006; Preston & Johnson, 2009).

Akathisia is defined as a compulsion to be in motion. Patients may tap their feet, shift their weight, or pace. In many cases it is difficult to distinguish whether the symptoms are caused by medication-induced EPS or worsening symptoms of psychosis. Severe akathisia may be interpreted as a worsening of the psychosis, whereas minor akathisia may be viewed as an increase in anxiety. Neuroleptic-induced akathisia is seen more frequently in younger patients and in patients using a higher dosage. Administration of anticholinergics generally resolves medication-induced akathisia. If anticholinergic therapy is not successful, the addition of a beta blocker or benzodiazepine may help control symptoms. Patients with medication-induced akathisia usually report a physical restlessness rather than emotional anxiety or agitation. If the akathisia is associated with worsening of the psychosis, increasing the dose of the antipsychotic therapy will improve the symptoms (Preston & Johnson, 2009).

The rehabilitation therapist should monitor patients for related changes in balance, posture, and involuntary movements and may be the first to observe these changes in motor function. The involuntary **choreoathetoid movements** in the extremities and the dystonia of the neck and trunk that are seen with EPS and TD can have long term detrimental effects on the motor performance necessary for performing functional tasks (e.g., speaking) and activities of daily living (e.g., eating and swallowing) (Laporta et al., 1990).

Recognizing the early clinical manifestations of TD and adjusting the dosage of antipsychotic medication is important in preventing permanent motor disturbances (Baldessarini, 2001; Benjamin & Munetz, 1994; Crismon et al., 2011; Crismon & Dornson, 2002; Markowitz & Morton, 2002; Meyer, 2011; Rooney & Johnson, 2000).

As part of patient care, the rehabilitation therapist should monitor the patient for therapeutic effects of antipsychotic medications and side effects such as EPS and TD. Because of the possible complications associated with antipsychotic therapy, long-term care facilities are required to use antipsychotic agents only when indicated and only with informed patient consent. Current guidelines recommend documenting regular attempts to titrate the dose of antipsychotics down to the lowest effective dose (Benjamin & Munetz, 1994; Markowitz & Morton, 2002; Munetz & Benjamin, 1988; Rooney & Johnson, 2000; Whall et al., 1983).

Several tools can help the rehabilitation therapist to monitor the patient for effects of antipsychotic medications. The Abnormal Involuntary Movement Scale (AIMS) is used when antipsychotic therapy is initiated and is repeated every 3 to 6 mo. The scale helps the rehabilitation therapist detect the initiation of or increase in involuntary movements in a patient early so that the prescribing physician can change the medication or reduce the dosage to reduce the incidence and severity of TD. The rehabilitation therapist uses the AIMS to monitor the patient's ongoing treatment and provides the results of the AIMS to the patient's physician and the consultant pharmacist for comparison with previous scores. The tool helps the physician and pharmacist evaluate the risks and benefits of continuing the antipsychotic medication and the effects of adjusting the dose. The form also requires documentation that the pharmacist and prescriber have attempted to reach the lowest effective dosage (Carl & Johnson, 2006).

The rehabilitation therapist can also use the Behavioral Intervention Monthly Flow Record to monitor antipsychotic effects. The therapist uses the form to track the patient on a daily basis and document behavior episodes (e.g., agitation, fighting, continuous crying), interventions (e.g., redirection, toileting, timeouts), intervention outcomes, and side effects. The record provides invaluable information that the physician can use to determine the consequences of behavioral interventions or medication effects and side effects (Carl & Johnson, 2006).

Anticholinergic Side Effects

Acetylcholine is a neurotransmitter that supports memory, learning, and concentration. The transmission of acetylcholine in the parasympathetic nervous system helps modulate the function of the heart, blood vessels, airways, and organs of the digestive system. Antipsychotic medications can block the effects of acetylcholine in the body, resulting in **anticholinergic** side effects. Anticholinergic side effects can significantly affect a patient's rehabilitation progress. The severity of anticholinergic side effects varies from agent to agent and depends on the extent of binding at the muscarinic acetylcholine receptors and inhibition of acetylcholine effects.

Anticholinergic side effects include sedation, dry mouth, constipation, urinary retention, slowed gastrointestinal motility, decreased gastric secretions, **bradycardia**, **orthostasis**, impaired cognition, blurred vision, and **mydriasis** (dilation of the pupil). Sedation and mental clouding significantly affect speech, language, and cognitive functioning. Sedation is especially problematic during the first and second weeks of therapy and immediately after a change in dosage, but the patient generally develops a tolerance to sedative effects. If sedation persists for more than 2 wk, the patient's physician should lower the dose and evaluate the patient's drug regimen for a possible drug interaction that may be contributing to the persistent sedation (Baldessarini, 2001; Crismon et al., 2011; Crismon & Dornson, 2002; Hall, 2001; Markowitz & Morton, 2002; Meyer, 2011; Rooney & Johnson, 2000).

During each rehabilitation session, the rehabilitation therapist should question the patient about the presence of any of the previously mentioned anticholinergic or sedative side effects as well as any new motor symptoms. The rehabilitation therapist should also monitor the patient for abnormal changes in heart rate (most notably tachycardia), symptoms of dizziness or orthostasis, or breathing problems, which can indicate heart arrhythmia. Finally, the rehabilitation therapist should monitor the patient for excessive drowsiness, symptoms of akathisia, or impaired cognition that interferes with learning and concentration during the treatment session (Crismon et al., 2011; Crismon & Dornson, 2002; Markowitz & Morton, 2002; Seale et al., 2007).

Neurocognitive Effects

Cognitive function can significantly affect the patient's ability to learn and participate in a rehabilitative session. Traditional antipsychotics can either impair or improve cognition. A patient's cognitive memory and attention skills can improve once antipsychotic therapy reduces positive symptoms such as hallucinations or delusions. Patients often complain of having trouble thinking, feeling fuzzy, memory problems, and trouble concentrating with initiation of antipsychotic therapy. Use of the newer antipsychotics can improve executive function, general cognitive function, memory, attention, and motor function over baseline. Haloperidol and clozapine both block the muscarinic receptors and can result in impaired memory (Guthrie, 2002b; Sumiyoshi et al., 2006).

Cardiac Side Effects

Both atypical and typical agents can prolong the length of the heart's contraction (prolonged QT interval) and can increase the risk of ventricular **fibrillation** and **torsades de pointes**, which may result in sudden cardiac death. This toxicity should be considered when choosing an antipsychotic for patients with underlying heart disease. The rehabilitation therapist should always monitor heart rate and rhythm when exercise therapy is initiated in patients on antipsychotic therapy. Other risk factors for QT prolongation include elderly age, liver disease, electrolyte abnormalities, and use of stimulant drugs. QT prolongation has been most often associated with the use of chlorpromazine (Thorazine), pimozide (Orap), haloperidol (Haldol; highest risk with intravenous use), paliperidone (Invega; highest risk with intravenous use), iloperidone, thioridazine (Mellaril), and ziprasidone (Geodon; highest risk with intravenous use). Mellaril and Geodon are associated with the highest incidence of QT prolongation, but parenteral administration of any of these agents increases risk. This risk increases when these antipsychotic agents are combined with other medications that cause QT prolongation such as **tricyclic antidepressants**, antiarrhythmics,

extended-spectrum quinolone antibiotics, and macrolide antibiotics (Dolder et al., 2008; Eon & Durham, 2009; Tanzi, 2009; Zemrak & Kenna, 2008).

Dysphagia

Dysphagia commonly occurs in patients taking antipsychotic medications. The most common side effects that increase the risk of dysphagia are sedation, anticholinergic effects, and EPS (extrapyramidal side effects or pseudoparkinsonism). EPS can cause dysphagia and has been associated with choking in patients who use antipsychotic agents. Antipsychotics cause choking in two ways. First, initiation of antipsychotic medication is associated with an acute blockade of dopamine and can cause acute episodes of laryngeal dystonia. This dystonia can be managed with parenteral anticholinergics. Second, late-onset choking is associated with swallowing or speech difficulties associated with TD, impaired esophageal motility, or medication-induced impairment of the gag reflex. These impairments can cause aspiration, which may lead to pneumonia. Dysphagia can result from anticholinergic-induced dry mouth (xerostomia) that makes it difficult for the patient to initiate a swallow, from abnormal peristalsis caused by anticholinergic effects on smooth visceral muscle, or from deglutitive inhibition caused by anticholinergic effects on the esophageal striated or smooth muscle. Sedation associated with the use of antipsychotics can impair mental or physical abilities and can result in decreased appetite and attention to eating (Campbell-Taylor, 1996, 2001; Carl & Johnson, 2006; Feinberg, 1997).

Metabolic Effects

Although they are safer to use in regard to movement disorders and are more effective in managing the negative, mood, and cognitive symptoms associated with psychosis, second-generation antipsychotics also have a side effect profile. Up to 50% of patients taking antipsychotics gain weight. This weight gain has been seen with the use of typical as well as atypical agents; however, more weight gain is associated with the use of the newer atypical antipsychotics. Risk of weight gain while using atypical agents appears to be higher in children than in adults. This increased weight gain can lead to the development of diabetes and dyslipidemia, thus increasing the risk of heart disease and stroke. Clozapine (Clozaril) and olanzapine (Zyprexa) are associated with the greatest weight gain, quetiapine (Seroquel) and risperidone (Risperdal) are associated with intermediate weight gain, and ziprasidone (Geodon) and aripiprazole (Abilify) are associated with the least weight gain. The rehabilitation therapist should monitor weight in all patients who receive antipsychotic therapy and should include in each patient's care plan a dietary plan for preventing weight gain (O'Keefe & Noordsy, 2002; Tom-Revzon & Lee, 2006).

The use of typical and atypical agents is also associated with elevated prolactin levels. The clinical consequences of hyperprolactinemia include galactorrhea, hypogonadism, menstrual irregularities, erectile dysfunction, loss of libido, and infertility. Hyperprolactinemia is more pronounced in postpubertal children and adolescents than in adults. The rehabilitation therapist should monitor patients for amenorrhea, oligomenorrhea, breast enlargement or engorgement, galactorrhea, decreased libido, erectile dysfunction, osteoporosis, and **hirsutism**. Clozapine (Clozaril) has the worst side effect profile (i.e., risk of seizures, anticholinergic effects, hypersalivation, myocarditis, and agranulocytosis) and requires pharmacist and prescriber registration with the manufacturer's Clozaril National Registry. Use of clozapine is reserved for patients who have failed other therapies (Masand, 2007; Nasrallah & Newcomer, 2004; Patel & Hlavinka, 2007; Tahir, 2007; Terri, 2008; Tom-Revzon & Lee, 2006).

Use of Antipsychotics During Pregnancy

Except clozapine (Clozaril), none of the antipsychotics are documented to be safe to use during pregnancy and are listed as category C medications (they may cause harm to the fetus, but studies are lacking; use only if therapy

benefits exceed this risk). More data about use during pregnancy are available for first-generation agents than for second-generation agents because first-generation agents have been in use longer. Use of butyrophenones such as haloperidol has not been documented to produce fetal malformations, but neonates may have withdrawal symptoms when exposed to these agents in the third trimester. Phenothiazines have not been associated with increased fetal malformations, but neonates can experience respiratory distress syndrome when exposed to these agents in the third trimester (Baylor & Patterson, 2009).

The second-generation agent clozapine (Clozaril) is considered category B, which means it is safe to use and has not been associated with fetal malformations. However, fetal overexposure can lead to floppy-infant syndrome and poor neonatal adaptation. A symptom of floppy-infant syndrome is abnormal hanging of the head and limbs. Neonates should also be tested for **agranulocytosis** after in utero exposure to Clozaril. No cases of fetal malformation have been reported with use of olanzapine (Zyprexa). However, this agent is associated with gestational diabetes, which increases risk to the fetus. If an antipsychotic is used during pregnancy, the lowest effective dose should be used in an effort to reduce EPS in the infant. Because data associated with the use of second-generation agents are limited, use of these agents during pregnancy cannot be recommended. The physician should monitor the mother and fetus closely when the mother uses antipsychotics during pregnancy (Baylor & Patterson, 2009).

PATIENT CASE 2

R.B., an 83-yr-old obese female who lives at a skilled-nursing facility, has a history of seizures and atrial fibrillation. R.B. enjoys singing and dancing in the day room on a weekly basis. R.B. has a long-standing history of schizophrenia and has threatened suicide in the past. Her physician placed her on clozapine (Clozaril) 300 mg to control her schizophrenia and behavioral problems. The staff at the skilled-nursing facility has noted that R.B is acting more sleepy than usual. R.B. also states that she is no longer interested in singing because her mouth and throat are dry and that she is now afraid to dance in the day room because she is afraid of falling. The physical therapist refers R.B. for a consultation with the medical director of the facility. During rounds, the medical director asks the physical therapist to comment on the change in R.B.'s behavior and motor function.

Question

What should the physical therapist consider when commenting on the change in R.B.'s behavior?

Answer

The physical therapist remembers that the change in function occurred after the addition of the medication clozapine (Clozaril). The therapist refers to table 5.1 for information about this medication and finds that it can cause serious agranulocytosis and is reserved for use only after other agents have been tried and found to be ineffective. The therapist also notes that the patient was started at a 300 mg dose of clozapine (Clozaril) and that starting this medication at a dose of 12.5 to 25 mg/day in 1 or 2 divided doses is recommended. Like all antipsychotic medications, clozapine dosage should be slowly titrated up to avoid side effects. The therapist also notes that this medication can cause seizures; R.B. has a history of seizures. In addition, R.B. is obese; weight gain is associated with this medication.

This medication can cause sedation as well as anticholinergic side effects such as dry mouth; these can affect R.B.'s ability to participate in singing activities and increase her risk of falls. R.B.'s medical disorders and the effects of this medication on activities important to her warrant consideration of a change in her antipsychotic medication.

Drug Interactions

Antipsychotic agents are metabolized by conjugation or by the oxidation via the liver's cytochrome P450 enzyme system. Agents that are metabolized by one primary path of the cytochrome P450 enzyme system are more likely to interact with other medications that are metabolized by the same pathway. Table 5.2 lists the CYP 450 metabolic pathways of the different antipsychotics (Johnson, 2001).

Drug interactions mediated by the same CYP 450 metabolic pathway can increase or decrease levels and effects of the antipsychotic, the other medication, or both. Such drug interactions can result in an increase in levels and the dose-related side effects of these medications or reduce the levels and effects of the medication. Antipsychotic drugs can interact with other medications that have sedative or anticholinergic properties (e.g., anesthetics, sedatives, **analgesics**, antihistamines, cold remedies, and alcohol), resulting in excessive sedation, respiratory depression, and potentiation of anticholinergic effects. The anticholinergic effects of clozapine (Clozaril) and thioridazine (Mellaril) can cause confusion and delirium, particularly when combined with other anticholinergics such as tricyclic antide-

Table 5.2   Metabolic Pathways for Liver Metabolism of Antipsychotic Medications

Cytochrome P450 pathway	Antipsychotics affected
CYP1A2	Clozapine (Clozaril), thioridazine (Mellaril), haloperidol (Haldol), olanzapine (Zyprexa), thiothixene (Navane)
CYP2D6	Phenothiazines: chlorpromazine (Thorazine), mesoridazine (Serentil), thioridazine (Mellaril), fluphenazine (Prolixin), perphenazine (Trilafon), trifluoperazine (Stelazine), risperidone (Risperdal), paliperidone (Invega), clozapine (Clozaril), olanzapine (Zyprexa)
CYP3A3/4	Quetiapine (Seroquel), clozapine (Clozaril), ziprasidone (Geodon)

pressants or antihistamines (Siegel & Hansten, 1993; Singer et al., 2003).

Antipsychotic drug interactions can be particularly important in patients with cardiovascular disease. Numerous interactions can occur when antipsychotics are used with antihypertensive agents that block alpha receptors. The alpha-adrenergic blocking properties of low-potency phenothiazines such as chlorpromazine (Thorazine) and thioridazine (Mellaril) can potentiate postural and orthostatic hypotension caused by these antihypertensives.

Thioridazine (Mellaril), clozapine (Clozaril), and pimozide (Orap) can prolong the length of time between contractions of the heart and can precipitate arrhythmias. Finally, some side effects can reduce the intended effects of other medications. Antipsychotic agents antagonize the effects of dopamine agonists and **levodopa** (L-dopa, Sinemet) used in patients with Parkinson's disease. Table 5.3 summarizes important drug interactions that are associated with use of antipsychotic medications (Siegel & Hansten, 1993; Singer, 2003).

Table 5.3   Drug Interactions With Antipsychotic Medications

Medication	Effect of interaction with antipsychotic
Aluminum antacids	Decreased antipsychotic levels due to complexation with drug in gastrointestinal tract
Amphetamines, anorexiants	Decreased weight loss, exacerbation of psychosis
Anticholinergics	Enhanced anticholinergic side effects of antipsychotics, decreased antipsychotic effects
Alpha blockers	Enhanced orthostasis and syncope
Barbiturates: phenobarbital	Decreased antipsychotic effects (induces metabolism of antipsychotics)
Benzodiazepines: diazepam (Valium)	Respiratory depression, stupor, ataxia, additive sedation
Caffeine	Increased levels of clozapine (Clozaril) and olanzapine (Zyprexa)
Caffeinated beverages	Reduced levels and effects of oral antipsychotic liquids (precipitation)
Carbamazepine (Tegretol)	Reduced (up to 50%) antipsychotic levels and effects when used with aripiprazole (Abilify), clozapine (Clozaril), risperidone (Risperdal), olanzapine (Zyprexa), quetiapine (Seroquel), or ziprasidone (Geodon)
Cigarettes	Reduced levels and effects of clozapine (Clozaril) (increased metabolism)
Cimetidine (Tagamet)	Increased levels, orthostasis, and sedation when used with quetiapine (Seroquel)
Clonidine (Catapres)	Increased hypotension
CYP3A4 inducers: carbamazepine (Tegretol), St. John's wort	Decreased levels of quetiapine (Seroquel)
CYP1A2 inhibitors: cimetidine (Tagamet), fluvoxamine (Luvox) Quinolone antibiotics: gatifloxacin (Tequin), moxifloxacin (Avelox)	Increased levels and effects of clozapine (Clozaril), haloperidol (Haldol), olanzapine (Zyprexa), thioridazine (Mellaril), or thiothixene (Navane)
CYP2D6 inhibitors: citalopram (Celexa), fluoxetine (Prozac), paroxetine (Paxil), sertraline (Zoloft), bupropion (Wellbutrin)	Increased levels and effects of clozapine (Clozaril), olanzapine (Zyprexa), phenothiazines, thioridazine (Mellaril), risperidone (Risperdal), and paliperidone (Invega)

› continued

Table 5.3   › *continued*

Medication	Effect of interaction with antipsychotic
CYP3A3/4 inhibitors : erythromycin, fluoxetine (Prozac), fluvoxamine (Luvox), grapefruit juice, ketoconazole (Nizoral), nefazodone (Serzone), ritonavir (Norvir), sertraline (Zoloft)	Increased effects of aripiprazole (Abilify), cimetidine (Tagamet), clozapine (Clozaril), quetiapine (Seroquel), and ziprasidone (Geodon); increased side effects of sedation and orthostasis
Disulfiram (Antabuse)	Increased antipsychotic levels and effects
Dopamine agonists used in Parkinson's disease	Reduced control of Parkinson's effects
Ethanol	Increased central nervous system depression, impaired psychomotor skills
Erythromycin	Increased levels and effects of clozapine (Clozaril) and quetiapine (Seroquel)
Fluoxetine (Prozac)	Increased levels and effects of haloperidol (Haldol) and phenothiazines, increased extrapyramidal side effects
Fluvoxamine (Luvox)	Increased levels and effects of clozapine (Clozaril) and olanzapine (Zyprexa), increased risk of seizures when used with clozapine (Clozaril)
Ketoconazole (Nizoral)	Increased levels of aripiprazole (Abilify), clozapine (Clozaril), quetiapine (Seroquel), and ziprasidone (Geodon)
Meperidine (Demerol)	Increased central nervous system depression, hypotension, sedation when used with antipsychotics
Mesoridazine (Serentil)	Decreased levels of risperidone (Risperdal)
Methyldopa (Aldomet)	Decreased antihypertensive effects
Metoclopramide (Reglan)	Increased extrapyramidal symptoms when used with antipsychotics
Nefazodone (Serzone)	Increased levels and effects of clozapine (Clozaril) and risperidone (Risperdal), increased sedation and orthostasis when used with quetiapine (Seroquel)
Paroxetine (Paxil)	Increased levels and effects of phenothiazine levels
Phenytoin (Dilantin)	Increased metabolism, decreased levels of antipsychotics; quetiapine (Seroquel) decreases levels and effects of phenytoin
Propranolol (Inderal)	Increased sedation and hypotension when used with antipsychotics
Quinidine	Increased levels and effects of phenothiazines and aripiprazole (Abilify)
Quinidine, procainamide	Prolongation of QT interval; arrhythmias when used with tricyclic antidepressants, thioridazine (Mellaril), mesoridazine (Serentil), or ziprasidone (Geodon)
Quinolone antibiotics: moxifloxacin (Avelox)	Increased levels and effects of clozapine (Clozaril) and olanzapine (Zyprexa)
Rifampin	Decreased levels of olanzapine (Zyprexa), clozapine (Clozaril), and quetiapine (Seroquel)
Ritonavir (Norvir)	Increased levels and effects of clozapine (Clozaril), aripiprazole (Abilify), quetiapine (Seroquel), and ziprasidone (Geodon)
Selective serotonin reuptake inhibitor antidepressants: citalopram (Celexa), fluoxetine (Prozac), paroxetine (Paxil), sertraline (Zoloft)	Increased extrapyramidal side effects and akathisia when combined with antipsychotics
Thioridazine (Mellaril)	Decreased levels of quetiapine (Seroquel)

Role of the Rehabilitation Therapist in Promoting Medication Adherence

Medication nonadherence is a common problem among patients with psychiatric disease. About 40% to 50% of patients with schizophrenia do not take their medications as prescribed. Many factors contribute to nonadherence, such as lack of a support system, lack of understanding about the illness and the importance of medication therapy, cognitive impairment, and social stigma associated with the disease and medications. In addition, pill burden or complexity of the medication regimen and inadequate or delayed response to medications can decrease medication adherence. Side effects of medications, including weight gain, **akinesia**, sexual dysfunction, and anticholinergic side effects (i.e., dry mouth, altered taste and smell, sedation, dizziness, orthostasis, and dysphagia) can cause patient distress. When asked which side effects are associated with moderate to severe distress, patients ranked the following side effects as the most distressing: akinesia, weight gain, anticholinergic side effects, sexual problems, muscle rigidity, and akathisia (Patel & Hlavinka, 2007). Methods for improving adherence include educating the patient and family about the illness and the importance and expected side effects of their medications, simplifying the patient's medication regimen using long-acting medications and once-daily dosing when possible, monitoring the frequency of medication refills, and following up with the patient when nonadherence is detected. Use of nonpharmacologic therapies (e.g., cognitive behavioral therapy) along with medication therapy can help patients maintain employment and healthy relationships (Patel & Hlavinka, 2007; Pierce et al., 2008; Terri, 2008; Weiden & Miller, 2001).

Rehabilitation Considerations

The schizophrenic patient also has movement disorders that can include tremors, tics, **ataxia**, or rapid or slow limb movements. Catatonia is the most severe movement disorder that can affect schizophrenics. These movement disorders can profoundly affect the patient. All of the disciplines in rehabilitation—physical therapy, occupational therapy, and speech–language pathology—can be involved in ameliorating these disorders. The speech–language pathologist may encounter oral motor deficits that can result in difficulties with articulation or dysphagia (Barch, 1997; Cohen & Docherty, 2004; Jacobson et al., 2007; Vogel et al., 2000).

The physical therapist and occupational therapist may identify impaired coordination, posture, and balance during the initial examination. The therapist must determine to what extent these impairments impede functional performance in activities of daily living. More importantly, the therapist must determine to what extent the movement dysfunction puts the patient at risk for falls. Data from the National Center for Injury Prevention and Control indicate that more than one third of individuals over 65 yr of age experience a fall each year. Twenty to thirty percent of these falls result in moderate to severe injuries such as hip fractures or head trauma that reduce mobility and increase the risk of premature death. During the history portion of the initial examination of a patient, the therapist must identify any factors, including the use of antipsychotic medications, that may negatively affect the central or peripheral sensory and motor systems or the cognitive function of the patient (Cameron & Monroe, 2007). To prevent falls, the therapist should monitor the patient's blood pressure before transfers from supine to sitting and especially before transfers from sitting to standing.

Rehabilitation therapists commonly use several self-reported standardized instruments to assess a patient's history of loss of balance and falls. Two such instruments include the Balance Efficacy Scale and the Activities-Specific Balance Confidence Scale. The Romberg Test (standing for 30 s with the feet together and the arms by the sides or folded across the chest) can be used to assess equilibrium. Rehabilitation therapists can also use several functionally oriented standardized tests to further assess the patient's balance, postural control, and gait. These include the Tinetti's Performance-Oriented Mobility Assessment, the Dynamic Gait Index, the Timed Up and Go Test, and the Berg Balance Test (Rose, 2003).

Balance-training interventions are effective in minimizing falls and improving functional performance (Rose, 2003). Deficits in the patient's flexibility should be identified and treated. Patients with balance problems and increased risk of falls often have tight ankle plantar flexors, hip flexors, and trunk musculature. Strength training the major muscle groups of the lower extremities and trunk also improves balance and reduces the risk of falls, especially in older adults (Chang et al., 2004).

Finally, installing appropriate assistive devices and making safety modifications in the patient's living environment are essential in preventing falls. The EPS of antipsychotic medications include pseudoparkinsonism, which can negatively affect gait and general motor performance. Collectively, EPS motor impairments create a risk for falls. The shuffling gait pattern creates a short stride length and a narrowed base of support, which contribute to potential loss of balance. The patient may also experience difficulty with sudden challenges to balance related to the narrow base of support and diminished postural control. A fall-prevention program should focus on initiating balance training early, gait training using appropriate assistive devices, and eliminating safety hazards in the patient's living environment. The rehabilitation therapist should also teach the patient to break complex motor tasks down into simpler tasks that can be executed more easily (Cameron & Monroe, 2007).

Summary

This chapter summarizes the actions and side effects of medications that are used to treat psychotic symptoms associated with schizophrenia or symptoms of agitation seen in other disease states such as bipolar disorder, major depression, cognitive disorders, and Alzheimer's disease. Being aware of changes in medications and being able to anticipate side effects that may affect the rehabilitation session are vital to keeping the patient safe and ensure that a therapy session is productive. In order to identify any side effects that may affect the risk and effectiveness of the rehabilitation session, the rehabilitation therapist should ask patients at each rehabilitation session whether they have started any new medications, changed the dosage of their medications, or developed any new symptoms since their last session. Many times these questions uncover concerns that a patient has or a lack of understanding about the side effects associated with medications. Educating the patient about methods for improving safety in daily activities can prevent falls and other adverse outcomes. Upon identifying new or worsening side effects or new-onset movement disorders, the therapist can communicate with the prescriber and other members of the health care team to positively affect patient care (Zagaria, 2008).

Medications Used to Treat Delirium, Dementia, and Alzheimer's Disease

The rehabilitation therapist will often encounter patients who have cognitive impairment and memory problems. Providing rehabilitation for these patients can be challenging because patients need cognition and memory in order to learn new motor skills and alternative approaches to completing activities of daily living (ADL). Cognitive impairment can range from mild impairment associated with normal effects of aging to severe and debilitating dementia such as Alzheimer's disease (AD). When evaluating a patient with altered cognition, the rehabilitation team should make an effort to determine whether the cause of the altered cognition is reversible. Reversible cognitive impairment may be caused by side effects of medications or adverse drug reactions, medication-associated delirium, or clinical conditions such as hypoglycemia, infection, malnutrition with dehydration, and depression. Irreversible cognitive impairment can be caused by several types of dementia, the most common of which is AD.

Reversible Cognitive Impairment Caused by Medications

A side effect of a medication is an effect that is not part of the intended effect and is usually undesired. Common side effects include sedation, cognitive impairment, constipation, and nausea. An adverse drug reaction (ADR) is an unintended or unexpected side effect associated with medication use that is severe enough to require alteration of the medication therapy. ADRs profoundly affect morbidity, mortality, and health care costs, especially in the older patient.

Incidence

ADRs occur globally. One study in the United Kingdom showed a prevalence of 6.5% in the United Kingdom. In more than 75% of the cases examined, the ADR directly led to the patient's hospital admission. The medications implicated in the ADR included aspirin, warfarin, diuretics, and nonsteroidal anti-inflammatory medications other than aspirin. Gastrointestinal bleeding was the most common reaction (Pirmohamed et al., 2004).

In 2000, 2.2 million ADRs were reported in the United States. These ADRs cost the U.S. health care system $85 billion and resulted in 106,000 deaths. When ranked with other disease states, ADRs are the fifth leading cause of death in the United States. Thirty-five percent of the ambulatory elderly will experience an ADR, and one third of these ADRs will be severe enough to require hospitalization. In a study of hospitalized elderly, the incidence of ADRs was 15.2/1000 person-years. More than 15% of patients had more than one ADR. Cardiovascular agents caused adverse events most frequently. The comorbid conditions most often associated with the ADR were congestive heart failure, diabetes, and cancer. More ADRs occurred in rural areas (Sikdar et al., 2012).

In a 4 yr period, two thirds of nursing home residents will experience an ADR and one out of seven of these the patients will require hospitalization. In an evaluation of ADR seen in nursing home patients, one third of the ADRs were associated with altered mental status and cognitive impairment; 20% of these patients experienced a fall related to the ADR (Caufield, 2007; Cummings & Benson, 1983; Mergenhagen & Arif, 2008).

Etiology and Pathophysiology

Risk factors for experiencing an ADR include taking more than five scheduled medications and taking an antibiotic, antipsychotic, or antidepressant medication. Elderly patients are at higher risk for experiencing an ADR because of the higher number of disease states seen in the older patient and the associated increase in the number of daily maintenance medications. Other risk factors for drug toxicity in the older patient include a reduced rate of medication metabolism and excretion and changes in body composition. As humans age, total body fat increases, which increases the risk of accumulation of fat-soluble drugs, and lean body mass and total body water decrease, which increases the risk for water-soluble toxicity. As humans age, brain mass decreases, cerebral blood flow decreases, motor coordination decreases, reaction time slows, and short-term memory becomes less efficient. The blood–brain barrier also becomes more permeable, allowing more medications to cross into the central nervous system and thus increasing risk of drug toxicity. Altered mental status, seen with many medications, is often related to the size of the dose; higher risk is seen in the older patient. Medication-induced delirium has many of the symptoms seen with dementia. Medication-induced changes in mental status should always be ruled out with a careful history of recent medication changes and an examination of whether these changes are related to the changes in mental status (Caufield, 2007; Cummings & Benson, 1983; Mergenhagen & Arif, 2008).

Rehabilitation Considerations

It is important for the rehabilitation therapist to be knowledgeable about the effects of medica-

tions on the rehabilitation process. The rehabilitation therapist needs to understand when to expect the onset of the medication's therapeutic effects in relation to the time of taking the dose so that rehabilitation can be scheduled to maximize the benefits of the medication. For example, the parkinsonian patient will be able to participate in exercise during the period in which his medication dose provides peak dopamine levels. The rehabilitation therapist should also be aware that effects of medication can be changed by particular therapeutic interventions. Full body warm whirlpool treatments, for example, may result in a drop in blood pressure due to the effects of vasodilation which can increase fall risk in patients on blood pressure medications. With the addition of any new medication, the therapist should monitor for side effects associated with the medication, as well as any new symptoms that may result from a drug interaction with the new medication. For example, adding an antipsychotic to a patient who is already receiving tricyclic antidepressant medications may increase the risk of extrapyramidal side effects in the patient. Side effects are more frequent in the elderly. This is particularly true in the elderly exhibiting liver or renal dysfunction. In addition, the elderly frequently have many medications (polypharmacy), thus increasing the chance for drug interactions leading to side effects that can interfere with rehabilitative efforts (Johnson, 2013).

Medication ADRs and Cognition

Many medications, if taken in excess, can cause neurotoxicity, resulting in disturbances in memory and attention span, poor concentration, and behavioral changes. In some instances medications taken in normal doses are associated with neurotoxicity. Medications with anticholinergic properties can elicit reversible cognitive impairment. Most anticonvulsants taken at doses to achieve therapeutic levels can mildly slow cognitive speed. Recurrent hypoglycemia is associated with insulin administration or oral hypoglycemic medications may result in brain damage. **Immunosuppressant** medications and steroids can exacerbate cognitive deficits and precipitate acute episodes of psychosis. Table 6.1 summarizes medications that commonly alter cognition and can contribute to patient fall risk (Caufield, 2007; Cummings & Benson, 1983; Mergenhagen & Arif, 2008).

Table 6.1   Medications That Alter Cognition and Increase Fall Risk

Medication class	Examples	Mechanism
Medications that can cause delirium		
Analgesics		
Nonsteroidal anti-inflammatory drugs	Ibuprofen (Motrin), naproxen (Naprosyn), ketorolac (Toradol)	Inhibits prostaglandin
Opiates	Morphine, meperidine (Demerol), propoxyphene (Darvon), pentazocine (Talwin)	Decreases activity of histamine receptors
Anticholinergic medications		
Antihistamines	Atropine, benztropine (Cogentin), diphenhydramine (Benadryl), scopolamine (Trans Scop patch)	Decreases activity of histamine and muscarinic receptors
Antidepressants		
Tricyclic antidepressants	Amitriptyline (Elavil), imipramine (Tofranil), doxepin (Sinequan)	Anticholinergic effects on histamine receptors
Selective serotonin reuptake inhibitors	Fluoxetine (Prozac), paroxetine (Paxil)	Increases levels of serotonin
Mirtazapine	Mirtazapine (Remeron)	Anticholinergic effects on histamine receptors
Skeletal muscle relaxants		
Cyclobenzaprine	Cyclobenzaprine (Flexeril)	Decreases muscle function, decreases levels of GABA
Sedative hypnotics		
Benzodiazepines	Temazepam (Restoril), diazepam (Valium), chlordiazepoxide (Librium), clonazepam (Klonopin)	Decreases levels of GABA
Corticosteroids		
Corticosteroids	Hydrocortisone (Solu-Cortef, Cortef), methylprednisolone (Solu-Medrol, Medrol), prednisone, dexamethasone (Decadron)	Increases levels of cortisol and endorphins
Dopamine agonists used in Parkinson's disease		
Dopamine agonists	Amantadine (Symmetrel), bromocriptine (Parlodel), levodopa (Levodopa, Sinemet), pramipexole (Mirapex), ropinirole (Requip)	Increases levels of dopamine
Medications that can cause cognitive decline		
Medication used in bipolar disorder		
Lithium	Eskalith	Decreases transmission of sodium and calcium
Typical antipsychotics		
Typical antipsychotics	Thioridazine (Mellaril), chlorpromazine (Thorazine), mesoridazine (Serentil), chlorprothixene (Taractan)	Anticholinergic effects

› continued

Table 6.1   › *continued*

Medication class	Examples	Mechanism
Anticonvulsants		
Anticonvulsants	Barbiturates, topiramate (Topamax), etho-suximide (Zarontin)	Decreases GABA levels, alters transmission of sodium and calcium
Cardiac medications		
Antiarrhythmics	Digoxin in doses >0.125 mg, amiodarone (Cordarone, Pacerone), disopyramide (Nor-pace)	Anticholinergic side effects, hypotension with bradycardia
Antihypertensive medications		
Antihypertensive medications	Diuretics (hydrochlorothiazide, furose-mide), clonidine (Catapres), methyldopa (Aldomet), propranolol (Inderal)	Increases loss of fluids and electrolytes with use of diuretics, urinary urgency and frequency, central depression of alpha receptors
Antineoplastic medications		
Antineoplastic medications	Vincristine (Oncovin), methotrexate (Trex-all), asparaginase (Elspar)	Direct neurotoxicity
Antibiotics		
Antibiotics	Fluoroquinolones (Cipro, Levaquin, Avelox), sulfonamides (Septra, Bactrim), metronidazole (Flagyl), nitrofurantoin (Mac-rodantin)	Increases action at the N-methyl-D-aspartate receptors, decreases activity of GABA, increases dopamine activity
Antidiabetics		
Antidiabetics	Insulin, first-generation sulfonylureas such as chlorpropamide (Diabinese), tolbuta-mide (Orinase) or tolazamide (Tolinase)	Hypoglycemia with associated depletion of glucose to the brain
Gastrointestinal agents		
Antispasmodics	Belladonna, hyoscyamine (Levsin)	Blocks histamine and muscarinic receptors
Histamine-2 blockers	Cimetidine (Tagamet), famotidine (Pepcid), ranitidine (Zantac)	Block histamine-2 reducing gastric acid production but may also block histamine-1 receptors causing sedation

GABA = gamma amino butyric acid.

Reversible Cognitive Impairment Caused by Medication-Associated Delirium

Medication-associated delirium is an acute confusional state associated with altered mood and inattention. The severity of these symptoms fluctuates and is not constant. Mood alterations associated with delirium can be characterized as hyperactive (including symptoms of agitation), hypoactive (including symptoms of lethargy), or mixed (including symptoms of agitation alternating with lethargy). Patients may have altered sleep cycles and symptoms of fear, apprehension, irritability, and anger. Patients with delirium often have difficulty focusing or shifting attention and their speech may be disorganized and irrational (Caufield, 2007; Mergenhagen & Arif, 2008).

PATIENT CASE 1

P.L. is a 75-yr-old female who lives with her daughter's family. Recently she has been more forgetful. For example, she misplaces her keys and sometimes repeats the same question several times. She seems sad, is not interested in going to her quilting class, and has been sleeping a lot. Her concurrent medical conditions include hypertension, diabetes, hyperlipidemia, and hyperthyroidism. Her medications include Synthroid 0.125 µg/day, lisinopril 20 mg/day, atenolol 25 mg/day, metformin 500 mg twice/day, and simvastatin 40 mg/day. P.L.'s daughter asks the physician whether her mother may be developing AD. Upon questioning, P.L. reveals that she has recently started taking Tylenol PM to help her sleep and over-the-counter Motrin IB for a nagging backache.

Question

What are some possible causes for P.L.'s change in mental status?

Answer

P.L. exhibits symptoms associated with depression (i.e., lack of interest in hobbies, changes in sleep patterns, and cognitive decline). She also has hypothyroidism. Her thyroid function should be evaluated because poorly controlled hypothyroidism can contribute to cognitive decline and cause symptoms of depression. She also has diabetes. Hypoglycemia can also contribute to cognitive changes, so her hemoglobin AIC and blood sugar testing results should also be reviewed.

Question

Could medication-associated delirium be contributing to P.L.'s symptoms?

Answer

Besides her medical conditions, her recent addition of a combination of over-the-counter products (Motrin IB and Tylenol PM) can be causing medication-associated delirium. Tylenol PM contains a very potent anticholinergic medication, diphenhydramine, which is commonly associated with delirium in the elderly. In addition, Motrin IB is a nonsteroidal anti-inflammatory drug that can cause acute confusion in the older patient. The toxicity of the combination of these medications can be additive and could be causing medication-induced delirium in P.L.

Incidence

More than 2 million geriatric patients experience medication-associated delirium each year. Delirium occurs in about 20% of hospitalized elderly patients. A study of hospitalized geriatric patients in Mexico reported an incidence of medication-induced delirium similar to that reported worldwide. In addition, the medication-induced delirium was generally associated with a longer hospital stay and greater mortality. Age, poor pain control, lower schooling levels, comorbidity, high glucose levels, and a hematocrit level less than 30% were associated with increased delirium (Berumen, 2003).

Etiology and Pathophysiology

Increased levels of dopamine appears to be the most common cause of delirium, but alterations in other neurotransmitters such as acetylcholine, gamma amino butyric acid (GABA), cortisol, endorphins, and serotonin can also lead to delirium. Decreases in acetylcholine can be associated with the use of anticholinergic drugs, hypoxia, anemia, hypotension, poor nutrition, infection, and surgery. Increases in dopamine can be caused by the use of dopamine agonists, infection, and surgery. Increases in cortisol and endorphins can be caused by administration of steroids or disruption in circadian rhythm. Increases in serotonin levels can be precipitated by use of antidepressant medications, infection, and hepatic encephalopathy. Decreases in GABA levels can occur with the use of benzodiazepines and in patients experiencing alcohol withdrawal. Other common causes of delirium include the following: the administration of corticosteroids such as **prednisone**, dexamethasone (Decadron), methylprednisolone (Medrol, Solu-Medrol), and hydrocortisone (Cortef, Solu-Cortef); the administration of dopamine agonists such as bromocriptine (Parlodel), levodopa (L-dopa, Sinemet), pramipexole (Mirapex), and ropinirole (Requip) used to treat Parkinson's disease; and the administration of sedatives such as diazepam (Valium) and propofol (Diprivan), a sedative commonly used in ventilated patients. Other medications that precipitate delirium include theophylline (Theo-Dur), cardiovascular drugs, histamine-2 blockers that reduce stomach acid such as cimetidine (Tagamet), fluoroquinolone antibiotics such as levofloxacin (Levaquin), and anticonvulsants such as phenytoin (Dilantin) (Caufield, 2007; Mergenhagen & Arif, 2008).

The drugs that most commonly cause delirium are sedative **hypnotics** such as benzodiazepines, opioid analgesics, and medications with anticholinergic effects. Pain medications such as the opioid analgesics and, in particular, morphine and meperidine (Demerol) can precipitate delirium. Other medications that increase the risk of delirium include nonsteroidal anti-inflammatory drugs such as ibuprofen (Motrin), anticholinergics such as diphenhydramine (Benadryl) and scopolamine (Trans Scop), tricyclic and selective serotonin reuptake inhibitor antidepressants, and the selective serotonin and norepinephrine reuptake inhibitor antidepressant mirtazapine (Remeron).

The severity of delirium increases with the size of the dose of the medications and the number of agents taken that have anticholinergic effects. Table 6.1 lists medications that commonly cause cognitive impairment and delirium and increase the risk of falls (Caufield, 2007; Mergenhagen & Arif, 2008).

Medication Therapy

Treating acute agitation in delirium includes using low doses of neuroleptics such as haloperidol (Haldol), quetiapine (Seroquel), and risperidone (Risperdal), and frequent patient assessments monitoring for resolution of symptoms. Once the delirium resolves, these medications should be discontinued to minimize their duration of therapy and possible risk for toxicity associated with the neuroleptic. Aripiprazole (Abilify), a new neuroleptic that affects dopamine and serotonin receptors, can also be used to treat acute agitation. Benzodiazepines such as diazepam (Valium) and lorazepam (Ativan) should not be used to treat agitation associated with delirium. In fact, they can worsen symptoms of agitation (Mergenhagen & Arif, 2008).

Rehabilitation Considerations

When using neuroleptics to treat delirium, patients should be monitored for sedation and

extrapyramidal side effects. Continuous electrocardiogram monitoring is needed to detect possible QT prolongation with arrhythmia. Reducing psychotropic medications to the lowest effective dose may help prevent delirium. A normal sleep–wake cycle and the orienting influence of family members may help reduce the risk of delirium in the older patient.

An unfortunate consequence of delirium is increased risk of falls. Patients without delirium who are at risk of falling include patients with gait disorders such as Parkinson's disease, **Lewy body dementia** (DLB), or stroke. The risk of falling in patients with dementia such as AD is three times that of the normal patient. Other risk factors for falling include muscle weakness, history of gait deficit, balance deficit, use of assistive devices, visual deficits, arthritis, depression, cognitive impairment, and age greater than 80 yr (Caufield, 2007; Cummings & Benson, 1983; Mergenhagen & Arif, 2008).

Of patients who are older and not in an institution, about 35% to 40% will fall in any given year; half of these cases are recurrent. The consequences of a fall, such as a hip fracture or subdural hematoma, can be serious. Fifty percent of patients who sustain a hip injury lose the ability to walk independently, and many of these patients develop a postfall anxiety syndrome that leads to decline in independent functioning and weakening of supporting muscles. Falls contribute to up to 40% of nursing home admissions (Caufield, 2007; Cummings & Benson, 1983; Mergenhagen & Arif, 2008).

Medications associated with falls include psychotropic medications (most strongly associated), analgesics, and anticholinergics. Anticholinergic effects that can increase the risk of falls include orthostasis, depression of the central nervous system, and agitation. One of the most commonly used anticholinergics is diphenhydramine (Benadryl), which is included in allergy treatments and sleep aids and is available over the counter. Even a single dose of diphenhydramine can have dramatic effects on cognitive function in elderly patients, resulting in decreased cognitive function, inattention, altered consciousness, altered motor activity, and altered sleep–wake cycle. These symptoms can occur within 48 h of administration of the dose. Use of diphenhydramine

(Benadryl) is not recommended in the elderly patient (Caufield, 2007). The therapist can help educate the patient about nonpharmacologic treatment of insomnia and the proper use of sedative–hypnotic agents. The pharmacist can help the rehabilitation specialist review the patient's medications to determine whether simplification is possible (Caufield, 2007).

Irreversible Cognitive Impairment (Dementia)

Age-associated cognitive impairment, which occurs in about 39% of older people, is associated with failure finding words, slower learning or concentration, and mild forgetfulness. Many of these patients do fine and are able to continue participating in daily activities. Dementia is defined as cognitive impairment that is associated with generalized mental deterioration over a prolonged period of time. The deterioration can occur in a number of areas such as orientation, perception, attention, language, visuospacial skills, memory, and cognition (i.e., calculation, abstraction, and judgment). The defining characteristic of dementia is memory difficulty (Rush Alzheimer's Disease Center, 2004). In dementia, the progressive decline in function is the result of damage or disease of the brain beyond that seen in normal aging that results in impaired language and attention skills. Higher executive functions are typically affected early in the disease process. As the dementia progresses, the patient can become disoriented to time, place, and person. Early recognition and accurate diagnosis of the type of dementia is important. Each form of dementia presents unique cognitive, memory, and behavioral difficulties and requires a different therapeutic approach (Barna & Hughes, 2009; Jacobson et al., 2007; Wick, 2008).

AD is the most common type of dementia. In AD, memory loss precedes impaired executive function. The patient has more difficulty with episodic memory than with other forms of declarative memory. Anomia is common, as are deficits in sensory and working memory. The patient with AD experiences early topographical disorientation, early short-term memory loss, and difficulty generating word lists. Behavior is socially appropriate in early disease, but agitation and misidentification occur in late disease.

Other common types of dementia include Lewy body dementia (DLB), vascular dementia, temporal dementia, and dementia associated with Parkinson's disease. Between 20% and 50% of dementia patients have mixed dementia. In patients with DLB, executive function and visuospacial orientation are impaired, language is slowed, and delusions and hallucinations can occur. In patients with vascular dementia, aphasia, apathy, and depression can occur. Frontotemporal dementia is characterized by early decline in executive function, decreased ability to concentrate, aphasia, and behavioral changes that include disinhibition, mania, and affective disorders (Elias et al., 2000; Emilien et al., 2004; Hilas & Ezzo, 2012; Perry et al., 2000).

Incidence

Of people over age 65 yr, 6% to 10% have dementia. The incidence of dementia increases with age. The most common form of dementia is AD, which affects 50% to 75% of patients with dementia. Currently, 4.5 million people in the United States live with AD; the projected incidence by the year 2050 is 14 million. AD, the sixth leading cause of death in the United States, causes almost 73,000 deaths annually. Although AD can be seen in patients as young as 40 yr of age, AD is primarily a disease of the elderly, with incidence highest in patients of advanced age. AD has an incidence of 3% in patients between the ages of 65 and 74 yr, 18% in patients between the ages of 75 and 84 yr, and 47% in patients over 85 yr of age.

DLB, the second leading cause of dementia, occurs in 15% to 25% of patients with dementia. Up to 40% of patients with AD have concomitant **Lewy bodies**. This overlap syndrome of DLB and AD is sometimes called the Lewy body variant of AD (LBV-AD). Signs and symptoms of LBV-AD also overlap those of DLB and AD. LBV-AD patients exhibit parkinsonian symptoms (with or without tremors) along with symptoms of dementia. Most of these patients are over 65 yr of age, and 60% of the patients are male. Patients typically survive approximately a decade after onset of symptoms (Barna & Hughes, 2009; Wick, 2008).

Vascular dementia, the third most common type of cognitive impairment, is impairment of memory and cognitive function associated with cardiovascular disease. **Vascular dementia** affects 30% of patients with dementia in the United States and often occurs after a stroke. Up to 60% of patients with AD are also affected by vascular dementia. Patients at risk for vascular dementia include males, people of Asian descent, and older people. Dementia can also be associated with Parkinson's disease (Hilas & Ezzo, 2012; Robishaw & Beadle, 2010).

Etiology and Pathophysiology

The leading hypothesis that describes the pathogenesis of AD is the **amyloid** cascade hypothesis. This hypothesis postulates that increased production of beta-amyloid protein amino acids causes deposition of the aggregated beta-amyloid protein amino acids on the neurons and the formation of neuritic plaques and neurofibrillary tangles. Neuritic plaques consist of beta-amyloid protein that is enclosed by a mass of damaged neurons. Neurofibrillary tangles are tight bundles of abnormal protein that accumulate with the neuronal cell. This increase in beta-amyloid protein deposits, neuritic plaques, and neurofibrillary tangles and associated cell damage trigger an inflammatory response associated with further oxidative injury of the neurons, resulting in atrophy of the cerebral cortex and widespread loss of basal neurons. Damage to the neurons results in depletion of acetylcholine, norepinephrine, and serotonin. Neurotoxic effects are also associated with excessive stimulation of the N-methyl-D-aspartate (NMDA) receptor by glutamine (Barna & Hughes, 2009).

Acetylcholine, the primary neurotransmitter associated with memory and cognition, acts on the nicotinic and muscarinic receptors. During the progression of AD and DLB, the **endogenous** levels of acetylcholine progressively decline. In DLB, a severe depletion of dopamine results in the parkinsonian symptoms seen with the disease. Levels and activity of other neurotransmitters are altered in AD as well. Monoamine oxidase-B (MAO-B) activity is increased and associated with increased **oxidative stress** and oxygen free radicals. A

decline also occurs in noradrenergic and serotonergic neurons in the **locus coeruleus** and raphe nuclei. Glutamate acts as an agonist on the NMDA receptor; activity of this receptor is required for memory, motor function, and perception. Levels of glutamate increase during the processes of learning and use of memory, and glutamate binds to the NMDA receptors. Stimulation of the NMDA receptors results in a change in membrane permeability and the influx of calcium into the neurons. Excessive stimulation of the glutamine receptors can result in overflow of calcium into the neuron and activation of catabolic enzymes (nucleases, proteases, and phospholipases), thus resulting in hypoxia, ischemia, abnormal phosphorylation of the neurofilaments, and destruction of the neuron. This, in turn, disrupts learning and memory. Neuropathologic changes occur principally in the entorhinal cortex and hippocampus and rapidly spread throughout the temporal lobe, and associated deficits in declarative memory occur (Boothby & Doering, 2004; Defilippi et al., 2002; Ho & Chagan, 2004; Mancano, 2004; Shirley, 2002).

Risk factors for AD include dementia in a close family member and the presence of the apolipoprotein E4 allele. Inheritance of the apolipoprotein E4 allele increases the risk for late-onset AD (i.e., onset in the fifth decade of life). Other risk factors for AD include alcohol abuse, diabetes, dyslipidemia, female sex, history of depression, hypertension, increased fat intake in the diet, infections, low level of education, metabolic syndrome, obesity, small head circumference, smoking, systemic inflammation, and thyroid dysfunction (Barna & Hughes, 2009; Defilippi et al., 2002; Jacobson et al., 2007; Mendez & Cummings, 2003; Shirley, 2002; Wick, 2008).

Vascular Dementia

Common causes of vascular dementia include large-artery infarctions, small-artery infarctions, hypoperfusion, and recurrent infarctions. Large-artery infarctions have been associated with vascular risk factors such as hypertension, diabetes, hyperlipidemia, and smoking and commonly occur after a stroke. Small-artery infarctions and hypoperfusion result in white matter lesions, which results in mild cognitive impairment and declines in executive function, new learning, and visual organization. Sixty percent of patients with AD also have vascular dementia (Hilas & Ezzo, 2012). Risk factors for the development of white matter lesions include advanced age, hypertension, chronic kidney disease, metabolic syndrome, microvascular retinopathy, low vitamin B_{12} levels, high homocysteine levels, and elevated C-reactive protein levels (a marker of inflammation). Vascular dementia is most commonly associated with cognitive impairment, in contrast to AD, which is associated with earlier and more significant memory impairment. Treating vascular dementia involves treating the underlying causes of the dementia, such as hypertension, hyperlipidemia, and diabetes, and modifying the patient's lifestyle to include exercise, diet, and weight management (Hilas & Ezzo, 2012; Robishaw & Beadle, 2010).

Lewy Body Dementia (DLB)

DLB, a progressive neurodegenerative disease, is the second leading cause of dementia and affects 15% to 25% of all patients with dementia. Lewy bodies, found in the neuronal cells in the cerebral cortex, are neurofilament proteins that become insoluble; Lewy **neuritis**, found in nerve cells, are synaptic protein aggregates. Neurofibrillary tangles and amyloid plaques that are markers used in diagnosing AD may also be seen in smaller numbers in DLB patients. Lewy bodies can also be found in lower numbers in the cerebral cortex of patients with AD. Key characteristics of DLB include fluctuating, recurrent, and progressive cognitive decline, spontaneous parkinsonian symptoms (occur in 70% of patients), and recurrent visual hallucinations that may be accompanied by delusions and apathy. As with AD, cognitive decline associated with DLB is due to a decrease in acetylcholine activity. DLB patients also experience parkinsonian motor dysfunction caused by dopamine depletion and have depleted norepinephrine levels (Hilas & Ezzo, 2012).

DLB patients are commonly very sensitive to neuroleptic medications, which can result in neuroleptic malignant syndrome. Because of this, use of antipsychotic medications should be avoided in these patients. The same medications that are used to treat AD are used to treat the cognitive impairment associated with DLB (Sonnett et al., 2006). The prominent cognitive changes seen in patients with DLB include impaired executive functioning, impaired attention, and visuospatial difficulties. Working memory, coincidental learning, cognitive reaction time, and attention are more impaired in the DLB patient than in the AD patient. The cognitive impairment includes fluctuations in attention. Inattention and periods of unresponsiveness can last for minutes or hours. Patients with DLB are at increased risk for falls associated with altered motor skills, cognition, and syncope. Severe dopaminergic loss in patients with DLB causes impaired execution of fine motor skills, mask face, stooped posture, and shuffling that is similar to that seen in Parkinson's disease but less severe. Symptoms fluctuate widely hourly and daily. Visual hallucinations often occur and cause serious confusion; patients frequently believe that a significant other is an imposter. DLB patients commonly experience apathy, depression, slowed thought processes, insomnia, and autonomic dysfunction, get lost easily, and lose thoughts midsentence. Treatment with neuroleptics actually worsens the parkinsonian symptoms and hallucinations and can cause life-threatening neuroleptic malignant syndrome (Emilien et al., 2004; Hilas & Ezzo, 2012; Mendez & Cummings, 2003; Sonnett et al., 2006).

Diagnosis of AD

Diagnostic criteria established by the National Institute of Neurological and Communicative Disorders and Stroke and the Alzheimer's Disease and Related Disorders Association have improved accuracy of diagnosis to greater than 90%. These criteria require a history of progressive cognitive deficits with no precipitating events for the diagnosis of AD. When patients with dementia are admitted to service, the physician and rehabilitation team should conduct a careful medication history to rule out other causes of dementia (e.g., head trauma, depression, stroke, subdural hematoma, and tumors) or drug use that can contribute to dementia symptoms. AD is classified as early onset (age of <65 yr) and late onset (>65 yr) and is subclassified by predominant symptoms (with delirium, with depressed mood, with delusions, with behavioral disturbances, and uncomplicated) (Defilippi et al., 2002; Reisberg et al., 1982; Shirley, 2002).

Early diagnosis and treatment is important in slowing down the cognitive decline seen with AD. Mild cognitive impairment (MCI), characterized by complaints about memory performance without a reduction in ADL functioning or diagnosis of dementia, may indicate that a patient is at risk for AD. MCI may present with impaired attention and executive function and disorders in affect and language. MCI patients perform more poorly on tasks of manual dexterity than do normally aging adults. When compared with normally aging adults, performance of patients with MCI declined faster on tasks of semantic and episodic memory and perceptual speed but not tasks of visuospacial ability. If preclinical identification of dementia is possible, early treatment, including pharmacological intervention, should be initiated. Several tests for assessing MCI are available. One assessment, the MCI Screen, reports 97% accuracy in differentiat-

ing between normal patients and patients with MCI (Defilippi et al., 2002; Emilien et al., 2004; Shankle et al., 2005).

Individuals with AD commonly experience decreased smell and changes in taste and appetite that can lead to weight loss. FMG Innovations developed an early-alert home-screening test for AD. It is a noninvasive, self-administered olfactory test that detects one of the early warning signs of AD (Nickerson & Sherman, 2007). Additional memory-screening tools include the Memory Impairment Screen and the Short Blessed Test. In the Memory Impairment Screen, patients are given the names of items in four categories and then are required to recall the names of each item after a short delay. The Short Blessed Test asks the patient to identify the year, month, and time of day; to count backward from 20; to recite the months of the year backward; and to recall a phrase. Memory impairment does not necessarily indicate that the patient has AD. The patient should always follow up with the physician to rule out reversible causes of impaired memory such as medications, hypothyroidism, depression, and hypoglycemia. Table 6.2 summarizes the tools

Table 6.2   Assessment Tools Used to Monitor Patients With Alzheimer's Disease

Tool	Type of assessment	Scoring and interpretation	Comments
Alzheimer's Disease Assessment Scale Cognitive Subscale	Cognitive function	0-70 scale. Higher scores indicate greater impairment.	FDA preferred method for assessing cognitive function in medication trials.
Mini Mental State Examination	Cognitive function	0-30 scale. Higher scores indicate greater impairment.	
Clinician's Interview-Based Impression of Change/Clinical Global Impression of Change	Global	7-point Likert scale. Higher scores indicate greater impairment.	FDA preferred method for assessing global function in medication trials.
Global Deterioration Scale for Assessment of Primary Degenerative Dementia (GDS)	Global	1-7 scale. Higher scores indicate greater impairment.	
Neuropsychiatric Inventory	Behavioral	10 items. Higher scores indicate greater frequency of symptoms and caretaker distress.	FDA preferred method for assessing behavioral function in medication trials.

Tool	Type of assessment	Scoring and interpretation	Comments
Progressive Deterioration Scale	Activities of daily living	0-100 scale/category.	10 categories rated by caregiver (e.g., dressing, eating independently, social interaction).
Mild Cognitive Impairment Screen	Cognitive screen	Series of 7 tests.	Tests measure memory, symbol fluency, and executive function. 97% accurate in identifying cognitive changes associated with normal aging.
Montréal Cognitive Assessment	Cognition	30 points possible.	Series of tests that helps differentiate cognitive changes associated with normal aging, mild cognitive impairment, and dementia. 26/30 considered normal. Takes 10 min. Involves alternative trailmaking, visuoconstructive skills, naming attention, sentence repetition, verbal fluency, abstraction, and delayed recall.
Cognitive Linguistic Quick Test	Cognition	Ratings of normal, mild, moderate, and severe impairment in each domain.	Takes 15-30 min. Measures 5 cognitive domains: attention, memory, executive function, language, and visuospatial skills. Involves 10 tasks, 5 of which have minimal language demands. Can be used in ages 18-89 yr in patients with known or suspected neurologic impairment.
Scales of Cognitive and Communication Ability for Neurorehabilitation	Cognitive and communicative deficits	8 scales.	Takes 30-45 min. Measures oral expression, orientation, memory, speech comprehension, reading comprehension, writing, attention, and problem solving. Used to identify cognitive and communication impairment, quantify severity of impairment, and develop patient-specific treatment goals and plans.
Environment and Communication Assessment Toolkit for Dementia Care	Cognitive and performance deficits	Identifies performance deficits and environmental barriers and identifies specific interventions and environmental adaptations that help improve the patient's independence and well-being.	Provides 300 specific recommendations for interventions and environmental modifications.

FDA = U.S. Food and Drug Administration.

commonly used to diagnose and monitor AD patients (Higuera et al., 2008; Nickerson & Sherman, 2007).

Dementia is further classified in stages of severity (progression). Determining the stage of dementia that the patient is currently in is critical in designing a therapeutic regimen. For example, the therapeutic goals and approach for a patient with AD staged as level III (early confusional stage) will greatly differ from those for a patient staged as level VI (moderately severe). Tools for cognitive assessment include the Alzheimer's Disease Assessment Scale, Mini Mental State Examination (MMSE), and the Global Deterioration Scale for Assessment of Primary Degenerative Dementia (GDS). The major tool used to stage the patient is the GDS, which clearly defines the levels of dementia on a seven-point scale. Other tests often use this scale to delineate levels of dementia. The Brief Cognitive Rating Scale derives a number that equals the staging on the GDS (Higuera et al., 2008; Nickerson & Sherman, 2007). Rehabilitation therapists can then use the Claudia Allen Crosswalk to reconcile the GDS staging levels and the Claudia Allen staging levels. The book *Understanding Cognitive Performance Modes* lists the Allen stages and gives examples of abilities and disabilities as well as functional goals for each stage (Allen, Blue, & Earhart, 1995).

The Alzheimer's Disease Assessment Scale has become the primary cognitive assessment tool accepted by the U.S. Food and Drug Administration (FDA) and is used in clinical drug trials to evaluate cognitive change. Outside of clinical trials, the MMSE and the Minimum Data Set are commonly used. The MMSE does not stage the patient but does help establish baseline function. The average expected decline in MMSE score is 2 to 4 points/yr. A decline of less than 2 to 4 points/yr indicates that medication treatment is successful. The Minimum Data Set was created to form a national database of nursing home residents across the country. The dementia-related changes in ADL are described as the four "late loss" ADLs which include the inability to get out of bed, to safely transfer from bed to a chair, to eat independently, and to toilet independently.

Another test, the St. Louis University Mental Status Test, has many of the components of the MMSE. However, the test differs when testing subjects who have a high school degree and those who do not. It also provides differentiation between patients with no cognitive impairment, older subjects with minimal cognitive impairment (MCI), and those with dementia (Defilippi et al., 2002; Shirley, 2002; Taylor, 2011). The Montréal Cognitive Assessment is also frequently used as a screening tool for mild dementia (Nasreddine et al., 2005). The Cognitive Linguistic Quick Test correlates well with the MMSE and is used extensively to test for Parkinson's associated dementia (Parashos et al., 2009). The Scales of Cognitive and Communication Ability for Neurorehabilitation tests oral expression, orientation, comprehension (reading and writing), and attention (Milman et al., 2008). The Environment and Communication Assessment Tool Kit for Dementia Care helps identify individual performance deficits, environmental barriers, and interventions and environmental adaptations. Tests that determine frontal lobe functioning (e.g., the Stroop test) should also be performed (Brush et al., 2011).

Rehabilitation Considerations

When assessing a patient with cognitive impairment, the therapist should take a careful medication history to rule out causes that may be addressed and improve cognition such as medication side effects, delirium associated with medication use, dehydration, or hypoglycemia. When reviewing medications, the therapist should note any recent changes in medications or medication dose and new use of over-the-counter (nonprescription) medications or herbal therapies in order to rule out reversible causes. Once reversible causes for cognitive impairment are ruled out, the therapist should determine the actual type and stage of dementia because therapeutic plans vary greatly depending on the specific diagnosis and the patient's stage of dementia. Assessment tools such as the Barthel ADL index, the Blessed Dementia Scale, or Functional Activities Questionnaire can be administered by any member of the rehabilitation team.

The primary manifestations of AD and other dementias include neuropsychiatric disturbances, cognitive impairments, and neurological deficiencies. The cognitive impairments include difficulties with sensory memory (as seen in impairments of selective or alternating attention span), arousal, processing speed, and concentration. Clinical processes such as orientation, memory, language, calculation ability, concentration, praxic capacity (i.e., ability to draw figures), visuospacial skills, hallucinations, anxiety, delusions, paranoia, apathy, despair, and executive functions are evident. The working memory components of phonological storage and articulatory rehearsal may be intact; however, the central executive function may be impaired. Speech may be fluent but empty in meaning (Barna & Hughes, 2009; Iversen et al., 2009).

The patient will get lost easily due to the impaired topographical memory secondary to impaired visuospacial abilities. Immediate memory is impaired less than is delayed recall. Deterioration of episodic and semantic memory occurs rapidly after onset; however, deterioration of working memory is more gradual. Naming difficulties occur more frequently in patients with AD than in those with vascular dementia (Lukatela et al., 1998). Episodic, semantic, and lexical therapies have been shown to be helpful in reducing anomia in patients with mild AD (Ousset et al., 2002). Because implicit learning is usually spared in AD, the patient may be responsive to priming as a therapeutic procedure for perceptual as opposed to conceptual implicit priming tasks (Fleischmann & Gabrieli, 1998).

Difficulties with acquiring new information are a hallmark of AD. Performance recall and recognition are impaired in both verbal and nonverbal situations. The AD patient may have difficulty with delayed recall after just a few minutes. Performance in delayed recall may be worse in patients with AD than in patients with Huntington's disease, Korsakoff's syndrome, or frontotemporal dementia (Emilien et al., 2004).

Neurological impairments can manifest in incontinence, difficulty walking, and the reoccurrence of primitive reflexes such as sucking.

These neurological deficiencies are usually evident in the later stages of the disease. The patient may have difficulty with ADL such as self-feeding. The patient may also exhibit carphologia (i.e., lint-picking behavior), wandering, sundowner's syndrome, and restlessness. Behavioral symptoms include paranoia, aggressiveness, sleep difficulties, phobias, and anxieties. As AD progresses, cognitive difficulties such as disorientation through time and space and impairment in remote memory and language increase. Psychological impairments, including paranoia and delusional behavior, also become more pronounced (Emilien et al., 2004).

Because medications are not curative, non-pharmacologic behavioral interventions are the mainstay of therapy for AD patients and their families. Modifying behavior, simplifying tasks, increasing physical exercise, and providing education and support for family members are very important in the multidisciplinary approach to managing the AD patient. Behavioral modification strategies include limiting wardrobe choices and accessories, encouraging showering instead of bathing, and eliminating unnecessary furniture and clutter to reduce fall risk. Simplifying tasks and demands can prevent confrontation and aggression (Barna & Hughes, 2009; Iversen et al., 2009).

The role of the therapist is to reduce the frequency of falls, increase motor skill and flexibility, and reduce mental decline. Non-pharmacologic interventions involve a wide variety of activities. Participating in mental activities reduces AD risk by up to 50%. People who participate in activities such as visiting a library or museum; reading a newspaper, books, or magazines; attending a concert, play, or musical; or writing letters reduce their risk for developing AD. Simple interventions such as mind games and exercises tend to stimulate cognitive functioning. Brain exercises and increased physical activity increase cerebral blood flow and oxygen consumption, resulting in improvements in cognition. Patients are encouraged to participate in activities that promote recall such as reminiscence activities, crossword puzzles, Sudoku, and computerized cognitive activities, which are now available through numerous websites. For example, Captain's Log offers computerized cognitive materials for traumatic brain injury, aphasia, and dementia. There are also numerous apps such as Lumosity that provide excellent cognitive exercises (Barna & Hughes, 2009; Iversen et al., 2009).

The rehabilitation team may work with different facilities to set up an appropriate program within the facility for the residents with dementia. An activities program that offers different activities for various diagnoses and stages can be extremely useful for this population. Active rehabilitation and activities tailored to the diagnosis and staging of the patients can help reduce behavioral outbursts, falls, and difficulty at the end of the day (sundowning); improve oral intake and gait; and promote more independent ADL functioning and self-feeding. A therapy–activities program identifies strengths, weaknesses, and staging for each individual. A therapy–activities program uses the physical therapist, occupational therapist, speech–language pathologist, and activities director to develop an ongoing, integrated program that meets the needs of the patient with more advanced disease. Additionally, a therapy–activities program provides a typical activity calendar for patients in early stages of dementia as well as a low-level sensory calendar designed to meet the needs of patients with more advanced disease (Camp, 1999; Bayles & Tomoeda, 2007; Brush & Camp, 1998; Eisner, 2001; Hopper et al., 2005; Mahendra et al., 2005; Sohlberg et al., 2005; Sohlberg & Mateer, 2001; Sohlberg & Turkstra, 2011).

Environmental manipulations are also a major part of therapeutic intervention. The AD patient requires a consistent, predictable environment and provides therapies and interventions that use the patient's intact nondeclarative memory systems to preserve and maintain the patient's current level of function as long as possible. Indirect interventions include assistive technology for cognition, simulated presence therapy, staff linguistic manipulations to improve patient understanding, and environmental manipulations (e.g., the placement of furniture, color of facility, reducing visual and auditory distractions, labeling rooms,

and increasing environmental adaptations for safety). Direct interventions for this population include reality orientation, spaced retrieval, metacognition training, errorless learning, priming, reminiscence therapy, Montessori therapy, chaining and chunking approaches, attention training, sensory stimulation, and imagery mnemonics. Treatment of patients with cortical dementia focuses on the spared nondeclarative memory system consisting of priming, procedural memory, conditioning, and habits (Bayles & Tomoeda, 2007; Brush & Camp, 1998; Camp, 1999; Eisner, 2001; Hopper et al., 2005; Mahendra et al., 2005; Sohlberg et al., 2005; Sohlberg & Turkstra, 2011).

Evidence shows that regular moderate exercise prevents disease and promotes health in the elderly. Regular exercise increases cardiac and respiratory endurance and tolerance to physical exertion, reduces cholesterol levels and inflammation, and increases insulin sensitivity. Consistent exercise may reduce the risk of AD and other types of dementia. Exercise may also moderate dementias by promoting the immune system and stimulating the cortex. A meta-analysis of 18 studies examining the effects of exercise on cognition showed that exercise training significantly benefits cognition, especially when exercise is performed for more than 30 min/session and is continued long term. Magnetic resonance imaging studies have demonstrated that exercise expands the dentate gyrus, a hippocampal subregion that is important for memory and is known to be adversely affected by aging. Exercise induces an increase in brain-derived neurotrophic growth factor in the hippocampus, increasing learning and memory. Exercise also increases levels of insulin-like growth factor, which assists in vascular remodeling in the adult brain (Pomerantz, 2008).

A balanced program of exercise should include activities that increase cardiovascular endurance, muscle strength, flexibility, balance, and neuromuscular control. In early-stage AD, group exercise programs are especially beneficial. The goal of an exercise program in early-stage AD is to improve and maintain psychomotor function that typically begins to deteriorate as the patient experiences decreased functional capabilities due to cognition and memory deficits. In this stage, gross motor function is either not affected or affected minimally. The rehabilitation specialist can determine which exercise-program setting is best for the patient with early-stage AD based on the patient's individual needs and the program design. In some instances a typical fitness center setting can be too overwhelming for the individual with AD. Exercising with a workout buddy or enrolling in a medical-based fitness program at a local hospital, private clinic, or community center may be more suitable. Because the onset of agitation and depression is common in the early stages of AD, exercising with a partner or in a group setting can also increase socialization and improve mood. The components of the exercise program should be performed in the same order and manner daily; this will greatly help the patient master the program. Patients with AD may forget that they exercised the day before, but due to intact procedural memory they usually are still able to execute with minimal verbal cueing the exercises that they learned in the past. Demonstration or physical guidance can be used if verbal cueing is unsuccessful. The rehabilitation specialist should use rote memory to help the patient acquire adaptive ADL mobility techniques in order to perform routine tasks safely. The specialist should also teach the patient to note visible cues for safety hazards, to recognize possible mistakes, and to use checklists to compensate for memory difficulties or identify problems. The patient also may be able to follow verbal and written directions with associated actions. The AD patient's nondeclarative memory systems should be used because these systems are spared (Allen, 1995; Bayles & Tomoeda, 2007; Brush & Camp, 1998; Camp, 1999; Eisner, 2001; Hopper et al., 2005; Mahendra et al., 2005; Sohlberg et al., 2005; Sohlberg & Turkstra, 2011).

In moderate-stage AD, the pathophysiology of the brain begins to affect the neuromuscular control of the body to a greater extent. Patients with moderate-stage AD exhibit agitation, restlessness, and wandering behavior. They are at risk for falls as well as elopement. Patients in the moderate stage are not aware of the

beginning, middle, and end of an activity. They recognize possessions with which they are familiar, remember information about several activities that are important to them, and are aware of social greetings. Therapy should focus on sequencing steps to accomplish familiar self-care routines, recognizing the need for assistance, performing mobility activities safely, using adaptive equipment effectively, establishing priorities for activities that are preferred, recognizing errors, and preserving social skills (Allen, Blue, & Earhart, 1995).

Patients with moderate-stage AD commonly exhibit gait and balance disturbances, decreased strength and mobility, and difficulty with performing routine ADLs. Better therapy results are achieved in patients who are able to attend to an activity for 5 min or more. The therapy program for patients with moderate-stage AD should be highly structured and relatively brief and should be performed in the same order each day. Simple exercises and functional activities that use images or demonstration rather than commands are typically more effective. Regular daytime exercise is likely to decrease the amount of restlessness and agitation that a patient with AD experiences in the early evening (sundowning). As in early-stage AD, treatment in moderate-stage AD should focus on the spared (i.e., nondeclarative) memory systems (Bayles & Tomoeda, 2007; Brush & Camp, 1998; Camp, 1999; Eisner, 2001; Hopper et al., 2005; Mahendra et al., 2005; Sohlberg et al., 2005; Sohlberg & Turkstra, 2011).

In the patient with late-stage AD, memory loss is severe and gait and balance disturbances typically prevent independent ambulation. In this stage, many patients begin using a wheelchair and become dependent on others for self-care and ADL. Physical and occupational therapy focus on addressing impairments in range of motion, strength, and balance that affect the patient's ability to participate in self-care and basic ADL. The speech–language pathologist should determine the proper diet with the patient. The rehabilitation team should work with the facility, nursing staff, and caregivers and provide training about preventing contracture, falls, and skin breakdown, problems that are common in late-stage AD. The rehabilitation specialist must train caregivers and nursing staff in transfers to ensure that the patient is moved in a manner that is safe to both the patient and the caregiver. The therapist should evaluate the patient's environment to maintain function and safety (Bayles & Tomoeda, 2007; Brush & Camp, 1998; Camp, 1999; Eisner, 2001; Hopper et al., 2005; Mahendra et al., 2005; Sohlberg et al., 2005).

Falls occur in approximately 30% of patients with AD. It is often difficult for the patient to move around objects in the environment. Decluttering the environment and removing trip hazards are important interventions in minimizing falls. Structured practice negotiating the remaining objects in the environment and therapy activities that improve balance and neuromuscular control are essential for improving the patient's understanding of where their body is in space. Improving the patient's ability to safely negotiate the living environment is especially important in patients with AD because these patients commonly pace and wander. The therapist may have to provide a majority of the effort to move from supine to sitting and sitting to supine and pivot from bed to wheelchair. The therapist should seek to control trunk stability with either adaptive equipment or a contact guard. One of the goals of treatment might be for the patient to sit in a chair without trunk support for 0.5 h. Another goal might be for the patient to answer yes or no questions in response to discomfort or comfort. Another might be to help the patient use universal gestures such as clapping hands to communicate with others. Again, nondeclarative memory systems should be used in rehabilitation teaching in the patient with AD (Allen, Blue, & Earhart, 1995; Bayles & Tomoeda, 2007; Brush & Camp, 1998; Camp, 1999; Eisner, 2001; Hopper et al., 2005; Mahendra et al., 2005; Sohlberg et al., 2005).

The occupational therapist works to increase the patient's ability to perform ADLs that enhance independence and functionality, including dressing, toileting, and eating. This results in a decrease in the burden of care for the caregiver. Self-feeding can be one of the most important variables in preventing aspi-

ration pneumonia in patients with dementia (Langmore et al., 1998). Tools for assessing an individual's functional ability to complete ADLs include the Canadian Occupational Performance Measure, the Functional Activities Questionnaire, the Cognitive Performance Test, and the Allen Cognitive Level Test.

The role of the speech–language pathologist in treating patients with dementia is to prolong cognitive linguistic functioning as long as possible. The speech–language pathologist also is concerned with the swallowing functions of the patient with dementia. This is particularly true in the early and middle stages of dementia. Several of the pragmatic language treatments may parallel aphasia therapy. In addition, the AD patient may present with swallowing apraxia and food agnosia (Gogia & Rastogi, 2009; Allen, Blue, & Earhart, 1995; Bayles & Tomoeda, 2007; Brush & Camp, 1998; Camp, 1999; Eisner, 2001; Mahendra et al., 2005; Sohlberg et al., 2005; Sohlberg & Turkstra, 2011).

The clinical pharmacist can help ensure that the medication dose of AD is titrated up to the maximum effective dose. Medications that have anticholinergic effects can impair memory and cognitive functioning, especially in the older patient, and the pharmacist should help caregivers avoid the use of anticholinergic medications in patients with AD. When counseling patients with AD, it is important to set realistic expectations for the effect of medications used to treat AD. In addition, the patient and family should be referred to support groups such as the Alzheimer's Association. Patients and families should be involved early in making decisions regarding durable power of attorney for health care and financial matters in order to avoid the difficulty and expense of petitioning for guardianship. The possibility of placement in a long-term facility should also be addressed well in advance so patients and families have time to select and apply to a facility and plan to pay for long-term care (Barna & Hughes, 2009).

Medication Therapy

Medications have no curative effect in AD or other dementias but can help slow the progression of the disease, reduce symptoms, improve quality of life, and potentially delay nursing home placement. Treatment should begin as soon as the diagnosis is made in an effort to preserve cognitive function (Boothby & Doering, 2004; Defilippi et al., 2002; Hilas & Ezzo, 2012; Ho & Chagan, 2004; Mancano, 2004; Shirley, 2002). As discussed previously, the physician or pharmacist should educate caregivers and family members and ensure that all have realistic expectations about the effect of AD medications.

Acetylcholine is an important chemical in brain function associated with memory. The acetylcholinesterase inhibitors are the cornerstone of medications used to treat AD and DLB. These medications enhance memory by preventing the enzymatic breakdown of acetylcholine and thus increasing its availability in the brain. Use of these agents has been noted to improve cognitive and motor functions (Boothby & Doering, 2004; Defilippi et al., 2002; Ho & Chagan, 2004; Hilas & Ezzo, 2012; Mancano, 2004; Shirley, 2002).

Glutamine is another chemical in the brain that is associated with memory and learning. Memantine (Namenda) regulates the action of glutamine on the brain's NMDA (N-Methyl-D-Aspartic acid) receptor. Memantine can also improve cognition, global function, and behavior when initiated in patients with mild AD. It can be used alone or in combination with the acetylcholine esterase inhibitor. In patients with moderate or severe-stage AD disease, an acetylcholine esterase inhibitor should be initiated in combination with memantine (Namenda). Extended-release products can be initiated at 7 mg/day and increased weekly by 7 mg to a maximum dose of 28 mg/day (Boothby & Doering, 2004; Defilippi et al., 2002; Ho & Chagan, 2004; Hilas & Ezzo, 2012; Mancano, 2004; Shirley, 2002).

Motor symptoms in patients with dementia may be treated with levodopa. However, these patients are at increased risk for dopaminergic side effects and hallucinations, even with low doses of dopamine. Agents used to treat motor symptoms of Parkinson's disease (i.e., dopamine agonists, amantadine, anticholinergics, and selegiline) should be avoided in patients with dementia because they are ineffective and are associated with increased risk for side effects. Baclofen may be used in these patients to improve symptoms of rigidity (Emilien et al., 2004; Jacobson et al., 2007; Mendez & Cummings, 2003; Taylor, 2011).

Acetylcholine Esterase Inhibitors

The acetylcholine esterase inhibitors increase levels of acetylcholine by inhibiting its metabolism by esterase enzymes. Use of acetylcholine esterase inhibitors has been shown to produce a modest increase in cognition lasting approximately 6 mo in one third to one half of patients with mild to moderate AD. These medications have also been shown to increase ADL functioning in behaviors such as walking, eating, and grooming. Improvements have been demonstrated in levels of anxiety, apathy, and aberrant motor behavior. Acetylcholine esterase inhibitors provide the greatest benefit when they are started early in the disease process and given for the long term. Use of acetylcholine esterase inhibitors is also suggested for other types of dementia including DLB, AD with cardiovascular disease, vascular dementia, and Parkinson's disease with dementia. These agents elicit a better response in patients with DLB than in those with AD, likely due to the preservation of the muscarinic receptors in DLB (Mendez & Cummings, 2003; Sonnett et al., 2006; Taylor, 2011).

Because acetylcholine esterase inhibitors are most effective at higher doses and exhibit a dose response, patient dosage should always be titrated up to the maximum dose. The titration should occur slowly to avoid gastrointestinal side effects, and these medications should be taken with food. The most common side effects include vomiting, diarrhea, abdominal pain, dizziness, and anorexia. If intolerable side effects occur, treatment should be discontinued for at least 1 wk and an alternative agent should be tried. Interruption of therapy for more than 1 wk requires restarting at the initial dose and gradually titrating. Because the acetylcholine esterase inhibitors differ in method of binding to acetylcholine esterase, the duration of action differs among agents. Tacrine (Cognex), donepezil (Aricept), and galantamine (Razadyne) bind via an anionic bond and have a very short duration of action. (Note that in 2004, Razadyne became the new name of the former, Reminyl.) Rivastigmine (Exelon), a carbamate ester, is hydrolyzed at a much slower rate, resulting in duration of action of up to 10 h. Because anticholinergic medications antagonize the effects of acetylcholine esterase inhibitors, concurrent use of anticholinergics should be avoided. The effects of these agents continue for at least 2 yr. After treatment for 1 to 2 yr, if doubt exists regarding the efficacy of the medication, therapy can be discontinued for 4 wk. If the patient's behavior does not change during the 4 wk period, the medication should be discontinued or another therapy may be considered. Table 6.3 summarizes the dosing and side effects of these medications (Defilippi et al., 2002; Shirley, 2002; Sucher & Mehlhorn, 2007; Taylor, 2011; Wick, 2008).

Tacrine (Cognex) was introduced in the 1980s. A short-half-life that requires dosing multiple times each day as well as liver toxicity have limited the use of this medication. It is no longer used on a routine basis and is now used as second line therapy after failure of other agents (Emilien et al., 2004; Iversen et al., 2009; Taylor, 2011).

Donepezil (Aricept) is effective in about 40% of patients with mild to severe AD. Peak concentrations occur 2 and 4 h after oral dose. It has a half-life of 70 h and a long duration that permits once/day dosing. Studies have demonstrated that donepezil improves cognitive functioning as well as ADL functioning in patients with mild to moderate dementia (Burns et al., 1999). Patients with moderate to severe AD also experience improvements in cognition, functioning, and behavior with this medication (Feldman et al., 2001). Patients in clinical trials have demonstrated improvements in cognitive functioning that have been maintained for several years (Iversen et al., 2009; Taylor, 2011).

Donepezil (Aricept) is used in doses of 5 to 15 mg to treat mild to moderate dementia and doses of 15 to 23 mg to treat moderate to severe dementia. In moderate to severe dementia, the combination of donepezil (Aricept) and memantine (Namenda) is recommended because the combination is significantly more efficacious than donepezil (Aricept) alone. Donepezil (Aricept) has an easy titration schedule. It starts at 5 mg once/day, and the dose may be increased to 10 mg once/day in 4 to 6 wk. A 23 mg dose that can be used to treat moderate to severe AD is now available. Donepezil (Aricept) also comes in orally disintegrating tablets, which provide easier administration in patients with swallowing disorders, and may be taken with or without food (Farlow et al., 2003; Iversen et al., 2009; Sucher & Mehlhorn, 2007; Taylor, 2011).

Galantamine (Razadyne), which is chemically related to codeine, acts directly on nicotinic receptors and has a cholinergic effect. It has a half-life of 5 to 7 h. Galantamine (Razadyne) must be given with meals. Galantamine (Razadyne) causes improvement or stabilization for about 9 mo longer than do other agents. Galantamine is well tolerated and has been shown to improve performance on memory tests (Defilippi et al., 2002; Shirley, 2002; Taylor, 2011).

Rivastigmine (Exelon) has a prolonged duration of action of 10 to 12 h and should be given with food. Rivastigmine (Exelon) is available as an oral solution or as a topical patch. The patch should be initiated in a dose of 4.5 mg applied once/day for the initial 4 wk and then increased to 9.5 mg/day. The patch should be applied to the upper or lower back or the upper arm or chest. Patients should change the location of the patch daily and not use the same spot twice within a 14 day period. The oral solution may be mixed with fluid and is stable unrefrigerated for up to 4 h after mixing. Significant improvements in cognition and ADL functioning in patients with mild to moderate AD are observed with doses of 12 mg/day (Emilien et al., 2004; Kayrak et al., 2008; Pavlis et al., 2007; Taylor, 2011).

NMDA and Glutamate Modulators

Memantine (Namenda) modulates the activation of the NMDA receptor by glutamine by binding to this receptor, promoting increased activation when glutamine levels are reduced and inhibiting excessive activation of the

See table 6.3 in the web resource for a full list of medication-specific indications, dosing recommendations, side effects, and other considerations.

Table 6.3 Medications Used to Treat Alzheimer's Disease

Medication	Side effects affecting rehab							Other side effects or considerations
Acetylcholine esterase inhibitors: First-line therapy for AD and DLB.								
Donepezil (Aricept)	Cog ++	S 0	A ++	Motor +	D +++	Com ++	F ++	Nausea, vomiting, abdominal pain, diarrhea, dyspepsia, anorexia. Start at the lowest dose and slowly titrate. Take with food.
Rivastigmine (Exelon) Capsules, oral solution, and transdermal patch	Cog ++	S 0	A ++	Motor +	D +++	Com ++	F ++	Nausea, vomiting, abdominal pain, diarrhea, dyspepsia, anorexia. Start at the lowest dose and slowly titrate, or use alternative dosage forms such as the transdermal patch. Take with food.
Galantamine (Razadyne) Tablets, oral solution, and extended-release capsules	Cog ++	S 0	A ++	Motor +	D +++	Com ++	F ++	Nausea, vomiting, abdominal pain, diarrhea, dyspepsia, anorexia. Start at the lowest dose and slowly titrate. Take with food.
Tacrine (Cognex)	Cog ++	S ++	A +	Motor ++	D +++	Com ++	F +++	Nausea, vomiting, abdominal pain, diarrhea, dyspepsia, anorexia. Monitor for hepatotoxicity. Not used as first-line therapy due to higher risk of hepatotoxicity and the requirement for frequent dosing. Second-line therapy for AD and DLB after failure of other acetylcholine esterase inhibitors.
N-methyl-D-aspartate antagonist: Adjunctive therapy in treatment of AD or DLB with acetylcholine esterase inhibitors.								
Memantine (Namenda)	Cog +++	S ++	A +++	Motor 0	D +++	Com ++	F ++	Diarrhea, constipation, altered mental status, sedation, urinary incontinence. Avoid concurrent use with dextromethorphan and other medications that affect the N-methyl-D-aspartate receptor (amantadine).

Cog = cognition; S = sedation; A = agitation or mania; Motor = discoordination; D = dysphagia; Com = communication; F = falls; AD = Alzheimer's disease; DLB = Lewy body dementia.

The likelihood rating scale for encountering the side effects is as follows: 0 = Almost no probability of encountering side effects. + = Little likelihood of encountering side effects. +/++ = Low probability of encountering side effects; however, probability increases with increased dosage. ++ = Medium likelihood of encountering side effects. +++ = High likelihood of encountering side effects, particularly with high doses. ++++ = Highest likelihood of encountering side effects; best to avoid in at-risk patients.

receptor when glutamine levels are excessive. Modulation of glutamine activity reduces resultant neuron death and alleviates symptoms associated with AD. Memantine (Namenda) is indicated for use as a sole therapy or for use in combination with one of the acetylcholine esterase inhibitors in the treatment of moderate to severe AD. Peak blood levels occur within 3 to 7 h of the dose and therapeutic results can be seen within 14 days of therapy initiation. It is eliminated by the kidneys, has no cytochrome P450 enzyme drug interactions, and has a half-life of 60 to 80 h. Lower doses should be used in patients with renal impairment. This agent should not be combined with medications that can increase urinary pH such as sodium bicarbonate because this can result in reduced elimination and increased levels and toxicity (Defilippi et al., 2002; Orgogozo et al., 2002; Reisberg et al., 2003; Shirley, 2002; Wilcock et al., 2002). Other important drug interactions with medications used to treat dementia are summarized in table 6.4.

PATIENT CASE 2

M.R. is a 79-yr-old woman who was recently diagnosed with Alzheimer's (AD) and who lives with her son and his family. M.R.'s concurrent diseases include diabetes and hypertension and she has had two strokes. Her medications include aspirin 325 mg/day, metformin 500 mg twice/day, lisinopril 20 mg/day, and Toprol XL 25 mg/day. She has residual hemiplegia from her most recent stroke and has been undergoing gait training and exercise training with the rehabilitation specialist. Her physician has prescribed an Exelon patch 9.5 mg to be applied daily along with Namenda 20 mg/day. Her son calls to

Table 6.4   Drug Interactions With Medications Used to Treat Alzheimer's Disease

Medications	Mechanism of drug interaction	Examples of interacting medications	Effects of interaction
Tacrine* (Cognex)	Cytochrome P450** CYP1A2 inhibition	Fluvoxamine (Luvox), cimetidine (Tagamet)	Increased levels and effects of tacrine, cholinergic side effects
Tacrine (Cognex)	Cytochrome P450** CYP1A2 inhibition	Theophylline (Theo-Dur, Theo-24)	Increased levels of theophylline, increased side effects of tachycardia, agitation, sleeplessness, and shakiness
Donepezil (Aricept)	Cytochrome P450** CYP2D6, CYP3A3/4 inhibition	Cholinergic agents and neuromuscular-blocking agents	Enhanced effects of donepezil, increased cholinergic side effects, increased neuromuscular blockade
Donepezil (Aricept)	Cytochrome P450** CYP2D6, CYP3A3/4 induction	Carbamazepine (Tegretol), phenytoin (Dilantin), rifampin, phenobarbital	Increased metabolism of donepezil, and therefore, decreased levels and effects of donepezil
Rivastigmine (Exelon)	Not metabolized	None	None
Galantamine (Razadyne)	Cytochrome P450** CYP2D6, CYP3A3/4 inhibition	Ketoconazole (Nizoral), paroxetine (Paxil), erythromycin	Inhibited metabolism and therefore, increased levels and effects of galantamine, increased cholinergic side effects
Memantine (Namenda)	Not metabolized	None	None

Anticholinergic medications antagonize the effects of medications used to treat AD and should be avoided. *Tacrine is seldom used due to high occurrence of hepatotoxicity. **Metabolized by the cytochrome P450 enzymes CYP2D6 and CYP3A3/4, which interact with many medications.

cancel his mother's therapy appointment and shares his concern about his mother's severe nausea, vomiting, and weakness. He reports that she has not been able to eat or drink anything in the past 48 h and is not able to participate in her scheduled physical therapy session.

Question

What advice can the therapist give M.R.'s son regarding her new medications?

Answer

The therapist realized that the initial dose of both the Exelon patch and the Namenda may be too high and contacted M.R.'s physician to report her symptoms. The physician instructed M.R.'s son to bring her into the office. Once M.R.'s symptoms were resolved, the physician initiated therapy at a lower dose and titrated dosage up slowly to avoid further gastrointestinal side effects. M.R.'s pharmacist instructed her to avoid any over-the-counter medications with anticholinergic effects (e.g., over-the-counter sleep aids, cold products, or antihistamines) because they interfere with the effectiveness of her AD medications. The physician instructed M.R.'s son to check with the pharmacist before starting any new medications or herbal therapies to ensure they do not interact with her current medications (Knudsen, 2007).

Standard Adjunctive Therapies for Patients with AD

Members of the American Association for Geriatric Psychiatry, the American Geriatrics Society, the American Association for Geriatric Psychiatry Expert Panel on Quality Mental Health Care in Nursing Homes, and the American Academy of Neurology developed consensus guidelines regarding treatment of behavioral and psychological symptoms in AD (Beier, 2007; Hilas & Ezzo, 2012; Zagaria, 2006). Behavioral symptoms can include physical aggression, screaming, restlessness, agitation, wandering, culturally inappropriate behaviors, sexual disinhibition, hoarding, cursing, and shadowing. Psycho-

logical symptoms include anxiety, depression, hallucinations, and delusions. Patients with delusions can believe that others are stealing, that they are in danger, that unwelcome guests are living in the house, that their family plans to abandon them, that their house is not their home, that their spouse is having an affair, that media figures are in the home, or that people are not who they claim to be. Hallucinations can include seeing things not seen by others, talking to people not there, hearing voices not heard by others, and feeling things on the skin that are not there.

Other causes of these symptoms (e.g., pain, medical illness) should first be eliminated. Then, nonpharmacologic methods should be used unless the patient poses a threat. After that, antipsychotic medications should be tailored to the individual patient and used to treat hallucinations, delusions, severe behavioral symptoms, and psychotic symptoms. Treatment should be given over a course of 12 wk and then be re-evaluated by the prescriber. If one agent is not effective after 4 to 6 wk, another agent should be tried. The prescriber should evaluate therapy for tapering or discontinuance not more than 6 mo after the patient is stabilized and every 6 mo thereafter. Caregivers should be educated about AD and the role of antipsychotic therapy to reduce the unnecessary use of antipsychotic medications (Beier, 2007; Zagaria, 2006).

Atypical antipsychotics such as olanzapine (Zyprexa) and risperidone (Risperdal) can be used to treat behavioral symptoms in patients with AD. Twenty percent of patients treated with these agents develop sedation and extrapyramidal side effects that require discontinuance. The FDA issued a black-box warning about using these agents in patients with dementia-related psychosis due to a potential increase in mortality. Alternatives to the antipsychotic medications that can be used to treat behavioral symptoms include carbamazepine (Tegretol) and valproic acid (Depakote). Selective serotonin reuptake inhibitors such as fluoxetine (Prozac) and paroxetine (Paxil) are the preferred agents for treating depression in patients with AD. Tricyclic antidepressants have significant anticholinergic effects and should be avoided. Short-acting benzodiazepines can be used short term to treat agitation (Beier, 2007; Zagaria, 2006).

Use of stimulant drugs such as methylphenidate (Ritalin), dextroamphetamine (Dexedrine), and dextroamphetamine–amphetamine (Adderall) has also been shown to result in mild improvement in cognitive functioning, particularly when the subject is fatigued (Iversen et al., 2009). Hydergine contains a combination of ergoloid mesylates and is another medication that can improve ADL and self-care in patients over 60 yr of age who exhibit declines in mental functioning (e.g., self-care, motivation, ADL functioning, and interpersonal and cognitive functioning). Use of Hydergine has also been shown to elevate mood in patients (Iversen et al., 2009).

Monoamine oxidase type B (MAO-B) activity is increased by the increased oxidative stress and oxygen free radicals accompanying AD. Selegiline (Eldepryl) is a selective MAO-B that is used to treat mild Parkinson's disease. Selegiline decreases the degradation of catecholamines in the brain and reduces the production of oxygen free radicals. A randomized placebo-controlled trial compared the effects of vitamin E alone, selegiline alone, and the effects of a combination of selegiline and vitamin E with the effects of a placebo over a 2 yr period in patients with AD. The combination of vitamin E and selegiline demonstrated no benefits, and the combination of these products is no longer recommended (Cummings, 2004; Defilippi et al., 2002; Sano et al., 1997; Shirley, 2002; Standaert & Young, 2001).

A relationship may exist between lipids, vascular changes in the brain, and dementia. Some evidence suggests that lipid-lowering agents such as the statins, which are used to treat hyperlipidemia, may be useful in lowering the risk of AD. An observational study conducted in England showed that patients who received statins had a substantially lower risk of developing dementia. More studies are needed to determine the usefulness of statin therapy in the treatment of AD (Elias et al., 2000; Jick et al., 2000; Shirley, 2002).

PATIENT CASE 2, *continued*

M.R.'s son brings an article about the effects of statin therapy on AD to his mother's next therapy session. He asks whether his mother should be on a statin.

Question
What should the therapist tell M.R.'s son about the use of statins in AD?

Answer
The role of statins in preventing dementia has not been established. However, in M.R.'s case, initiation of a statin would be appropriate for her for several reasons. She is diabetic, which increases the risk of high cholesterol and cardiovascular risk. She has had two strokes, and the most recent stroke guidelines recommend initiating statin therapy in patients who have had a stroke. The therapist should advise M.R.'s son to ask her physician whether his mother could benefit from statin therapy.

Alternative Therapies for Patients with AD

Therapies such as vitamin E, ginkgo biloba, coenzyme Q, estrogen supplementation, and nonsteroidal anti-inflammatory drugs have also been studied for their anti-inflammatory effects in AD. Earlier trials of gingko biloba showed promise in younger patients, but a recent trial indicated that the agent is not effective in the older patient with AD. Gingko biloba acts as a scavenger for free radicals and has been used to treat dementia. Two large double-blind studies conducted in Germany evaluated the use of gingko biloba 120 mg twice/day in patients with mild to moderate AD and found significant improvement in cognitive functioning. However, gingko biloba carries an increased risk of bleeding and should be avoided in patients taking **anticoagulants** (Barrett-Connor & Kritz-Silverstein, 1993; Mendez & Cummings, 2003; Mulnard et al., 2000; Shirley, 2002; Stewart et al., 1997; Van Dongen et al., 2000).

Researchers believed that nonsteroidal anti-inflammatory drugs such as ibuprofen (Motrin) reduced the immune reaction triggered by beta-amyloid protein, neurofibrillary tangles, and neuritic plaques and studied these agents to determine whether they could prevent AD. This immune reaction appears to be mediated by alpha-antichymotrypsin, interleukin-1, interleukin-6, and tissue necrosis factor. Ginkgo biloba, nonsteroidal anti-inflammatory drugs, and coenzyme Q all increase the risk of bleeding and use of these agents is no longer recommended. Estrogen supplementation is also no longer recommended due to an associated increased risk of uterine cancer (Brinton, 2004; Le Bars et al., 1997).

Vitamin E, a fat-soluble vitamin that acts as an antioxidant as well as an anti-inflammatory agent, was studied for its effects in patients with AD. A recent meta-analysis found that doses of vitamin E greater than 400 IU/day may increase mortality. The patient or caregiver should speak with the physician and carefully weigh the benefits and risks before initiating any of these alternative therapies (Berman & Brodaty, 2004; Sucher & Mehlhorn, 2007).

Many members of the lay public have been interested in the development of cognitive enhancers that increase cognitive performance in otherwise healthy individuals or stave off cognitive decline with aging. Increases in cognitive performance are the result of increases in motivation and attention. Attention is part of sensory memory, which is the foundation of other memory systems. Many of the medications used to treat cortical and subcortical dementias, attention deficit–hyperactivity disorder, and stroke increase motivation and attention. Caffeine is widely consumed as a stimulant in order to improve cognitive functioning. Nicotine has also been shown to improve attention and memory. Several food extracts (i.e., vitamins B_6, B_{12}, and E, ginkgo biloba, folate, lecithin, and neurosteroids) are also reported to increase cognition. Most of the studies have proved to be inconclusive. Nootropic agents (food supplements and herbal products used in Europe that include nefiracetam, oxiracetam, and piracetam) have been used as cognitive enhancers for a number of disorders such as post-concussion syndrome and dementia (Iversen et al., 2009).

Homotaurine is a synthetic form of a natural compound found in seaweed. This product interferes early in the amyloid cascade by binding with amyloid and preventing the formation of plaque. Studies conducted in Europe and the United States failed to document efficacy, and some were concerned about the possibility of the formation of abnormal aggregation of taurine. The use of homotaurine may actually worsen symptoms of AD. This product is now being marketed as a nutriceutical called Vivimind (50 mg tablets to be taken twice/day) that costs the patient $1800/yr. The Alzheimer's Disease Foundation has taken a strong stand against the use of this product for treating AD (Swanson, 2009).

Research Medications

Two new therapies currently being studied are the first disease-modifying therapies for AD. Tramiprosate (Alzhamed) is believed to reduce the deposition of amyloid in the brain by binding to soluble beta-amyloid peptides. Flurbiprofen (Ansaid) reduces levels of the toxic amyloid peptide 42 by about 70%. Amyloid peptide 42 is thought to cause cell death in the brain and initiate formation of plaques in the brain. It modulates the action of gamma-secretase enzymes to produce shorter amyloid peptides that are less likely to clump together.

A serotonin-4 receptor agonist is also being studied for use in combination with donepezil in patients with mild AD. Studies show improvement in the encephalograph of patients receiving the combination therapy compared with patients receiving a placebo. Finally, the use of intravenous gamma globulin has been studied in very small groups of patients and has resulted in stabilization and cognitive improvement in patients with AD. The intravenous gamma globulin is believed to bind to the beta-amyloid, thus helping to clear the protein from the brain and blocking the toxic effects of beta-amyloid (Belden, 2007). The development of a vaccine to produce antibodies against beta-amyloid plaques in AD patients is also an area of research.

Summary

This chapter introduces reversible and irreversible causes of cognitive impairment. Reversible causes include fluid and electrolyte imbalances, hypoglycemia, ADR, and delirium secondary to medication use. Reversible causes should always be looked for and addressed in a patient with altered cognition. Irreversible causes of cognitive impairment include several types of dementia, including AD. This chapter summarizes medication and nonpharmacologic therapies for treating dementia and describes appropriate tools and parameters for monitoring patients with cognitive impairment.

Medications Used to Treat Anxiety, Anxiety Disorders, and Insomnia

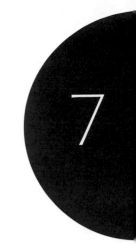

7

In clinical practice, the rehabilitation therapist will care for patients with anxiety, anxiety disorders, and insomnia. This chapter introduces concepts associated with anxiety, defines anxiety disorders, and describes how these disorders and insomnia affect patient progress in rehabilitation. This chapter also reviews medications used to treat these disorders and recommends how to enhance rehabilitation and reduce risk of falls in patients with anxiety and insomnia and in patients taking these medications.

Anxiety Disorders

Anxiety is a normal reaction that helps people cope with the stresses of daily life and difficult situations. Symptoms of anxiety include chest pain, lightheadedness, diarrhea, tachycardia, sweating, cold hands and feet, trembling, muscle tremors, impaired concentration, paresthesias (tingling of the skin), attention difficulties, sleep difficulties, and derealization (sense of unreality). Anxiety disorders are characterized by anxiety that is irrational or excessive. Anxiety disorders include generalized anxiety disorder (GAD), panic disorder, obsessive–compulsive disorder (OCD), post-traumatic stress disorder (PTSD), and specific phobias (Saljoughian, 2006).

Incidence

Anxiety disorders affect 40 million adults in the United States. Specific phobias affect 19 million Americans; the incidence of specific phobias in women is twice that in men. Social phobia affects 15 million Americans. PTSD affects 7.7 million adults. GAD affects almost 7 million Americans; the incidence of GAD in women is twice that in men. Approximately 25% of the elderly with chronic illness are diagnosed with GAD (Ayers et al., 2009). Panic disorder affects about 6 million adults. OCD, which affects more than 2 million adults, usually appears in childhood or early adulthood (Saljoughian, 2006).

Etiology and Pathophysiology

Medical conditions associated with anxiety include alcoholism, delirium, pulmonary embolism, postconcussion syndrome, cardiac arrhythmia, Cushing's disease, angina, and drug withdrawal syndrome. Anxiety often accompanies psychiatric and neurologic diseases such as Parkinson's disease, stroke, neurodegenerative diseases, and dementia (Jacobson et al., 2006). Most anxiety disorders (i.e., GAD, panic disorder, OCD, and social phobias) have a genetic component. PTSD is triggered after a patient witnesses an event involving death or serious injury to himself or others. Medications and foods that can cause or worsen anxiety include caffeine, nicotine, alcohol, cocaine, appetite suppressants, amphetamines, asthma medications, nasal decongestants, and corticosteroids (Preston et al., 2008).

GAD involves chronic and exaggerated worry that is generalized and not associated with a trigger. This worry is associated with physical symptoms of fatigue, headache, muscle tension, muscle aches, difficulty swallowing, twitching, irritability, sweating, and hot flashes. GAD is associated with difficulty concentrating and sleeping. Abnormal functioning of the neurotransmitters gamma amino butyric acid (GABA), serotonin, and norepinephrine is associated with GAD. This disorder is treated with medication therapy (Saljoughian, 2006).

Panic disorder is associated with panic attacks, which are defined as episodes of sudden fear due to stressors. Symptoms associated with a panic attack include pounding heart, sweating, weakness, faintness, or dizziness. Sometimes the patient believes he is having a heart attack, losing his mind, or on the verge of dying. These symptoms usually peak within 10 min, but attacks can last longer. Many patients try to avoid the place or situation associated with the first attack; this may interfere with daily activities. When this severely restricts the patient from going out into public, the panic disorder is called **agoraphobia** (fear of crowds). Patients with panic disorder develop intense anxiety between panic attacks and worry about when the next one will occur. Panic disorder is treated with psychotherapy and medications (Matthew & Hoffman, 2009; Saljoughian, 2006).

The symptoms of OCD include persistent, unwanted thoughts (obsessions) or repetitive, ritualistic behaviors (compulsions; e.g., hand washing, checking, counting, or silently repeating words) that cause extreme distress and interfere with daily life. Severe OCD can interfere with a patient's ability to earn a living. OCD is related to low levels of serotonin activity in the brain. This disease responds to psychotherapy and medication therapy (Matthew & Hoffman, 2009; Saljoughian, 2006).

Posttraumatic stress disorder (PTSD) is an anxiety disorder that follows a traumatic event. The most common causes of PTSD are combat, motor vehicle accidents, and sexual abuse. Acute stress disorder occurs immediately after the traumatic event, whereas PTSD may not occur until the patient experiences a triggering event that involves recurrence of at least part of the initial traumatic event. Response to the triggering event includes nightmares and flashbacks that interfere with sleep and work, disrupt daily activities, and cause the patient to avoid situations or places. Symptoms include difficulty sleeping, irritability, outbursts of anger, difficulty concentrating, hypervigilance, and an exaggerated startle response. These patients avoid any reminders of the event and may not be able to recall parts of the event itself. Eighty to ninety percent of patients with PTSD have other psychiatric illnesses. This disorder can be accompanied by substance abuse, alcohol abuse, depression, or other anxiety disorders. It may last for months or may be chronic and last for years. Treatment includes cognitive–behavioral therapy and medication. Post-combat stress disorder, also called shell shock, is a short-term condition similar to PTSD in which the soldier presents with tremor, nervous exhaustion, and an inability to function normally (Chavez, 2006; Eaton-Maxwell et al., 2010).

Another type of anxiety disorder can result from traumatic brain injury associated with a concussion or contusion resulting from an accident, trauma, or even use of a firearm in warfare. Traumatic brain injury may result in impaired cognition (e.g., attention difficulties, memory problems, and difficulty in concentrating) or in physical and behavioral changes that may manifest immediately or up to 1 wk after the injury (Eaton-Maxwell et al., 2010).

Patients with social phobia have a persistent, chronic, and intense fear of being watched or judged by others and are embarrassed or humiliated by their own actions. This fear may interfere with daily activities or work. They may worry for weeks before a future event. The phobia may be associated with specific tasks such as speaking in front of others or may be so generalized that it interferes with being around others. Patients may experience blushing, profuse sweating, trembling, nausea, and difficulty speaking. Patients may be involved in substance abuse in an attempt to treat the disorder themselves. This disorder can be successfully treated with psychotherapy or medication (Eaton-Maxwell et al., 2010; Saljoughian, 2006).

Specific phobias include fears of certain specific things such as heights (altophobia), darkness (lygophobia), fire (pyrophobia), water (aquaphobia), and flying (aviatophobia). These phobias are usually treated with psychotherapy (Saljoughian, 2006).

Rehabilitation Considerations

The behavioral signs of anxiety include hyperalertness, irritability, uncertainty, apprehensiveness, difficulty with memory or concentration, and sleep disturbances. Recognizing these clinical manifestations will help the clinician adjust the patient's treatment session and refer the patient to the appropriate health care practitioner for treatment to alleviate the anxiety (Cameron & Leventhal, 2003; Eaton-Maxwell et al., 2010).

Anxiety influences the cognitive functions of attention and perception. The anxious patient also tends to focus on the negative aspects of the symptoms, resulting in rumination. Anxiety can also influence information processing, problem solving, and anxiety regulation. For example, in the ill patient with anxiety, response to new information is processed with an attitude that is excessively self-protective rather than appropriate for the situation. The rehabilitation patient may view past success in treatment in an unrealistically negative manner. The patient may also have difficulty processing instructions in therapy. The patient with high levels of anxiety may be hypervigilant in watching for potential threats and may erroneously interpret ambiguous stimuli as negative and threatening (Cameron & Leventhal, 2003).

Medications used to treat anxiety can also alter cognition. Benzodiazepines often have amnesic side effects that include difficulty in processing new information and storing the information in memory as well as consolidating information in memory. Chronic therapy with benzodiazepines may be associated with deficits in sustained attention and visuospacial impairment that are insidious and not recognized by the patient (Iverson et al., 2009).

Cognitive Behavioral Therapy

Anxiety disorders such as panic disorder, OCD, phobias, PTSD, and social phobia benefit from cognitive–behavioral therapy. Cognitive therapy helps patients change thinking patterns that prevent them from overcoming their fears. Behavioral therapy helps patients change their reactions to anxiety-provoking situations. In behavioral therapy, a person who is fearful of a situation is exposed to that situation in order to confront and help overcome that fear. A patient with OCD may participate in exposure and response-prevention therapy in which the patient is exposed to a stressful trigger and is asked to refrain from engaging in the usual ritualistic response behavior for a specified length of time. This is repeated until the anxiety associated with the exposure diminishes and is not associated with the old, ritualistic behavior. Cognitive behavioral therapy used in combination with medication therapy provides better results than does medication therapy alone (Iverson et al., 2009; Saljoughian, 2006).

Exercise and Anxiety

A mounting body of evidence shows that regular exercise is an important component in the management of anxiety. Patients with anxiety disorder or panic attacks may be fearful of exercise or other therapeutic interventions. Because panic attacks can occur during rehabilitation sessions, the clinician should be alert to the physical signs of such an episode (tachycardia, increased blood pressure, shortness of breath, dizziness, hyperventilation, sweating, nausea, chest pain, lump in the throat, muscle tension, and dry mouth) (Goodman et al., 2003).

Prudent use of antianxiety medications can benefit rehabilitation because the patient may be more relaxed and cooperative. Rehabilitation exercise may best be scheduled for 2 to 4 h after oral administration, when the medication reaches its peak blood level; however, at that time the patient may be too sedated. Preexisting cognitive difficulties exacerbated by medicine-induced sedation may put the patient at risk during some exercises. The reduced cognition, generalized weakness, and poor eyesight and hearing of some elderly can combine with the sedation associated with antianxiety medications to increase the risk of falls. The rehabilitation therapist should provide balance training and adaptations to the patient environment to reduce the risk of falls in patients receiving antianxiety medications (Ciccone, 2007; Garuti et al., 2003).

Beta blockers may be used to treat panic disorders. Side effects of beta blockers can include dizziness and reduced heart rate and blood pressure. The reduction in blood pressure can result in orthostatic hypotension, which can put the patient at risk for an episode of syncope and a related fall. The decrease in heart rate and contraction force can decrease the patient's maximal exercise capacity. The rehabilitation therapist must be aware that resting heart rate and exercising heart rate will be reduced in a patient using beta blockers and must not overtax the patient's heart by trying to reach

age-adjusted maximal target heart rates (Peel & Mossberg, 1995).

Medication Therapy

Approximately 50% of patients with an anxiety disorder are prescribed an antidepressant or other antianxiety medication. Abnormal functioning of the neurotransmitters GABA, serotonin, and norepinephrine is associated with GAD, and this disorder is treated with medication therapy. Medications used to treat GAD include selective serotonin reuptake inhibitors (SSRI), benzodiazepines, and buspirone (Buspar) (Saljoughian, 2006). Table 7.1

 See table 7.1 in the web resource for a full list of medication-specific indications, dosing recommendations, and side effects.

Table 7.1   Medications Used to Treat Anxiety Disorders

Medication	Side effects affecting rehab							Other side effects or considerations			
Tricyclic antidepressants (TCAs): Amitriptyline is used to treat PTSD; clomipramine is used to treat OCD; imipramine is used to treat panic disorder, GAD, and PTSD.											
Amitriptyline (Elavil)	Cog ++++	S ++++	A 0	Motor ++	D ++++	Com ++++	F ++++	Weight gain +++	Seizure +++	Cardiac +++	Sexual ++
Clomipramine (Anafranil)	Cog ++++	S ++++	A 0	Motor ++	D ++	Com ++++	F ++	Weight gain ++	Seizure ++++	Cardiac +++	Sexual +
Imipramine (Tofranil)	Cog +++	S +++	A +	Motor ++	D +++	Com +++	F ++++	Weight gain ++	Seizure +++	Cardiac +++	Sexual ++
Selective serotonin reuptake inhibitors (SSRIs): Used to treat OCD, panic disorder, PTSD, and social phobia; fluvoxamine is used to treat OCD only.											
Fluvoxamine (Luvox)	Cog 0/+	S 0/+	A +	Motor +	D +++	Com 0/+	F 0	Weight gain 0	Seizure 0	Cardiac 0	Sexual 0
Fluoxetine (Prozac)	Cog 0/+	S 0/+	A +	Motor 0	D 0/+	Com 0/+	F 0	Weight gain 0/+	Seizure ++	Cardiac 0/+	Sexual +++
Paroxetine (Paxil)	Cog +	S +	A +	Motor 0	D +	Com +	F +	Weight gain 0	Seizure 0	Cardiac 0	Sexual +++
Sertraline (Zoloft)	Cog 0/+	S 0/+	A +	Motor 0	D +++	Com +	F 0	Weight gain 0	Seizure 0	Cardiac 0	Sexual +++
Citalopram (Celexa)	Cog 0	S +	A 0/+	Motor 0	D +++	Com 0	F 0	Weight gain 0	Seizure ++	Cardiac 0	Sexual +++
Selective serotonin and norepinephrine reuptake inhibitors (SSNRIs): Used to treat GAD.											
Venlafaxine (Effexor)	Cog +	S +	A 0/+	Motor 0	D +	Com +	F +	Weight gain 0	Seizure ++	Cardiac +	Sexual ++

Medication	Side effects affecting rehab							Other side effects or considerations			
Monoamine oxidase inhibitor (MAOIs): Used to treat PTSD.											
Phenelzine (Nardil)	Cog	S	A	Motor	D	Com	F	Weight gain	Seizure	Cardiac	Sexual
	++	++	0/+	0	+	++	+	+	+	+	+++
Benzodiazepines: Clonazepam is used to treat social phobia and GAD; alprazolam is used to treat panic disorder and GAD; lorazepam is used to treat panic disorder; diazepam is used to treat GAD. Benzodiazepines carry risk of dependence and addiction.											
Clonazepam (Klonopin)	Cog	S	A	Motor	D	Com	F	Fatigue, ataxia, headache, nausea, risk of dependence and withdrawal symptoms. Half-life is 23 h.			
	+	+	++	++	++	++	+				
Alprazolam (Xanax)*	Cog	S	A	Motor	D	Com	F	Fatigue, ataxia, headache, nausea, risk of dependence and withdrawal symptoms. Half-life is 12 h.			
	+	+	++	++	0/+	+	+				
Lorazepam (Ativan)*	Cog	S	A	Motor	D	Com	F	Fatigue, ataxia, headache, nausea, risk of dependence and withdrawal symptoms. Half-life is 14 h. Use short term to avoid dependence or addiction.			
	+++	+++	++	+++	++	++	+++				
Diazepam (Valium)	Cog	S	A	Motor	D	Com	F	Fatigue, ataxia, headache, nausea, risk of dependence and withdrawal symptoms. Half-life is 43 h. Use short term to avoid dependence or addiction.			
	++++	++++	++	+++	++	++++	++++				
Azapirone: Used to treat GAD.											
Buspirone (Buspar)	Cog	S	A	Motor	D	Com	F	Sedation, ataxia, low risk of dependence. Half-life is 2-3 h.			
	+	+	0	0	+	+	+				

*Higher risk of dependence and withdrawal symptoms.

Cog = cognition; S = sedation; A = agitation or mania; Motor = discoordination; D = dysphagia; Com = communication; F = falls; GAD = generalized anxiety disorder; OCD = obsessive–compulsive disorder; PTSD = posttraumatic stress disorder.

The likelihood rating scale for encountering the side effects is as follows: 0 = Almost no probability of encountering side effects. 0/+ = Low probability of encountering side effects but increased with use of higher doses. + = Little likelihood of encountering side effects. +/++ = Low probability of encountering side effects; however, probability increases with increased dosage. ++ = Medium likelihood of encountering side effects. +++ = High likelihood of encountering side effects, particularly with high doses. ++++ = Highest likelihood of encountering side effects; best to avoid in at-risk patients.

Weight is associated with weight gain and increased cardiovascular risk. Sexual is associated with sexual side effects.

summarizes medications used to treat anxiety disorders.

Benzodiazepines are the medications most frequently used to treat GAD and insomnia. These medications can have anxiolytic, muscle relaxant, anticonvulsant, hypnotic, and sedative effects on the patient. The prescribing physician chooses a benzodiazepine based on the medication's rate of absorption, onset of action, length of action, side effects, and drug interactions. The prescriber should initiate the benzodiazepine at a low dose and slowly titrate it up to an effective dose. Because these medications are metabolized by the liver, doses should be decreased in patients with liver disease. Prolonged treatment with benzodiazepines is associated with increased risk of accidents and psychomotor retardation, and cognitive decline and is not recommended (Baldessarini, 2001).

Buspirone (Buspar), a non-benzodiazepine antianxiety medication, functions as a partial agonist for serotonin receptors and provides antidepressant and anxiolytic effects. It also has weak actions on the dopamine receptors.

Because it does not affect the central nervous system neurotransmitter GABA, it causes minimal sedation. Side effects are also minimal and may include drowsiness, dry mouth, dizziness, fatigue, headache, and insomnia. It can be used in the long-term management of anxiety disorders and is not associated with the development of tolerance or addiction (Charney, 2001; Matthew & Hoffman, 2009; Saljoughian, 2006).

Benzodiazepines such as diazepam (Valium) are not beneficial in treating PTSD and may actually worsen symptoms of depression. Antidepressants are commonly used to treat PTSD. The antidepressants most often used include SSRIs and the selective serotonin and norepinephrine reuptake inhibitors (SSNRIs) venlafaxine (Effexor) and nefazodone (Serzone). Although nefazodone effectively reduces nightmares associated with PTSD, it is used less often because hepatotoxicity is associated with its use. It may take 4 to 6 wk to see the onset of effects of these antidepressants and up to 9 mo to see the full effects. The patient and family must understand this in order to ensure that the patient adheres to the medication and allows an adequate trial period (Chavez, 2006; Taylor & Cates, 2008). Adding a second-generation antipsychotic may be beneficial in patients with psychotic symptoms that are not responsive to antidepressant therapy. Prazosin (Minipress), an alpha-blocking agent that can reduce norepinephrine levels, has been shown to reduce nightmares in PTSD. In patients with concurrent bipolar disorder, adjunctive use of anticonvulsants has improved symptoms of intrusive thoughts, flashbacks, nightmares, and insomnia (Chavez, 2006; Taylor & Cates, 2008).

Side Effects of Medications

The side effects of benzodiazepines are related to the size of the dose. The most common side effects include sedation, dizziness, weakness, and unsteadiness. Less common side effects include fatigue, drowsiness, amnesia, memory impairment, confusion, disorientation, depression, unmasking of depression, disinhibition, euphoria, suicide ideation or attempt, ataxia, **asthenia**, extrapyramidal symptoms, seizures, tremor, vertigo, vision changes, slurred speech,

respiratory depression, apnea, worsening of sleep apnea, worsening of obstructive pulmonary disease, gastrointestinal symptoms (nausea, change in appetite, constipation), and changes in liver function. In patients with chronic obstructive pulmonary disease or dementia, anxiety should be treated with SSRI or buspirone (Buspar) to avoid the negative effects on respiratory function or cognitive awareness associated with benzodiazepines (Ayers et al., 2009). Abrupt discontinuance of benzodiazepines can result in symptoms of mild to moderate withdrawal, which include nightmares, restlessness, rebound anxiety, and insomnia. Symptoms of severe withdrawal include **psychosis**, seizures, and death (Preston et al., 2008).

Side effects of benzodiazepines that can affect participation in rehabilitation sessions include sedation, ataxia, slowed thought, balance problems, difficulty concentrating, reduced visual accommodation, weakness, and drowsiness. Incoordination and dysarthria may also be present. Balance assessments, balance training, and environmental modifications such as removing trip hazards are important measures for patients who are susceptible to falls. Benzodiazepines can cause dysphagia due to the side effects of motor incoordination, sedation, and diminished concentration and gastrointestinal side effects of heartburn, nausea, vomiting, diarrhea, constipation, gastrointestinal pain, anorexia, taste alterations, and dry mouth. Chronic benzodiazepine use can cause significant pharyngeal phase dysphagia, including cricopharyngeal incoordination, hypopharyngeal incoordination, and aspiration. Pharyngeal dysphagia may be diminished by ceasing use of the medication (Alvi, 1999; Carl & Johnson, 2006).

Drug Interactions

Adverse drug reactions associated with benzodiazepines are dose related and are potentiated when these medications are combined with other sedating medications. Use of other central nervous system depressants such as alcohol or even over-the-counter sedative products should be discouraged in patients taking benzodiazepines because the resulting significant increases in sedation and cognitive impairment can increase risk of falls, delirium, respiratory depression, immobility, confusion, incontinence, and coma. The prudent rehabilitation therapist will recognize these symptoms during treatment and immediately notify the prescriber if these symptoms worsen. Table 7.2 summarizes important drug interactions involving benzodiazepines (Cumming & Le

Table 7.2 Drug Interactions With Benzodiazepines and Resultant Effects

Interacting medication	Benzodiazepine medication	Effect on benzodiazepine
Alcohol		
Alcohol use	Chlordiazepoxide (Librium), diazepam (Valium)	Decreased clearance and increased effects
Alcohol treatment: disulfiram (Antabuse)	Chlordiazepoxide (Librium), diazepam (Valium)	Decreased clearance and increased effects
Antacids		
Cimetidine (Tagamet)	Alprazolam (Xanax), chlordiazepoxide (Librium), clorazepate (Tranxene), diazepam (Valium)	Decreased clearance and increased effects
Omeprazole (Prilosec)	Diazepam (Valium)	Decreased clearance and increased effects
Anti-infectives		
Itraconazole (Sporanox)	Alprazolam (Xanax), diazepam (Valium), triazolam (Halcion), zolpidem (Ambien), zaleplon (Sonata)	Decreased clearance and increased effects
Isoniazid (INH)	Diazepam (Valium)	Decreased clearance and increased effects
Ketoconazole (Nizoral)	Alprazolam (Xanax)	Decreased clearance and increased effects
Protease inhibitor: ritonavir (Norvir)	Alprazolam (Xanax), diazepam (Valium), triazolam (Halcion), zolpidem (Ambien), zaleplon (Sonata)	Decreased clearance and increased effects
Rifampin	Diazepam (Valium)	Increased clearance and decreased effects
Asthma medication		
Theophylline	Alprazolam (Xanax)	Decreased clearance and increased effects
Antidepressants		
Fluoxetine (Prozac)	Diazepam (Valium)	Decreased clearance and increased effects
Fluvoxamine (Luvox)	Alprazolam (Xanax)	Decreased clearance and increased effects
Nefazodone (Serzone)	Alprazolam (Xanax), diazepam (Valium), triazolam (Halcion), zolpidem (Ambien), zaleplon (Sonata)	Decreased clearance, doubled drug levels, increased effects
Cardiac medication		
Diltiazem (Cardizem)	Alprazolam (Xanax), diazepam (Valium), triazolam (Halcion), zolpidem (Ambien), zaleplon (Sonata)	Decreased clearance and increased effects
Oral contraceptives		
Oral contraceptives	Alprazolam (Xanax), chlordiazepoxide (Librium), diazepam (Valium)	Decreased clearance and increased effects

Couteur, 2003; Iverson et al., 2009; Jacobson et al., 2007; Matthew & Hoffman, 2009).

PATIENT CASE 1

M.Z. is an 88-yr-old female who is seeing a rehabilitation therapist for strength training and assistance with ambulation after recently being hospitalized with pneumonia. M.Z. recently lost her spouse of 50 yr and has been having symptoms of anxiety and insomnia. Her physician prescribed diazepam (Valium) 5 mg 3 times/day for her anxiety and flurazepam (Dalmane) 15 mg at bedtime for insomnia. During her rehabilitation session, M.Z. complains that she is always tired and is having difficulty walking. She also states that she has no appetite, that her mouth is dry all the time, and that she occasionally feels like she is choking when she attempts to eat. She is afraid to drive home feeling the way she does.

Question
Could M.Z.'s symptoms be related to one of her new medications?

Answer
After reviewing the profiles of both Valium and Dalmane, the therapist concludes that M.Z.'s symptoms could be related to her new medications. Both Valium and Dalmane have long half-lives and are converted in the body to metabolites that also cause sedation. Because of this, neither of these medications should be used in the elderly patient. The therapist explains M.Z.'s symptoms to her physician and recommends that the physician discontinue these medications and instead use shorter-acting medications that do not have active metabolites. A possible alternative regimen is temazepam (Restoril) 7.5 mg for sleep only if needed combined with buspirone (Buspar) 1 mg twice/day for anxiety symptoms if needed. The prescriber instructs M.Z. to discontinue her medications and makes an appointment to see her later that day. The therapist arranges for M.Z.'s neighbor to pick her up from her therapy session and to take her to see the physician.

Insomnia

Insomnia is defined as difficulty falling asleep (sleep latency), difficulty staying asleep, waking up too early, or not getting restful, restorative sleep. Acute insomnia, defined as insomnia that lasts up to a few weeks, is usually the result of emotional or physical stress. Chronic insomnia, defined as difficulty sleeping for at least 3 nights/wk for more than 1 mo, is often associated with medical or psychological disorders. Symptoms of insomnia include lack of energy, problems with memory or concentration, and sleepiness. Insomnia may also result in symptoms of headache, tachycardia, and nausea. Consequences of insomnia, which include reduced daytime functioning along with fatigue and a lack of concentration, can negatively affect the patient's ability to participate in rehabilitation activities (Dopheide & Kushida, 2005; Knudsen, 2008).

Incidence

Estimates of the incidence of insomnia vary due to differing definitions of insomnia. As a result, estimates of worldwide incidence vary from 10% to 40%. For example, insomnia may be defined as experiencing symptoms at least 3 nights/wk, as difficulty maintaining sleep, or as waking up repeatedly. In any case, insomnia is a major health issue worldwide (Mai & Buysse, 2008). Insomnia affects at least 50 million people, or one third of adults, in the United States. Ten percent of the population suffers from impaired daytime function due to insomnia. Insomnia occurs most frequently in women, especially during pregnancy and after menopause, and the elderly. Older people tend to nap during the day and frequently complain of waking earlier than planned (Dopheide & Kushida, 2005; Hulisz & Duff, 2009; Passarella & Duong, 2008; Sherwood & Rey, 2007).

Etiology and Pathophysiology

Sleep is regulated in the hypothalamus and pineal glands in the brain. Most adults need 7 to 8 h of sleep per night, but needs are individualized and can vary from 5 to 10 h. Sleep can be divided into two states: rapid eye movement (REM) and non-REM. Non-REM comprises four stages that progress toward REM sleep. Stage 1 is early sleep (alpha rhythm), which is the stage between wakefulness and sleep. Stage 2, which makes up the largest percentage of time asleep, is intermediate sleep. Stages 3 and 4 are deep sleep (delta rhythm); these are the restorative stages of sleep. REM sleep comes after stages 1 through 4 of non-REM sleep. In the REM stage, rapid eye movements and variations in blood pressure, heart rate, and respiratory rate occur. During this stage dreams can be recalled upon waking. REM sleep is vital for consolidating memory and sustaining life. A complete sleep cycle lasts for 1.5 to 2 h and repeats 4 to 5 times each night. The amount of time spent in stage 2 and REM sleep increases with each sequential sleep cycle. As people get older, it takes longer to fall asleep, more sleep time is spent in stage 1 (early-stage sleep), and less time is spent in stages 3 and 4 (deep or delta-wave sleep) (Charney, 2001; Knudsen, 2008).

Medications, medical conditions, and dietary intake of caffeine can cause insomnia. The prescriber should identify and address these factors before treating a patient's insomnia with medications. Medical conditions that can contribute to insomnia include depression, anxiety, asthma, bipolar disorder, chronic pain, chronic obstructive pulmonary disease, gastroesophageal reflux disease, congestive heart failure, thyroid disease, pain, sleep apnea, snoring, multiple sclerosis, incontinence, neurological problems such as restless-leg syndrome, and withdrawal from alcohol, pain medications, or sedatives. Medications that can cause insomnia include alcohol, antihypertensives such as alpha agonists and beta blockers, atomoxetine, bitter orange, caffeine, diuretics, cocaine, dopamine agonists used to treat Parkinson's disease, ginseng, guarana, lipid-lowering agents, modafinil, nicotine, oral contraceptives, respiratory medications such as beta agonists or theophylline, thyroid supplements, SSRI antidepressants, steroids, stimulants, and sympathomimetics found in diet aids or decongestants (Baldessarini, 2001; Carl & Johnson, 2006; Dopheide & Kushida, 2005; Hulisz & Duff, 2009; Jarvis et al., 2008; Passarella & Duong, 2008; Sherwood & Rey, 2007).

Rehabilitation Considerations

Cognitive–behavioral therapy can be helpful in managing insomnia. Such therapy includes stimulus-control therapy, promoting good sleep hygiene, sleep-restriction therapy, and employing relaxation techniques such as yoga, music, or meditation. Stimulus-control therapy helps the patient associate the bedroom with sleep. Patients are instructed to go to bed only when tired and to use the bedroom only for sleeping or intimacy (not for watching television or reading). The patient should be educated on methods for improving sleep hygiene before starting medications to treat insomnia. These instructions should include the following for improving sleep: Avoid daytime naps, create a comfortable sleep environment (e.g., eliminate noise and light, set a comfortable temperature), take medications that cause insomnia in the morning, avoid heavy meals and limit fluid intake before bedtime, and avoid the use of caffeine, nicotine, and alcohol just before going to bed. Regular exercise can help reduce insomnia, but patients should avoid exercise or other stressful activities just before bedtime. Setting a regular time to go to sleep and wake up is also important in promoting good sleep habits. Finally, sleep-restriction therapy is a behavioral therapy that may help promote sleep efficiency by temporarily inducing sleep deprivation (Hulisz & Duff, 2009; Jarvis et al., 2008; Passarella & Duong, 2008; Sherwood & Rey, 2007).

The use of antihistamines, sedatives, and hypnotics to treat insomnia can affect a patient's progress in rehabilitation. These agents can place the patient at risk for aspiration and falls and can impair cognition and communication, which can potentially reduce rehabilitation success. When engaging the patient in rehabilitation exercises and functional training, the rehabilitation therapist should be aware of the medications the patient is using (Ciccone, 2007). The therapist must be certain that the patient is able to demonstrate the steps and sequences involved in performing safe transfers and maintaining a safe gait. For example, it is not uncommon for a patient with memory difficulties to forget to lock the wheels on the wheelchair before attempting to go from sitting to standing. It is also likely that the therapist needs to closely monitor the patient's compliance with home exercises and minimize complex or confusing instructions. It is important to educate caregivers on methods of verbal cueing and other strategies in order to maintain patient safety while participating in therapeutic activities and in activities of daily living (Passarella & Duong, 2008).

Medication Therapy

Benzodiazepines and benzodiazepine agonists are the medications most commonly prescribed to treat insomnia. Benzodiazepine hypnotics induce sleep by binding to the GABA receptors on postsynaptic neurons in the central nervous system and inhibiting neuronal excitation by increasing neuronal chloride permeability. Benzodiazepines shorten the onset of sleep but increase stage 2 sleep and increase REM latency. Adverse effects include dizziness and impaired memory. Medications used to treat insomnia can also have residual effects the next day, called hangover effects, which can impair cognition and communication, result in ataxia and discoordination, and significantly affect the patient's ability to participate in the rehabilitation session. The hangover effect is more pronounced in agents with a long half-life. Short-acting benzodiazepines can cause anterograde amnesia. Abrupt discontinuance of benzodiazepines and other medications used to treat insomnia can cause withdrawal symptoms of anxiety, rebound insomnia, tachycardia, and diarrhea. Table 7.3 summarizes medications used to treat insomnia (Charney, 2001; Curtis & Jermain, 2002; Knudsen, 2008; Passarella & Duong, 2008).

 See table 7.3 in the web resource for a full list of medication-specific dosing recommendations, time to onset, half-life, duration, and drug interactions.

Table 7.3　Medications Used to Treat Insomnia

Medication	Duration	Drug interactions or comments
Benzodiazepines		
Clorazepate (Tranxene) Triazolam (Halcion)	Short	CYP3A4 inhibitors such as ketoconazole (Nizoral), clarithromycin (Biaxin), itraconazole (Sporanox), nefazodone (Serzone), ritonavir (Norvir), and nelfinavir (Viracept) increase triazolam (Halcion) levels.
		CYP3A4 inducers (rifampicin) decrease triazolam (Halcion) levels.
Estazolam (Prosom) Temazepam (Restoril)	Intermediate	CYP3A4 inhibitors such as ketoconazole (Nizoral), clarithromycin (Biaxin), itraconazole (Sporanox), nefazodone (Serzone), ritonavir (Norvir), and nelfinavir (Viracept) increase estazolam (Prosom) levels.
Flurazepam (Dalmane) Quazepam (Doral)	Long	CYP2B6 inhibitors (orphenadrine) increase quazepam (Doral) levels and effects.
		Avoid both of these sleep agents in the elderly.
Nonbenzodiazepines		
Zaleplon (Sonata)	Ultrashort	CYP3A4 inhibitors such as ketoconazole (Nizoral), clarithromycin (Biaxin), itraconazole (Sporanox), nefazodone (Serzone), ritonavir (Norvir), and nelfinavir (Viracept) increase zaleplon (Sonata) levels.
		CYP3A4 inducers (rifampicin) decrease zaleplon (Sonata) levels.
Eszopiclone (Lunesta) Zolpidem (Ambien; Ambien CR)	Intermediate	CYP3A4 inhibitors such as ketoconazole (Nizoral), clarithromycin (Biaxin), itraconazole (Sporanox), nefazodone (Serzone), ritonavir (Norvir), and nelfinavir (Viracept) increase zolpidem (Ambien) and eszopiclone (Lunesta) levels.
		CYP3A4 inducers (rifampicin) decrease zolpidem (Ambien) and eszopiclone (Lunesta) levels.

Medication	Duration	Drug interactions or comments
Melatonin agonist		
Ramelteon (Rozerem)	Short	CYP3A4 inhibitors such as ketoconazole (Nizoral), clarithromycin (Biaxin), itraconazole (Sporanox), nefazodone (Serzone), ritonavir (Norvir), and nelfinavir (Viracept) increase ramelteon (Rozerem) levels.
		CYP3A4 inducers (rifampicin) decrease ramelteon (Rozerem) levels.
		CYP2C9 inhibitors such as fluconazole (Diflucan), miconazole, and valproic acid (Depakote) and CYP1A2 inhibitors such as fluoroquinolones, fluvoxamine (Luvox), and verapamil (Isoptin) increase ramelteon (Rozerem) levels.
First-generation antihistamines		
Diphenhydramine (Benadryl) Doxylamine (Unisom)	Long	Avoid use of both in elderly due to altered cognition and fall risk.
Herbals		
Valerian	Short	Avoid with other sedatives.
		Paradoxical stimulation can occur with long-term use.
		Binds with gamma amino butyric acid receptors; may be associated with hepatotoxicity.
Chamomile tea	Short	Avoid in ragweed allergy.
		May increase anticoagulant effects of warfarin (Coumadin).
		Avoid using with other sedatives.
Melatonin	Short	Take sustained-release product 1-2 h before bedtime.
		May alter menstrual cycle.
		May increase anticoagulant effect of warfarin (Coumadin).
Treatment of nightmares and insomnia associated with posttraumatic stress disorder		
Prazosin (Minipress)	Intermediate	Avoid taking with other medications that can decrease blood pressure.

The benzodiazepines triazolam (Halcion) and temazepam (Restoril) have short half-lives. Tolerance to these agents may occur quickly, increasing the risk of rebound insomnia. The hypnotic medication flurazepam (Dalmane) has a long half-life of 2 to 3 h and active metabolites that extend its overall half-life to 47 to 100 h. Quazepam (Doral) also has a prolonged half-life associated with the parent drug (25 h) and active metabolites that extend its overall half-life to 84 h. Such a prolonged half-life can result in prolonged sedation, impaired cognition, and decline in quality of life and can impair the patient's ability to complete functions of daily life. These products can contribute to significant dysphagia (Campbell-Taylor, 1996, 2001). Prolonged use of benzodiazepines can result in significant esophageal dysphagia (Carl & Johnson, 2006) and can increase the risk of falls. Therefore, use of benzodiazepines in the elderly patient is not recommended. These medications appear on the Beer's list, which lists medications that should not be used in the elderly patient due to increased risk of adverse effects (Baldessarini, 2001; Carl & Johnson, 2006; Charney, 2001; Curtis & Jermain, 2002; Iverson et al., 2009; Knudsen, 2008).

Benzodiazepine receptor agonists such as zolpidem (Ambien), zaleplon (Sonata), and eszopiclone (Lunesta) also promote sleep by promoting the binding of the central neurotransmitter GABA on the GABA receptors, thus inhibiting neuronal excitability through increased chloride permeability. These agents cause less rebound insomnia and less hangover effect than do the benzodiazepines. Zolpidem (Ambien) does not affect the normal sleep cycle but is associated with sleepwalking and sleep-related eating disorders. Zolpidem (Ambien) and eszopiclone (Lunesta) have a rapid onset and improve both sleep latency and sleep maintenance. Eszopiclone (Lunesta) is associated with an unpleasant taste and can cause headache and dry mouth. Zaleplon (Sonata) has a rapid onset and duration of action. It improves sleep latency without causing hangover effects and can be taken any time up until 4 h before wake time. Patients should take these products on an empty stomach to avoid delays in onset of absorption and effects (Baldessarini, 2001; Carl & Johnson, 2006; Halas, 2006; Passarella & Duong, 2008).

Ramelteon (Rozerem) is a melatonin receptor agonist, which is a new classification of medications used to treat insomnia. Rozerem targets the melatonin receptors MT1 and MT2, located on the hypothalamus, that are believed to be involved in the sleep–wake cycle. This product does not affect GABA receptors and, unlike benzodiazepines and benzodiazepine receptor agonists, is not a controlled substance. The recommended dose is 8 mg 30 min before bedtime; no dosage reduction is required for the elderly patient. Because ramelteon (Rozerem) is metabolized by the CYP1A2 enzymes of the liver, it should be used with caution in patients with liver impairment. This product reduces sleep latency and increases the duration of sleep. Side effects include somnolence, fatigue, and dizziness. It is not associated with rebound insomnia. High-fat meals can delay absorption and onset (Charney, 2001; Curtis & Jermain, 2002; Iverson et al., 2009; Knudsen, 2008; Passarella & Duong, 2008).

PATIENT CASE 2

E.D. is a 79-yr-old woman who is referred for rehabilitation therapy after a recent hospitalization stay that was complicated by ventilator-associated pneumonia and respiratory failure. She has a history of Type 2 diabetes, hypertension, and emphysema. She is very weak after the long hospitaliza-tion and is referred for strengthening exercises and gait training. She appears tired, has difficulty understanding instructions, and fatigues very quickly in her first session. The rehabilitation specialist learns that she has not slept well since her discharge from the hospital. E.D. asks if there are any sleeping medications that are not addictive that she could ask her physician to prescribe.

Question
How should the therapist respond to E.D.'s inquiry?

Answer
The therapist should provide education to E.D. on maintaining appropriate sleep hygiene with non-pharmacologic interventions. Such interventions include going to bed only when tired and using the bedroom only for sleeping or intimacy (not for watching television or reading). Steps for improving sleep include avoiding daytime naps, creating a comfortable sleep environment (e.g., eliminating noise and light, setting a comfortable temperature), taking medications that cause insomnia in the morning, avoiding heavy meals and limiting fluid intake before bedtime, and avoiding use of caffeine, nicotine, and alcohol just before going to bed. Regular exercise can help reduce insomnia, but patients should avoid exercise or other stressful activities just before bedtime. Setting a regular time to go to sleep and wake up is also important in promoting good sleep habits. Most prescription medications used to treat insomnia are benzodiazepines or related agents that work at the benzodiazepine receptor, and their long-term use can result in dependence. However, a newer prescription medication called Rozerem works at the melatonin receptor and does not result in dependence. Rozerem targets the melatonin receptors MT1 and MT2, located on the hypothalamus, which are believed to be involved in the sleep–wake cycle. In addition, herbal tea, such as chamomile tea, and over-the-counter melatonin may be tried prior to starting a prescription medication.

Antihistamines

Patients frequently use over-the-counter antihistamines when self-medicating for symptoms of insomnia. Diphenhydramine (Benadryl) or doxylamine (Unisom) is often the major components in over-the-counter sleep aids. These agents have a pronounced and prolonged sedative effect that results from strong binding to the muscarinic acetylcholine receptors and the histamine-1 receptors. Patients with glaucoma should not use these agents. When used at night, these agents are associated with the hangover effect of sedation the next morning. Other anticholinergic effects include dizziness, dry mouth, and constipation. These products can contribute to significant dysphagia (Campbell-Taylor, 1996, 2001). Because the elderly are significantly more susceptible to the sedating effects of first-generation antihistamines, use of these agents in the elderly is not recommended. Diphenhydramine is included on the Beer's list (Asperheim, 2002; Charney, 2001; Cumming & Le Couteur, 2003; Curtis & Jermain, 2002; Garuti et al., 2003; Knudsen, 2008; Peel & Mossberg, 1995).

Herbal Products

Valerian, an herbal product that interacts with GABA receptors, has been used for insomnia. Side effects include dizziness, nausea, headache, and gastrointestinal distress. Melatonin, an over-the-counter herbal that affects the melatonin receptors, is also used to treat insomnia. Side effects associated with melatonin use include headache, nausea, depression, nightmares and vivid dreams, irritability, abdominal cramps, and dizziness. It also may worsen depression and decrease sex drive (Cumming & Le Couteur, 2003; Garuti et al., 2003; Knudsen, 2008).

Summary

This chapter summarizes the incidence, symptoms, and pathophysiology associated with anxiety disorders and insomnia and reviews the medications used to treat these disorders. Treatment of anxiety disorders can include medication, behavioral therapy, cognitive therapy, or lifestyle changes such as improved diet, reduced intake of stimulants such as caffeine and nicotine, regular exercise, relaxation techniques, and improved sleep. Relaxation techniques, stress-reduction techniques, and massage techniques can be helpful in decreasing anxiety. Herbal and aroma therapies have also been used (Carl & Johnson, 2006; Kirkwood & Melton, 2002; Saljoughian, 2006).

At the beginning of each rehabilitation session, the therapist should ask the patient about any changes in medication use. Changes may necessitate appropriate interventions such as education, altering the structure of the rehabilitation session, or even contacting the patient's prescriber (Cumming & Le Couteur, 2003; Garuti et al., 2003; Knudsen, 2008; Peel & Mossberg, 1995).The rehabilitation therapist should be aware that potential side effects of medications used in treatment of anxiety and insomnia include drowsiness, ataxia, and decreased excitability of skeletal muscle and that these effects can negatively influence the patient's rehabilitation process and activities of daily living (Asperheim, 2002). Collectively, these potential side effects can increase the risk for falls. The clinician should assess the patient's balance, muscle strength, and gait to determine whether any changes in psychomotor performance are evident. In addition, changes in weight or mentation may indicate dysphagia or withdrawal symptoms associated with abrupt discontinuance of benzodiazepines.

Patients should avoid long-term use of sedatives and most antianxiety medications because of these adverse effects and the potential for dependence. Rehabilitation therapists should educate patients and caregivers about the use of cognitive and behavioral therapies to assist in the treatment of these anxiety and sleep disorders, and other therapies such as biofeedback and stress reduction should be initiated in rehabilitation (Ciccone, 2007). Deep-breathing exercises, positive imagery, regular physical activity, calming music, therapeutic massage, and good sleep hygiene should be implemented to assist the patient with symptoms of insomnia (Cumming & Le Couteur, 2003; Garuti et al., 2003; Knudsen, 2008; Peel & Mossberg, 1995).

PART III

Medications Used to Treat Neurologic and Movement Disorders

The chapters in part III deal with neurologic and movement disorders. Topics discussed in this section include seizure disorders, spasticity and muscle spasm, Parkinson's disease, and movement disorders associated with skeletal muscle disease and demyelinating neuromuscular disease.

Chapter 8 introduces the types of seizure disorders and explains how seizures are classified based on etiology, pathophysiology, and signs and symptoms. Prognosis, associated cognitive impairment and learning disabilities, and ease of controlling and preventing seizures vary widely among different types of seizures. Many new medications have been introduced and are now used to treat seizures. This chapter outlines recommended treatments based on type of seizure as well as the effects of medication use on cognitive function, muscle function, and nutritional status. The chapter also discusses side effects that can affect rehabilitation and important drug interactions associated with seizure medications. The rehabilitation therapist should especially be aware of side effects associated with a life-threatening rash that can progress to Stevens-Johnson syndrome

and liver failure. Finally, this chapter discusses methods for reducing a patient's seizure risk during the therapy session and recommended measures the rehabilitation therapist should take if a patient experiences a seizure during a therapy session.

Chapter 9 differentiates symptoms associated with spasticity from those seen with muscle spasm. Presence of spasticity or muscle spasm can significantly interfere with a patient's ability to complete activities of daily living, and the severity of these symptoms varies with acute illness or injury. Spasticity can be associated with many chronic diseases such as cerebral palsy. This chapter reviews medications and nonpharmacologic interventions that are used to manage spasticity. Muscle spasm often follows acute injury; this chapter also reviews common medication combinations and nonpharmacologic treatments used to manage pain and spasm associated with injury.

Chapter 10 discusses Parkinson's disease and related treatments of the motor symptoms of the disease. It also reviews recommended therapies for managing nonmotor symptoms such as Parkinson's-associated dementia, orthostatic hypotension, urinary retention, gastrointestinal side effects, dysphagia, disorders of speech and voice, and psychiatric symptoms such as depression, psychosis, agitation, and insomnia.

Chapter 11 discusses amyotrophic lateral sclerosis, multiple sclerosis, and myasthenia gravis and the recommended medication and nonpharmacologic therapies used to manage these conditions. Amyotrophic lateral sclerosis, also known as Lou Gehrig's disease, is an adult-onset, idiopathic, progressive disease that involves degeneration of anterior horn cells and upper and lower motor neurons, leading to progressive muscle weakness and fasciculations. Multiple sclerosis is a chronic autoimmune disease of the central nervous system characterized by inflammation, demyelination, and axonal injury. Impaired axonal transmission affects the brain, spinal cord, and optic nerves. Multiple sclerosis includes exacerbations of muscle weakness, imbalance, incoordination, spasticity, fatigue, bladder and bowel difficulties, vision loss, altered sensory patterns (hyperesthesia), cognition impairment, and neuropathic pain. Myasthenia gravis is a relatively rare autoimmune disorder affecting the skeletal muscles that is characterized by weakness and fatigue that are relieved by periods of rest. The disorder typically follows a slow, progressive course that is characterized by periods of remission and **exacerbation**.

Chapter 12 reviews additional clinical conditions that result in disorders of movement, including essential tremor, subcortical dementias (including dementias accompanied by motor symptoms), Huntington's disease, Wilson's disease, and restless-leg syndrome. This chapter discusses medications used to treat movement disorders and provides methods for optimizing therapy sessions and improving patient outcomes while providing rehabilitation therapy. The chapter also provides a good review of medication-induced movement disorders and guidance on how to prevent these disorders and how to treat them once they occur.

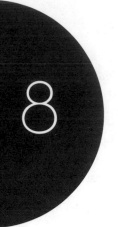

Medications Used to Treat Seizure Disorders

In clinical practice, the rehabilitation specialist will care for patients with **seizure** disorders. This chapter introduces the pathophysiology and etiology of seizure disorders (seizures, convulsions, and epilepsy), discusses medications used to treat seizures, and reviews methods for reducing risk of seizure during the rehabilitation session. It also reviews the appropriate action the rehabilitation specialist should take if a patient experiences a seizure during a therapy session.

Classification of Seizures

The International Classification of Epileptic Seizures classifies the four major types of seizures—partial, generalized, unclassified, and status epilepticus—and their subtypes. The seizures are organized based on whether the source of the seizure is localized (partial or focal) or distributed (generalized). Partial seizures are subdivided based on the extent of the victim's consciousness. If the seizure does not affect the victim's consciousness, it is called a simple partial seizure. If it does, it is called a complex partial (psychomotor) seizure. All generalized seizures involve a loss of consciousness and are labeled according to the effect on the victim's body. These include absence (petit mal), myoclonic, clonic, tonic–clonic (grand mal), **tonic**, and **atonic** seizures (Guthrie, 2006; Iversen et al., 2009; Pesaturo et al., 2011; Wolff & Graves, 2006).

Common epileptic syndromes in children include **febrile** seizures, neonatal seizures, infantile spasms, **Lennox-Gastaut syndrome**, and childhood and adolescent absence epilepsy. Table 8.1 summarizes classifications of seizures and associated treatments (Guthrie, 2006; Iversen et al., 2009; Pesaturo et al., 2011; Wolff & Graves, 2006).

Seizures, Convulsions, and Epilepsy

Seizures are specific events caused by sudden, abnormal, and excessive electrical discharge in the brain. Convulsions, which may or may not occur with seizures, are violent, involuntary contractions of the voluntary muscles. Epilepsy is defined as the occurrence of two or more unprovoked, recurrent seizures (Guthrie, 2006; Iversen et al., 2009; Pesaturo et al., 2011).

Incidence

Worldwide incidence of epilepsy varies depending on whether the episode is characterized as acute symptomatic or unprovoked. The incidence of acute symptomatic episodes, which tend to occur more often in men than in women, is 29 to 39 per 100,000 people per year. Cardiovascular disease, traumatic brain injury, infarct, drug withdrawal, and metabolic insults are the most common causes of acute symptomatic episodes. The incidence of single unprovoked seizures is 23 to 61 per 100,000 person years. Single unprovoked seizures are more common in males than in females and

Table 8.1   Classification of Seizures and Treatments

Classification	Symptoms	Medication therapies
Type I: Partial seizures. Focal seizures that originate in one hemisphere and involve asymmetric symptoms; 60% of new seizures are partial seizures.		
Simple	No impairment of consciousness. Can involve motor symptoms, special **somatosensory** symptoms, or psychic symptoms.	Phenobarbital, primidone (Mysoline), gabapentin (Neurontin), lamotrigine (Lamictal), topiramate (Topamax), tiagabine (Gabitril), oxcarbazepine (Trileptal), levetiracetam (Keppra), zonisamide (Zonegran), felbamate (Felbatol)
Complex	40% of seizures. Preceded by an aura and followed by alterations in behavior. Can involve seemingly purposeful behavior such as speech or walking. Followed by **postictal** confusion and no recollection of what happened.	Phenytoin (Dilantin), fosphenytoin (Cerebyx), phenobarbital, carbamazepine (Tegretol), valproic acid (Depakene), gabapentin (Neurontin), lamotrigine (Lamictal), topiramate (Topamax), tiagabine (Gabitril), oxcarbazepine (Trileptal), levetiracetam (Keppra), zonisamide (Zonegran), felbamate (Felbatol)
Type II: Generalized seizures. Nonfocal; can involve bilateral, symmetrical symptoms accompanied by a loss of consciousness.		
Absence	Sudden lapse of consciousness accompanied by minor jerking, abnormal motor movements, lip smacking, and a blank stare	Lamotrigine (Lamictal), ethosuximide (Zarontin), valproic acid (Depakene), levetiracetam (Keppra)
Myoclonic	Shock-like muscle contractions	Clonazepam (Klonopin), lamotrigine (Lamictal), levetiracetam (Keppra), topiramate (Topamax), valproic acid (Depakene), zonisamide, (Zonegran)
Clonic	Rigidity of muscles	Levetiracetam (Keppra)
Tonic	Muscle contraction	Topiramate (Topamax), levetiracetam (Keppra)
Tonic–clonic (classic grand mal)	Loss of consciousness, violent convulsions of the trunk and extremities, increased salivation, loss of bladder and bowel control, and a period of postictal confusion	Topiramate (Topamax), lamotrigine (Lamictal), phenytoin (Dilantin), fosphenytoin (Cerebyx), phenobarbital, valproic acid (Depakene), carbamazepine (Tegretol), gabapentin (Neurontin), levetiracetam (Keppra)
Atonic	Sudden loss of muscle tone	Levetiracetam (Keppra)
Infantile spasms	Sudden stiffening of the body, typically after waking	Levetiracetam (Keppra)
Type III: Unclassified seizures. Seen primarily in infants; are not well characterized.		
Type IV: Status epilepticus (usually tonic–clonic) seizures		
Status epilepticus	Last >30 min; a medical emergency. Caused by tumor, infection of the central nervous system, drug abuse, or febrile seizures.	Diazepam (Valium), lorazepam (Ativan), phenytoin (Dilantin), fosphenytoin (Cerebyx)

are seen mostly in individuals younger than 12 mo of age or older than 65 yr. The standardized mortality ratios (SMR) for single unprovoked seizures is 2.5 to 4.1. Mortality is highest in infants and patients with symptomatic seizures (Hauser & Beghi, 2008).

Epilepsy affects 2% of the US population, or more than 3 million Americans. Seventy five percent of epilepsy cases are classified as primary, and the remaining cases result from another disorder of the central nervous system (CNS). Among all ages, the most common risk factors for epilepsy include CNS infection, stroke, and head trauma. Epilepsy is the third most common serious neurological disease in the elderly; dementia and stroke are the most and second most common, respectively. Ten percent of stroke patients experience a seizure within the first 24 to 48 h after the stroke occurs, but only a small percentage develop epilepsy. Current data indicate that 77 out of 100,000 seniors have epilepsy, and incidence increases to 159 out of 100,000 in patients over 80 yr of age. The three most common causes of seizures in seniors are medication or alcohol withdrawal, stroke, and electrolyte disorders (French et al., 2004; Talati et al., 2009; Zagaria, 2008).

Each year 150,000 pediatric patients experience a seizure for the first time, and 30,000 are diagnosed with epilepsy. Four to ten percent of children have recurrent seizures by 18 yr of age. Most seizures in children are attributable to high fever, infection, syncope, head trauma, hypoxia, toxins, and cardiac arrhythmias. Fever is the most common cause of seizures in children between the ages of 6 mo and 5 yr. These episodes typically occur within the first 24 h of a fever. Seizures from infancy to early school age are also commonly caused by CNS infections, electrolyte or metabolic disorders, toxic ingestions, and CNS tumors. Adolescents experience first-time seizures associated with ingestion of toxic substances, use of illicit drugs or alcohol, brain tumors, and excessive use of video games (Goodman et al., 2003; Guthrie, 2006).

Etiology and Pathophysiology

The nerve cells in the brain transmit impulses using CNS neurotransmitters released into the synapse by the ion transport systems. Normal neurotransmitter release and activity requires adequate oxygen, glucose, amino acids, and the ions sodium, potassium, chloride, and calcium. CNS neurotransmitters that enhance excitability and propagation of neuronal activity include glutamate, aspartate, acetylcholine, norepinephrine, purines, peptides, cytokines, and steroid hormones. Those that inhibit central nerve transmission include gamma amino butyric acid (GABA) and dopamine. Seizures are associated with changes in electrical discharge in the brain that result in neuronal membrane instability. This instability can be caused by abnormalities of potassium conduc-

tance, defects in voltage-sensitive ion channels, and deficiencies in enzymes called ATP-ases that are linked to ion transport through membranes (Gidal et al., 2002; McNamara, 2001; Rogers & Cavezos, 2011; Welty, 2002).

Medical conditions that can cause seizures include hypoxia, brain injury, alcohol intoxication and withdrawal, brain tumors, endocrine disorders, head trauma, intracranial masses, CNS infections, stroke, ingestion of toxic substances or poisons, liver failure, renal failure, hypoglycemia, electrolyte disorders, fever, heat stroke, Alzheimer's disease, degenerative brain disorders, and pneumonia. Patients who are malnourished due to alcoholism, cognitive disorders, or cancer are at increased risk for electrolyte disorders that can cause seizures (Goodman et al., 2003; Weinberg, 2008).

Seizures can also occur as a result of medications. The medications most commonly associated with seizures include bronchodilators such as the beta agonists and theophylline, insulin, isoniazid, and lidocaine. Many antipsychotics and antidepressants can also cause seizures. The pain medications tramadol (Ultram) and meperidine (Demerol) carry higher risk of seizures. Finally, medications that cause electrolyte disorders (e.g., diuretics, aminoglycoside antibiotics, steroids, amphotericin B, and many chemotherapy agents) can also cause seizures (Carl & Johnson, 2006; Zagaria, 2008).

Rehabilitation Considerations

Patients with epilepsy can have decreased attention, reduced concentration, and increased distractibility. Patients may have difficulty dividing attention among several stimuli and difficulty sustaining attention for a period of time. Anticonvulsants can worsen these effects. Attention deficits complicate rehabilitation instruction because the patient may be so distractible that they have difficulty paying attention to instructions (Motamedi & Meader, 2008). In these instances the therapist can use procedural learning methods that emphasize performing many repetitions of step-by-step tasks until the tasks become automatic. The therapist should then progress the procedural learning methods to the point of introducing new variables to the task or environment so that the patient is able to execute the task under more than one set of constraints. The therapist should also initially focus on eliminating distractions in the treatment area and establishing the patient's attention before the initiation of the task. The use of eye contact, tactile cues, and verbal cues can help focus the patient's attention on a specific psychomotor task (Ciccone, 2007; Goodman et al., 2003; Schachter et al., 2008; Vingerhoets, 2008).

The patient may experience decreased sensory memory as a result of attention difficulties. Sensory memory difficulties can affect both short-term and long-term memory performance as well as processing speed. The patient also may not be able to make the necessary psychomotor adjustments to environmental variables. For example, the patient may have trouble ambulating through a doorway without hitting the doorjamb. In this instance, the patient has the psychomotor ability to perform the task but requires strategies for increasing focus on the primary task. A brief pause as the patient approaches the doorway followed by verbal cueing may be sufficient to allow the patient to successfully cross the doorway without bumping into the doorjamb. If verbal cueing is insufficient, the use of tactile cueing may help promote a higher degree of focus. Finally, the therapist must keep rehabilitation activities interesting and functional in nature. A patient who has a high degree of interest in the task at hand typically demonstrates better focus, concentration, and overall attention to the task.

Memory is usually associated with the temporal and frontal lobes. Patients with medial temporal lobe epilepsy have memory difficulties. Left temporal lobe epilepsy is associated with deficits with verbal memory. Reduced learning of word lists and stories is associated with temporal lobe epilepsy (Ciccone, 2007; Goodman et al., 2003; Schachter et al., 2008; Vingerhoets, 2008).

The patient may also be sensitive to light, sound, or time of day and may react when placed in a busy rehabilitation environment. Rescheduling therapy at a time of day when these problems are minimized can be helpful. When a patient experiences seizure activity the same time each day, the timing of the seizures may be related to the dosage schedule of the medication or a recurrent external stimulus that is present at that time of day. Some factors that may trigger a seizure are stress, poor nutrition, missed medication, skipping meals, flickering lights, illness, fever, allergies, lack of sleep, heat with humidity, and emotions such as anger, worry, and fear. Many individuals with epilepsy experience a higher frequency of seizures when they take large doses of caffeine (Ciccone, 2007; Goodman et al., 2003).

Medication Therapy

Anticonvulsant medications increase the threshold of central neuronal stimulation, thus decreasing neuronal firing and associated seizures. They reduce neuronal stimulation by increasing the effects of the inhibitory central neurotransmitter GABA, decreasing the excitatory effects of glutamate or aspartate, or decreasing sodium and calcium channel transport at the cell membrane site of the neuron. The mesial–temporal structures of the brain may learn to potentiate and generate seizure activity independent of the epileptogenic focus in a process called kindling. Anticonvulsants are used to reduce kindling in seizure disorders; they are also used to reduce frequency of mood cycling in bipolar disorder (Carl & Johnson, 2006; Farooq et al., 2009; Gidal et al., 2002; McNamara, 2001; Rogers & Cavezos, 2011; Welty, 2002).

Medications used for epilepsy can be traced back to the middle of the 19th century, when bromides were introduced. Phenobarbital was introduced in 1912 and became the medication of choice for many years. Phenytoin (Dilantin), which was used to manage primary tonic–clonic seizures and partial seizures, was introduced in 1938, and carbamazepine (Tegretol), which was used to treat partial seizures, was introduced in 1974. When ethosuximide (Zarontin) became available in 1960, it became the drug of choice for absence seizures. Diazepam (Valium), a benzodiazepine that was introduced in 1968, is still used to treat status epilepticus seizures. Valproic acid (Depakote) was introduced in 1978. In the 1990s several new medications were introduced, including topiramate (Topamax), lamotrigine

(Lamictal), zonisamide (Zonegran), levetiracetam (Keppra), gabapentin (Neurontin), tiagabine (Gabitril), and oxcarbazepine (Trileptal). Levetiracetam (Keppra) has a unique mechanism of action and is used in multiple seizure disorders, including generalized tonic–clonic, absence, myoclonic, Lennox-Gastaut syndrome, and refractory epilepsy in children and adults. It decreases the kindling effect by suppressing brain-derived neurotrophic factor and neuropeptides Y and increasing levels of hippocampal Y1 and Y5-like receptors. It is also used in psychiatric disorders such as generalized anxiety disorder, panic disorder, stress disorders, mood and bipolar disorders, autism, and Tourette's syndrome. Another newer agent, felbamate (Felbatol), carries a warning from the U.S. Food and Drug Administration (FDA) due to hepatotoxic effects and risk of aplastic anemia; it is now a second-line agent (Carl & Johnson, 2006; Farooq et al., 2009; Garnett, 2005; Magill-Lewis, 2006; Rogers & Cavezos, 2011).

A new agent called eslicarbazepine (Stedesa) is currently being studied for the adjunctive treatment of partial onset seizures and is pending FDA approval. It is chemically related to carbamazepine and oxcarbazepine and acts as a voltage-regulated sodium channel blocker that inhibits sodium channel release of neurotransmitter. It reduces seizure activity at a rate similar to that of carbamazepine or oxcarbazepine. It is dosed at 800 mg or 1200 mg once/day. It is metabolized in the liver and eliminated through the kidneys and has a half-life of 20 to 24 h; dosage should be reduced in patients with renal impairment. The most commonly encountered side effects include dizziness, somnolence, headache, nausea, diplopia, abnormal coordination, and vomiting. Most side effects occur early in therapy upon initiation or dose titration. Because eslicarbazepine can reduce the drug levels and effectiveness of oral contraceptives, patients should be counseled to use a second form of contraception while taking this agent (Talati et al., 2009).

Another antiepileptic agent approved in 2011 for adjunctive treatment of partial onset seizures is lacosamide (Vimpat). This agent, which is available in oral and intravenous (IV) formulations, is initiated at doses of 50 mg twice/day; dosage may be increased at weekly intervals by 100 mg/day to an effective dose of 200 to 400 mg/day. The maximum daily dose for patients with severe renal impairment (< 30 mls/min) is 300 mg/day. IV Vimpat should be diluted in IV saline or in IV 5% dextrose solution and administered over 30 to 60 min. Mixed solutions are stable in the refrigerator for 24 h. The most commonly encountered side effects include dizziness, diplopia, ataxia, vomiting, nausea, vertigo, and blurred vision. Other side effects reported include cardiac arrhythmia, syncope, suicidal or psychotic reactions, and allergic reactions. Other than a 20% increase in ethinyl estradiol in patients concurrently using oral contraceptives containing this medication, no significant drug interactions have been identified (Rogers & Cavezos, 2011).

Vigabatrin (Sabril) is another anticonvulsant that affects the GABA receptor and was approved in 2009 for the treatment of infantile spasms; it has been used in Europe for this indication since 1989. Adrenocorticotropic hormone has been the traditional agent of choice for the treatment of infantile spasms, but some of the new guidelines list Vigabatrin 100 to 150 mg/kg/day as an alternative first-line therapy in the treatment of infantile spasms associated with tuberous sclerosis. A major side effect associated with Vigabatrin is bilateral concentric visual defects; therefore, prescribers must participate in an FDA-required Risk Evaluation and Mitigation Strategy program that mandates ophthalmic examination every 3 mo and efficacy assessment every 2 to 4 wk. Common adverse effects identified in seven studies include drowsiness (15%-28%), behavioral problems such as irritability (18%-33%), and hypotonia (12%-33%). Another important consideration that requires further study is differences in cognitive development that occur when this agent is used versus when steroid therapy is used (Rogers & Cavezos, 2011; Pesaturo et al., 2011).

The prescribing physician chooses an anticonvulsant based on the patient's type of seizure, concurrent disease states, and potential side effects and potential drug interactions.

The physician should initiate therapy with a low dose and slowly titrate up until efficacy is achieved. To prevent breakthrough seizures when transitioning a patient from one anticonvulsant to another, the medications are cross-tapered: The new drug is titrated up slowly while the dose of the existing is slightly reduced. Once a therapeutic dose of the new drug is achieved, the older agent is tapered off. The goal is to control the seizures at the lowest possible dose. In many instances the medication selected is used to treat the seizure disorder as well as ameliorate a secondary diagnosis. Many newer anticonvulsants are now being used to treat pain disorders and as mood stabilizers in depression and bipolar illness. Table 8.1 summarizes the classifications of seizures and the anticonvulsants used for each seizure type. Table 8.2 summarizes dosing and side effects associated with each anticonvulsant (Carl & Johnson, 2006; Farooq et al., 2009; Rogers & Cavezos, 2011).

 See table 8.2 in the web resource for a full list of medication-specific indications, dosing recommendations, side effects, and toxicities.

Table 8.2 Medications Used to Treat Seizures

Medication	Side effects affecting rehab							Toxicities
First-generation agents								
Benzodiazepines: Used to treat status epilepticus seizures. Enhances effects of GABA.								
Lorazepam (Ativan)	Cog +++	S +++	A ++	Motor +++	D ++	Com ++	F +++	Ataxia, sedation, headache, fatigue, nausea, dependence. Half-life is 14 h.
Diazepam (Valium)	Cog ++++	S ++++	A ++	Motor +++	D ++	Com ++++	F ++++	Ataxia, sedation, headache, fatigue, nausea, dependence, active metabolite. Half-life is 43 h.
Hydantoins: Used to treat status epilepticus, tonic–clonic, and partial complex seizures. Blocks sodium channels and decreases calcium uptake, reducing central neurotransmission.								
Phenytoin (Dilantin)	Cog ++	S ++	A 0	Motor ++	D +++	Com +++	F ++	Liver ++ Hematologic +++ Renal ++ Rash (Stevens-Johnson) +++ Anticonvulsant hypersensitivity syndrome, gingival hyperplasia, hirsutism, acne, coarsening of features, hepatic failure, lymphadenopathy, osteomalacia
Fosphenytoin (Cerebyx)	Cog ++	S ++	A 0	Motor +++	D +++	Com +++	F ++	Sedation, headache, cerebellar signs (e.g., ataxia, dysarthria, nystagmus)
Barbiturates: Used to treat partial simple and tonic–clonic seizures. Increase chloride channels and GABA.								
Phenobarbital	Cog +++	S +++	A ++	Motor +++	D +++	Com +++	F +++	Liver +++ Hematologic +++ Renal 0 Rash (Stevens-Johnson) +++ Anticonvulsant hypersensitivity syndrome (phenobarbital), sedation, lethargy, decreased cognition, decreased attention, hyperactivity, depression, nystagmus, ataxia, skin rash
Primidone (Mysoline)	Cog +++	S +++	A ++	Motor +++	D +++	Com +++	F +++	Sedation, lethargy, decreased cognition, decreased attention, hyperactivity, depression, nystagmus, ataxia, skin rash

› continued

Table 8.2 › *continued*

Medication	Side effects affecting rehab							Toxicities			

Miscellaneous agents

Valproic acid: Used to treat partial, tonic–clonic, myoclonic, and absence seizures. Blocks sodium channels and increases calcium-dependent potassium conductance, reducing central neurotransmission.

Medication	Cog	S	A	Motor	D	Com	F	Liver	Hematologic	Renal	Rash (Stevens-Johnson)
Valproic acid (Depakote)	++	++	++	++	++	++	++	+++	+++	0	+++

Anticonvulsant hypersensitivity syndrome, weight gain, hepatotoxicity, dyspepsia, pancreatitis (potentially life threatening), alopecia, tremor, thrombocytopenia, platelet dysfunction, rash, hair loss

Ethosuximide (Zarontin): Partial complex agent of choice in treatment of absence seizures. Blocks calcium channels.

Medication	Cog	S	A	Motor	D	Com	F	Liver	Hematologic	Renal	Rash
Ethosuximide (Zarontin)	++	++	++	++	++	++	++	0	+++	+++	+

Leukopenia, headache, dizziness, dyskinesia, bradykinesia, blood dyscrasias (rare), rash (rare)

Iminostilbene (Tegretol): Used to treat partial complex and tonic–clonic seizures. Blocks sodium channels and decreases calcium uptake, reducing central neurotransmission.

Medication	Cog	S	A	Motor	D	Com	F	Liver	Hematologic	Renal	Rash (Stevens-Johnson)
Carbamazepine (Tegretol)	++	++	+	++	++	++	+++	+++	+++	+++	+++

Anticonvulsant hypersensitivity syndrome, blurred vision, benign leukopenia, cardiac arrhythmias, congestive heart failure, syndrome of inappropriate antidiuretic hormone (rare), aplastic anemia (rare); genetic testing required before initiation in Asians (high risk of AHS)

Second-generation agents

Felbamate (Felbatol): Second-line agent for partial simple and partial complex seizures not treated with other agents. Blocks NMDA receptors and modulates GABA.

Medication	Cog	S	A	Motor	D	Com	F	Liver	Hematologic	Renal	Rash
Felbamate (Felbatol)	++	+	+++	++	+++	+	++	++++	++++	0	++

Anticonvulsant hypersensitivity syndrome, headache, fatigue, somnolence, dizziness, insomnia, nausea, vomiting, anorexia, dyspepsia, diarrhea

Gabapentin (Neurontin): Add-on therapy for partial complex and tonic–clonic seizures. Binds to glutamate synapses and increases GABA turnover.

Medication	Cog	S	A	Motor	D	Com	F	Liver	Hematologic	Renal	Rash
Gabapentin (Neurontin)	++	++	+	+++	0	++	+++	0	0	+++	+

Peripheral edema, tremor, dizziness, fatigue, ataxia, drowsiness, weight gain, behavioral changes

Lamotrigine (Lamictal): Add-on therapy for partial, absence, tonic–clonic, and myoclonic seizures in children >2 yr. Blocks sodium channels and inhibits presynaptic release of glutamate and aspartate.

Medication	Cog	S	A	Motor	D	Com	F	Liver	Hematologic	Renal	Rash (Stevens-Johnson)
Lamotrigine (Lamictal)	++	0	++	+	0	++	++	+	0	+	+

Anticonvulsant hypersensitivity syndrome.

Teratogenic; avoid in pregnancy (causes cleft palate).

Medication	Side effects affecting rehab							Toxicities			

Levetiracetam (Keppra): Used to treat partial, atonic, tonic, clonic, tonic–clonic, myoclonic, and absence seizures. Decreases brain-derived neurotrophic factor and NPY and increases Y1 and Y5 receptors to reduce kindling.

	Cog	S	A	Motor	D	Com	F	Liver	Hematologic	Renal	Rash
Levetiracetam (Keppra)	+++	+++	0	+++	+	++	+++	0	+	+++	+

Somnolence, tiredness, dizziness, upper-respiratory infections.

Pyridoxine may decrease psychiatric side effects.

Oxcarbazepine (Trileptal): Used to treat simple seizures; used as adjunctive therapy in children with partial seizures. Blocks sodium channels and decreases calcium uptake.

	Cog	S	A	Motor	D	Com	F	Liver	Hematologic	Renal	Rash
Oxcarbazepine (Trileptal)	++	++	0	+++	+++	++	+++	+	0	0	+++

Anticonvulsant hypersensitivity syndrome, hyponatremia, nausea, rash.

Active metabolite of carbamazepine; fewer side effects than carbamazepine.

Tiagabine (Gabitril): Used to treat partial seizures; used in children >12 yr as add-on therapy for complex partial seizures. Blocks reuptake of GABA and enhances GABA activity.

	Cog	S	A	Motor	D	Com	F	Liver	Hematologic	Renal	Rash
Tiagabine (Gabitril)	++	++	++	+++	++	+++	+++	+	0	0	++

Confusion, difficulty speaking, mild sedation, paresthesias, irritability, weakness, dizziness, nervousness

Topiramate (Topamax): Used to treat partial, tonic, myoclonic, and tonic–clonic seizures; used in children >2 yr as add-on therapy for refractory complex seizures. Blocks sodium channels.

	Cog	S	A	Motor	D	Com	F	Liver	Hematologic	Renal	Rash
Topiramate (Topamax)	++	++	++	+++	+	+++	++	0	0	+++	++

Language impairment, behavioral changes, weight loss, altered taste, metabolic acidosis, kidney stones, hypohidrosis

Zonisamide (Zonegran): Used to treat partial and myoclonic seizures; used in children >16 yr as adjunct therapy for myoclonic seizures. Mechanism is unknown.

	Cog	S	A	Motor	D	Com	F	Liver	Hematologic	Renal	Rash (Stevens-Johnson)
Zonisamide (Zonegran)	++	++	++	++	++	+++	++	+++	+++	+++	+++

Anticonvulsant hypersensitivity syndrome, behavioral changes, weight loss, kidney stones, rash, hypohidrosis

Recently approved agents and agents pending approval

Eslicarbazepine (Stedesa): Adjunctive treatment for partial onset seizures. Sodium channel blocker.

	Cog	S	A	Motor	D	Com	F	Toxicities
Eslicarbazepine (Stedesa)	++	+++	0	+++	++	+++	+++	Dizziness, somnolence, headache, nausea, diplopia, abnormal coordination, vomiting.

Can reduce the drug levels and effectiveness of oral contraceptives.

› continued

Table 8.2 › *continued*

Medication	Side effects affecting rehab							Toxicities
Vigabatrin (Sabril): Used to treat refractory complex partial seizures in adults; alternative first-line therapy in treatment of infantile spasms associated with tuberous sclerosis. Enhances GABA activity.								
Vigabatrin (Sabril)	Cog +++	S +++	A ++	Motor +++	D +	Com +++	F +++	Drowsiness, behavioral problems, irritability, hypotonia, impaired cognitive development. Risk Evaluation and Mitigation Strategy program mandates ophthalmic examination every 3 mo and efficacy assessment every 2-4 wk.
Lacosamide (Vimpat): Adjunctive therapy in partial onset seizures. Inhibits sodium channels and acts on CRMP-2, a microtubule binding protein involved in neurotransmission.								
Lacosamide (Vimpat)	Cog +	S 0	A +	Motor ++	D +++	Com ++	F +++	Dizziness, diplopia, ataxia, vomiting, nausea, vertigo, blurred vision, cardiac arrhythmia, syncope, suicidal or psychotic reactions, allergic reactions

Cog = cognition; S = sedation; A = agitation or mania; Motor = discoordination; D = dysphagia; Com = communication; F = falls; GABA = gamma amino butyric acid; CRMP = collapsin response mediator protein; NPY = neuropeptide Y; AHS = anticonvulsant hypersensitivity syndrome.

The likelihood rating scale for encountering the side effects is as follows: 0 = Almost no probability of encountering side effects. + = Little likelihood of encountering side effects. +/++ = Low probability of encountering side effects; however, probability increases with increased dosage. ++ = Medium likelihood of encountering side effects. +++ = High likelihood of encountering side effects, particularly with high doses. ++++ = Highest likelihood of encountering side effects; best to avoid in at-risk patients.

PATIENT CASE 1

Y.P. is a 32-yr-old female who was recently discharged from the hospital after a motor vehicle accident. In the accident she sustained a head injury and associated seizures, rib fractures, and a hip fracture, for which she underwent surgery. She was referred to a physical therapist for assistance with ambulation and strength and gait training. Y.P.'s medication list includes the following: phenytoin (Dilantin) 300 mg/day, alprazolam (Xanax) 0.25 mg 3 times/day for anxiety, and temazepam (Restoril) 30 mg at bedtime as needed for insomnia. The physical therapist asks Y.P. how her medications are working for her. She responds tearfully that she is tired all of the time, cannot concentrate, and now has difficulty eating.

Question

What risk factors should the physical therapist address when planning Y.P.'s therapy sessions?

Answer

Y.P. is experiencing sedation and altered cognition because each of her three medications has sedative side effects. The physical therapist could discuss with Y.P.'s physician whether she needs to continue taking Xanax on a scheduled basis or whether she could take it only as needed, and could ask whether Y.P. still needs Restoril for insomnia. The speech language pathologist should perform a swallow evaluation and examination of the mouth to determine possible issues contributing to Y.P.'s dysphagia. Many side effects of phenytoin and benzodiazepines can contribute to dysphagia. Dilantin can cause inflammatory changes in the mouth (mucositis), sedation, ataxia, dry mouth, and decreased appetite. Benzodiazepines can alter taste perception, cause xerostomia, decrease concentration, increase coordination difficulties, and cause gastrointestinal upset that can contribute to dysphagia. The therapist should counsel Y.P. to avoid over-the-counter medications such as antihistamines that can worsen these effects and to avoid alcohol while taking these medications.

Use of Anticonvulsants in Pediatrics

Drug absorption and clearance rates continuously change throughout the neonatal period and childhood. Therefore, medication levels should be closely monitored and dosage should be frequently adjusted in order to maintain therapeutic effects. Children often require higher doses per body weight than adults. Levels do not fluctuate as dramatically during late childhood and adolescence, although dosing may need to be adjusted after growth spurts (Guthrie, 2006; Rogers & Cavezos, 2011).

Febrile seizures may be associated with sepsis or bacterial meningitis. Treatment is patient specific and involves identifying and treating the underlying cause and using **antipyretics** and cooling measures to control the fever. Neonatal seizures, which are associated with a high risk of morbidity and mortality, may be caused by CNS infections, hypoxia, electrolyte disorders, or **pyridoxine** deficiency. Fifteen percent of patients with neonatal seizures are mentally retarded, and 45% of patients with neonatal seizures have cerebral palsy. Infantile spasms, which present in patients less than 1 yr of age, consist of rapid, jackknife flexor or extensor spasms that occur in clusters. Of children with infantile spasms, 67% have underlying CNS disorders such as congenital brain malformation or tuberous sclerosis and 90% to 95% suffer from mental retardation. Treatment includes administration of adrenocorticotropic hormone or prednisone (Guthrie, 2006).

Lennox-Gastaut syndrome is a severe form of epilepsy with a poor prognosis. It is associated with mental retardation in 78% to 96% of patients and involves multiple types of seizures. Valproic acid (Depakote) is used as a first-line treatment. A child with this disorder requires multiple anticonvulsants, such as lamotrigine (Lamictal), topiramate (Topamax), or felbamate (Felbatol), as a last resort and must adhere to a ketogenic diet. Childhood and juvenile absence epilepsy usually occurs between 4 to 12 yr of age; the absence seizures are frequent and recurrent. Treatment options include ethosuximide (Zarontin) or valproic acid (Depakote). Patients usually outgrow this seizure disorder (Guthrie, 2006).

Status epilepticus seizures, which occur for at least 30 continuous minutes, are a medical emergency. Treatment involves protecting the airway, providing cardiac and respiratory support, checking and replacing electrolytes and glucose, and checking for and treating drug toxicity. Parenteral benzodiazepines such as diazepam (Valium) or lorazepam (Ativan) and simultaneous loading doses of either phenytoin (Dilantin) or fosphenytoin are administered. If these two agents are unsuccessful, phenobarbital is then administered (Guthrie, 2006; Rogers & Cavezos, 2011).

Side Effects

Common side effects of anticonvulsants include slowed cognitive function, lethargy, nausea, headaches, irritability, skin rashes, sedation, decreased reaction time, nystagmus, ataxia, dysphagia, and dysarthria. Patient tolerance to sedation generally develops after 7 to 10 days of therapy, but sedation can reoccur with changes in dosage. Continued sedation can indicate that the dose needs to be lowered or can indicate the presence of a drug interaction. Anticonvulsant medications such as phenytoin (Dilantin) and carbamazepine (Tegretol) can cause toxicity to the cerebellum even at therapeutic doses. Long-term use of phenytoin has been associated with atrophy of the cerebellum, resulting in skeletal muscle dysfunction, ataxia, and pronounced oropharyngeal dysphagia. Medication-induced ataxia may negatively influence overall coordination in functional activities and performance during gait and may increase the risk for falls. The rehabilitation therapist should implement coordination and functional-training exercises in order to address fall risks and persistent deficits in motor performance (Carl & Johnson, 2006; Gidal et al., 2002).

Use of anticonvulsants can cause dysphagia associated with side effects of sedation, discoordination, gastrointestinal upset, **gingival hyperplasia**, mucosal injury, and gastrointestinal side effects. Anticonvulsants associated with weight gain include gabapentin (Neurontin), valproic acid (Depakene), phenytoin (Dilantin), and lamotrigine (Lamictal). Anticonvulsants associated with weight loss include felbamate (Felbatol), topiramate (Topamax), and zonisamide (Zonegran) (Alvi, 1999; Campbell-Taylor, 1996, 2001; Carl & Johnson, 2006; Feinberg, 1997; Gidal et al., 2002; McNamara, 2001; Rogers & Cavezos, 2011; Welty, 2002).

Because anticonvulsants can be associated with serious skin and mucosal toxicities, the rehabilitation specialist should monitor the skin and protect the skin integrity of patients who use these agents. This includes eliminating the use of therapeutic modalities that could worsen the skin problem. Anticonvulsant hypersensitivity syndrome (AHS) is a delayed adverse drug reaction that is associated with the use of aromatic anticonvulsants. Other names for AHS include drug hypersensitivity syndrome, drug-related eosinophilia with systemic symptoms, Dilantin hypersensitivity reaction, phenytoin syndrome, Kawasaki-like syndrome, mononucleosis-like syndrome, and phenobarbital hypersensitivity syndrome. AHS is caused by the metabolism of aromatic anticonvulsants to arene oxides that cause cell death by directly binding to macromolecules or by acting as antigens. AHS has most often been reported with use of phenytoin (Dilantin), carbamazepine (Tegretol), and phenobarbital, but it has also occurred with use of lamotrigine (Lamictal) and valproic acid (Depakene). Patients with AHS can encounter the same toxicity with other aromatic anticonvulsant medications. Other aromatic anticonvulsants that should be avoided in patients with a history of AHS include felbamate (Felbatol), oxcarbazepine (Trileptal), and zonisamide (Zonegran) (Bohan et al., 2007; Rogers & Cavezos, 2011).

Symptoms of AHS include fever, rash, and evidence of systemic organ involvement (most often the liver). The rash is most often maculopapular, sometimes exfoliative, and may progress to Stevens-Johnson syndrome or toxic epidermal necrolysis (TEN). Symptoms can include **sloughing** off of the skin, gastrointestinal mucosa, eosinophilia, **thrombocytopenia**, neutropenia, elevated transaminases, elevated C-reactive protein, and lymphadenopathy. This side effect can contribute to significant difficulty swallowing and dysphagia when the gastrointestinal mucosa is involved. These may also be accompanied by facial swelling, cough, glossitis, congested throat, inflamed conjunctiva, and myocarditis. Treatment includes discontinuing medication and administering steroids (Alvi, 1999; Bohan et al., 2007; Feinberg, 1997).

Drug Interactions

The FDA warns against concurrently using lamotrigine (Lamictal) and valproic acid (Depakote) because this combination may increase the incidence of Stevens-Johnson syndrome or toxic epidermal **necrolysis**. Risk is increased when dose is increased too rapidly or when large daily doses are used (Carl & Johnson, 2006; Rogers & Cavezos, 2011; Welty, 2002).

Most anticonvulsants are metabolized by the cytochrome P450 enzyme systems of the liver. Table 8.3 summarizes the significant drug interactions involved with the anticonvulsants. In addition, the medication levels of phenytoin (Dilantin) and carbamazepine (Tegretol) suspensions are lowered significantly when these agents are administered concurrently with enteral nutrition (tube feedings) because the enteral product binds the medication. Clinicians should generally hold tube feeding for 1 h before and 1 h after administration in patients receiving enteral feedings (Carl & Johnson, 2006; Gidal et al., 2002; McNamara, 2001; Welty, 2002).

PATIENT CASE 2

H.L. is a 3-yr-old male who was diagnosed with Lennox-Gastaut syndrome. He is mentally retarded and has multiple types of seizures. He has received valproic acid and topiramate (Topamax) for the past 2 yr, but his seizures are not well controlled. His physician added lamotrigine (Lamictal) to his regimen 2 wk ago. He has followed a ketogenic diet for the past 2 yr. His mother notices that he is not eating his favorite foods and that he has a rash on his trunk, which is red and has raised welts. The inside of his mouth and throat is also inflamed. She asks the therapist whether the rash is an indication that her son is allergic to Lamictal.

Question

How should the therapist advise H.L.'s mother?

Answer

The therapist tells H.L.'s mother that H.L. is possibly experiencing a very serious side

Table 8.3 Drug Interactions and Monitoring of Anticonvulsants

Anticonvulsant	Interacting medications	Drug interaction
Phenytoin (Dilantin)	Anticonvulsants: felbamate (Felbatol), oxcarbazepine (Trileptal), topiramate (Topamax), valproic acid (Depakene)	Increased levels and effects of phenytoin
	Anti-infective: doxycycline (Vibramycin)	Decreased effects of doxycycline
	Anti-infectives: fluconazole (Diflucan), isoniazid (INH), metronidazole (Flagyl), rifampin, Septra, chloramphenicol	Increased effects of phenytoin
	Anti-infective: rifampin	Decreased effects of phenytoin
	Asthma medication: theophylline	Decreased levels of phenytoin and theophylline
	Cardiac medication: amiodarone (Cordarone, Pacerone)	Increased levels and effects of phenytoin
	Cardiac medication: digoxin (Lanoxin)	Decreased levels and effects of digoxin
	Cardiac medication: disopyramide (Norpace)	Decreased levels of disopyramide
	Cardiac medications: quinidine	Decreased levels and effects of quinidine
	Antacids: cimetidine (Tagamet), omeprazole (Prilosec)	Increased levels and effects of phenytoin
	Antacid: sucralfate (Carafate)	Decreased levels and effects of phenytoin
	Oral contraceptives	Decreased effects of contraceptives
Carbamazepine (Tegretol)	Anticonvulsants: phenobarbital, primidone (Mysoline), felbamate (Felbatol)	Decreased levels and effects of carbamazepine
	Anti-infectives: danazol (Danocrine), erythromycin, clarithromycin (Biaxin), isoniazid (INH), ketoconazole (Nizoral), itraconazole (Sporanox)	Increased levels and effects of carbamazepine
	Antidepressant: fluoxetine (Prozac)	Increased levels of carbamazepine
	Cardiac medications: diltiazem (Cardizem), verapamil (Isoptin, Calan)	Increased levels and effects of carbamazepine
	Asthma medication: theophylline	Increased levels of carbamazepine
	Cancer chemotherapy: cisplatin (Platinol), doxorubicin (Adriamycin)	Decreased levels of carbamazepine
Ethosuximide (Zarontin)	Anticonvulsants: carbamazepine (Tegretol), phenytoin (Dilantin), primidone (Mysoline), phenobarbital, valproic acid (Depakene)	Decreased levels and effects of ethosuximide
	Anti-infectives: nevirapine (Viramune), ritonavir (Norvir)	
Felbamate (Felbatol)	Anticonvulsant: carbamazepine (Tegretol)	Decreased levels of felbamate
Gabapentin (Neurontin)	Antacids: space 2 h from administration of gabapentin	Decreased levels of gabapentin

› continued

Table 8.3　›continued

Anticonvulsant	Interacting medications	Drug interaction
Lamotrigine (Lamictal)	Anticonvulsants: phenytoin (Dilantin), carbamazepine (Tegretol)	Decreased levels and effects of lamotrigine
	Anticonvulsant: valproic acid (Depakene)	Increased levels and effects of lamotrigine
Levetiracetam (Keppra)	No known drug interactions	
Oxcarbazepine (Trileptal)	Anticonvulsants: phenytoin (Dilantin), phenobarbital, carbamazepine	Decreased levels and effects of oxcarbazepine
Valproic acid (Depakene)	Anticonvulsants: phenobarbital, phenytoin (Dilantin), lamotrigine (Lamictal)	Decreased levels and effects of valproic acid
Phenobarbital	Carbamazepine (Tegretol)	Decreased levels and effects of phenobarbital
	Valproic acid (Depakene)	Increased levels and effects of phenobarbital
Topiramate (Topamax)	Anticonvulsants: carbamazepine (Tegretol), phenytoin (Dilantin), valproic acid (Depakene)	Decreased levels and effects of topiramate
Tiagabine (Gabitril)	Anticonvulsants: phenytoin (Dilantin), phenobarbital, carbamazepine	Decreased levels and effects of tiagabine
	Valproic acid (Depakene)	Increased levels and effects of tiagabine
Valproic acid (Depakene)	Anti-infective: meropenem (Merrem)	Decreased levels and effects of valproic acid
	Antidepressants: amitriptyline (Elavil), nortriptyline (Pamelor)	Decreased levels and effects of valproic acid
	Anticonvulsants: phenytoin (Dilantin), phenobarbital, carbamazepine (Tegretol), topiramate (Topamax)	Decreased levels and effects of valproic acid
Zonisamide (Zonegran)	Anticonvulsants: phenytoin (Dilantin), phenobarbital, carbamazepine	Decreased levels and effects of zonisamide

effect caused by a drug interaction between valproic acid and the Lamictal that was recently added. The therapist calls H.L.'s physician, who instructs H.L.'s mother to discontinue the Lamictal and to come to the office immediately so that the rash can be evaluated and treated.

Summary

This chapter summarizes the different types of seizure disorders and reviews the medications that are commonly used to treat them. This chapter also discusses ways the rehabilitation specialist can tailor therapy sessions and environment to minimize risk and optimize effectiveness for patients who experience seizures. At the beginning of each session, the therapist should review any changes in the patient's use of medications, herbals, or caffeine. In many instances, altered cognition and motor function associated with medication use are initially detected during rehabilitation sessions. Educating the patient and family and communicating appropriately with the patient's prescriber can be invaluable in optimizing patient care.

Medications Used to Treat Spasticity and Muscle Spasm

9

In clinical practice, the rehabilitation therapist will care for patients with symptoms of spasticity and symptoms of muscle spasm. This chapter summarizes the pathophysiology associated with these disorders and introduces the medications used to treat them. This chapter also reviews methods used to address these patient's needs in the rehabilitative session and explains how medication effects can affect rehabilitation.

Muscle relaxants are used to treat spasticity and muscle spasm. Spasticity is caused by injury to the central nervous system (CNS; brain or spinal cord). Muscle spasms, on the other hand, are associated with musculoskeletal injury or compression of a spinal nerve root in the peripheral nervous system (Satkunam, 2003).

Spasticity

Spasticity is characterized by an abnormal increase in muscle tone or muscle stiffness that is associated with pain and that interferes with speech and movement. Spasticity is usually caused by damage to nerve pathways in the brain and spinal cord that are associated with movement. Spasticity can be associated with disorders such as cerebral palsy, stroke, head trauma, and amyotrophic lateral sclerosis (ALS), as well as metabolic diseases such as phenylketonuria. Patients with spasticity may exhibit symptoms such as **clonus**, hypertonicity, scissoring, contractures, and deep-tendon reflexes. Severity of spasticity can range from mild to severe and can directly affect activities of daily living (National Institute of Neurological Diseases and Stroke, 2011).

Incidence

Spasticity affects approximately 12 million people worldwide. The rate of spasticity varies based on the medical condition of the patient. For example, 80% of patients with cerebral palsy have spasticity. The incidence of spasticity may vary in patients with disorders such as traumatic brain injury based on the nature and severity of the injury (Hudson, 2008).

Spasticity affects about half a million Americans with conditions such as multiple sclerosis, cerebral palsy, stroke, or traumatic brain or spinal cord injury. Patients report associated symptoms of stiffness and decreased range of motion. Abnormal posture, pain, inability to sleep, and limitation in activities of daily living (e.g., eating, writing, dressing, walking, sitting, and standing) most negatively affect quality of life. Pain and contracture associated with spasticity can result in isolation, depression, and anxiety and can interfere with the patient's ability to work (Mullarkey, 2009; Satkunam, 2003; VanDenburgh et al., 2010).

Etiology and Pathophysiology

Spasticity is hypertonicity related to injury or disease involving the brain or spinal cord. Spasticity of spinal origin results from spinal cord injury or multiple sclerosis (an autoimmune disorder associated with demyelination in both the brain and spinal cord). Spasticity of cerebral origin can be caused by stroke, traumatic brain injury, cerebral palsy, and other upper motor neuron lesions. Spasticity can be classified as focal (isolated, local motor disturbance affecting a single body part), regional (motor disturbance involving a large region of the body), or generalized (motor disturbance involving widespread bodily regions). Focal spasticity is commonly seen poststroke, whereas spasticity associated with spinal cord injury or multiple sclerosis is more diffuse. Spasticity can be associated with gait disturbances, speech problems, clonus, and uncontrollable muscle spasm (Merello et al., 1994; Mullarkey, 2009; Satkunam, 2003; VanDenburgh, 2010).

Muscle tone, which is controlled by the descending motor systems, results from a balance between the inhibitory effects on stretch reflexes mediated by the dorsal **reticulospinal tract** and the facilitatory effects on extensor tone mediated by the medial reticulospinal tract and the **vestibulospinal tract**. The neurophysiology of spasticity is related to an overactive stretch reflex that these higher centers cannot dampen. These higher centers normally inhibit excessive activation of the muscle spindle (a proprioceptor in muscle that is highly sensitive to stretch and the rate of stretch imposed) through descending influences. However, in the case of an upper motor neuron lesion, cortical control to inhibit excessive stretch reflex is lost. As a result, the muscle spindle fires directly onto the alpha motor neuron at the spinal cord level, causing excessive excitability of the skeletal muscle and no inhibition from the brain. This spasticity is characterized by involuntary forceful contraction of the affected muscles. The muscle contraction is often so strong that the weak antagonists to the spastic muscle cannot overcome the force of the spastic muscle in order to bring the joint into a neutral position (Merello et al., 1994; Mullarkey, 2009; Satkunam, 2003; VanDenburgh, 2010).

Rehabilitation Considerations

The spasticity that results from an upper motor neuron lesion can present a rehabilitation paradox. High levels of spasticity negatively influence neuromuscular control and functional performance, but the increased muscle tone can provide stability during functional activities. For example, a patient with spastic hemiplegia may use the increased muscle tone in a weak lower extremity to bear weight during gait. Reducing this increased tone with treatment might unmask the underlying weakness and prevent weight bearing. Spasticity should be treated gradually in order to enable the patient to adequately reduce spasticity without negatively affecting functional performance in instances when the patient is using the increased tone to increase stability during functional performance (Ciccone, 2007; Houglum et al., 2005; Magee, 2007; Satkunam, 2003).

Posture can play an important role in controlling spasticity. The rehabilitation therapist should teach patients not to assume certain postures that promote spasticity. Keeping the head in a neutral position (i.e., good postural alignment) can prevent the activation of strong postural reflexes in the trunk and extremities. Good posture training and positioning techniques are essential in minimizing spasticity, hastening recovery, and minimizing contracture. The rehabilitation therapist should emphasize therapeutic activities that promote the development of proximal stability in the trunk so that the patient will have a good base of support to work from during tasks that require distal mobility (e.g., reaching tasks). In addition, the therapist should promote therapeutic activities that emphasize progressive weight bearing through the affected upper and lower extremities. Weight-bearing postures can decrease tone and provide excellent sensory input that promotes contraction of the muscles surrounding the affected joints (Ciccone, 2007; Magee, 2007; Satkunam, 2003).

Spasticity often leads to contracture because the muscle is habitually in the shortened position and can result in upper-body deformities (e.g., adducted or internally rotated shoulder, flexed elbow, pronation of the forearm, flexion of the wrist, clench fist, and thumb-in-hand deformity). Preventing and treating contractures is of paramount importance, and a variety of positioning and splinting techniques can be implemented. Techniques such as low-load prolonged stretching, soft-tissue manipulation, joint mobilization, splinting, and serial casting may be used to address the shortened soft tissue that causes joint contracture. Preheating tissue using thermal agents (e.g., moist heat, shortwave diathermy, and ultrasound) before stretching can also help increase soft-tissue extensibility when combined with passive stretching, soft-tissue mobilization, and joint-mobilization techniques. However, before using thermal agents, the rehabilitation therapist must assess the patient's thermal sensation and local circulation in the region to be treated to determine whether the patient is at risk of sustaining burns due to impaired sensation or blood flow that is inadequate to dissipate the heat. The therapist should emphasize therapeutic interventions that focus on slow, sustained stretching of the spastic agonist muscle and restoring neuromuscular control in the weakened antagonist muscle. Contracture management may also involve serial casting or splinting the limb into a position that inhibits reflex. Various forms of electrical stimulation can also be used to decrease spasticity and improve neuromuscular control as late as 5 yr poststroke (Ciccone, 2007; Magee, 2007; Satkunam, 2003; Sullivan & Hedman, 2004). The rehabilitation therapist should also be aware of the many factors that can potentially increase spasticity, such as pressure ulcers, ingrown toenails, constipation, urinary tract infections, or a poor fit in a brace or wheelchair (Satkunam, 2003).

The rehabilitation therapist may also deal with spasticity in the pediatric population. Cerebral palsy is the most common upper motor neuron lesion the pediatric rehabilitation specialists will encounter. About 75% of patients with cerebral palsy experience spasticity (Wilson-Howle, 1999). The disease is a nonprogressive CNS disorder that is caused by damage to the developing CNS before, during, or soon after birth. Cerebral palsy occurs in 2 to 3 per 1,000 live births in the United States, and it is estimated that 764,000 children and adults in the United States have cerebral palsy (Cameron & Monroe, 2007; Kopec, 2008).

In addition to altered muscle tone, children with cerebral palsy typically show delayed postural reactions, persistence of primitive reflexes, delayed motor development, and impaired motor function. Motor impairment may be accompanied by disturbances of sight, hearing, cognition, communication, and behavior (Bjornson et al., 2003; Leary et al., 2006). Motor impairment may also contribute to nutritional deficiencies resulting from cricopharyngeal and other forms of dysphagia (Biltzer, 1997). The level of disability associated with cerebral palsy varies. Some individuals with the disease are completely dependent and others lead a nearly normal life. Most children with mild to moderate cerebral palsy have normal life spans, and their level of disability depends on the severity of their condition. Spasticity in patients with cerebral palsy may be accompanied by hypertonicity, clonus, hyperreflexia, decreased motor planning, loss of selective motor control, weakness, poor endurance, and, less commonly, athetosis, chorea, dystonia, and ataxia (Kopec, 2008).

One challenge in managing spastic cerebral palsy is reducing spasticity in order to improve functional performance, prevent contracture, and allow for personal hygiene. In addition to the physical therapy techniques of splinting, bracing, orthosis, and assistive technology, medications and surgical interventions can be used to treat spasticity. Skeletal muscle relaxants such as baclofen (Lioresal), diazepam (Valium), dantrolene (Dantrium), clonidine (Catapres), tizanidine (Zanaflex), and botulinum toxin can help control spasticity (Albright et al., 2003; Milanov & Georgiev, 1994). Surgical procedures such as dorsal rhizotomy, muscle-lengthening procedures, or muscle releases (e.g., hip adductors, iliopsoas, and hamstrings) can also be employed to manage spasticity (Cameron & Monroe, 2007; Kopec, 2008).

Medication Therapy

The pharmacological treatment of spasticity generally involves oral medications that modify the centrally mediated inhibitory effect on the final common pathway. The final common pathway comprises the motor neuron originating in the spinal cord or brainstem, the axon, and all of the muscle fibers that the motor neuron innervates (Purves et al., 2001). The Ashworth Scale and Modified Ashworth Scale, which quantify the patient's level of spasticity, can be used to monitor effects of treatment and detect worsening of symptoms (Albright et al., 2003; Milanov & Georgiev, 1994; Mullarkey, 2009).

Gamma amino butyric acid (GABA) is a central neurotransmitter that plays an important role in the control of spasticity. Medications commonly used to treat spasticity include the skeletal muscle relaxants baclofen (Lioresal) and dantrolene sodium (Dantrium) and benzodiazepines such as diazepam (Valium), clonidine (Catapres), gabapentin (Neurontin), and tizanidine (Zanaflex). In addition to oral medications, Botox injections and phenol injections can change the final common pathway by blocking the nerve (Ahsan et al., 2000). Table 9.1 summarizes the medications used to treat spasticity (Satkunam, 2003).

Baclofen

Baclofen (Lioresal) is a synthetic agonist of the neurotransmitter GABA. Baclofen reduces the release of excitatory neurotransmitters at the spinal cord, thus reducing spinal reflex action, clonus, and frequency of flexor spasm and improving joint range of motion. Baclofen can be administered orally for mild to severe spasticity. The goal of treatment is to reduce flexor and extensor spasticity without increasing weakness. Baclofen is the treatment of choice for spasticity associated with spinal cord injury, multiple sclerosis, or cerebral palsy. Of patients treated with baclofen, spasticity improves in 70% to 87% and spasm improves in 75% to 96% (Wise & Conklin, 2004; Zhang et al., 2002). Baclofen can improve speech, reduce symptoms of dysphagia associated with spasticity, and improve esophageal reflux symptoms (Albright et al., 2003; Bjornson et al., 2003; Koek et al., 2003; Leary et al., 2006; Lidums et al., 2000; Omari et al., 2006; Rietman & Geertzen, 2007; Vittal & Pasricha, 2006).

Baclofen is well absorbed orally but is 30% protein bound and has low lipid solubility. It does not readily cross the blood–brain barrier into the CNS. Adverse effects of oral baclofen include drowsiness during the first week of medication use; this drowsiness typically resolves as the dosage is adjusted. Additional reported side effects include muscle weakness, ataxia, orthostatic hypotension, fatigue, headache, nausea, and dizziness; confusion and hallucinations have been reported in the elderly and those with history of stroke. Abrupt discontinuation may result in a rebound increase in spasticity, **rhabdomyolysis**, disorientation, hallucination, and seizures (Kopec, 2008).

Intrathecal baclofen can be used in individuals with severe spasticity that is not treatable with oral therapy. Intrathecal baclofen provides long-term delivery of the medication into the intrathecal space bypassing the blood–brain barrier and offers improved bioavailability compared with the oral form. Intrathecal baclofen attains effective concentrations in the cerebrospinal fluid while reducing plasma baclofen concentrations 100 fold. This reduction in plasma baclofen concentrations results in a reduction of many of the side effects associated with its oral use. Intrathecal baclofen is administered via a programmable pump that is implanted in the patient's abdominal wall. The pump delivers the drug directly to the subarachnoid space of a specific level of the spinal cord (Ciccone, 2007; Walker et al., 2000).

Common adverse effects of intrathecal baclofen include chronic constipation, hypotonia, somnolence, headache, vomiting, and paresthesias. Complications that can occur with intrathecal administration include pump malfunction, local **seroma**, **hematoma**, or infection at the pump implantation site. In addition, the catheter can become kinked or blocked, resulting in interrupted therapy. Pump failure or problems with the catheter can precipitate withdrawal symptoms. Mild withdrawal symptoms can include pruritus, agitation, **diaphoresis**, and increased muscle tone (Peng et al., 1998). Symptoms can progress to seizures, hallucinations, delirium, rhabdomyolysis, and death if therapy is abruptly interrupted. Patients receiving intrathecal baclofen should be educated about the early symptoms of withdrawal and should have oral baclofen available for

See table 9.1 in the web resource for a full list of medication-specific indications, dosing recommendations, side effects, and other considerations.

Table 9.1   Medications Used to Treat Spasticity and Muscle Spasm

Medication	Side effects affecting rehabilitation							Other side effects or considerations
Agents used to treat spasticity								
Baclofen (Lioresal)	Cog ++	S +++	A ++	Motor +++	D ++	Com ++	F +++	Oral: Initial sedation, muscle weakness, ataxia, orthostatic hypotension, fatigue, headache, nausea, dizziness; confusion and hallucinations reported in elderly or those with history of stroke. Intrathecal: Chronic constipation, hypotonia, somnolence, headache, vomiting, paresthesias. Eliminated by the kidneys; reduce dose with renal dysfunction. Abrupt discontinuance results in rebound increase in spasticity, rhabdomyolysis, disorientation, hallucination, and seizures.
Dantrolene (Dantrium)	Cog ++	S +++	A ++	Motor +++	D +++	Com ++	F +++	Drowsiness, dizziness, nausea, diarrhea, dysphagia. Dose-limiting hepatotoxicity; test baseline liver function and monitor throughout therapy. Hyperkalemia when combined with verapamil, increased risk for hepatotoxicity when combined with estrogens, and increased CNS depression when combined with other CNS depressants. Avoid combining with MAOI.
Clonidine (Catapres)	Cog +	S +++	A 0	Motor +	D +	Com +	F ++	Hypotension, dizziness, sedation, gastrointestinal upset. Gradually taper off when discontinuing therapy to avoid rebound effects. Additive sedation when used with other CNS depressants. May be administered as an epidural injection, daily patch, or orally.
Tizanidine (Zanaflex)	Cog ++	S +++	A 0	Motor +	D ++	Com ++	F +++	Sedation, hypotension, dizziness, gastrointestinal upset. Starting with a very low dose and titrating slowly may reduce or eliminate side effects such as sedation, xerostomia, and dizziness. Monitor liver-function tests. Therapy should be scheduled 2 h after the dose, when peak effects are seen with this medication.
Gabapentin (Neurontin)	Cog ++	S +++	A ++	Motor +++	D 0	Com ++	F +++	Sedation, fatigue, dizziness, ataxia, peripheral edema. No known drug interactions. Adjust dose for renal insufficiency.

› continued

Table 9.1 › *continued*

Medication	Side effects affecting rehabilitation							Other side effects or considerations
Agents used to treat focal spasticity								
Botulinum toxin (Botox, Myobloc)	Cog 0	S 0	A 0	Motor ++	D ++	Com 0	F ++	Pain on injection, muscle soreness, bruising, excessive weakness in injected and adjacent muscles, rash, fever, possible changes in gait.
Phenol injection	Cog 0	S 0	A 0	Motor ++	D 0	Com +	F ++	Peripheral edema, wound infection, skin sloughing, pain, chronic dysesthesias. No known drug interactions.
Agent used to treat spasticity or muscle spasm								
Diazepam (Valium)	Cog +++	S +++	A ++	Motor +++	D +++	Com ++	F +++	Sedation, impaired memory, decreased attention, ataxia, weakness, constipation, urinary retention, worsened depression, impaired cognition, tolerance, dependence, withdrawal symptoms of anxiety, agitation, restlessness, irritability, tremor, nausea, hyperpyrexia, seizures. Enhances the effects of other CNS depressants, including alcohol. May block the action of levodopa. Cimetidine, disulfiram, omeprazole, isoniazid, oxcarbazepine, ticlopidine, topiramate, ketoconazole, itraconazole, probenecid, fluoxetine, fluvoxamine, erythromycin, propranolol, imipramine, ciprofloxacin, and valproic acid prolong action by inhibiting elimination of diazepam. Rifampin, phenytoin, phenobarbital, St. John's wort, carbamazepine, and dexamethasone decrease levels and effects.
Agents used to treat muscle spasm								
Carisoprodol (Soma)	Cog ++	S +++	A 0	Motor +++	D ++	Com ++	F ++	Headaches, dizziness, drowsiness, facial flushing, insomnia, coordination problems. Abuse potential. Potentiates effects of opiates, allowing reduction in opiate dosage. Metabolized by CYP2C19 to meprobamate.
Chlorzoxazone (Parafon Forte)	Cog ++	S ++	A 0	Motor ++	D ++	Com ++	F ++	Stomach upset, drowsiness, dizziness, light-headedness, weakness, hepatotoxicity. Additive hepatotoxicity when used with acetaminophen (Tylenol).
Cyclobenzaprine (Flexeril)	Cog ++++	S ++++	A 0	Motor +++	D ++	Com ++	F ++++	Somnolence, confusion, dizziness, paresthesias, seizures, arrhythmias. Avoid using with MAOIs, SSRIs, guanethidine, and other CNS depressants. Combining with tramadol (Ultram) or bupropion increases seizure risk. Combining with topiramate (Topamax) increases risk of heat stroke. Chemical structure like that of tricyclic antidepressants. Limit use to no more than 3 wk.

Medication	Side effects affecting rehabilitation							Other side effects or considerations
Metaxalone (Skelaxin)	Cog ++	S ++	A ++	Motor ++	D ++	Com ++	F ++	Nausea, vomiting, headache, irritability. CYP450 enzyme metabolism and drug interactions.
Methocarbamol (Robaxin, Skelex)	Cog ++++	S ++++	A ++	Motor +++	D ++	Com ++	F +++	Somnolence, dizziness, vertigo, syncope, muscular incoordination, stomach upset, flushing, blurred vision, fever, skin rash, pruritus, bradycardia, jaundice, mood changes, slow heart rate, fainting, clumsiness, difficulty urinating. Additive sedation when taken with other CNS depressants. Metabolized by demethylation, so no significant drug interactions exist. May cause discoloration of urine (black, blue, or green).
Orphenadrine citrate (Norflex)	Cog ++	S +++	A ++	Motor ++	D ++	Com ++	F ++++	Dry mouth, dizziness, drowsiness, restlessness, insomnia, constipation, urine retention, orthostatic hypotension, euphoria. Anticholinergic agent closely related to diphenhydramine (Benadryl). Avoid combining with other anticholinergic agents.

Cog = cognition; S = sedation; A = agitation or mania; Motor = discoordination; D = dysphagia; Com = communication; F = falls; CNS = central nervous system; MAOI = monoamine oxidase inhibitor; SSRI = selective serotonin reuptake inhibitor.

The likelihood rating scale for encountering the side effects is as follows: 0 = Almost no probability of encountering side effects. + = Little likelihood of encountering side effects. +/++ = Low probability of encountering side effects; however, probability increases with increased dosage. ++ = Medium likelihood of encountering side effects. +++ = High likelihood of encountering side effects, particularly with high doses. ++++ = Highest likelihood of encountering side effects; best to avoid in at-risk patients.

emergency use. Early identification of pump malfunction leading to overdose is important in preventing toxicity such as increased seizures, respiratory depression, decreased cardiac function, and coma. Overdose may be associated with incorrect programming of the pump or restarting therapy after an interruption that results in a patient's loss of developed tolerance to the medication (Dario & Tomei, 2004; Gallichio, 2004; Kopec, 2008; Mullarkey, 2009; Satkunam, 2003; Tsereng et al., 1998).

Clonidine

Clonidine (Catapres), a centrally acting selective alpha-2 adrenergic agonist used in the management of hypertension, is effective in treating spasticity associated with spinal cord injury and traumatic brain injury. It is available in oral form and as a transdermal patch, but use is limited because it increases the risk of hypotension. Other adverse effects include sedation and gastrointestinal upset (Kopec, 2008; Mullarkey, 2009).

Tizanidine

Tizanidine (Zanaflex), a centrally acting alpha-2 adrenergic agonist, binds to central alpha-2 receptors and reduces decreasing excitatory input to alpha motor neurons, thus improving spasm and clonus. This medication can be useful as a first-line treatment for spasticity related to spinal cord injury, stroke, and multiple sclerosis. When compared with oral baclofen, tizanidine is more effective and has fewer adverse effects. Risk of severe muscle weakness is lower in patients using this medication than in those using diazepam (Valium) and baclofen, and risk of hypotension is lower in patients using this medication than in those using clonidine (Gallichio, 2004; Kopec, 2008).

Diazepam

Diazepam (Valium), one of the oldest treatments for spasticity associated with cerebral palsy, increases binding of GABA to its receptor, thus enhancing the inhibitory effects of GABA and reducing spinal reflexes. It is approved by the U.S. Food and Drug Administration for the management of spasticity caused by upper neuron disorders and may improve passive range of motion, reduce hyperreflexia, and reduce spasm. Diazepam is particularly helpful in children with cerebral palsy and spasticity associated with spinal cord injury. It possesses anxiolytic, anticonvulsant, hypnotic, sedative, skeletal muscle relaxant, and amnestic properties (Kopec, 2008; Mullarkey, 2009).

Although it is as effective as baclofen, diazepam causes more sedation, which limits its clinical use. Adverse effects are more pronounced in the first 2 wk of therapy. Other adverse effects include impaired memory, decreased attention, ataxia, weakness, constipation, and urinary retention. Use of benzodiazepines such as diazepam can also cause or worsen depression.

The rehabilitation therapist should assess and monitor the patient's balance because the side effects of dizziness and decreased psychomotor performance may increase the patient's risk of falls. Patients taking diazepam will likely exhibit confusion and have some difficulty following directions and participating in psychomotor tasks. Other adverse effects can include slurred speech and dysphagia. Chronic use of benzodiazepines can result in significant pharyngeal phase dysphagia, notably cricopharyngeal incoordination, hypopharyngeal incoordination, and aspiration (Carl & Johnson, 2006; Kopec, 2008). Valium is not intended for long-term, chronic use in the treatment of spasticity because its strong sedative effect causes drowsiness, decreased psychomotor performance, dizziness, reflex tachycardia, and potential for tolerance and physical dependence. Additive effects of sedation, ataxia, and confusion occur when diazepam is combined with other CNS depressants (e.g., antipsychotics, antidepressants, and alcohol) (Ciccone, 2007; Walker et al., 2000).

Dantrolene Sodium

Dantrolene sodium (Dantrium) prevents full muscle contraction by interfering with the release of calcium from the **sarcoplasmic reticulum** of the skeletal muscle cell, thereby reducing muscle tone, clonus, and spasm. Calcium is needed for the **actin** and **myosin** cross-bridging that results in muscle contraction. Dantrium is unique in that it acts at the skeletal muscle level whereas other agents act at the spinal cord level. It is used to manage hypertonicity related to upper motor neuron lesions and to treat severe spasticity seen in patients with stroke, advanced multiple sclerosis, traumatic spinal cord lesions, and cerebral palsy. Dantrium is also used to treat neuroleptic malignant syndrome and **malignant hyperthermia** associated with the use of anesthesia and neuromuscular-blocking agents (Ciccone, 2007; Gallichio, 2004; Mullarkey, 2009).

During the first 7 to 10 days of use, Dantrium may cause drowsiness, dizziness, nausea, and diarrhea. Side effects can also include dysphagia. Because dantrolene sodium acts peripherally (i.e., at the muscle level), it does not have adverse effects on the CNS. Dantrolene is associated with dose-limiting hepatotoxicity, and hepatitis that may be fatal has been reported. Baseline liver-function tests in patients using dantrolene sodium are needed, and these liver-function tests should be monitored regularly throughout therapy (Kopec, 2008).

Gabapentin

Gabapentin (Neurontin), originally developed as an anticonvulsant, is used to treat neuropathic pain and to decrease spasticity. It enhances the effects of GABA, decreases alpha motor neuron firing, and reduces spasticity. This medication is used to reduce spasticity associated with multiple sclerosis and spinal cord injury, especially in individuals who experience significant pain with their spasticity (Ciccone, 2007). Peak concentration occurs 2 to 4 h after ingestion; therapy sessions should be scheduled to coincide with peak blood levels. Adverse side effects include sedation, fatigue, dizziness, and ataxia (Ciccone, 2007).

PATIENT CASE 1

S.B. is a 50-yr-old woman with multiple sclerosis. S.B. is able to live independently in a wheelchair-accessible apartment. In the recent past, she has been able to ambulate short distances in her small apartment but has required the use of a wheelchair for longer distances in the community. She demonstrates spastic hemiplegia (left greater than right). Over the past 6 wk her spasticity has increased to the point that it has negatively affected her performance in activities of daily living and she must use her wheelchair at all times. Transfers to and from S.B.'s wheelchair have become unsafe because of the increased spasticity. In the past, S.B.'s spasticity has been successfully managed with oral baclofen 15 mg 4 times/day. Although S.B. asks her therapist for her opinion, S.B. understands that her physician must make the final decision on whether increasing her baclofen dose would better control the spasticity.

Question

What factors should S.B.'s therapist consider when answering her question regarding her medication?

Answer

S.B.'s spasticity has been consistently well controlled with baclofen in the recent past. The dose appears to be sufficient. Many individuals with spasticity require 40 to 80 mg/day, and some require a much higher dose (Satkunam, 2003). S.B.'s history suggests a sudden decline in function that must be addressed. S.B. mentions to her rehabilitation therapist that she is experiencing some common clinical manifestations of urinary tract infection (increased urinary urgency and frequency, fever, chills, and unexplained fatigue). The therapist notifies S.B.'s physician, who makes a diagnosis of urinary tract infection. S.B.'s physician prescribes antibiotics to treat the urinary tract infection. Over the course of the next several weeks, the patient notes a gradual decrease in spasticity and returns to her previous level of function. Factors that can increase spasticity are not always related to insufficient dosages of medication. Urinary tract infections, constipation, ingrown toenails, pressure ulcers, and poorly fitting braces or wheelchairs can cause noxious stimuli that increase spasticity (Satkunam, 2003).

Phenol Injections

Phenol injections have been used as a focal treatment for spastic muscles. Phenol injections, which can be administered **perineurally** or intramuscularly, cause chemical denervation of the muscle and thus address hypertonicity (Gallichio, 2004). Injections of phenol can be used to block large nerves to specific spastic muscles. Depending on the concentration of the medication, injection site, and individual differences in response to this medication, patients may have sustained positive effects that last from several weeks to years (O'Brien et al., 1996). Side effects can include peripheral edema, wound infection, skin sloughing, pain, and chronic dysesthesias. With dysesthesias, the patient may experience an unpleasant or abnormal touch sensation such as burning, wetness, itching, electric shock, and pins and needles, which may be accompanied by a feeling of pain. This side effect is more common in the diabetic population (Satkunam, 2003).

Botulinum Toxin

Botulinum toxin (Botox, Myobloc) is an extremely potent neurotoxin produced by the bacterium *Clostridium botulinum*. Administration of botulinum toxin in systemic doses may result in widespread paralysis, including paralysis of the respiratory muscles that can be serious or fatal. Despite this, botulinum toxin can be safely used as a focal injection to treat specific spastic muscles. Botulinum toxin binds to the presynaptic acetylcholine vesicles at the neuromuscular junction of skeletal muscles and prevents the release of acetylcholine from the presynaptic terminals into the neuromuscular junction, thus preventing neuromuscular transmission and muscle contraction. When Botox is injected into a muscle, it causes selective paralysis of the muscle. This paralysis may begin within several days after the injection and may last 1 to 6 mo (Gallichio, 2004). The induced muscle paralysis is not permanent because the body develops collateral sprouting of new nerve endings from the same axon in which Botox disabled the presynaptic terminal. The new terminals grow into the muscle and provide the muscle with a new source of acetylcholine, thereby restoring dystonia in the muscle. Botox takes effect in approximately 7 days and can last for 3 to 4 mo, but duration of effects can vary from less than 1 mo to 6 mo. For this reason, repeated injections are required (Brin, 1997).

Type-A botulinum is marketed as Botox and is better tolerated than the type B product (Myobloc), which is used in patients with cervical dystonia. Compared with the type A product, the type B product causes more intense anticholinergic effects such as dry mouth, dysphagia, and voiding difficulties. Botulinum toxin injection is typically reserved for smaller muscles that can be selectively targeted. Diffusion to other muscles depends on the dose, volume, dilution, and number of injections administered. The rehabilitation specialist should counsel patients to expect a change in gait and to take precautions to prevent accidental fall and injury (Gallichio, 2004; Kopec, 2008; Ozcakir & Sivrioglu, 2007).

Research shows that Botox effectively reduces localized spasticity after upper motor neuron lesions (e.g., stroke). This reduction in spasticity can be very beneficial when the rehabilitation therapist is trying to prevent or treat contracture associated with spasticity. Botox injection may allow for more effective limb positioning, stretching, splinting, and serial casting techniques in therapy. Botox has been used to treat severe spasticity in the hemiplegic upper extremity after stroke (Gallichio, 2004; Ozcakir & Sivrioglu, 2007).

The rehabilitation therapist should use the time that spasticity is effectively reduced (typically a 3 mo period) to normalize muscle length in order to facilitate effective muscle function and to allow the patient to complete activities of daily living such as personal hygiene and dressing. However, the rehabilitation thera-pist must also realize the functional limitations that may result from blocking the final common pathway to the muscle. Functional consequences often occur when a muscle goes from spastic paralysis to flaccid paralysis. The therapist must target other muscle groups that can assist in function and employ adaptive and compensatory techniques. It also provides an opportunity for the rehabilitation therapist to train the weak antagonists to the spastic muscles without excessive resistance from the spastic muscle(s). For example, when the spastic wrist and finger flexors are injected with Botox, the weak, inhibited wrist and finger extensors can be trained (Ciccone, 2007; Gallichio, 2004).

Botox has been used to treat a variety of speech–language pathology disorders, including spastic dysphonia and dysphagia. Spastic dysphonia is one of the most severe neurologic voice disorders. The voice is produced by hyperadduction of the vocal cords, and the false cords may be closed. As a result, the patient's voice sounds strangled (Boone & McFarlane, 2000; Ciccone, 2007; Satkunam, 2003). Injections of Botox are the primary method of treating spastic dysphonia. Botox may be injected into the thyroarytenoid (posterior end) with absorption also into the lateral cricoarytenoid. The patient may experience several weeks of coughing, breathiness, and mild symptoms of aspiration. The patient usually returns to the rehabilitation therapist for voice therapy after a few weeks. The combination of Botox injections and voice therapy usually results in a functional voice for up to 6 mo. Increasing phonatory tightness may indicate that continued injections are needed (Boone & McFarlane, 2000). Botox may also be injected into the laryngopharynx to treat bilateral vocal cord paralysis, vocal tics, stuttering, and arytenoid rebalancing and to prevent posterior glottic stenosis and recurrent vocal fold granuloma, ventricular dysphonia, puberphonia, and dysphagia. Botox can also be used as an adjunct to voice therapy for disorders such as adductor spasmodic dysphonia. Chapter 24 discusses the use of Botox in treating dysphagia (Cunningham & Teller, 2004; Murry & Woodsen, 1995).

Muscle Spasm

Skeletal muscle spasm is involuntary muscle tension that is the result of orthopedic musculoskeletal injury or compression of a spinal nerve root (peripheral nervous system). For example, a patient who has sustained a whiplash injury in a motor vehicle accident may experience a continuous tonic muscle contraction in the upper trapezius that limits range of motion and causes pain. Researchers believe that the purpose of this hyperexcitability of skeletal muscle, often called muscle guarding, is to stabilize the affected joint or body part.

Incidence

The exact incidence of muscle spasm worldwide or in the United States is unknown because musculoskeletal spasm is a clinical manifestation of underlying musculoskeletal conditions. For example, cervical spasm commonly occurs as a result of a whiplash injury to the neck, and low-back spasm commonly occurs as a result of musculoskeletal injury to the lumbar spine. The incidence of cervical spasm associated with whiplash is 3.8/1,000 people in the United States. Forty to 70% of the population will experience clinically significant neck pain (Hunter & Freeman, 2008). Approximately 80% of the population in the United States will experience an episode of lower back pain at some time during a lifetime (Rubin, 2007). Muscle relaxants are prescribed for approximately 1% of Americans with spasm in the spinal regions or the extremities (Dillon et al., 2004).

Etiology and Pathophysiology

The neurophysiology of muscle spasm is related to the pain spasm cycle. After acute injury, chemical mediators such as prostaglandin, **bradykinin**, histamines, and substance P are released to the injured area. These chemical mediators cause chemical irritation to free nerve endings and increase the nociceptive (pain) input to the spinal cord, which in turn stimulates the alpha motor neuron to fire excessively and causes hyperexcitability of the affected skeletal muscle (spasm). Prolonged spasm often decreases blood flow to the area,

causing ischemia and further muscle spasm. The use of transcutaneous electrical stimulation can decrease nociceptive (painful) stimuli to the spinal cord, which can result in less nociceptive input or stimulation of firing of alpha motor neurons. Removing the pain shuts down the pain spasm cycle.

PATIENT CASE 2

E.F. is a 42-yr-old male employed as a long-distance mover. While lifting a heavy box, E.F. felt a muscle strain in the lower part of his back. He immediately went home and put ice on his back and stayed home from work for several days, hoping to gain relief from the muscle spasm in his back. He finally went to a physician, who recommended continued rest for a while and prescribed chlorzoxazone (Parafon Forte) as a muscle relaxant. E.F. has been taking this muscle relaxant with extra strength Tylenol to control his pain and muscle spasm. E.F. began experiencing fatigue and dizziness and on several occasions came very close to falling. Because E.F. knew that using this medication could result in drowsiness, he was not significantly worried about the side effect. However, he has recently been experiencing nausea and vomiting, abdominal pain, and has lost his appetite. His wife noticed today that his skin and eyes have developed a yellow color and insisted that he call his physician for an appointment.

Question

Are his symptoms related to the medications that E.F. is taking for his muscle spasm and pain?

Answer

E.F. was not concerned about these symptoms and did not relate them to his medications. His wife, on the other hand, was very concerned and called the doctor. The doctor told her that these symptoms were serious and related to his medication and that E.F. should come into the office to be seen right away. After examining E.F., the physician diagnosed medication-induced hepatotoxicity. E.F.'s decision to combine

Tylenol with the Parafon Forte resulted in a significant drug interaction that further increased risk of developing hepatotoxicity. E.F. was instructed to stop both medications and use local heat to the area of spasm. He was instructed to always check with his physician or pharmacist prior to adding an over-the-counter medication alongside prescribed medications to avoid serious drug interactions in the future. E.F.'s symptoms of hepatotoxicity were completely resolved two weeks after discontinuing these medications.

Rehabilitation Considerations

Side effects of most of the muscle relaxants used to treat spasm include sedation, dizziness, dry mouth, and gastrointestinal upset. Drowsiness and dizziness can also increase the risk of falls and may interfere with rehabilitation by impairing the patient's ability to follow instructions and participate in the therapy session. The clinician should educate the patient about the possibility of these symptoms and ensure the patient's safety during gait training and exercise sessions, especially when the patient is in early stages of taking these medications. These medications can also cause dysphagia and may affect the anticipatory, oral preparatory, and oral phases of swallowing. Xerostomia may interfere with formation and passage of a food bolus during the pharyngeal and esophageal phases of swallowing. The use of polysynaptic inhibitors should be limited to the short term, and long-term use should be avoided to prevent adverse side effects, tolerance, and dependency (Carl & Johnson, 2006; Chou et al., 2004; Ciccone, 2007).

Medication Therapy

Anti-inflammatory medications can help eliminate the chemical irritation that causes nociceptive input. Pain medications can help eliminate the painful stimuli that enter the spinal cord and stimulate the increased alpha motor neuron firing. Muscle relaxants can be used to decrease alpha motor neuron firing directly. At times a combination of medications is necessary to address the underlying pathophysiology in a comprehensive manner. For example, patients with severe back pain related to a lumbar disc herniation have a great deal of inflammation around the affected nerve root, muscle spasm throughout the low back on the affected side, severe pain, and paresthesias (e.g., burning, numbness) in the low back or nerve root distribution (e.g., sciatica). A common initial treatment for lumbar disc herniation is the prescription of **opiate** pain medication to treat the severe pain, muscle relaxants to treat the muscle spasm, and a steroid dose pack to decrease inflammation. These medications in combination can be highly effective in calming the pain, spasm, and inflammation, allowing the patient to move forward with rehabilitation (Chou et al., 2004; Ciccone, 2007).

Medications used for the above conditions include the benzodiazepine diazepam (Valium) and the polysynaptic inhibitors, which include carisoprodol (Soma), chlorzoxazone (Parafon Forte), cyclobenzaprine (Flexeril), metaxalone (Skelaxin), methocarbamol (Robaxin), and orphenadrine citrate (Norflex). The polysynaptic inhibitors decrease polysynaptic reflex activity at the spinal cord level. They block the afferent input at the dorsal horn of the spinal cord, where all sensory input is received before interacting at the alpha motor neuron. This prevents the firing of the alpha motor neuron to the muscle and decreases muscle spasm. Research shows that the polysynaptic inhibitors are more effective than placebo in decreasing muscle spasm. Table 9.1 summarizes dosing and side effects of these medications (Chou et al., 2004; Ciccone, 2007).

Summary

Spasticity and musculoskeletal spasm are commonly seen in rehabilitation patients. This chapter summarizes medications used to treat spasticity and muscle spasm. The rehabilitation therapist should be familiar with the physiologic action of the medications, timing medications for peak effect, and the side effects that can affect the rehabilitation process. The rehabilitation therapist should alter therapy sessions to maximize patient safety and minimize risks associated with these side effects.

Medications Used to Treat Parkinson's Disease

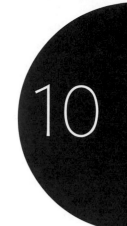

The rehabilitation therapist may encounter patients with Parkinson's disease in clinical practice. This chapter summarizes signs and symptoms associated with Parkinson's disease and reviews how this disease can affect rehabilitation. It also reviews medications used to treat Parkinson's disease and explains how these medications can affect the patient's cognition, behavior, and motor function. Finally, the chapter provides recommendations for altering rehabilitation sessions to accommodate the needs of patients with Parkinson's disease.

Parkinson's Disease

Parkinson's disease (PD) is the second most common neurological disorder in patients over 65 yr of age (Alzheimer's disease is first) and the third most common diagnosis presented in neurology clinics (after headache and seizures). In the United States, costs associated with caring for patients with PD exceed $6 billion annually (Chen et al., 2009).

PD involves a progressive degeneration of the **substantia nigra** neurons and fibers projecting into the neostriatum and globus pallidus along with a profound depletion of the central neurotransmitter dopamine and a relative increase in acetylcholine activity. This results in extrapyramidal motor dysfunction. Loss of 70% to 80% of substantia nigra neuronal activity occurs before the initial symptoms of PD appear. Dysfunction associated with the dopamine receptors results in loss of motor control and can contribute to significant disability in many patients. This disability usually

occurs 10 to 15 yr after initial diagnosis (Chen, 2002; Chen et al., 2009; Chen & Swope, 2007; Lertxundi et al., 2008; Nelson et al., 2002; Standaert & Young, 2001; Weintraub et al., 2008a).

PD is characterized by bradykinesia (slowed movement), tremors at rest, muscle rigidity, and postural instability. A unilateral tremor of the hand or foot, called resting tremor, is the first symptom of PD in about 70% of patients. It is called resting tremor because it is evident when the patient is relaxed and subsides with purposeful movement. Hand tremors can cause a back-and-forth rubbing of the thumb and forefinger known as pill rolling. Rigidity is an increased muscle resistance to passive movement and may cause aching and muscle cramps. Other motor symptoms include posture that is stooped and flexed forward, decreased arm swing, dystonia, festination (accelerated gait), akinesia (absence of movement), freezing (intermittent akinesia), turning en bloc (i.e., lack of truncal rotation when turning), shuffling gait, and micrographia. Drug-induced parkinsonism, which should always be ruled out when making a diagnosis of PD, can be caused by many medications, including typical antipsychotics (e.g., phenothiazines, butyrophenones, risperidone), certain **antiemetics** (e.g., metoclopramide, prochlorperazine, promethazine), and certain antihypertensives (e.g., reserpine and methyldopa) (Factor & Weiner, 2008; Kyle & Kyle, 2007; Lew, 2007).

Nonmotor symptoms are grouped into four categories: cognitive, sleep, sensory, and autonomic. Cognitive symptoms include slowed reaction times, fatigue, dementia, psychosis, anxiety, depression, apathy, and anhedonia. Cognitive impairment occurs in 85% of patients within 15 yr of diagnosis, and 30% to 50% of patients develop PD dementia. Sleep disturbances include daytime somnolence, insomnia, rapid eye movement sleep disorder, sleep apnea, and restless-leg syndrome. Sensation changes include olfactory dysfunction (occurs in 70%-100% of patients), pain, paresthesias, impaired proprioception, and impaired sensitivity to visual contrast. One of the first symptoms of PD is a loss of smell. Autonomic symptoms include orthostatic hypotension, urinary incontinence, constipation and gastric dysmotility, dysphagia with choking, hypersalivation, **hypophonia**, temperature intolerance, and altered sexual function. Medications used to treat the motor symptoms of PD can worsen the nonmotor symptoms of PD. For example, levodopa or dopamine agonists can worsen hallucinations or orthostatic hypotension in the PD patient (Weintraub et al., 2008a; Wood, 2011).

Incidence

Accurately identifying the incidence of PD worldwide is difficult because many studies use different methods to calculate incidence. A number of studies have come up with a similar incidence of 16 to 19/100,000 people. Most incidence studies have also shown that PD is more prevalent in males than in females (Twelves et al., 2002). PD affects more than 1 million people in the United States and commonly affects people over age 50 yr. It affects 1.5% of people over age 60 yr and 4% to 5% of people over age 85 yr. Of all cases of PD, 90% are sporadic and 10% are of genetic origin. Risk of developing PD is two- to threefold higher in patients with a first-degree relative with PD (Chen, 2002; Chen et al., 2009; Kyle & Kyle, 2007; Langston et al., 2007; Weintraub et al., 2008a).

Etiology and Pathophysiology

Researchers have long known that PD is a chronic, progressive disease of the subcortical gray matter in the basal ganglia. Recent studies have documented that PD also involves extranigral pathways and connections between the autonomic basal ganglia, spinal cord, and neocortex of the brain. PD involves a loss of dopaminergic neurons in the substantia nigra and is characterized by the presence of insoluble protein inclusions called Lewy bodies or Lewy dendrites. These Lewy bodies and **dendrites** contain misfolded alpha-synuclein protein. In the premotor stage of PD, Lewy bodies and dendrites are found in the brainstem (locus coeruleus, medulla oblongata, raphe nuclei, and olfactory bulb) and are associated with development of symptoms of anxiety, depression, and impaired olfaction. As PD progresses, the Lewy pathology of the nerves spreads to the midbrain (particularly the substantia nigra); this is associated with development of motor symptoms seen with PD. As PD advances, the Lewy body pathology spreads to the cortex; this is associated with many of the behavioral and cognitive symptoms seen in patients with PD (Chen, 2012).

PATIENT CASE 1

J.B. is a 55-yr-old male with a 1 yr history of PD. J.B.'s speech is dysarthric but his language patterns are normal. J.B.'s initial symptoms included loss of smell and impaired cognition, which involved reduced processing speed and reduced attention span. J.B. also began to experience resting tremors in his hands. Since then he has begun to lose some of his facial expressions. The most prominent symptom, however, seems to be depression. J.B. asks the rehabilitation therapist how his depression is related to PD. He also asks whether his symptoms of resting tremors and loss of facial expression are associated with his disease.

Question

How should the rehabilitation therapist respond to J.B.'s questions?

Answer

The rehabilitation therapist should tell J.B. that patients with PD can experience depression due to changes in the level of the chemical messenger **dopamine** in the brain. The therapist should also tell him that the resting **tremors** and loss of facial expression (masked facies) are normal symptoms associated with his disease (Carl & Johnson, 2006; Chen, 2012). The therapist should contact J.B.'s prescriber to facilitate additional education from the prescriber regarding J.B.'s disease.

Rehabilitation Considerations

Therapy may include physical therapy, occupational therapy, speech–language pathology, psychosocial support, medication therapy, and surgery for the drug-refractory patient. One goal of individualized therapy is to maintain mental and physical function as long as possible. The rehabilitation therapist focuses heavily on improving motor control and postural stability necessary in reaching tasks, gait, transfers, and activities of daily living (Chen, 2002; Chen et al., 2009; Morris et al., 2008; Nelson et al., 2002; Standaert & Young, 2001; Trail et al., 2008).

Bradykinesia is the hallmark of PD. One test of motor speed includes the Grooved Peg Board Test, a timed manipulative-dexterity task that evaluates the patient's ability to place pegs into the holes of a peg board. This simple test provides a reliable index of brain damage and severity of the disease and identifies patients who have difficulty with manual dexterity and fine-motor movements. PD patients generally function within normal limits on tests of apraxia. A relationship appears to exist between PD motor symptoms and cognition. Cognition is usually normal when the predominant motor symptom is tremor, and cognition is usually impaired when the predominant motor symptom is rigidity and bradykinesia. Understanding the relationship between motor functioning and cognition can help the rehabilitation therapist more accurately treat the PD patient (Yorkston et al., 2004).

Patients with PD have problems with functional movement, including bradykinesia, tremor, rigidity, and impaired postural reflexes. Risk of falling is increased in these patients; physical therapy can help prevent falls. On-off phenomenon is a term used to describe fluctuations in the control of motor symptoms in patients treated with the PD medication, levodopa. As the disease progresses the duration of motor control (termed the "on" state) becomes shortened and the "wearing off" of the effects at the end of the dosage period occurs progressively earlier. In the "off" state the patient becomes very stiff, slow, and may be unable to move for a few minutes (termed freezing). In some patients this off state is predictable, occurring several hours after a dose of levodopa and the patient can plan their activities accordingly. In other patients, the off period occurs less predictably and can result in increased risk for falls. Adjustments in a patient's medication regimen used to correct this on-off phenomenon are described later in the chapter. Freezing of gait is observed as the severity of PD increases. Additionally, freezing of gait occurs more often when the patient attempts turning movements and is associated with falls. Medications may improve stride length in the PD patient. However, dysphagia, falling, freezing of gait, and postural instability may not respond to dopamine enhancing medications and can be disabling (Chen, 2012).

The rehabilitation therapist must be proactive in preventing contracture and disuse atrophy and must work toward improving the neuromuscular control necessary for functional activities. Use of the following strategies can also enhance motor performance: rhythmical auditory feedback; rocking the body to stimulate weight shifting necessary for gait; drills that require the patient to step over tape lines on the floor; and the use of quick head movements, music, clapping, verbal cueing, and self-talk. The rehabilitation therapist may schedule the patient's rehabilitation treatment to coincide with the peak effects of medications in order to help the patient maintain motor control and function during the therapy session. The use of rhythmic auditory stimulation has been shown to improve gait and motor performance (Brunt et al., 2008).

Each year, 68% of patients with PD experience a fall. Medications can significantly improve movement disorders in PD, but side effects of medications can also impair motor function. Medications used in patients with PD may also increase the risk of falls caused by postural hypotension, cognitive difficulties, reduced muscle strength, or blurred vision. The physical therapist should evaluate the patient's home environment and make recommendations for enhancing safety and preventing falls. For example, PD patients commonly have difficulty stepping over the edge of the bathtub. Installing grab bars and training the caregiver in the use of verbal cueing can be beneficial. Functional activities that involve visual cueing and feedback are more effective than noncued or traditional therapeutic exercise programs. For example, visual cueing during gait training improves stride length and minimizes time spent in double-leg stance. Verbal instruction sets using cognitive strategies have been shown to improve walking speed, amplitude of arm swing, and step length (Behrman et al., 1998). Because the patient likely has episodes of motor freeze-ups, it can be helpful for the therapist to evaluate the patient's home environment to determine where these events are likely to occur (e.g., narrow passageways) and to either modify the environment or train the family member in cueing the patient. Occupational therapists can help the patient carry out tasks of daily living such as brushing teeth, tying shoes, and self-feeding. Speech–language pathologists can assist with dysphagia, hydrophonia and impaired cognition by providing specific treatment plans to assist the patient in performance of ADL (Kyle & Kyle, 2007; Morris et al., 2008).

The rehabilitation therapist should monitor patients with a history of cardiac irregularities because levodopa therapy may increase risk of cardiac arrhythmias, especially during physical exertion. Furthermore, the therapist should monitor the patient during positional changes to minimize orthostatic hypotension related to the medication. The therapist should also be aware that patients with PD respond to submaximal exercise tests with greater heart rate and increased oxygen consumption regardless of medication use. This is an important concept in prescribing exercise for and monitoring this patient population (Protas et al., 1996).

Some of the earliest symptoms of PD are related to voice and speech. In hypokinetic dysarthria, the major speech symptom, voice is characterized by monotone, reduced volume, and hoarseness or breathlessness. The patient can also experience reduced facial expressiveness and bodily gestures, which can influence the listener's perception of the speaker's communication skills (Sapir et al., 2008). The patient's vocal difficulties can be attributed to laryngeal dysfunction such as vocal fold bowing, laryngeal tremor, or incomplete vocal fold closure. The patient with PD may also develop respiratory dysfunction, resulting in reduced vital capacity and changed intraoral air pressure. Articulatory disorders may also be seen in this population, and PD may affect the rate of articulation. Sensory difficulties play an important role in exacerbating the patient's articulatory difficulties (Sapir et al., 2008; Zweig & Elliott, 2008).

Studies have indicated that transcortical or transdermal stimulation of the motor cortex concurrent with exercise of the associated muscles may be of therapeutic value in treatment of speech, voice, and swallowing disorders in PD. In the study of Pagni and colleagues (2003), such therapy allowed a reduction of 50% in drug dosage. For training of the motor nerves concurrent with the electrical stimulation of the motor cortex to be successful, the patient must cognitively engage in the training of the motor nerves during completion of the prescribed motor tasks. Training in self-perception, internal cueing, and amplitude regulation is part of the Lee Silverman voice treatment. The rehabilitation therapist concerned with voice, speech, and swallowing should become familiar with this treatment modality. Research on pallidotomy and thalamotomy as they relate to speech has provided inconsistent results (Sapir et al., 2008).

Maintaining adequate nutrition in patients with PD is especially challenging because of symptoms that limit the patient's ability to chew, swallow, and eat independently. The clinical dietitian can provide the patient with teaching and provide assistance in developing a patient-specific diet plan. The speech–language pathologist can assist the patient with problems encountered in chewing, swallowing, cognition, and communication. **Gastroparesis** is often seen in patients with prominent on-off symptoms. Prokinetic medications can be of assistance in treatment of gastroparesis but may also interfere with the action of PD medications that enhance motor function. Olfactory losses, which can affect taste, smell, and appetite, are seen in 90% of patients with PD and can negatively affect nutritional status (Chen, 2012). In PD patients with gastroparesis or gastroesophageal reflux disease, alternative methods of providing nutrition such as jejunal feedings after surgical jejunostomy may be considered (Quigley, 2008). Calcium and vitamin D supplementation (with or without or sunlight exposure) is important in preventing osteoporosis and bone fracture and should be incorporated into the therapeutic plan for patients with PD (Chen, 2002; Nelson et al., 2002; Standaert & Young, 2001).

A vast majority of patients with PD experience difficulties with dysphagia. Swallowing difficulties, along with voice and speech difficulties, may be one of the first signs of PD. An important symptom that contributes to dysphagia in PD patients is sialorrhea (drooling). The drooling and saliva-management problems are the result of dysfunctional swallowing, not of abnormal salivation. The rehabilitation specialist, especially the speech–language pathologist, must notify the team and the patient's physician about the patient's symptoms of dysphagia in a timely fashion so that appropriate interventions are used to maintain safe and adequate nutrition in the patient (Fuh et al., 1997; Gallena et al., 2001; Quigley, 2008).

Dysphagia in the PD population is observed in all phases of the swallow. The oral phase can be affected by reduced oral transit times, lingual tremor, drooling, lingual pumping, piecemeal **deglutition**, premature spillage, delayed lingual onset, prolonged ramp-like posture, and reduced lingual strength and motion. Difficulties during the pharyngeal phase include valleculae and pyriform pooling, laryngeal dysfunction, swallow delay, decreased hypolaryngeal elevation, aspiration, laryngeal closure difficulties, reduced peristalsis, and increased transit time. Esophageal difficulties may include reduced esophageal peristalsis (Fuh et al., 1997; Gallena et al., 2001; Sapir et al., 2008; Yorkston et al., 2004).

A large proportion of PD patients experience some form of cognitive difficulty. Cognitive difficulties have been reported at all stages of the disease. Even in early-stage PD, patients experience impaired executive functioning and difficulties with cognitive slowing. Cognitive slowing (bradyphrenia) is characteristic of PD that increases as the disease becomes more severe (York & Alvarez, 2008). Executive function comprises working memory, inhibition and shifting, and attention. Patients with PD may require assistance in areas of safety, financial planning, driving, and occupational performance (York & Alvarez, 2008).

The cognitive problems that occur most frequently are difficulties with recall memory, executive functioning, verbal fluency, and attention, as well as impaired visuospatial functioning. These cognitive disorders are associated with disorders of prefrontal cortex caused by dopamine deficiency. Concurrent processing of cognitive information is also impaired and attributed to dopamine deficiency. Visuospatial difficulties in PD include problems with visual discrimination, visuospatial processing, visual attention, visuomotor abilities, and body spatial orientation. On the other hand, visuosensory functions and visual-recognition skills appear to be intact in the PD population (York and Alvarez, 2008). In general, PD patients have more difficulty with recall memory than with recognition memory (York & Alvarez, 2008). Patients with PD also perform better on frontal lobe tasks such as shifting, verbal fluency, and psychomotor speed when treated with levodopa therapy (Marder & Jacobs, 2008). Difficulty with verbal fluency, one of the earliest signs of PD, results from impaired executive function rather than language impairment. Patients with PD demonstrate impaired recall of events in the immediate past (Marder & Jacobs, 2008).

Medication Therapy

Medication therapies for PD aim to correct the imbalance between dopamine and **acetylcholine** activity. They accomplish this by enhancing the activity of dopamine through dopamine or dopamine substitutes (agonists) or by inhibiting the breakdown of dopamine by metabolism. Medications used to treat PD fall into six categories: anticholinergics, dopamine agonists, levodopa with or without carbidopa, catechol-O-methyl-transferase inhibitors, monoamine oxidase-B inhibitors, and N-methyl-D-aspartate receptor inhibitors. The coming sections discuss these medications in detail. Medication therapy should be initiated once functional impairment is evident. Medications should be initiated at a low dose and slowly titrated up to the lowest effective dose. Medications should always be tapered before discontinuance (Chen, 2002; Chen et al., 2009; Ciccone, 2007; Langston et al., 2007; Nelson et al., 2002; Rascol et al., 2003; Standaert & Young, 2001).

The American Academy of Neurology developed guidelines for initiating medication therapy for PD and maximizing the long-term effectiveness of dopamine-enhancing medications in the treatment of PD. These guidelines recommend initiating treatment of the first PD symptoms with medications such as selegiline (Eldepryl, Zelapar) or amantadine (Symmetrel) in an effort to delay the use of dopamine in early PD. Amantadine (Symmetrel) should be tried before selegiline (Eldepryl, Zelapar) if the patient is having dyskinesia, is elderly, or has cognitive dysfunction (Langston et al., 2007).

Once PD advances, dopamine-enhancing medications such as levodopa (Sinemet) or dopamine agonists such as bromocriptine (Parlodel), ropinirole (Requip), pramipexole (Mirapex), apomorphine (Apokyn), and rotigotine (Neupro) should be used. Levodopa (Sinemet) is preferred for symptoms of bradykinesia, whereas a dopamine agonist is preferred for symptoms of dyskinesia. When significant off time of the control of motor effects between doses of levodopa is observed, the American Academy of Neurology recommends first adding entacapone (Comtan) or rasagiline (Azilect) to the levodopa therapy. If these agents fail to reduce levodopa off time, another dopamine agonist should be added to the levodopa therapy (Langston et al., 2007). Table 10.1 classifies the medications used to treat PD and lists the side effects commonly associated with each agent that may affect rehabilitation.

Scheduling the patient's therapy session to coincide with peak medication effects (during on effects) can enhance the patient's neuromuscular control during therapy interventions and functional training tasks. Peak effects of products containing levodopa such as Sinemet differ with each patient and medication dosage form and can vary with diet and protein intake. The therapist should ask the patient or family member when peak effects occur in relationship to time of medication administration. Peak effects usually occur 1 h after taking an oral immediate-release dose. Rapid-dissolving medications have a faster onset of 10 to 15 min, and subcutaneous medications have a shorter onset of 15 to 30 min. Long-acting products have a more delayed onset; peak effects occur 1 to 4 h after administration of the dose. Peak effects achieved with the long-acting product improve motor function for several hours. For example, scheduling rehabilitation at least 1 h after the morning long-acting dose of levodopa maximizes motor performance and reduces fatigue levels. Avoiding drug interactions with food or other medications is important in optimizing medication effects and avoiding toxicity. Table 10.2 lists important drug interactions involving agents used to treat PD (Chen, 2002; Chen et al., 2009; Langston et al., 2007; Nelson et al., 2002; Standaert & Young, 2001).

Dopamine Enhancers

Dopamine-enhancing medications include the levo isomer of dopamine (levodopa, L-dopa), levodopa combined with carbidopa (Sinemet), and medications that act on the dopamine receptor, enhancing dopamine effects. Other classes of medications enhance the effects of dopamine by decreasing its metabolism. Dopamine enhancers include dopamine agonists, catechol-O-methyl-transferase inhibitors, and monoamine oxidase-B inhibitors (Chen, 2002; Chen et al., 2009).

Levodopa and Levodopa—Carbidopa (Sinemet)   For more than 30 yr, levodopa has been the gold standard of PD therapy. Levodopa, which is manufactured in the body from the dietary amino acid tyrosine, is the precursor to the catecholamines dopamine, norepinephrine, and epinephrine. Levodopa crosses the

See table 10.1 in the web resource for a full list of medication-specific indications, dosing recommendations, and side effects.

Table 10.1 Medications Used to Treat Parkinson's Disease

Medication	Side effects affecting rehab							Other side effects or considerations
Anticholinergics: Used as single therapy to treat tremor in early PD, especially in younger patients.								
Benztropine (Cogentin)	Cog ++	S ++	A ++	Motor ++	D ++	Com ++	F ++	Side effects common to all agents: Nausea, vomiting, diarrhea, constipation, dry mouth, dry eyes, cognitive impairment, sedation, ataxia, urinary retention, tachycardia, nervousness, depression, psychosis
Procyclidine (Kemadrin)	Cog ++	S ++	A ++	Motor ++	D ++	Com ++	F ++	
Trihexyphenidyl (Artane)	Cog ++	S ++	A ++	Motor ++	D ++	Com ++	F ++	
N-methyl-D-aspartic acid receptor inhibitor: Used as single therapy in early PD to treat mild symptoms of bradykinesia and rigidity; used as adjunctive therapy with levodopa to reduce levodopa-induced dyskinesias.								
Amantadine (Symmetrel)	Cog ++	S 0	A ++	Motor 0	D ++	Com ++	F +++	Hypotension, dizziness, edema, livedo reticularis, seizures, heart failure, suicide attempts, confusion, hallucinations, nausea, constipation, gastrointestinal bleeding, vomiting, dry mouth
Levodopa enhancers: Gold standard treatment of advanced PD. Initiation is delayed as long as possible by using alternative therapies to prolong its effectiveness in advanced PD.								
Carbidopa–levodopa (Sinemet) Immediate- or sustained-release product (Parcopa) Orally disintegrating tablets: 25/100 mg and 25/250 mg	Cog +++	S +++	A +++	Motor +++	D +++	Com ++	F ++++	Anorexia, nausea, vomiting, dry mouth, gastrointestinal bleeding, constipation, somnolence, hallucinations, delusions, sleep disturbances, choreiform movements, dystonia, bradykinesia, cardiac irregularities, orthostatic hypotension, mental changes, depression, dementia, sleep attacks (rare)
Carbidopa–levodopa–entacapone combination (Stalevo 50: 12.5/50/200 mg; Stalevo 100: 25/100/200 mg; Stalevo 150: 37.5/150/200 mg; Stalevo 200: 50/200/200 mg)	Cog ++	S +++	A ++	Motor +++	D ++	Com ++	F +++	

› continued

Table 10.1 ›*continued*

Medication	Side effects affecting rehab							Other side effects or considerations
Levodopa enhancer: Used in combination with levodopa or Sinemet to provide enhanced levels of dopamine and reduce nausea and vomiting associated with levodopa therapy.								
Carbidopa (Lodosyn)	Cog +++	S +++	A ++	Motor +	D +++	Com ++	F ++	Confusion, constipation, diarrhea, dizziness, drowsiness, dry mouth, headache, loss of appetite, nausea, taste changes, trouble sleeping, stomach upset, urinary tract infection, vomiting
Direct dopamine receptor agonists: Used in early PD to postpone use of levodopa; used in combination with levodopa to reduce the needed dose and prolong the effects of levodopa.								
Bromocriptine (Parlodel)	Cog +++	S +++	A +++	Motor +++	D +++	Com ++	F +++	Nausea, dyskinesia, hallucinations, confusion, on–off phenomenon, dizziness, vomiting, hypotension, constipation, retroperitoneal fibrosis (rare), impulse-control disorders, visual changes, insomnia, depression, sleep attacks
Pramipexole (Mirapex)	Cog +++	S +++	A +++	Motor +++	D +++	Com ++	F ++++	Side effects common to both: Hallucinations, dizziness, somnolence, anorexia, nausea, vomiting, dry mouth, gastrointestinal bleeding, constipation, edema, compulsive behaviors, confusion, sleep attacks
Ropinirole (Requip)	Cog +++	S +++	A ++	Motor ++	D +++	Com ++	F ++++	
Apomorphine (Apokyn): Adjunct therapy used to treat freezing episodes associated with advanced PD. Administered as subcutaneous injection. Use antiemetic therapy with administration to prevent nausea and vomiting.								
Apomorphine (Apokyn)	Cog +++	S +++	A +++	Motor ++	D ++	Com +	F +++	Irritation at the injection site, yawning, dyskinesias, nausea, vomiting, somnolence, dizziness, rhinorrhea, hallucinations, edema, chest pain, sweating, flushing, pallor, orthostasis, impulse-control disorders, sleep attacks. Administered as subcutaneous injection. Use antiemetic therapy with administration to prevent nausea and vomiting.
Rotigotine (Neupro) transdermal patch: Useful for patients who cannot swallow; provides better control of motor symptoms with decreased off time and doubled on time of dopamine effects.								
Rotigotine (Neupro) transdermal patch	Cog ++	S +++	A +	Motor +	D ++	Com +	F ++	Reactions at application site, nausea, vomiting, dizziness, somnolence, sleep attacks
Inhibitors of enzymatic breakdown of dopamine: MAO-B inhibitors used in early, untreated PD to provide relief of symptoms, delay need for initiation of levodopa, extend mobility, and reduce freezing of gait. When used with levodopa in later PD, it can reduce the dosage requirement for levodopa and attenuate the wearing-off phenomenon.								
Rasagiline (Azilect)	Cog +++	S +	A +++	Motor +++	D ++	Com +	F ++++	Dyskinesia, arthralgias, depression, dyspepsia, falls, hallucinations, diarrhea, nausea, vomiting, constipation, weight loss, postural hypotension, headache, dizziness, drowsiness, dry mouth, flu-like symptoms, sleeplessness, stuffy nose, ecchymosis with higher doses

Medication	Side effects affecting rehab	Other side effects or considerations
Selegiline (Eldepryl; Zelapar—rapidly dissolving tablet)	Cog S A Motor D Com F +++ 0 +++ +++ +++ ++ ++++	Anorexia, gastrointestinal upset, gastrointestinal bleeding, dry mouth, constipation, orthostasis, hypertension, chest pain, syncope, arrhythmia, extrapyramidal symptoms, dyskinesias, delusions, insomnia, agitation, confusion, hallucinations, depression. Zelapar has fewer side effects than oral tablet.

Inhibitors of enzymatic breakdown of dopamine: COMT inhibitor used to prolong levodopa effects, enhance motor function, and reduce off time. Not effective as monotherapy; use with levodopa.

Medication	Side effects affecting rehab	Other side effects or considerations
Entacapone (Comtan)	Cog S A Motor D Com F +++ 0 +++ ++++ +++ +++ ++++	Diarrhea, exacerbation of levodopa side effects, bright-orange urine, anorexia, nausea, vomiting, dry mouth, gastrointestinal bleeding, constipation, confusion, extrapyramidal symptoms, dyskinesias, hyperkinesias, dizziness, abdominal pain, hypotension, syncope, hallucinations, rhabdomyolysis (rare)
Tolcapone* (Tasmar)	Cog S A Motor D Com F +++ +++ +++ ++++ +++ +++ ++++	Explosive diarrhea, dyskinesia, nausea, sleep disorders, dystonia, excessive dreaming, anorexia, muscle cramps, orthostasis, somnolence, confusion, dizziness, headache, urine discoloration. Exacerbates side effects of levodopa. Hepatotoxicity; monitor liver-function tests. Discontinue if liver-function test results are twice normal levels. Fatal hepatotoxicity is rare.

*Use limited due to hepatotoxicity with this medication.

Cog = cognition; S = sedation; A = agitation or mania; Motor = discoordination; D = dysphagia; Com = communication; F = falls; COMT = catechol-O-methyl-transferase; MAO-B = monoamine oxidase-B; PD = Parkinson's disease.

The likelihood rating scale for encountering the side effects is as follows: 0 = Almost no probability of encountering side effects. + = Little likelihood of encountering side effects. +/++ = Low probability of encountering side effects; however, probability increases with increased dosage. ++ = Medium likelihood of encountering side effects. +++ = High likelihood of encountering side effects, particularly with high doses. ++++ = Highest likelihood of encountering side effects; best to avoid in at-risk patients.

Table 10.2   Drug Interactions in Medications Used to Treat Parkinson's Disease

Medication	Interacting medication classes and examples	Effects of interaction
Anticholinergics		
Benztropine (Cogentin)	Antihistamines: diphenhydramine (Benadryl), promethazine (Phenergan) Tricyclic antidepressants: amitriptyline (Elavil)	Increased anticholinergic side effects such as dry mouth, nausea, vomiting, decreased gastric secretions, decreased gastric motility, sedation, confusion, and ataxia
	Central nervous system depressants: Benzodiazepine: diazepam (Valium) Opioid: morphine Antipsychotic: chlorpromazine (Thorazine)	Enhanced sedation, confusion, and ataxia

› continued

Table 10.2 ›continued

Medication	Interacting medication classes and examples	Effects of interaction
Procyclidine (Kemadrin)	Antihistamine: diphenhydramine (Benadryl), promethazine (Phenergan) Tricyclic antidepressant: amitriptyline (Elavil)	Increased anticholinergic side effects such as dry mouth, nausea, vomiting, decreased gastric secretions, decreased gastric motility, sedation, confusion, and ataxia
	Central nervous system depressants: Benzodiazepines: diazepam (Valium) Opioids: morphine Antipsychotic: chlorpromazine (Thorazine)	Enhanced sedation, confusion, and ataxia
Trihexyphenidyl (Artane)	Antihistamines: diphenhydramine (Benadryl), promethazine (Phenergan) Tricyclic antidepressant: amitriptyline (Elavil)	Increased anticholinergic side effects such as dry mouth, nausea, vomiting, decreased gastric secretions, decreased gastric motility, sedation, confusion, and ataxia
	Central nervous system depressants: Benzodiazepine: diazepam (Valium) Opioid: morphine Antipsychotic: chlorpromazine (Thorazine)	Enhanced sedation, confusion, and ataxia
Dopamine enhancers		
Amantadine (Symmetrel)	Antipsychotics: haloperidol (Haldol), olanzapine (Zyprexa)	Increased extrapyramidal symptoms, dry mouth, confusion, nausea, vomiting, and constipation
	Antiemetics: metoclopramide (Reglan), promethazine (Phenergan)	Increased extrapyramidal symptoms, dry mouth, confusion, nausea, vomiting, and constipation
Carbidopa–levodopa (Sinemet)	Antipsychotics: haloperidol (Haldol), olanzapine (Zyprexa)	Increased extrapyramidal symptoms, dry mouth, confusion, nausea, vomiting, and constipation
	Antiemetics: metoclopramide (Reglan), promethazine (Phenergan)	Increased extrapyramidal symptoms, dry mouth, confusion, nausea, vomiting, and constipation
	Food	Increases levodopa levels by 50%; peaks by 25%
	Iron	Binds to levodopa in stomach; space by 2 h. Decreases absorption of and effects of levodopa.
	Antihypertensive: methyldopa (Aldomet)	Decreased effects of levodopa; methyldopa blocks central conversion of levodopa to dopamine
Direct dopamine receptor agonists		
Bromocriptine (Parlodel)	Antiemetics: metoclopramide (Reglan), promethazine (Phenergan)	Increased extrapyramidal symptoms, dry mouth, confusion, nausea, vomiting, and constipation
Pramipexole (Mirapex)	Antipsychotics: haloperidol (Haldol), olanzapine (Zyprexa) Antiemetics: metoclopramide (Reglan), promethazine (Phenergan)	Increased extrapyramidal symptoms, dry mouth, confusion, nausea, vomiting, and constipation

Medication	Interacting medication classes and examples	Effects of interaction
Ropinirole (Requip)	Antipsychotics: haloperidol (Haldol), olanzapine (Zyprexa) Antiemetics: metoclopramide (Reglan), promethazine (Phenergan)	Increased extrapyramidal symptoms, dry mouth, confusion, nausea, vomiting, and constipation
Apomorphine (Apokyn)	Serotonin antagonists: ondansetron, granisetron, dolasetron, palonosetron, alosetron	Contraindicated due to profound hypotension and loss of consciousness
	Dopamine antagonists: amoxapine (Asendin), metoclopramide (Reglan), promethazine (Phenergan) Antipsychotics: phenothiazine, butyrophenone, and thiothixene classes	Antagonizes effects of apomorphine
	Antihypertensive agents and vasodilators: calcium channel blockers and nitrates, including isosorbide (Isordil) Calcium channel blockers: nifedipine, diltiazem Beta blockers: metoprolol, propranolol, nitroglycerin Isosorbide	Increased risk of hypotension, falls, bone and joint injury, and myocardial infarction
	Medications that prolong the QT interval: levofloxacin, quinidine, erythromycin	Additive effects of QT prolongation and arrhythmias
Rotigotine (Neupro)	No known drug interactions	

Monoamine oxidase-B inhibitors

Selegiline (high dose >20 mg/day; Eldepryl; Zelapar—oral disintegrating tablet)	Foods with high tyramine content (aged, fermented, pickled, and smoked foods, including cheeses, meats, fish, and wines)	Hypertension, headache, vomiting, tachycardia, and intracerebral hemorrhage
	MAOI antidepressants: isocarboxazid (Marplan), phenelzine (Nardil), tranylcypromine (Parnate)	In high doses: not selective for MAO-B, higher risk for drug and food interactions with MAO-A inhibitor antidepressants
	Tricyclic antidepressants: clomipramine (Anafranil), imipramine (Tofranil)	Excessive serotonin levels: mania, excitation, hyperpyrexia, and convulsions
	Serotonergic drugs: meperidine (Demerol) is absolutely contraindicated due to high risk of serotonin syndrome Other agents that increase risk: buspirone (Buspar), citalopram (Celexa), dextromethorphan, escitalopram (Lexapro), fluoxetine (Prozac), mirtazapine (Remeron), nefazodone (Serzone), paroxetine (Paxil), sibutramine (Meridia), tramadol (Ultram), trazodone (Desyrel), venlafaxine (Effexor)	Serotonin syndrome: agitation, confusion, hypomania, myoclonus, rigidity, hyperreflexia, incoordination, sweating, shivering, tremor, seizures, and coma
	Foods with high tyramine content (aged, fermented, pickled, and smoked foods, including cheeses, meats, fish, and wines)	Hypertension, headache, vomiting, tachycardia, and intracerebral hemorrhage

› continued

Table 10.2   › *continued*

Medication	Interacting medication classes and examples	Effects of interaction
Rasagiline (Azilect)	Serotonergic drugs: meperidine (Demerol) is absolutely contraindicated due to high risk of serotonin syndrome Other agents that increase risk: buspirone (Buspar), citalopram (Celexa), dextromethorphan, escitalopram (Lexapro), fluoxetine (Prozac), mirtazapine (Remeron), nefazodone (Serzone), paroxetine (Paxil), sibutramine (Meridia), tramadol (Ultram), trazodone (Desyrel), venlafaxine (Effexor)	Serotonin syndrome: agitation, confusion, hypomania, myoclonus, rigidity, hyperreflexia, incoordination, sweating, shivering, tremor, seizures, and coma
COMT inhibitors		
Entacapone (Comtan)	MAOI antidepressants: isocarboxazid (Marplan), phenelzine (Nardil), tranylcypromine (Parnate)	Contraindicated due to increased toxicity of these nonselective MAOI
	Sympathomimetic drugs metabolized by COMT: dextroamphetamine (Dexedrine), phenylephrine, diethylpropion (Tenuate), dopamine, ephedrine, fenoldopam (Corlopam), isometheptene (Midrin), methylphenidate (Ritalin), pseudoephedrine (Sudafed), methyldopa (Aldomet), nadolol (Corgard)	Increased heart rate, arrhythmias, and hypertension
	Agents that interfere with biliary excretion of Comtan: erythromycin, rifampin, cholestyramine (Questran)	Increased levels and effects of entacapone (Comtan)
	Iron	Decreased absorption of entacapone (Comtan); space administration by 2 h
	MAOI antidepressants: isocarboxazid (Marplan), phenelzine (Nardil), tranylcypromine (Parnate)	Contraindicated due to increased toxicity of these nonselective MAOI
Tolcapone (Tasmar)	Sympathomimetic drugs metabolized by COMT: dextroamphetamine (Dexedrine), phenylephrine, diethylpropion (Tenuate), dopamine, ephedrine, fenoldopam (Corlopam), isometheptene (Midrin), methylphenidate (Ritalin), pseudoephedrine (Sudafed), methyldopa (Aldomet), nadolol (Corgard)	Increased heart rate, arrhythmias, and hypertension
	Iron	Decreased absorption and effects of tolcapone (Tasmar); space administration by 2 h

COMT = catechol-O-methyl-transferase; MAOI = monoamine oxidase inhibitor.

blood–brain barrier, where it is converted to dopamine by the enzyme dopa decarboxylase. The therapeutic effects of levodopa therapy include improvements in tremor, bradykinesia, and rigidity. Levodopa improves functioning in activities of daily living as well as motor symptoms by 50%, whereas a 30% improvement is seen with the use of dopamine agonists (Hou & Lai, 2008; Jacobson et al., 2007).

Although levodopa reduces symptoms associated with PD, its use can also be associated with the development of motor complications, including involuntary muscle movements (**dyskinesia**), involuntary muscle spasms (dystonia), freezing of gait, and increased on-off phenomena (increased symptoms seen at end of the dosing interval). The severity of these motor complications is related to the size of the dose and dependent on the length of time the patient is treated with levodopa; the longer the patient is treated and the higher the cumulative dose, the greater the severity of on-off phenomena. In order to delay the development of motor complications, the initiation of treatment with levodopa is reserved for more advanced stages of the disease and other agents are used in early PD (Chen et al., 2009; Hou & Lai, 2008; Jacobson et al., 2007).

Approximately 80% of patients receiving levodopa therapy exhibit some form of dyskinesia. The dyskinesias, which usually occur after the patient has been on levodopa therapy for more than 3 mo, may be caused by an overstimulation of dopamine in the basal ganglia. Dyskinesias associated with use of levodopa include movement disorders such as choreoathetoid movements, dystonia, **myoclonus**, and tics or tremors. The time to onset of dyskinesia may range from 3 mo to as long as 3 yr. Goals of treatment are to ameliorate the motor dysfunction (e.g., **bradykinesia**, cogwheel rigidity, resting tremor) and not cause further motor impairments related to medication-induced dyskinesia. A common side effect of levodopa related to inconsistent absorption is peak-dose dyskinesia, which is characterized by chorea-like jerks, restlessness, and writhing movements and likely caused by medication overcorrection resulting in excessive dopamine peak levels and effects (Chen et al., 2009; Hou & Lai, 2008; Jacobson et al., 2007).

Sinemet, a combination of levodopa and carbidopa, was introduced to minimize the dose of levodopa administered to patients. Decarboxylase is an enzyme that breaks down levodopa outside the central nervous system and does not cross the blood–brain barrier. Carbidopa protects levodopa from enzymatic destruction by decarboxylase until it crosses the blood–brain barrier, thus increasing levodopa levels in the brain and reducing the size of the levodopa dose needed. The earlier a patient is treated with levodopa and the higher the dose used, the more rapid the development of the motor complication known as on–off phenomenon. The use of the combination product Sinemet can improve motor function in patients treated with levodopa by 50%

(Chen et al., 2009; Faulkner, 2006; Iversen et al., 2009; Kyle & Kyle, 2007).

Carbidopa–levodopa (Sinemet) is available as sustained-release or immediate-release products. With immediate-acting oral disintegrating tablets, the onset of effects occurs within 30 min. These tablets should not be chewed or swallowed. Sustained-release products were introduced to provide more prolonged levels of dopamine and to reduce on–off symptoms. Onset of effects of the sustained release product occurs 1 h after the dose and effects peak in 30 to 120 min after the dose is taken. Peak blood levels achieved are 30% lower in patients taking the sustained-release Sinemet compared with achieved peak levels in patients taking the same dose of immediate-release Sinemet. Because the effects of the medication are related to achieved peak effects, the size of the dose should be increased by 30% when converting a patient from the immediate-release product to the sustained-release product. When a patient is being treated with sustained-release Sinemet (with the delayed achievement of peak levels), immediate peak levels with onset of therapeutic effects can be achieved with supplemental or booster doses of the immediate-release product. Sinemet dosage should always be tapered before discontinuance to prevent withdrawal effects of confusion, rigidity, and fever (Chen et al., 2009; Faulkner, 2006; Iversen et al., 2009; Kyle & Kyle, 2007).

The timing of the Sinemet dose in relationship to meals and protein intake can affect the absorption, onset, and duration of effects of the medication. Doses should be given at least 30 min before meals or at least 60 min after meals. Patients should avoid high-fat meals, which delay stomach emptying and thereby decrease absorption. Iron supplements should be spaced 2 h from Sinemet administration to prevent a reduction in Sinemet absorption (Chen et al., 2009; Faulkner, 2006; Iversen et al., 2009; Kyle & Kyle, 2007).

Levodopa tends to become less effective the longer it is administered. If levodopa is administered for more than 4 yr, the effect of the medication diminishes. After several years the patient may experience increased on-off fluctuation of therapeutic effects; these symptoms can be managed with more continuous dopamine stimulation. This may be achieved by initiating controlled-release formulations, increasing dosage or frequency, or adding other medications such as dopamine agonists or catechol-O-methyl-transferase inhibitors to the levodopa product (Chen et al., 2009; Faulkner, 2006; Iversen et al., 2009; Kyle & Kyle, 2007).

The therapeutic effects of levodopa are also shortened in advanced PD. This is called end of dose akinesia and is usually seen as dystonia or akinesia that occurs in the morning upon waking. The rehabilitation therapist should observe the PD patient closely during therapy sessions and ask if any new symptoms have occurred prior to each therapy session. Patients should be closely monitored for changes in motor effects during the initiation of therapy or during periods of medication adjustment to determine whether medications are achieving sustained therapeutic effects. These can be especially evident during therapy sessions. New symptoms or decreased control of symptoms should always be reported to the patient's prescriber as they may warrant a change in medication therapy (Chen et al., 2009; Faulkner, 2006; Iversen et al., 2009; Kyle & Kyle, 2007).

Prescribing physicians may temporarily hold the PD medications of patients exposed to long-term levodopa therapy to address developed tolerance to levodopa therapy; this interruption in therapy is referred to as a drug holiday. During the holiday the body can recover from drug tolerance that reduces levodopa effects and from levodopa-induced side effects. After the drug holiday, the patient may be reintroduced to levodopa at a lower dose. Patients on drug holidays may exhibit severe motor deficiencies associated with the withholding of their medications and therefore require rehabilitation to maintain mobility as much as possible. Drug holidays are used sparingly because the reduction of medications may lead to patient immobility and associated complications such as pneumonia and pulmonary embolism (Chen et al., 2009; Faulkner, 2006; Iversen et al., 2009; Kyle & Kyle, 2007).

Food–Drug Interactions With Levodopa   The half-life of levodopa is 1.5 h. Therapeutic effects usually begin approximately 30 min after levodopa is taken and may last 6 to 8 h. Levodopa is administered 3 or more times/day throughout the waking day. The type and amount of food in the stomach affect the absorption rate of levodopa. Patients should avoid consuming too much protein around the time of levodopa administration because protein can compete with levodopa for transport across the blood–brain barrier and thereby decreases absorption, decreasing achieved levels and therapeutic effects. To improve absorption, patients should take this medication on an empty stomach with a full glass of water whenever possible (Chen et al., 2009; Faulkner, 2006; Iversen et al., 2009; Kyle & Kyle, 2007).

Side Effects of Levodopa   Side effects associated with levodopa therapy include gastrointestinal effects of nausea, vomiting, and anorexia associated with stimulation of the **chemoreceptor** trigger zone. Using Sinemet doses that provide at least 70 mg of carbidopa/day can minimize these side effects. Other side effects can include abdominal pain, constipation, gastrointestinal bleeding, dry mouth, elevated liver enzymes, and black discoloration of the saliva, urine, and sweat. Taking the medication with meals may reduce gastrointestinal upset. Levodopa therapy can cause dysphagia due to associated side effects of nausea, anorexia, vomiting, xerostomia, changes in taste sensation, constipation, dyskinesias, and extrapyramidal symptoms (e.g., uncontrollable movements of the tongue, mouth, and jaw; teeth clinching or grinding; and difficulty opening the mouth). Use of levodopa can also result in decreased attention span, lightheadedness, clumsiness, and abnormal thinking, which can reduce attention to eating and interfere with motor skills involved in eating (Alvi, 1999; Campbell-Taylor, 1996, 2001; Feinberg, 1997).

Cardiovascular and psychiatric side effects can also occur with Sinemet therapy. Cardiovascular side effects include orthostatic hypotension and elevated homocysteine levels (an atherosclerotic risk factor). Elevated homocysteine levels are often treated with folic acid supplementation. Psychiatric side effects include agitation, confusion, **euphoria**, hallucinations, sleep disorders, psychosis, and hypersexuality. Reducing dosage or using long-acting formulations of levodopa–carbidopa (Sinemet) may reduce these side effects (Chen et al., 2009; Faulkner, 2006; Iversen et al., 2009; Kyle & Kyle, 2007).

PATIENT CASE 2

A.E. is a 75-yr-old woman with a 3 yr history of PD who recently started taking Sinemet. Her initial dose of Sinemet was increased from 10/100 mg 3 times/day to 25/100 mg 3 times/day because she was experiencing severe nausea and vomiting. Her symptoms of nausea and vomiting have subsided, but her continued symptoms of bradykinesia and rigidity prompted the physician to adjust her Sinemet dose to 25/250 3 times/day. A.E. is currently receiving home care physical therapy after a recent open reduction internal fixation of her right hip to treat a hip fracture that resulted from a fall in her home. A.E. reported that the fall occurred about 1 h after having her breakfast and taking her morning dose of Sinemet. She explained that she was getting up from the kitchen table when she immediately got very light-headed and fell to the ground, striking her right hip against the floor. The physical therapy evaluation reveals that she has mild bradykinesia, mild cogwheel rigidity in the extremities, and unilateral pill rolling of the fingers of the left hand. A.E. noted that her episodes of freeze-ups (akinesia) have decreased since her Sinemet dosage was increased. A.E. is able to ambulate with her walker using a partial weight-bearing gait on the right. She continues to experience lightheadedness when getting up from bed or from a seated position and is very fearful of having another fall.

Question
How should the rehabilitation therapist address A.E.'s concerns?

Answer
A.E.'s recent increase in Sinemet dosage did reduce the bradykinesia, rigidity, and akinesia that she was experiencing. However, her history indicated that she was experiencing orthostatic hypotension. During A.E.'s physical therapy evaluation, the physical therapist monitored A.E.'s blood pressure immediately before and after positional changes and confirmed that orthostatic hypotension was occurring. Orthostatic hypotension is one of the most frequently occurring side effects of Sinemet. A.E. continued to be at risk for another fall, especially because her recent surgery complicated her gait performance. The therapist consulted with A.E.'s prescribing physician, who adjusted her medication dosage to sustained-release Sinemet 25/250 3 times/day. This significantly reduced her symptoms of lightheadedness and orthostasis. The physical therapist educated A.E. about orthostatic hypotension and the need for slow positional changes to allow blood pressure to adapt. The therapist also recommended that A.E. perform some active range-of-motion exercises for the ankles and knees before going from sitting to standing positions. The therapist monitored A.E.'s blood pressure at follow-up visits to verify that orthostatic hypotension was no longer occurring. Patient education and adjustment of her medication to a sustained release dosage form resolved A.E.'s orthostatic hypotension and reduced her risk of another fall.

Anticholinergics

Anticholinergics, which balance dopamine and acetylcholine activity in the brain, may be used in combination with other PD medications. Anticholinergic drugs are used in initial treatment of PD, especially in younger patients in whom tremor is predominant. Centrally acting anticholinergics include benztropine (Cogentin), trihexyphenidyl (Artane), and procyclidine (Kemadrin). These agents should not be used in patients with angle-closure glaucoma or prostatic hypertrophy (Chen, 2002; Chen et al., 2009; Kyle & Kyle, 2007; Langston et al., 2007).

Side effects are dose related (i.e., increased with higher doses) and include altered cognition, orthostasis, blurred vision, dry eyes, dry mouth, drowsiness, confusion, memory impairment, tachycardia, constipation, and urinary retention. Because orthostatic hypotension can occur, the rehabilitation therapist should monitor the patient's heart rate and blood pressure in supine, sitting, and standing positions and especially before the patient changes positions. Anticholinergics can worsen the dysphagia that is already present in PD patients, thus affecting swallow function and cognition. Anticholinergic medications are not well tolerated in older patients and should be used with caution. When discontinuing anticholinergic therapy, tapering is required to prevent severe agitation and confusion (cholinergic syndrome) (Chen, 2002; Chen et al., 2009; Kyle & Kyle, 2007; Langston et al., 2007).

N-Methyl-D-Aspartate Receptor Inhibitors

Amantadine (Symmetrel) enhances dopamine effect and blocks glutamate action at the N-methyl-D-aspartate receptors in the brain. This medication is effective in early disease as monotherapy for treating mild symptoms of bradykinesia and rigidity and may be used as adjunctive therapy with levodopa in more advanced PD. The effectiveness of this agent wears off (tachyphylaxis) within 3 mo of initiation, but effectiveness can be restored by discontinuing the drug for a few weeks (i.e., a drug holiday). Amantadine is also useful in combination with levodopa because it alleviates levodopa-induced dyskinesias. Dosing is initiated at 100 mg/day and titrated up on a weekly basis to 400 mg/day. Because the drug is eliminated renally, dosage should be reduced in patients with creatinine clearance less than 50 ml/min (Chen, 2002, 2012; Chen & Swope, 2007; Kyle & Kyle, 2007; Nelson et al., 2002; Standaert & Young, 2001).

Side effects are mild and include vivid dreams and nightmares (occur with initial use and fade with continued use), confusion, hallucinations, dizziness, insomnia, nausea, orthostatic hypotension, dry skin, skin rash or mottling (livedo reticularis), and ankle edema. The rehabilitation therapist should monitor the patient for side effects that may interfere with rehabilitation. For example, orthostatic hypotension or dizziness can increase the patient's fall risk, impaired cognition associated with sleep deprivation and insomnia can interfere with patient learning and performance in rehabilitation, and altered mental status or gastrointestinal side effects such as nausea can contribute to dysphagia. Use of this agent should be tapered upon discontinuance to reduce withdrawal symptoms (Chen, 2002; Chen & Swope, 2007; Kyle & Kyle, 2007; Nelson et al., 2002; Standaert & Young, 2001).

Dopamine Receptor Agonists

Direct dopamine receptor agonists have been used for more than 10 yr as an alternative to early initiation of levodopa and as adjunctive therapy in more advanced disease. These agents bind directly to the dopamine receptor, thus enhancing the action of dopamine, and effectively treat tremors, rigidity, and bradykinesia. Patients with early PD who receive these agents have about half the risk of developing complications of dyskinesia, freezing, and wearing off compared with patients receiving levodopa. The five dopamine receptor agonist agents currently available include bromocriptine (Parlodel), ropinirole (Requip), pramipexole (Mirapex), apomorphine (Apokyn), and rotigotine (Neupro). Pergolide (Permax) is a dopamine agonist that was removed from the market in 2007 due to associated increased risk of valvular heart disease (Chen et al., 2009; Kyle & Kyle, 2007).

Dopamine agonists directly stimulate striatal dopamine and do not require enzymatic activation. They are less effective than levodopa, but they have a longer half-life that results in prolonged effects and fewer fluctuations in striatal action. They are used in early PD in an effort to postpone the use of levodopa. Use of dopamine agonists is associated with a lower incidence of dyskinesia but a higher incidence of psychiatric side effects. Dosage of these agents must be titrated over several weeks to prevent the dose-related side effects of nausea and orthostasis. Patients with a history of dementia should be started at half the normal dose and titrated up very slowly. Dopamine agonists differ from levodopa in that their absorption is not impaired by intake of dietary protein around the time of medication administration. Once levodopa therapy is initiated, use of dopamine agonists can reduce the needed levodopa dose by 30%. Reducing the needed levodopa dose benefits the patient by reducing the development of tolerance to the effects of levodopa associated at onset of on-off symptoms. Bromocriptine 10 mg is equivalent to ropinirole 4 mg, rotigotine 4 mg, or pramipexole 1 mg. The dosage of these agents should be slowly tapered before discontinuance to avoid neuroleptic malignant syndrome (Chen et al., 2009; Hopfer-Deglin & Hazard Vallerand, 2010; Kyle & Kyle, 2007).

Bromocriptine (Parlodel), an ergot derivative, is less effective than the other agents, but its use can reduce the needed levodopa dose by 20%. Erythromycin, clarithromycin (Biaxin), and nefazodone (Serzone) can increase bromocriptine levels by inhibiting its metabolism and should be avoided in patients receiving bromocriptine. Bromocriptine (Parlodel) has been associated with development of fibrosis in the cardiac valves, lungs, and retroperitoneum. Routine monitoring by chest X-ray is recommended for patients being treated with this medication (Chen et al., 2009; Hopfer-Deglin & Hazard Vallerand, 2010; Kyle & Kyle, 2007).

Pramipexole (Mirapex) can be used as monotherapy, but when used with levodopa it can reduce the needed levodopa dose by 25% to 30%. Because it is eliminated renally, the dose should be reduced in patients with creatinine clearance less than 60 ml/min. Cimetidine (Tagamet), ranitidine (Zantac), triamterene (Dyrenium), diltiazem (Cardizem), verapamil (Isoptin), **quinidine**, and quinine can increase levels of pramipexole (Mirapex) and should be avoided in patients receiving pramipexole (Mirapex) (Chen et al., 2009; Kyle & Kyle, 2007; Lo et al., 2007).

Ropinirole (Requip), when used with levodopa, can reduce the needed levodopa dose by 30%. It is metabolized by the liver enzymes CYP1A2. Concurrent use of the fluoroquinolone antibiotics levofloxacin (Levaquin) and moxifloxacin (Avelox) should be avoided because they can increase levels of ropinirole (Requip). This agent is also used to treat restless-leg syndrome (Chen et al., 2009; Kyle & Kyle, 2007; Lo et al., 2007).

Apomorphine (Apokyn) is used as adjunct therapy for treating freezing episodes associated with advanced PD. It is administered via subcutaneous injection. Antiemetic therapy should be used with apomorphine (Apokyn) administration to prevent nausea and vomiting (Chen, 2012; Chen et al., 2009; Kyle & Kyle, 2007; Lo et al., 2007).

Rotigotine (Neupro) is administered through a transdermal patch. Skin irritation is the most common side effect. It can also cause nausea, somnolence, and dizziness. It is useful for patients who cannot swallow and carries the advantage of once/day dosing and a simple titration schedule. This product provides better control of motor symptoms through decreased off time and doubled on time effects. It has a half-life of 5 to 7 h. A delay of onset of 3 h occurs after applying a new patch, but blood levels are maintained through the entire 24 h period. Rotigotine is metabolized by multiple CYP450 liver enzymes rather than just one type of enzyme, which reduces the risk of clinically significant drug interactions. The patch should be applied daily to clean, dry, healthy skin on the front of the abdomen, thigh, hip, **flank**, shoulder, or upper arm. The patch should be applied immediately after opening, pressed in place for 20 to 30 s, and worn continuously for a 24 h period. If adhesion is a problem, the patient can use first aid tape to anchor the patch to the skin. Rotating the application site daily is recommended, and the patch should not be applied to the same area of skin more often than every 14 days. If applying to a hairy area, the patient should shave the area at least 3 days before applying the patch. Because the back layer of the patch is aluminum, the patient should avoid contact with excessive heat through heating pads, electric blankets, and saunas. To prevent burns, the patch should be removed before cardioversion or magnetic resonance imaging (Chen et al., 2009; Kyle &

Kyle, 2007; Lo et al., 2007; Talati et al., 2007; Tanzi, 2007).

The dopamine agonists do not typically produce dyskinesias and generally have fewer side effects than other agents. Side effects can include edema, dizziness, **somnolence**, insomnia, confusion, yawning, visual hallucinations, psychosis, and hypersexual behavior. Orthostatic hypotension can occur with the first dose. The prescriber, pharmacist, and other health care providers should counsel patients about sudden and overpowering somnolence (sleep attacks) that can occur without warning and warn them to exercise caution and to avoid driving, operating heavy machinery, or working at heights if taking these medications (Carl & Johnson, 2006; Chen, 2002; Schwartz, 2003).

Catechol-O-Methyl-Transferase Inhibitors

When levodopa is given with carbidopa, an increase in metabolism of levodopa by the enzyme catechol-o-methyl-transferase (COMT) occurs. Entacapone (Comtan) and tolcapone (Tasmar) inhibit this metabolism by COMT, resulting in a 50% increase in levels of levodopa. This change in bioavailability results in less off time and 1 to 2 h more of on time, resulting in improved symptoms (Chen, 2012).

COMT inhibitors are generally not effective as monotherapy for PD and are usually used as concurrent therapy with levodopa. COMT inhibitors prolong levodopa action by increasing dopamine in the brain. They enhance motor function and reduce off time when combined with levodopa. The resultant increase in dopamine levels can also result in increased dopamine side effects. Side effects associated with these agents include hallucinations and dyskinesias that may necessitate a decrease in the levodopa dose (Hou & Lai, 2008; Jacobson et al., 2007). Because tolcapone (Tasmar) carries a high risk of hepatotoxicity, its use is generally restricted to patients who have failed alternative therapies (Chen, 2002; Chen et al., 2009; Standaert & Young, 2001).

These agents can also inhibit the metabolism of other medications that are metabolized by COMT. Combining these agents with catecholamine medications such as epinephrine, iso-proterenol (Isuprel), dobutamine (Dobutrex), and methyldopa (Aldomet) can result in excessive levels of catecholamines and subsequent symptoms of agitation, insomnia, hypertension, increased heart rate, and arrhythmias (Chen, 2002; Nelson et al., 2002; Standaert & Young, 2001).

Monoamine Oxidase-B Inhibitors

Monoamine oxidase (MAO) inhibitors are used in early PD as monotherapy, and their use can delay the need to use levodopa. They may also be used in combination with other products as adjunctive therapy in more advanced stages of PD. MAO is an enzyme found in the body in two isomers: type A and type B. Type A is found in the intestinal tract and peripheral tissues, whereas type B is found predominantly in the brain. MAO-B inhibitors are selective and block the breakdown of dopamine in the brain without inhibiting the breakdown of MAO-A found in other tissues. Because of this selectivity, MAO-B inhibitors do not carry the risk of many of the food and drug interactions and toxicities seen with the nonselective MAO inhibitors (which inhibit MAO-A and MAO-B) used to treat depression (Fernandez & Chen, 2007).

Selegiline (Eldepryl, Zelapar), a first-generation MAO-B inhibitor, is chemically related to amphetamine. Its amphetamine-derived metabolites are responsible for neurotoxic side effects as well as cardiovascular side effects. The oral tablet is poorly absorbed (only 8% is bioavailable) and requires higher doses for therapeutic effects. Use of higher doses (>20 mg/day) decreases the agent's selectivity for MAO-B and places the patient at risk for the side effects and drug interactions seen with MAO-A inhibitors. When selegiline is initiated in patients with early, untreated disease it can relieve symptoms, delay the need for initiation of levodopa, extend mobility, and reduce freezing of gait. When used with levodopa it can reduce the dosage requirement for levodopa and attenuate the wearing off phenomenon. It is initiated at doses of 2.5 mg/day and gradually increased to 5 mg twice/day. It should be administered no later than 12 p.m. to decrease symptoms of insomnia and vivid dreams (Fernandez & Chen, 2007).

Selegiline (Zelapar) is available as a rapidly absorbed oral disintegrating tablet (ODT) that has an onset of 10 to 15 min. It should be dissolved on the tongue rather than swallowed. It is directly absorbed into the bloodstream through the tongue and therefore bypasses first-pass hepatic metabolism, thus increasing bioavailability and decreasing levels of amphetamine metabolites and associated side effects. Because food decreases the peak concentration and total concentrations of the drug by 60%, patients should take the medication on an empty stomach and avoid the intake of food and liquid for at least 5 min before and after the dose. Use of selegiline ODT (Zelapar) decreases the time that the patient experienced off symptoms by 2.2 h/day. The dose is started at 1.25 mg/day for 6 wk and then may be increased to 2.5 mg/day. Emsam is a transdermal patch form of selegiline that is not used in PD but is used in higher doses to treat depression (Antonopoulos & Kim, 2007; Chen, 2002; Chen et al., 2009; Fernandez & Chen, 2007).

Rasagiline (Azilect), a second-generation MAO-B inhibitor, is an irreversible inhibitor of MAO used as a monotherapy in early PD or as adjunct therapy in more advanced cases. Rasagiline is 15 times more selective for MAO-B and has inactive metabolites. In addition, the bioavailability of rasagiline is four times greater than that of selegiline. Rasagiline has a half-life of 3 h, and peak effects occur 1 h after the dose. It is excreted by the kidneys and in the feces (Fernandez & Chen, 2007; Kyle & Kyle, 2007).

Studies indicate that the use of this product may actually slow the progression of PD (Parkinson Study Group, 2004). In the TEMPO (Rasagiline Mesylate [TVP-1012] in Early Monotherapy for Parkinson's Disease) study, Azilect at doses of 1 or 2 mg was more effective than a placebo. Azilect 1 mg significantly reduced daily off time by 1.18 h compared with the placebo (0.4 h) and increased on time without dyskinesia by 0.85 h. This study indicated that this agent may also have a neuroprotective effect. In the LARGO (Lasting effect in Adjunct therapy with Rasagiline Given Once daily) study, which involved 687 patients with more advanced PD, Azilect was as equally effective as entacapone when compared with a placebo

(Chen et al., 2009; Fernandez & Chen, 2007; Iversen et al., 2009; Kyle & Kyle, 2007; Lo et al., 2007).

Side effects of rasagiline (Azilect) include diarrhea, dizziness, drowsiness, dry mouth, flu-like symptoms, headache, joint pain, lightheadedness, sleeplessness, stomach upset, and stuffy nose (Fernandez & Chen, 2007; Kyle & Kyle, 2007).

Serotonin syndrome can occur when selegiline or rasagiline are combined with meperidine (Demerol). Risk of serotonin syndrome is related to the dose used. Serotonin syndrome can cause confusion, agitation, restlessness, rigidity, hyperreflexia, shivering, fever, myoclonus, diaphoresis, nausea, diarrhea, autonomic instability, flushing, coma, and even death (Chen, 2012; Fernandez & Chen, 2007; Kyle & Kyle, 2007).

Hypertensive crisis is associated with extremely high blood pressure and is the most serious side effect associated with the use of the MAO inhibitors. Rehabilitation therapists should check the patient's blood pressure and teach patients who are taking MAO inhibitors to check their own blood pressure with symptoms of headache, palpitations, diaphoresis, dizziness, neck stiffness, chest constriction, nausea, or vomiting (Chen, 2002; Fernandez & Chen, 2007; Kyle & Kyle, 2007; Nelson et al., 2002; Standaert & Young, 2001).

Strategies for Managing Dyskinesia and Dystonia

Strategies for treating dyskinesia and dystonia as recommended by the American Academy of Neurology involve manipulating the levels of dopamine throughout the day and include using shorter- or longer-acting formulations, adjusting the doses based on meals and protein intake, and adding other agents that have a longer duration of action on the dopamine receptors. Table 10.3 summarizes strategies for managing dyskinesia and dystonia (Chen, 2012; Langston et al., 2007).

Deep Brain Stimulation

Deep brain stimulation (DBS) involves implanting a neurostimulator device in the patient's chest and electrodes at a target site in the brain. DBS of the globus pallidus interna or

Table 10.3   Strategies for Managing Dyskinesia and Dystonia

Symptom	Strategy
Dyskinesia	Decrease the levodopa dose.
	Add a dopamine agonist.
	Add amantadine.
Wearing off time	Use smaller, more frequent doses of levodopa or use the sustained-release formulation.
	Add one of the following: COMT inhibitor, dopamine agonist, monoamine oxidase-B inhibitor, or amantadine.
	Adjust the dose time to avoid concurrent food and to avoid concurrent intake of dietary protein intake
Delayed onset of effects	Take Sinemet on an empty stomach or use the dissolving tablet.
	Take an immediate-release formulation along with the sustained-release formulation.
	Add a COMT inhibitor.
	Adjust the dose time to avoid concurrent food and to avoid concurrent intake of dietary protein intake
Freezing gait	Increase the dose of Sinemet.
	Add a dopamine agonist or selegiline.
	Reduce number of medications.
	Use nonpharmacologic techniques.
Unpredictable off-symptoms	Change long acting dosage therapy to smaller, immediate release formulations of Sinemet throughout the day.
	Add a dopamine agonist or apomorphine.
	Increase the Sinemet dose.
Peak-dose dyskinesia	Reduce the levodopa dose.
	Use lower, immediate-release formulations of Sinemet more frequently.
	Add an immediate-release Sinemet dose to the sustained-release dose.
	Add a COMT inhibitor, dopamine agonist, or amantadine.
Dystonia	Take sustained release Sinemet at bedtime.
	Take the morning dose earlier.
	Add a dopamine agonist at bedtime.
Nonmotor side effects	Reduce dose or discontinue the offending agent.

COMT = catechol-O-methyl-transferase.

the subthalamic nucleus may alleviate severe dyskinesias that do not respond to medication adjustment. DBS may also alleviate motor complications such as wearing off, dyskinesia, and medication failure as well as severe tremor and rigidity. DBS does not help alleviate balance and gait problems, impaired cognition, depression, falling, speech problems, or other nonmotor symptoms (e.g., confusion, hallucinations, hypotension, psychosis, and somno-

lence). Patients with dementia or atypical PD (PD not responsive to levodopa therapy) are not good candidates for DBS (Chen, 2012).

Medication Management of Nonmotor PD Effects

The following sections and table 10.4 summarize treatment strategies for managing nonmotor PD side effects, including orthostasis, urinary retention, gastrointestinal side effects,

Table 10.4   Management of Nonmotor Symptoms of Parkinson's Disease

Symptoms	Therapeutics interventions
Orthostatic hypotension	Increase intake of fluids, salt, and caffeine.
	Use support hose and physical counter maneuvers (e.g., toe-raising, leg crossing, thigh contracting, bending at the waist).
	Use of fludrocortisone (Florinef) or sympathomimetics such as ephedrine, pseudoephedrine (Sudafed), methylphenidate (Ritalin), and the herbal yohimbine.
Insomnia	Use melatonin or clonazepam (Klonopin) after instituting good sleep hygiene through cognitive behavioral therapy, relaxation techniques, biofeedback, and massage.
Urinary incontinence	Use of tamsulosin (Flomax), terazosin (Hytrin), tolterodine (Detrol), oxybutynin (Ditropan), darifenacin (Enablex), or solifenacin (Vesicare).
	Use of behavioral therapy, pelvic floor and bladder exercises, neuromodulation with sacral nerve stimulation, and surgery for bladder augmentation.
Erectile dysfunction	Use of sildenafil (Viagra), vardenafil (Levitra), tadalafil (Cialis).
Depression	Use of SSRIs (selective serotonin reuptake inhibitors) or SSNRIs (selective serotonin and norepinephrine reuptake inhibitors).
	Avoid tricyclic antidepressants or monoamine oxidase-A inhibitors.
Psychotic symptoms	Eliminate PD medications in the following order (starts with the agent with the highest likelihood of causing altered cognition and lists agents in order of risk): anticholinergics, selegiline, amantadine, dopamine agonists, and levodopa.
	Quetiapine (Seroquel) is the antipsychotic of choice if one is required.
Dementia	Eliminate PD medications in the following order (starts with the agent with the highest likelihood of causing altered cognition): anticholinergics, selegiline, amantadine, tricyclic antidepressants, sedatives, dopamine agonists, and levodopa.
	Short-term use of rivastigmine (Exelon) may be trialed after ruling out Lewy body dementia.
Anxiety	Rule out motor fluctuation as a cause of anxiety.
	Use cognitive behavioral therapy and good sleep hygiene.
	Use buspirone (Buspar) 5 mg 3 times/day short term.
Nausea and vomiting	Avoid the phenothiazine antiemetics promethazine (Phenergan), prochlorperazine (Compazine), and metoclopramide (Reglan); these agents antagonize PD medications.
	Use a serotonergic agent such as ondansetron (Zofran) 4 mg every 6 h as needed.
Hiccups	Use of baclofen (Lioresal) 5-20 mg 3-4 times/day.
Impaired voice	Use of clonazepam (Klonopin) 0.25-0.5 mg/day.
Sialorrhea	Use of glycopyrrolate (Robinul) 1-2 mg up to 4 times/day.
	Apply scopolamine patch (Transderm Scop) 1.5 mg every 3 days.
	Inject Botox into the parotid and submandibular glands.

PD = Parkinson's disease.

dysphagia, and psychiatric symptoms (Chen et al., 2009).

Orthostatic Hypotension   Up to 50% of patients with PD experience orthostatic hypotension, which is defined as a decrease in blood pressure of at least 10 mm Hg upon changing positions (i.e., standing from sitting or lying down). Symptoms associated with orthostatic hypotension include blurred vision, dizziness, fainting, weakness, lightheadedness, and syncope, which can contribute to fall risk in the PD patient. All medications used to treat PD, and in particular those that increase dopamine levels, can cause orthostatic hypotension. This side effect is potentiated with use of other medications such as antihypertensive agents, diuretics, anticholinergics, antipsychotics, and antidepressants. When orthostasis occurs, the therapist should alert the prescriber and pharmacist of the symptoms. The pharmacist can assist with a review of the patient's medication regimen to identify any medications with anticholinergic effects, as these should be the first agents to be discontinued. Additional interventions that may be helpful include wearing elastic stockings, increasing salt and caffeine intakes, avoiding high temperatures, avoiding sudden changes in posture, and avoiding alcohol. Medications that may be prescribed to treat orthostasis not corrected by these interventions include fludrocortisone 0.1 to 0.3 mg/day, midodrine 2.5 to 10 mg/day, or the nonsteroidal anti-inflammatory drug indomethacin (Indocin) titrated to improvement of symptoms (Chen, 2012; Chen et al., 2009; Wood, 2011).

Urinary and Sexual Dysfunction   Sixty percent of patients with PD have urinary dysfunction. Treatments include behavioral therapy, physical therapy that focuses on the pelvic floor, neuromodulation with sacral nerve stimulation, and surgery for bladder augmentation. Medications such as bladder-selective antimuscarinics (e.g., darifenacin [Enablex] and solifenacin [Vesicare]) and nonselective antimuscarinics (e.g., oxybutynin [Ditropan] and tolterodine [Detrol]) may also be beneficial in controlling symptoms. The use of antimuscarinics is limited by the side effects of confusion, dry mouth, and dysphagia. Intradetrusor injection of botulinum toxin A has emerged as a well-tolerated, effective treatment that is repeated every 6 mo. These injections reduce urinary urgency, frequency, and micturitions during the day and night. Less commonly, patients may develop neurogenic failure to empty the bladder, which is usually managed by daily intermittent straight catheterization (Chen, 2012). The use of phosphodiesterase-5 inhibitors (e.g., sildenafil [Viagra]) or mechanical devices may help patients with sexual dysfunction (Chen et al., 2009; Weintraub et al., 2008a).

Psychiatric Symptoms   Antidepressants without significant anticholinergic effects (e.g., selective serotonin reuptake inhibitors or selective serotonin and norepinephrine reuptake inhibitors) can help patients with psychiatric disorders associated with PD (Weintraub et al., 2008b). Psychotic symptoms occur in 40% of patients treated with dopamine-enhancing therapies for motor symptoms associated with PD. Psychotic symptoms most often seen include visual hallucinations or persecutory delusions. Because treatment of the psychosis with typical antipsychotic medications can antagonize the effects of the PD medications, anticholinergic medications should first be discontinued and then doses of the following medications should be reduced in the order listed: MAO-B inhibitors, amantadine, dopamine agonists, COMT inhibitors, and dopamine prior to adding an antipsychotic agent. If adjustment of these medications is not effective in resolving psychotic symptoms the patient's prescriber may consider the careful addition of quetiapine (Seroquel) or clozapine (Clozaril). Quetiapine (Seroquel) is the preferred agent when an antipsychotic agent is needed in patients with PD. If quetiapine (Seroquel) is ineffective, the use of clozapine (Clozaril) can be considered. When used in low doses, clozapine (Clozaril) has been shown to reduce psychotic symptoms in PD without worsening the symptoms of PD. Its use requires enrollment of the prescriber and pharmacist in the Clozaril registry because of serious side effects such as neutropenia that require special monitoring of blood cell counts (Lertxundi et al., 2008; Weintraub et al., 2008c).

Dementia   The presence of dementia in PD patients complicates pharmacotherapy because medications used to treat motor symptoms of PD tend to exacerbate cognitive difficulties. One strategy is to eliminate the medications from the patient's regimen in the order of their tendency to alter cognition: anticholinergics, selegiline, amantadine, tricyclic antidepressants, sedatives, dopamine agonist, and levodopa. An additional strategy might be to reduce dopaminergic agents to the lowest effective dose. Short-term use of cholinesterase inhibitors such as rivastigmine may provide moderate benefit for cognition for up to 6 mo without affecting motor function. Dementia with Lewy bodies is characterized by hallucinations and, often, fluctuations in cognition. When psychosis appears early in PD before introducing dopaminergic therapy, Lewy body dementia should be ruled out as a possible alternative diagnosis to PD (Chen & Swope, 2007; Marder & Jacobs, 2008; Weintraub et al., 2008c).

Insomnia and Anxiety Sleep abnormalities occur in 80% to 90% of PD patients. One half of patients report excessive daytime sleepiness, which may be caused by the dopamine-enhancing medications used to treat their PD motor symptoms. Interventions should include patient education regarding good sleep habits (e.g., avoiding caffeinated beverages, heavy metals, and exercise before bedtime; avoiding using the bedroom for activities other than sleeping, such as reading or watching television; and avoiding sleeping during the day). In addition, clonazepam and melatonin may help promote sleep (Chen et al., 2009). Sleep attacks may occur in patients on dopamine agonists and may require a change in therapy. Anxiety may be associated with fluctuation of motor symptoms; this cause should be ruled out before adding an antianxiety agent. Buspirone (Buspar) may help alleviate anxiety not corrected with nonpharmacologic therapies (Carl & Johnson, 2006; Langston et al., 2007; Marder & Jacobs, 2008; Weintraub et al., 2008c).

Gastrointestinal Disorders The management of gastrointestinal side effects of PD medications such as nausea, vomiting, constipation, slowed gastric emptying, and gastrointestinal reflux can present a challenge. Initial interventions for managing these symptoms include assessing the patient's drug regimen for anticholinergic medications that should be discontinued if possible, optimizing dietary intake of fiber and fluids, and adding appropriate **laxatives** to treat constipation. Many medications used to treat nausea and vomiting are structurally related to the **phenothiazines** and can cause dopamine blockade and antagonism of the dopamine agonists used to treat PD. Serotonin antagonists such as ondansetron should be used as an alternative to these phenothiazines. Metoclopramide (Reglan) is a **prokinetic** agent used to promote gastrointestinal motility and gastric emptying. Because this agent also blocks central dopamine and can antagonize the action of PD medications, it should be avoided in PD patients. Chapter 24 provides additional information on managing constipation, nausea, vomiting, gastroesophageal reflux, and slowed gastric emptying (Fuh et al., 1997; Gallena et al., 2001; Lertxundi et al., 2008; Wood, 2010).

Dysphagia Dysphagia, or difficulty swallowing and eating, affects an estimated 82% of patients with PD. Dysphagia in many with PD is not identified and can lead to silent aspiration, aspiration pneumonia, and weight loss in the PD patient (Fuh et al., 1997; Gallena et al., 2001; Hunter et al., 1997). Up to 50% of patients with impaired swallowing are unaware of it. Sialorrhea or drooling can also occur in patients with PD due to impaired swallowing rather than overproduction of saliva; this can increase the risk of aspiration. Interventions for dysphagia include assessment by a speech–language pathologist for patient-specific recommendations, training the patient to eat in an upright position, tucking the chin to the neck, eating smaller bites at a slower rate followed by a cough, and using a thickening agent in liquids. Interventions for sialorrhea include repositioning the patient from a forward head-tilt posture, assessing medications that can contribute to swallowing, treatment with botulinum toxin A, or sublingual use of atropine eye drops. In addition to sialorrhea and impaired swallowing, gastroparesis and impaired gastrointestinal transit of food as well as a decrease in ability to self feed can negatively impact appetite and food intake and can contribute to decline in the PD patient's nutritional status. Chapter 24 includes additional information on managing dysphagia (Wood, 2010).

Speech and Voice Hiccups associated with PD medications can occur. Chlorpromazine (Thorazine), the agent commonly used to treat hiccups, should not be used in patients with PD because it antagonizes the dopamine-enhancing effects of PD medications. Baclofen (initiated at 5 mg 3 times/day and increased gradually to 20 mg 3 to 4 times/day) may be an option for treating hiccups in the patient with PD (Lertxundi et al., 2008). Clonazepam (dosed at 0.25-0.5 mg/day) has been reported to significantly improve speech in individuals with PD and hypokinetic dysarthria. Levodopa therapy can also assist with speech impairment (DeLetter et al., 2005; Fox et al., 2008; Sapir et al., 2008).

PATIENT CASE 3

R.U. is a 70-yr-old female with a 25 yr history of PD. Her other medical problems include atrial fibrillation, a history of stroke and deep vein thrombosis, hypertension, depression, and hyperlipidemia. She is referred to therapy for gait training with a rolling walker and assistance with self-feeding. R.U. has lost 20 lb (9.1 kg) in the past 3 mo and has no appetite. She also does not have the strength to ambulate safely and has fallen 3 times in the past 3 mo. Her medication list includes Sinemet sustained release 25/250 mg twice/day, Sinemet immediate release 25/100 up to 4 times/day as needed, Coumadin 2 mg/day for stroke prevention and atrial fibrillation, simvastatin 20 mg/day for high cholesterol, Toprol XL 50 mg/day for blood pressure, paroxetine (Paxil) 20 mg/day for depression, and Detrol LA 4 mg/day for urinary incontinence.

Question

What are some risk factors for dysphagia identified in R.U.?

Answer

PD itself carries symptoms that can contribute to dysphagia, and tremors, rigidity, bradykinesia, and akathisia can all affect the motor function necessary for manipulating food and eating. Additional symptoms that can affect eating and swallowing include delayed gastric emptying, olfactory deficits, and drooling. Medication therapies that R.U. is taking also can contribute to dysphagia. Sinemet can also cause xerostomia and dyskinesias that can affect motor functions needed for feeding. Detrol LA has high anticholinergic activity and can cause confusion, xerostomia, delayed gastric emptying, orthostasis, and constipation.

Summary

This chapter summarizes symptoms of PD and provides information on the use of medications in managing motor and nonmotor symptoms. The rehabilitation team should monitor the patient's response to these medications and provide valuable feedback to the prescriber regarding achievement of desired effects as well as side effects that can influence rehabilitation. Therapy sessions should include patient education regarding appropriate use of medications and information on fall prevention. Improved motor function as a result of rehabilitation therapy may allow a reduction in parkinsonian medications. The rehabilitation team must collaborate to assist the prescriber in adjusting the patient's therapy.

Patients should be counseled not to abruptly stop taking their medications and should be educated about possible side effects that should be communicated to the team. Many times, side effects can be minimized by altering the medication dose, changing the frequency of the dose, or changing the dosage form. Patients should be educated about possible drug and food–drug interactions that can affect the medication's onset, side effects, and duration of effects. Pharmacists can also assist the rehabilitation team by providing recommendations for altering the medication regimen to minimize its complexity and promote patient adherence to a more simplified regimen. Patients should be taught to consult with the pharmacist for help selecting safe over-the-counter medications and herbal products. Providing information about support groups and PD organizations to the PD patient and family can also assist in optimizing patient outcome (Kyle & Kyle, 2007).

Medications Used to Treat Amyotrophic Lateral Sclerosis, Multiple Sclerosis, and Myasthenia Gravis

The rehabilitation therapist will commonly care for patients with neurologic disorders. This chapter provides an overview of amyotrophic lateral sclerosis, multiple sclerosis, and myasthenia gravis and describes both pharmacologic and nonpharmacologic therapies used to treat these disorders. This chapter also describes the effects of these disease states and associated medication therapies on rehabilitation.

Amyotrophic Lateral Sclerosis

Amyotrophic lateral sclerosis (ALS; also known as motor neuron disease, Charcot's disease, and Lou Gehrig's disease) is an adult-onset, **idiopathic**, progressive disease characterized by degeneration of anterior horn cells and upper and lower motor neurons that leads to progressive muscle weakness and **fasciculations** (Ciccone, 2007; Jacobson et al., 2007).

Incidence

The incidence of ALS is relatively consistent worldwide across Caucasian populations. Whether ethnic variation exists remains unknown. Some studies have suggested that the disease occurs less frequently in Hispanic and African American individuals (Cronin et al., 2007).

ALS, the most common neurodegenerative disease of the motor neuron system, affects approximately 6/100,000 people. The ratio of affected males to females is 2.5:1. The risk of developing ALS is twice as high in smokers as it is in nonsmokers. The age of onset of classic ALS is approximately 65 yr.

Etiology and Pathophysiology

Etiology may be multifactorial and may involve viral, autoimmune, genetic, and neurotoxic factors. Researchers theorize that neurotoxicity results from abnormalities of calcium and amino acids involving glutamate neurotransmission. Classic ALS involves the loss of motor neurons in multiple sections of the body, including lower motor neurons in the anterior horn of the spinal cord and in the brainstem, corticospinal upper motor neurons of the precentral gyrus, and prefrontal motor neurons. This motor loss leads to progressive muscle weakness and wasting (atrophy), stiffness (spasticity), abnormally active reflexes, and cognitive impairment, especially executive dysfunction. Reinnervation occurs when neurons are lost, but the new neuron connections are larger and more easily fatigued than the normal neuron connections. This eventually causes progressive weakness and associated muscle atrophy. The affected muscles are categorized into four regions: bulbar (i.e., muscles of the face, mouth, and throat), cervical (i.e., muscles of the back of the head, neck, shoulders, upper back, and upper extremities), thoracic (i.e., muscles of the chest, abdomen, and the middle portion of the spinal muscles), and lumbosacral (i.e., muscles of the lower back, groin, and lower extremities). The disease usually starts with one section of the body and progressively spreads, resulting in respiratory failure and death about 3 to 5 yr from the onset of symptoms (Mendez & Cummings, 2003; Vogel et al., 2000). If the disease affects only the lower body it is called progressive muscular atrophy, and if the disease affects only the upper body it is called primary lateral sclerosis. The life span of patients whose disease is limited to the upper or lower body is usually longer (decades rather than years) than the life span of patients with classic ALS (Armon, 2010; Ciccone, 2007; Jacobson et al., 2007).

Rehabilitation Considerations

The majority of ALS patients have muscular weakness in the upper extremity at onset. As classic ALS progresses, it affects both the upper and lower extremities. The bulbar symptoms include dysphagia and dysarthria. Upper motor neuron symptoms include stiffness, spasticity, abnormal reflexes, loss of dexterity, strained voice, and increased lingual and labial tone. Lower motor neuron symptoms include twitching muscles, foot drop, breathing difficulties, muscle atrophy, breathy voice, and fasciculation of the lip, tongue, and soft palate. Spinal symptoms include upper and lower extremity functions. Upper motor neuron symptoms include increased tone in the arms and legs, weakness, and slow movement. Lower motor neuron symptoms include muscle atrophy and weakness. Weakness, muscle cramps, difficulties with speech and swallowing, and unsteadiness accompany upper or lower motor dysfunction. The patient also can experience dysphagia symptoms, including food spilling out of the mouth, salivary issues, and difficulty with mastication. Speech problems usually include dysarthria, hypernasality, and prosody difficulties. The patient may exhibit cognitive problems such as frontoexecutive symptoms of memory and verbal learning. Emotional labiality, including involuntary laughing or crying and depression, may be present (Armon, 2010; Ciccone, 2007; Jacobson et al., 2007).

Treatment of ALS includes education, mechanism-specific treatment, and adaptive or supportive treatment. Rehabilitation requires a multidisciplinary approach focused on managing the problem the individual exhibits, such as muscle weakness, muscle spasms and cramping, and depression. The rehabilitation team needs to manage significant disability associated with ALS such as the inability to perform activities of daily living, eat safely, or breathe without assistance (Yorkston et al., 2004).

The rehabilitation program is based on the impairments and functional limitations found during the patient's physical examination. The patient with ALS usually presents with a combination of upper motor neuron and lower motor neuron signs and symptoms. Pathology of the lower motor nerve results in weakness in the distal muscle groups of one arm or leg. In the early stages of ALS, strength is commonly impaired in the knee flexors and hip extensors. As strength deficits in the lower extremity progress from mild to moderate, the lack of strength begins to limit safe and efficient gait. The early phase of ALS therapy focuses on using appropriate assistive devices, conserving energy, and using nonexhaustive (submaximal) functional training to promote safe and efficient mobility and performance of activities of daily living. Because ALS has a degenerative effect on motor neurons, strength significantly declines as the patient approaches the moderate stage of ALS. At this stage, the diseased motor neurons can no longer control the muscle fibers that they innervate (Armon, 2010).

Patient mobility declines significantly during the moderate stage of ALS. At the earlier part of this stage, gait and balance disturbances usually necessitate the use of a wheelchair when traveling long distances. By the end of this stage, almost all patients are wheelchair dependent. During this stage, ability to perform activities of daily living declines and pain increases. The pain is often associated with muscle cramping and spasticity, which are associated with the upper motor neuron symptoms. The therapist must focus on preventing contractures and skin breakdown by using appropriate positioning, range-of-motion interventions, and pressure-relief techniques (Drory et al., 2001).

Patients in the late stage of ALS are wheelchair dependent, are 100% dependent on others for all activities of daily living, and have extreme weakness of the extremity, trunk, and neck muscles. Respiratory compromise, dysarthria, and dysphagia typically become progressively worse throughout the final stage of the disease. The survival rate after the onset of early signs and symptoms of ALS is approximately 3 yr, unless the patient uses a mechanical ventilator to sustain breathing (Havercamp et al., 1995).

Controversy exists among rehabilitation professionals regarding the use of exercise in patients with ALS. Professionals agree that patients should not exercise to the point of fatigue. In patients with slow-developing ALS, exercise programs of submaximal intensity may be beneficial, especially in the early stages of ALS. As the disease progresses, the patient should learn work simplification and energy conservation (Yorkston et al., 2004). For example, as the patient's muscle weakness progresses to the point where impaired upper-extremity strength and trunk control create functional limitation and disability, the use of a motorized or tilt-in-space wheelchair is an appropriate method of simplifying work and conserving energy (Drory et al., 2001).

The patient with ALS is at risk for falls related to weakness in the distal muscles (e.g., foot drop), spasticity, weakness of proximal muscles throughout the trunk, and impaired postural control. Use of medications such as riluzole (Rilutek) can cause postural hypotension and further increase the risk of falls. In this case the clinician should monitor the patient's blood pressure in supine, sitting, and standing positions and should instruct the patient to avoid changing positions suddenly. The patient should engage in remedial exercise to increase circulation before changing positions. Correct wheelchair positioning is essential. The rehabilitation therapist must constantly reassess the patient's ability to move safely and incorporate methods of fall prevention into the care plan for the patient with ALS as the degenerative disease continues to progress (Drory et al., 2001).

The patient with ALS may eventually lose meaningful speech and may depend on augmentative communication devices. The patient's respiratory difficulties may necessitate a trachcostomy and eventually a ventilator.

The inability to swallow safely may result in an altered diet and eventually alternative means of hydration and nutrition, such as a percutaneous endoscopic gastrostomy tube. Functions in activities of daily life may be compromised. The rehabilitation therapist needs to work with the patient and caregivers in order to help the physician effectively manage the disorder (Drory et al., 2001).

Medication Therapy

Historically, pharmacological management of ALS has revolved around relieving patient symptoms. Medications are administered to control symptoms of spasticity, muscle cramps, and fatigue. Pharmacological intervention has been limited because the damage to motor neurons is irreversible. Currently, no medication halts the course of the disease.

The use of riluzole (Rilutek), a glutamate pathway antagonist released in 1995 by the U.S. Food and Drug Administration (FDA), does not change the course of the disease but may delay tracheostomy and prolong survival time (Ciccone, 2007; Jacobson et al., 2007; Vogel et al., 2000). In two double-blind placebo-controlled trials, this agent prolonged median tracheostomy-free survival by 2 to 3 mo in patients younger than 75 yr with definite or probable ALS. Riluzole inhibits the release of glutamate from axons and reduces excitatory activity of glutamate on adjacent neurons, thus slowing the loss of motor neuron cells. Dosing is 50 mg twice/day, and side effects include **hypertonia**, fatigue, depression, dizziness, somnolence, paresthesias, postural hypotension, gastrointestinal disturbance, and hypertension. These side effects can increase the patient's risk of falls (Armon, 2010; Vogel et al., 2000; Yorkston et al., 2004).

Additional treatments manage symptoms of spasticity, **sialorrhea**, respiratory secretions, depression, emotional lability, and anxiety. Table 11.1 summarizes the medications commonly used to treat ALS. Spasticity may be treated with agents such as baclofen (Lioresal) and tizanidine (Zanaflex); sialorrhea may be alleviated with anticholinergics such as amitriptyline (Elavil) or trihexyphenidyl (Artane), pseudoephedrine (Sudafed), injection of botulinum toxin type B into the salivary glands, and irradiation of the salivary gland. Hydration, humidifying the room air, and using mucolytics such as guaifenesin (Robitussin) may help manage respiratory secretions. Mechanical suction devices may be needed to remove secretions. Antidepressants such as the selective serotonin reuptake inhibitor citalopram (Celexa) can be used to manage depression, and anxiolytics such as lorazepam (Ativan) can be used to manage anxiety. A combination of dextromethorphan and quinidine, recently approved by the FDA, has shown efficacy in ameliorating involuntary laughter and crying (the expression of pseudobulbar affect). Table 11.1 summarizes medication therapy used to treat ALS (Armon, 2010).

PATIENT CASE 1

S.B. is a 55-yr-old male who was diagnosed with ALS 11 mo ago. He initially complained of difficulty walking due to tightness in his calves. Several months later he began experiencing progressive weakness throughout both lower extremities and the trunk and developed a right foot drop. Recently, S.B. began having trouble writing, developed weakness of the right hand and arm, and began experiencing diffuse muscle twitches accompanied by painful muscle cramps. S.B.'s reflexes were hyperactive and his therapist observed fasciculations in the right leg. S.B.'s occupational therapist recently fit S.B. for an electric wheelchair in order to improve his mobility throughout his home. S.B.'s physical therapist trained his caregivers in transfers and in remedial, low-grade range-of-motion and strengthening exercises that will help S.B. prevent contractures and maintain the strength necessary for performing transfers and activities of daily living for as long as possible. The speech–language pathologist is using neuromuscular electrical stimulation and diet modifications to allow S.B. to continue with oral intake and delay the use of a feeding tube for as long as possible. When S.B. was first diagnosed with ALS 11 mo ago, his neurologist prescribed riluzole (Rilutek)

50 mg by mouth every 12 h, 1 h before a meal, or 2 h after a meal. S.B. recently expressed concern to his neurologist that the medication is not working because all of his symptoms are steadily worsening.

Question
What is an appropriate response to S.B.'s concerns?

Answer
The rehabilitation therapist notified S.B.'s neurologist about his recent changes in response to his medication and facilitated a follow-up appointment with his neurologist. The neurologist provided further education to S.B. and his caregivers about the expected progression of the disease. He explained that riluzole is not curative and that the goal of the drug therapy is to slow the progression of the disease in order to improve S.B.'s quality of life as long as possible. Unfortunately, most individuals affected by ALS live for only 12 to 18 mo after diagnosis, provided the patient receives good supportive care and therapy services. The neurologist further explained that the therapy services in place would improve S.B.'s survival time and quality of life. He also explains that S.B. will likely require respiratory care, including assisted ventilation, as the disease progresses. Finally, the neurologist prepares S.B. and his family for the eventuality that maintaining nutrition will become more challenging when swallowing becomes more difficult and that this will likely necessitate the use of a feeding tube. The neurologist also educates the family about the importance of hospice care as the disease approaches the late stage.

Riluzole (Rilutek), the only medication approved by the FDA for slowing the progression of ALS, is indicated for the treatment of patients with ALS. Researchers believe that the drug reduces levels of glutamate, a chemical messenger in the brain that is often present in higher levels in individuals with ALS. Although the use of riluzole is not curative, it has been

See table 11.1 in the web resource for a full list of medication-specific indications, dosing recommendations, side effects, and other considerations.

Table 11.1 Medications Used to Treat Amyotrophic Lateral Sclerosis

Medication	Side effects affecting rehab							Other side effects or considerations
Disease-modifying agent: Used to inhibit glutamate release and slow neuronal damage and loss of function.								
Riluzole (Rilutek)	Cog ++	S +++	A ++	Motor +++	D ++	Com ++	F +++	Hypertonia, fatigue, depression, dizziness, somnolence, paresthesias, postural hypotension, gastrointestinal disturbance, hypertension
Antispasticity agents								
Baclofen (Lioresal)	Cog ++	S +++	A ++	Motor +++	D ++	Com ++	F +++	Oral: Initial sedation, muscle weakness, ataxia, orthostatic hypotension, fatigue, headache, nausea, dizziness; confusion and hallucinations reported in the elderly or those with history of stroke. Intrathecal: Chronic constipation, hypotonia, somnolence, headache, vomiting, paresthesias.
Tizanidine (Zanaflex)	Cog ++	S +++	A ++	Motor +++	D ++	Com ++	F +++	Sedation, hypotension, dizziness, gastrointestinal upset. Starting with a very low dose and titrating slowly may reduce or eliminate side effects such as sedation, xerostomia, and dizziness.
Agent used to treat emotional liability								
Dextromethorphan–quinidine 20/10 mg (Nuedexta)	Cog +	S +	A 0	Motor +	D ++	Com 0	F +	Diarrhea, dizziness, cough, vomiting, asthenia, peripheral edema, flatulence. Avoid with medications that increase serotonin levels.
Agents used to treat sialorrhea								
Pseudoephedrine (Sudafed)	Cog +	S 0	A ++	Motor +	D ++	Com 0	F ++	Difficulty urinating, dizziness, headache, nausea, nervousness, restlessness, sleeplessness, stomach irritation
Trihexyphenidyl (Artane)	Cog ++	S ++	A ++	Motor ++	D ++	Com ++	F ++	Mild nausea, vomiting, dry mouth, blurred vision, dizziness, dry eyes, constipation, nervousness, cognitive impairment, sedation, urinary retention, abdominal pain, diarrhea, dyspepsia, ataxia, confusion
Botulinum toxin type B	Cog +	S ++	A +	Motor ++	D +++	Com +	F +	Anxiety, back pain, dizziness, drowsiness, dry eyes, dry mouth, flu-like symptoms, headache, increased cough, indigestion, nausea, neck pain, reactions at injection site (pain, redness, swelling, or tenderness), runny nose, sensitivity to light, sweating, stomach upset, weakness of the muscles at or near injection site
Mucolytic agent								
Guaifenesin (Robitussin)	Cog +	S +	A 0	Motor +	D +	Com 0	F +	Dizziness, drowsiness, stomach upset

Cog = cognition; S = sedation; A = agitation or mania; Motor = discoordination; D = dysphagia; Com = communication; F = falls.

The likelihood rating scale for encountering the side effects is as follows: 0 = Almost no probability of encountering side effects. + = Little likelihood of encountering side effects. +/++ = Low probability of encountering side effects; however, probability increases with increased dosage. ++ = Medium likelihood of encountering side effects. +++ = High likelihood of encountering side effects, particularly with high doses. ++++ = Highest likelihood of encountering side effects; best to avoid in at-risk patients.

shown to extend survival time or time to tracheostomy. This case emphasizes that the clinician must understand and communicate this information as well as the pathophysiology and prognosis of ALS so that the patient's expectations for this drug therapy will be realistic.

Multiple Sclerosis

Multiple sclerosis (MS) is a chronic autoimmune disease of the central nervous system characterized by inflammation, **demyelination**, and axonal injury accompanied by impaired axonal transmission that affects the brain, spinal cord, and optic nerves. Multiple lesions damage the protective coat (myelin) of the nerve, inhibiting neurotransmission in the brain and spinal cord. Clinical presentation of MS includes exacerbated muscle weakness, imbalance, incoordination, spasticity, fatigue, bladder and bowel difficulties, vision loss, altered sensory patterns (hyperesthesia), cognitive impairment, and neuropathic pain. Symptoms can also include tremor, incoordination, ataxia, dysarthria, visual disturbances (**nystagmus**, optic neuritis, **diplopia**), fatigue, acute or chronic neuropathic pain (**trigeminal neuralgia**, **dysesthesias**), and affective lability. Although any part of the central nervous system may be affected, the sites most commonly affected are the optic nerves (resulting in visual deficits), spinal cord (resulting in sensory and motor weakness of the arms and legs), and brainstem (resulting in dysarthria, dizziness, vertigo, and diplopia) (Gawronski et al., 2010; Guthrie, 2005; Litzinger & Litzinger, 2009; Tanzi, 2010; Vogel et al., 2000).

Incidence

Researchers generally believe that a genetic factor influences the incidence of MS worldwide. MS is prevalent in temperate zones in the north and south hemispheres. MS is seen more frequently in cold climates above 40° latitude and is most common among Caucasians and persons of Northern European descent. The north–south gradient is a way of describing the variation in incidence of MS based on geographical climate and migration patterns of Europeans. In addition to the usual north–south gradient, some European countries result in variations in incidence in small geographic areas. The incidence of MS is lowest in individuals of African American ancestry. However, environment has been shown to influence the incidence among individuals in the same ethnic class (Rosati, 2001).

MS affects 2.5 million people worldwide. In the United States, between 250,000 and 350,000 people are diagnosed with MS, and 200 new diagnoses are made each week. MS ranks third in causes of disability, behind trauma and arthritis. Onset of symptoms usually occurs between the ages of 20 and 50 yr. The disease affects females almost three times more often than males, and onset occurs later in males than in females. Indicators of a better prognosis include female sex, onset of illness before age 35, involvement of only one brain region, no brainstem involvement (denoted by nystagmus and tremor), and a complete recovery after an attack. MS reduces life expectancy by 5 to 10 yr, and median onset of death is 30 yr after diagnosis (Guthrie, 2005; Kurtzke & Wallin, 2000; Litzinger & Litzinger, 2009; Sobieraj, 2010).

Etiology and Pathophysiology

The proposed causes of MS include an autoimmune response that attacks neural tissue, a slow-acting latent viral infection that triggers an autoimmune response, or environmental factors. Other proposed causes include malfunction of the immune system, genetics, susceptible blood–brain barrier, diet, vitamin deficiencies, and allergic reactions, which all lead to a resultant inflammatory response. The inflammation causes stripping of the myelin covering of the neuron, damage to the axon, and damage to the oligodendrocytes (cells that produce myelin). The demyelinated axons increase sodium channels, which reduces neurotransmission. Lost myelin is found in multiple lesions and is replaced with scar tissue (sclerosis) (Kurtzke & Wallin, 2000; Litzinger & Litzinger, 2009).

Diagnosis is made by clinical symptoms after excluding other causes and requires at least two documented exacerbations separated by at least 30 days. Cerebral spinal fluid (CSF) testing and using magnetic resonance imaging to detect lesions can help diagnose the disease when clinical symptoms are absent. Four categories of MS exist: relapsing–remitting MS (RRMS), secondary progressive MS (SPMS), primary progressive MS (PPMS), and progressive relapsing MS (PRMS). Patients with RRMS alternate between periods of relapse (recurrence of symptoms for longer than 48 h in absence of fever) and remission (periods free of symptoms). If left untreated, RRMS progresses to SPMS after 10 to 15 yr. SPMS is characterized by continuous progression of symptoms with or without any periods of relapse. In PPMS, which occurs in about 10% of patients with MS, patients show steady decline in symptoms and experience no relapses. PRMS, which affects 5% of patients with MS, is characterized by steady progression of the disease with periods of exacerbations (Kurtzke & Wallin, 2000; Litzinger & Litzinger, 2009).

Rehabilitation Considerations

Despite the benefits derived from medications, the MS patient will still experience residual neurologic damage. Numerous studies have addressed the positive effect of multidisciplinary rehabilitation on the MS patient (Grasso et al., 2005; Khan et al., 2008; Lo & Triche, 2008). The rehabilitation methods used depends on the phase of the patient's disease. For example, in a patient with static residual disability, therapy would focus on treating the symptoms and rehabilitating the patient to maximal function and gait. Rehabilitation in the acute relapse phase involves medical and physical supportive assistance that helps the MS patient deal with new impairments and functional limitations.

The rehabilitation therapist's role in treating pain in patients with MS includes assessing pain quality and intensity and providing nonpharmacologic methods of pain reduction, such as the use of transcutaneous electrical stimulation. In one study, use of this method led to a significant decrease in pain scores on a visual analog scale in the upper extremities of patients with pain related to MS (Chitsaz et al., 2009).

The motor symptoms of the patient with MS typically include decreased muscle strength and decreased muscular endurance due to impaired nerve conduction in the central nervous system. The weakness can be found throughout the muscular system but is usually most profound in the trunk and lower extremities. Additional impairments that contribute to decreased functional performance include spasticity, tremor, ataxia, and impaired balance. Mild spasticity may result in a loss of fine motor control; however, pronounced spasticity in the major muscle groups can impede neuromuscular control and result in joint contracture. The rehabilitation therapist should evaluate the patient's gait for both safety and efficiency. As MS progresses, the patient will experience increased fatigue upon exertion. Using the appropriate assistive device can minimize fatigue and episodes of loss of balance during gait. For example, the use of forearm crutches is a common intervention that assists with balance and provides additional support as the performance of the trunk and lower extremity muscles begins to decrease. The rehabilitation therapist should educate the patient about energy conservation and strategies for avoiding heat exposure and excessive exertion as the disease progresses. Patients who live in warmer climates will benefit from using air conditioning to avoid heat-related fatigue, which is common in this patient population. The rehabilitation therapist should also educate the patient and caregivers about positioning techniques that help prevent joint contracture and skin breakdown (Kurtzke & Wallin, 2000; Litzinger & Litzinger, 2009).

Visual difficulties occur in approximately 85% of patients with MS. The patient can also experience a decrease in touch, pain, vibration, and position senses. This combined with cerebellar difficulties such as disequilibrium, dizziness, and vertigo can exacerbate fall risk in the patient (Kurtzke & Wallin, 2000; Litzinger & Litzinger, 2009).

Approximately 50% to 70% of patients with MS experience cognitive decline, which can vary considerably from patient to patient. These cognitive disorders are subcortical; therefore, patients experience difficulties with memory retrieval, conceptual reasoning, and information processing, whether the stimulus is auditory or visual. Visual and verbal retrieval strategies may be impaired. Working memory may be impaired, thus necessitating multiple learning trials. When given adequate time to process, the patient's performance matches that of controls. The rehabilitation therapist should break down instructions into smaller segments and speak slowly. Cognitive rehabilitation treatments should focus on sensory memory components such as attention and processing speed, both with and without environmental distractions (DeLuca, 1999). MS can also affect frontoexecutive functions such as abstract reasoning, set shifting, attention, planning, and organization. Patients with MS may also experience depression, apathy, or euphoria. Depression may exacerbate the already slow processing speed of the patient. General intelligence and nondeclarative memory functions such as priming and implicit memory generally remain intact. As such, the rehabilitation therapist should consider using therapeutic procedures such as spaced retrieval (Mendez & Cummings, 2003).

The speech of the MS patient may be characterized by **dysarthria**. The rate of speech may be slow, and the patient may have prosody difficulties. Hypernasality and a strained vocalization may be present, and speech may be monotone. The patient may also suffer from anomia. Verbal fluency, word-list generation, and confrontational naming may be affected in this population (Mendez & Cummings, 2003).

Fatigue, one of the hallmarks of MS, can affect the patient socially and vocationally. Moderate, nonexhausting conditioning exercises may be of assistance to the MS patient. Exercise prescription should be based on the findings of the physical examination and the patient's tolerance to exercise. Strength training at submaximal levels (i.e., 50% or less of maximum contraction force) is commonly recommended. The rehabilitation therapist must monitor the patient for fatigue and take measures to prevent heat stress because both can exacerbate symptoms if not controlled. The level of aerobic exercise that has therapeutic benefits varies from patient to patient based on the stage of the disease, level of mobility, and exercise tolerance. Increased lower-body strength and endurance has been observed in patients who participate in aquatic-therapy programs. Water temperature should be less than 85 °F to prevent heat stress (Gehlsen et al., 1984). In all stages of MS, the rehabilitation therapist should implement therapy aimed at maintaining and improving joint range of motion and muscle length in order to prevent or treat contractures that interfere with activities of daily living.

The therapist should also periodically reevaluate the patient to determine whether the patient needs additional adaptive equipment in order to carry out activities of daily living and essential functional tasks. In patients who are experiencing decreased functional performance and decreased stability during gait, the use of compensatory adaptive equipment or assistive devices (e.g., canes, forearm crutches, and walkers) can greatly improve safety and efficiency of gait. Patients in the later stages of MS may require specialized splinting or bracing. In instances in which a wheelchair becomes necessary for patient mobility, the rehabilitation therapist should fit the patient for a wheelchair that will address their specific needs and should instruct the patient in transfer techniques and wheelchair mobility as well as pressure-relief techniques that help prevent skin breakdown. The rehabilitation therapist should instruct the patient in gait and mobility using principles of motor learning, matching the type and level of feedback to the patient's cognitive status and taking care to not overwhelm the patient with feedback and tasks. If learning the whole task is too complex for the patient, breaking the task into component parts can be helpful.

Because the patient's cognitive status is influenced by frontal lobe impairment, executive functions such as planning and carrying out activities are impaired. The patient requires structured cueing, chaining, and chunking activities in small steps. External memory aids can also be of assistance to the MS patient. Numerous software programs are available online. For example, Captain's Log offers a number of programs that address sensory, working, and declarative memories. Also, iPad users have a variety of cognitive apps available such as Lumosity (Yorkston et al., 2004).

Medication Therapy

Treatment of MS has changed dramatically in the past two decades. In the past, pharmacological interventions focused on modifying symptoms. Recently introduced immunosuppressant medications modify the course of the disease by limiting the number and severity of relapsing or remitting symptoms. Six injectable medications are currently approved for disease-modification treatment of MS: interferon beta-1a (Avonex and Rebif), interferon beta-1b (Betaseron), glatiramer acetate (Copaxone), natalizumab (Tysabri), and mitoxantrone (Novantrone). These medications have shown positive effects on learning and memory. The medications are typically given in the relapsing–remitting stage to reduce early axonal damage. In addition, fingolimod (Gilenya), the first oral medication for preventing relapses in MS, was recently approved. Table 11.2 summarizes medications used to treat MS (Feret, 2009; Gawronski et al., 2010; Litzinger & Litzinger, 2009; Rosenzweig et al., 2010; Tanzi, 2010).

 See table 11.2 in the web resource for a full list of medication-specific indications, dosing recommendations, side effects, and other considerations.

Table 11.2   Medications Used to Treat Multiple Sclerosis

Medication	Side effects affecting rehab							Other side effects or considerations
Immunomodulators used to treat RRMS								
Interferon beta-1a (Avonex)	Cog 0	S 0	A 0	Motor 0	D 0/+	Com 0	F 0	Flu-like symptoms with injection, depression, mild anemia, allergic reaction, elevated liver enzymes. RRMS; antagonizes effects of proinflammatory cytokines; downregulates T-cell activity.
Interferon beta-1a (Rebif)	Cog 0	S 0	A 0	Motor 0	D 0/+	Com 0	F 0	Flu-like symptoms with injection, depression, low white and red cell counts, allergic reaction. RRMS; enhances suppressor T-cell activity; reduces cytokines.
Interferon beta-1b (Betaseron)	Cog 0	S 0	A 0	Motor 0	D 0/+	Com 0	F 0	Flu-like symptoms with injection, depression, low white count, allergic reaction, elevated liver enzymes. RRMS; antagonizes effects of proinflammatory cytokines; downregulates T-cell activity.
Glatiramer acetate (Copaxone)	Cog 0	S 0	A +	Motor 0	D 0/+	Com 0	F +	Reactions at injection site, vasodilation, chest pain, anxiety, shortness of breath, flushing for 15-30 min after injection. RRMS; interferes with activation of myelin-based, protein-reactive T-cells; affects T-cell differentiation.

› *continued*

Table 11.2 › *continued*

Medication	Side effects affecting rehab							Other side effects or considerations
Mitoxantrone (Novantrone)	Cog 0	S 0	A 0	Motor 0	D +++	Com 0	F 0	Blue-green urine for 24 h, bone marrow suppression, hair loss, nausea, bladder infections, mouth ulcers. Monitor for liver and heart toxicity. RRMS; inhibits cells that destroy myelin in the CNS.

New oral agents: Cladribine is used to treat PPMS; fingolimod, laquinimod, and teriflunomide are used to treat RRMS and SPMS.

Medication	Cog	S	A	Motor	D	Com	F	Other side effects or considerations
Cladribine (Leustatin)* (IV only)	0	0	0	0/+	0	0	0	Decreased white blood cell and lympho-cyte counts, peripheral neuropathy (rare). PPMS; damages CD4 cells.
Fingolimod (Gilenya)	0	0	0	++	0	0	++	Reduction of lymphocytes by 20%-30%, increased risk of infection, maculopapular rash, macular edema resulting in loss of vision, decreased pulmonary function, increased liver enzymes. Restricted by FDA REMS due to risk of bradycardia. Baseline electrocardiography is needed; ophthalmologic exams required at baseline and after 3-4 mo. Teratogenic. RRMS, SPMS; reduces lymphocyte migration into the CNS.
Laquinimod**	0	0	0	0	0	0	0	Increased erythrocyte sedimentation rate, increased liver enzymes. RRMS, SPMS; reduces action of T-helper cells.
Teriflunomide (Aubagio)	0	0	0	+++	+++	0	+++	Hepatic enzyme elevation and hepatic dysfunction, neutropenia, rhabdomyoly-sis, trigeminal neuralgia, paresthesias, limb pain, arthralgias, nausea, diarrhea, alopecia, urinary tract infection. RRMS, SPMS; blocks pyrimidine and cell synthesis; reduces T-cell activation and cyclooxygenase activity.

Monoclonal antibodies: Natalizumab and alemtuzumab are used to treat RRMS; rituximab is used to treat RRMS and PPMS.***

Medication	Cog	S	A	Motor	D	Com	F	Other side effects or considerations
Natalizumab (Tysabri)	0	0	0	++	0	0	0	Headache, fatigue, urinary tract infection, respiratory infection, depression, joint pain, chest discomfort. Restricted by FDA manufacturer REMS. Allergic reactions occur within 2 h of infu-sion; monitor for progressive multifocal leukoencephalopathy. RRMS; blocks access of lymphocytes into CNS.

Medication	Side effects affecting rehab							Other side effects or considerations
Alemtuzumab (Campath)*	Cog 0	S 0	A 0	Motor +	D ++	Com 0	F 0	Infusion reactions (rigors, fever, nausea, vomiting, rash, and hypotension) occur in 90%; pretreat with 1 g of methylprednisolone before infusion. Other side effects include increased infections, reduced T- and B-cell counts, and Graves' disease (27% of patients). RRMS; targets CD52 on lymphocytes and monocytes, reducing number of circulating T-cells.
Daclizumab (Zenapax)*	Cog 0	S 0	A 0	Motor 0	D ++	Com 0	F 0	Mouth ulcers, photosensitivity with rash, formation of antibodies causing discontinuance, reduced lymphocyte count, lymphadenopathy, transient increase in bilirubin. RRMS, SPMS; targets interleukin-2 on activated lymphocytes, reducing IL CD24 complexation; reduces T-cell activation.
Rituximab (Rituxan)*	Cog ++	S ++	A 0	Motor 0	D ++	Com ++	F ++	Infusion reactions (chills, headache, nausea, pruritus, pyrexia, and fatigue) occur in 75%; pretreat with diphenhydramine and acetaminophen 30-60 min before infusion. Other side effects include increased urinary tract infections, sinusitis, throat irritation, and nasopharyngitis. RRMS, PPMS; depletes CD20+ pre-B- and B-cells.

Steroids: Used as short-term treatment of acute exacerbations of RRMS and PPMS.

Medication	Side effects affecting rehab							Other side effects or considerations
Methylprednisolone (Solu-Medrol)	Cog ++	S 0	A ++	Motor ++	D 0	Com +	F ++	Increased appetite, psychosis, bloating, acne, insomnia, headache, muscle weakness, hyperglycemia, altered mental status.
Prednisone	Cog ++	S 0	A ++	Motor ++	D 0	Com +	F ++	RRMS, PPMS; decreases inflammatory cytokines; decreases activation of T-lymphocytes; decreases migration of lymphocytes into the CNS.

*Available but not approved for multiple sclerosis. **Not available. ***Immunize prior to initiation. Avoid in patients with congestive heart failure. Monitor for reactivation of latent infection such as hepatitis, tuberculosis, or fungal infections (e.g., histoplasmosis).

Cog = cognition; S = sedation; A = agitation or mania; Motor = discoordination; D = dysphagia; Com = communication; F = falls; PPMS = primary progressive multiple sclerosis; RRMS = relapsing–remitting multiple sclerosis; SPMS = secondary progressive multiple sclerosis; REMS = risk evaluation and mitigation strategies; IL = interleukin; CNS = central nervous system; FDA = Food and Drug Administration.

The likelihood rating scale for encountering the side effects is as follows: 0 = Almost no probability of encountering side effects. 0/+ = Low probability of encountering side effects but increased with increased dosage. + = Little likelihood of encountering side effects. +/++ = Low probability of encountering side effects; however, probability increases with increased dosage. ++ = Medium likelihood of encountering side effects. +++ = High likelihood of encountering side effects, particularly with high doses. ++++ = Highest likelihood of encountering side effects; best to avoid in at-risk patients.

Beta interferon (Avonex, Rebif, Betaseron) and glatiramer (Copaxone) are considered first-line therapies for treatment of RRMS and have been shown to decrease relapses by 30%. Researchers believe that beta interferon works by suppressing T-helper cell response and reducing T-cell migration across the blood–brain barrier. The rehabilitation therapist should teach patients methods for reducing pain and discomfort associated with these injections (e.g., using antipyretic medications to reduce flu-like symptoms, injecting medications at room temperature, icing or warming the injection site before and after the injection, avoiding shaking the vial, and rotating the site of injection with each injection) and tell them that the flu-like symptoms associated with these injections usually resolve with time. The prescribing physician selects which agent to use based on side effects and the patient's concurrent disease states and preference.

Interferon beta-1a is administered by intramuscular injection 3 times/wk, whereas interferon beta-1b is administered by subcutaneous injection every other day (Gawronski et al., 2010; Guthrie, 2007a). Glatiramer (Copaxone), which is thought to interfere with T-cell activation and differentiation, is administered by subcutaneous injection daily. Side effects of glatiramer include formation of masses and irritation at the injection site and depression. It does not cause flu-like symptoms and is an alternative to interferon beta when this side effect is troublesome (Gawronski et al., 2010; Litzinger & Litzinger, 2009; Ryan, 2007; Tanzi, 2010).

Natalizumab (Tysabri) is a human monoclonal antibody that antagonizes alpha-4-integrin of the adhesion molecule and very late activating antigen on leukocytes. Its action blocks the migration of T-cells across the blood–brain barrier. This agent reduces relapse rates and slows disease progression. In one study, this agent reduced relapses by 56% and reduced lesions on magnetic resonance imaging by 87% when compared with beta interferon. Unfortunately, the agent is considered a second-line therapy in the treatment of RRMS because it increases the risk of multifocal leukoencephalopathy, a potentially fatal infection caused by the JC (John Cunningham) polyomavirus, which causes permanent demyelination. The drug was withdrawn from the market in 2005, and the agent is available only through an FDA-approved manufacturer's REMS (Risk Evaluation and Mitigation Strategy) program (Bennett, 2007; Gawronski et al., 2010; Rosenzweig et al., 2010).

Mitoxantrone (Novantrone) is an immunosuppressant that is chemically related to the antineoplastic antibiotics doxorubicin (Adriamycin) and daunorubicin (Daunomycin). It causes breakage of deoxyribonucleic acid (DNA) and prevents topoisomerase DNA repair of rapidly dividing cells, including leukocytes and other blood components of the immune system. This reduces antigen presentation and destruction, decreases inflammatory action of the cytokines, and reduces migration of the white blood cells. The use of cumulative doses of greater than 100 mg/m^2 of this agent increases the risk of cardiotoxicity. Use of this medication can also cause severe bone marrow suppression. Because of its associated toxicities, it is a second-line agent that is used when other agents fail to treat worsening RRMS, SPMS, and PRMS (Bennett, 2007; Gawronski et al., 2010; Litzinger & Litzinger, 2009; Rosenzweig et al., 2010; Ryan, 2007; Tanzi, 2010).

Fingolimod (Gilenya), a new agent in a new class of medications, is the first oral medication introduced for treating MS. Fingolimod reduces the onset of symptoms, frequency of exacerbations, and onset of disability associated with the disease. It is dosed at 0.5 mg once/day, and food does not affect its absorption or effects. It is a structural analog of a substance called sphingosine-1-phosphate (SIP) and affects SIP-1 receptors on T- and B-lymphocytes. SIP receptors are found in the immune, cardiovascular, and central nervous systems. Fingolimod is believed to reduce migration of lymphocytes into the central nervous system by blocking SIP receptors 1, 2, 4, and 5, thus preventing lymphocytes from leaving the lymph nodes and reducing circulating lymphocytes. Reduction of lymphocytes reduces the autoimmune reaction to the axonal myelin sheath seen with MS. Because this agent can reduce heart rate and atrioventricular conduction, patients should be monitored for bradycardia for 6 h after the initial dose. The prescriber should take a baseline electrocardiogram before initiating this medication. It can lower the heart rate of patients concurrently using atenolol (Tenormin), and concurrent use of ketoconazole (Nizoral) can interfere with the metabolism of fingolimod and increase its blood levels and toxicity. This medication is teratogenic; therefore, adequate contraception should be provided to females of child-bearing age. Because of these toxicities, this agent may be prescribed and dispensed only in compliance with a REMS monitoring program established by the manufacturer and FDA (Gawronski et al., 2010; Sobieraj, 2010; Tanzi, 2010).

Four additional agents have been developed for treating MS and are in various stages of FDA approval: cladribine (Leustatin), laquinimod, dimethyl fumarate (BG-12), and teriflunomide (Aubagio). Three of these agents are oral formulations, and two of the oral formulations are given once daily. These options are expected to greatly enhance adherence in patients with MS and Aubagio is now approved and available in oral form (Gawronski et al., 2010; Litzinger & Litzinger, 2009; Ryan, 2007; Tanzi, 2010).

Cladribine (Leustatin) is a purine analog that acts by damaging DNA resulting in cell death, which has a preferential action on CD4 cells. Oral, subcutaneous, and intravenous formulations of cladribine have been studied. It is expected to be used to reduce symptoms of patients with SPMS and PPMS and to be the first agent approved for use in these classes of MS. Laquinimod, an oral agent that has effects on T-helper cells, is being studied for use in patients with RRMS and SPMS. Teriflunomide (Aubagio), an oral agent that has anti-inflammatory and antiproliferative properties, is now approved for use in patients with RRMS and SPMS. It is the active metabolite of leflunomide (Arava), an agent currently being used in the treatment of rheumatoid arthritis. Dimethyl fumarate (BG-12) is an oral agent that induces T-helper-2-like cytokines to cause apoptosis in activated T-cells. It also causes down regulation of intracellular adhesion molecules, thus reducing migration of lymphocytes into the central nervous system (Bainbridge, 2007; Bennett, 2007; Gawronski et al., 2010).

In addition, three monoclonal antibody agents that are approved for other indications are now being studied for use in the MS patient. They include alemtuzumab (Campath), daclizumab (Zenapax), and rituximab (Rituxan). Alemtuzumab (Campath) is a humanized monoclonal antibody currently approved for use in patients with chronic lymphocytic leukemia. It targets CD52 on lymphocytes and monocytes, causing extended reduction in circulating T-cells. It has been shown to be effective in treating patients with RRMS and SPMS. Daclizumab (Zenapax) is a humanized monoclonal antibody that antagonizes interleukin-2 on activated lymphocytes. It is currently approved for preventing kidney rejection in transplantation and has been shown to be effective in treating patients with RRMS and SPMS (Bennett, 2007). Rituximab (Rituxan) is a chimeric monoclonal antibody approved for use in the treatment of non-Hodgkin's lymphoma and rheumatoid arthritis. It has been shown to be effective in treating patients with PPMS and RRMS. These are avoided in patients with congestive heart failure and require immunization prior to use. They can reactivate latent infections (see table 11.2) (Cree, 2006; Gawronski et al., 2010; Litzinger & Litzinger, 2009; Ryan, 2007; Tanzi, 2010).

Some have hypothesized that infection can trigger acute exacerbations of MS (Bennett, 2007; Guthrie, 2005, 2007a; Rosenzweig et al., 2010). Treatment of acute exacerbations of MS usually involves a short course of corticosteroids. High-dose intravenous methylprednisolone (Medrol) or high-dose oral prednisone are generally used to treat acute exacerbations (Guthrie, 2007b). The following interventions can be used to minimize the adverse effects of steroids. Drinking chocolate milk or eating candy can minimize metallic taste. Short-acting benzodiazepines can minimize insomnia (the patient should avoid over-the-counter antihistamines because they worsen taste alterations). Gastrointestinal upset can be minimized by avoiding spicy foods, caffeine, and nonsteroidal anti-inflammatory drugs such as ibuprofen. Headaches and body aches should be treated with **acetaminophen**.

In addition to the disease-modifying therapies, other medications are used to manage symptoms associated with MS. Table 11.3 lists supportive therapies (Litzinger & Litzinger,

Table 11.3 Medications Used to Manage Symptoms of Multiple Sclerosis

Symptom	Medications
Impaired walking ability	Fampridine-SR (Ampyra)
Impaired balance and coordination	Meclizine (Antivert), prochlorperazine (Compazine), promethazine (Phenergan)
Spasticity	Baclofen (Lioresal), botulinum toxin, clonazepam (Klonopin), clonidine (Catapres), dantrolene (Dantrium), tiagabine (Gabitril), tizanidine (Zanaflex)
Tremor	Clonazepam (Klonopin), propranolol (Inderal), gabapentin (Neurontin), primidone (Mysoline)
Fatigue	Amantadine (Symmetrel), selective serotonin reuptake inhibitor antidepressants, methylphenidate (Ritalin), 4-amino pyridine
Urinary incontinence	Desmopressin (DDAVP), oxybutynin (Ditropan), propantheline (Banthine), tolterodine (Detrol), tricyclic antidepressants (e.g., amitriptyline, nortriptyline)
Irritable bowel	Dicyclomine (Bentyl)
Constipation	Docusate (Colace), senna–Colace (Senokot), magnesium products (milk of magnesia)
Neuropathic pain	Gabapentin (Neurontin), pregabalin (Lyrica), duloxetine (Cymbalta), tricyclic antidepressants
Sensory alterations	Duloxetine (Cymbalta), gabapentin (Neurontin), pregabalin (Lyrica), tricyclic antidepressants
Depression	Selective serotonin reuptake inhibitors, tricyclic antidepressants, selective serotonin and norepinephrine reuptake inhibitors (e.g., duloxetine [Cymbalta], venlafaxine [Effexor])

2009). Adrenocorticotropic hormone may be given to shorten recovery, but it is usually not used unless a corticosteroid cannot be administered. Other immunosuppressant medications used less frequently in the treatment of MS include methotrexate, azathioprine (Imuran), cyclophosphamide (Cytoxan), and cyclosporine (Neoral, Sandimmune) (Iversen et al., 2009; Ryan, 2007).

The prescribing physician may consider a number of medications to treat the patient's spasticity. The drug of choice is baclofen (Lioresal), which impairs neural transmission from the spinal cord to the skeletal muscles, resulting in reduced flexor and extensor spasms. Tizanidine (Zanaflex) is also frequently used to decrease spasticity. It is as effective as baclofen and causes less weakness but causes extreme sedation. The benzodiazepines diazepam (Valium) and clonazepam (Klonopin), though used less frequently, can be used to treat nocturnal spasms not responding to the other agents. Dantrolene (Dantrium) is used as a last resort for treating spasticity. This medication is

typically prescribed for severe spasticity when the combination of baclofen and diazepam is not effective. Finally, botulinum toxin can be given intramuscularly for focal target areas of spasticity (Gawronski et al., 2010; Litzinger & Litzinger, 2009; Ryan, 2007; Tanzi, 2010).

Dalfampridine (Ampyra; formally called Fampridine-SR) is a new oral medication that is indicated for improving walking ability in patients with MS. It is a sustained-release tablet that is dosed at 10 mg twice/day. Comprising 4-aminopyridine, it enhances impulse conduction in nerve fibers. This medication acts as a voltage-dependent blocker of potassium channels, which increases neuronal excitability, potentiates synaptic and neuronal transmission, and relieves conduction blockade in the demyelinated axons. This agent enters the open potassium channels and remains trapped for an extended period of time in the closed channels. This allows for prolonged potassium channel blockade, which results in a greater-than-normal influx of calcium and, thus, enhanced neuroneural and neuromuscular transmission. In addition, potassium channel blockade results in immune modulation, thus reducing the hypersensitivity response to myelin protein seen in patients with MS (Perez, 2009; Rosenzweig et al., 2010).

MS patients with psychiatric difficulties can benefit from psychotropic medications, particularly antidepressants. However, MS patients may be more sensitive to the side effects of these medications. Support groups and psychotherapy may also be of assistance. Medications used to increase cognitive functioning in patients with MS are donepezil (Aricept), amantadine (Symmetrel), 4-aminopyridine (treats cognitive fatigue), and interferon (treats cognitive deterioration) (Cohen et al., 2002).

PATIENT CASE 2

J.E. is a 32-yr-old woman who is married and has one child. She was recently diagnosed with RRMS. Her physician prescribed interferon beta-1b (Betaseron) 0.25 mg subcutaneously every other day. She was referred for physical therapy due to her complaints of altered sensation in her upper and lower extremities, muscle weakness, fatigue, and unsteadiness on her feet. Most notably, she complains of tripping over her right foot because she is not able to sufficiently lift the foot to clear the floor during gait (early stages of foot drop). She begins physical therapy 4 wk after beginning the interferon beta-1b therapy. During her initial physical therapy examination, she reports that she has not taken the medication for the past 2 wk because she was experiencing flu-like symptoms along with intermittent episodes of nausea, vomiting, mood swings, and a heightened sense of smell. All symptoms are worst first thing in the morning. J.E. notes that she previously enjoyed a large cup of coffee every morning but now cannot tolerate the smell of coffee because it makes her nauseous. She further reports that she has been living on saltines and ginger ale, which seem to be the only things that settle her stomach. Finally, she states that she took some ibuprofen to treat the flu-like symptoms, which have since resolved.

Question

What is an appropriate intervention for the rehabilitation therapist to make at this time?

Answer

Beta-interferons, including interferon beta-1b (Betaseron), are first-line treatments for patients with RRMS. Flu-like symptoms are one of the most common side effects of interferon beta-1b therapy. However, J.E.'s morning symptoms of nausea, vomiting, mood swings, and heightened senses of smell are a cause for concern. The physical therapist was concerned that J.E. may be experiencing morning sickness that commonly begins in the fourth through sixth week of pregnancy. The physical therapist contacted J.E.'s physician, and the physician examined J.E. later that day. J.E.'s pregnancy test was positive. The physician was pleased that J.E. discontinued the beta-interferon injections after just 2 wk because this medication is contraindicated during pregnancy. Interferon beta-1b (Betaseron) should not be used during pregnancy or by any woman who is trying to become pregnant. Women taking this medication should use birth control measures at all times. J.E.'s physician also recommended that she discontinue the use of ibuprofen and that she use acetaminophen as a pain reliever. J.E. resumed an 8 wk course of physical therapy and had good overall results. Neuromuscular electrical stimulation and therapeutic exercise were used to restore dorsiflexion strength in the right ankle to a functional level. A molded ankle foot orthosis was not necessary at the time. Balance training, low-grade strengthening, and a stretching program were effective in improving J.E.'s functional performance. J.E. was also counseled on energy-conservation and relaxation techniques. At a follow-up appointment 6 mo later, J.E. reported having a healthy baby boy.

This case highlights how important it is for the rehabilitation therapist to know the expected side effects of a medication and decipher side effects that are not consistent with the known side effects of the medication. A thorough history and systems review is essential in screening out other medical conditions (e.g., pregnancy) that contraindicate the use of a medication. Communication with the prescriber and pharmacist is essential when the patient complains of symptoms that are inconsistent with the known side effects of a medication.

Myasthenia Gravis

Myasthenia Gravis (MG) is a relatively rare autoimmune disorder affecting the skeletal muscles that is characterized by weakness and fatigue that are relieved by periods of rest. The disorder typically follows a slow, progressive course that is characterized by periods of remission and exacerbation (Shah, 2011).

Incidence

The worldwide incidence of MG varies widely due to differences in methodology of data collection. It is estimated that MG occurs in 5.3/1 million person years. Reports show that the incidence of MG has increased over the past 50 yr. Researchers believe that the increase is attributable to improved identification techniques (Carr et al., 2010). In the United States, the incidence of MG is approximately 1/200,000 people. It typically affects women in their twenties and thirties and men in their fifties and sixties. Remission of symptoms can occur early in the course of the disease.

Etiology and Pathophysiology

MG is an autoimmune disease in which antibodies develop in the nicotinic postsynaptic acetylcholine receptor at the neuromuscular junction of skeletal muscle, resulting in the destruction of these receptors. Edrophonium chloride (Tensilon) is an injectable medication used to diagnose MG. This disease does not affect smooth muscle receptors. Symptoms of weakness and fatigue occur after 30% of available receptors are destroyed. In addition, abnormalities in the thymus occur in 75% of patients. **Hyperplasia** of the thymus occurs in 85% of these patients and thymoma occurs in 15% of these patients. The thymus is the central organ in T-cell-mediated immunity and is believed to be the site of the formation of these antibodies. About 15% to 20% of MG patients develop myasthenic crisis; most episodes occur within the first 2 yr of diagnosis. Myasthenic crisis is characterized by body limpness; slackness of the face, jaw, and neck along with the inability to support the head; inability to manage respiratory secretions; and inability to generate adequate ventilation, resulting in respiratory compromise. Concurrent illness or some medications can exacerbate weakness, quickly precipitating a myasthenic crisis and rapid respiratory compromise (Awwad & Mal'uf, 2010; Shah, 2011).

Rehabilitation Considerations

Approximately 50% of patients with MG present with drooping of the eyelid (ptosis). This symptom eventually occurs in 90% of patients and can result in double vision. Bulbar muscle weakness can result in dysphagia and flaccid dysarthria, resulting in unintelligible speech. In approximately 85% of patients the weakness is generalized and affects the limb musculature. Weakness of palatal muscles can result in a nasal twang to the voice and nasal regurgitation of food and especially liquids. Chewing may become difficult. Severe jaw weakness may cause the jaw to hang open; the patient may sit with a hand on the chin for support. Swallowing may become difficult and aspiration may occur with fluids, giving rise to coughing or choking while drinking. Weakness of neck muscles is common; neck flexors are usually affected more severely than are neck extensors (Awwad & Mal'uf, 2010; Shah, 2011).

Certain limb muscles are more commonly affected than others. For example, upper-limb muscles are more likely to be affected than are lower-limb muscles. In the upper limbs, deltoids and extensors of the wrist and fingers are affected most. Triceps are more likely than biceps to be affected. In the lower extremities, commonly affected muscles include the hip flexors, quadriceps, and hamstrings. Involvement of foot dorsiflexors or plantar flexors is less common (Awwad & Mal'uf, 2010; Shah, 2011).

The rehabilitation therapist should be aware that symptoms typically fluctuate throughout the course of the day and can vary from day to day. The therapist should also be alert for the onset of a myasthenic crisis, which is evidenced by increasing muscle weakness, respiratory distress, and more difficulty with talking, chewing, or swallowing than usual. Therapy sessions should be planned for the time of day when the patient has the most energy. The therapist should teach the patient energy-conservation techniques and should implement submaximal, nonexhaustive functional exercises. The patient with MG needs greater recovery time as the intensity of exercises or exertion increases. The therapist should closely monitor the patient's therapy program and overall activity level and progress or regress sessions based on the patient's response to treatment and exercise tolerance. Patients with mild MG have been shown to tolerate higher levels of strength training, provided they are monitored closely for fatigue and are given adequate rest between bouts of exercise (Lohi et al., 1993). Environmental stressors such as excessive exposure to heat or cold should also be avoided in order to prevent exacerbations.

The rehabilitation therapist must monitor the patient's respiratory function, including negative inspiratory force, vital capacity, and tidal volume, because respiratory impairment is a serious complication of MG. Weak pharyngeal muscles may collapse the upper airway, and respiratory muscle weakness may produce acute respiratory failure. This is a true neuromuscular emergency, and immediate intubation may be necessary. Patients with MG may experience difficulty chewing and swallowing because of oropharyngeal weakness. It may be difficult for the patient to chew meat or veg-

etables because of weakness of the masticatory muscles. If dysphagia develops, it is usually most severe when the patient consumes thin liquids due to weakened pharyngeal muscles. Liquids should be thickened in order to avoid nasal regurgitation or frank aspiration (Shah, 2011).

Medication Therapy

Medications used to treat MG include the acetylcholinesterase inhibitors pyridostigmine (Mestinon) and neostigmine (Prostigmin). These medications increase acetylcholine levels, which facilitates stimulation of muscular activity and thus results in decreased weakness. These medications can cause increased neuromuscular blockade when combined with aminoglycosides (amikacin, gentamicin, and tobramycin), anesthetics, or neuromuscular-blocking agents and potentiate effects of antiarrhythmics. Anticholinergics antagonize the gastrointestinal effects of these acetylcholinesterase inhibitors, and atropine antagonizes the antimuscarinic effects of these agents. Side effects of these medications include excessive salivation and gastrointestinal disturbances (Awwad & Mal'uf, 2010; Shah, 2011).

Immunosuppressant therapy may be initiated in patients whose symptoms are not ameliorated by acetylcholinesterase inhibitors. The use of immunosuppressants such as corticosteroids (prednisone), azathioprine (Imuran), mycophenolate mofetil (CellCept), cyclosporine (Neoral, Sandimmune), cyclophosphamide (Cytoxan), and rituximab (Rituxan) may modulate the antibody action on the acetylcholine receptors. Corticosteroids are often used as the major pharmacological intervention in the treatment of MG. Immunosuppressants can improve bulbar muscular strength and endurance, thus improving dysarthria and general speech intelligibility. Long-term use of corticosteroids, however, can result in mental confusion and impaired memory. Use of immunosuppressant therapy can also increase the patient's risk for infection. Table 11.4 summarizes medications used to treat MG (Awwad & Mal'uf, 2010; Shah, 2011).

See table 11.4 in the web resource for a full list of medication-specific indications, dosing recommendations, side effects, and other considerations.

Table 11.4 Medications Used to Treat Myasthenia Gravis

Medication	Side effects affecting rehab							Other side effects or considerations
Acetylcholine esterase inhibitors: Used to increase acetylcholine levels in myasthenia gravis and improve motor function.								
Neostigmine (Prostigmin)	Cog +	S +	A 0	Motor ++	D ++	Com ++	F ++	Excessive salivation, abdominal cramps, miosis, diarrhea, urinary urgency, sweating, nausea, vomiting, increased lachrymal and bronchial secretions, nicotinic effects of muscle cramps and fasciculation, malaise, vertigo
Pyridostigmine (Mestinon)	Cog +	S +	A 0	Motor ++	D ++	Com ++	F ++	
Ambenonium chloride (Mytelase)	Cog +	S +	A 0	Motor ++	D ++	Com ++	F ++	
Immunosuppressant: Used to treat symptoms not controlled with acetylcholine esterase inhibitors.								
Prednisone	Cog ++	S 0	A ++	Motor ++	D 0	Com +	F ++	Increased appetite, psychosis, bloating, acne, insomnia, headache, muscle weakness, hyperglycemia, confusion. Initial deterioration with high dose therapy; initiate under medical supervision.
Infusion of antibodies: Used as acute treatment of myasthenic crisis.								
Immune globulin intravenous (Gamimune, Gammagard, Sandoglobulin)	Cog ++	S ++	A 0	Motor ++	D ++	Com +	F ++	Back pain, chills, cough, diarrhea, ear pain, fatigue, flushing, headache, muscle cramps, nausea, reactions at injection site (pain, swelling, muscle stiffness, or redness), sore throat, stuffy nose, weakness, allergic reactions. Best used in crisis management or before surgery.
Immunosuppressants: Used to modulate antibody action on acetylcholine receptors and treat symptoms not controlled with acetylcholine esterase inhibitors.								
Azathioprine (Imuran)	Cog 0	S 0	A 0	Motor 0	D ++	Com 0	F 0	Mild nausea or vomiting, diarrhea, fever, malaise, myalgias, increased risk of infection, leukopenia, thrombocytopenia
Cyclosporine A (Neoral, Sandimmune)	Cog 0	S 0	A ++	Motor +++	D +++	Com +	F +++	Acne, dizziness, flushing, headache, increased hair growth, nausea, runny nose, sleeplessness, stomach discomfort, vomiting, renal dysfunction tremor, hirsutism, hypertension, gum hyperplasia
Cyclophosphamide (Cytoxan, Neosar)	Cog 0	S 0	A 0	Motor 0	D ++	Com 0	F 0	Nausea, vomiting, alopecia, leukopenia, thrombocytopenia, interstitial nephritis
Mycophenolate mofetil (CellCept, Myfortic)	Cog +	S +	A +	Motor +++	D +++	Com +	F +++	Anxiety, back pain, constipation, cough, diarrhea, dizziness, headache, loss of appetite, mild stomach pain, mild tiredness or weakness, nausea, tremor, trouble sleeping, upset stomach, vomiting, diarrhea, leukopenia, sepsis, increased risk of infection

Medication	Side effects affecting rehab							Other side effects or considerations
Rituximab (Rituxan)*	Cog ++	S ++	A 0	Motor 0	D ++	Com ++	F ++	Infusion reactions (chills, headache, nausea, pruritus, pyrexia, and fatigue) occur in 75%; pretreat with diphenhydramine and acetaminophen 30-60 min before infusion. Other side effects include increased urinary tract infections, sinusitis, throat irritation, and nasopharyngitis. Avoid in congestive heart failure.

*Can reactivate latent infections; immunize prior to initiation.

Cog = cognition; S = sedation; A = agitation or mania; Motor = discoordination; D = dysphagia; Com = communication; F = falls.

The likelihood rating scale for encountering the side effects is as follows: 0 = Almost no probability of encountering side effects. + = Little likelihood of encountering side effects. +/++ = Low probability of encountering side effects; however, probability increases with increased dosage. ++ = Medium likelihood of encountering side effects. +++ = High likelihood of encountering side effects, particularly with high doses. ++++ = Highest likelihood of encountering side effects; best to avoid in at-risk patients.

PATIENT CASE 3

F.H. is a 55-yr-old college tennis coach who has just been diagnosed with MG. His primary-care doctor referred him to a neurologist after hearing his complaints of a 3 mo history of double vision, ptosis, generalized muscle weakness, and balance difficulties. A positive Tensilon test and a positive blood test for acetylcholine (ACH) antibodies confirmed the clinical diagnosis of MG. The neurologist prescribed prednisolone 60 mg/day and pyridostigmine (Mestinon) 60 mg 4 times/day. F.H. was also referred to physical therapy to address his generalized muscle weakness and balance difficulties that were interfering with his tennis coaching and participation in a men's doubles tennis league. F.H. noted that the early-stage MG symptoms he was experiencing improved for about 3 h after each dose of his medication. However, he had to miss several rehabilitation sessions due to what he described as a stomach bug. He complained of abdominal cramps, nausea, diarrhea, and vomiting.

Question

What is an appropriate intervention for the rehabilitation therapist to make at this time?

Answer

F.H. is experiencing gastrointestinal symptoms that are frequent side effects of pyridostigmine (Mestinon). The physical therapist asked F.H. several questions about the timing of his medication, how he took his medication, and whether he took the medication on a full or empty stomach. F.H. replied that he has recently experienced some difficulty swallowing pills first thing in the morning and that he has been crushing the tablets and mixing the medication into applesauce before taking it about 1 h before breakfast. The physical therapist explained to the neurologist and pharmacist the gastrointestinal symptoms that F.H. was experiencing and how he was taking his medication. Both the pharmacist and neurologist recommended that F.H. discontinue crushing the tablet and that he take the medication 1 h later in the morning with food or milk. A speech–language pathology consult was also ordered to evaluate the patient's new complaint of difficulty swallowing. The neurologist and pharmacist also stated that the patient could take the pyridostigmine (Mestinon) in syrup form in the future if the speech–language pathology consult indicated that this was necessary.

About 1 wk later F.H. noted significant improvement in the gastrointestinal symptoms and continued improvement in the MG symptoms. He was able to successfully participate in low-grade aerobic training on a treadmill and a low-resistance strength-training program. Taking the medication with food and milk 1 h after waking allowed him to swallow the medication with greater ease. Based on the speech–language pathology evaluation, the syrup form of this medication was not necessary at the time. After 6 wk of physical therapy, F.H. returned to light-duty tennis coaching and to participating in recreational-level doubles tennis once/wk.

This case highlights the importance of properly administrating medication. In this case, crushing the Mestinon tablets likely destroyed the medication's sustained-release matrix and contributed to F.H.'s gastrointestinal symptoms. The case also illustrates the importance of a multidisciplinary approach to solving issues related to medication side effects.

Medications that can exacerbate MG and precipitate myasthenic crisis include antibiotics such as aminoglycosides, ciprofloxacin, erythromycin, and ampicillin; beta blockers such as propranolol (Inderal) and timolol (Timoptic) eye drops; lithium; magnesium; procainamide (Pronestyl); verapamil (Calan, Verelan, Isoptin); quinidine; chloroquine; prednisone; and anticholinergics such as antihistamines, trihexyphenidyl (Artane), procyclidine (Kemadrin), and amitriptyline (Elavil). Neuromuscular-blocking agents, including vecuronium and curare, should be used cautiously in patients with MG in order to avoid prolonged neuromuscular blockade (Awwad & Mal'uf, 2010; Shah, 2011).

Plasmapheresis or plasma exchange can be used to reduce the antibodies and immune complexes from the blood in preparation for surgery, to reduce postoperative respiratory problems, or in treatment of myasthenic crisis. This treatment improves symptoms within days and lasts 6 to 8 wk. An alternative therapy used is intravenous gamma globulin. Thymectomy (surgical removal of the thymus) may induce remission, especially if thymoma is present (Shah, 2011).

Summary

This chapter summarizes the rehabilitation considerations, medications, and nonpharmacologic therapies that are used in the care of patients with ALS, MS, and MG. The table format provides easy access to information on medications, including dosing, side effects, and drug interactions that the rehabilitation therapist must be aware of when caring for these patients.

Medications Used to Treat Other Movement Disorders

In clinical practice, the rehabilitation therapist will care for many patients with movement disorders. Changes in motor function frequently occur with the normal aging process. These changes can be associated with declines in visual, vestibular, and proprioceptive function, motor and psychomotor slowing, and an increase in postural sway. Movement disorders affect the patient's speed, fluency, quality, and ease of movement. Abnormal fluency or speed of movement (dyskinesia) may involve excessive or involuntary movement (e.g., tics) or slowed or absent voluntary movement (hypokinesia). Movement disorders can cause ataxia (lack of coordination, often producing jerky movements) and dystonia (causes involuntary movement and prolonged muscle contraction). Movement disorders such as Parkinson's disease, stroke-related movement disorders, essential tremor, and dyskinesias (orofacial and neuroleptic induced) occur with increased frequency after age 65 yr (Emilien et al., 2004; Jacobson et al., 2007; Mendez & Cummings, 2003).

This chapter reviews essential tremor, subcortical dementias with movement disorders such as Lewy body dementia and vascular dementia, **progressive supranuclear palsy**, restless-leg syndrome, Huntington's disease, and Wilson's disease, as well as the medications used to treat these disorders. It also reviews movement disorders that can be caused or exacerbated by medication use (Spillantini et al., 2006) and how movement disorders can affect the patient's rehabilitation session.

Essential Tremor

Tremor is usually classified by the behaviors that activate the tremor and include resting tremor and action tremor. **Resting tremors** occur in the absence of voluntary muscle contraction. During resting tremor, the tremulous body part must be supported against gravity. Causes of resting tremor include use of neuroleptics, Parkinson's disease, alcoholic degeneration, and multiple sclerosis. **Action tremors** include tremors associated with voluntary muscle contraction. These can include postural (tremor present while voluntarily maintaining a posture), kinetic (tremor present during voluntary movement), and isometric (tremor associated with muscle contraction against a rigid, stationary object) tremors. Common causes of action tremor include essential tremor (ET), tremor associated with medication use, and tremor associated with **thyrotoxicosis**, hypoglycemia, multiple sclerosis, or drug withdrawal (Chen, 2002).

Incidence

The true incidence of ET worldwide is unclear because many individuals fail to seek medical attention for this disorder. The general worldwide incidence of ET is reported to be 1.2% for individuals over 70 yr of age. The high incidence of ET in identical twins suggests that a genetic factor contributes to the incidence. In the study of Lorenz and colleagues (2004), ET occurred in 93% of the identical twins studied.

ET is an action tremor and can include postural or kinetic tremor. The mean onset age of ET is 45 yr; bimodal peak onsets occur in the thirties and then in the sixties. Incidence of ET increases with increasing age, and it occurs at the same frequency in both sexes. Estimated overall incidence worldwide of ET is around 18/100,000 persons. About 1.4 million people aged 65 or older have ET (Chen, 2002; Jacobson et al., 2007).

Etiology and Pathophysiology

About 50% of patients with ET report a positive family history and there is an autosomal dominant mode of inheritance with familial ET. In children of parents with ET, the risk of developing the movement disorder is increased fivefold if the parent developed ET later in life and tenfold if the parent developed the syndrome early in life. Researchers believe that ET is associated with cerebellar dysfunction associated with alterations in gamma amino butyric acid (GABA) and adrenergic systems (Chen, 2002).

Rehabilitation Considerations

Onset of ET is insidious and usually begins with bilateral postural or kinetic tremor that affects the upper extremities. ET can interfere with activities of daily living. As the disease progresses, the tremor increases in amplitude and the tremors can be seen in other parts of the body (e.g., the head and trunk) and can be heard in the voice. Patients with ET that involves the head display a "no, no" movement of the head. Oropharyngeal regions may be affected and can result in tremor of the voice, tongue, and muscle of the soft palate, thus affecting speech and swallowing. This can be a challenge for the speech–language pathologist working to improve the patient's voice abilities.

The goal of therapy is to improve the patient's functional ability and quality of life. Treatments involve physical therapy, occupational therapy, and speech and language interventions as well as pharmacological, psychological, and behavioral therapies (Chen, 2002; Jacobson et al., 2007). The physical therapist may focus

on improving posture and trunk stability. The occupational therapist may focus on improving the patient's eating skills, such as holding a knife or fork and drinking from a cup.

Medication Therapy

When new onset or worsening of tremor is noted, the rehabilitation team should ask the pharmacist to carefully review the patient's medication list in order to identify any recent medication changes that may cause or exacerbate the tremor. If the patient is taking a medication that is known to contribute to tremor, the rehabilitation therapist should ask the prescriber whether the patient's medication regimen can be changed (Carl & Johnson, 2006; Emilien et al., 2004; Mendez & Cummings, 2003). Table 12.1 lists medications that are commonly used to treat ET. Table 12.4, later in this chapter, lists medications that can cause tremors (Chen, 2002; Cheng et al., 2006; Jacobson et al., 2007).

Subcortical Dementia

Patients with subcortical dementia exhibit movement disorders known as extrapyramidal symptoms. Subcortical dementias include dementias associated with Parkinson's disease, Lewy body dementia (DLB), vascular dementia (VD), progressive supranuclear palsy (PSP), and corticobasal degeneration (CBD). VD and DLB may be either cortical or subcortical in nature. Patients with Huntington's disease or Wilson's disease, who also have symptoms of dementia, are considered to have subcortical dementias (Emilien et al., 2004; Mendez & Cummings, 2003).

Incidence

Most incidence studies categorize dementia by diagnosis rather than by whether the dementia is cortical or subcortical. The incidence studies discussed here report international statistics. Alzheimer's disease is the leading cause of dementia, and DLB is the second leading cause. DLB occurs in 15% to 25% of patients with dementia. Most patients are over 65 yr of age,

See table 12.1 in the web resource for a full list of medication-specific indications, dosing recommendations, side effects, and other considerations.

Table 12.1 Medications Used to Treat Essential Tremor, Subcortical Dementias, Huntington's Disease, and Wilson's Disease

Medication	Side effects affecting rehab							Other side effects or considerations
Treatment of ET: Beta blockers								
Propranolol (Inderal)	Cog ++	S ++	A 0	Motor ++	D +	Com +	F ++	Bradycardia, heart block, orthostasis, fatigue, dizziness.
Metoprolol (Lopressor, Toprol)	Cog +	S +	A 0	Motor ++	D +	Com +	F ++	Avoid using with cocaine, amphetamines, and decongestants such as pseudoephedrine medications that increase sympathetic tone—increase in heart rate and arrhythmia may occur.
Treatment of ET: Anticonvulsants								
Primidone (Mysoline)	Cog +++	S +++	A ++	Motor +++	D +++	Com +++	F +++	Sedation, lethargy, decreased cognition, decreased attention, hyperactivity, depression, nystagmus, ataxia, skin rash
Gabapentin (Neurontin)	Cog ++	S ++	A +	Motor +++	D 0	Com ++	F +++	Peripheral edema, tremor, dizziness, fatigue, ataxia, drowsiness, weight gain, behavioral changes
Treatment of ET: Benzodiazepines								
Clonazepam (Klonopin)	Cog +	S +	A ++	Motor ++	D ++	Com ++	F +	Sedation, impaired cognition, dysphagia, ataxia, headache, fatigue, nausea.
Diazepam (Valium)	Cog ++++	S ++++	A ++	Motor +++	D ++	Com ++++	F ++++	Avoid combining with alcohol. Risk of dependence or addiction.
Lorazepam (Ativan)	Cog +++	S +++	A ++	Motor +++	D ++	Com ++	F ++	
Treatment of ET: Botulinum toxin								
Botulinum toxin type A—focal injection	Cog 0	S 0	A 0	Motor ++	D +++	Com +	F +	May cause paralysis or motor dysfunction adjacent to injection site
Treatment of cognitive symptoms of DLB: Acetylcholine esterase inhibitors								
Tacrine* (Cognex)	Cog ++	S ++	A +	Motor ++	D +++	Com ++	F +++	Dysphagia secondary to nausea, vomiting, abdominal pain, diarrhea, dyspepsia, anorexia.
Donepezil (Aricept)	Cog ++	S 0	A ++	Motor +	D +++	Com ++	F ++	Decrease dose of donepezil for liver or renal disease.
Rivastigmine (Exelon)	Cog ++	S 0	A ++	Motor +	D +++	Com ++	F ++	Decrease dose of galantamine for severe renal disease or for liver disease.
Galantamine (Razadyne)	Cog ++	S 0	A ++	Motor +	D +++	Com ++	F ++	

› continued

Table 12.1 › *continued*

Medication	Side effects affecting rehab							Other side effects or considerations
Treatment of motor symptoms of DLB or PSP: Muscle relaxant								
Baclofen (Lioresal)	Cog ++	S +++	A ++	Motor +++	D ++	Com ++	F +++	Oral: Initial sedation, muscle weakness, ataxia, orthostatic hypotension, fatigue, headache, nausea, dizziness; confusion and hallucinations reported in the elderly or those with history of stroke. Intrathecal: Chronic constipation, hypotonia, somnolence, headache, vomiting, paresthesias.
Treatment of psychotic symptoms of DLB: Second-generation antipsychotics								
Clozapine (Clozaril)	Cog ++++	S ++++	A ++	Motor +	D ++++	Com ++++	F ++++	Weight gain ++++ Seizure ++++ Cardiac +++ Sexual + Use requires enrollment in Risk Evaluation and Mitigation Strategy program for monitoring for agranulocytosis. Use limited to failure of other agents.
Quetiapine (Seroquel)	Cog ++	S ++	A +	Motor ++	D +	Com ++	F +++	Weight gain ++ Seizure 0 Cardiac ++ Sexual + High risk for orthostasis and falls.
Aripiprazole (Abilify)	Cog +	S +	A +	Motor +	D +	Com +	F ++	Weight gain + Seizure 0 Cardiac + Sexual +
Treatment of vascular dementia								
Medications and lifestyle changes	Treat underlying causes of hypertension and hyperlipidemia with medications and lifestyle changes (i.e., weight loss, diet therapy, exercise, and smoking cessation).							
Treatment of motor symptoms of PSP: Tricyclic antidepressant								
Amitriptyline (Elavil)	Cog ++++	S ++++	A 0	Motor ++	D ++++	Com ++++	F ++++	Weight gain +++ Seizure +++ Cardiac +++ Sexual ++ Not recommended in elderly due to high sedative and anticholinergic effects that increase falls risk. Elderly or adolescents may require lower doses.
Treatment of motor symptoms of CBD or DLB: Dopamine agonists								
Carbidopa–levodopa (Sinemet)	Cog +++	S +++	A +++	Motor +++	D +++	Com ++	F ++++	Nausea, vomiting, headache, drowsiness, nightmares. Avoid high-protein meals near bedtime, which can decrease absorption. Take on an empty stomach. Avoid driving or operating machinery.
Bromocriptine (Parlodel)	Cog +++	S +++	A +++	Motor +++	D +++	Com ++	F +++	Nausea, dyskinesia, hallucinations, confusion, on–off phenomenon, dizziness, drowsiness, vomiting, visual disturbance, insomnia, depression, hypotension, constipation, retroperitoneal fibrosis (rare), impulse-control disorders

Medication	Side effects affecting rehab							Other side effects or considerations
Pramipexole (Mirapex)	Cog +++	S +++	A +++	Motor +++	D +++	Com ++	F +++	Nausea, fainting spells, lightheadedness, sweating, flushing, xerostomia, sleep attacks.
Ropinirole (Requip)	Cog +++	S +++	A +++	Motor +++	D +++	Com ++	F +++	Avoid using alcohol and driving or operating machinery. Treat xerostomia with sugarless gum or drinking water.
Treatment of motor symptoms of Huntington's disease								
Tetrabenazine (Xenazine)	Cog ++	S ++	A ++	Motor +++	D ++	Com ++	F +++	Akathisia, depression, parkinsonism, dizziness, drowsiness, fatigue, nervousness, anxiety
Initial chelation therapy for WD: Used to remove excess copper.								
D-penicillamine (Cuprimine)	Cog 0	S 0	A 0	Motor +++	D ++	Com +	F +++	Drug-induced lupus, myasthenia gravis, neuropathies (peripheral, sensory, and motor), reversible optic neuritis, gastrointestinal upset, tinnitus, diarrhea, nausea, vomiting, loss of appetite, loss of taste, oral ulcerations, bone marrow depression, proteinuria that can lead to renal failure, dystonia, skin reactions, respiratory fibrosis, pneumonitis
Trientine (Syprine)	Cog 0	S 0	A 0	Motor ++	D 0	Com 0	F ++	Abnormal muscle contractions or spasms, lupus, muscle weakness, severe allergic reactions, skin reactions. Used in patients with intolerance to penicillamine therapy.
Maintenance therapy for WD: Used to maintain healthy levels of copper after successful chelation therapy.								
Zinc acetate (Galzin)	Cog 0	S 0	A 0	Motor 0	D 0/+	Com 0	F 0	Gastric upset; take with food.

*Only used after other agents have failed, second line therapy.

Cog = cognition; S = sedation; A = agitation or mania; Motor = discoordination; D = dysphagia; Com = communication; F = falls; CBD = corticobasal degeneration; DLB = Lewy body dementia; ET = essential tremor; PSP = progressive supranuclear palsy; WD = Wilson's disease.

Sexual is associated with sexual side effects.

The likelihood rating scale for encountering the side effects is as follows: 0 = Almost no probability of encountering side effects. 0/+ = Low probability of encountering side effects but increased with increased dosage. + = Little likelihood of encountering side effects. +/++ = Low probability of encountering side effects; however, probability increases with increased dosage. ++ = Medium likelihood of encountering side effects. +++ = High likelihood of encountering side effects, particularly with high doses. ++++ = Highest likelihood of encountering side effects; best to avoid in at-risk patients.

and approximately 60% of the patients are male. Survival rate is approximately a decade after onset. Large, community-based studies including postmortem examination are generally not available. Current data, however, appear to verify that incidence of DLB is higher than that of pure VD but not as high as any vascular contribution to dementia (Heidebrink, 2002).

After Parkinson's disease and DLB, PSP is the third most common form of degenerative Parkinsonism. PSP occurs in 1.3/100,000 people, and the mean age of onset is typically 63 yr. VD occurs in approximately 4% to 12% of patients with Parkinson's disease. CBD is a progressive disease of unknown etiology that occurs in the elderly and manifests in higher cortical dysfunction, neuropsychiatric difficulties, and motor abnormalities. CBD is more common in females and is not thought to be inherited. The mean age of onset is 63 yr and the duration is 8 yr.

Etiology and Pathophysiology

Patients with subcortical dementia exhibit extrapyramidal symptoms associated with impairment of dopamine activity in the central nervous system. Patients with subcortical dementias also typically have normal language and abnormal (e.g., dysarthria) speech patterns. The patient's posture is typically stooped (Emilien et al., 2004; Mendez & Cummings, 2003).

Rehabilitation Considerations

The rehabilitation specialist should be aware that patients with dementia learn best or respond to treatment differently based on the presence or absence of certain cortical involvements. For example, patients with intact declarative memory systems learn best through trial and error. On the other hand, patients with declarative memory difficulties but spared procedural memory (i.e., those with Alzheimer's disease) learn best through errorless learning techniques such as vanishing cues (e.g., backward chaining) and spaced retrieval (Sohlberg & Turkstra, 2011).

Medication Therapy

Table 12.1 summarizes medication therapies used to treat subcortical dementias. The sections that follow provide additional details about each disorder.

Lewy Body Dementia (DLB)

In DLB, acetylcholine dysfunction results in symptoms of dementia and severe dopaminergic loss causes impaired execution of fine motor skills, mass face, stooped posture, and shuffling that is similar to that seen with Parkinson's disease. Symptoms widely fluctuate hourly and daily. Tremors occur less frequently in DLB than in Parkinson's disease. The DLB patient exhibits parkinsonian symptoms (with or without tremors), psychosis (including visual hallucinations), sleep disorders, and fluctuating attention. Patients with DLB are at increased risk for falls as a result of syncope and altered motor skills and cognition (Crystal, 2010; Jacobson et al., 2007; Mendez & Cummings, 2003; Sonnet et al., 2006).

Acetylcholinesterase inhibitors are used to treat cognitive disorders associated with DLB. Parkinsonian symptoms in patients with DLB are treated with carbidopa–levodopa (Sinemet) or baclofen (Lioresal). Psychotic symptoms are treated with second-generation antipsychotic agents that have reduced effects on dopamine, including clozapine (Clozaril), quetiapine (Seroquel), or aripiprazole (Abilify) (Sonnet et al, 2006).

Progressive Supranuclear Palsy

Progressive supranuclear palsy (PSP) (or the Steele-Richardson-Olszewski syndrome) is a degenerative disease associated with abnormal tau protein accumulation in the supranuclear portion of the brain that affects cognition, eye movements, and posture. The tau protein is important in maintaining neuronal morphology through microtubule binding. Abnormalities of this protein are seen in several neurodegenerative diseases in which the normally soluble tau protein collects into insoluble protease-resistant helical filaments called neurofibrillary tangles. Pathologically, PSP is defined by the accumulation of neurofibrillary tangles in the supranuclear portion of the brain. The accumulation of the phosphorylated tau protein differs in rate, localization, and pattern and these differences may account for the variation in clinical phenomena seen in patients with PSP. The exact triggers for the conversion from normal tau to the aggregate form are not completely understood.

Patients with PSP have difficulty with gaze, pseudobulbar palsy, axial rigidity, and dementia and have frequent falls that are secondary to difficulty looking down. Cognitive changes are mild in the early stages of the disorder. Later stages involve a frontal subcortical dementia similar to DLB and Parkinson's disease. The patient is apathetic, forgetful, and mentally slow with frontal executive functioning disability. Subsequently, categorization and set shifting is impaired. The patient also exhibits difficulty with memory, information retrieval, and acquired knowledge. The patient's speech is dysarthric and hypophonic. Linguistically, the patient shows difficulty with verbal fluency, reading, and writing (Eggenberger & Vanek, 2010). Early-onset dysphagia, incontinence, and falls are predictive of early mortality. Mortality is generally caused by pneumonia.

Problems with oral stage swallowing are more common in patients with PSP than in those with Parkinson's disease. Oral stage difficulties include uncoordinated lingual movements, difficulties with soft palate elevation, and premature spillage. Pharyngeal phase difficulties include difficulties with epiglottic inversion and pooling in the valleculae. Generally, the degree of dysphagia increases as the patient's cognition decreases. The speech–language pathologist may need to consider implementing alternative diets or liquids. Compensatory strategies or therapeutic interventions used depend on the patient's cognitive status (Eggenberger & Vanek, 2010).

No effective medication treatment exists for patients with PSP. Medication therapies may be employed to alleviate symptoms associated with the disease, but these therapies are generally ineffective. Acetylcholinesterase inhibitors that are used to treat Alzheimer's disease are generally not used because they may exacerbate motor symptoms and interfere with the patient's motility (Eggenberger & Vanek, 2010).

Low doses of amitriptyline (Elavil) and bromocriptine (Parlodel) have been associated with some improvement in motor function. Antidepressants such as trazodone (Desyrel) have been used to treat symptoms of depression (Eggenberger & Vanek, 2010; Mendez & Cummings, 2003; Yorkston et al., 2004).

Parkinsonian symptoms are not responsive to levodopa, but some of the motor sequences in eating and swallowing may improve with administration of dopamine medications. The specialist should also be aware that difficulties with valleculae pooling and esophageal motility may result in irregular or compromised absorption of medication. The rehabilitation therapist should consider the timing of the medications when teaching eating and swallowing activities because medications may affect oral and pharyngeal functions as well as those of the upper extremity (Eggenberger & Vanek, 2010; Yorkston et al., 2004).

Vascular Parkinsonism

In vascular parkinsonism (VD), parkinsonian symptoms result from vascular disease. There is no resting tremor. In VD the lower extremity blood vessels are usually more affected than those in the upper extremities. The disorder is typically symmetrical and the course of the disease is more rapid than that of Parkinson's disease. This disorder also causes incontinence, pseudobulbar affect, and dementia. VD patients are more prone to postural instability, gait difficulties, and falls (Robishaw & Beadle, 2010). Pharmacological treatment of the disorder focuses on medications that reduce risk factors for cardiovascular disease such as hyperlipidemia, hypertension, and smoking. Motor symptoms associated with VD are not responsive to levodopa (Jacobson et al., 2007; Mendez & Cummings, 2003).

Corticobasilar Degeneration (CBD)

In most cases, patients with CBD exhibit the triad of rigidity, apraxia, and akinesia. CBD patients first present with motor difficulties and cognitive dysfunction and then exhibit asymmetric limb clumsiness. The most common symptoms are unilateral rigidity of the limb or bradykinesia, ideomotor apraxia, asymmetric limb clumsiness, postural imbalance, unilateral limb dystonia, and tremor. Ideomotor apraxia is characterized by difficulty in sequencing, timing, spatial organization, and movement. The patient may also exhibit pseudobulbar palsy along with dysarthria and dysphagia. Myoclonic movements may precede dystonic postures. Approximately 50% of CBD patients exhibit alien limb sensation (Jacobson et al., 2007; Mendez & Cummings, 2003).

Approximately 36% of patients with CBD exhibit dementia. Patients exhibit difficulty learning, psychomotor slowing, and difficulties with insight. The patient may have cortical visuomotor difficulties, an inability to attend to a stimulus, and the inability to direct limbs based on visual guidance. All of these ataxic disorders complicate rehabilitative efforts. The patient with CBD may also exhibit depression, anxiety, disinhibition, agitation, and delusions.

Medications used to treat CBD include dopamine agonists or levodopa (medications used in

Parkinson's disease) to treat dystonia. Patient response to levodopa or dopamine agonists is generally poor. Clonazepam (Klonopin) is a benzodiazepine used to treat kinetic tremor and myoclonus. Botox injections are used to relieve painful focal dystonia (Jacobson et al., 2007).

Symptoms of orthostatic hypotension are treated with sodium and volume repletion, elastic stockings, elevation of the head at night, and medication therapy. Medications used to treat orthostatic hypotension include fludro-cortisone (Florinef), indomethacin (Indocin), clonidine (Catapres), ephedrine, and intranasal desmopressin (DDAVP). Urinary incontinence can be treated with anticholinergic medications such as oxybutynin (Ditropan) or propantheline (Banthine), and symptoms of impotence may improve with the use of yohimbine or sildenafil (Viagra) (Mendez & Cummings, 2003).

Huntington's Disease

Huntington's disease (HD; also called Huntington's chorea) is an inherited, autosomal dominant, degenerative neurologic disease. Dementia associated with HD is considered a subcortical dementia.

Incidence

The worldwide incidence of HD has declined secondary to genetic counseling and family support systems. The incidence of HD is 7/100,000 people. Children of parents with the disease have a 50% chance of developing the disease as well. Sex does not seem to play a role in incidence. Age of onset is approximately 35 to 40 yr in 90% of HD patients. The juvenile variant of HD, the onset of which occurs before age 20 yr, is a more aggressive form of the disease. If the disorder originates later in life (35-40 yr), the symptoms are less severe. Death usually occurs 15 to 20 yr after onset (DeRuiter & Holston, 2009; Neumiller et al., 2009).

Etiology and Pathophysiology

HD is caused by a deficiency in the neurotransmitter GABA in the basal ganglia that results in over-activity of dopaminergic systems. HD is characterized by chorea, psychiatric and behavioral changes, and cognitive decline. Chorea is defined as rapid, jerky, repetitive movements, particularly seen in the limbs and face. HD can present with positive movement disorders such as chorea and dystonia as well as negative motor symptoms such as bradykinesia and apraxia. In later stages, bradykinesia and spasticity symptoms predominate and positive symptoms are less evident. The HD patient may have forehead chorea (eyebrow movements), difficulties with gait and posture, facial apraxia, and difficulty with lingual protrusion. The patient has difficulties with involuntary movements as well as difficulty planning, sequencing, and executing voluntary movements. These motor difficulties lead to difficulties with speech and swallowing. The most common emotional symptoms of HD are irritability and depression (DeRuiter & Holston, 2009; Neumiller et al., 2009).

Rehabilitation Considerations

The HD patient experiences cognitive decline early in the course of the disorder. In fact, cognitive testing may reveal mild cognitive disorders years before the motor symptoms appear. Cognitive decline is progressive; short-term memory and visuospatial function are affected early in the disease and full dementia develops later in the disease. The HD patient will have cognitive difficulties in concentration and in the acquisition of new information. Impaired verbal fluency, visuospatial deficits, impaired attention, delayed recall, deficiencies in digit span, impaired object recall, deficient memory requiring effortful processing, decreased procedural learning, and faulty memory-retrieval strategies are all part of the cognitive dysfunction in the HD patient. The HD patient has more difficulty retrieving information and less difficulty storing memories, and performs better on recognition tasks than on recall tasks. In HD, recall is improved by priming (e.g., previous exposure to the material), encoding enrichment (e.g., embedding the material to be recalled in a story), and semantic retrieval cues (e.g., telling the patient the category in which the target word belongs). HD patients also have difficulty with skill and procedural learning (e.g., mirror writing) (Mendez & Cummings, 2003, p. 293). These cognitive difficulties complicate the patient's attempts to compensate for their motor difficulties, which impairs the patient's rehabilitative efforts.

Patients with HD usually have language difficulties involving naming or auditory comprehension and difficulties with connected speech. The HD patient has decreased syntactic complexity, phrase length, and articulatory agility and increased paraphasic errors. Because HD is considered a frontal or subcortical dementia, many of the approaches used in disorders such as Alzheimer's disease are inappropriate for use in the HD patient. For example, the procedural memory system is spared in patients with Alzheimer's disease, whereas the HD patient has difficulties with procedural memory activities. HD patients do better with predictable, scripted activities to compensate for the lack of procedural memory abilities. The patient's dysarthria may respond to prosody drills and establishment of appropriate rate. More severe dysarthria may require alphabet boards, conversational starters, or a yes–no system (Yorkston et al., 2004).

Patients may exhibit poor judgment and difficulty concentrating as they lose cognitive function. Typical behavioral symptoms include depression, agitation, mania, sexual disorders, and anxiety. Development of increased suspicion and personality changes occur 2 to 5 yr after onset of HD. Eight percent of HD patients have suicidal ideation (Jacobson et al., 2007; Yorkston et al., 2004).

Swallowing problems in patients with HD are usually described as a combination of uncontrolled and rapid swallowing patterns, excessive belching, involuntary movements of the respiratory system, and glottic penetration. The occupational therapist or speech–language pathologist may incorporate changes in posture to assist with swallowing into the patient's therapeutic plan. In addition to posture changes, the use of assistive devices such as a built-up spoon, dietary changes, or instruction in compensatory strategies (e.g., rate of eating) may assist the patient with HD with eating and swallowing. The patient may eventually require alternate routes of feeding such as enteral feeding using a PEG (percutaneous endoscopic gastrostomy) tube or enteral feeding via a jejunostomy tube (J-tube) (Jacobson et al., 2007; Yorkston et al., 2004).

Medication Therapy

Medication therapy in HD is not curative but rather is intended to manage symptoms; management of chorea is the major focus. Tetrabenazine (Xenazine) depletes monoamines, dopamine, serotonin, norepenephrine, and histamine from nerve terminals. Peak levels occur 1–1.5 h after a dose. Use of tetrabenazine (Xenazine) may worsen behavioral and cognitive disorders. Tetrabenazine carries a warning regarding depression and increased suicide ideation. The U.S. Food and Drug Administration regulates the prescribing and dispensing of this medication through a REMS (Risk Assessment and Mitigation Strategy) program. Table 12.1 summarizes medication therapies used in the treatment of HD. Table 12.2 summarizes the numerous drug interactions involved in the use of tetrabenazine (Xenazine) (DeRuiter & Holston, 2009; Neumiller et al., 2009).

Table 12.2   Drug Interactions With Tetrabenazine (Xenazine)

Medication class	Examples of medication	Adverse events	Effects on rehab
Antiarrhythmics	Amiodarone (Cordarone), disopyramide (Norpace), dofetilide (Tikosyn), procainamide (Pronestyl), quinidine, sotalol (Betapace)	QT prolongation (ventricular arrhythmias and torsades de pointes)	Increased risk of falls and arrhythmia associated with exercise
Antipsychotics	Chlorpromazine (Thorazine), haloperidol (Haldol), olanzapine (Zyprexa), paliperidone (Invega), risperidone (Risperdal), ziprasidone (Geodon)	QT prolongation (ventricular arrhythmias and torsades de pointes)	Increased risk of falls and arrhythmia associated with exercise

› *continued*

Table 12.2 › *continued*

Medication class	Examples of medication	Adverse events	Effects on rehab
Gastrointestinal agents	Cisapride (Propulsid)	QT prolongation (ventricular arrhythmias and torsades de pointes)	Increased risk of falls and arrhythmia associated with exercise
Antibiotics	Levofloxacin (Levaquin), moxifloxacin (Avelox), azithromycin (Zithromax), clarithromycin (Biaxin)	QT prolongation (ventricular arrhythmias and torsades de pointes)	Increased risk of falls and arrhythmia associated with exercise
Antineoplastics	Lapatinib (Tykerb), sunitinib (Sutent)	QT prolongation (ventricular arrhythmias and torsades de pointes)	Increased risk of falls and arrhythmia associated with exercise
Analgesics	Methadone	QT prolongation (ventricular arrhythmias and torsades de pointes)	Increased risk of falls and arrhythmia associated with exercise
Antianginal agents	Ranolazine (Ranexa)	QT prolongation (ventricular arrhythmias and torsades de pointes)	Increased risk of falls and arrhythmia associated with exercise
Phosphodiesterase inhibitors	Vardenafil (Levitra)	QT prolongation (ventricular arrhythmias and torsades de pointes)	Increased risk of falls and arrhythmia associated with exercise
Antipsychotics	Chlorpromazine (Thorazine), haloperidol (Haldol), olanzapine (Zyprexa), paliperidone (Invega), risperidone (Risperdal), ziprasidone (Geodon)	Neuroleptic malignant syndrome	Potentially fatal side effect associated with high fever, rigidity, and muscle hypertonicity; increased risk of falls
Antipsychotics	Chlorpromazine (Thorazine), haloperidol (Haldol), olanzapine (Zyprexa), paliperidone (Invega), risperidone (Risperdal), ziprasidone (Geodon)	Extrapyramidal symptoms, tardive dyskinesia	Increased motor tremor, dyskinesia, ataxia, dystonia associated with increased risk of falls, reduced motor abilities, dysphagia with aspiration
Monoamine oxidase inhibitor antidepressants	Isocarboxazid (Marplan), phenelzine (Nardil), tranylcypromine (Parnate), rasagiline (Azilect), selegiline (Emsam)	Elevated catecholamines (hypertensive crisis, cardiac arrhythmias)	Increased blood pressure, arrhythmia, increased risk of falls, cardiac events, stroke
Antihypertensives	Reserpine	Elevated catecholamines (hypertensive crisis, cardiac arrhythmias)	Increased blood pressure, arrhythmia, increased risk of falls, cardiac events, stroke
CYP2D6 inhibitors	Fluoxetine (Prozac), paroxetine (Paxil), quinidine (Quinaglute)	Elevated levels and effects of tetrabenazine; toxicity: akathisia, depression, extrapyramidal symptoms, dizziness, drowsiness, fatigue, nervousness, anxiety	Impaired cognition and ability to learn, impaired motor function, increased risk of falls, dysphagia associated with aspiration
Central nervous system depressants	Opiates, benzodiazepines, ethanol, antipsychotics, antidepressants, antihistamines, anticholinergics	Increased sedation, decreased motor function, cognitive impairment	Impaired cognition, impaired ability to learn and ambulate, increased risk of falls or injury

PATIENT CASE 1

S.R. is a 52-yr-old male with an 8 yr history of HD. In the past, S.R.'s chorea was mild and was not interfering with his functional activities and activities of daily living. Over the past 3 mo, the choreic movements have worsened to the point of interfering with daily functions, including walking with a rolling walker. Over the past 6 wk S.R.'s physician has gradually increased the dose of tetrabenazine to 60 mg/day, which is effectively controlling the chorea. S.R. is now able to ambulate with his rolling walker. S.R. is receiving outpatient physical therapy 3 times/wk at 9:00 a.m. The therapist notes that S.R.'s chorea is reduced significantly but that S.R. is too drowsy to participate in therapy.

Question

At this point, what interventions should the rehabilitation therapist make on S.R.'s behalf?

Answer

When the therapist asked S.R. when he takes his morning dose of tetrabenazine, S.R. reported that he regularly takes the medication at 7:30 a.m. The therapist concluded that S.R. likely was unusually drowsy because the drug concentration reaches peak levels 1 to 1.5 h after administration. The therapist rescheduled S.R.'s therapy for 11:00 a.m. Because the chorea was still well controlled and drowsiness was less of a problem, S.R. was able to participate in therapy. The therapist also educated S.R. and his caregivers about other frequently occurring side effects, such as depression and difficulty swallowing, that require physician notification and adjustment of the medication regimen.

This case illustrates how important it is for the therapist to understand when peak drug concentration occurs and how to schedule therapy sessions accordingly. The rehabilitation therapist is often the first to recognize side effects that warrant prescriber notification because the therapist sees the patient on a more regular basis than does the prescriber. This case also highlights the importance of patient education in early recognition of other frequently occurring side effects associated with tetrabenazine.

Wilson's Disease

Wilson's disease (WD), also known as **hepatolenticular degeneration**, is a rare autosomal, recessive, familial metabolic disorder. In WD copper accumulates in tissues; this manifests as neurological or psychiatric symptoms and liver disease. It is treated with medication that reduces copper absorption or removes the excess copper from the body, but occasionally a liver transplant is required. WD is also associated with subcortical dementia. In adults, the symptoms of WD include dysarthria, ataxia, flapping wrist tremors, and shoulder tremors followed by parkinsonian symptoms, dystonia, and spasticity. Approximately 50% of adult patients with WD have ataxia and other cerebellar disorders. WD patients also exhibit dysphagia, drooling, intentional tremors, and dysarthria. Juvenile WD patients exhibit parkinsonian rigidity and bradykinesia or a hyperkinetic syndrome with athetosis.

Incidence

WD has been reported in many countries around the world at an incidence of 1/30,000 people worldwide (Walshe & Cox, 1998). In general, the incidence is similar from country to country except in localities with inbred populations in which incidence is increased. Onset generally peaks in the early twenties. Juvenile WD is usually diagnosed between six and 20 years of age. Adult WD is usually diagnosed after 40 years of age. Time from onset to death is between 4 and 12 yr. WD affects males and females at the same rate.

Etiology and Pathophysiology

WD is due to mutations in the Wilson disease protein (ATP7B) gene. A single abnormal copy of the gene is present in 1 in 100 people, who then do not develop any symptoms (they are carriers). If a child inherits the gene from both parents, the child has a higher risk of developing Wilson's disease.

Rehabilitation Considerations

Symptoms include mental slowness, inertia, and poor concentration. As a result, juvenile WD patients typically do not do well in school. Progression of the disease results in frontal executive difficulties and personality changes. Patients with WD exhibit mild dementia that is accompanied by disinhibition, apathy, withdrawal, irritability, and explosive, antisocial, and hysterical behavior. These patients may act schizophrenic or paranoid. Due to frontal lobe difficulties, these patients may have difficulty with abstraction and forming concepts. Dysarthria is a hallmark of WD. As the disease progresses, the patient may eventually become mute. The speech pattern of patients with WD is a mixed spastic, ataxic, and hypokinetic dysarthria. Speech is characterized by a lack of precision in articulation, irregular articulatory breakdown, prolonged intervals, slow rate, low pitch, harsh voice, and monopitch. Musculoskeletal impairments worsen in the moderate to severe stage of WD. These impairments include muscle atrophy, contractures, deformities, osteomalacia, and pathologic fractures (Smeltzer & Bare, 2000).

PATIENT CASE 2

T.J. is a 21-yr-old male who has recently developed difficulty with eating and swallowing. T.J. asked his physician for a referral to a speech–language pathologist. By the time of the appointment, T.J. noticed that his speech has also begun to deteriorate. The speech–language pathologist told him that he had also developed dysarthria, and soon the symptoms of tremors and drooling emerged. As T.J. began to work on his speech and dysphagia, the speech–language pathologist noted that T.J.'s mental powers were decreasing and that he was beginning to act childish. T.J. attempted to rationalize his childish behavior by stating that he was "just a child at heart."

Question

Does T.J. need to be concerned about the rapid onset of these additional symptoms? Can these symptoms be traced to a single disorder?

Answer

Yes, the patient needs to be concerned about the progressive nature of these symptoms. The rehabilitation specialist may be the first professional to identify symptoms and therefore needs to recognize changing symptoms and report these changes to the patient's physician as soon as possible. T.J. was given a urine copper test, which identified increased amounts of copper, and was placed on D-penicillamine (Cuprimine). In addition, he restricted his intake of foods containing copper and of tap water, which may have been in copper tubing. T.J. noticed that some of his cognitive abilities seemed to improve with this regimen.

Medication Therapy

Timely treatment with copper-chelating therapy can decrease the progression of WD and toxic effects on the liver and central nervous system. Copper-chelating therapies include D-penicillamine (Cuprimine), triethylenetetramine (Trientine), and zinc. Dementia can be partially reversible if medications are initiated early in the course of the disease. Some studies show that pharmacological intervention can positively affect the ability of the patient to communicate clearly. D-penicillamine (Cuprimine) mobilizes copper throughout the body tissues and facilitates renal excretion. Side effects of this medication include nausea, vomiting, reduced sense of smell, and spontaneous bruising. Patients are placed on a low-copper diet and avoid foods such as shellfish, liver, nuts, chocolate, dried fruit, and mushrooms. Triethylenetetramine (Trientine) may be prescribed for patients who are not able to tolerate Cuprimine therapy. Zinc can be used as maintenance therapy once the patient is treated with Cuprimine or Trientine. Therapies used to manage other symptoms include anticholinergics, baclofen (Lioresal), GABA antagonists, levodopa to treat motor symptoms, anticonvulsants to treat seizures, and antipsychotics to treat symptoms of psychosis. Patients with a history of WD need to be followed throughout their lives, but if WD is caught early and treated patients can have a normal life span. Table 12.1 summarizes medications used to treat WD (Mendez & Cummings, 2003; Vogel et al., 2000).

Restless-Leg Syndrome

Restless-leg syndrome (RLS) is another movement disorder that can contribute to sleep disorders and can affect the patient's ability to participate in rehabilitation. RLS is characterized by an uncomfortable sensation deep in the leg accompanied by the urge to move the leg. The discomfort has been described as water flowing in the legs, bugs in the bones, or electricity in the legs. RLS may involve other body parts in addition to the legs. Symptoms begin or worsen during rest or inactivity and are synchronous with the slowing of cerebral cortical activity. A similar movement disorder seen in sleep is periodic limb movements of sleep (PLMS). PLMS are periodic, single movements that occur every 20 to 40 s during sleep and can include the rhythmic extension of the big toe, dorsiflexion of the ankle, or flexion at the knee and hip. PLMS symptoms can be associated with RLS, narcolepsy, and obstructive sleep apnea. Eighty percent of patients with RLS have five or more PLMS each hour of sleep. RLS and PLMS can affect the patient's rehabilitation progress by disrupting sleep, can result in decreased cognition during the day and daytime drowsiness, and can interfere with activities of daily living (DeSimone & Petrov, 2009; Ryan & Slevin, 2006).

To be diagnosed with RLS, the patient must meet all four essential diagnostic criteria: 1) urge to move legs, sometimes involving disturbing sensations in the arms and torso; 2) motor restlessness during inactivity (lying down or sitting); 3) relief with movement; and 4) worsening symptoms in the evening or at night. Clinical features that support the diagnosis include positive family history, positive response to dopamine agonists, sleep disturbances, and the presence of PLMS. Other diag-

noses with similar symptoms include nighttime leg cramps (which are focal and unilateral), akathisia (which does not correlate with rest or time of day), deep vein thrombosis (which is associated with decreased peripheral pulses, ulceration, and altered leg-hair distribution), and peripheral neuropathies associated with diabetes (which are characterized as numbness or tingling pain and are not associated with time of day) (DeSimone & Petrov, 2009; Ryan & Slevin, 2006).

Incidence

RLS is classified as primary (idiopathic) or secondary (resulting from causes associated with iron deficiency). Incidence of RLS is basically the same in the United States as it is internationally. One study that examined the incidence of RLS in France estimated a prevalence of 8.5%; RLS was more prevalent in women (10.8%) than in men (5.8%). Prevalence increased with age until the age 64 yr, where it declined for both sexes (Tison et al., 2005). In the United States, RLS occurs in 10% to 15% of the population and affects 10 million adults and 1.5 million children and adolescents. Women are twice as susceptible as men, and the disease is more common in older adults (DeSimone & Petrov, 2009; Ryan & Slevin, 2006).

Etiology and Pathophysiology

The complete pathophysiology of RLS and PLMS has not yet been established. Both RLS and PLMS are associated with enhanced spinal cord excitability, which is believed to be associated with decreased levels of the central neurotransmitter dopamine. Proteins involved with transport of dopamine also exhibit the circadian rhythms seen with RLS and PLMS. In addition, iron is a cofactor for tyrosine hydroxylase (a rate-limiting enzyme for dopamine synthesis), which may explain how iron deficiency can contribute to symptoms of secondary RLS (DeSimone & Petrov, 2009; Ryan & Slevin, 2006).

Primary RLS is more common in people under 40 yr of age. Sixty percent of patients with primary RLS report a familial history.

This hereditary form of RLS has an autosomal, dominant inheritance pattern, is associated with early onset, and worsens during pregnancy. RLS is strongly associated with concurrent anxiety disorders, panic disorders, or depression (DeSimone & Petrov, 2009; Iversen et al., 2009; Jacobson et al., 2007; Preston et al., 2008; Ryan & Slevin, 2006). The onset of symptoms of primary RLS is insidious.

The onset of symptoms of secondary RLS is more abrupt, and therapy targets correcting the iron deficiency. Causes can include pregnancy (RLS occurs in up to 19% of pregnant women) and renal failure (RLS occurs in up to 50% of patients with end-stage renal disease). Serum and CSF (cerebral spinal fluid) iron levels vary in a circadian manner. Serum levels decrease 30% to 50% during the night, and **ferritin** levels in the brain decrease 68% during this period of time (DeSimone & Petrov, 2009; Ryan & Slevin, 2006).

Rehabilitation Considerations

Patients can find relief with counter stimulus such as massage, exercise, stretching, and taking hot or cold baths. Patients also report that participating in activities that maintain alertness (e.g., playing video games or doing crossword puzzles) and maintaining good sleep hygiene reduce the severity of symptoms. Using biofeedback and relaxation techniques at bedtime and avoiding alcohol, nicotine, and caffeine may improve symptoms. Medications that may worsen symptoms of RLS include antidepressants such as selective serotonin reuptake inhibitors (SSRI), tricyclic antidepressants (TCAs), and lithium, all of which enhance serotonin transmission and decrease dopamine transmission. Histamine-2 blockers such as cimetidine (Tagamet) and ranitidine (Zantac) also can worsen RLS symptoms. Patients should schedule sedentary activities for the morning, when RLS is least symptomatic (DeSimone & Petrov, 2009; Ryan & Slevin, 2006).

Medication Therapy

Intermittent RLS, which is usually mild, is usually managed with nonpharmacologic therapies, whereas patients with daily RLS symptoms are treated with pharmacologic therapies. Medications used to treat Parkinson's disease, such as levodopa and dopamine agonists, enhance dopamine transmission and effectively reduce symptoms of primary RLS and PLMS. In addition, anticonvulsants such as gabapentin, carbamazepine, and valproic acid have been used to treat RLS. These agents augment GABA activity in the central nervous system, thus reducing nerve impulse transmission at the spinal cord level and affecting release of dopamine and serotonin. Clonazepam (Klonopin) is a benzodiazepine that has been effectively used to treat RLS. Opioids such as propoxyphene, oxycodone, and tramadol are second-line agents that reduce PLMS associated with arousal but are associated with adverse effects and dependence issues that limit their usefulness. (Propoxyphene was withdrawn from the U.S. market in 2010 because adverse cardiac events have been associated with its use.) Treatment of secondary RLS includes treating the iron deficiency with iron supplementation. Table 12.3 summarizes the medications commonly used to treat RLS.

Medication-Induced Movement Disorders

Many medications can cause or worsen movement disorders, many of which are life threatening. Medications that change the level of the neurotransmitters dopamine and norepinephrine can affect motor function. Medications most frequently associated with altered dopamine or norepinephrine levels that have the potential to induce movement disorders include antipsychotics, antidepressants, lithium, and medications that are used to treat Parkinson's disease. Most drug-induced movement disorders are related to the size of the dose, and many can occur as the result of additive effects when the medication is combined with other agents or of drug interactions that increase levels and effects of the medication. For example, seizures may occur when the dose of histamine-2 blockers, antacids, or many beta-lactam antibiotics is not adjusted

See table 12.3 in the web resource for a full list of medication-specific indications, dosing recommendations, and side effects.

Table 12.3 Medications Used to Treat Restless-Leg Syndrome

Medication	Side effects affecting rehab							Other side effects or considerations
Iron replacement therapy: Used to treat iron deficiency causing RLS.								
Ferrous sulfate	Cog	S	A	Motor	D	Com	F	Take with food to minimize stomach upset.
Ferrous gluconate	0	0	0	0	++	0	0	High risk of constipation; take a laxative with iron.
Ferrous fumarate								Separate administration from products containing calcium, magnesium, or aluminum to ensure that iron is absorbed. Separate from products containing tetracycline to prevent decreased absorption of iron and tetracycline.
Dopamine precursor								
Carbidopa–levodopa (Sinemet, Sinemet CR, Parcopa)	Cog +++	S +++	A +++	Motor +++	D +++	Com ++	F ++++	Nausea, vomiting, headache, drowsiness, nightmares. Avoid high-protein meals, which can decrease absorption, near bedtime. Take on an empty stomach. Avoid driving or operating machinery.
Dopamine agonists: First-line treatment for severe RLS.								
Ropinirole (Requip)	Cog +++	S +++	A +++	Motor +++	D +++	Com ++	F +++	Nausea, fainting spells, lightheadedness, sweating, flushing, xerostomia, sleep attacks. Contact physician if sleep attack occurs.
Pramipexole (Mirapex)	Cog +++	S +++	A +++	Motor +++	D +++	Com ++	F +++	Take with or without food with glass of water. Avoid alcohol and driving or operating machinery.
Anticonvulsants: Used to relax blood vessels and treat symptoms of mild to moderate RLS.								
Gabapentin (Neurontin)	Cog ++	S ++	A +	Motor +++	D 0	Com ++	F +++	Somnolence, dizziness, nausea, constipation, peripheral edema, tremor, dizziness, fatigue, ataxia, drowsiness, weight gain, behavioral changes. Contact physician for symptoms of allergy or for worsened mood or suicidal thoughts.
	Adjust dose for renal insufficiency.							
Carbamazepine (Tegretol)	Cog ++	S ++	A +	Motor ++	D ++	Com ++	F +++	Ataxia, blurred vision, drowsiness, agitation, disequilibrium, dizziness, cardiac arrhythmias, congestive heart failure. Avoid using alcohol and driving or operating machinery. Genetic testing required prior to initiation in Asians due to increased risk of AHS.
Benzodiazepines: Used to treat insomnia and anxiety associated with RLS.								
Clonazepam (Klonopin)	Cog +	S +	A ++	Motor ++	D ++	Com ++	F ++	Daytime sleepiness, cognitive impairment, nausea, constipation, diarrhea, fainting spells, confusion, depression, headache, dependence.
Alprazolam (Xanax)	Cog +	S +	A ++	Motor ++	D ++	Com ++	F ++	Avoid using alcohol and driving or operating machinery.

› continued

Table 12.3 › *continued*

Medication	Side effects affecting rehab							Other side effects or considerations
Opioids: Used to treat pain associated with severe RLS not relieved by Tylenol or nonsteroidal anti-inflammatory drugs.								
Oxycodone (OxyIR)	Cog ++	S ++	A 0	Motor +++	D ++	Com ++	F ++	Constipation, urinary retention, sleepiness, itching, dizziness, xerostomia.
Oxycodone SR (Oxycontin)	Cog ++	S ++	A 0	Motor +++	D ++	Com ++	F ++	Take with food for symptoms of nausea or vomiting.
Methadone (Dolophine)	Cog ++	S ++	A 0	Motor +++	D ++	Com ++	F ++	Treat xerostomia with sugarless gum or hard candy or by increasing water intake. Tolerance and potential abuse limit usefulness.
Tramadol (Ultram)	Cog ++	S ++	A 0	Motor ++	D ++	Com ++	F ++	Avoid using alcohol and driving or operating machinery; avoid with medications that increase serotonin. Headache can occur with tramadol.

Cog = cognition; S = sedation; A = agitation or mania; Motor = discoordination; D = dysphagia; Com = communication; F = falls; RLS = restless-leg syndrome; AHS = anticonvulsant hypersensitivity syndrome.

The likelihood rating scale for encountering the side effects is as follows: 0 = Almost no probability of encountering side effects. 0/+ = Low probability of encountering side effects but increased with increased dosage. + = Little likelihood of encountering side effects. +/++ = Low probability of encountering side effects; however, probability increases with increased dosage. ++ = Medium likelihood of encountering side effects. +++ = High likelihood of encountering side effects, particularly with high doses. ++++ = Highest likelihood of encountering side effects; best to avoid in at-risk patients.

in patients with renal impairment. Movement disorders can significantly affect the patient's ability to participate in rehabilitation sessions.

The rehabilitation therapist may be the first to notice a new movement disorder and should be aware of the most serious disorders caused by medication use. To ensure optimal patient care, the therapist should alert the prescriber in a timely manner to a new movement disorder that may require dose adjustment or discontinuance of a medication. The sections that follow describe some of the more common drug-induced movement disorders. Table 12.4 summarizes medications that commonly cause movement disorders.

Drug-Induced Parkinsonism

Drug-induced parkinsonism is also called extrapyramidal side effects or pseudoparkinsonism. Drug-induced parkinsonism is typically the result of exposure to neuroleptics (antipsychotics). This disorder most often occurs with use of high-potency typical (first-generation) antipsychotics because these agents work primarily by decreasing dopamine levels. Risk increases when these agents are used in high doses, but this disorder can also occur with the use of newer atypical agents, especially when

given in high doses or parenterally. Atypical antipsychotics such as clozapine (Clozaril), olanzapine (Zyprexa), and quetiapine (Seroquel) also affect serotonin levels and have reduced effects on dopamine, thus resulting in fewer parkinsonian side effects. These side effects are usually reversible when medication dosage is decreased or when the patient changes to another antipsychotic medicine. Other medications that can induce extrapyramidal side effects include benzamides such as metoclopramide (Reglan); antihypertensives such as reserpine, methyldopa (Aldomet), and calcium channel blockers; lithium (Eskalith); high-dose diazepam (Valium); the chemotherapy agent cytosine arabinoside (Ara-C); and the anticonvulsant valproic acid (Depakene) when used long term (Mendez & Cummings, 2003).

Akathisia

The patient with akathisia feels restless and desires to keep moving. The patient may pace the floor or repeatedly cross and uncross their legs. This disorder, which is particularly evident in the lower extremities, occurs with the use of antidepressants such as SSRI, atypical and typical antipsychotics, and calcium channel

Table 12.4 Medication-Induced Movement Disorders

Movement disorder	Medications	Corrective action
Extrapyramidal symptoms	Antipsychotics: metoclopramide (Reglan), lithium (Eskalith)	Reduce dose or discontinue medication.
	Antihypertensives: reserpine, methyldopa (Aldomet), calcium channel blockers	Add an anticholinergic in the short term.
	Chemotherapy: cytosine arabinoside (Ara-C)	
	Anticonvulsants: long-term valproic acid (Depakene), high-dose diazepam (Valium)	
Akathisia	Antidepressants, antipsychotics, calcium channel blockers	Reduce dose of the offending medication and add propranolol or a benzodiazepine.
		Avoid anticholinergic medications.
Dystonia	Antipsychotics, abrupt withdrawal of anticholinergic therapy	Discontinue or reduce dose of antipsychotic.
		Administer parenteral anticholinergic medications such as benztropine (Cogentin) or trihexyphenidyl (Artane).
Serotonin syndrome	Combining any of these serotonin-enhancing medications: citalopram, fluoxetine, fluvoxamine, paroxetine, duloxetine, venlafaxine, isocarboxazid, phenelzine, selegiline, tranylcypromine, linezolid (Zyvox)	Discontinue the offending medications.
	With any of these: amitriptyline, imipramine, doxepin, trazodone, mirtazapine, buspirone, morphine, tramadol, triptans used to treat migraines, meperidine, cocaine, cyclobenzaprine, ergot alkaloids, fentanyl, lithium, methadone, methamphetamine, metoclopramide, ondansetron, St. John's wort, valproic acid, dextromethorphan (a cough suppressant used in over-the-counter cough syrups), L-tryptophan, tyramine-rich foods	Administer Lorazepam (Ativan) for behavioral symptoms, cyproheptadine (Periactin) for autonomic symptoms, nitroglycerin for chest pain, propranolol (Inderal) to control heart rate and blood pressure.
Neuroleptic malignant syndrome	Antipsychotic therapies	Discontinue the antipsychotic.
		Treat with bromocriptine 30 mg/day or dantrolene 400 mg/day.
Tremor	Alcohol (chronic)	Discontinue the offending medication or reduce dose.
	Antiarrhythmics: amiodarone (Cordarone), mexiletine (Mexitil), procainamide (Pronestyl)	
	Anticonvulsants: carbamazepine (Tegretol), phenytoin (Dilantin) valproic acid (Depakene)	
	Selective serotonin reuptake inhibitors	
	Tricyclic antidepressants	
	Antipsychotics	
	Bronchodilators: albuterol, salmeterol (Serevent, Advair)	
	Corticosteroids: prednisone, methylprednisolone	
	Cyclosporine (Neoral, Sandimmune)	
	Sympathomimetics: amphetamine, cocaine, ephedrine, methylphenidate (Ritalin), pseudoephedrine (Sudafed), weight-reduction preparations	
	Heavy metals: arsenic, manganese, lead, mercury	
	Metoclopramide (Reglan), caffeine, theophylline (Theodur), nicotine, reserpine, thyroid supplements, lithium (Eskalith) combined with antidepressants	

blockers. Patients who have drug-induced parkinsonism have a greater risk of developing akathisia. The preferred treatment for akathisia is lowering the dose of the offending medication. Administration of propranolol (Inderal) or a **benzodiazepine** such as lorazepam (Ativan) can also reduce the severity of the symptoms. Anticholinergic medications such as benztropine (Cogentin) or trihexyphenidyl (Artane) that are used to reduce drug-induced parkinsonism do not reduce akathisia (Jacobson et al., 2007).

Dystonia

Dystonias are muscle contractions primarily of the neck and face. They are usually seen after acute exposure to neuroleptic medications (antipsychotics) or with abrupt discontinuation of anticholinergic medications. The risk of developing dystonia increases with the use of high-potency typical antipsychotics or with parenteral use of any of the antipsychotics. Dystonias have a rapid onset and can occur after a single dose of the offending medication. Acute dystonia may be treated with parenteral benztropine (Cogentin) or diphenhydramine (Benadryl). An oral anticholinergic is then administered temporarily while the neuroleptic dose is reduced or the patient is placed on an atypical antipsychotic. The oral anticholinergic should be discontinued after symptoms improve in order to avoid side effects such as constipation, urinary retention, and delirium (Jacobson et al., 2007).

Tardive Dyskinesia

Tardive dyskinesia (TD) is an irreversible disorder of the involuntary movements caused by chronic use of antipsychotic medications. Onset is usually insidious and occurs after at least 1 yr of antipsychotic use. Symptoms include mouth movements such as lip smacking, sucking, and puckering; tongue protrusion and involuntary tongue movements; choreoathetoid movements of the fingers or toes; and slow, writhing movements of the trunk. These movements increase during waking hours and subside during sleep. The patient may speak unintelligibly and with a reduced rate of articulation.

TD results from the long-term blockade of dopamine-2 receptors in the nigrostriatal pathway, which causes the receptors to become supersensitive and to up-regulate. TD may be seen with use of all types of antipsychotics, but incidence is lower with the use of atypical antipsychotics (which affect serotonin and dopamine) than with the use of older typical antipsychotics (which primarily affect dopamine). The major risk factors for TD are prolonged use of antipsychotic medications and the use of anticholinergic medication with an antipsychotic. Factors that increase risk include affective disorder, **ethanol** use, diabetes, female sex, advanced age, and degenerative brain disease. Reducing neuroleptic medication dose to the minimum effective dose and reducing adjunct use of anticholinergics can reduce the risk of TD. No effective treatment of TD exists, but propranolol (Inderal) and nifedipine (Procardia) have been helpful in alleviating symptoms of TD. The best approach for detecting extrapyramidal symptoms early and preventing TD is carefully monitoring patients on antipsychotics using a tool such as the Abnormal Involuntary Movement Scale (AIMS) (Ciccone, 2007; Jacobson et al., 2007; Preston et al., 2008).

Neuroleptic Malignant Syndrome

Neuroleptic malignant syndrome (NMS) is a rare but potentially fatal side effect associated with the use of antipsychotic (neuroleptic) medications, and occurs in about 1% of patients treated with neuroleptic medications. NMS is a medical emergency and is believed to be associated with acute dopamine blockade at the hypothalamus and basal ganglia as a result of neuroleptic exposure or abrupt withdrawal of dopamine agonists. Symptoms of NMS can develop rapidly and are similar to those seen with serotonin syndrome: fever, muscle rigidity (often extreme, lead-pipe, or cogwheel rigidity; not seen with serotonin syndrome), autonomic instability, fluctuating consciousness, and elevated creatinine kinase levels. White cell count and liver enzymes may also be elevated. The patient may exhibit delirium, **catatonia**, tremors, dystonia, myoclonus, and bradykinesia. Risk factors for the development of NMS include a rapid increase in antipsychotic dosage and parenteral administration of antipsychotics. Patient risk factors include male sex, younger age, and concurrent affective disorders, agitation, or mental retardation. Treatment of NMS includes discontinuing the antipsychotic and treatment with a dopamine agonist such as bromocriptine 30 mg/day or dantrolene 400 mg/day. Complications of NMS can include pneumonia, pulmonary embolism, cardiac arrest, and renal failure (Ciccone, 2007; Jacobson et al., 2007).

Serotonin Syndrome

This syndrome, which can result in movement disorder, is thought to be caused by overstimulation of the postsynaptic nerve due to excessive levels of serotonin. It usually results from a drug interaction involving a medication that increases serotonin levels such as SSRI antidepressants and medications that increase serotonin levels such as lithium, trazodone (Desyrel), L-tryptophan, buspirone (Buspar), morphine, tramadol (Ultram), or sumatriptan (Imitrex) or tyramine-rich foods. Common offending agents include monoamine oxidase inhibitors, SSRI and other antidepressants, and linezolid (Zyvox), which is an antibiotic with weak monoamine oxidase inhibition. Most cases of serotonin syndrome associated with Zyvox involve the concurrent use of an SSRI antidepressant (Huang & Gortney, 2006; Kishel & Palkovic, 2006; Narita, Tsuji, & Yu, 2007).

Severe cases of serotonin syndrome are usually seen when monoamine oxidase inhibitors are combined with meperidine (Demerol), dextromethorphan (a cough suppressant used in over-the-counter cough syrups), or SSRI (Grimsley, 1998). Unfortunately, many health care professionals are not aware of which medications can cause serotonin syndrome and the causative agents of adverse drug effect frequently are not identified. Table 12.4 lists some of the medications that can cause serotonin syndrome (Brown, 2010).

Onset of symptoms of serotonin syndrome is rapid and occurs within 6 h of adding a drug, changing a dosage, or overdose. Symptoms of serotonin syndrome include cognitive impairment (disorientation and confusion); behavioral changes such as agitation, akathisia, and delirium; neuromuscular findings including

clonus, myoclonus, incoordination, peripheral hypertonicity, ataxia, tremor, hyperreflexia, and shivering; and autonomic dysfunction including fever, tachycardia, mydriasis, diaphoresis, hyperactive bowel sounds, and diarrhea. Patients with cardiac disease or **coronary artery disease** are at increased risk for this side effect. Pharmacological treatment involves discontinuing the offending medications, which usually results in resolution of symptoms within 24 h. In severe cases, the administration of lorazepam (Ativan) may help alleviate behavioral changes and cyproheptadine (Periactin) may help alleviate autonomic symptoms. Antihypertensive agents such as nitroglycerin may be needed to manage cardiac ischemia, and beta blockers such as propranolol (Inderal) may be needed to manage hypertension and tachycardia (Brown, 2010; Grimsley, 1998; Huang & Gortney, 2006; Jacobson et al., 2007; Kishel & Palkovic, 2006; Narita et al., 2007).

Summary

Numerous movement disorders can directly affect rehabilitation. This chapter summarizes how these disorders can affect rehabilitation therapy progress and introduces the reader to treatment modalities of ET (essential tremor), subcortical dementias associated with movement disorders (i.e., DLB [Lewy body dementia], VD [vascular dementia], HD ([Huntington's disease], and WD [Wilson's disease]). In addition, the chapter summarizes how restless-leg syndrome (RLS) and associated therapies can impact the rehabilitation progress. Finally, the chapter reviews the most common medication-induced movement disorders (i.e., drug-induced parkinsonism, akathisia, dystonia, TD [tardive dyskinesia], NMS [neuroleptic malignant syndrome], and serotonin syndrome). The rehabilitation therapist should be aware of how medications can affect the patient's rehabilitation and how certain medications may cause or exacerbate movement disorders. The rehabilitation therapist should develop a collaborative relationship with the patient's physician and the consulting pharmacist in the workplace in order to understand and potentially ameliorate the patient's movement disorder and produce more functional activities.

Medications Used to Treat Pain and Substance-Use Disorders

Part IV comprises three chapters. Chapter 13 introduces the pathophysiology associated with various types of pain and reviews how pain is classified, assessed, and treated. The chapter discusses tools for assessing pain in patients who cannot communicate effectively and barriers that lead to inadequate management of pain as well as the importance of involving the patient and family in the development of a pain-management treatment plan. This chapter reviews commonly encountered conditions associated with acute pain, discusses the impact of failure to control pain on rehabilitation success, and discusses pharmacologic and nonpharmacologic treatments commonly used to manage acute pain. Pain medications are classified based on the severity and type of pain. Tables in the chapter provide a comparison of the relative potency, time to onset of effect, and duration of action of opiate medications as well as guidelines for titrating doses, converting oral doses to equivalent parenteral doses, and safely converting from one opiate medication to an equivalent dose of another opiate. The chapter also discusses providing long-acting pain medication for ongoing pain along with short-acting pain medications to manage breakthrough pain. Important concepts such as dependence, addiction, tolerance, and pseudoaddiction are also defined.

Chapter 14 reviews common syndromes associated with chronic pain and explains how therapy for managing chronic pain differs from treatment of acute pain. Chronic pain is often a complication of inadequate management of acute pain and is often accompanied by symptoms of hopelessness and depression that limit performance in activities of daily living and impair cognitive processes. This chapter reviews chronic pain syndromes the rehabilitation therapist may encounter in practice, including migraine headaches, neuropathic pain resulting from stroke, neuromuscular disease, and neurologic disorders. The chapter reviews medications as well as nonpharmacologic therapies used to manage these pain disorders.

Chapter 15 reviews substance-use disorders, including abuse of prescription drugs, alcohol, and illicit drugs, and the effect of these disorders on rehabilitation. This chapter also provides an overview of medications commonly used to treat substance-use disorders, methods for monitoring patients with substance-use disorders, and methods for appropriately altering rehabilitation sessions. The rehabilitation therapist should understand the symptoms associated with substance-use disorders as well as symptoms of withdrawal in order to effectively monitor the patient and ensure that rehabilitation sessions are safe and effective.

13 Medications Used to Treat Pain

The rehabilitation therapist will care for many patients who have pain. This chapter introduces the types of pain, explains how pain can affect the rehabilitation session, and provides methods for assessing and managing pain. This chapter also discusses the different classes of medications used to treat pain along with side effects of these medications and how they can affect rehabilitation. Special emphasis is placed on how the therapist can alter rehabilitation sessions to ensure safety and optimize therapy for patients being treated with pain medications.

Classification of Pain

According to the International Association for the Study of Pain, **pain** is defined as an unpleasant sensory and emotional experience associated with actual or potential tissue damage. Pain is subjective, and the relationship between the pain the patient experiences and associated tissue damage can be highly variable. The patient's reported level of pain should always guide therapy, even if the reported pain and associated behaviors do not seem to match (Carl & Johnson, 2006; Strassels et al., 2007).

Pain is classified by the tissue from which it originates and can be classified as either nociceptive or neuropathic. Nociceptive pain is generally associated with injury to structural tissue or organs. It usually results from pressure, temperature, or chemical stimuli. **Nociceptive** pain is further divided into somatic and visceral pain. Somatic pain originates from muscles, ligaments, skin, or bone and is usu-

ally proportional to the degree of tissue injury. This pain is characterized as constant aching and throbbing and can usually be traced to a specific site. Visceral pain, on the other hand, is characterized as dull, crampy pain that may be difficult to localize. It is commonly called referred pain (i.e., the pain originates in one area but is felt in a different area). Nociceptive pain, with the exception of arthritis pain, is generally self-limiting (Carl & Johnson, 2006; Strassels et al., 2007).

Neuropathic pain is characterized as burning, shooting, shocking, or tingling and may be accompanied by numbness or paresthesias. Neuropathic pain is more difficult to control, and use of several medications and modalities may be required to obtain relief. This type of pain can severely restrict ambulation and prevent patient participation in activities of daily life and in rehabilitation. This pain is caused by central or peripheral nerve dysfunction. Central nerve pain is seen with poststroke syndromes, whereas peripheral neuropathic pain is associated with diabetic neuropathy or postherpetic **neuralgia**. This pain is typically disproportional to the degree of tissue damage. The patient may also experience heightened sensitivity (hyperalgesia) and allodynia (pain caused by a nonpainful stimulus) (Carl & Johnson, 2006; Strassels et al., 2007).

Pain can be acute, chronic, or, in many cases, a combination of both. Treatment of acute pain often fails to address chronic pain, such as neuropathic pain, that the patient had before the acute injury. Distinguishing between acute and chronic pain can be difficult because acute pain often lasts longer than expected (Hutchinson, 2007; Strassels et al., 2007).

Incidence

Management of postoperative pain is considered to be suboptimal worldwide. In one European study, only 45% of patients received information regarding postoperative pain from an anesthesiologist, more than 70% of hospitals did not have an acute pain-management unit, and only 28% of anesthesiologists were satisfied with the pain-management procedures in their hospital (Puig et al., 2001). Each year, 73 million Americans undergo surgery and experience acute pain associated with the experience. Of all patients undergoing surgery, 80% reported they had postoperative pain and 20% of these patients described their pain as severe. Inadequate management of postoperative pain can cause patients to avoid movement and ambulation, which can result in deep vein thrombosis, pulmonary embolism, coronary ischemia, myocardial infarction, pneumonia, poor wound healing, reduced immune response, and chronic pain syndrome (Hutchinson, 2007; Strassels et al., 2007).

Acute pain generally subsides with healing of the tissues. Acute pain is accompanied by rapid heart rate, increased breathing, elevated blood pressure, sweating, anxiety, and dilated pupils. Accompanying anxiety can stimulate prostaglandins, thus intensifying pain, and reduce production of endorphins that help control nerve cell sensitivity to pain. Inadequate treatment of pain can increase catabolic demand, decrease ambulation, and result in shallow breathing and suppression of cough. These can extend length of stay and lead to hospital readmission and patient dissatisfaction (Hutchinson, 2007).

Chronic pain, defined as pain that lasts longer than 3 to 6 mo, affects 20% of adults in developed countries and 75 million Americans. The cost of chronic pain in the United States is more than $100 billion annually. The repeated stimulation of nerve cells can change the structure of nerve cells and fibers. Chronic pain can lead to depression, appetite loss, disturbed sleep, weight loss, decreased energy, fatigue, and impaired ability to complete daily activities. Chronic pain can last for years and frequently goes unrecognized by the practitioner because the patient may accept chronic pain as normal and fail to discuss their chronic pain with their physician. In many patients, the neuropathic component associated with chronic pain is frequently missed or inappropriately treated. Complete elimination of chronic pain, especially if it is neuropathic, may not be possible. In this instance, the goal is to achieve a pain level that allows the patient to accomplish daily functions and maintain a good quality of life (Caufield, 2006; Hutchinson, 2007).

Pain is often seen in the older adult. Approximately 50% of elderly adults who live independently and 80% of nursing home residents experience pain that affects functional abilities. Geriatric patients who are hospitalized report frequent episodes of pain, and many of these patients are dissatisfied with the management of their pain. The consequences of poor pain management can include anxiety, insomnia, depression, malnutrition, delirium, attentional and memory problems, and reduced functional mobility and ability to perform activities of daily living. Poor pain management can negatively affect patient rehabilitation (Aegis, 2010; Jacobson et al., 2007).

Etiology and Pathophysiology

Pain transmission involves many neural pathways and neurotransmitters in both the central and peripheral nervous systems. The initial step in pain transmission is transmission, in which a noxious stimulus activates pain receptors (nociceptors). The nociceptors release sensitizing substances such as prostaglandins. Anti-inflammatory medications such as nonsteroidal anti-inflammatory drugs (NSAIDs) and corticosteroids that reduce prostaglandin production can reduce pain experienced at this step. The next step is transduction, in which an action potential is transmitted from the point of origin to the spinal cord via afferent nerve fibers. Which afferent nerve fibers are involved depends on the type of pain transmitted. Sharp, well-localized pain is transmitted rapidly along myelinated A-delta fibers covered by myelin, whereas dull, aching, and poorly localized pain travels more slowly along the unmyelinated C-fibers. The action potential travels to the dorsal horn of the spinal cord, where pain neurotransmitters such as glutamate and substance P are released. Opioids can reduce transmission of pain at the transduction step. The next step is perception, during which the signal travels up through ascending pathways to the brain and pain becomes a conscious experience. Distraction techniques and biofeedback interventions work well to reduce pain perception during this step. The final step is modulation, in which the brain sends inhibitory stimuli through descending pathways to the spinal cord to inhibit the pain sensation. This inhibition is accomplished through endogenous opioids, serotonin, norepinephrine, and gamma amino butyric acid (GABA). Antidepressants that increase norepinephrine and serotonin and anticonvulsants that increase GABA activity work at this step to control pain response (Hulisz & Moore, 2007).

Rehabilitation Considerations

Pain is consistently undertreated in the United States for a multitude of reasons. Documented barriers to providing effective pain relief include deficiencies in education of health professionals, the prescriber's fear of prosecution, and attitudes and beliefs of the health care worker, prescriber, patient, and family. Another factor is the patient's inability to communicate the presence of pain. Patients who are confused, demented, sedated, or mechanically ventilated have difficulty communicating their needs. Patients of different cultures and ages perceive and communicate the presence of pain in different ways. The most prevalent barriers for effectively managing pain in elderly patients involve psychocultural biases, fears of side effects or addiction, loss of independence, and concerns about cost. Many elderly patients and family members believe that pain is a normal part of the aging process or think that seeking pain relief indicates that they are weak or a bad patient. As a result, many older patients are extremely reluctant to report pain. Seniors have difficulty effectively communicating their need for pain relief due to dynamics of family roles and interactions, guilt about burdening

the family, fear of loss of independence, and embarrassment about their inability to tolerate pain. Elderly patients may have sensory impairments, dementia, and distractibility that may also impede communication (Phillips, 2007; Zagaria, 2009).

Failure to understand the concepts of tolerance, dependence, addiction, and pseudoaddiction can contribute to ineffective management of pain. Tolerance, which refers to the body's compensatory adjustment to the effects of a medication, may necessitate increasing the dose over time to maintain pain relief. Patients receiving opiates long term commonly require increased doses to achieve the same level of pain relief. Dependence, which can occur with the use of many medications, can occur as the body's compensatory mechanisms adjust to the presence of medications used chronically. This is why medications used chronically (e.g., beta blockers and antidepressants) should not be discontinued abruptly. Withdrawal symptoms that occur after use of opioids is abruptly discontinued include anxiety, irritability, chills, abdominal pain, hot flashes, joint pain, **lacrimation**, diaphoresis, nausea, and vomiting. The rehabilitation therapist should be aware of symptoms of withdrawal in patients who have been on opiate pain medications, question the patient regarding their use of pain medications, and facilitate communication with the prescriber in the event that withdrawal symptoms occur (Iversen et al., 2009). Addiction is the most frequently misunderstood concept concerning opiate use. Fear of addiction contributes to under-prescribing by physicians, under-administration by nurses or family members, and poor compliance by patients. Most patients stop taking pain medication once the pain stops. Patients who are addicted develop a psychological dependence on the opiate and their control over their drug use is impaired. They compulsively use and crave the drug and continue to use the drug inappropriately in ways that can cause self-harm. Patients who use opiates as prescribed, who have stable pain control, and who are willing to use additional methods to relieve their pain are unlikely to become addicted. Incidence of iatrogenic addiction is less than 1%. Fear of addiction should not interfere with the appropriate use of these agents to adequately control pain. *Pseudoaddiction* is a term used to describe patients whose pain has been undertreated and who develop drug-seeking behaviors, ask for pain medications more frequently, report continued pain without relief, and even shop for a doctor in an attempt to obtain pain relief. Once the pain in these patients is adequately treated, these behaviors disappear. The patient and prescriber can prevent pseudoaddiction by developing good communication and trust, mutually participating in developing a pain-treatment plan that provides adequate pain relief, and using nonpharmacologic interventions in addition to pain medications (Carl & Johnson, 2006; Strassels et al., 2007).

Members of the rehabilitation team should teach patients and family members about each of these concepts. Spouses or caregivers should be part of the discussion when the health care team formulates pain-treatment plans and evaluates them for effectiveness. Fear of associated cost of therapy should always be discussed because many older patients are on fixed incomes and feel that they cannot afford medications or interventions that help manage their pain. When asking patients about pain, the therapist should use more than one term to describe pain and use terms that are appropriate for the patient's level of literacy. For instance, some patients state they are not having pain but admit to being sore or hurting. Educating the patient and caregivers about the therapy plan is critical in allaying fears, particularly the frequently held fear of addiction. A pain contract between prescriber and patient that outlines the expectations of both in the therapeutic plan can be an effective tool in developing a pain plan. In addition, physicians and patients with a history of opiate abuse whose pain is not controlled by alternative therapy should discuss and agree on a clear plan for opiate tapering and discontinuation before initiating opiate therapy (Carl & Johnson, 2006; Strassels et al., 2007).

Initial Pain History

When initiating care of a patient with pain, members of the rehabilitation team should conduct an initial pain history to identify any acute and chronic pain in the patient. The following questions can be used to elicit valuable information from the patient and family (Carl & Johnson, 2006; Strassels et al., 2007).

- Are you having any pain now? On the pain scale of 1 to 10, how severe is your pain now? What is your usual level of pain?
- Where do you feel your pain? Please describe exactly where your pain is located.
- Does it spread or radiate to other places in your body? If so, where? Are you having any numbness, tingling, or weakness with this pain?
- What initially triggered your pain? When did the pain first begin to affect your activities?
- How often do you experience your pain on average: per day, per week, per month?
- What activities bring on the pain? How long does the pain last?
- Is the pain getting better, staying the same, or getting worse?
- What tests have you had in the past to evaluate your pain?
- What do you do to help relieve your pain at home?
- Are you taking any medication for pain now? Does this medication help your pain?
- What medications did you take for your pain in the past? Why did you stop taking these medications?

Ongoing Pain Assessment

Treatment of pain is based on initial history and assessment, development of a therapeutic plan, and subsequent routine pain assessment. Pain goals should be individualized for each patient, established with active communication and input from the patient and family, and include frequent reassessments of how well the patient's pain is being controlled. When conducting a pain reassessment, members of the rehabilitation team should ask about the severity (using a pain scale), location, and duration of the pain; a description of pain; any identified triggers for the pain; and the degree to which pain is relieved after medication is administered or nonpharmacologic interventions are made. A pain goal of zero is usually not appropriate or achievable and can lead to overmedication and associated side effects. Health care team members, including the surgeon, should establish an appropriate and achievable goal before any surgical procedure and educate the patient and family about the expected level of pain. Performing a follow-up reassessment, communicating with the prescriber about the degree of pain control, and using interventions for managing pain are important because under-treating acute pain can result in chronic pain (Aegis, 2010; Hulisz & Moore, 2007; Jacobson et al., 2007).

The pain assessment determines the patient's current level of pain and the frequency, intensity, origin (i.e., neuropathic, visceral, or somatic), and quality (e.g., aching, burning, stabbing, or crampy) of the pain. Health team members should assess the patient's level of pain initially and at regular intervals using a visual rating scale. One such scale is the Wong-Baker Faces Scale, with which patients quantify their level of pain via numeric rating or matching their feelings to the facial expressions on the scale. Many institutions consider pain assessment to be the fifth vital sign (along with blood pressure, pulse, temperature, and respiratory rate) and require assessment and documentation of pain level during each shift. Other assessment tools include the Discomfort Scale for Dementia of the Alzheimer's Type; the Checklist of Nonverbal Pain Indicators; the Face, Legs, Activity, Cry, and Consolability Scale; the Pain Assessment in Advanced Dementia Scale; the Assessment of Discomfort in Dementia protocol; the Quality of Life Scale from the American Chronic Pain Association; the Verbal Numeric Scale; the Visual Analog Scale; and the Numeric Pain Intensity Scale (Aegis, 2010; Phillips, 2007).

Because many clinicians believe that assessing pain in the cognitively impaired patient is impossible, pain in these patients is often undertreated. Untreated or inadequately treated pain can lead to behavioral disturbances, particularly in the patient with cognitive impairment. As cognitive function declines, the patient's ability to use a scale to describe their pain also declines. Cognitively impaired patients may have difficulty with the complex task of choosing a number, description, or facial expression that directly correlates with their level of pain. It is also very difficult for a patient with impaired cognition to use the Visual Analog Scale, which quantifies level of pain on a scale of no pain to the most pain imaginable. The Wong-Baker Faces Scale may also be ineffective. Some critics have suggested that the scale assesses emotion, which can be influenced by sex and culture, rather than pain. A patient may misinterpret the smiling face as a way to show approval of the way his pain is being managed rather than to show that he does not have pain. A patient with severe cognitive impairment may point to the face that he likes the best rather than relate it to his level of pain. Use of a pain map, a picture of a person, or a doll can help the patient describe the location of the pain (Phillips, 2007; Zagaria, 2009).

The American Geriatrics Society has identified certain behaviors that may indicate pain in cognitively impaired patients. These include facial expressions, negative verbalizations, movements consistent with agitation, changes in interpersonal interactions, changes in activity patterns or routines, and changes in mental status. The pain scale for cognitively impaired nonverbal adults is a six-item scale, and is a reliable and practical tool that can be used in clinical practice for assessing pain behaviors in cognitively impaired and cognitively intact elderly adults. Behaviors that may indicate pain include the following: nonverbal expressions of pain such as moans, groans, grunts, cries, gasps, and sighs; facial grimaces and winces; bracing during movement; restlessness; rubbing an area; and verbal complaints (Phillips, 2007; Zagaria, 2009).

Because not all patients respond to the same strategies, the rehabilitation therapist needs to be familiar with a number of tools.

Nonpharmacologic interventions can include implantable devices and surgical interventions, alternative medicine, psychosocial interventions, and rehabilitation techniques. Implantable devices and surgical interventions may include brain surgery, intraspinal drug delivery, and spinal cord stimulation. Alternative medicine may include biofeedback, aromatherapy, acupuncture, homeopathic medicine, hypnotherapy, massage, manipulation, music therapy, herbal therapy, dietary supplements, reflexology, relaxation training, tai chi, Reiki therapy, and yoga (Aegis, 2010; Cameron & Monroe, 2007).

Psychosocial interventions may include assertiveness training, relaxation training, biofeedback, behavioral interventions that teach the patient how to respond to pain, body mechanics, and cognitive–behavioral treatment. In cognitive–behavioral treatment, the patient is educated about pain and their reaction to pain. Patients should receive instruction in skills for coping with pain. Engaging in activities that distract the patient from centering on the pain, such as playing cards or board games, can also help (Aegis, 2010).

Rehabilitation techniques can include increasing activity with the goal of improving quality of life and maintaining ability to complete ADLs. Aquatic therapy may help the patient increase activity during the session while minimizing pain. Diathermy reduces pain by transmitting electromagnetic radiation to painful tissue. Cold packs may modulate swelling and reduce pain by numbing nerve endings and constricting blood vessels. Hot packs can deliver superficial heat and reduce pain in nonacute conditions. Effects of heat therapy include increased delivery of oxygen and nutrients to the site and decreased joint stiffness, pain, and muscle spasm. Electrical stimulation may be used to block pain signals. The rehabilitation therapist may also teach the patient work-simplification and energy-conservation techniques that eliminate or reduce pain in certain situations. The patient typically begins an exercise program to improve fitness and reduce pain. Elderly patients may resist exercise due to a fear of falling. The rehabilitation therapist needs to assure the patient that the proposed exercises are safe (Aegis, 2010).

The rehabilitation therapist may use massage to reduce swelling, muscle tension, and spasms and to relieve pain or may use myofascial release therapy to increase motion and decrease pain. Orthosis such as splints, braces, and casts can help protect injured tissue and promote healing.

The rehabilitation therapist and physician should also strongly consider using nonpharmacologic methods of pain management such as transcutaneous electrical nerve stimulation (TENS), cold therapy, thermal therapy, and low-level laser therapy. Sensory-level TENS is the use of electrical stimulation to depolarize sensory nerves for the purpose of decreasing pain by blocking pain impulses at the spinal cord level. Motor-level TENS is the use of electrical stimulation to depolarize motor nerves and pain nerve fibers to decrease pain through the activation of endogenous opiates. Sensory-level TENS should be used on patients who are currently using opioid pain medication. Motor-level TENS is less effective because its mechanism of pain relief involves producing and releasing endogenous opiates, to which the patient has likely developed a tolerance. The use of TENS can significantly reduce the necessary dosage of opioid pain medications (Sluka, 2001).

Medication Therapy

Preventing pain is easier than regaining control of pain. This principle applies to both acute and chronic pain. Mild, intermittent pain can be treated with analgesic medications on an as-needed basis. More severe or consistent pain should be treated with scheduled, around-the-clock dosing of short- or long-acting pain medications. The use of long-acting products should be accompanied by the use of a short-acting (breakthrough) medication for managing intermittent pain. This approach is beneficial because the patient spends less time in pain, the doses of analgesic can be lower if pain is not allowed to increase or become severe, fewer side effects occur with lower doses, the patient experiences less anxiety about the return of pain, the patient is less concerned about obtaining relief when needed, and the patient's overall activity increases. The rehabilitation therapist can help ensure that the patient receives a short-acting pain medication within 1 h of the scheduled session in order to provide optimal pain control during the exercise session. If the patient is on long-acting pain medication for pain control and anticipates experiencing pain with the activities of the session, a short-acting (breakthrough) pain medication should be administered before the session to facilitate patient participation (Acute Pain Management Guidelines Panel, 1992; Gutstein & Akil, 2001; Jacobson et al., 2007; Jacox et al., 1994; Max et al., 1999; Roberts & Morrow, 2001).

The World Health Organization (WHO) classifies pain medications into three categories: nonopioid analgesics that include aspirin, acetaminophen (Tylenol), and NSAIDs such as ibuprofen (Motrin); narcotics, such as morphine, which are now called opioids (after the first narcotic, opium); and adjuvant analgesics that are used in combination with the previously mentioned agents to enhance their effects. Adjuvant medications include antiemetic agents such as promethazine (Phenergan) that are used to control nausea associated with opiate use, tricyclic antidepressants such as amitriptyline (Elavil) that are used to treat neuropathic pain, and topical therapies such as lidocaine patches or capsaicin.

Step 1 Medications Used to Treat Mild Pain

The WHO analgesic ladder assigns analgesics to three steps. Step 1 agents are used to treat the least-intense pain and step 3 agents are used to treat the most severe pain. Step 1 agents include acetaminophen (Tylenol), aspirin, and NSAIDs such as ibuprofen (Motrin). These agents may be combined with an adjuvant analgesic used to treat atypical (neuropathic) pain such as gabapentin (Neurontin) and are often combined with less-potent opiates to augment pain action (Bone et al., 2002). Table 13.1 summarizes the dosing, side effects, and drug interactions of step 1 medications.

Aspirin   Aspirin, one of the oldest nonnarcotic medications used for pain, is derived from willow bark and was used in Native American medicine. Aspirin is used to treat inflammation, pain, and fever in adults. Aspirin use in children has been associated with **Reye syndrome** and it is no longer used in the pediatric population. Aspirin is very effective but is generally not used chronically to manage pain because it can cause dose-related gastrointestinal bleeding and ulceration. In addition, tinnitus can also occur with chronic, high-dose use. Patients requiring low-dose aspirin for antiplatelet therapy should take enteric-coated baby aspirin. Patients on daily aspirin therapy for antiplatelet therapy (e.g., for reducing cardiovascular risk) should not concurrently use NSAIDs, which may block the cardioprotective effects of aspirin (Carl & Johnson, 2006; Strassels et al., 2007).

Acetaminophen   Acetaminophen (Tylenol) is a centrally acting analgesic that produces mild analgesia and can be used to treat mild pain. It does not block prostaglandin action, reduce inflammation, or impair platelet function. Because it does not block prostaglandins, it does not have the adverse effects of gastrointestinal bleeding or ulceration seen with aspirin or NSAIDs. It is the safest agent for treating mild pain in elderly patients and treating patients on oral anticoagulants such as warfarin (Coumadin). A dose of 650 mg of acetaminophen provides the analgesic equivalent of 200 mg of ibuprofen or 650 mg of aspirin (Carl & Johnson, 2006).

Patients who take acetaminophen or medications which contain acetaminophen should be taught not to take more than 2600 mg/day. Although the maximum daily dose was 4000 mg in the past, in 2009 the U.S. Food and Drug Administration (FDA) advisory panel recommended lowering the maximum daily dose to 2600 mg and decreasing the recommended single dose from 1000 mg to 650 mg because significant hepatotoxic effects can occur with

See table 13.1 in the web resource for a full list of medication-specific indications, dosing recommendations, side effects, and drug interactions.

Table 13.1 Step 1 Medications Used to Treat Mild Pain

Medication	Side effects affecting rehab							Other side effects or considerations
Acetaminophen: Used to reduce fever and relieve pain.								
Acetaminophen (Tylenol)	Cog 0	S 0	A 0	Motor 0	D 0	Com 0	F 0	Hepatotoxicity with daily doses >3000 mg. Avoid use in patients with hepatic disease. Do not take with combination products containing acetaminophen (Percocet, Lortab, Norco, Ultracet).
NSAID nonselective inhibitors of cyclo-oxygenase 1 and 2: Used to reduce fever and inflammation and relieve pain.								
Diclofenac (Voltaren; Cataflam EC; Voltaren XR—sustained release) Combined with misoprostol to protect gastrointestinal tract. Arthrotec: 50/200 mg, 75/200 mg (Voltaren, Cataflam)	Cog +	S 0	A 0	Motor 0	D ++	Com +	F +	Gastrointestinal upset, dyspepsia, xerostomia, oral ulceration, glossitis, gastrointestinal mucosal hemorrhage, abrupt acute renal insufficiency, fluid retention, worsening of congestive heart failure, memory loss, confusion, dizziness, headache. Reversible inhibition of platelet aggregation with NSAIDs lasts 1-3 days. Increased bleeding risk when used with oral anticoagulant warfarin (Coumadin). Do not combine with aspirin. Antagonizes effects of antihypertensives.
Diflunisal (Dolobid)	Cog +	S 0	A 0	Motor 0	D ++	Com +	F +	
Etodolac (Lodine, Lodine XL)	Cog +	S 0	A 0	Motor 0	D ++	Com +	F +	
Fenoprofen (Nalfon)	Cog +	S 0	A 0	Motor 0	D ++	Com +	F +	
Flurbiprofen (Ansaid)	Cog +	S 0	A 0	Motor 0	D ++	Com +	F +	
Ibuprofen (Motrin, Advil)	Cog +	S 0	A 0	Motor 0	D ++	Com +	F +	
Indomethacin (Indocin, Indocin SR)	Cog ++	S 0	A 0	Motor 0	D ++	Com +	F ++	
Ketoprofen (Orudis)	Cog +	S 0	A 0	Motor 0	D ++	Com +	F +	
Ketorolac (Toradol)	Cog +	S 0	A 0	Motor 0	D ++	Com +	F +	
Meclofenamate (Meclomen)	Cog +	S 0	A 0	Motor 0	D ++	Com +	F +	

› continued

Table 13.1 › *continued*

Medication	Side effects affecting rehab							Other side effects or considerations
Mefenamic acid (Ponstel)	Cog	S	A	Motor	D	Com	F	
	+	0	0	0	++	+	+	
Meloxicam	Cog	S	A	Motor	D	Com	F	
(Mobic)	+	0	0	0	+	+	+	
Nabumetone	Cog	S	A	Motor	D	Com	F	
(Relafen)	+	0	0	0	++	+	+	
Naproxen	Cog	S	A	Motor	D	Com	F	
(Aleve, Naprosyn)	+	0	0	0	++	+	+	
Naproxen sodium (Anaprox, Naprelan— sustained release)								
Oxaprozin	Cog	S	A	Motor	D	Com	F	
(Daypro)	+	0	0	0	++	+	+	
Piroxicam	Cog	S	A	Motor	D	Com	F	
(Feldene)	+	0	0	0	++	+	+	
Sulindac	Cog	S	A	Motor	D	Com	F	
(Clinoril)	+	0	0	0	++	+	+	
Tolmetin	Cog	S	A	Motor	D	Com	F	
(Tolectin)	+	0	0	0	++	+	+	

Cog = cognition; S = sedation; A = agitation or mania; Motor = discoordination; D = dysphagia; Com = communication; F = falls; NSAID = nonsteroidal anti-inflammatory drug; EC = enteric coated.

The likelihood rating scale for encountering the side effects is as follows: 0 = Almost no probability of encountering side effects. 0/+ = Low probability of encountering side effects but increased with increased dosage. + = Little likelihood of encountering side effects. +/++ = Low probability of encountering side effects; however, probability increases with increased dosage. ++ = Medium likelihood of encountering side effects. +++ = High likelihood of encountering side effects, particularly with high doses. ++++ = Highest likelihood of encountering side effects; best to avoid in at-risk patients.

use of higher doses or use in high-risk patients, including those with hepatic disease, renal disease, chronic alcohol use, or malnutrition. Toxicities associated with chronic overuse include hepatic necrosis along with associated abdominal pain, jaundice, coagulopathy, encephalopathy, nausea, vomiting, renal failure, and even death (Strassels et al., 2007).

Non-Steroidal Anti-Inflammatory Drugs Nonsteroidal anti-inflammatory drugs (NSAIDs) are particularly effective in treating acute or chronic nociceptive pain. NSAIDs inhibit the central and peripheral synthesis of prostaglandins, thus reducing inflammation and fever. Prostaglandins act as messengers in the process of inflammation and fever. They block the inflam-

matory action of prostaglandins peripherally at the site of injury, block leukocyte migration, and inhibit the release of lysosomal enzymes associated with inflammation. Fever is mediated by elevated levels of prostaglandin E2, which signals to the hypothalamus to increase the body's thermal set point. NSAIDs block the effects on prostaglandin E2 and can reduce fever. Many NSAIDs are available without a prescription for treatment of intermittent pain. NSAIDs used for the treatment of chronic pain should be started at a low dose and titrated up each week until analgesia or the maximum dose is reached. The prescriber and patient should be aware that the maximal effects of chronic NSAID therapy may not be seen for 2 to 6 wk (Carl & Johnson, 2006; Strassels et al., 2007).

Most NSAIDs are nonselective inhibitors of cyclooxygenase (COX) and inhibit both COX 1 and COX 2. COX catalyzes the formation of prostaglandins and thromboxane from arachidonic acid. Because thromboxane is an important factor in platelet aggregation, NSAIDs can also prolong bleeding with surgery or injury. Reversible inhibition of platelet aggregation with NSAIDs lasts 1 to 3 days. Patients using a COX 2 inhibitor should not concurrently use a COX 1 inhibitor because combination therapy increases toxicity and causes the loss of the gastrointestinal protective effect of the COX 2 agent (Carl & Johnson, 2006; Strassels et al., 2007).

NSAIDs can have significant side effects, including effects on the gastrointestinal tract, liver, and kidney and on cognition. The gastrointestinal side effects of NSAIDs are related to the inhibition of prostaglandins, which have a protective effect on the mucosa of the stomach. Prostaglandin inhibitors such as NSAIDs block this protective effect and increase the patient's risk for gastrointestinal damage from stomach acid. NSAIDs and salicylates such as aspirin can also be associated with dysphagia because they can cause xerostomia, oral ulceration, glossitis, **dyspepsia**, peptic ulcers, and gastrointestinal mucosal hemorrhage. If an NSAID is necessary for relieving pain in patients with risk for gastrointestinal bleeding, COX 2-selective celecoxib (Celebrex) may be considered because it provides equianalgesic effects with reduced gastrointestinal toxicity. Several COX 2-selective NSAIDs have been removed from the market because they increase the risk of myocardial infarction or stroke. NSAIDs (aside from low-dose aspirin) are associated with a doubled risk of symptomatic heart failure in patients without a history of cardiac disease and a more than 10-fold increase in heart failure in patients with a history of cardiac disease. The use of NSAIDs in patients with congestive heart failure has been associated with increased hospital admissions due to acute decompensated heart failure. NSAIDs can cause nephrotoxicity and should not be used with other agents that impair kidney function. Abrupt acute renal insufficiency with oliguria and retention of sodium and water due to blockade of intrarenal vasodilatory prostaglandins can also occur with NSAID use. Patients with renal insufficiency, congestive heart failure, dehydration, or advanced age are at increased risk for this side effect. NSAIDs can also affect central nervous system function and can be associated with memory loss, confusion, dizziness, and headache. This risk is increased with the use of high-potency agents such as indomethacin (Indocin), with the use of higher doses or sustained-release products, and in the elderly or patients with hepatic or renal insufficiency (Carl & Johnson, 2006; Strassels et al., 2007).

PATIENT CASE 1

W.T. is an 82-yr-old female who was recently placed on Indocin SR 75 mg/day for pain in her knee due to osteoarthritis. Her knee replacement is scheduled in 3 wk. Five days after W.T. starts this medication, the rehabilitation therapist notes that W.T. is extremely confused and has significant ankle swelling. The therapist checks W.T.'s blood pressure, finds that it is 180/90, and calls W.T.'s physician, who instructs W.T.'s daughter to take W.T. to the emergency room. The emergency room nurse reviews W.T.'s medication list: Zocor 20 mg/day for hyperlipidemia, Coumadin 2.5 mg/day for a history of atrial fibrillation, Cardizem CD 120 mg/day for hypertension, Hydrodiuril 25 mg/day for hypertension, and Indocin SR 75 mg/day for knee pain. W.T. has elevated blood pressure, significant pedal edema, and blood in her stool. Laboratory work reveals that W.T. has a significantly elevated serum creatinine level, anemia, and an elevated INR (International Normalized Ratio) of greater than 10 (normal is 2-3). W.T. is diagnosed with coagulopathy, acute renal failure, fluid overload, and a gastrointestinal bleed.

Question

What drug interaction was most likely the cause of W.T.'s coagulopathy and gastrointestinal bleeding?

Answer

When a patient who was stable on a drug regimen suddenly develops signs of toxicity, a good rule of thumb is to question the patient to see whether their drug regimen has recently changed. In most instances, the drug most recently added either caused the side effect or caused a drug interaction with another medication to cause the effect. In this instance, the recent addition of Indocin, an NSAID, should be considered the most likely cause of W.T.'s bleeding. The drug interaction of Indocin with the anticoagulant Coumadin caused the coagulopathy (denoted by the high INR of >10) and the gastrointestinal bleeding. Patients on Coumadin therapy should avoid NSAIDs, which can cause gastrointestinal bleeding even in patients not on anticoagulants, particularly when used in high doses or in older patients.

Question

What medication was most likely the cause of W.T.'s fluid overload and elevated blood pressure?

Answer

NSAIDs such as Indocin can cause fluid retention and can antagonize the effects of medications used to reduce blood pressure, such as the Hydrodiuril and Cardizem that W.T. was taking.

Question

What medication is most likely the cause of W.T.'s new-onset confusion?

Answer

NSAIDs can cause changes in mental status and confusion, particularly when used in high doses or in the older patient. The Indocin likely caused W.T.'s confusion.

Question

What medication is most likely the cause of W.T.'s acute renal failure, denoted by her elevated serum creatinine level?

Answer

NSAIDs such as Indocin inhibit production of prostaglandins and provide inflammatory and analgesic effects. Patients like W.T. who are older often have reduced renal function associated with the aging process, and their bodies rely on prostaglandin's effect of vasodilation to maintain blood flow to the kidneys. Acute inhibition of prostaglandins associated with the use of NSAIDs can block the action of these prostaglandins, resulting in poor blood flow to the kidneys and resultant acute renal failure. The use of NSAIDs is common, and many NSAIDs are available without prescription. Patients who are older, and in particular patients with hypertension, congestive heart failure, or gastrointestinal bleeding, should take NSAIDs only at the advice of their physician and should be carefully monitored for side effects and drug interactions such as those mentioned in this case.

Opioid Analgesics

Opioids are classified by the WHO as either weak or strong. Step 2 pain medications are weaker opioids that are used to treat moderate or intermittent pain; these are often combined with step 1 pain medications. Step 3 pain medications are stronger opioids and are used to treat severe pain that is sustained (Carl & Johnson, 2006; Hartrick et al., 2009; Metzger, 2009).

Opioid analgesics inhibit pain by binding to mu, delta, and kappa receptors in and outside the nervous system. They may be classified as agonists, agonist–antagonists, or antagonists based on their interactions with these receptors. Examples of pure mu agonists include codeine, morphine, hydromorphone (Dilaudid), oxycodone, methadone (Dolophine), and fentanyl (Duragesic). Because opioids that are mu agonists have no ceiling effect, pain effects increase with increased doses (Carl & Johnson, 2006; Hartrick et al., 2009; Metzger, 2009).

Mu agonists provide analgesia but also affect mood and reward behavior. Agents that act on the kappa receptors produce less respiratory depression and miosis and are more often associated with **dysphoria**. Agents with mixed activity of kappa receptor agonists and mu-receptor antagonists provide pain relief without associated respiratory depression and potential for abuse. Such agents, called agonist–antagonists, include pentazocine (Talwin), butorphanol (Stadol), and nalbuphine (Nubain). These agents have a ceiling effect (i.e., effects do not increase past a certain point despite increases in dose) and the ability to precipitate withdrawal symptoms in patients receiving opioids. These products carry a high incidence of confusion and hallucinations, especially in the elderly or in patients with renal impairment (Carl & Johnson, 2006; Hartrick et al., 2009; Metzger, 2009).

Buprenorphine (Subutex, Suboxone) is a partial agonist that is used as a maintenance medication to assist the opioid dependent patient in maintaining abstinence from opioids. Buprenorphine may be prescribed only by certified physicians in office-based treatment programs. Opioid antagonists include naloxone (Narcan) and naltrexone (ReVia). These agents bind to the opioid receptors but do not provide analgesia, thus blocking the effects of opioids (Zichterman, 2007). They are used in treatment of opioid overdose.

Step 2 Medications Used to Treat Moderate Pain Weak opioid agents are used if mild pain is not controlled with step 1 agents or if the patient presents with moderate rather than mild pain. The use of agents such as acetaminophen or NSAIDs alone is ineffective in patients with moderate or severe pain. NSAIDs or acetaminophen have been combined with opioid analgesics to provide more potent pain control in patients who require intermittent therapy for intermittent pain or for breakthrough therapy in combination with a long-acting opioid product (Carl & Johnson, 2006; Hartrick et al., 2009; Metzger, 2009).

When combination products containing acetaminophen, such as hydrocodone with acetaminophen (Norco, Vicodin, Lortab), tramadol with acetaminophen (Ultracet), or oxycodone with acetaminophen (Percocet) are prescribed, caution must be taken to avoid exceeding the maximum daily acetaminophen dose. There is often overuse of acetaminophen due to supplementation of these products with over-the-counter acetaminophen. Because the daily dosing limits of acetaminophen limit the number of pills that the patient can take each day, the use of these combination products alone may not control more severe pain. Patients using these products should be cautioned to not supplement them with over-the-counter products containing acetaminophen and to not increase the dose of these products on their own. Forty-two percent of cases of acute liver failure are associated with acetaminophen overdose, and 63% of unintentional acetaminophen overdoses are associated with combination products of opiates plus acetaminophen. Because of these risks, the FDA is considering removing these combination products from the market and many institutions are removing these combination products from their formularies (Carl & Johnson, 2006; Strassels et al., 2007; Zichterman, 2007).

Tramadol (Ultram) is available as a combination product with acetaminophen (Ultracet) and as an extended-release product (Ultram-ER). Tramadol binds to mu receptors and inhibits norepinephrine and serotonin reuptake and is useful in treating neuropathic pain. It should be titrated slowly over several weeks in order to minimize side effects of nausea and vomiting; therefore, it is less useful in managing acute pain. Its use has been associated with increased risk of seizures and serotonin syndrome. Tramadol should not be combined with monoamine oxidase inhibitors (MAOI) or tricyclic antidepressants (TCA), which can enhance the risk of this toxicity. The FDA recently advised prescribers to use this agent with caution in patients with history of substance abuse or psychiatric illness because of the increased risk for suicide and overdose in this patient population (Carl & Johnson, 2006; Strassels et al., 2007; Zichterman, 2007).

Several opiates are not recommended for use because of increased risk for toxicity or lack of potency. These include propoxyphene, codeine, and meperidine. Products containing propoxyphene have recently been removed from the market because of increased risk for cardiac death, particularly in the elderly patient, and increased risk of falls in the elderly. Codeine is a prodrug, and its analgesic effects require conversion to its active metabolite morphine. Ten percent of this agent is converted in the liver to the active metabolite morphine. However, the amount of analgesia provided is minimal; 30 mg of codeine provides the analgesia equivalent to 1 mg of morphine. Concurrent use of medications that inhibit CYP2D6 metabolism, such as phenothiazines, haloperidol, fluoxetine, and paroxetine, further reduce the efficacy of codeine. This product should not be used in patients with renal insufficiency. In addition, codeine is highly constipating, which prevents dosage increases to provide pain relief (Carl & Johnson, 2006; Strassels et al., 2007; Zichterman, 2007).

Meperidine is another agent that has decreased potency but increased risk of toxicity. It provides only one tenth of the analgesic effects provided by morphine. Its short duration of action requires more frequent administration to control pain. It also is metabolized to a neurotoxic metabolite (normeperidine) that increases the risk of seizures in patients with poor renal function and older patients and when used in high doses. When combined with MAOI meperidine can trigger hypertensive crisis, and when combined with selective serotonin reuptake inhibitor (SSRI) antidepressants, it can precipitate serotonin syndrome. Both of these adverse effects can be life threatening. Because of these concerns most facilities have removed this product from their formularies (Carl & Johnson, 2006; Hartrick et al., 2009; Metzger, 2009; Zichterman, 2007).

Step 3 Medications Used to Treat Severe Pain

Patients presenting with severe pain should start scheduled doses of a strong opioid, and dose should be titrated up until the patient's pain goal is met. Table 13.2 compares the relative potencies of the opiates, the onset and duration of action of the different dosage forms, and methods of administration (Brenton-Wood, 2009; Carl & Johnson, 2006; Hartrick et al., 2009; Metzger, 2009).

Morphine is a pure mu agonist that has two active metabolites: morphine 3-glucuronide and morphine 6-glucuronide. The 3-glucuronide metabolite is a neuroexcitatory agent that is associated with myoclonus, hyperalgesia, and confusion. The 6-glucuronide metabolite is two to four times as potent as morphine and contributes to the analgesic effects of morphine. Because these metabolites are renally eliminated, the use of morphine in patients with renal insufficiency can be associated with a buildup of these active metabolites and can be associated with respiratory depression and oversedation. Morphine also induces histamine release, which can result in hypotension and pruritus and commonly causes nausea and vomiting (Zichterman, 2007).

Hydromorphone (Dilaudid) is five to seven times more potent than morphine but has no active metabolite and does not cause histamine release, making it safer to use in patients with renal insufficiency when appropriately dosed. When converting from intravenous (IV) to oral (PO) doses, the dose must be increased fivefold for equivalent effects (see table 13.2) (Carl & Johnson, 2006; Hartrick et al., 2009; Metzger, 2009).

Oxycodone is more potent than hydrocodone and does not cause the histamine release and nausea commonly seen with morphine. It is available alone in immediate-release (Oxy IR) and sustained-release (OxyContin) products and as combination products with acetaminophen (Percocet, Tylox) and aspirin (Percodan). Oxycodone is metabolized by CYP2D6 enzymes to an active metabolite (oxymorphone), which is now available as an oral sustained-release product (Opana-ER) (Zichterman, 2007).

Fentanyl is 100 times more potent than morphine and is dosed in micrograms (μg) (1 mg is equivalent to 1,000 μg). It acts at the mu receptor, does not cause histamine release, and causes less sedation and constipation than is seen with morphine. It has a short duration of 30 to 60 min and is available as a transdermal patch (Duragesic), oral transmucosal lozenge (Actiq), and buccal tablet (Fentora). It is used parenterally in administration of patient-controlled analgesia (PCA) and in the intensive-care setting. It has no active metabolite and is safe to use in patients with renal dysfunction (Carl & Johnson, 2006; Hartrick et al., 2009; Metzger, 2009; Zichterman, 2007).

Methadone is a mixture of levorotary and dextrorotary isomers that result in different

Table 13.2 Opioid Medications Dosage Equivalencies and Pharmacokinetic Action

Medication	IV/IM/SC*	Oral*	IV to PO**	Time to onset and peak effects	Duration (h)
Morphine immediate release	10 mg	30 mg	3	Oral: Onset is 45 min; peak is 1-2 h. SC: Onset is 0.5-1 h; peak is 1 h. SL: Onset is 15 min; peak is 30 min. IV: Onset is 15-30 min; peak is 30 min.	3-4
Morphine sustained release (MS Contin, Oramorph, Roxanol SR)	10 mg	30 mg	3	Oral: Onset is 4 h; peak is 4-8 h.	12
Morphine 24 h sustained release (Kadian, Avinza)	10 mg	30 mg	3	Oral: Onset is 4 h; peak is 4-8 h.	24
Oxymorphone sustained release (Opana ER)	1 mg	10 mg	10	Oral: Onset is 4 h; peak is 4-8 h.	12
Hydromorphone (Dilaudid)	1.5 mg	7.5 mg	5	Oral: Onset is 45 min; peak is 1-2 h. IM, SC: Onset is 0.5-1 h. IV: Onset is 5 min.	3-4
Hydrocodone (Vicodin, Lortab)	N/A	30 mg	N/A	Oral: Onset is 45 min; peak is 1-2 h.	3-5
Oxycodone immediate release (Oxyfast, Roxycodone, Percocet)	N/A	15-20 mg	N/A	Oral: Onset is 45 min; peak is 1-2 h.	3-5
Oxycodone long-acting (OxyContin)	N/A	15-20 mg	N/A	Oral: Onset is 4 h; peak is 4-8 h.	12
Fentanyl (Actiq, Oracet)	0.1 mg	N/A	N/A	IV: Onset is 5 min. Buccal: Onset is 5-15 min.	1-2
Fentanyl (Duragesic patch)	25 µg patch = 90 mg/day of oral morphine			Onset is 12-16 h; peak is 12-72 h.	72
Tapentadol (Nucynta)	N/A	50 mg	N/A	Onset is 45 min; peak is 1.25 h.	6
Methadone (Dolophine)	10 mg	20 mg	2	Oral: Onset is 45 min; peak is 1-2 h.	6-8
Meperidine (Demerol)	75 mg	300 mg	4	Oral: Onset is 45 min; peak 1-2 h. IM, SC: Onset is 0.5-1 h. IV: Onset is 15-30 min.	2-3
Codeine	130 mg	200 mg	15	Oral: Onset is within 45 min; peak is 1-2 h.	3-4

*These columns list equivalent doses of each opioid.

**Conversion factor used to convert IV dosing to oral dosing.

IM = intramuscular; IV = intravenous; N/A = not applicable; SC = subcutaneous; SL= sublingual; PO = oral dose; µg = microgram.

pharmacologic actions. The levo isomer confers opioid activity, and the dextro isomer antagonizes the N-methyl-D-aspartate (NMDA) receptor and inhibits reuptake of norepinephrine and serotonin. The NMDA receptor plays a role in the development of opioid tolerance and may increase pain relief in patients who were taking other opioids. Switching to methadone may be beneficial for patients who require high doses of opioids which are causing intolerable side effects, and can assist the patient in reducing the dose of opioid needed to provide pain relief. Methadone has a long half-life of 24 h, but the half-life can range from 12 to 190 h in different patients. The duration of analgesia is shorter than the half-life and necessitates dosing every 4 to 6 h initially and then every 6 to 12 h once steady state is achieved. Because of the extended half-life and delayed steady state, life-threatening sedation and respiratory depression can occur 3 to 5 days after initiation. Methadone is **lipophilic** and tends to collect in fat tissue, thus extending time until elimination. It is metabolized by CYP3A4 and CYP2D6. High doses can cause QT prolongation and torsades de pointes. Methadone is also used to assist patients in maintaining opioid abstinence. Doses of greater than 40 mg should be reserved for patients who are being treated in opiate-detoxification and maintenance programs. Although methadone costs less than some of the other long-acting analgesics, the use of methadone for analgesia should be reserved for prescribers who are well versed in its pharmacokinetics and potential toxicities in order to avoid adverse events (Zichterman, 2007).

Tapentadol (Nucynta, 2009), a new class II opioid analgesic used to treat moderate to severe pain, is a centrally acting synthetic analgesic that is thought to produce effects through mu-opioid agonist activity and inhibition of norepinephrine reuptake. Its onset of action is 1.25 h and its half-life is about 4 h. It is metabolized by glucuronidation to an inactive metabolite and is excreted in the urine. Dosing should start at 50 to 100 mg every 4 to 6 h as needed on day 1. A second dose may be administered more than 1 h after initial dose. The maximum dose on day 1 is 700 mg. After day 1, the medication is dosed at 50 to 100 mg

every 4 to 6 h as needed. Dosage should be decreased in the elderly and in patients with moderate liver disease. Nucynta is as equally effective as oxycodone but has fewer gastrointestinal side effects. Common (>10%) side effects include dizziness, somnolence, nausea, and vomiting; less-common (1%-10%) side effects include fatigue, insomnia, constipation, xerostomia, and pruritus. Nucynta should not be used in patients with significant respiratory depression, acute or severe bronchial asthma, **hypercapnia**, paralytic ileus, or severe liver or renal impairment or patients who are taking MAOI or who have taken them within the past 14 days. Nucynta can potentiate respiratory depression in patients who are taking other mu-opioid analgesics, general anesthetics, phenothiazines, tranquilizers, sedatives, hypnotics, or other central nervous system depressants (including alcohol). In addition, this agent may inhibit serotonin reuptake, and serotonin syndrome may occur with concomitant use of medications that increase serotonin levels such as SSRIs (selective serotonin reuptake inhibitors), SSNRIs (selective serotonin-norepinephrine reuptake inhibitors), TCAs (tricyclic antidepressants), MAOIs (monoamine oxidase inhibitors), or triptans such as sumatriptan (Imitrex) used to treat migraines (Hartrick et al., 2009; Metzger, 2009; Tanzi, 2009).

Initiation and Dosing of Opiates Used to Treat Severe Pain   To start a patient on an opioid, an immediate-acting opiate should be initiated and administered on a scheduled basis to prevent periods of untreated pain. The daily dose should be titrated up in increments of no more than 25% until pain relief is achieved. If pain is expected to continue for a prolonged period, the dose of the short-acting product can be converted to an equivalent dose of a long-acting agent. In addition to scheduled administration of a long-acting agent, the patient should have a regimen for treating breakthrough pain as needed. The usual dose for breakthrough pain is 10% to 25% of the long-acting dose; this dose is administered at an interval appropriate for its duration of action. Members of the health care team should monitor breakthrough pain doses and provide the information to the prescriber so that appropriate changes in the patient's scheduled maintenance doses can be made to provide optimal pain control. A dose of the short acting breakthrough medication should be administered about 1 h before exercise sessions to minimize associated pain and improve the patient's ability to participate (Carl & Johnson, 2006; Hartrick et al., 2009; Metzger, 2009).

Table 13.2 provides a summary of commonly used opioids. Each horizontal row includes agent-specific information on conversion factors to use to calculate equivalent doses of parenteral and oral doses to assist the prescriber in transitioning from intravenous to oral therapy or vice versa. The table also provides pharmacokinetic information on each agent such as the onset of action based on the route of administration and the associated duration of action of each agent. The vertical dosing column provides equivalent doses of the different opioids. For example, 10 mg of intravenous morphine provides the same pain relief as 1.5 mg of intravenous hydromorphone (Carl & Johnson, 2006; Hartrick et al., 2009; Metzger, 2009).

If the patient needs to be converted from one opioid to another, the prescriber should follow several principles listed below for calculating a dose of the new opioid product that is equivalent to the dose of the current therapy:

• To convert from one opioid to another, calculate the total daily dose of the current opiate and the total daily dose of the new drug using the comparative strength ratio provided in the chart. Decrease the calculated equianalgesic dose by 25% before converting to the new agent.

• Use the IV (intravenous):PO (by mouth) ratio when converting to a different route. If converting from parenteral to oral, multiply the total daily dose by the conversion factor to get an equivalent oral dose. If converting from oral to parenteral, divide the daily dose by the conversion factor to obtain the parenteral dose.

• To calculate an appropriate breakthrough dose of a short-acting product, divide the strength of the sustained-release product by four and administer the breakthrough dose at an appropriate frequency as determined

by the duration of action listed for the agent. For example, if Oxycontin 100 mg twice/day is being administered, a breakthrough dose equivalent to 25 mg of oxycodone every 3 to 4 h as needed should be provided.

• Once a pain regimen has been implemented, dosing should be titrated as needed based on pain scores and daily breakthrough medication requirements.

PATIENT CASE 2

W.P. is a 69-yr-old male who underwent a resection of oral cancer 2 mo ago and is undergoing 6 cycles of chemotherapy with radiation. He was referred to therapy for problems with uncontrolled pain and weakness. He has lost 20 lb (9 kg) in the past 2 mo. The therapist reviews W.P.'s medication list, which includes Nicotine 21 mg patch/day for smoking cessation, Duragesic 100 µg patch every 72 h for pain, Oxy IR 20 mg by mouth every 3 h as needed for breakthrough pain, phenergan (Promethazine) 25 mg by mouth every 6 h as needed for nausea and vomiting, aspirin 81 mg by mouth/day, Toprol XL 50 mg by mouth/day for blood pressure, lisinopril 20 mg by mouth/day for blood pressure, and atorvastatin (Lipitor) 10 mg by mouth/day for high cholesterol.

Question

What barriers might prevent successful rehabilitation in W.P.?

Answer

W.P.'s pain is unrelieved despite high doses of opiates. Such unrelieved pain is a significant barrier to rehabilitation progress. Medications provided in patch form may not be reliably absorbed in patients with inadequate fat tissue or who place the patches inappropriately and are not effective in treating the acute pain that W.P. is experiencing. The rehabilitation therapist should take a thorough pain history to identify whether W.P. is experiencing neuropathic pain that his opiate regimen is not addressing. The therapist should notify

W.P.'s physician about his uncontrolled pain, and additional orders for controlling W.P.'s pain should be obtained.

W.P. has experienced significant weight loss and has many risk factors for dysphagia, which can result in weakness, weight loss, immunosuppression, and increased risk of infection and aspiration. Surgery and radiation of the mouth and chemotherapy can all contribute to eating and swallowing disorders. Alignment of dentition, inflammatory reactions, and stomatitis associated with the chemotherapy and radiation therapies can contribute to difficulty chewing and swallowing. Radiation damage to the saliva glands may significantly contribute to xerostomia as well.

Medication therapy can add to the risk of dysphagia. Opiate pain medications can contribute to xerostomia, sedation, impaired motor function, slowed gastrointestinal transit, and a high likelihood of severe constipation. A scheduled bowel regimen should be initiated and should include adequate intake of fluid and fiber, exercise, and a laxative such as Senokot-S that acts as a bowel stimulant and stool softener. The promethazine prescribed for nausea has anticholinergic side effects that can contribute to dysphagia by potentiating dry mouth and sedation. Promethazine is a phenothiazine derivative that can be associated with extrapyramidal side effects such as dystonia and tremor and can cause orthostasis, which can increase fall risk and cognitive impairment. These, in turn, can interfere with W.P.'s ability to understand rehabilitation instructions.

Side Effects of Opioid Analgesics   The most common side effects associated with the opioid analgesics include respiratory depression, peripheral vasodilatation, orthostatic hypotension, constipation, sedation, nausea, and vomiting. Less-common side effects include respiratory depression, mental confusion, drowsiness, pruritus, myoclonus, dry mouth, urinary retention, altered cognitive function, dysphoria, euphoria, sleep disturbance, and sexual dysfunction. The combination of ortho-

static hypotension, mental confusion, altered cognitive function, and sleep disturbance can put the patient at significant risk for falls. These side effects can also directly affect the patient's ability to perform activities of daily living and follow directions in therapy. Opioid analgesics can cause or worsen dysphagia through their side effects of sedation, constipation, gastrointestinal upset (nausea and vomiting), dry mouth, impaired gastrointestinal secretions, and reduced esophageal and gastrointestinal motility. Table 13.3 summarizes strategies for managing side effects associated with opiate use (Hartrick et al., 2009; Iversen et al., 2009; Metzger, 2009).

Constipation, which is associated with opioid binding to opioid receptors in the gastrointestinal tract, can result in decreased peristalsis and decreased intestinal secretions. Constipation does not resolve with time, and unresolved constipation can result in anorexia, abdominal pain, abdominal distention, nausea, and vomiting, which may progress to **adynamic ileus**. Patients placed on chronic opioid therapy should also be placed on a bowel regimen with the goal of maintaining a comfortable bowel movement every other day. Patients should avoid straining associated with a bowel movement, which can result in cardiac events. Adequate hydration and exercise should also be encouraged as approved by the patient's physician. The bowel regimen should include taking in adequate amounts of water each day (at least 2 to 3 qt [1.9-2.8 L] if the patient has no fluid restrictions), increasing physical activity and incorporating exercise when possible, and using a daily laxative such as Senokot-S that softens the stool and stimulates gastrointestinal motility. Opiate-induced constipation should be treated with scheduled rather than as-needed (PRN) laxative use. The rehabilitation team should educate the caregivers that the patient should have a bowel movement without straining every 24-48 h. The team should educate caregivers regarding the components of the patient's approved bowel regimen and about the physical mobility and prescribed level of exercise for the patient.

In patients on thickened liquids who do not maintain adequate levels of hydration the speech–language pathologist can help by

Table 13.3   Side Effects and Management of Opiate (Narcotic) Analgesics

Side effects	Recommended management measures
Constipation	**Preventative measures:** Use a prophylactic stimulant laxative plus a stool softener (senna and docusate 2 tablets every morning); increase intakes of fluid and dietary fiber; increase exercise. **Treatment:** Assess cause and treat; rule out obstruction; titrate laxative to maximal dose with goal of 1 unforced stool every 1-2 days; consider adding nonopioid analgesic to allow reduction of opiate dose. **Treatment of persistent constipation:** Reassess for cause; check for impaction; consider adding another laxative; administer Fleets, saline, or tap water enema; consider adding prokinetic medication (metoclopramide); consider adding neuraxial analgesics or neuroablative techniques to lower opiate dose.
Respiratory depression	Cautiously use reversing agents such as naloxone (Narcan) after attempting to stimulate patient, adjust patient's position. May need to readminister the dose of reversing agent several times depending on duration of action of the opiate.
Nausea	**Preventative measures:** Make antiemetics available when prescribing opiates (prochlorperazine, metoclopramide). **Treatment:** Assess cause and treat; consider adding nonopioid analgesic to allow opiate dose reduction. **Treatment of persistent nausea:** Use around-the-clock antiemetics for 1 wk and then change to administration on a PRN (as needed) basis as needed; add serotonin antagonist such as ondansetron (Zofran); reassess cause; change opioid; consider adding neuraxial analgesics or neuroablative techniques to lower opiate dose.
Sedation	**Preventative measures:** Start opioid at low doses and titrate up slowly in increments of no more than 25%. **Treatment of persistent sedation:** Assess for other causes; decrease opioid dose (use lower dose more frequently) or change to another opioid; consider adding a nonopioid agent to allow opioid dose reduction; consider adding methylphenidate or dextroamphetamine; consider adding neuraxial analgesics or neuroablative techniques to lower opiate dose.
Delirium	Assess for other causes (e.g., hypercalcemia, central nervous system metastasis, other psychoactive medications); consider adding nonopioid to lower dose of opioid; consider changing opioid; consider use of haloperidol (Haldol).
Motor or cognitive impairment	Usually seen with dose changes and titration. Start with low doses and slowly titrate to minimize these side effects.
Opioid toxicity syndrome	Associated with very high doses of opioid, renal impairment, dehydration, and debilitation. Symptoms include hyperalgesia, altered mental status, and myoclonus. Managed by rotating opioid or temporarily replacing use of opioid with nonopioid management.

working to remove thickened liquids from the patient's diet in order to increase the intake of thin liquids. Patients notoriously dislike thickened liquids, and avoidance results in lack of hydration. Upgrading the patient to thin liquids if possible can significantly affect the patient's level of hydration. As discussed previously, opioid use can also cause or exacerbate dysphagia symptoms.

The rehabilitation therapist can help ensure that the patient adheres to their prescribed bowel regimen and this can have a marked influence on the patient's rehabilitation performance. The occupational therapist may incorporate toileting into the therapy session to increase the probability that the patient will follow through on maintaining regular bowel movements. The patient on chronic opioid therapy may be hesitant to go through the effort of trying to defecate because of their pain level or medication-induced sedation (Carl & Johnson, 2006; Hartrick et al., 2009; Metzger, 2009).

Opioids stimulate the chemoreceptor zone in the brain, inhibit peristalsis, and can increase vestibular sensitivity, causing nausea and vomiting. Nausea and vomiting are usually transient and occur in the first 48 h of therapy. Patients should be told that the effects are short term, and an antiemetic should be available for the patient in case one is needed. Other measures for controlling nausea and vomiting include maintaining a clean and odor-free environment, properly caring for the mouth, maintaining hydration, and providing foods with low potential for causing nausea such as dry toast, crackers, ginger ale, cola, baked potatoes, and rice (Campbell-Taylor, 1996, 2001).

Sedation occurs with opiate initiation and dosage increases and is usually transient. Patients develop tolerance to this side effect within the first few days or weeks. The physician, pharmacist, and other team members should educate patients and family about this side effect and should advise patients to not drive or perform activities that require alertness until the effect resolves and to not use alcohol. Persistent sedation may indicate that the dose needs to be lowered (usually by 25%) or may be the result of a drug interaction with another central nervous system depressant (Carl & Johnson, 2006; Hartrick et al., 2009; Metzger, 2009).

Respiratory depression occurs as a result of the opioid attaching to the mu2-opioid receptors in the medulla. Opioid respiratory depression is associated with sedation, mental clouding, decreased rate and depth of respiration, and decreased oxygen saturation. Risk of respiratory depression increases when patients with pulmonary disease are treated with opioids, when opioids are initiated in opioid-naive patients, and when opioids suddenly relieve chronic pain (**neurolysis**). Respiratory depression and the resulting symptoms can be particularly serious in this population. The rehabilitation therapist needs to modify the patient's exercise regimen to account for any depressed respiratory responses. In these instances, the rehabilitation therapist should monitor the patient's vital signs before and after exertion and ensure that the patient has adequate time to recover between bouts of exercise (Carl & Johnson, 2006; Hartrick et al., 2009; Metzger, 2009).

The rehabilitation therapist needs to be particularly aware of complications due to respiratory depression when engaging patients on opioids in exercise. The patient may experience a lack of oxygen (hypoxia) or excess carbon dioxide (hypercapnia). Initial symptoms of an increase in carbon dioxide can be increased blood pressure, skin flushing, hand flapping, confusion, lethargy, and headache. Severe hypercapnia can result in hyperventilation, panic, unconsciousness, and death. Symptoms of hypoxia include shortness of breath, headache, nausea, euphoria, fatigue, memory loss, inattentiveness, lack of judgment, and decreased motor coordination. Rapid-onset hypoxia can result in seizures, coma, and death. The rehabilitation therapist should have oxygen readily available for use when caring for patients who are using opioids. An antagonist such as naloxone (Narcan) can be used to arouse breathing if verbal or physical stimulation are ineffective, but this agent should be used cautiously because it can precipitate severe withdrawal symptoms and loss of analgesia. The rehabilitation therapist should contact medical personnel immediately when patients exhibit signs of respiratory depression (Cameron & Monroe, 2007; Ciccone, 2007).

Administration of a short-acting pain medication can help the patient participate in the rehabilitation session. The rehabilitation therapist may have access to the patient on an ongoing basis and can assess the patient's responses to pain, medication side effects, and physical activity. These observations can significantly help the physician manage the patient's pain. The rehabilitation therapist also needs to work with the physician to ensure that the patient is receiving enough medication to prevent pain but not enough medication to cause side effects such as respiratory depression (Carl & Johnson, 2006).

Opiate-associated cognitive impairment may last from a few days up to 2 wk and can include difficulty concentrating, mental clouding, mood changes, or hallucinations. Electrolyte imbalances, hypoxia, or drug interactions may potentiate confusion or delirium.

Reducing dosage or changing to an alternative opioid may be effective in managing persistent confusion. Seizures can occur with use of high doses of opioids and in patients with renal or liver failure. Meperidine (Demerol) is associated with a high risk of seizures when used in high doses, in the elderly, or in the renally impaired patient due to the accumulation of the metabolite normeperidine. In the geriatric patient, pharmacokinetic changes involving the liver (decreased size, blood supply, enzymatic activity, and synthesis of plasma proteins) and kidney (decreased blood flow and tubular function) increase drug levels and increase rates of drug toxicity. Therefore, agents with shorter half-lives (i.e., oxycodone, hydromorphone, and morphine) are preferred in the elderly patient (Carl & Johnson, 2006; Hartrick et al., 2009; Metzger, 2009).

The therapist should also monitor the patient for withdrawal symptoms initiated by sudden discontinuance of opiates such as anorexia, diarrhea, fever, insomnia, appetite loss, stomach cramps, sweating, yawning, restlessness, tremor, tachycardia, depression, muscle spasms, weakness, nausea, and vomiting. The rehabilitation therapist can be of assistance by notifying the patient's physician about persistent sedation or symptoms of withdrawal (Carl & Johnson, 2006; Hartrick et al., 2009; Metzger, 2009).

Routes of Administration of Opioids   Oral administration of pain medications is preferred whenever possible because it is safer, more effective, more convenient, and less expensive. Immediate-release tablets of hydromorphone, oxycodone, or oxymorphone may be crushed. Liquid formulations of morphine, hydromorphone, oxycodone, and methadone are available for patients who cannot swallow tablets. Administering the medication by rectal, intravenous, subcutaneous, or intraspinal routes can be considered in patients who are unable to take oral medications. Buccal and oral transmucosal fentanyl products such as Actiq and Fentora are approved for managing breakthrough cancer pain and have an onset of 5 to 15 min (Carl & Johnson, 2006; Hartrick et al., 2009; Metzger, 2009).

Sustained-release products such as OxyContin, MS Contin, and Opana ER should not be split or crushed; doing so destroys the time-release mechanism and can cause a potentially lethal overdose. Controlled-release morphine capsules (Kadian and Avinza) can be opened and sprinkled on soft food for patients who cannot swallow capsules. Intermediate-release products can be administered rectally (Carl & Johnson, 2006; Hartrick et al., 2009; Metzger, 2009). Rectal administration of long-acting products every 12 h is commonly used in palliative care. Rectal absorption is variable and depends on rectal placement. Higher blood levels and effects are obtained if the product is placed past the rectal sphincter because first-pass metabolism is avoided and the product is absorbed directly into the bloodstream (Gutstein & Akil, 2001; Jacox et al., 1994; Max et al., 1999).

When oral or parenteral routes of administration are not appropriate, transdermal fentanyl (Duragesic) can be used in patients with stable (non-escalating), severe pain. Because the fentanyl patch (Duragesic) has a slow onset of action (12-18 h) and a long half-life (17-21 h), it cannot be used in patients with rapidly escalating pain. When initiating fentanyl patch therapy, an immediate-acting pain medication should be administered to provide pain relief for at least 12 to 18 h until onset of pain relief from the fentanyl patch (Duragesic) occurs. Dosage of the patch should be titrated no more often than every 96 h to allow assessment of achieved pain control once drug levels have reached a steady state. If a patient is to be discharged from an acute care facility on fentanyl patch (Duragesic), the patch should be initiated early enough in the admission to ensure that the dose has been adequately titrated before discharge. Blood levels decrease by one half 17 h after patch removal. The patient should take care to remove the old patch before placing a new patch to prevent accidental overdose. The patient should also have access to adequate breakthrough pain medication. As a general rule, a breakthrough agent that is equivalent in strength to oral morphine 10 mg every 3 to 4 h should be available for each 25 µg increment of the fentanyl (Duragesic) patch (Carl &

Johnson, 2006; Hartrick et al., 2009; Metzger, 2009). Heat can increase absorption of fentanyl from the patch and result in overdose. Fever greater than 104 °F can speed delivery by one third and contribute to overdose. Patients should not apply heating pads directly to the patch. Patients should dispose of transdermal patches by folding the patch with the sticky side in and placing in a secure area away from pets and children. Active product remains in *used* patches removed after 72 h of use. Used patches have been associated with cases of lethal drug overdose in which drug abusers chewed patches, applied multiple patches to the skin, and inserted patches rectally (Carl & Johnson, 2006; Hartrick et al., 2009; Metzger, 2009).

Intravenous administration of opiate medication provides more rapid onset of effects but shorter duration of action than oral administration. Subcutaneous administration is associated with a slower onset and lower peak levels than intravenous administration. Intramuscular administration of opiates is painful and is not recommended. Intravenous PCA (patient controlled analgesia) has proven to be an excellent method of managing patients with acute pain such as postoperative patients. Better control of pain is achieved because the patient can control the timing of the dosing of their breakthrough analgesic based on their own assessment of their pain. This results in fewer total doses over a shorter period of time, more rapid recovery to an ambulatory status and ability to participate in rehabilitative exercise, and improved rates of recovery from the surgical procedure. Use of continuous narcotic infusions using a basal rate in patients receiving PCA therapy is not recommended immediately after surgery or in opiate-naive patients. However, PCA is very useful for maintaining analgesia in patients admitted on chronic opioid therapy, such as patients with chronic cancer pain who have established opioid tolerance and who cannot take their usual oral pain therapy immediately before or after surgery because of their NPO (nothing by mouth) status (Carl & Johnson, 2006; Hartrick et al., 2009; Metzger, 2009).

Patient safety is a primary concern. Studies that examined adverse events associated with the use of PCA therapy identified a high risk of programming errors and miscalculation of drug concentrations. Unauthorized PCA administration by family members, visitors, and health professionals (referred to as PCA by proxy) may result in oversedation and has resulted in patient death. Patients and family should understand that they should not do PCA by proxy. The Institute for Safe Medication Practices and the United States Pharmacopeia made several recommendations for improving safety in the use of PCA, including using barcode technology; educating staff, patients, and family about PCA therapy; using smart pump technology; using a single standard concentration for each medication given by intravenous PCA; establishing patient-selection criteria for the use of PCA; using standardized, preprinted order forms to guide prescribing; and requiring that two clinicians double-check pump setting and medications before initiation. Additional recommended practices involve verifying PCA settings with each shift change, verifying whether the connections are for intravenous or epidural lines, and reassessing PCA settings if the patient complains of pain. Table 13.4 lists the recommended starting dose of opiates administered by PCA (Gutstein & Akil, 2001;

Table 13.4   Intravenous Patient-Controlled Analgesia Dosing of Opioid (Narcotic) Analgesics

Medication	Starting dose	Dosing range	Lockout dose	Lockout range
Morphine 1 mg/ml	1 mg	0.5-2.5 mg	8 min	5-10 min
Hydromorphone 0.2 mg/ml (Dilaudid)	0.2 mg	0.05-0.4 mg	8 min	5-10 min
Fentanyl 50 µg/ml	10 µg	10-50 µg	6 min	5-8 min

Adapted from AHCPR Pub. No. 92-0032 (1992).

Hutchinson, 2007; Jacox et al., 1994; Max et al., 1999).

Analgesics administered via epidural catheters provide significantly better postoperative pain relief than intravenous therapy. Opioids administered via the intrathecal or epidural routes are usually associated with less confusion, constipation, respiratory depression, and other side effects because much lower doses are required. Seventy percent of patients have adequate pain control without additional treatment modality or epidural catheter replacement. Epidural analgesia may be associated with motor block, numbness, nausea, and vomiting. Intraspinal opioids can cause histamine release, resulting in hypotension and pruritus, which is usually managed with administration of diphenhydramine (Benadryl). Urinary retention can also occur with use of intraspinal opioids due to increased smooth muscle tone, bladder spasm, and increased bladder sphincter tone and may require urinary catheterization. Intraspinal products should always be compounded with preservative-free products to prevent neurotoxic damage that can result in paralysis. The risk of neuraxial hematoma is increased with placement of epidural catheters in patients receiving anticoagulant therapy and guidelines have been developed to hold parenteral anticoagulant doses for at least 12 h before and after manipulation or insertion of these catheters (Ghafoor et al., 2007; Viscusi, 2007). Table 13.5 provides information about intraspinal dosing of pain medications (Gutstein & Akil, 2001; Jacox et al., 1994; Max et al., 1999).

Postoperative analgesia can also be administered via iontophoresis. This is a system of drug delivery that applies low-level electrical current to a similarly charged drug solution and drives the medication through the skin to underlying tissue. Iontophoresis can be used to deliver medications locally or systemically.

A noninvasive, credit card-size device has been developed that delivers fentanyl via iontophoresis. This system delivers preprogrammed doses into systemic circulation. The adhesive device is placed on the patient's upper arm or chest and is accessed when the patient presses a recessed button twice in 3 s. This triggers the microprocessor to activate low-intensity direct electrical current, thus transferring 40 µg of fentanyl across the skin and into the circulation over a period of 10 min. In one study, the fentanyl iontophoresis transdermal delivery system provided pain control similar to that of intravenous PCA therapy but led to fewer errors and less inhibition of ambulation. Side effects associated with this therapy include nausea, vomiting, erythema at the site of application, and headache. Before initiation, the patient should be titrated to an acceptable level of

Table 13.5   Dosing Guidelines for Intraspinal (Epidural and Intrathecal) Opioid Analgesics

Medication	Intermittent single doses	Continuous infusion doses	Time to onset (min)	Duration (h)
Epidural administration				
Morphine	1-6 mg	0.1-1.0 mg/h	30	6-24
Fentanyl	0.025-0.1 mg	0.025-0.1 mg/h	5	4-8
Clonidine		0.3 mg/h		
Hydromorphone (Dilaudid)	0.8-1.5 mg	0.15-0.3 mg/h	5-8	4-6
Subarachnoid (intrathecal) administration				
Morphine	0.1-0.3 mg	N/A	15	8-34
Fentanyl	0.005-0.025	N/A	5	3-6

N/A = Not applicable.

Adapted from: AHCPR Pub. No. 92-0032 (1992).

analgesia (Viscusi, 2007). Additional information on the use of iontophoresis use in delivery of medications can be found in the appendix.

Adjuvant Analgesics   Adjuvant analgesics are used in combination with other analgesics to enhance analgesic efficacy and treat concurrent symptoms that exacerbate pain or alone as an analgesic to treat atypical pain such as neuropathic pain. These agents include anticonvulsants, tricyclic antidepressants, psychostimulants, muscle relaxants, neuroleptics, antihistamines, corticosteroids, benzodiazepines, **antispasmodics**, and oral or parenteral local anesthetics and antiarrhythmics. Antidepressants and anxiolytics can improve pain control through direct effects on neurotransmitters and by reducing depression or anxiety associated with pain. Neuropathic pain is usually treated with anticonvulsants and the antidepressants that inhibit norepinephrine and serotonin. Adjuvant analgesics such as the tricyclic antidepressant amitriptyline (Elavil) and older antihistamines such as hydroxyzine (Vistaril) and promethazine (Phenergan) have high anticholinergic effects and can potentiate the sedative and constipating effects of the opioids. Use of these agents in the older patient is not recommended because increased orthostasis sedation, confusion, and arrhythmia can increase risk of falls (Finnerup et al., 2005; Jann & Slade, 2007; Wiffen et al., 2005).

Patients with advanced-stage cancer may be treated with psychostimulants such as methylphenidate and dextroamphetamine to increase energy and decrease opioid-induced sedation (Eidelman et al., 2007; Swarm et al., 2007; Toth, 2009). Topical agents such as Lidoderm patch and diclofenac patch or topical gel can also provide analgesic relief. Topical NSAIDs provide blood levels similar to those seen with oral agents. A recent FDA warning states that liver-function tests of patients receiving topical NSAIDs should be checked periodically during the first 6 wk of initiation and throughout therapy to identify hepatotoxic effects. Table 13.6 summarizes medications commonly used as adjuvant analgesic therapy (Ciccone, 2007; Iversen et al., 2009; Jacobson et al., 2007; Preston et al., 2008).

Medications Used to Treat Neuropathic Pain

Neuropathic pain is described as burning or shooting pain and is usually associated with **postherpetic neuralgia**, migraine headache, arthritis, compression fracture, diabetic neuropathy, peripheral neuropathy, and malignant nerve infiltration. Neuropathic pain may lead to continuous or stimulus-evoked pain. Allodynia (pain after light touch) can also develop. The extent of nerve damage may not be proportional to the neuropathic pain experienced. Twenty-eight percent of patients with multiple sclerosis experience neuropathic pain, whereas 8% of stroke patients and 5% of patients with traumatic nerve injuries experience neuropathic pain. When patients do experience neuropathic pain, it can be difficult to manage. Approximately one half of patients with neuropathic pain obtain pain relief using medications (Iversen et al., 2009). TCAs (tricyclic antidepressants), SSNRI (selective serotonin-norepinephrine reuptake inhibitor), and SSRI (serotonin-norepinephrine reuptake inhibitor) antidepressants, topically applied capsaicin, and anticonvulsants are the agents most frequently used to treat neuropathic pain. Table 13.6 summarizes the medications used to treat neuropathic pain (Dworkin et al., 2007; Hulisz & Moore, 2007; Montfort et al., 2010; Teague, 2007; Westanmo et al., 2005).

Research into other devices for reducing or eliminating neuropathic pain is ongoing. For example, rehabilitation specialists may use low-level laser therapy and light therapy to reduce pain and increase microcirculation without medication and medication side effects. The protocol typically calls for patients with chronic pain to be treated for at least 30 min 3 times/wk for approximately 1 mo. For patients with acute conditions, treatment can be given up to 3 times/day. In every instance, the patient receives other skilled therapeutic interventions along with the infrared light therapy.

Anticonvulsants   Anticonvulsants are useful in treating neuropathic pain (described as lancinating, shock like, shooting, lightning-like,

See table 13.6 in the web resource for a full list of medication-specific indications, dosing recommendations, and side effects.

Table 13.6 Adjuvant Analgesic Medications

Medication	Side effects affecting rehab							Other side effects or considerations
Corticosteroids: Used to reduce inflammation.								
Dexamethasone (Decadron)	Cog ++	S 0	A ++	Motor ++	D ++	Com +	F ++	Gastrointestinal upset and ulceration, hyperglycemia, confusion, increased risk of infection
Prednisone	Cog ++	S 0	A ++	Motor ++	D ++	Com +	F ++	Gastrointestinal upset and ulceration, hyperglycemia, confusion, increased risk of infection
Anticonvulsants: Used to treat neuropathic pain. Monitor for liver, hematologic, and renal changes, as well as rash. Anticonvulsant hypersensitivity syndrome can lead to Stevens-Johnson syndrome.								
Carbamazepine (Tegretol)	Cog ++	S ++	A +	Motor ++	D ++	Com ++	F +++	Liver +++ Hematologic +++ Renal +++ Rash +++ Sedation, hypersensitivity reactions, gastrointestinal upset, appetite changes, slowed cognitive function, lethargy, nausea, headaches, irritability, skin rashes, decreased reaction time, nystagmus, ataxia, dysphagia, dysarthria; genetic testing in Asians required to reduce risk of AHS
Phenytoin (Dilantin)	Cog ++	S ++	A 0	Motor ++	D +++	Com +++	F ++	Liver ++ Hematologic +++ Renal ++ Rash ++ Sedation, hypersensitivity reactions, gastrointestinal upset, appetite changes, slowed cognitive function, lethargy, nausea, headaches, irritability, skin rashes, decreased reaction time, nystagmus, ataxia, dysphagia, dysarthria
Clonazepam (Klonopin)	Cog +	S +	A 0	Motor 0	D 0/+	Com +	F +	Sedation, gastrointestinal upset, appetite changes
Gabapentin (Neurontin)	Cog ++	S ++	A +	Motor +++	D 0	Com ++	F +++	Liver 0 Hematologic 0 Renal +++ Rash + Sedation, gastrointestinal upset, appetite changes, ataxia, gait changes, tremor, dizziness, fatigue, ataxia, drowsiness, behavioral changes, peripheral edema, weight gain
Keppra (Levetiracetam)	Cog +++	S +++	A 0	Motor +++	D +	Com ++	F +++	Liver 0 Hematologic + Renal +++ Rash + Somnolence, tiredness, dizziness, upper-respiratory infections. Pyridoxine decreases psychiatric side effects.
Lamotrigine (Lamictal)	Cog ++	S 0	A ++	Motor +	D 0	Com ++	F ++	Liver + Hematologic 0 Renal + Rash + Anticonvulsant hypersensitivity syndrome, insomnia, rash that can progress to Stevens-Johnson syndrome. Avoid in pregnancy.

› continued

Table 13.6 › *continued*

Medication	Side effects affecting rehab							Other side effects or considerations
Pregabalin (Lyrica)	Cog ++	S ++	A +	Motor +++	D 0	Com ++	F +++	Liver 0 Hematologic 0 Renal +++ Rash + Dizziness, somnolence, dry mouth, edema, blurred vision, weight gain, difficulty with concentration and attention
Topiramate (Topamax)	Cog ++	S ++	A ++	Motor +++	D +	Com +++	F ++	Liver 0 Hematologic 0 Renal +++ Rash ++ Dizziness, somnolence, dry mouth, edema, blurred vision, weight gain, difficulty with concentration and attention, language impairment, behavioral changes, weight loss, altered taste, metabolic acidosis, kidney stones, hypohidrosis
Valproic acid (Depakene)	Cog ++	S ++	A ++	Motor ++	D ++	Com ++	F ++	Liver ++ Hematologic +++ Renal 0 Rash +++ Tremor, dyspepsia, weight gain, anticonvulsant hypersensitivity syndrome, hepatotoxicity, pancreatitis, alopecia, thrombocytopenia, sedation, appetite changes, gastrointestinal upset, rash, AHS

Tricyclic Antidepressants: Used to treat neuropathic pain.

Medication	Cog	S	A	Motor	D	Com	F	Other side effects or considerations
Amitriptyline (Elavil)	++++	++++	0	++	++++	++++	++++	Impaired cognition, sedation, seizure risk, cardiac arrhythmia, sexual dysfunction, orthostasis, gastrointestinal upset.
Desipramine (Norpramin)	++	++	+	++	++	++	+	Desipramine and nortriptyline preferred agents due to lower sedation, cardiac, and anticholinergic effects.
Doxepin (Sinequan)	++++	++++	++	++	++	+++	++++	
Imipramine (Tofranil)	+++	+++	+	++	+++	+++	++++	
Nortriptyline (Pamelor)	+++	++	0	++	++	++	+	
Trazodone (Desyrel)	++++	++++	0	++	++	+++	+++	

Norepinephrine serotonin reuptake inhibitor antidepressants: Used to treat neuropathic pain.

Medication	Cog	S	A	Motor	D	Com	F	Other side effects or considerations
Duloxetine (Cymbalta)	+	0	+	0	++	0	+	Somnolence, nausea, dry mouth, decreased appetite, constipation; jitteriness and insomnia at higher doses
Venlafaxine (Effexor)	+	+	0/+	+	+	+	+	

Muscle relaxants: Used to treat spasticity.

Medication	Cog	S	A	Motor	D	Com	F	Other side effects or considerations
Baclofen (Lioresal)	++	+++	++	+++	++	++	+++	Oral: Initial sedation, muscle weakness, ataxia, orthostatic hypotension, fatigue, headache, nausea, dizziness; confusion and hallucinations reported in the elderly or those with history of stroke. Abrupt discontinuation may result in rebound (increased spasticity, rhabdomyolysis, disorientation, hallucination, seizures). Intrathecal: Chronic constipation, hypotonia, somnolence, headache, vomiting, paresthesias.

Medication	Side effects affecting rehab							Other side effects or considerations
Antihistamines: Used to treat anxiety, nausea, and insomnia.								
Hydroxyzine (Vistaril)	Cog ++	S ++	A ++	Motor ++	D ++	Com ++	F ++	Dry mouth, sedation, orthostasis, confusion, impaired cognition
Promethazine (Phenergan)	Cog ++	S ++	A ++	Motor ++	D ++	Com ++	F ++	
Local anesthetics and antiarrhythmics: Used to treat neuropathic pain.								
Lidocaine	Cog +++	S +++	A +	Motor +++	D ++	Com ++	F +++	Sedation, gastrointestinal upset, confusion, tremor, ataxia, seizures
Tocainide (Tonocard)	Cog +++	S +++	A +	Motor +++	D ++	Com ++	F +++	
Psychostimulants: Used to decrease sedation.								
Dextroamphet-amine	Cog ++	S 0	A ++	Motor ++	D ++	Com +	F ++	Tremor, xerostomia, altered taste, decreased appetite
Methylpheni-date (Ritalin)	Cog ++	S 0	A ++	Motor ++	D ++	Com +	F ++	

Cog = cognition; S = sedation; A = agitation or mania; Motor = discoordination; D = dysphagia; Com = communication; F = falls; AHS = anticonvulsant hypersensitivity syndrome.

The likelihood rating scale for encountering the side effects is as follows: 0 = Almost no probability of encountering side effects. + = Little likelihood of encountering side effects. +/++ = Low probability of encountering side effects; however, probability increases with increased dosage. ++ = Medium likelihood of encountering side effects. +++ = High likelihood of encountering side effects, particularly with high doses. ++++ = Highest likelihood of encountering side effects; best to avoid in at-risk patients.

or stabbing), neuralgias, tumor encroachment on a nerve (brachial or lumbosacral plexus), or neuropathic pain not relieved by tricyclic antidepressants. The anticonvulsants act at many sites that may be involved with pain transmission. They inhibit sodium and calcium channels, potentiate the action of GABA, and inhibit glutamate receptors. These actions decrease neuronal excitation and enhance inhibition of the pain signal. Gabapentin (Neurontin) and pregabalin (Lyrica), which are second-generation anticonvulsants, are commonly used to treat neuropathic pain because they are better tolerated and have fewer drug interactions than the first-generation anticonvulsants (Dubinsky et al., 2004; Hulisz & Moore, 2007; Jann & Slade, 2007; Rosenstock et al., 2004; Teague, 2007).

Gabapentin (Neurontin) binds to alpha-2 delta subunits of voltage-gated calcium channels, inhibiting the release of excitatory neurotransmitters. Effective doses for treatment of neuropathic pain are 1800 to 3600mg/day. This agent must be titrated over 6 to 8 wk to ensure safe and effective dose titration. Patients should be tapered over 1 wk if discontinuance is necessary (Finnerup et al., 2005; Jann & Slade, 2007; Wiffen et al., 2005).

Pregabalin (Lyrica) also binds to alpha-2 delta subunits of voltage-gated calcium channels, inhibiting the release of excitatory neurotransmitters. Effective doses for treatment of neuropathic pain are 300 to 600 mg/day. This agent can be administered twice/day, and less time is required to titrate it to an effective dose compared with gabapentin. Improvements in fatigue, insomnia, and pain were noted when pregabalin was used to treat fibromyalgia. This agent should be tapered over 1 wk if discontinuance is necessary (Blommel & Blommel, 2007; Hulisz & Moore, 2007; Jann & Slade, 2007; Teague, 2007).

Antidepressants TCA have been used for years to treat pain due to their ability to increase the amount of circulating inhibitory pain. The neurotransmitter serotonin acts at the terminals of endogenous pain-modulating pathways that originate in the medulla and synapse at every level of the spinal cord. Tricyclic antidepressants prevent the reuptake of norepinephrine and serotonin at the central nervous system synapses; as a result, more serotonin is available to inhibit pain transmission. The analgesic activity of TCA is independent of their antidepressant activity, and their pain effects have a faster onset (days versus weeks) and occur at lower doses than their antidepressant effects. Desipramine (Norpramin) and nortriptyline (Pamelor) are generally the preferred TCA for treating neuropathic pain due to their lower incidence and extent of anticholinergic, cardiotoxic, and sedative effects (Hulisz & Moore, 2007; Jann & Slade, 2007; Preston et al., 2008).

A newer group of antidepressants is the SSNRIs (selective serotonin and norepinephrine reuptake inhibitors), also called the dual reuptake inhibitors. Duloxetine (Cymbalta) inhibits reuptake of both norepinephrine and serotonin, thus providing increased levels at the receptor site and improved modulation of pain. These agents do not act on the histamine or muscarinic receptors and provide pain relief without the anticholinergic side effects associated with the use of TCAs (tricyclic antidepressants). Duloxetine (Cymbalta) is commonly used to treat neuropathic pain, diabetic neuropathy, and pain associated with fibromyalgia. This agent has balanced effects on both neurotransmitters at low doses, whereas other SSNRIs such as venlafaxine (Effexor) preferentially affect serotonin levels at low doses. Although they are effective antidepressants, the SSRIs preferentially affect serotonin and are not used to treat pain (Hulisz & Moore, 2007; Jann & Slade, 2007; Moultry & Poon, 2009; Westanmo et al., 2005).

Topical Therapy

Topical capsaicin therapy provides relief to some patients by depleting substance P in the peripheral sensory neurons. Substance P is thought to be one of the principal chemical mediators of pain impulses from the periph-

ery to the central nervous system. Products containing capsaicin include Zostrix, Zostrix HP, Capzasin P, R-Gel, Capsin, and No Pain HP. Topical Capsaicin should be applied to the affected area no more than 3 to 4 times/day, and contact with the eyes, contact lenses, and broken or irritated skin should be avoided. Use of gloves or an applicator during application is recommended. The person administrating this agent should wash their hands immediately and thoroughly after each application. Adverse effects include transient burning, stinging, and erythema of area of application. Cough and respiratory irritation can also occur (Carl & Johnson, 2006).

Other topical therapies include a transdermal lidocaine 5% (Lidoderm) patch applied for 12 h/day and the topical NSAID diclofenac (Voltaren) in 1% gel or topical patch 1.3% (Flector). Dosing cards for measuring the dose and applying the gel to the treatment area are provided with the gel. The patches, which are applied directly to the area of pain, should be worn for up to 12 h and then removed. Medication patches should not be worn while bathing, showering, or swimming and can be secured using medical tape if they fall off. The used patch or dose should be folded in half and thrown away in an area that children or pets cannot access. Topical NSAIDs provide blood levels similar to those seen with oral agents. A recent FDA warning states that liver-function tests of patients receiving topical NSAIDs should be checked periodically during the first 6 wk of initiation and throughout therapy to identify hepatotoxic effects (Dubinsky et al., 2004).

Summary

This chapter summarizes the different types of pain and the medications used to treat pain. It also discusses tools for assessing pain and monitoring the effectiveness of pain management and covers important side effects and drug interactions involving pain medications. The rehabilitation team should use a cadre of strategies, both pharmacologic and nonpharmacologic, when managing pain.

Medications Used to Treat Chronic Pain Syndromes

The rehabilitation therapist will often provide therapy to patients with chronic pain syndromes. An estimated 50 million Americans are partially or totally disabled as a result of pain, and the associated cost to the U.S. economy is several billion dollars annually. As many as one third of Americans experience chronic pain at some point in life and many take prescription medications, nonprescription medications, and even alternative therapies such as herbals and homeopathic pain remedies to relieve their pain (Gibson, 2010). The rehabilitation therapist should understand the pathophysiology associated with chronic pain syndromes, how this pain affects rehabilitation, and how to adjust therapy sessions to meet the needs of patients experiencing chronic pain. This chapter discusses the rehabilitative and traditional medication therapies used to treat migraine headache, fibromyalgia, trigeminal neuralgia, cancer pain, amputation pain (phantom limb pain), central pain syndromes, and complex regional pain syndromes.

Migraine Headache

Migraines are characterized by throbbing pain, usually located on one side of the head, accompanied by nausea, vomiting, and sensitivity to light and sound. The migraine has three phases: the preheadache phase, the headache phase, and the postdromal phase. The preheadache phase includes the premonitory phase and migraine aura. This phase, which may precede the attack by hours or days, is seen in 20% to 60% of patients. The headache phase presents with throbbing, pulsatile pain in the frontotemporal region that can last from 4 to 72 h. Accompanying symptoms can include nausea, vomiting, autonomic symptoms, nasal congestion, and lacrimation. The postdromal phase consists of fatigue and irritability that lasts from 24 to 48 h. On average, a patient with migraines experiences 1.5 attacks/mo. Attacks usually last for 24 h, but 20% of patients report attacks that last 2 to 3 days (Demaagd, 2008a; Feliu et al., 2007).

Incidence

According to the World Health Organization, migraine headache accounts for 1.4% of disability-adjusted life years worldwide and is in the top 20 causes of disability worldwide (Leonardi et al., 2005). In the United States, 29.5 million people suffer from migraines. Cost associated with migraines is estimated to be $23 billion/yr. Females are three times more likely to have migraine headaches than are males, and migraines are most prevalent in people aged 20 to 45 yr. Many females experience migraine attacks associated with their menstrual cycle. Eighty percent of patients report a family history of the disorder. Migraine can be associated with concurrent depression, bipolar disease, fibromyalgia, irritable bowel syndrome, overactive bladder, sleep disorders, obsessive–compulsive disorder, and anxiety disorders (Demaagd, 2008a; Feliu et al., 2007).

Etiology and Pathophysiology

Researchers believe that migraine is associated with an imbalance of central serotonin and that low levels of serotonin lead to activation of the trigeminovascular system. When this system is activated by external or internal triggers, inflammatory peptides such as calcitonin gene-related peptide, substance P, neurokinin A, and nitric oxide are released. These peptides cause a perivascular inflammatory response at the trigeminal nucleus caudalis in the brainstem and in the cervical cord area. These pain data are transmitted to the thalamus and cortex, resulting in cortical sensitization and the symptoms associated with migraine. Common triggers include chemicals found in foods or medications and psychological and physical factors (Demaagd, 2008a; Feliu et al., 2007).

Rehabilitation Considerations

Nonpharmacologic interventions for treating migraine include biofeedback and behavioral therapy such as relaxation and stress-management techniques. Physical interventions include acupuncture, application of heat or cold, impulse magnetic field therapy, **photic** stimulation, exercise, and chiropractic manipulations. Keeping a headache diary may help patients identify possible triggers and develop preventative strategies (Demaagd, 2008a; Feliu et al., 2007).

Medication Therapy

Medications recommended for use in abortive therapy of migraines include nonsteroidal anti-inflammatory drugs (NSAIDs) and medications that increase serotonin levels (e.g., ergot alkaloids and triptans). Table 14.1 summarizes medications used to abort migraine attacks. Agents that have been used in the past but are no longer first line include aspirin, acetaminophen, barbiturates, opiates, and the combination product Midrin. NSAIDs have anti-inflammatory effects on the vasoactive peptide-induced inflammation that occurs during migraine. Ergot alkaloids, including ergotamine tartrate and dihydroergotamine mesylate, were the first agents introduced for treatment of migraine. These agents act on the serotonin, dopamine, and norepenephrine receptors. These agents should not be used in patients with heart disease. *Ergotism* is a term that describes ischemic complications of major body systems, including the heart, associated with prolonged use or overuse of ergot products. Retroperitoneal fibrosis can also occur (Demaagd, 2008b; Feliu et al., 2007).

The triptans (5-hydroxytryptamine), which are serotonin receptor agonists, are now the agents of choice for abortive management of migraine, especially in patients nonresponsive to or intolerant of NSAID therapy. The mechanism of action of the triptans is similar to that of the ergot products, but the triptans are more selective for the serotonin 1b,1d receptor and do not interact with the adrenergic and dopaminergic receptors. Action at these serotonin receptors includes **vasoconstriction** of the intracranial blood vessels, inhibition of the release of vasoactive neuropeptides, and blocking of the transmission of pain signals. All of the triptans are effective and differ in bioavailability, onset and duration of action, and method of metabolism in and excreted from the body (Demaagd, 2008a).

Preventative therapy for migraine is used to reduce the frequency and severity of attacks in patients who experience 2 or more migraines/wk. Preventative agents include beta blockers, tricyclic antidepressants, and some anticonvulsants. Table 14.2 summarizes medications used to prevent migraine headache (Demaagd, 2008b; Feliu et al., 2007).

Fibromyalgia

Fibromyalgia is a disorder characterized by chronic muscle pain and joint pain, extreme fatigue, and tenderness in certain areas. Symptoms of fibromyalgia include burning, throbbing, aching, or tenderness upon pressure. Common sites include the shoulders, back, neck, jaw, hip joints, arms, and legs. Many patients experience overwhelming fatigue. Other common symptoms include insomnia, early-morning stiffness, restless-leg syndrome, headache, poor concentration, numbness and tingling in the extremities, irritable bowel syndrome, pelvic pain, painful menstruation, and

See table 14.1 in the web resource for a full list of medication-specific indications, dosing recommendations, side effects, and drug interactions.

Table 14.1 Medications Used in Abortive Therapy for Migraine Headache

Medication	Side effects affecting rehab							Other side effects or considerations
NSAIDs								
Ibuprofen (Motrin, Advil)	Cog +	S 0	A 0	Motor 0	D ++	Com +	F +	Gastrointestinal upset, dyspepsia, xerostomia, oral ulceration, glossitis, gastrointestinal mucosal hemorrhage, abrupt acute renal insufficiency, fluid retention, worsening of congestive heart failure, memory loss, confusion, dizziness, headache.
Naproxen (Aleve)	Cog +	S 0	A 0	Motor 0	D ++	Com +	F +	Reversible inhibition of platelet aggregation with NSAIDs lasts for 1-3 days. Increased risk of bleeding when used with oral anticoagulant warfarin (Coumadin). Do not combine with aspirin. Antagonizes effects of antihypertensives.
Ergot alkaloids								
Dihydroergotamine mesylate (DHE 45 injection, Migranal nasal spray)	Cog +	S +	A 0	Motor ++	D ++	Com +	F +	Nausea, vomiting, muscle cramps, tingling in the extremities, difficulty swallowing, chest discomfort, nasal congestion, depression, fatigue, ischemic complications of major body systems including the heart, retroperitoneal fibrosis. Avoid use in patients with heart disease.
Ergotamine tartrate	Cog +	S +	A 0	Motor ++	D ++	Com +	F +	Increased effects of vasodilation occur when used with beta blockers, grapefruit juice, or nicotine. Do not take with a macrolide antibiotic (e.g., erythromycin or clarithromycin), HIV protease inhibitor (e.g., ritonavir, nelfinavir, indinavir, amprenavir, or saquinavir), or azole antifungal (e.g., ketoconazole [Nizoral] or itraconazole [Sporanox]). Do not take sumatriptan and dihydroergotamine within 24 h of each other.
Sympathomimetic								
Isometheptene 65 mg–dichloralphenazone 100 mg–acetaminophen 325 mg (Midrin)	Cog 0	S 0	A ++	Motor ++	D +	Com 0	F ++	Dizziness, allergic reactions, skin rash. Space administration at least 14 days from last dose of monoamine oxidase inhibitors (e.g., isocarboxazid [Marplan], phenelzine [Nardil], selegiline [Eldepryl, Emsam], or tranylcypromine [Parnate]). Avoid concurrent use of tricyclic antidepressants (e.g., amitriptyline [Elavil], nortriptyline [Pamelor], doxepin [Sinequan], or desipramine [Norpramin]).

› continued

Table 14.1 › continued

Medication	Side effects affecting rehab							Other side effects or considerations

Serotonin receptor agonists (triptans): Sumatriptan, rizatriptan, zolmitriptan, and eletriptan have fast onset; naratriptan and frovatriptan have slow onset and are long duration.

Medication	Cog	S	A	Motor	D	Com	F	Other side effects or considerations
Sumatriptan (Imitrex)	++	++	0	+++	++	+	+++	Dizziness, paresthesias, somnolence, asthenia, fatigue, flushing sensations, myalgias, transient increases in blood pressure, nausea, vomiting, ischemic side effects.
Rizatriptan (Maxalt, Maxalt MLT)	++	++	0	+++	++	+	+++	Avoid concurrent use of selective serotonin reuptake inhibitors, norepinephrine and serotonin reuptake inhibitors, or antidepressants; can result in serotonin syndrome.
Zolmitriptan (Zomig)	++	++	0	+++	++	+	+++	Avoid use in patients with cardiac disease.
Naratriptan (Amerge)	++	++	0	+++	++	+	+++	
Almotriptan (Axert)	++	++	0	+++	++	+	+++	
Frovatriptan (Frova)	++	++	0	+++	++	+	+++	
Eletriptan (Relpax)	++	++	0	+++	++	+	+++	

Cog = cognition; S = sedation; A = agitation or mania; Motor = discoordination; D = dysphagia; Com = communication; F = falls; NSAID = nonsteroidal anti-inflammatory drug; HIV = human immunodeficiency virus.

The likelihood rating scale for encountering the side effects is as follows: 0 = Almost no probability of encountering side effects. + = Little likelihood of encountering side effects. +/++ = Low probability of encountering side effects; however, probability increases with increased dosage. ++ = Medium likelihood of encountering side effects. +++ = High likelihood of encountering side effects, particularly with high doses. ++++ = Highest likelihood of encountering side effects; best to avoid in at-risk patients.

 See table 14.2 in the web resource for a full list of medication-specific indications, dosing recommendations, and side effects.

Table 14.2 Medications Used to Prevent Migraine Headache

Medication	Side effects affecting rehab							Other side effects or considerations

Beta blockers

Medication	Cog	S	A	Motor	D	Com	F	Other side effects or considerations
Propranolol (Inderal)	+++	+++	0	++	+	+	+++	Bradycardia, decreased blood pressure, sexual dysfunction. Do not abruptly discontinue.
Nadolol (Corgard)	++	++	0	+	+	+	++	Avoid combining with sympathomimetics; can cause hypertension and increased heart rate.
Timolol (Blocadren)	++	++	0	+	+	+	++	
Atenolol (Tenormin)	++	++	0	+	+	+	++	
Metoprolol (Toprol)	++	++	0	+	+	+	++	

Tricyclic antidepressants

Medication	Cog	S	A	Motor	D	Com	F				
Amitriptyline (Elavil)	++++	++++	0	++	++++	++++	++++	Weight gain +++	Seizure +++	Cardiac +++	Sexual ++

Not recommended in elderly due to high sedative and anticholinergic effects that increase risk of falls.

Medication	Side effects affecting rehab							Other side effects or considerations
Nortriptyline (Pamelor)	Cog +++	S ++	A 0	Motor ++	D ++	Com ++	F +	Weight gain + / Seizure ++ / Cardiac ++ / Sexual ++ Preferred tricyclic antidepressant in elderly due to low anticholinergic and sedative effects.
Doxepin (Sinequan)	Cog ++++	S ++++	A 0	Motor ++	D +++	Com ++++	F ++	Weight gain ++ / Seizure +++ / Cardiac ++ / Sexual ++
Desipramine (Norpramin)	Cog ++	S ++	A +	Motor ++	D ++	Com ++	F ++	Weight gain + / Seizure ++ / Cardiac ++ / Sexual ++ Prolongs QT interval and increases risk of arrhythmia.
Monoamine oxidase inhibitor antidepressant								
Phenelzine (Nardil)	Cog ++	S ++	A 0/+	Motor 0	D +	Com ++	F +	Weight gain + / Seizure + / Cardiac + / Sexual +++ Tyramine-rich foods and beverages should be avoided starting on day 1 and for 2 wk after discontinuance.
Selective serotonin reuptake inhibitor antidepressants								
Fluoxetine (Prozac)	Cog 0/+	S 0/+	A +	Motor 0	D 0/+	Com 0/+	F 0	Weight gain 0/+ / Seizure ++ / Cardiac 0/+ / Sexual +++ 20% incidence of nausea; take with food. 20% incidence of insomnia; take in morning.
Anticonvulsants								
Topiramate (Topamax)	Cog ++	S ++	A ++	Motor +++	D +	Com +++	F ++	Dizziness, somnolence, dry mouth, edema, blurred vision, weight gain, difficulty with concentration and attention, language impairment, behavioral changes, weight loss, altered taste, metabolic acidosis, kidney stones, hypohidrosis
Valproic acid (Depakene)	Cog ++	S ++	A ++	Motor ++	D ++	Com ++	F ++	Weight gain, hepatotoxicity, dyspepsia, rash, pancreatitis that can be life threatening, alopecia, tremor, thrombocytopenia, platelet dysfunction, hair loss, anticonvulsant hypersensitivity syndrome
Calcium channel blocker								
Verapamil (Calan)	Cog ++	S ++	A 0	Motor +	D +	Com +	F ++	Decreased heart rate, decreased blood pressure, sexual dysfunction
Nonsteroidal anti-inflammatory drugs								
Naproxen (Aleve, Naprosyn)	Cog +	S 0	A 0	Motor 0	D ++	Com +	F +	Gastrointestinal upset, xerostomia, oral ulceration, glossitis and gastrointestinal mucosal hemorrhage, abrupt acute renal insufficiency, fluid retention, worsening of congestive heart failure, memory loss, confusion, dizziness, headache
Ketoprofen (Orudis)	Cog +	S 0	A 0	Motor 0	D ++	Com +	F +	

Cog = cognition; S = sedation; A = agitation or mania; Motor = discoordination; D = dysphagia; Com = communication; F = falls.

The likelihood rating scale for encountering the side effects is as follows: 0 = Almost no probability of encountering side effects. 0/+ = Low probability of encountering side effects but increased with increased dosage. + = Little likelihood of encountering side effects. +/++ = Low probability of encountering side effects; however, probability increases with increased dosage. ++ = Medium likelihood of encountering side effects. +++ = High likelihood of encountering side effects, particularly with high doses. ++++ = Highest likelihood of encountering side effects; best to avoid in at-risk patients.

depression. Diagnostic criteria include muscle and joint pain above and below the waist and on both sides of the body for at least 3 mo along with pain at 11 of 18 tender points (Morin, 2009; Nickerson, 2009).

Incidence

Chronic pain is common. The worldwide prevalence of chronic pain is 7.3% to 12.9%, and the worldwide prevalence of fibromyalgia ranges from 0.5% to 5% (Neumann & Buskila, 2003). In the United States, fibromyalgia affects 2% to 4% of the population and is the second most common disorder (after osteoarthritis) seen by rheumatologists. Fibromyalgia occurs 7 times more frequently in women than in men and primarily affects women between 30 and 50 yr of age. Patients with autoimmune disorders such as lupus or rheumatoid arthritis are more likely to be affected (Morin, 2009; Nickerson, 2009).

Etiology and Pathophysiology

The cause of fibromyalgia is unknown, but symptoms may be traced to a triggering event such as an injury or a stressful event. Researchers believe that fibromyalgia is associated with increased levels of substance P. Levels of serotonin, norepinephrine, dopamine, and growth hormone may also be disturbed in patients with fibromyalgia (Morin, 2009).

Rehabilitation Considerations

Ninety percent of patients with fibromyalgia seek alternative pain-relief therapies such as alternative medicine, massage therapy, chiropractic manipulation, and acupuncture. The patient's therapeutic plan should also include biofeedback and cognitive behavioral therapy. Nonpharmacologic treatments include muscle relaxation, sleep, and exercise therapy that stretches muscles and improves muscle strength (Nickerson, 2009).

Medication Therapy

Medications that have been used to treat fibromyalgia include tricyclic antidepressants, selective serotonin reuptake inhibitors, norepinephrine and serotonin reuptake inhibitors (NSRI), tramadol (Ultram), and the anticonvulsants gabapentin (Neurontin) and pregabalin (Lyrica). Antidepressant agents that increase both norepinephrine and serotonin such as tricyclic antidepressants and NSRI provide more effective relief in patients with chronic pain syndromes than do selective serotonin reuptake inhibitors, which increase serotonin levels only. The U.S. Food and Drug Administration has approved three medications for use in treating fibromyalgia: the anticonvulsant pregabalin (Lyrica), the NSRI duloxetine (Cymbalta), and milnacipran (Savella). Table 14.3 summarizes the medications used to treat fibromyalgia (English et al., 2010; Morin, 2009; Nickerson, 2009).

Trigeminal Neuralgia

Trigeminal neuralgia (also called tic douloureux) produces sudden, severe, recurrent, unilateral face pain. The pain, which patients describe as unilateral, shock-like, stabbing pain, results from the stimulation of cutaneous areas, teeth, or oral mucosa innervated by the trigeminal nerve and is triggered by activities such as shaving, brushing the teeth, chewing, swallowing, and talking.

Incidence

Few cases of trigeminal neuralgia are reported in the United States, United Kingdom, France, Germany, Italy, Spain, and Japan. However, more cases exist than previously thought. Epidemiologists estimate that more than 800,000 cases occur per year in these seven countries (Bombourg, 2012). Incidence of trigeminal neuralgia is highest in patients between 50 and 70 yr of age, and 60% of patients affected are female.

Etiology and Pathophysiology

The majority of cases are caused by compression of the trigeminal nerve by an anomalous loop of artery or vein, which results in nerve demyelination. Pain attacks are triggered by neuronal hypersensitivity, altered peripheral nerve sensitivity, and increased sensitivity to cold and mechanical stimuli.

See table 14.3 in the web resource for a full list of medication-specific indications, dosing recommendations, and side effects.

Table 14.3 Medications Used to Treat Fibromyalgia

Medication	Side effects affecting rehab							Other side effects or considerations
Anticonvulsant: Inhibits voltage-dependent calcium channels.								
Pregabalin (Lyrica)	Cog ++	S ++	A +	Motor +++	D 0	Com ++	F +++	Dizziness, somnolence, dry mouth, edema, blurred vision, weight gain, difficulty with concentration and attention, angioedema, hypersensitivity, peripheral edema
Selective serotonin and norepinephrine reuptake inhibitor antidepressants: Inhibits serotonin and norepinephrine reuptake.								
Duloxetine (Cymbalta)	Cog +	S 0	A +	Motor 0	D ++	Com 0	F +	Nausea, dry mouth, constipation, somnolence, hyperhidrosis, decreased appetite, increased suicide risk (children, adolescents, and young adults), hepatotoxicity, orthostasis, serotonin syndrome, neuroleptic malignant syndrome, hypomania, seizures, urinary retention, hyponatremia, altered glucose levels. May interact with CYP1A2 and CYP2D6 inhibitors.
Milnacipran (Savella)	Cog +	S +	A +	Motor 0	D ++	Com +	F +	Nausea, dry mouth, dizziness, hot flushing, constipation, insomnia, hyperhidrosis, vomiting, palpitations, increased heart rate, increased blood pressure, increased suicide risk (children, adolescents, and young adults), hepatotoxicity, orthostasis, serotonin syndrome, neuroleptic malignant syndrome, hypomania, seizures, urinary retention, hyponatremia. Avoid concurrent use of alcohol.

Cog = cognition; S = sedation; A = agitation or mania; Motor = discoordination; D = dysphagia; Com = communication; F = falls.

The likelihood rating scale for encountering the side effects is as follows: 0 = Almost no probability of encountering side effects. 0/+ = Low probability of encountering side effects but increased with increased dosage. + = Little likelihood of encountering side effects. +/++ = Low probability of encountering side effects; however, probability increases with increased dosage. ++ = Medium likelihood of encountering side effects. +++ = High likelihood of encountering side effects, particularly with high doses. ++++ = Highest likelihood of encountering side effects; best to avoid in at-risk patients.

Rehabilitation Considerations

If pharmacotherapy fails, the physician may consider treatment with surgical decompression of the nerve or nerve ablation (Matthews & Horton, 2007).

Medication Therapy

Anticonvulsants are used to treat this pain related to trigeminal neuralgia. First-line therapies include carbamazepine (Tegretol) and oxcarbazepine (Trileptal), and second-line therapies include gabapentin (Neurontin), lamotrigine (Lamictal), and phenytoin (Dilantin).

Cancer Pain

Pain in the cancer patient can be a mixture of acute pain related to the disease itself and pain related to therapeutic interventions such as surgery, diagnostic procedures, intravenous line insertion, radiation, and chemotherapy. Mucositis associated with chemotherapy or radiation is a frequent cause of somatic pain and can be associated with dysphagia and a decline in nutritional intake. Chapter 18 discusses therapies used to manage mucositis. Patients with cancer may experience chronic pain as their disease progresses, and tumor encroachment or chemotherapy may cause neuropathic pain. Chemotherapy can also damage the nervous system and lead to resultant neuropathic pain. Chapter 18 lists chemotherapy agents that are commonly associated with neuropathic pain (Eidelman et al., 2007; Swarm et al., 2007; Toth, 2009).

Incidence

Approximately 30% of newly diagnosed cancer patients report pain, whereas almost 80% of patients with advanced cancer report pain. A number of international studies note that the management of cancer pain is not optimal (Levy, 1996). Between 65% and 85% of patients with cancer experience pain that is classified as moderate to severe. Moderate to severe pain occurs in 80% to 90% of patients with bone cancer and oral cancer, 65% to 80% of patients with genitourinary cancer, 50% to 55% of patients with breast cancer, and 40% to 50% of patients with lung cancer. Moderate to severe pain occurs less frequently in patients with hematologic cancers such as lymphoma and leukemia (Eidelman et al., 2007; Swarm et al., 2007; Toth, 2009).

Etiology and Pathophysiology

For full information, please refer to chapter 18.

Rehabilitation Considerations

Nonpharmacologic therapies for managing cancer pain include both physical and cognitive modalities. Physical interventions include instruction in positioning, the use of assistive devices for gait and functional activities, massage, acupuncture, therapeutic exercise, and relaxation exercises. Cognitive modalities include imagery, hypnosis, distraction training, relaxation techniques, coping techniques, graded task assignments, setting goals, pacing

and prioritizing, cognitive–behavioral training, consulting with pain or palliative specialists, and spiritual care (Swarm et al., 2007).

Interventional therapies for managing cancer pain can be considered adjuvant therapies to systemic analgesia. Afferent visceral pain nerve fibers pass through the paravertebral sympathetic ganglia. Blocking visceral sympathetic ganglia can help control visceral cancer pain. Pancreatic cancer and upper-abdominal malignancies are associated with severe pain and nausea. Neurolytic celiac plexus block using alcohol or phenol can provide long-term pain relief in these patients. Superior hypogastric nerve block can provide analgesia in patients with malignancies of the cervix, uterus, ovaries, vagina, testes, prostate, bladder, descending colon, and rectum. Pain related to head and neck cancer can be treated with nerve blocks of the trigeminal, mandibular, maxillary, or glossopharyngeal nerves. Adverse effects associated with this procedure include orthostasis and diarrhea that resolve spontaneously in 1 to 2 days, hematoma, or infection at the injection site. Paraplegia occurs in 1/700 procedures. Finally, osteoporosis, multiple myeloma, or metastatic tumor can cause spinal compression fractures. Percutaneous vertebroplasty, which introduces polymethacrylate bone cement into the compressed vertebral body using large bore needles, is used to stabilize the compressed vertebra. This procedure provides excellent pain relief in 80% to 90% of patients with painful compression fractures associated with osteoporosis and 50% to 85% of patients with compression fractures associated with metastasis or tumor (Eidelman et al., 2007; Swarm et al., 2007; Toth, 2009).

Medication Therapy

Neuropathic pain can be treated with a tricyclic antidepressant such as nortriptyline or desipramine or an NSRI antidepressant such as duloxetine (Cymbalta) or venlafaxine (Effexor) (Swarm et al., 2007). Pain associated with inflammation can be treated with NSAIDs or glucocorticoids. Bone pain can be managed with initiation of NSAIDs that is then titrated to effective relief. Local bone pain can be treated with local radiation therapy or nerve block. Diffuse bone pain can be relieved with bisphosphonate therapy such as pamidronate (Aredia) or with radioisotope therapy. Short-term treatment with a corticosteroid such as intravenous methylprednisolone (Solu-Medrol) or oral prednisone can be effective in patients experiencing nerve compression or inflammation (Swarm et al., 2007). Spinal administration of analgesics may help manage cancer pain. Table 14.4 summarizes medications used to manage pain in cancer patients.

 See table 14.4 in the web resource for a full list of medication-specific indications, dosing recommendations, and side effects.

Table 14.4 Pain Medications and Adjuvant Analgesic Medications Used in Cancer Patients

Medication	Side effects affecting rehab							Other side effects or considerations
Opiates: Used to treat visceral and somatic pain, adjunct to other agents for severe neuropathic pain.								
Oxycodone (Oxycontin)	Cog ++	S ++	A +	Motor +++	D ++	Com ++	F +++	Constipation, nausea, vomiting, sedation, respiratory depression, impaired cognition and communication, increased motor discoordination, increased risk of fall risks. Intraspinal dosing reduces side effects.
Morphine (MS Contin)	Cog ++	S ++	A +	Motor +++	D ++	Com ++	F +++	Constipation, nausea, vomiting, sedation, respiratory depression, impaired cognition and communication, increased motor discoordination, increased risk of falls. Intraspinal dosing reduces side effects.
Hydromorphone (Dilaudid)	Cog ++	S ++	A +	Motor +++	D ++	Com ++	F +++	
Fentanyl (Duragesic)	Cog ++	S ++	A +	Motor +++	D ++	Com ++	F +++	Morphine is hydrophilic and spreads easily to CSF when given by intraspinal route; hydromorphone is hydrophilic and has intermediate spread to CSF when given by intraspinal route; and fentanyl is lipophilic and has low spread to CSF when given by intraspinal route. Itching occurs due to histamine release with intraspinal dosing; treat with diphenhydramine (Benadryl).
Corticosteroids: Used to reduce inflammation and pain.								
Dexamethasone (Decadron)	Cog ++	S 0	A ++	Motor ++	D ++	Com +	F ++	Gastrointestinal upset and ulceration, hyperglycemia, confusion, increased risk of infection
Prednisone	Cog ++	S 0	A ++	Motor ++	D ++	Com +	F ++	Gastrointestinal upset and ulceration, hyperglycemia, confusion, increased risk of infection
Anticonvulsants: Used to treat neuropathic pain.								
Carbamazepine (Tegretol)	Cog ++	S ++	A +	Motor ++	D ++	Com ++	F +++	Liver +++ Hematologic +++ Renal +++ Rash +++ Sedation, hypersensitivity reactions, gastrointestinal upset, appetite changes, slowed cognitive function, lethargy, nausea, headaches, irritability, skin rashes, decreased reaction time, nystagmus, ataxia, dysphagia, dysarthria, aplastic anemia; genetic testing required in Asians (increased risk of AHS)

> *continued*

Table 14.4 › *continued*

Medication	Side effects affecting rehab							Other side effects or considerations
Phenytoin (Dilantin)	Cog ++	S ++	A 0	Motor ++	D +++	Com +++	F ++	Liver ++ Hematologic +++ Renal ++ Rash +++
								Sedation, hypersensitivity reactions, gastrointestinal upset, appetite changes, slowed cognitive function, lethargy, nausea, headaches, irritability, skin rashes, decreased reaction time, nystagmus, ataxia, dysphagia, dysarthria, AHS
Clonazepam (Klonopin)	Cog +	S +	A ++	Motor ++	D ++	Com ++	F +	Sedation, gastrointestinal upset, appetite changes, ataxia, headache, fatigue, dependence
Gabapentin (Neurontin)	Cog ++	S ++	A +	Motor +++	D 0	Com ++	F +++	Liver 0 Hematologic 0 Renal +++ Rash +
								Sedation, gastrointestinal upset, appetite changes, ataxia, gait changes, tremor, dizziness, fatigue, ataxia, drowsiness, behavioral changes, peripheral edema, weight gain
Keppra (Levetiracetam)	Cog +++	S +++	A 0	Motor +++	D +	Com ++	F +++	Liver 0 Hematologic + Renal +++ Rash +
								Somnolence, tiredness, dizziness, upper-respiratory infections. Pyridoxine decreases psychiatric side effects.
Lamotrigine (Lamictal)	Cog ++	S 0	A ++	Motor +	D 0	Com ++	F ++	Liver + Hematologic 0 Renal + Rash +
								Anticonvulsant hypersensitivity syndrome, rash that can progress to Stevens-Johnson syndrome, insomnia; avoid in pregnancy
Pregabalin (Lyrica)	Cog ++	S ++	A +	Motor +++	D 0	Com ++	F +++	Liver 0 Hematologic 0 Renal +++ Rash +
								Dizziness, somnolence, dry mouth, edema, blurred vision, weight gain, difficulty with concentration and attention
Topiramate (Topamax)	Cog ++	S ++	A ++	Motor +++	D +	Com +++	F ++	Liver 0 Hematologic 0 Renal +++ Rash ++
								Dizziness, somnolence, dry mouth, edema, blurred vision, weight gain, difficulty with concentration and attention, language impairment, behavioral changes, weight loss, altered taste, metabolic acidosis, kidney stones, hypohidrosis
Valproic acid (Depakene)	Cog ++	S ++	A ++	Motor ++	D ++	Com ++	F ++	Liver ++ Hematologic +++ Renal 0 Rash +++
								Tremor, dyspepsia, weight gain, anticonvulsant hypersensitivity syndrome, hepatotoxicity, pancreatitis, alopecia, thrombocytopenia, sedation, appetite changes, gastrointestinal upset, rash

Medication	Side effects affecting rehab							Other side effects or considerations
Tricyclic antidepressants: Used to treat neuropathic pain.								
Amitriptyline (Elavil)	Cog ++++	S ++++	A 0	Motor ++	D ++++	Com ++++	F ++++	Weight gain +++ Seizure ++++ Cardiac +++ Sexual + Not recommended in elderly. Impaired cognition, sedation, risk of seizure, cardiac arrhythmia, sexual dysfunction, orthostasis, gastrointestinal upset.
Desipramine (Norpramin)	Cog ++	S ++	A +	Motor ++	D ++	Com ++	F ++	Weight gain + Seizure ++ Cardiac ++ Sexual ++ Prolongs QT interval. Impaired cognition, sedation, risk of seizure, cardiac arrhythmia, sexual dysfunction, orthostasis, gastrointestinal upset.
Doxepin (Sinequan)	Cog ++++	S ++++	A 0	Motor ++	D +++	Com ++++	F ++	Weight gain ++ Seizure +++ Cardiac +++ Sexual ++ Impaired cognition, sedation, risk of seizure, cardiac arrhythmia, sexual dysfunction, orthostasis, gastrointestinal upset
Imipramine (Tofranil)	Cog +++	S +++	A +	Motor ++	D +++	Com +++	F ++++	Weight gain ++ Seizure +++ Cardiac +++ Sexual ++ Impaired cognition, sedation, risk of seizure, cardiac arrhythmia, sexual dysfunction, orthostasis, gastrointestinal upset
Nortriptyline (Pamelor)	Cog ++	S ++	A 0	Motor ++	D ++	Com ++	F +	Weight gain + Seizure ++ Cardiac ++ Sexual ++ Impaired cognition, sedation, risk of seizure, cardiac arrhythmia, sexual dysfunction, orthostasis, gastrointestinal upset
Trazodone (Desyrel)	Cog ++++	S ++++	A 0	Motor ++	D ++	Com +++	F +++	Weight gain + Seizure ++ Cardiac + Sexual + Impaired cognition, sedation, risk of seizure, cardiac arrhythmia, sexual dysfunction, orthostasis, gastrointestinal upset
Norepinephrine and serotonin reuptake inhibitor antidepressants: Used to treat neuropathic pain.								
Duloxetine (Cymbalta)	Cog +	S 0	A +	Motor 0	D ++	Com 0	F +	Nausea, dry mouth, constipation, somnolence, hyperhidrosis, decreased appetite, increased suicide risk (children, adolescents, and young adults), hepatotoxicity, orthostasis, serotonin syndrome, neuroleptic malignant syndrome, hypomania, seizures, urinary retention, hyponatremia, altered glucose levels. May interact with CYP1A2 and CYP2D6 inhibitors.
Venlafaxine (Effexor)	Cog +	S +	A 0/+	Motor 0	D +	Com +	F +	Somnolence, nausea, dry mouth, decreased appetite, constipation; jitteriness and insomnia at higher doses

› continued

Table 14.4 › *continued*

Medication	Side effects affecting rehab							Other side effects or considerations
Muscle relaxant: Used to treat spasticity.								
Baclofen (Lioresal)	Cog ++	S +++	A ++	Motor +++	D ++	Com ++	F +++	Oral: Initial sedation, muscle weakness, ataxia, orthostatic hypotension, fatigue, headache, nausea, dizziness; confusion and hallucinations reported in the elderly or those with history of stroke. Abrupt discontinuation may result in rebound increase in spasticity, rhabdomyolysis, disorientation, hallucination, and seizures. Intrathecal: Chronic constipation, hypotonia, somnolence, headache, vomiting, paresthesias.
Antihistamines: Used to relieve anxiety, nausea, and insomnia.								
Hydroxyzine (Vistaril)	Cog ++	S ++	A ++	Motor ++	D ++	Com ++	F ++	Dry mouth, sedation, orthostasis, confusion, impaired cognition
Promethazine (Phenergan)	Cog ++	S ++	A ++	Motor ++	D ++	Com ++	F ++	Dry mouth, sedation, orthostasis, confusion, impaired cognition
Anesthetics: Used to treat neuropathic pain.								
Lidocaine	Cog +++	S +++	A +	Motor +++	D ++	Com ++	F +++	Sedation, gastrointestinal upset, confusion, tremor, ataxia, seizures
Tocainide (Tonocard)	Cog +++	S +++	A +	Motor +++	D ++	Com ++	F +++	
Psychostimulants: Used to decrease sedation.								
Dextroamphetamine	Cog ++	S 0	A ++	Motor ++	D ++	Com +	F ++	Tremor, xerostomia, altered taste, decreased appetite
Methylphenidate (Ritalin)	Cog ++	S 0	A ++	Motor ++	D ++	Com +	F ++	

Cog = cognition; S = sedation; A = agitation or mania; Motor = discoordination; D = dysphagia; Com = communication; F = falls; CSF = cerebral spinal fluid; AHS = anticonvulsant hypersensitivity syndrome.

The likelihood rating scale for encountering the side effects is as follows: 0 = Almost no probability of encountering side effects. + = Little likelihood of encountering side effects. +/++ = Low probability of encountering side effects; however, probability increases with increased dosage. ++ = Medium likelihood of encountering side effects. +++ = High likelihood of encountering side effects, particularly with high doses. ++++ = Highest likelihood of encountering side effects; best to avoid in at-risk patients.

PATIENT CASE 1

W.O. is a 56 yr-old male with a history of mouth cancer who recently underwent an extensive surgical resection of his tumor and just received his second cycle of chemotherapy. He is also receiving radiation treatments. He is admitted for cancer rehabilitation services after a recent hospitalization for neutropenic fever. The patient has thrush and difficulty in swallowing. He received 2 mg of morphine via IV every 4 h as needed for pain along with 1-2 tablets of Percocet orally every 4 h as needed for pain while in the hospital. The rehabilitation therapist completing his admission history notes his hospital pain scores were consistently 10 out of 10 on the pain scale, reflecting inadequate pain relief.

Question
What type of pain does this patient have?

Answer
The patient has chronic pain which may be due to his cancer and radiation treatments,

acute pain associated with his surgery, and acute thrush infection in his mouth.

Question

What is the role of taking a medication history in managing this patient's pain?

Answer

It is important when treating a patient with chronic pain to know what medications he received prior to his hospital admission to manage his pain. It is also important to identify any neuropathic pain issues that require a different type of medication than somatic or acute pain from the surgery and infection.

PATIENT CASE 1, continued

Upon questioning the patient, the therapist learns that the patient was taking Oxy-Contin 80 mg by mouth 3 times/day at home along with OxyIR 20 mg every 3 h as needed for breakthrough pain. He also was receiving 800 mg of Gabapentin 3 times/day for nerve pain associated with his cancer. His pain levels were 2-3 on a pain scale of 1 to 10 at home on this regimen.

Question

How should this information impact his plan for pain management during his rehabilitation?

Answer

His hospital pain regimen provided only a small fraction of the opioid dose the patient was receiving prior to his admission, and did not address his neuropathic pain. This explains his continued high level of pain during his recent hospitalization.

Question

How should the therapist intervene to help this patient with his pain?

Answer

The information regarding W.O.'s home pain medications should be immediately communicated to the physician so that his pain regimen can be appropriately adjusted.

Amputation Pain

The majority of lower-extremity amputations result from poorly controlled diabetes and vascular disease. These conditions account for over 74% of amputations. They can also can lead to the need for amputation of the contralateral limb within 5 yr in 50% of amputees (Adams et al. 1999). Traumatic injury accounts for 23% of all amputations. Most upper-extremity amputations are the result of traumatic injury. A small number (3%) of all amputations are the result of congenital limb anomalies or malignancy that requires amputation (Adams et al., 1999). Potential postamputation complications include wound separation, infection, and bleeding at the surgical incision on the residual limb. Additional complications include joint contracture, bone spurs, formation of scar tissue, skin graft problems, phantom limb sensations, and phantom limb pain. The term *phantom pain* describes the patient's perception of pain from the area of the body that was amputated. The pain commonly is perceived as originating from the most distal segment of the amputated extremity. The reported pain sensations vary but may include burning, shooting, stabbing, boring, squeezing, and throbbing pain. In some instances the patient may describe the pain as similar to intermittent electric shocks. The pain sensations can interfere with activities of daily living, functional activities, sleep, and the patient's overall quality of life (Ziegler-Graham et al., 2008).

Incidence

The incidence of amputation in the United States is estimated to be more than 1/200 individuals (Adams et al., 1999). It is further estimated that more than 1.6 million people are living with limb loss (Ziegler-Graham et al., 2008). Approximately 135,000 amputations are performed each year in the United States alone (Adams et al., 1999). The number of people living with an amputation is expected to more than double from 1.6 million to 3.6 million by 2050, largely due to the rapidly increasing incidence of diabetes and peripheral vascular disease.

Pain typically begins within the first few days after amputation and is usually intermittent rather than constant. A patient-controlled analgesia pump that delivers narcotic pain medication can be used to control initial pain immediately after surgical amputation. Phantom pain occurs in 60% to 80% of patients post-amputation. The phantom pain begins to subside within the first year after amputation in many patients but persists in others. Weather changes, pressure on the remaining part of the limb, or emotional stress can aggravate phantom pain symptoms (Parkes, 1973). Research has found that persistent phantom limb pain is more likely to occur in patients with rigid or compulsively self-reliant personalities, with illness or severe pain lasting more than 1 yr before amputation, and with severe residual limb pain during first month after operation (Parkes, 1973). Patients who do not have residual limb complications (e.g., infection, poor healing, contracture) that persist for more than 13 mo and those who are employed at 13 mo post-amputation are less likely to develop severe phantom limb pain (Flor et al., 2006; Parkes, 1973; Robinson et al., 2004).

Etiology and Pathophysiology

Post-amputation, most patients remain aware of the surgically removed portion of the limb through a phenomenon known as phantom sensation. Although the limb or a portion of it was amputated, the sensory system continues to report sensation and pain from that area (Flor et al., 2006; Parkes, 1973; Robinson et al., 2004). This sensation can lead to anxiety and depression because it constantly reminds the patient of the loss of the limb. Phantom pain can be a troubling and challenging impairment to manage following an amputation.

Imaging scans note brain activity in the area that correlates to the phantom pain and the missing limb (Flor et al., 2006). After amputation, areas of spinal cord and brain lose sensory input from the missing limb and adjust to this detachment in unpredictable ways. This is believed to result in an inability of the central nervous system (CNS) to accurately localize pain (Jensen et al., 1985).

Researchers believe that a number of other factors contribute to phantom pain, including damaged nerve endings, scar tissue at the site of the amputation, and the physical memory of pre-amputation pain in the affected area. The level of pain that the patient experiences before and immediately after amputation appears to influence the severity of phantom limb pain. The CNS often keeps sending the reverberating pain message even after the limb and sensory nerves have been severed. If this happens for a long period of time, the neuropathic pain becomes more chronic and more challenging to treat. Neuromas, or abnormal growths on a damaged nerve ending on the residual limb, can also contribute to phantom limb pain. Finally, a poorly fitted prosthesis can lead to increased pain, wounds, and infection. A properly fitted prosthesis is essential (Cameron & Monroe, 2007; Chan et al., 2007; Flor et al., 2006; Jensen et al., 1985; Parkes, 1973; Ramachandran & Altschuler, 2009; Robinson et al., 2004).

Rehabilitation Considerations

It is important to differentiate between pain originating from the surgical incision on the residual limb and true phantom pain that the patient perceives as being in the area of the body that was amputated (i.e., distal to the residual limb). Most patients have a certain degree of both types of pain, and interventions vary for each. For example, local treatment of the residual limb area using physical therapy modalities to decrease pain, control edema, and promote healing of the surgical incision can reduce residual limb pain. After amputation, the rehabilitation therapist should encourage patients to maintain good care of the residual limb, use positioning and exercise techniques to prevent contracture, participate in activities that take the mind off the amputation and associated phantom pain, increase overall activity level without violating the healing constraints of the residual limb, use relaxation techniques, and comply with the recommendations of their medical providers for controlling residual limb pain and phantom pain. Good pre-amputation and post-amputation pain management is essential in minimizing the likelihood of chronic phantom limb pain (Cameron & Monroe, 2007; Chan et al., 2007; Ramachandran & Altschuler, 2009; Ziegler-Graham et al., 2008).

The healing surgical incision can be a source of pain post-amputation. Adequate healing of the surgical incision wound is essential to recovery from amputation. Goals of initial treatment include controlling edema in the residual limb, preventing infection, and developing a residual limb that will serve as a good base for the prosthesis. Compressive limb dressings known as shrinker socks are used to help shape the residual limb and prepare it for prosthesis fitting. Elastic compressive limb dressings also serve to reduce pain. In some instances the patient develops a neuroma near the surface of the residual limb. This can be especially painful and create the sensation of local pain or phantom pain. If necessary, the neuroma can be removed surgically. Pain in the area of the residual limb can be reduced through the use of massage techniques, which provide sensory input into the area that may desensitize the area or serve as a counterirritant and override the pain impulses. Exercise of the contralateral limb (overflow effect), relaxation techniques, and transcutaneous electrical nerve stimulation have all been used to decrease pain at the residual limb (Cameron & Monroe, 2007; Flor et al., 2006; Parkes, 1973; Robinson et al., 2004).

Transcutaneous Electrical Nerve Stimulation

Transcutaneous electrical nerve stimulation is a commonly used nonpharmacologic method of managing pain in patients who have undergone amputation. Electrical impulses from a portable, battery-powered electrical-stimulation device are delivered to the patient through electrodes in order to desensitize the area and override pain impulses. Although the technique is not curative, it is a good nonpharmacologic method of relieving pain and has no adverse side effects (Black et al., 2009). Transcutaneous electrical nerve stimulation is considered a first-line therapy because it is noninvasive, inexpensive, and generally helpful in decreasing pain in this patient population. The patient can be trained to use the device so that it can be used at home on an as-needed basis (Chabal et al., 1998; Sluka, 2001).

Mirror Box

A mirror box contains mirrors that create the illusion that an amputated limb exists. The mirror box has two openings, one for the intact limb and one for the residual limb. The technique allows the patient to perceive the missing limb by focusing on the reflection of the contralateral limb during specific exercises that they perform with the unaffected side. The patient visualizes movement of the amputated part (perception) through the reflection from the mirror. The patient is instructed in performing symmetrical exercises while watching the intact limb move and imagining that they are actually observing the missing limb moving. Researchers believe that this perception allows the patient's sensory cortex to reconfigure. This technique has been used to relieve phantom pain in a significant number of people and has been integrated into many post-amputation rehabilitation programs (Chan et al., 2007; Ramachandran & Altschuler, 2009).

Medication Therapy

The anticonvulsants gabapentin (Neurontin) and carbamazepine (Tegretol) have been used to treat the neuropathic pain associated with phantom limb pain. These agents stabilize the misfiring of damaged nerves and slow the transmission of neuropathic pain. One study of a 6 wk trial of gabapentin (Neurontin) for treating phantom limb pain showed a 3-point reduction in pain on a visual analog scale (10-point scale) (Bone et al., 2002). Tricyclic antidepressants have also been used to relieve neuropathic pain in the treatment of phantom limb pain. Medications such as amitriptyline and nortriptyline (Pamelor) have been used because they block the reuptake of serotonin and norepenephrine, resulting in inhibition of relayed pain signals. These medications can also improve mood and help the patient achieve more restful sleep (Robinson et al., 2004). Opioids can be used immediately post-surgery to control pain, but long-term use is typically discouraged because they have limited effectiveness on neuropathic pain and because patients may develop dependence (Gutstein & Akil, 2001). Injection of local anesthetics or steroids into the residual limb has been used to treat neuromas that may contribute to phantom pain. Successful local treatment with these medications can prevent or delay the need for surgery to remove the neuroma (Cameron & Monroe, 2007).

Central Pain Syndromes

Central pain is chronic pain associated with lesions of the nervous system that is often intractable and that results in damage to the peripheral nervous pathways. Common causes of central pain are stroke, trauma, multiple sclerosis, or spinal cord compression. Pain associated with spinal cord injury may be delayed in onset and may be associated with damage to the center of the spinal cord (syringomyelia). Three types of central pain exist: spontaneous and steady pain associated with deafferentation of sensory nerves in the CNS, spontaneous neuralgic pain that is usually burning, and pain that is evoked from external stimuli and presents as allodynia or hyperalgesia. Some pain is associated with brush-evoked allodynia (brush pain) and wind-up pain (pain caused by repeated prickling of the skin) (Finnerup et al., 2005; Matthews & Horton, 2007; Moultry & Poon, 2009).

Incidence

The average reported prevalence of chronic pain after spinal cord injury is about 65%; one third of these patients experience severe pain. However, incidence reported by individual studies varies widely. Incidence of pain in patients undergoing inpatient rehabilitation can be as high as 90% (Siddall et al., 2003).

Etiology and Pathophysiology

Strokes cause the majority of central pain originating in the brain. Onset of pain may occur 1 to 2 mo after stroke or may be delayed up until 6 yr after the CVA (cerebral vascular accident). Researchers believe that central pain is caused by a chemical imbalance between glutamate and gamma amino butyric acid (GABA). Central pain is characterized by steady and evoked pain along with symptoms of muscle pain, dysesthesias, hyperpathia, allodynia, intermittent shooting or lancinating pain, circulatory pain, and peristaltic or visceral pain (Finnerup et al., 2005; Matthews & Horton, 2007).

Multiple sclerosis pain is also common; 30% to 80% of patients with multiple sclerosis experience chronic pain. Patients may experience centrally mediated neuropathic pain associated with direct neurologic damage due to demyelination (onset of this pain occurs in early-stage disease and progresses) or musculoskeletal pain associated with decreased mobility. Central nerve pain can be precipitated by light touch, temperature changes, physical activity, and emotional stress. This pain is described as exhausting, shooting, burning, cramping, heavy, and aching. Interferon therapy used in MS is also associated with muscle pain and headache (Finnerup et al., 2005; Matthews & Horton, 2007).

Rehabilitation Considerations

Centrally mediated neuropathic pain is challenging to treat and treatment is best achieved through a multidisciplinary approach that includes rehabilitation specialists, physicians, pharmacists, pain psychologists, and vocational counselors, The rehabilitation therapist focuses on functional restoration and pain management. It is important that the rehabilitation team teach the patient self-management techniques for controlling pain. The use of transcutaneous electrical stimulation (TENS) is one such technique that allows the patient to manage their chronic pain with a portable device that can be used as needed. Instructing the patient in stress management, deep breathing exercises, and regular exercise and physical activity are important interventions to assist with pain management and to maintain and improve function. An interdisciplinary approach has been shown to be more effective in managing chronic pain, preventing unnecessary emotional and physical impairment, and controlling medical costs (Harden & Cole, 1998).

PATIENT CASE 2

T.W. is a 38-yr-old female who is married and has two children. She was diagnosed with relapsing–remitting multiple sclerosis 6 yr ago. She has been taking interferon beta-1b (Betaseron) 0.25 mg subcutaneously every other day for the past 6 yr. She is receiving physical therapy for altered sensation in her upper and lower extremities, muscle weakness, fatigue, and unsteadiness on her feet. She now complains of severe muscle pain that is interfering with her movement, shooting pains, and headache. She is also having increasing difficulty with spasticity.

Question

What are some possible sources of T.W.'s pain? What are some treatment options for managing her pain and spasticity?

Answer

Interferon can cause muscle pain, but because she has been on this therapy for years it is unlikely that her medication is causing her pain. Her symptoms are likely associated with central pain disorder, a neuropathic pain disorder that can be treated with anticonvulsants or tricyclic antidepressants. NSAIDs or opioid therapy may relieve her muscle pain. An oral agent or intrathecal baclofen therapy can be used to treat her symptoms of spasticity.

Medication Therapy

Agents that effectively and immediately treat acute central pain include intravenous lidocaine (provides relief for up to 45 min), ketamine (provides relief for up to 30 min), and propofol (provides relief for up to 3 h). Effective long-term treatment of central pain includes anticonvulsants and antidepressants, which relieve dysesthetic extremity pain. Lidocaine patches, applied for 12 h/day, are also considered first-line therapy. NSAIDs and muscle relaxants such as methocarbamol (Robaxin) can relieve musculoskeletal pain. Short-acting opiates should also be initiated. Other agents that may help control pain include capsaicin (Zostrix), methylprednisolone for optic neuritis, clonidine (Catapres), and mexiletine (Mexitil). Spasticity, which occurs in 75% of patients with multiple sclerosis, is treated with baclofen (Lioresal) and tizanidine (Zanaflex). Baclofen may be continuously administered via an intrathecal pump. Botulinum injections are used to treat focal spasticity. Use of diazepam (Valium) and dantrolene (Dantrium) can be considered in patients who are unresponsive to other therapy. Table 14.5 summarizes medications used to manage central pain syndromes (Cheng et al., 2006a; Finnerup et al., 2005; Matthews & Horton, 2007).

Implanted intrathecal (subarachnoid) drug delivery systems (IDDS) are used for long-term management of persistent, severe pain despite conventional therapy. Medications commonly administered through IDDS include opioids, local anesthetics, clonidine, baclofen (Lioresal), and ziconotide (Prialt). Guidelines have been developed for the safe administration of pain medications using IDDS. The two IDDS available in the United States allow continuous delivery of medication at fixed rates and bolus dosing. If the patient requires a different dose, the concentration of the solution is changed and the device is refilled. Intrathecal pumps are typically implanted in the lower abdomen just beneath the surface of the skin (Cheng et al., 2006b; Ghafoor et al., 2007; Matthews & Horton, 2007).

Cerebral spinal fluid (CSF) plays an important role in distributing and eliminating medications administered intrathecally. CSF is replaced 3 to 4 times each day at a rate of 0.3 to 0.4 ml/min. Epidural and intrathecal medications must diffuse from the CSF and penetrate the spinal cord to produce analgesia. The spinal cord comprises grey and white matter; lipids compose 80% of the white matter. Lipophilic opioids such as fentanyl and sufentanil preferentially move through the white matter and are rapidly cleared into the plasma. Gray matter is host to the synaptic activity in the spinal cord though neuronal axons and dendrites. Hydrophilic opioids such as morphine and hydromorphone move into the grey matter. Side effects of opioids administered intrathecally include urinary retention, nausea, vomiting, and pruritus. Long-term

See table 14.5 in the web resource for a full list of medication-specific indications, dosing recommendations, side effects, and drug interactions.

Table 14.5 Medications Used to Manage Central Pain Syndromes

Medication	Side effects affecting rehab	Other side effects or considerations
Tricyclic antidepressant: Used to treat pain related to the spinal cord. Inhibits reuptake of serotonin and norepinephrine.		
Amitriptyline (Elavil)	Cog ++++, S ++++, A 0, Motor ++, D ++++, Com ++++, F ++++	Weight gain +++, Seizure +++, Cardiac +++, Sexual ++ Not recommended in elderly due to high sedative and anticholinergic effects that increase risk of falls.
Anticonvulsant: Used to treat pain related to the spinal cord or multiple sclerosis. Inhibits sodium channels.		
Lamotrigine (Lamictal)	Cog ++, S 0, A ++, Motor +, D 0, Com ++, F ++	Liver +, Hematologic 0, Renal +, Rash + Insomnia, rash that can progress to Stevens-Johnson syndrome. Titrate slowly to avoid rash or more severe skin reactions (i.e., TEN and Stevens-Johnson). Anticonvulsant hypersensitivity syndrome (AHS). Avoid in pregnancy. Teratogenic; causes cleft palate.
Muscle relaxants: Used to treat pain related to multiple sclerosis.		
Baclofen (Lioresal)	Cog ++, S +++, A ++, Motor +++, D ++, Com ++, F +++	Oral: Initial sedation, muscle weakness, ataxia, orthostatic hypotension, fatigue, headache, nausea, dizziness; confusion and hallucinations reported in the elderly or those with history of stroke. Intrathecal: Chronic constipation, hypotonia, somnolence, headache, vomiting, paresthesias. Eliminated by the kidneys; reduce dose with renal dysfunction. Abrupt discontinuance results in rebound increase in spasticity, rhabdomyolysis, disorientation, hallucination, and seizures.
Dantrolene (Dantrium)	Cog ++, S +++, A ++, Motor +++, D +++, Com ++, F +++	Drowsiness, dizziness, nausea, diarrhea, dysphagia. Dose-limiting hepatotoxicity. Hyperkalemia with verapamil, increased hepatotoxicity with estrogens, increased central nervous system depression with other central nervous system depressants. Avoid combining with monoamine oxidase inhibitors.
Muscle relaxant: Used to treat pain related to multiple sclerosis. Alpha-2 adrenergic receptor agonist; increases presynaptic transmission of excitatory neurotransmitters.		
Tizanidine (Zanaflex)	Cog ++, S +++, A 0, Motor +, D ++, Com ++, F +++	Sedation, hypotension, dizziness, gastrointestinal upset. Starting with a very low dose and titrating slowly may reduce or eliminate side effects such as sedation, xerostomia, and dizziness. Monitor liver-function tests at baseline and throughout therapy.

Medication	Side effects affecting rehab							Other side effects or considerations

Muscle relaxant: Used to treat pain related to multiple sclerosis. Decreases impulses from the spinal cord to skeletal muscle.

Medication	Cog	S	A	Motor	D	Com	F	Other side effects or considerations
Methocarbamol (Robaxin)	++++	++++	++	+++	++	++	+++	Somnolence, dizziness, vertigo, syncope, muscular incoordination, stomach upset, flushing, blurred vision, fever, skin rash, pruritus, bradycardia, jaundice, mood changes, slowed heart rate, fainting, clumsiness, difficulty urinating, discoloration of urine (e.g., black, blue, or green). Additive sedation with other central nervous system depressants. Metabolized by demethylation; no significant drug interactions.

Anticonvulsants: Used to treat pain related to multiple sclerosis or trigeminal neuralgia. Blocks sodium channels.

Medication	Cog	S	A	Motor	D	Com	F	Other side effects or considerations
Carbamazepine (Tegretol)	++	++	+	++	++	++	+++	Liver +++ Hematologic +++ Renal +++ Rash (Stevens-Johnson) +++ Ataxia, blurred vision, drowsiness, agitation, disequilibrium, dizziness, benign leukopenia, cardiac arrhythmias, congestive heart failure, anticonvulsant hypersensitivity syndrome, hepatic failure (rare), syndrome of inappropriate antidiuretic hormone (rare), aplastic anemia (rare). Dosage adjustments may be needed after first 3-5 wk due to induction of its own metabolism. Genetic testing required for Asians (risk of AHS).
Oxcarbazepine (Trileptal)	++	++	0	+++	+++	++	+++	Liver + Hematologic 0 Renal 0 Rash (Stevens-Johnson) +++ Hyponatremia, nausea, rash, anticonvulsant hypersensitivity syndrome

Anticonvulsants: Used to treat pain related to multiple sclerosis or trigeminal neuralgia. Activates gamma amino butyric acid receptors. Gabapentin also decreases glutamate.

Medication	Cog	S	A	Motor	D	Com	F	Other side effects or considerations
Diazepam (Valium)	++++	++++	0	+++	++	++++	++++	Sedation, impaired memory, inattention, ataxia, weakness, constipation, urinary retention, depression, dependence. Enhances the effects of other central nervous system depressants, including alcohol. Diazepam may block the action of levodopa. Many medications interact with diazepam (see chapter 8).
Gabapentin (Neurontin)	++	++	+	+++	0	++	+++	Sedation, peripheral edema, tremor, dizziness, fatigue, ataxia, drowsiness, weight gain, behavioral changes. Adjust dose for renal insufficiency. No known drug interactions.

Local anesthetic: Used to treat pain related to multiple sclerosis.

Medication	Cog	S	A	Motor	D	Com	F	Other side effects or considerations
Lidocaine 5% topical patch (Lidoderm)	+	+	+	+	+	+	+	Confusion, nervousness, lightheadedness, euphoria, tremors, blurred vision, vomiting, hypotension

Cog = cognition; S = sedation; A = agitation or mania; Motor = discoordination; D = dysphagia; Com = communication; F = falls; TEN = toxic epidermal necrolysis; AHS = anticonvulsant hypersensitivity syndrome.

The likelihood rating scale for encountering the side effects is as follows: 0 = Almost no probability of encountering side effects. + = Little likelihood of encountering side effects. +/++ = Low probability of encountering side effects; however, probability increases with increased dosage. ++ = Medium likelihood of encountering side effects. +++ = High likelihood of encountering side effects, particularly with high doses. ++++ = Highest likelihood of encountering side effects; best to avoid in at-risk patients.

adverse effects include sweating, gynecomastia, decreased libido, impotency, menstrual irregularities, hypogonadism, hypocorticism, growth hormone deficiency, fluid retention, and edema. High-dose intrathecal opioids can produce myoclonus, hyperalgesia, paranoia, Meniere's disease, nystagmus, **polyarthralgia**, sedation, and respiratory depression (Cheng et al., 2006b; Ghafoor et al., 2007; Matthews & Horton, 2007).

Local anesthetics administered intrathecally penetrate the CSF to block the conduction of nerve impulses by binding to receptor sites on the sodium channel. Lipid-soluble anesthetics are more potent, and lower concentrations are required to produce analgesia equivalent to that of agents that are less lipid soluble. Bupivacaine can be administered alone or, when given concurrently with morphine, can reduce the amount of morphine required for analgesia. Adverse effects associated with bupivacaine are dose related and occur with doses greater than 45 mg/24 h. They include paresthesias, motor and sensory blockade, arterial hypotension, diarrhea, and urinary retention (Cheng et al., 2006a; Ghafoor et al., 2007; Matthews & Horton, 2007).

Clonidine is a centrally acting alpha-2 adrenergic antagonist that is administered as adjunct therapy in combination with intrathecal morphine to treat neuropathic pain. Pain relief is associated with inhibitory interaction with pre- and postsynaptic afferent fibers in the dorsal horn of the spinal cord. Adverse effects associated with intrathecal clonidine include sedation, hypotension, dry mouth, and bradycardia (Cheng et al., 2006a; Ghafoor et al., 2007; Matthews & Horton, 2007).

Ziconotide (Prialt) is a highly selective reversible blocker of calcium channels in the spinal ganglion. It suppresses transmission of pain in the dorsal horn from type A mechanoreceptive and type C nociceptive neuronal input. Adverse effects are related to high initial doses or rapid dose escalation and include severe dizziness, nausea, memory loss, nystagmus, confusion, loss of word-finding ability, psychosis, gait imbalance, constipation, and urinary retention (Cheng et al., 2006a; Ghafoor et al., 2007; Matthews & Horton, 2007).

Baclofen is a GABA receptor agonist used to control spasticity. GABA receptors are found in laminae I to III in the dorsal horn of the spinal cord. Baclofen increases potassium conductance to cause hyperpolarization of second-order neurons and inhibits calcium channel conductance across voltage-gated calcium channels. Baclofen can be combined with an opioid when pain management is needed and works best to control chronic pain. Adverse effects include weakness, hypotonia, sedation, constipation, impaired erection, loss of sphincter control, and respiratory depression (Cheng et al., 2006a; Ghafoor et al., 2007; Matthews & Horton, 2007).

Complications of intrathecal therapy include postoperative subarachnoid hemorrhage accompanied by symptoms of back pain, loss of sensation, lower-extremity weakness, and bowel and bladder incontinence. This complication requires immediate surgery to prevent permanent neurologic injury. Risk of this complication can be minimized by ensuring that anticoagulants, antiplatelet therapy, and NSAIDs are discontinued or adjusted before the procedure. Guidelines have been developed to prevent bleeding complications associated with insertion of catheters for intrathecal therapy. The antiplatelet drugs abciximab (ReoPro) and eptifibatide (Integrilin) used in cardiac catheterization should be avoided within 4 wk of intrathecal catheter insertion. In addition, the antiplatelet medication ticlopidine (Ticlid) should be held for 14 days and the antiplatelet medications clopidogrel (Plavix) and prasugrel (Effient) should be held for 7 days before catheter insertion. Anticoagulants such as enoxaparin (Lovenox) and dalteparin (Fragmin) should be held for 24 h before surgery; use can resume 8 to 12 h after the procedure. The oral anticoagulant warfarin (Coumadin) should be held for 4 to 5 days before surgery to achieve an INR (international normalized ratio) of less than 1.5; use can resume immediately after the procedure (Ghafoor et al., 2007).

Another complication of intrathecal therapy is catheter-tip inflammatory masses. These masses are reabsorbed over time, but if spinal cord compression develops surgical removal is needed to prevent permanent paralysis. Using appropriate concentrations of intrathecal medication solutions helps reduce the risk of developing these masses. Infection is another complication that can occur. Infection usually involves the pocket site but can also be associated with contamination of the compounded solution or improper aseptic technique when accessing the reservoir port (Cheng et al., 2006a; Ghafoor et al., 2007; Matthews & Horton, 2007).

Abrupt cessation of therapy due to a missed refill or pump malfunction can be associated with severe pain or life-threatening withdrawal symptoms. Symptoms of baclofen withdrawal include muscle rigidity, high fever, labile blood pressure, and lethargy that may progress to rhabdomyolysis, multisystem organ failure, disseminated intravascular coagulation, and death. These symptoms are treated with intravenous benzodiazepines, dantrolene, oral baclofen, and restoration of the intrathecal therapy as soon as possible. Symptoms of opioid withdrawal include malaise, anxiety, **myalgias**, insomnia, dehydration, fever, and recurrence of pain. Withdrawal is treated with administration of opiates (Ghafoor et al., 2007).

Complex Regional Pain Syndrome

Complex regional pain syndrome (CRPS) is also known as algodystrophy, shoulder–hand syndrome, posttraumatic dystrophy, Sudeck's atrophy, and reflex sympathetic dystrophy. The pain that is associated with nerve injury typically occurs in one or more extremities but can affect any area of the body. It can occur spontaneously or result from a minor or major injury. Early diagnosis is important in providing treatment and preventing spread to other parts of the body and incapacitation. If left untreated CRPS can result in deformity and chronic pain and require long-term treatment. However, if it is caught early, physical therapy and sympathetic nerve blocks can prevent disease progression (Brenton-Wood, 2009; Marlowe, 2007).

Incidence

The estimated international incidence of CRPS is 26.2/100,000 person years. CRPS occurs more often in females than in males and most often occurs in females older than 60 yr of age. The upper extremity is involved more often than the lower extremity, and most cases are caused by fracture (de Mos et al., 2006). In the United States, CRPS occurs in approximately 1% to 15% of patients with peripheral nerve injury. The incidence after fractures and contusions ranges from 10% to 30%; however, many times the pain cannot be traced to an identifiable nerve injury (Parillo & O'Conner, 2011). Onset of CRPS usually occurs in patients between 25 and 55 yr of age and is often precipitated by surgery, fracture, immobilization, sprain, crush injury, or stroke with motor involvement. Most patients are not able to work or complete normal activities of daily living. Patients with CRPS often have concurrent depression, anxiety, and phobias (Brenton-Wood, 2009; Marlowe, 2007).

Etiology and Pathophysiology

CRPS is a chronic pain condition resulting from dysfunction in the central or peripheral nervous system. Changes in skin color, texture, and temperature of the skin over the affected limb or body part may be noted. The development of intense burning pain, skin sensitivity, sweating, and swelling is common. CRPS is often triggered by a previous musculoskeletal or nerve injury and occurs when the initial transmission of pain and response to injury do not terminate normally, perhaps due to ineffective clearance of the inflammatory mediators in the periphery. The pain triggers another response, establishing a cycle of pain and swelling. The continued pain response increases sympathetic tone in the area associated with increased amounts of vasoconstricting catecholamines, resulting in edema and altered perfusion in the affected limb. This results in burning pain in the extremity and mottling of the skin. The patient becomes increasingly more protective of the limb or body part leading to decrease functional use and increased hypersensitivity.

Symptoms of CRPS involve abnormal function of the sympathetic nervous system such as changes in blood flow, sweating, movement disorders, swelling or edema, muscle atrophy or dystrophy, hyperalgesia, allodynia, and osteopenic bone changes. Neuropathic pain (e.g., burning, shooting, pricking) deep within a limb is a common complaint. Up to 50% of patients have deficits in temperature and tactile perception. Autonomic symptoms include swelling or edema, blue or purple and paled discoloration of the skin, abnormal sweating, and altered skin temperature. More than one half of patients with CRPS have edema in the affected limb and a difference in temperature (at first a warmer temperature and then cooler) between the affected limb and the unaffected limb. Motor symptoms occur as well: 75% of patients report weakness of the limb and 50% report tremor of the limb. Patients can also lose perception of the limb and exhibit limb neglect. Decreased hair and nail growth and osteopenia may occur in the affected limb (Brenton-Wood, 2009; Marlowe, 2007).

Rehabilitation Considerations

Nonpharmacologic therapies include physical and occupational therapy, psychological counseling, behavioral therapy, and interventional pain therapy. Rehabilitation is usually focused on gradually restoring normal sensory function. Therapy starts with gentle movement of the affected limb, progresses to weight bearing, and then progresses to resumption of normal function of the affected limb. Activities include desensitization techniques, range-of-motion activities, low-grade strengthening activities, stress loading, aerobic conditioning, postural training, ergonomics, movement therapy, and vocational and functional rehabilitation (Brenton-Wood, 2009; Marlowe, 2007).

Behavioral therapy can include patient and family education, relaxation training, encouraging constructive self-talk, realistic pain-limited reactivation, addressing cognitions underlying fear of movement, increasing social support, and identifying comorbid psychiatric illnesses. Interventional pain therapy can include nerve blocks with anesthetics or steroids, epidural blocks, intrathecal infusions, neurostimulators, spinal cord stimulation, and sympathetic nerve resection (Brenton-Wood, 2009; Marlowe, 2007).

Medication Therapy

Pharmacologic therapies include analgesics for treating mild to moderate pain; opiates or pharmacologic nerve blocks for treating moderate to severe pain; steroids, NSAIDs, and immunomodulators for treating chronic inflammation or edema; antianxiety or antidepressant therapy for treating psychiatric symptoms or insomnia; anticonvulsants for treating neuropathic pain; and bisphosphonates for treating osteopenia (Brenton-Wood, 2009; Marlowe, 2007; Teague, 2007).

Anti-inflammatory medications used include NSAIDs and short courses of corticosteroids such as prednisone 30 mg/day for 12 wk and then tapered. Anticonvulsants include gabapentin (Neurontin) and carbamazepine (Tegretol). Antidepressants that are helpful in treating neuropathic pain include tricyclic antidepressants and the NSRI duloxetine (Cymbalta) and venlafaxine (Effexor). Opiates are generally not helpful in treating CRPS (Gutstein & Akil, 2001; Hartrick et al., 2009).

The administration of the N-methyl-D-aspartate receptor agonist ketamine in anesthetic doses over a period of 5 days has resulted in remission of symptoms for month to years. Midazolam (Versed) is concurrently administered to manage the psychiatric side effects of ketamine (Brenton-Wood, 2009; Marlowe, 2007; Teague, 2007).

Alpha adrenergic-blocking agents can also provide pain relief. Direct application of clonidine (Catapres) topical patch to the painful area resulted in decreased hyperalgesia to cold and mechanical stimuli. Oral terazosin (Hytrin) can provide vasodilation and pain improvement. Nifedipine (Procardia XL) 60 mg/day controls vasoconstriction and improves pain. Intranasal calcitonin doses of 100 to 300 U/day help regulate bone metabolism and improve pain in patients with CRPS (Brenton-Wood, 2009; Marlowe, 2007; Teague, 2007).

Bisphosphonates such as alendronate (Fosamax) 40 mg/day for 8 wk and intravenous pamidronate (Aredia) decrease bone remodeling and reduce pain in patients with CRPS.

Topical therapies that also help relieve CRPS pain include topical lidocaine 5% patches administered 12 h/day and topical capsaicin (Zostrix) (Brenton-Wood, 2009; Marlowe, 2007; Teague, 2007).

Summary

This chapter discusses several chronic pain syndromes, including migraine, fibromyalgia, trigeminal neuralgia, cancer pain, phantom pain associated with amputation, CRPS (complex regional pain syndrome), and central pain syndromes that are associated with stroke, spinal cord damage, and multiple sclerosis. This chapter also provides information regarding pharmacologic and nonpharmacologic treatments that may be used in patients with chronic pain and includes a discussion on surgically implanted devices.

Medications Used to Treat Substance-Use Disorders

In clinical practice, the rehabilitation therapist will provide care for some patients with a history of substance-use disorders. This chapter introduces substance-use disorders, provides an overview of the medications used to treat these disorders, and summarizes how these disorders can affect rehabilitation. This chapter also discusses methods the rehabilitation therapist can use to monitor patients with substance-use disorders and methods for appropriately altering rehabilitation sessions.

Definition of Substance-Use Disorder

Substance-use disorder (SUD) is a complex behavioral disorder and is defined as excessive, repeated use of a substance such as nicotine, alcohol, or a medication. SUD is usually accompanied by the development of tolerance to a substance accompanied by withdrawal symptoms associated with discontinuing its use. In contrast to most patients taking these substances, patients with SUD develop a loss of control over the amount taken that leads to overuse with an accompanying preoccupation with obtaining the substance. This preoccupation results in impaired social and occupational functioning. *Substance-use disorder* is a more precise term than *substance abuse*, which the public uses to describe the use of any illegal substance. Medical practitioners also use the term *substance abuse*, but this term indicates a

pattern of overuse of a substance that produces significant adverse results (Kenna, 2007a).

In 2001, the Office of National Drug Control Policy estimated costs associated with substance-use disorders to be $143.4 billion annually in the United States. A survey conducted in 2004 found that 53% of inmates were diagnosed with substance abuse or dependence and 69% of inmates admitted to using illicit drugs regularly. In comparison, it is estimated that 2% of the general population suffers from substance-use disorder. A 2005 survey found that 74% of inmates were diagnosed with a mental illness and concurrent substance dependence or abuse (Kenna, 2007b). In 2000, the National Institute on Alcohol Abuse and Alcoholism estimated costs associated with alcohol-use disorders to be almost $185 billion annually in the United States. Finally, nicotine abuse, in the form of cigarette smoking, is the leading behavioral risk factor in the world for premature morbidity and mortality. Almost 25% of deaths in the United States are attributable to nicotine abuse (Kenna, 2007a). Chapter 22 discusses medications used to assist in smoking cessation. This chapter discusses medications and treatments used to treat SUD that involve alcohol or drugs.

Alcohol-Abuse Disorders

Approximately 80,000 deaths each year are attributable to alcohol. Alcohol abuse is the third leading lifestyle-related cause of death in the United States (Centers for Disease Control and Prevention, 2012).

Incidence

In 2004, 50% of Americans were current users of alcohol, and 55 million of them engaged in binge drinking (5 or more drinks at a time). In 2004, 17 million Americans were heavy drinkers, defined as engaging in binge drinking 5 or more times per month; the highest prevalence of binge drinking was found in persons between 18 and 25 yr of age. Ten percent of the U.S. population is dependent on alcohol (Kenna, 2007a). Alcohol use can also be a significant problem in the elderly population; this may reflect difficulty coping with life changes such as retirement and the loss of loved ones. Even small doses of alcohol on a daily basis may increase the risk of drug interactions and additive side effects in the elderly. This is because of age-related pharmacokinetic changes and the higher number of medications that can be used for treatment of chronic disease in the elderly. Because of these factors, toxicity, drug interactions, and adverse drug reactions tend to occur more frequently in the elderly, particularly when they are combined with the use of alcohol (Carl & Johnson, 2006).

Etiology and Pathophysiology

Alcohol activates gamma amino butyric acid-mediated inhibition of the central nervous system (CNS). Concurrent use of benzodiazepines, tricyclic antidepressants, opioids, and monoamine oxidase inhibitor (MAOI) antidepressants can increase the CNS depression associated with alcohol impairing cognition and motor function and can also result in respiratory depression (Sproule, 2002).

Significant alcohol abuse or alcoholism can be associated with a number of comorbidities such as depression, falls, amnesia, anxiety, trauma, **neuropathy**, insomnia, anorexia, malnutrition, and cirrhosis. Elderly persons with alcohol difficulties may not be identified easily because they may be retired and isolated socially. The rehabilitation therapist should rule out alcohol difficulties, particularly in patients who frequently experience

falls or have malnutrition issues (Jacobson et al., 2007).

PATIENT CASE 1

S.J. is a 74-yr-old alcoholic. He has been living in a skilled-nursing facility for the past 15 mo and has not had access to alcohol. During lunch hour one day, the speech–language pathologist attempts to evaluate S.J. for possible dysphagia. However, the pathologist is having difficulty performing the evaluation because S.J. refuses to sit down. Instead, S.J. runs around and steals packets of sugar and then hides in the corner of the dining room with his back to the others and quietly opens the packets. Once he finishes eating the sugar, he laughs almost uncontrollably and begins to run around the dining room again, looking for and stealing more packets of sugar.

Question

The speech–language pathologist is bewildered by S.J.'s behavior and frustrated that she cannot get him to sit down for the evaluation. Why is S.J. exhibiting this behavior?

Answer

S.J.'s alcoholic past can explain his behavior. In his mind, S.J. is stealing drinks and running off to a corner to consume his alcohol in a hidden fashion. The sugar in the packets may help remind S.J. of alcohol. The speech–language pathologist spoke with a nurse who had considerable experience dealing with alcoholics. The nurse provided very direct and consistent instructions and suggested a reinforcement structure that solved the problem.

Rehabilitation Considerations

Alcohol, opioids, sedative hypnotics, and stimulants all present dependence, abuse, intoxication, and withdrawal issues. Hallucinogens and phencyclidine present dependence, abuse, and intoxication issues but not withdrawal issues. The rehabilitation therapist should be aware that substance-related disorders can mimic other disorders, such as delirium, psychotic disorders, and mood disorders. In addition, disorders related to alcohol and sedative–hypnotic substances can mimic dementia, amnesia, and anxiety disorders, and disorders related to stimulants can mimic anxiety disorders (Preston et al., 2008; Sproule, 2002).

SUD can lead to cognitive disorders, withdrawal, intoxication, and mood disorders (Jacobson et al., 2007). Impaired cognition, mental clouding, and sedation can present a significant safety risk for the patient and can complicate the therapeutic process. For example, the patient may show decreased ability to follow instructions during therapy sessions, low motivation, and impaired psychomotor performance. SUD can result in restricted function in activities of daily life (ADL) and can be associated with compulsive behaviors and symptoms of tolerance or withdrawal (Jacobson et al., 2007). Associated inability to function in ADL increases the burden of care for caregivers.

Patients with SUD may have accompanying psychiatric problems and substance-related difficulties. For example, antisocial personality disorder and depression disorders are frequently found in patients with substance abuse. Remediating the substance-related difficulties may actually precede the development of these psychiatric problems (Epstein et al., 1994).

Upon admission to rehabilitation services patients should be screened for substance-use disorders. Several tools are available for screening and identifying SUD. One can use simple questions to screen for problems with alcohol use. For example, asking a man "During the past year, on how many occasions have you had five or more drinks?" (or asking a woman "During the past year, on how many occasions have you had four or more drinks?") may identify whether further inquiry is needed. A second tool called CAGE consists of 4 questions: 1) Have you ever felt you should <u>C</u>ut down on your drinking? 2) Have people <u>A</u>nnoyed you by criticizing your drinking? 3) Have you ever felt bad or <u>G</u>uilty about your drinking? and 4) Have you ever felt that you needed a drink first thing in the morning (<u>E</u>ye opener) to steady your nerves or get rid of a hangover? (Kenna, 2007a; Sproule, 2002).

Tools that screen for drug abuse include the Drug Abuse Screening Test (DAST), which is a 28-question screen; the DAST-10, which is an abbreviated 10-question screen; and the CRAFFT, which is intended for use in adolescents. CRAFFT is a mnemonic acronym of the first letters of key words in the screening questions. Laboratory urine testing can also confirm use of alcohol or drugs (Sproule, 2002).

Patients should also be monitored for symptoms of acute intoxication and for symptoms of acute alcohol withdrawal syndrome. Early withdrawal symptoms peak 24 h after alcohol cessation, although withdrawal can also emerge several days after cessation of alcohol use. Symptoms of withdrawal can resolve in a few hours or persist for up to 2 wk. Symptoms of alcohol withdrawal syndrome can range from mild tremor to delirium, hallucinations, seizures, and death (Jacobson et al., 2007). The effects of alcohol withdrawal in the elderly are similar to the effects of alcohol withdrawal in the middle-aged patient. The rehabilitation therapist may suspect acute withdrawal if a patient exhibits unexplained symptoms of respiratory depression, hypotension, hypertension, trauma, seizure, ataxia, arrhythmia, psychiatric disorders, or other changes in mental status (Jacobson et al., 2007).

In an alert patient who is acutely intoxicated, referral to the acute care setting for supportive and protective management may be indicated. The physician and members of the health care team should assess the hydration status, electrolyte levels, and nutritional status of patients being treated for alcohol intoxication or withdrawal. Patients who have lost fluids from vomiting, sweating, or hyperthermia may need intravenous fluid replacement. Magnesium deficiency is commonly seen in alcoholic patients. Thiamine deficiency is also common. Thiamine can be administered as 100 mg IM for the initial dose and then 100 mg 3 times/day for 3 to 4 wk. Thiamine should be administered before dextrose is administered in order to prevent **Wernicke's encephalopathy**, which includes symptoms of ataxia, acute confusion, and ophthalmoplegia. Long term impairment of cognition following Wernicke's encephalopathy is termed the Wernicke-Korsakoff syndrome (Kenna, 2007a; Sproule, 2002).

A short-acting benzodiazepine such as lorazepam (Ativan) 1 to 2 mg or haloperidol (Haldol) 2 to 5 mg intravenously can be used to treat acute violent behavior or severe agitation associated with acute alcohol withdrawal. Benzodiazepines are the preferred agents for managing these symptoms. Antipsychotic agents should be used with caution because they can lower seizure threshold, and patients experiencing alcohol withdrawal are already at risk for developing seizures.

The most reliable tool for assessing the extent of withdrawal and guiding treatment is the Clinical Institute Withdrawal Assessment of Alcohol—Revised (CIWA-Ar), which is a 10-item scale used for grading the severity of withdrawal symptoms. A maximum of 67 points can be assigned; a score of 8 or less indicates mild withdrawal, a score of 9 to 15 indicates moderate withdrawal, and a score of 16 or more indicates severe withdrawal. This tool also provides guidelines for managing withdrawal symptoms based on the continued reassessment of the severity of symptoms.

The Sedation Agitation Scale can be used in combination with the CIWA-Ar to determine the appropriate benzodiazepine dosing for managing symptoms. Long-acting benzodiazepines are frequently used because their sedative effects fluctuate less and they are easier to wean with a self-tapering effect. Patients who have liver disease or are elderly should be treated with short-acting benzodiazepines in order to prevent oversedation and adverse events (Kenna, 2007b).

Patients with less severe symptoms are managed with a symptom-triggered regimen of benzodiazepine administration, whereas those with more severe symptoms are usually managed with fixed-schedule regimens. Table 15.1 summarizes treatment strategies for managing acute alcohol withdrawal syndrome. In addition, beta blockers may be used to manage severe hypertension or other autonomic hyperactivity symptoms (Kenna, 2007a; Sproule, 2002).

Predictors of complications associated with acute alcohol withdrawal include the duration of alcohol consumption, number of previous alcohol detoxifications, number of episodes of withdrawal-associated delirium, and history of seizures associated with withdrawal.

Table 15.1   Medication Protocol Used to Treat Acute Alcohol Withdrawal Using CIWA-Ar Scoring

Medication	Indications	Dosing	Considerations
Chlordiazepoxide (Librium) Diazepam (Valium) Lorazepam (Ativan)	Symptom-triggered regimen protocol for treating acute alcohol withdrawal	Dosed to control symptoms until CIWA-Ar score is 8-10 for a period of 24 h.	Long-acting benzodiazepines. Available in IV and IM forms. Lorazepam is appropriate to use in elderly and patients with hepatic impairment.
Fixed-schedule regimen for lorazepam (Ativan) as listed in doses based on CIWA-Ar score of mild, moderate, or severe.*			
Lorazepam (Ativan)	Used for **mild** symptoms (CIWA-Ar score <10, SBP >150 mm Hg or DBP >90 mm Hg, HR >100 beats/min, temperature >100 °F)	1-2 mg by mouth every 4-6 h as needed for 1-3 days; titrate dose to control symptoms. In addition to scheduled doses, provide as needed to achieve CIWA-Ar score of 8-10.	Rapid onset of action. Can be administered orally, IV, or IM.

› continued

Table 15.1 ›continued

Medication	Indications	Dosing	Considerations
Lorazepam (Ativan)	Used for **moderate** symptoms (CIWA-Ar score 11-15, SBP 150-200 mm Hg or DBP 100-140 mm Hg, HR >110-140 beats/min, temperature 100-101 °F, presence of tremors, insomnia, and agitation)	Days 1 and 2: 2-4 mg by mouth 4 times/day; titrate dose to control symptoms. Days 3 and 4: 1-2 mg by mouth 4 times/day; titrate dose to control symptoms. Day 5: 1 mg by mouth twice/day; titrate dose to control symptoms. In addition to scheduled doses, provide as needed to achieve CIWA-Ar score of 8-10.	Rapid onset of action. Can be administered orally, IV, or IM.
Lorazepam (Ativan)	Used for **severe** symptoms (CIWA-Ar score >15, SBP >200 mm Hg or DBP >140 mm Hg, HR >140 beats/min, temperature >101 °F, presence of tremors, insomnia, and agitation)	1-2 mg IV every h while patient is awake for 3-5 days and titrate dose; end point is sedation. In addition to scheduled doses, provide as needed to achieve CIWA-Ar score of 8-10.	Rapid onset of action. Can be administered orally, IV, or IM.
Alternative protocols for benzodiazepine allergy or contraindication			
Carbamazepine (Tegretol)	Alternative treatment protocol for acute alcohol withdrawal in patients with benzodiazepine allergy or contraindication	Day 1: 600-800 mg by mouth. Taper to 200 mg over 5 days.	Consider drug interactions listed in table 9.3. Nonaddictive. Causes relatively little cognitive impairment.
Gabapentin (Neurontin)	Alternative treatment protocol for acute alcohol withdrawal in patients with benzodiazepine allergy or contraindication	400 mg by mouth 3 times/day for 3 days, then 400 mg twice/day for 1 day, then 400 mg for 1 day.	Consider drug interactions listed in table 9.3. Nonaddictive. Causes relatively little cognitive impairment.
Adjunctive therapies			
Clonidine (Catapres)	Adjunctive therapy for mild to moderate adrenergic hyperactivity associated with acute alcohol withdrawal	0.1 mg up to every 2 h. Maximum dose of 1 mg in 24 h.	
Atenolol (Tenormin)	Beta blocker used as adjunctive therapy for adrenergic hyperactivity associated with acute alcohol withdrawal	50 mg by mouth/day.	
Carbamazepine (Tegretol)	Used to treat adrenergic hyperactivity and seizures associated with acute alcohol withdrawal	800 mg by mouth on day 1, taper down to 200 mg/day over 5 days.	
Haloperidol (Haldol)	Neuroleptic used to treat agitation, hallucinations, and delirium associated with acute alcohol withdrawal	0.5-5 mg by mouth/IV/IM every h. Maximum dose of 100 mg/day.	Rapid onset of action.

CIWA-Ar = Clinical Institute Withdrawal Assessment of Alcohol; DBP = diastolic blood pressure; HR = heart rate; IM = intramuscular; IV = intravenous; SBP = systolic blood pressure. *refer to CIWA-Ar for dosing recommendations for diazepam or chlordiazepoxide use. The *CIWA-Ar* is not copyrighted and may be reproduced freely: www.chce.research.va.gov/apps/PAWS/support_site/howto/ciwar.html.

Risk of seizures and delirium associated with alcohol withdrawal increase as CIWA-Ar scores increase. Alcohol-withdrawal delirium (delirium tremens), a severe manifestation of alcohol withdrawal, usually peaks at 72 to 96 h after cessation of alcohol intake and carries a mortality rate of 5%. The rate of seizures associated with alcohol withdrawal can be as high as 15% (Kenna, 2007a; Sproule, 2002). Seizures are treated with the administration of benzodiazepines, carbamazepine (Tegretol), or gabapentin (Neurontin) (Jacobson et al., 2007).

Long term complications associated with alcohol dependency include impaired cognitive abilities long after the period of alcohol withdrawal ends. Symptoms may include amnesia, apraxia, and impaired abstract reasoning. Patients with alcoholic dementia typically do not demonstrate the language deficits (anomia) found in Alzheimer's patients; rather, they more typically exhibit peripheral neuropathy, ataxia, and cerebellar atrophy. The rehabilitation therapist must be aware that alcohol-related dementia affects the entire body, not just the brain itself. Patients with alcohol-related dementia often have balance deficits. Balance training and gait training are commonly used to address ataxia and pre-

vent falls. Therapeutic activities that focus on improving the coordination necessary for self-care and safety when performing ADL are also commonly used to address the general lack of coordination found in this patient population (Jacobson et al., 2007; Poldrugo, 2006).

The patient with a history of long term alcohol abuse may also develop peripheral neuropathies, which can cause decreased proprioceptive feedback and lead to poor coordination and poor balance. Neuropathy also contributes to the development of wounds and infection in the insensate areas. The rehabilitation therapist should instruct the patient to practice good foot care and to regularly inspect the skin for damage that they are unable to perceive due to the neuropathy. The cognitive and motor symptoms found in the patient with alcoholic dementia are the result of damage to the frontal cortex, thalamus, pons, and cerebellum. Acamprosate (Campral) combined with alcohol abstinence may be useful in preventing future deterioration (Jacobson et al., 2007; Poldrugo, 2006).

Medication Therapy

A number of medications can help the alcoholic patient maintain abstinence from alcohol. Table 15.2 summarizes medications used for this

 See table 15.2 in the web resource for a full list of medication-specific indications, dosing recommendations, and side effects.

Table 15.2   Maintenance Medications Used to Assist With Alcohol Abstinence After Treatment of Acute Alcohol Withdrawal

Medication	Side effects affecting rehab							Other side effects or considerations
Disulfiram (Antabuse): Acetaldehyde dehydrogenase inhibitor used as maintenance therapy to promote alcohol abstinence in patients with alcohol dependence. FDA approved.								
Disulfiram (Antabuse)	Cog +	S +	A +	Motor ++	D +	Com +	F ++	Optic neuritis, peripheral neuropathy, hepatitis (rare), skin eruptions, mild drowsiness, fatigue, garlic taste, occasional psychotic reactions with high doses
Naltrexone (Depade, ReVia): Opioid antagonist used as maintenance therapy to promote alcohol abstinence in patients with alcohol dependence. FDA approved.								
Naltrexone (Depade, ReVia)	Cog ++	S ++	A ++	Motor +++	D +	Com +++	F ++	Nausea, dizziness, fatigue, vomiting, increased risk of depression and suicide, somnolence, hepatotoxicity with high doses. Withdrawal symptoms: Tearfulness, nausea, restlessness, abdominal cramps, bone or joint pain, myalgia, nasal symptoms.

› continued

Table 15.2 › *continued*

Medication	Side effects affecting rehab							Other side effects or considerations			
Acamprosate (Campral): Maintenance therapy used to promote alcohol abstinence in patients with alcohol dependence. N-methyl-D-aspartate modulator; may interact with glutamate and GABA to restore balance in patients with alcohol dependence. FDA approved.											
Acamprosate (Campral)	Cog +	S +	A 0	Motor 0	D +	Com +	F +	Diarrhea, dyspepsia, dizziness, dry mouth, itching, weakness, neuropathy in hands, feet, or legs			
Buspirone (Buspar): Antianxiety agent; serotonin 1A partial agonist and dopamine-2 antagonist used to promote alcohol abstinence in patients with alcohol dependence and generalized anxiety disorder. Not FDA approved.											
Buspirone (Buspar)	Cog +	S +	A 0	Motor 0	D +	Com +	F +	Weight gain 0 Half-life is 2-3 h	Seizure 0	Cardiac 0	Sexual 0
Fluoxetine (Prozac), Sertraline (Zoloft): Selective serotonin reuptake inhibitors used to promote abstinence in patients with alcohol dependence with later onset or with severe dependence and family history of alcoholism. Not FDA approved.											
Fluoxetine (Prozac)	Cog 0/+	S 0/+	A +	Motor 0	D 0/+	Com 0/+	F 0	Weight gain 0/+	Seizure ++	Cardiac 0/+	Sexual +++
Sertraline (Zoloft)	Cog 0/+	S 0/+	A +	Motor 0	D +++	Com +	F 0	Weight gain 0	Seizure 0	Cardiac 0	Sexual +++
Ondansetron (Zofran): Serotonin antagonist used to promote abstinence in patients with alcohol dependence with early onset history. Not FDA approved.											
Ondansetron (Zofran)	Cog +	S +	A 0	Motor ++	D +	Com +	F ++	Headache, malaise, fatigue, constipation, dizziness, rash. Can increase QT prolongation and arrhythmias when combined with antiarrhythmics, tricyclic antidepressants, antipsychotics, anesthetics, or diuretics.			
Topiramate (Topamax): GABA inhibitor and glutamate antagonizer used to promote abstinence in patients with alcohol dependence and history of heavy drinking. Not FDA approved.											
Topiramate (Topamax)	Cog ++	S ++	A ++	Motor +++	D +	Com +++	F ++	Monitor for changes in renal function and for rash. May cause language impairment, behavioral changes, weight loss, altered taste, metabolic acidosis, kidney stones, hypohidrosis.			
Aripiprazole (Abilify): Partial D2 agonist, serotonin 1A partial agonist, and serotonin 2A antagonist used to promote abstinence in patients with alcohol dependence. Not FDA approved.											
Aripiprazole (Abilify)	Cog +	S +	A 0	Motor +	D +	Com +	F +	Weight gain +	Seizure 0	Cardiac +	Sexual +
Quetiapine (Seroquel): Serotonin 1A and 2, dopamine 1 and 2, histamine 1, and adrenergic A1 and A2 receptor antagonist used to promote abstinence in patients with alcohol dependence and sleep disorder. Not FDA approved.											
Quetiapine (Seroquel)	Cog ++	S ++	A 0	Motor ++	D +	Com ++	F +++	Weight gain ++ High risk for orthostasis and falls	Seizure 0	Cardiac ++	Sexual +

Cog = cognition; S = sedation; A = agitation or mania; Motor = discoordination; D = dysphagia; Com = communication; F = falls; FDA = U.S. Food and Drug Administration; GABA = gamma amino butyric acid.

Sexual = increased risk of sexual side effects.

The likelihood rating scale for encountering the side effects is as follows: 0 = Almost no probability of encountering side effects. 0/+ = Little likelihood of encountering side effects, but increased likelihood with use of higher doses. + = Little likelihood of encountering side effects. +/++ = Low probability of encountering side effects; however, probability increases with increased dosage. ++ = Medium likelihood of encountering side effects. +++ = High likelihood of encountering side effects, particularly with high doses. ++++ = Highest likelihood of encountering side effects; best to avoid in at-risk patients.

purpose that are approved and not approved by the U.S. Food and Drug Administration.

Disulfiram (Antabuse) has been used for many years as a method for maintaining abstinence from alcohol use. Disulfiram increases the production of acetaldehyde when patients consume alcohol, which results in the "Antabuse reaction": nausea, vomiting, palpitations, hypotension, flushing, headache, sweating, dizziness, shortness of breath, confusion, and blurred vision. Disulfiram (Antabuse) is dosed at 250 mg/day at bedtime starting 12 to 24 h after the initiation of abstinence. The prescriber and appropriate members of the health care team should monitor the patient's liver enzymes while the patient is using Antabuse. Common side effects include sedation, a metallic or garlic taste, sexual dysfunction, and psychosis (Kenna, 2007a; Sproule, 2002).

The Antabuse reaction can also occur when disulfiram is used in combination with over-the-counter mouthwashes and cough syrups that contain alcohol. Disulfiram should not be combined with the antibiotic metronidazole (Flagyl) because acute confusion may occur. More serious side effects such as bradykinesia, heart failure, myocardial infarction, hypotension, and seizures can occur in patients taking high doses of this medication or patients with previous cardiac difficulties. Patients with cardiomyopathy, arrhythmia, congestive heart failure, or coronary artery disease should not take this agent. Patients with renal disease, elevated liver enzymes, peripheral neuropathy, pulmonary disease, or impulsive behaviors are also at increased risk for serious toxicity and should not take disulfiram. Because this medication increases dopamine levels, schizophrenia and mania can be associated with its use. Disulfiram therapy is most effective when used in patients who have a stable home life and who adhere to therapy and can be used to improve adherence in high-risk social situations in which alcohol is served (Jacobson et al., 2007; Kenna, 2007a).

Naltrexone (Vivitrol) blocks the actions of endorphins across the mu-opioid receptors when alcohol is consumed. It decreases the craving for alcohol and helps the patient maintain abstinence (Preston et al., 2008).

Naltrexone should be used in conjunction with a comprehensive alcohol-treatment program, adjunctive counseling, and cognitive behavioral therapy. Naltrexone is usually dosed at 50 mg/day, but doses of 25 to 150 mg/day have been effectively used. Studies show that this agent is most effective in patients with poor cognitive status and a strong craving for alcohol and that it requires high adherence. Naltrexone therapy is most likely to benefit patients who have a family history of alcoholism, who began drinking at an early age, and who abuse other drugs. This medication is generally well tolerated and has been successfully used to reduce alcoholic binges in the elderly. Naltrexone has also been used successfully in the treatment of traumatic brain injury. The results have indicated improvements in mobility, speech, and overall functional independence measurement scores (Calvanio et al., 2000).

Naltrexone (Vivitrol) is contraindicated in patients with liver disease or patients who are taking or dependent on opioids. Patients should be off opioids for at least 7 to 10 days before initiating naltrexone. Patients using this medication should wear a medical emergency identifier because any attempt to overcome the opiate-blocking effects of naltrexone to treat acute pain can result in a fatal overdose. Acute pain in these patients should be managed with an intravenous nonsteroidal anti-inflammatory drug (NSAID) such as ketorolac (Toradol), conscious sedation with a benzodiazepine such as midazolam (Versed), or a general anesthetic (Kenna, 2007a; Sproule, 2002).

The rehabilitation therapist should be aware that patients using disulfiram (Antabuse) or oral naltrexone (Vivitrol) may stop using these medications and start drinking again. Therefore, even though the patient may have a prescription for medications that help decrease alcohol use, a noncompliant patient may still be consuming alcohol.

Acamprosate (Campral) antagonizes the glutamate N-methyl-D-aspartate receptor thereby attenuating postsynaptic hyperexcitability during alcohol withdrawal. This product works best in patients who are highly motivated to stop drinking, who are able to be abstinent for at least one week, and who do not live alone.

This medication is initiated after the patient has been abstinent for a minimum of 4 days and is dosed at 666 mg 3 times/day. Side effects include diarrhea, nausea, and bloating. It does not cause sedation. It should not be used in patients with renal insufficiency (creatinine clearance <30 ml/min) (Kenna, 2007a; Poldrugo, 2006).

Several other disorders are associated with neurotoxicity to alcohol. Wernicke's encephalopathy is associated with thiamine deficiency. Symptoms include ataxia, confusion, and problems with ocular motor movement, such as nystagmus. Wernicke-Korsakoff syndrome is characterized by anterograde amnesia, disinhibition, apathy, perseveration, and confabulatory speech. Alcoholic hallucinations are characterized by delusions and auditory hallucinations. Cerebellar degeneration presents with ataxia and **dysmetria**, in which the patient will overshoot or undershoot their desired location (Jacobson et al., 2007).

Drug-Abuse Disorders

The next section discusses the different forms of drug-abuse disorders. The early part of this section deals with opioid use, intoxication, withdrawal, and maintenance. The latter part of this section discusses abuse of prescription drugs, benzodiazepines, antipsychotics, and illicit drugs. Drug-abuse disorders are, unfortunately, problems the rehabilitation therapist will encounter frequently.

Opioid-Use Disorder

Opioids, which are used to treat moderate to severe pain, include fentanyl, oxymorphone, hydromorphone, morphine, meperidine, hydrocodone, and oxycodone (Preston et al., 2008). Opioids are usually selected based on the patient's age, pain severity, the presence of major organ failure, and the presence of coexisting disease (Carl & Johnson, 2006). The rehabilitation therapist frequently encounters patients who are taking opiates for pain relief. The relief of pain may allow the rehabilitation therapist to engage the patient in a more aggressive program of rehabilitation. The therapist should work with the physician,

nurse, or pharmacist to determine peak levels of medication and should schedule the patient for treatment at a time when the medication is at peak levels (Ciccone, 2007). The side effects of opiates such as impaired cognition, impaired motor function, and sedation and respiratory depression may complicate participation with rehabilitation and treatment success (Davis et al., 2002).

Opioid Intoxication

Less than 1% of hospitalized patients exhibit addiction to opiates. Typically, when the pain stops, the patient stops using the medication. This situation may be different in settings where the patient may not be assessed and monitored as readily. Physical dependence on opiates occurs when the body adapts to the presence of opioid. Dependence on opiates is revealed when an antagonist is given or the opioid is withdrawn (Carl & Johnson, 2006). Acute opioid intoxication may present with stupor, depressed respiration, constipation, hypothermia, and bradycardia. Opioid intoxication is characterized by symptoms of euphoria, dysphoria, apathy, motor retardation, sedation, slurred speech, impaired attention, and **miosis**. Naloxone (Narcan), an opioid antagonist used to treat opioid overdose and resultant respiratory depression, is given intravenously at doses of 0.4 to 2 mg every 3 min in conjunction with supportive therapy. Response to this medication typically occurs within several minutes (Davis et al., 2002; Kenna, 2007a; Preston et al., 2008; Sproule, 2002).

Opioid Withdrawal

Symptoms of acute opioid withdrawal include lacrimation, anxiety, insomnia, yawning, sweating, and **rhinorrhea**, followed by pinpoint pupils, tremor, gooseflesh, chills, anorexia, shallow breathing, and muscle cramps. About 24 h after opiate discontinuance, signs of withdrawal include increased heart rate, increased blood pressure, dilated pupils, and elevated respiration and temperature. Onset of acute withdrawal is opiate dependent; it can occur within a few hours to 2 to 3 days and can peak at 2 to 3 days. Opiate withdrawal is not life threatening and resolves within 10 days (Kenna, 2007a; Sproule, 2002).

Withdrawal symptoms can be treated with one of the following: naltrexone (ReVia, Vivitrol) induction and maintenance, methadone (Dolophine) at tapered doses, buprenorphine (Subutex), clonidine (Catapres), or anesthesia-assisted detoxification. The therapy of choice is methadone. Methadone 10 mg is given every 4 h to a maximum dose of 40 to 50 mg in the first 24 h. The total methadone daily dose given on day 1 is given in 2 divided doses on day 2, and the daily dose is decreased by 5 mg/day each day thereafter to the smallest dose that controls symptoms (Davis et al., 2002; Kenna, 2007a; Preston et al., 2000; Sproule, 2002).

Buprenorphine (Subutex), another agent used to treat withdrawal symptoms, can be administered on either a flexible-dosing or a fixed-dosing schedule and can be initiated in an inpatient or outpatient setting. Buprenorphine may be dosed in a 3 day, 5 day, 7 day, or 10 day inpatient protocol that starts at 4 to 12 mg and tapers over the specified time period. In addition, buprenorphine may be dosed in an 8 day outpatient regimen that starts at 4 to 8 mg and tapers down over the 8 days. Clonidine (Catapres), another agent, can be dosed at 0.1 mg 3 to 4 times/day for 5 days and then is taken on an as-needed basis. Alternatively, clonidine can be dosed at 0.1 to 0.2 mg every 8 h (maximum dose of 1.2 mg/day) until day 7, when naltrexone is introduced as the maintenance regimen for maintaining abstinence. In anesthesia-assisted ultrarapid detoxification, the patient receives anesthesia for 4 to 6 h after receiving naloxone intravenously or naltrexone 50 mg orally (Kenna, 2007a; Sproule, 2002).

Opioid Maintenance Therapies

Methadone is used as maintenance therapy in doses of 40 to 120 mg/day; greater success is achieved with daily doses of 60 mg or greater. It may take up to 6 wk to determine the optimal dose; dosage should be adjusted no more often than every 4 to 5 days. Peak effects of methadone occur in 2 to 4 h and last for 8 to 60 h. Because pain relief from methadone lasts for only 4 to 8 h, great potential for overdose exists if this agent is being dosed for relief of pain. Symptoms of methadone overdose include shallow or difficult breathing; extreme lethargy; sleepiness; blurred vision; inability to talk, think, or walk normally; and feeling dizzy, faint, or confused. Methadone is still the main treatment for heroin addiction and is safe to use during pregnancy. Concurrent use of fluvoxamine (Luvox), nefazodone (Serzone), and carbamazepine (Tegretol) should be avoided as these agents can reduce methadone clearance and increase risk of methadone toxicity (Sproule, 2002).

Buprenorphine (Buprenex) is a partial agonist of the mu opioid receptor. It is combined with naloxone (Narcan) in a product called Suboxone. Suboxone is designed for initiation of opioid abstinence therapy in an outpatient (office-based) setting. Physicians must complete education and receive special certification to prescribe this product. It is available in a 0.3 mg/ml injectable dosage form and in 2 mg and 8 mg sublingual tablets. Initiation helps patients switch from the opiate of abuse to Suboxone as quickly as possible while minimizing withdrawal symptoms. Patients take the first dose of 4 mg when withdrawal signs first appear and subsequent doses are taken based on withdrawal symptoms, cravings, and adverse effects. Symptoms are alleviated 20 to 40 min after a dose (Johnson et al., 2003; Lintzeris et al., 2003).

Side effects of Suboxone include cold or flu-like symptoms, nausea, vomiting, sweating, sleeping difficulties, and constipation. The levels and effects of the medication can be altered when the medication is combined with medications that induce or inhibit CYP3A4 metabolism, such as anticonvulsants (phenytoin, carbamazepine, valproic acid, phenobarbital, clonazepam) and several HIV (human immunodeficiency virus) antiretroviral therapies. The concurrent use of these agents should be avoided. The dose of Suboxone should be reduced in patients with hepatic impairment (Kenna, 2007a).

Prescription-Drug Abuse

In 2004, over 7 million people in the United States took prescription drugs for recreational use; 4.4 million used pain relievers, 1.6 million used tranquilizers, 1.2 million used stimulants, and 330,000 used sedatives. During this period of time abuse of prescription drugs increased in Americans aged 18 to 25 yr; many of these individuals abused oxycodone or hydrocodone products (Kenna, 2007b).

Abuse of Benzodiazepines

Benzodiazepines are medications that are prescribed for anxiety and often are associated with overuse and long-term use. Elderly female patients who have a low level of education and a history of emotional difficulties are at higher risk to develop physical dependence to benzodiazepines. The shorter the action and more rapid onset of effects associated with a benzodiazepine, the higher the potential for symptoms of withdrawal and subsequent overuse. Short-acting benzodiazepines include midazolam (Versed) and triazolam (Halcion). Intermediate-acting agents include alprazolam (Xanax), lorazepam (Ativan), oxazepam (Serax), and temazepam (Restoril) (Sproule, 2002). The long-acting benzodiazepines include chlordiazepoxide (Librium), clorazepate (Tranxene), diazepam (Valium), and flurazepam (Dalmane). Symptoms of withdrawal from benzodiazepines include fatigue, dizziness, anxiety, tremors, insomnia, difficulty concentrating, instability, delirium, hallucinations, and seizures (Jacobson et al., 2007).

Acute overdose of benzodiazepines is treated in the acute care setting with flumazenil (Romazicon), which inhibits the binding of the benzodiazepine to the receptor, thus reversing the benzodiazepine's effect of CNS depression. This medication can be effective in cases of oversedation accompanied by respiratory depression and can be particularly important in treating intentional and unintentional overdose. Unfortunately, benzodiazepines are often combined with alcohol; this combination can result in profound oversedation and respiratory depression (Carl & Johnson, 2006). Benzodiazepines are often combined with stimulants such as cocaine or methamphetamine and are used by patients with SUD to attenuate the side effects of stimulant (Kenna, 2007a).

When discontinuing a patient from long term benzodiazepine therapy the physician may choose to slowly taper off the medication with or without concurrently initiating a **barbiturate** or anticonvulsant such as carbamazepine (Tegretol), gabapentin (Neurontin), or valproate (Depakene) to mitigate the withdrawal symptoms (Kenna, 2007a; Sproule, 2002). Selective serotonin reuptake inhibitor antidepressants may help the patient maintain abstinence from benzodiazepines once therapy is discontinued.

Chronic use of benzodiazepines is associated with sedation, cognitive difficulties, depression, anxiety, falls, and ataxia. Patients with a history of chronic use of benzodiazepines may present with symptoms of dementia (psychomotor slowing and incoordination, inattention) and amnesia. These symptoms typically abate after withdrawal of the medication. The symptoms vary depending on the particular drug involved. The patient withdrawing from use of a short-term benzodiazepine may exhibit rebound insomnia, blurred vision, headaches, vertigo, incontinence, weakness, joint pain, and chest pain (Carl & Johnson, 2006).

Chronic use of benzodiazepines may also result in significant pharyngeal phase dysphagia, which is characterized by hypopharyngeal incoordination, cricopharyngeal incoordination, and aspiration. Ceasing use of the medication may reduce pharyngeal phase dysphagia (Carl & Johnson, 2006). Rehabilitation therapists are not trained in pharmacology and therefore may not always identify medications causing or exacerbating the patient's dysphagia. However, the prudent therapist does understand that medications play a critical role in causing or exacerbating dysphagia. The prudent therapist understands that identifying these medications by collaborating with the pharmacist and physician to identify the causative medication and alter therapy can affect the therapist's success in remediation of the dysphagia (Carl & Johnson, 2006).

PATIENT CASE 2

S.A. is a 55-yr-old female who works very long hours at a local accounting firm. Recently, S.A. began to feel as though food is getting stuck in her throat and esophagus. She tried eating slowly and cutting her food into small pieces, but this did not seem to solve the problem. Subsequently, S.A. underwent a dysphagia evaluation with an SLP. The SLP suggested a number of compensatory strategies and therapeutic interventions, but none of the interventions seem to be improving S.A.'s situation.

Question

What should the SLP do to help improve the patient's situation?

Answer

The SLP reviewed the patient's medical history again and discovered that the patient had been taking benzodiazepines for more than 5 yr to "relax." The SLP sought the advice of the facility's consultant pharmacist who explained that chronic use of benzodiazepines can lead to cricopharyngeal dysfunction and esophageal dysmotility. The pharmacist called the patient's physician and suggested alternatives to the current medication regimen. The patient was placed on a non-benzodiazepine medication for her anxiety, and her dysphasia symptoms slowly subsided.

The rehabilitation therapist can help reduce use of benzodiazepines by instructing the patient in relaxation techniques and developing a program of regular exercise for the patient. Patients who exercise regularly report a 20% reduction in anxiety symptoms compared with those who do not exercise (Herring et al., 2010).

Abuse of Antipsychotics

The neurotransmitter dopamine has been identified as important in reinforcing the abuse of drugs. Administrating dopamine antagonists or blocking the dopamine receptor in the nucleus accumbens decreases self-administration of alcohol. The dopamine antagonists haloperidol (Haldol), olanzapine (Zyprexa), and clozapine (Clozaril) reduce cravings for alcohol and increase abstinence from alcohol use. Neuroleptics upregulate dopamine-2 receptors and reduce positive symptoms of schizophrenia; they also can reduce substance abuse. Use of quetiapine (Seroquel) for treating cocaine, alcohol, benzodiazepine, and opiate dependence has been investigated in studies involving small numbers of patients (Hanley & Kenna, 2008).

Antipsychotics have recently emerged as substances of abuse. Colloquial labels for quetiapine (Seroquel) include quell, Susie-Q, and baby heroin. Quetiapine (Seroquel) has been implicated in the majority of case reports on antipsychotic abuse in the literature. People who are incarcerated have feigned psychiatric symptoms in order to obtain this medication. Intranasal snorting of quetiapine (Seroquel) tablets has also been reported in patients with a history of substance abuse. Some users reportedly liquefy quetiapine (Seroquel) tablets and administer the product intravenously alone or in combination with other products (Hanley & Kenna, 2008). Some postulate that psychotropic agents are used for their anxiolytic and sedative properties in place of benzodiazepine and barbiturates, which are more closely controlled and difficult to obtain. Others propose that these agents attenuate the symptoms of withdrawal from other drugs of abuse (Hanley & Kenna, 2008).

Illicit-Drug Abuse

In 2004, 19 million Americans used illicit drugs; 14.6 million used marijuana, approximately 2 million used cocaine (467,000 used crack cocaine), 1.4 million used methamphetamine, an estimated 929,000 used hallucinogens, about 450,000 used ecstasy, and about 166,000 used heroin. Hallucinogens such as lysergic acid diethylamide or phencyclidine are usually not associated with withdrawal or dependence (Kenna, 2007b; Preston et al., 2008).

Cocaine and Amphetamine Abuse

Potential for abuse of medications such as amphetamines and cocaine is high. These substances increase dopamine and norepinephrine and cause symptoms such as hyperexcitability and euphoria. Concurrent use of MAOI antidepressants should be avoided as they can increase amphetamine and cocaine levels, resulting in increased, dangerously high blood pressure. Other medications that should be avoided with amphetamines or cocaine include fluoxetine (Prozac) and antipsychotic medications. Fluoxetine (Prozac) is an antidepressant that can reduce amphetamine clearance and increase effects. Concurrent use of virtually all antipsychotics can block dopamine effects and can decrease amphetamine effects (Sproule, 2002).

Bromocriptine 2.5 mg 3 times/day has been used to treat withdrawal from and cravings for cocaine. Otherwise, treatment is supportive and consists of closely monitoring the patient's cardiac and neurological status. Cocaine-induced seizures can be treated with benzodiazepine or barbiturates. Antipsychotics can lower the seizure threshold and should not be used to manage symptoms. Cardiotoxicity is increased when alcohol and cocaine are combined. Medications used to reduce cravings and promote abstinence include antidepressants, baclofen (Lioresal) 20 mg 3 times/day, topiramate (Topamax) 100 mg twice/day, quetiapine (Seroquel) 400 mg/day, tiagabine (Gabitril) 24 mg/day, buprenorphine (Buprenex) 16 mg/day, and bupropion (Wellbutrin) sustained-release tablets 150 mg twice/day (Kenna, 2007b; Preston et al., 2008).

Marijuana Abuse

Acute intoxication associated with use of marijuana rarely requires treatment. Severe anxiety can be treated with benzodiazepines such as lorazepam (Ativan). Selegiline (Eldepryl), an MAOI that inhibits dopamine metabolism, may also be helpful in treating dependence. Bupropion (Wellbutrin, Zyban) may be helpful in treating withdrawal associated with marijuana discontinuation (Kenna, 2007b).

Table 15.3 lists psychoactive medications that are commonly abused and summarizes the mechanisms of addiction, associated symptoms of tolerance and withdrawal, effects of prolonged use, and treatments.

Table 15.3   Effects of Abuse of Psychoactive Medications and Indicated Treatments

Drug	Mechanism	Tolerance and withdrawal	Effects of prolonged use	Treatment
Alcohol	Inhibits N-methyl-D-aspartate, glutamate, and calcium channels; enhances GABA	Tolerance due to increased hepatic metabolism, down-regulation of GABA receptors, and upregulation of glutamine receptors. Withdrawal symptoms: Shaking, weakness, agitation, headache, dizziness, vomiting, paresthesias, insomnia, seizures, delirium tremens.	Altered prefrontal cortex, nutritional deficits along with associated cognitive impairment and decreased brain volume	FDA approved: disulfiram (Antabuse), naltrexone (ReVia), acamprosate (Campral). Not FDA approved: topiramate (Topamax), aripiprazole (Abilify), quetiapine (Seroquel).
Benzodiazepines, sedatives	GABA agonists	Rapid development of tolerance due to downregulation of GABA receptors	Memory impairment	Switch to long-acting benzodiazepine or anticonvulsant and taper.
Opiates	Mu and delta opioid agonists disinhibit GABA and increase dopamine response	Tolerance due to downregulation of receptors. Withdrawal symptoms: Watery eyes, runny nose, yawning, sweating, restlessness, chills, cramps, muscle aches.	Altered receptors; altered adaptations in reward, learning, and stress responses	Methadone (Dolophine), buprenorphine (Subutex), naltrexone (ReVia), buprenorphine–naltrexone (Suboxone)
Cannabinoids	Activates cannabinoid receptors and increases dopamine in mesolimbic dopamine pathway	Tolerance develops rapidly to effects of tachycardia, increased appetite, dry mouth, euphoria, and sensory intensification. Withdrawal is rare.	Cognitive impairment, impaired ability to form memories, may trigger mental illness	Not FDA approved: selegiline (Eldepryl)

Drug	Mechanism	Tolerance and withdrawal	Effects of prolonged use	Treatment
Cocaine	Blocks dopamine transport and inhibits dopamine reuptake	Withdrawal symptom: Depression	Cognitive deficits, impaired motor function, decreased reaction time, increased cardiovascular events and stroke	Not FDA approved: bromocriptine (Parlodel), disulfiram (Antabuse), tiagabine (Gabitril), topiramate (Topamax), baclofen (Lioresal)
Methamphetamine, amphetamine	Increases dopamine release, inhibits dopamine reuptake, alters dopamine receptors	Tolerance develops rapidly. Withdrawal symptoms: Fatigue, depression, sleep disorders, anxiety, craving for the drug.	Sleep disturbances, anxiety, decreased appetite, metabolic changes, cognitive and memory impairment, declining dentition (meth mouth)	Non FDA approved: bromocriptine (Parlodel), amantadine (Symmetrel), quetiapine (Seroquel), topiramate (Topamax)
Methylenedioxymethamphetamine (Ecstasy)	Increases serotonin release and inhibits reuptake	Withdrawal symptoms: Depression, insomnia	Damage to serotonin brain systems that results in behavioral and physiologic changes, permanent memory impairment, paranoia, depression, panic attacks	Supportive measures
Inhalants	Enhances GABA effects	Withdrawal symptom: Seizures	Changes in dopamine binding that result in decreased cognitive function, psychiatric disorders	Supportive measures
Hallucinogens	Different agents may affect function of serotonin, glutamate, or acetylcholine receptors	Tolerance develops rapidly. No withdrawal symptoms.	Acute psychotic flashbacks	Supportive measures
Gamma hydroxybutyrate	Alters dopamine transmission in basal ganglia, affects GABA receptors	Insomnia, anxiety, sweating. No antidote known for overdose.	Amnesia, hypotonia, sleep disorders	Supportive measures
Antipsychotics	Antagonizes dopamine, histamine, and adrenergic receptors	Physical tolerance develops. Used in inmates as alternative to benzodiazepine.	Somnolence, dry mouth, constipation, orthostasis, weight gain, neuroleptic malignant syndrome, dyskinesia	Supportive measures
Dextromethorphan	High doses convert to dextromethorphan, an N-methyl-D-aspartate antagonist	Dependence and withdrawal are not well documented.	Dissociation, hallucinations, tachycardia, agitation, ataxia, psychosis	Supportive measures

FDA = U.S. Food and Drug Administration; GABA = gamma amino butyric acid.

Summary

This chapter summarizes the different types of SUD and their effects on rehabilitation and introduces the medication therapies commonly used to treat SUD. The rehabilitation therapist can play a major role in identifying patients with substance abuse and referring them for appropriate treatment. The specialist may be the first professional to identify the symptoms of substance abuse in a patient who, for example, has had repeated falls, a history of chronic pain, dysphagia, or sedation. The rehabilitation specialists should work with the physician and pharmacist to reduce the substance abuse in the patient, educate the patient and the patient's caregivers about risk factors for substance abuse, and provide rehabilitation to reduce the negative effects of substance abuse.

Medications Used to Treat Disorders of the Immune System

Part V provides information on disorders that affect the immune system and includes chapters on infections, arthritis and other rheumatic disease, and cancer. Chapter 16 overviews the infections most commonly encountered in the patient undergoing rehabilitation, including urinary tract infections, skin and soft-tissue infections, respiratory infections such as pneumonia, infections of the blood, and bone infections such as those associated with surgery or diabetic foot infections. This chapter reviews the stages of wound healing and discusses methods for minimizing risk of skin breakdown in patients who are nonambulatory. This chapter also reviews recommendations for using antibiotic therapies and other treatments for infection and discusses concepts of infection control that the rehabilitation therapist must use to prevent the spread of infection to other patients and caregivers.

Chapter 17 reviews osteoarthritis, gout, and rheumatoid arthritis disorders and associated treatments. Patients with arthritis and gout have limited ability to ambulate and participate in therapy sessions. This chapter discusses medications used on a chronic basis to control inflammation and reduce deformity and pain associated with these clinical conditions. It also presents methods the therapist can use for appropriately timing pain therapies before therapy sessions to optimize patient success in rehabilitation. The chapter also discusses therapeutic effects, important side effects, and significant drug interactions associated with the use of these medications that the therapist should be aware of in planning therapy and monitoring the patient during therapy.

Chapter 18 introduces the treatment of different types of cancer and supportive therapies that are commonly used in these patients. A complete discussion of the different types of cancer is beyond the scope of this text. However, this chapter provides a brief overview of important concepts involved in cancer treatment and reviews the therapies most commonly used. The chapter also presents important principles involved in monitoring patients receiving chemotherapy medication combinations and immunotherapy, and provides guidance in the adjustment of therapy sessions and modification of the rehabilitation environment to maintain patient safety and optimal outcomes. The chapter discusses using supportive medication therapies to manage side effects associated with radiation or chemotherapy such as nausea and vomiting, anemia, neutropenia, and mucositis. A section also discusses cancer-associated fatigue. The chapter explains how cancer and cancer treatment affect immune status and risk for infection and reviews signs and symptoms of neutropenia fever, a life-threatening complication of cancer treatment. Finally, the chapter discusses how cancer and its treatments can affect activities of daily living and the patient's ability to participate in rehabilitation as well as how supportive medications can improve the patient's quality of life.

16

Medications Used to Treat Infections

In clinical practice, the rehabilitation therapist will care for many patients who have infections. Infections can be caused by **bacteria**, **viruses**, **parasites**, **prions**, or **fungus**. This chapter introduces the terminology and concepts associated with diagnosis, treatment, and prevention of infections. In addition, the chapter discusses the treatment of bacterial infections frequently encountered in patients undergoing rehabilitative therapy, including urinary tract infections, skin and wound infections, bone and joint infections, pulmonary infections, and antibiotic-associated diarrhea, also called *Clostridium difficile* (*C. difficile*) diarrhea. This chapter also reviews important practices in infection control that are necessary for protecting patients and the rehabilitation therapist from the spread of infectious disease.

Classification of Bacteria

Bacteria are usually classified by their **morphology** (size and shape when viewed under the microscope) and by their staining characteristics when stain is added in the laboratory. Common classifications include gram positive (stain red), gram negative (do not stain), cocci (spherical in shape), and bacilli or rods (elongated in shape). The major classifications are gram-positive cocci, gram-negative cocci, gram-positive bacilli, and gram-negative bacilli. Bacteria are further classified by other laboratory testing methods and are classified by fermentation characteristics and whether they are aerobic (require oxygen for growth) or anaerobic (can grow without oxygen). Strict

aerobes require oxygen for growth, whereas oxygen rapidly kills anaerobes. Aerobes and anaerobes can survive in close proximity to each other. Facultative anaerobes can survive in both conditions by growing aerobically and then switching to anaerobic metabolism in the absence of oxygen. Anaerobic bacteria commonly cause formation of abscesses. Table 16.1 summarizes classifications of common bacteria.

Normal Protective Bacteria

The presence of bacteria does not constitute infection. The presence of bacteria without any inflammatory host reaction is termed colonization. Some bacteria normally found in different parts of the body, called normal flora, protect the host from being colonized by more pathogenic bacteria that are associated with more serious infections. In addition, normal flora such as bacteria in the gastrointestinal tract serve important functions in the processing of nutrients and maintaining immune function. When this normal flora is eliminated by the use of antibiotics, more pathogenic bacteria may take its place, increasing the risk for a secondary infection. An example of this is antibiotic-associated diarrhea (*C. difficile* diarrhea) that occurs when most of the bowel bacteria are killed, thus allowing overgrowth of *C. difficile* bacteria that produces a toxin and resultant diarrhea. Another example is vaginal tract infections that frequently occur after antibiotic use. The antibiotic kills the normal flora of the vaginal tract, allowing overgrowth of fungus in the vaginal tract and leading to associated

Table 16.1   Normal Location, Transmission, and Associated Infections of Common Bacteria

Class	Bacteria	Morphology	Oxygen requirements	Normal location	Method of transmission	Associated infections
Gram-positive cocci	*Staphylococcus* sp.	Cocci, grapelike clusters	Facultative anaerobic	Skin, nares	Direct contact, endogenous spread, aerosolized spread	Skin, soft-tissue, bone, or joint infections; endocarditis; food poisoning
	Streptococcus sp.	Cocci, pairs or chains	Facultative anaerobic	Oropharynx, skin	Direct contact, endogenous spread, aerosolized spread	Skin infection, **pharyngitis**, endocarditis, toxic shock syndrome
	Streptococcus pneumoniae (pneumococcus)	Diplococci, lancet-shaped	Facultative anaerobic	Oropharynx, sinus	Aerosolized spread	Pneumonia, otitis, sinusitis, meningitis
	Enterococcus	Cocci, pairs or chains	Facultative anaerobic	GI tract	Direct contact, endogenous spread	Urinary tract infection, GI tract infection, catheter-related infection
Gram-positive bacilli	*Clostridia*	Rods, spore forming	Anaerobic	GI tract, soil	Skin opening, ingestion, endogenous spread	Tetanus, antibiotic-associated diarrhea, gangrene, botulism
	Corynebacterium	Rods, non-spore-forming	Facultative anaerobic	Skin	Skin opening	Catheter-related infection, diphtheria
	Listeria	Rods, non-spore-forming	Facultative anaerobic	GI tract	Animals, food products, ingestion	Meningitis
	Lactobacillus (lactic acid bacteria that convert lactose to lactic acid)	Rods	Facultative anaerobic or microaerophilic	GI tract, vaginal tract	Endogenous spread	Protect normal function. Supplements can cause bacteremia in patients with compromised GI tract or sepsis.
	Actinomyces	Irregular, filamentous, sulfur granules	Anaerobic	GI tract	Endogenous spread	Skin and soft-tissue infections
Gram-negative cocci	*Neisseria*	Cocci, kidney bean-shaped	Microaerophilic	Pharynx, sex organs	Sexual contact, aerosolized spread	Meningitis, pelvic inflammatory disease, gonorrhea
	Haemophilus	Coccobacillary, pleomorphic	Facultative anaerobic	Respiratory tract	Endogenous spread, aerosolized spread	Respiratory infection, otitis, meningitis, sinusitis

› *continued*

Table 16.1   › continued

Class	Bacteria	Morphology	Oxygen requirements	Normal location	Method of transmission	Associated infections
Gram-negative rods	Enterobacteriaceae (*Escherichia coli, Klebsiella, Salmonella, Shigella*)	Rods	Facultative anaerobic	GI tract, vaginal tract	Endogenous spread, fecal–oral contact	Diarrhea, urinary tract infection, wound infection, food poisoning
	Bacteroides	Rods	Anaerobic	GI tract	Endogenous spread	Abscess, abdominal infection
	Pseudomonas	Rods	Aerobic	Water, soil	Endogenous spread, breach of protective barriers (e.g., skin, respiratory tract)	Infection in immuno-compromised hosts, wound infection, respiratory infection
	Vibria (Cholerae)	Rods, curved	Microaerophilic	Contaminated food or water	Ingestion	Diarrhea
	Campylobacter	Rods, curved	Microaerophilic	Contaminated food or water	Ingestion	Diarrhea, bacteremia
	Legionella	Rods, poorly stained	Microaerophilic	Contaminated water or air conditioner vents	Inhalation of aerosolized bacteria	Pneumonia

GI = gastrointestinal.

symptoms of itching and discomfort. Infection occurs when bacteria deposit and multiply in tissue and cause an associated inflammatory reaction in the host. Table 16.1 summarizes the normal flora found in the body that protects the host from colonization by pathogenic bacteria and risk of infection.

Antibiotic Resistance

Widespread and inappropriate use of antibiotics, such as in treatment of the common cold, has resulted in the development of more resistant bacteria (National Institute of Allergy and Infectious Disease, 2000). An important variable in the development of antimicrobial **resistance** is the ability of the infectious organism to adapt to new conditions. These **microbes** are generally unicellular and possess a small number of genes. A mutation of a single gene can influence their ability to produce disease. In addition, microbes can reproduce and evolve very rapidly. As a result, the mutation that allowed the microbe to survive the antibiotic can easily predominate. Microbes can also acquire genetic material called plasmids, which can be encoded for drug resistance.

Nosocomial Infections

Nosocomial infections are usually defined as infections that occur as a result of treatment in a health care facility. The incidence rate of nosocomial infections, which occur in 5% of all acute-care hospitalizations, is 5 infections/1,000 patient days. This equates to 2 million cases of health care-associated infections (HAIs)/yr. In the United States, HAIs are associated with doubled morbidity and mortality and cause 70,000 deaths annually. HAIs cost the U.S. health care system $4.5 billion/yr. Centers for Medicare and Medicaid Services will not reimburse for infections acquired in the hospital because any costs associated with these infections are preventable when appropriate infection-control practices are used (Centers for Medicare and Medicaid Services, 2011; Knox, 2009).

HAIs are caused by a number of **iatrogenic** risk factors, including pathogens on the hands of medical personnel, invasive procedures, and overuse of antibiotics. Patients at increased risk for development of a HAI include those with severe illness, those with prolonged hospital stays, and those who are immunocompromised due to their disease (e.g., diabetes, cancer) or the medications they are treated with (e.g., chemotherapy, steroids) (Gerberdin, 2002; Mylotte et al., 2000a).

Common HAIs include bloodstream infections (28% of HAIs; Raad & Maki, 2007), ventilator-associated pneumonia (21% of HAIs; Fine et al., 1997), urinary tract infections (15% of HAIs; Hershkovitz et al., 2002; Nicolle et al., 2005; Wu & Baguley, 2005), pneumonia (12% of HAIs; Houck et al., 2004; Schmitt, 2005), gastrointestinal infections such as *C. difficile* infection (10% of HAIs), skin and soft-tissue infections (10% of HAIs; Singhal, 2006), and surgical-site infections (7% of HAIs; Kingsley, 2001). Resistant pathogens that commonly cause HAIs include methicillin-resistant *Staphylococcus aureus* (*Staph. aureus*), vancomycin-resistant *Enterococcus*, *Acinetobacter baumannii*, and *C. difficile* (Centers for Medicare and Medicaid Services, 2011; Knox, 2009).

These infections can be transmitted through direct contact. For example, a clinician who touches a patient and then cares for another patient without washing her hands carries the bacteria from the first patient to the second. This common cause of infection inspired the "wash your hands" campaigns and the use of contact precautions in health care facilities (McGuicken et al., 2004). Indirect contact can also transmit infection. For example, a patient may use a piece of equipment that was not properly sanitized after an infected

patient used the equipment, thus coming into contact with the pathogen. Viral or bacterial pathogens can also be spread through airborne transmission. For example, an infected patient may sneeze or cough and another person may subsequently breathe the pathogen in. Patients should be taught and encouraged to use cough etiquette (i.e., covering the cough or sneeze and appropriately using disposable tissue) in order to reduce risk of transmission. In addition, certain infections that have a high likelihood of airborne transmission necessitate isolation of infected patients, use of droplet precautions, and use of face masks to protect patients and staff from infection. Patients with drug-resistant infections such as tuberculosis, methicillin-resistant *Staph. aureus*, and vancomycin-resistant *Enterococcus* must be isolated from other patients, and staff members should use appropriate personal protective equipment to reduce spread of the pathogen to other patients or staff (Haley et al., 1985). Equipment and the patient's room must be disinfected using special methods, termed infection control methods, in order to prevent the spread of these types of infection (Cameron, 2003; Mylotte et al., 2001). Infection control methods and concepts are further discussed at the end of this chapter.

Urinary Tract Infections

Urinary tract infections (UTIs), one of the most common bacterial infections, are the most common nosocomial infection diagnosed in patients in hospital or long-term care settings. Lower-tract infections include **cystitis**, **urethritis**, **prostatitis**, and **epididymitis**. Pyelonephritis is a UTI involving the kidneys and is classified as an upper-tract UTI (Howes, 2010; Inge, 2010; Petri, 2011).

Incidence

UTIs are common worldwide. Risk for developing a urinary tract infection is increased in the elderly population. A representative study of long-term care facilities in Ireland reported that more than 11% of all patients had signs and symptoms of infection. Approximately 35% of patients were over 85 yr of age. The most common infection (40%) was UTI (Cotter et al., 2012). UTIs, which are responsible for 8 million patient visits annually, occur at some point in life in 20% of females but less than 0.1% of males. Men experience UTIs more frequently as they get older, when prostate enlargement can result in obstruction and subsequent UTI. Catheter-associated UTIs make up 40% of nosocomial infections in the hospital setting and lead to 15% of nosocomial bacteremia (infection in the blood) in hospitalized patients. In 2008, Centers for Medicare and Medicaid Services stopped paying for the care of catheter-associated UTI, which can add anywhere from $800 to $2,800 to the cost of a hospital admission, because such infections are considered to be preventable. Hospitals and long-term facilities throughout the United States have implemented programs to prevent catheter-associated UTI (Howes, 2010; Inge, 2010; Petri, 2011).

Etiology and Pathophysiology

Uncomplicated UTIs occur when infection is not associated with or caused by an obstruction of the urinary tract. Complicated UTIs are associated with some type of obstruction, such as a kidney stone, prostatic hypertrophy, or indwelling catheter. Indwelling catheters are a risk factor for developing UTI and bacteremia associated with UTI. Therefore, current recommendations include the removal of urinary catheters as soon as possible and the use of condom catheters in males who require catheters. National patient safety guidelines require that health care professionals exert continuous efforts to remove indwelling urinary catheters as soon possible to reduce catheter-associated UTI and associated sepsis (Hooton et al., 2010; Howes, 2010; Inge, 2010; Petri, 2011).

UTIs are associated with the presence of significant amounts of bacteria in the urine and are associated with symptoms of **dysuria**, urgency, frequency, nocturia, and suprapubic heaviness. Gross hematuria may also be seen. Infection of the upper tract is associated with flank pain, costovertebral tenderness, abdominal pain, fever, nausea, vomiting, and malaise. Elderly patients with UTI often present with

altered mental status, change in eating habits, or gastrointestinal symptoms. Patients with indwelling catheters or neurologic disorders will not exhibit symptoms with lower-tract infection but will exhibit symptoms with upper-tract UTI. Symptoms of acute bacterial prostatitis include fever, urinary retention, urinary frequency, dysuria, nocturia, and perineal, sacral, or suprapubic pain. The prostate is swollen, tender, warm, and indurated in patients with acute bacterial prostatitis. Symptoms of chronic bacterial prostatitis include voiding difficulties, low-back pain, and perineal and suprapubic discomfort. However, many men with chronic prostatitis have no symptoms (Howes, 2010; Inge, 2010; Petri, 2011).

Diagnosis of UTI is made if a bacterial count of more than 100,000 bacteria/ml in the urine is accompanied by a white blood cell count of more than 10 white blood cells/mm^3 in the urine. **Hematuria** may or may not be present. Elevated protein counts in the urine are also common with UTI. Presence of numerous epithelial cells in the urine sample indicates that the sample was contaminated by the skin during collection. Clean-catch urine samples are frequently contaminated when urine hits the skin before collection. Therefore, use of the midstream method is more reliable. With this method, the urethral opening is cleaned, the initial 30 ml of urine is voided, and the sample of urine is then collected. Other more reliable methods of collecting urine samples include catheterization using aseptic technique or suprapubic bladder aspiration (Gupta et al., 2011; Hooton et al., 2010; Howes, 2010; Inge, 2010; Petri, 2011).

UTIs are most often caused by contamination of the urinary tract with fecal bacteria. UTIs are commonly associated with wiping from back to front in females or with sexual activity. The most common cause of UTI is the gram-negative bacterium *Escherichia coli* (*E. coli*), which is the bacterium most commonly found in the intestine. The prescriber usually selects and initiates antibiotics empirically rather than waiting for culture and sensitivity results for the bacteria isolated. Therapy is then altered if necessary once culture and sensitivity results are available. Patients with severe UTI or with infections caused by more resistant bacteria may need parenteral therapy with a combination of antibiotics such as an extended spectrum penicillin (e.g. piperacillin/tazobactam [Zosyn]) with an aminoglycoside (e.g. tobramycin). Table 16.2 summarizes empiric selection (initial selection before cul-

tures are available) of antibiotics for UTI as recommended by Infectious Diseases Society of America guidelines. Table 16.3 summarizes side effects and dosing of antibiotics commonly used to treat UTI (Gupta et al., 2011; Hooton et al., 2010; Howes, 2010; Inge, 2010; Petri, 2011).

Table 16.2   Empiric Treatment of Urinary Tract Infections (Presumptive Therapy Before Culture Results) as Recommended By Infectious Diseases Society of America

Diagnosis	Common pathogens	Treatment	Comments
Acute uncomplicated cystitis	*Escherichia coli, Staphylococcus saprophyticus*	Trimethoprim–sulfamethoxazole (Septra, Bactrim) 1 DS tablet every 12 h for 3 days. Ciprofloxacin (Cipro) 250-500 mg every 12 h for 3 days. Nitrofurantoin (Macrodantin) 100 mg every 12 h for 3 days.	3-day therapy more effective than single-dose therapy.
Lower-tract urinary tract infection in pregnancy	*Escherichia coli, Staphylococcus saprophyticus*	Amoxicillin–clavulanate (Augmentin) 500 mg every 12 h for 7 days. Cephalexin (Keflex) every 6 h for 7 days. Trimethoprim–sulfamethoxazole (Septra, Bactrim) 1 DS tablet every 12 h for 7 days.	Avoid trimethoprim–sulfamethoxazole in third trimester of pregnancy.
Recurrent urinary tract infections	*Escherichia coli, Staphylococcus saprophyticus*	Nitrofurantoin 50 mg once/day for 6 mo. Trimethoprim 100 mg once/day for 6 mo. Trimethoprim–sulfamethoxazole (Septra, Bactrim) 1 single-strength tablet/day for 6 mo.	Recurrent is defined as multiple symptomatic urinary tract infections. Use long-term prophylactic therapy (6 mo).
Acute pyelonephritis (uncomplicated)	*Escherichia coli*	Trimethoprim–sulfamethoxazole (Septra, Bactrim) 1 DS tablet every 12 h for 14 days. Ciprofloxacin (Cipro) 250-500 mg every 12 h for 14 days.	Can be treated as outpatient. (No obstruction.)
Acute pyelonephritis (complicated)	*Escherichia coli, Proteus mirabilis, Klebsiella pneumoniae, Pseudomonas aeruginosa, Enterococcus faecalis*	Ciprofloxacin (Cipro) 500 mg every 12 h for 14 days. Piperacillin–tazobactam (Zosyn) 3.375 mg IV every 6 h plus gentamicin IV for initial therapy.	If severe, may need IV therapy initially; can complete 14 days with oral therapy as outpatient (Associated with obstruction.)
Prostatitis	*Escherichia coli, Klebsiella pneumoniae, Proteus sp., Pseudomonas aeruginosa*	Trimethoprim–sulfamethoxazole (Septra, Bactrim) 1 DS tablet every 12 h for 4-6 wk. Ciprofloxacin (Cipro) 500 mg every 12 h for 4-6 wk.	Acute prostatitis may require IV therapy initially. Chronic prostatitis may require longer treatment or surgery.

DS = double strength; IV = intravenous.

See table 16.3 in the web resource for a full list of medication-specific indications, dosing recommendations, side effects, and other considerations.

Table 16.3 Treatment of Urinary Tract Infections Once Cultures are Available as Recommended by Infectious Diseases Society of America

Medication	Side effects affecting rehab							Other side effects or considerations
Sulfonamides: Most sulfonamides are no longer used because humans have developed resistance, but trimethoprim–sulfamethoxazole is effective against UTI caused by most aerobic enteric bacteria other than *Pseudomonas aeruginosa.*								
Trimethoprim–sulfamethoxazole (Bactrim, Septra)	Cog ++	S 0	A ++	Motor ++	D +	Com ++	F ++	Rash, allergy, folate deficiency, leukopenia, thrombocytopenia, hemolytic anemia with G6PD deficiency, elevated liver enzymes, Stevens-Johnson syndrome, tremors, nervousness, myoclonus, aseptic meningitis, ataxia, peripheral neuritis, insomnia, delirium, arthralgias, myalgias, hallucinations, depression, nervousness, acute psychosis, metabolic acidosis, hypoglycemia, hepatotoxicity, decreased creatinine clearance, renal failure, interstitial nephritis, crystalluria. Increases effect of warfarin (Coumadin). Decreases effects of oral contraceptives. Increases drug levels of amantadine, dapsone, digoxin, methotrexate, phenytoin (Dilantin), rifampin, and zidovudine (AZT). Decreases cyclosporine levels. Leukopenia with use of azathioprine; hyperkalemia with use of potassium-sparing diuretics; increased folate loss with use of methotrexate.
Quinolone antibiotics: Effective treatment for pyelonephritis and prostatitis.								
Ciprofloxacin (Cipro)	Cog +++	S 0	A ++	Motor +++	D +++	Com ++	F +++	Taste perversion, abnormal dreams, vision changes, confusion, behavior changes, hallucinations, speech disorders, arthralgias, myalgias, bone marrow suppression, dysphagia, glossitis, gastritis, nausea, vomiting, stomatitis, *Clostridium difficile* colitis, altered coordination and gait, exacerbation of myasthenia gravis, allergic reactions, liver dysfunction, renal dysfunction, drug fever, rash that can lead to Stevens-Johnson syndrome, headache, abdominal pain, pain in the feet and extremities, dizziness, insomnia, malaise, seizures, Achilles tendon rupture or tendinitis, increased risk of arrhythmia and cardiac arrest. Increases risk for QT prolongation, arrhythmia, and cardiac arrest. Increases effects of warfarin (Coumadin).
Levofloxacin (Levaquin)	Cog +++	S 0	A ++	Motor +++	D +++	Com ++	F +++	

Medication	Side effects affecting rehab							Other side effects or considerations
								Absorption is decreased when taken with aluminum, magnesium, antacids containing calcium, or iron or zinc supplements.
								Increased effects on the central nervous system when used with nonsteroidal anti-inflammatory drugs or probenecid.
								Increases levofloxacin levels.
								Avoid use in children and pregnant women; causes tooth discoloration and cartilage abnormalities.

Penicillins: Because 25% of *Escherichia coli* that cause UTI are resistant to amoxicillin, empiric use of Augmentin has replaced amoxicillin.

Medication	Cog	S	A	Motor	D	Com	F	Other side effects or considerations
Amoxicillin—clavulanic acid (Augmentin) Ampicillin–sulbactam (Unasyn) (IV)	+	+	+	++	++	+	+	Drug fever, rash, increased liver enzymes, nausea, vomiting, diarrhea, allergic reaction, *Clostridium difficile* colitis, bone marrow depression, dizziness, insomnia, confusion, agitation, convulsions, behavioral changes, serum sickness reactions, Stevens-Johnson skin reactions, tooth discoloration. More gastrointestinal upset and diarrhea with use of ampicillin–sulbactam than with use of amoxicillin. Increased rash when used with allopurinol.

Cephalosporin: First-generation cephalosporin useful for treatment of UTI. Effective against *Escherichia coli* (the most common cause of UTI) but does not cover *Enterococcus*.

Medication	Cog	S	A	Motor	D	Com	F	Other side effects or considerations
Cephalexin (Keflex)	+	+	+	+	++	+	+	Drug fever, rash, dyspepsia, gastritis, abdominal pain, allergic reactions, skin reactions, dizziness, hallucinations, fatigue, confusion, agitation, diarrhea, interstitial nephritis, bone marrow suppression. No drug interactions identified.

Urinary antiseptics

Medication	Cog	S	A	Motor	D	Com	F	Other side effects or considerations
Nitrofurantoin (Macrodantin)	0	0	0	++	+	0	++	Stomach upset, acute hypersensitivity reactions with pneumonitis (reversible), chronic irreversible reactions (chronic hepatitis, peripheral neuropathy, interstitial fibrosis of lung). Absorption is decreased when used with antacids containing aluminum, magnesium, or calcium. Probenecid can increase nitrofurantoin levels. Avoid use in pregnant women within 1-2 wk of delivery, nursing mothers, those with kidney disease, and those with creatinine clearance <30 ml/min.

› *continued*

Table 16.3 › *continued*

Medication	Side effects affecting rehab							Other side effects or considerations
Trimethoprim	Cog	S	A	Motor	D	Com	F	Folate deficiency, nausea, vomiting, glossitis, bone marrow depression, skin reactions.
	0	0	0	0	++	0	0	
								Increased leukopenia when used with azathioprine, nystagmus when used with phenytoin, hyperkalemia when used with potassium-sparing diuretics, and hyponatremia when used with thiazide diuretics.
								Increases levels of amantadine, dapsone, digoxin, methotrexate, phenytoin, rifampin, and zidovudine.
								Increases effects of warfarin (Coumadin).
								Low potential for allergic reaction.

Cog = cognition; S = sedation; A = agitation or mania; Motor = discoordination; D = dysphagia; Com = communication; F = falls; UTI = urinary tract infection; G6PD = glucose-6-phosphate dehydrogenase.

The likelihood rating scale for encountering the side effects is as follows: 0 = Almost no probability of encountering side effects. + = Little likelihood of encountering side effects. +/++ = Low probability of encountering side effects; however, probability increases with increased dosage. ++ = Medium likelihood of encountering side effects. +++ = High likelihood of encountering side effects, particularly with high doses. ++++ = Highest likelihood of encountering side effects; best to avoid in at-risk patients.

Rehabilitation Considerations

UTIs are commonly seen in the elderly patient because of increased risk of urinary retention and prostate enlargement in males leading to obstruction. UTIs are especially prevalent in patients with urinary catheters. Indwelling catheters are a risk factor for developing UTI and bacteremia associated with UTI. Therefore, urinary catheters should be removed as soon as possible and condom catheters should be used in males who require catheters. Symptoms of UTI that can interfere with therapy include nausea, vomiting, vertigo, and urinary urgency. Urinary urgency also places the patient at risk for falls. The rehabilitation therapist should be alert to any UTI symptoms the patient experiences and promptly notify the patient's physician of these symptoms in order to treat the UTI and prevent the development of more serious infections such as urosepsis (a serious infection in the blood resulting from a urinary tract infection) (Hooton et al., 2010; Howes, 2010; Inge, 2010; Petri, 2011).

Medication Therapy

The medication therapy used to treat UTI depends on the patient's age and associated risk factors such as concurrent disease. Common empiric therapy is used to cover the most common cause of UTI: gram-negative bacteria and *E. coli* in particular because it is the most common bacteria in the colon and rectal area. More resistant pathogens include fungi (25%) and *Enterococcus* (10%). *Enterococcus* is a sphere-shaped (cocci), gram-positive bacterium that is part of the normal flora of the colon. The widespread use of vancomycin has resulted in the emergence of vancomycin-resistant *Enterococcus* (VRE). Up to 28% of *Enterococcus* is now vancomycin resistant (Knox, 2009). VRE is spread person to person and through contaminated surfaces. VRE can live on surfaces for up to 1 wk and can be easily washed off the hands and killed with hospital disinfectant. Table 16.3 summarizes antibiotics commonly used to treat UTI (Duerden et al., 1997; Howes, 2010; Inge, 2010; Knox, 2009; Petri, 2011).

PATIENT CASE 1

B.A. is an 83-yr-old female who was admitted to the hospital from the nursing home with impaired speech and weakness on the right side. She was diagnosed with acute cerebral vascular accident (CVA). On day 5 of admission she spikes a fever to 101 °F and the urine in her Foley bag is dark and has a foul odor. Laboratory test results are as follows: urine culture (obtained from her Foley) is pending, gram stain shows many gram-negative bacilli and multiple white blood cells, and two sets of blood cultures are pending.

Question

What risk factors for a UTI does B.A. have?

Answer

The presence of the Foley catheter, B.A.'s age and sex, and the neurological impairment from the CVA are all risk factors for a UTI.

Question

What likely pathogen should treatment cover?

Answer

The most common pathogens for UTI are gram-negative enteric bacteria (50%) and *E. coli*.

Question

What is an appropriate empiric regimen of treatment for B.A. until culture results are available?

Answer

If B.A. is not currently on antibiotic therapy, an antibiotic that covers *E. coli* would be a good choice. Because of her age and the possibility of renal dysfunction, a low-dose quinolone antibiotic such as Cipro 250 mg twice/day would be a good initial choice.

Question

What measures should be recommended to reduce B.A.'s risk of infection?

Answer

The most effective way to reduce B.A.'s risk of infection is to remove her Foley catheter. Nursing should discuss with B.A.'s physician whether the Foley is still needed or whether it can be removed.

Skin and Soft-Tissue Infections

Infections of the skin and soft tissues are commonly seen in hospital and community settings, and the rehabilitation specialist will often encounter patients with these infections. Recently, health care institutions have seen an increasing number of isolates of methicillin-resistant *Staph. aureus* (MRSA). **MRSA** is a leading cause of nosocomial infections and community-acquired infections and is the second leading cause of nosocomial infections in the elderly. MRSA is spread through person-to-person contact or contamination of environmental surfaces. Appropriate hand washing with **antibacterial** soap can easily remove this pathogen from the hands. All health care professionals should wash hands before and after eating, after using the restroom, before and after coming into contact with a patient or patient equipment, before and after handling medications, and when entering and leaving a patient's room or patient-care area. When washing the hands, one should wet both hands with warm water, apply a bactericidal soap, rub the front and back of the hands from the fingertips up to the wrists for at least 20 s, rinse the hands with warm water, dry both hands with a clean paper towel, and discard the paper towel. Some strains of MRSA have developed intermediate or high resistance to vancomycin, which has been the standard IV antibiotic used to treat MRSA for the past 30 yr. Such resistance mandates the use of more expensive antibiotics, which adds cost burden to the health care system (Alzen et al., 2007; Knox, 2009; Pailaud et al., 2005; Stevens et al., 2005).

Most MRSA strains isolated from patients with community-acquired MRSA infections have been microbiologically distinct from those endemic in health care settings, suggesting that some of these strains may have developed in the community due to resistance developed by methicillin-susceptible *Staph. aureus* strains. Community-acquired MRSA infection most commonly presents as relatively minor skin and soft-tissue infections, but if left untreated it may develop into severe, invasive disease such as pneumonia, necrotizing fasciitis, severe osteomyelitis, or sepsis. Colonization with MRSA can be prolonged, and patients who are initially cleared of MRSA after decolonization therapy have reported a high frequency of subsequent recolonization. Several regimens have successfully been used to decolonize patients carrying MRSA in their nares; these include topical mupirocin alone or in combination with orally administered antibiotics (e.g., rifampin in combination with trimethoprim–sulfamethoxazole or ciprofloxacin) plus the use of an antimicrobial soap for bathing. A 5-day regimen of baths with chlorhexidine soap and nasal therapy with mupirocin is commonly used to reduce colonization of MRSA. All health care workers should follow strict contact precautions for preventing the spread of MRSA infection to other areas of the body or other persons. These precautions include washing their hands after coming in contact with a lesion and immediately washing any clothing or washcloths that come in contact with the lesion or drainage from the lesion. All health care workers should use contact precautions indefinitely when providing treatment for previously infected and known colonized patients in view of the common problem of recolonization (Liu, 2011; Stevens et al., 2005).

Recently, incidence of community-associated, methicillin-resistant staphylococcal skin infections has increased. These infections can be difficult to eradicate. Community-associated MRSA infections can be treated with oral clindamycin, minocycline, or trimethoprim–sulfamethoxazole for 7 to 10 days. Clindamycin is the agent of choice for pregnant females who have a suspected community-acquired MRSA skin infection. Oral linezolid (Zyvox) may be used to treat infections that do not respond to these antibiotics; however, it is very expensive (Liu, 2011; Stevens et al., 2005).

Incidence

The incidence of MRSA has increased dramatically worldwide. However, incidence of MRSA varies widely among countries. For example, the prevalence of MRSA in the United States, Southern European countries, and Japan is between 20% and 60%, whereas the incidence of MRSA in Scandinavian countries and the Netherlands is less than 5%. In the past decade, the prevalence of MRSA in Germany has dramatically increased from less than 2% to more than 20%. MRSA is clearly a global health care problem (Hain & Hain, 2012).

Etiology and Pathophysiology

The skin is a very effective barrier that serves as a primary defense against bacterial infections. The skin comprises the epidermis, the dermis (directly under the epidermis), and the subcutaneous fat layer (just under the dermis). Beneath the subcutaneous layer is the fascia, which separates the skin from underlying muscle, and the deep fascia, which forms sheets for the muscle. The skin and subcutaneous tissues are normally very resistant to infection. Skin is relatively dry, the epidermis is continually replaced via shedding of the outer layer along with any bacteria, and secretions by the sebaceous glands inhibit bacterial and fungal growth. Skin infection usually occurs when bacterial concentration is increased on the skin, the skin remains wet, blood supply to the skin is reduced, or skin damage allows bacterial penetration. Common types of skin infection include folliculitis, **furuncles** and **carbuncles**, cellulitis, diabetic wound infections, pressure sores, and surgical wound infections.

Folliculitis, Furuncles, and Carbuncles

Folliculitis is a superficial infection surrounding the hair follicles. Pruritic erythematous papules occur within 48 h of contact with the pathogenic bacteria and evolve into pustules that form a head in several days. Folliculitis caused by gram positive organisms such as staphylococcus or streptococcus is treated with warm saline compresses and topical antibiotics such as mupirocin (Bactroban), clindamycin, or erythromycin. Furuncles and carbuncles can be treated with moist heat to promote drainage and an oral antibiotic such as dicloxacillin, clindamycin, or erythromycin for 7 to 10 days. Folliculitis caused by *Pseudomonas*, a gram negative bacterium found in water and soil, can be associated with inadequate chlorination of whirlpools or hot tubs (Danziger et al., 2002; Stevens et al., 2005).

Furuncles or boils, which are extensions of folliculitis that extend into the dermis, commonly occur where the skin is subject to moisture or friction. These lesions usually drain spontaneously; however, surgical drainage may be required in lesions that do not drain spontaneously. Carbuncles are several boils that coalesce and extend to the subcutaneous tissue. These lesions are commonly associated with chills, fever, and malaise. Infection can spread to the bloodstream, which may require IV treatment with antibiotics such as vancomycin or linezolid (Zyvox) if it is caused by MRSA (Danziger et al., 2002; Stevens et al., 2005).

Lymphangitis

Lymphangitis, which is the inflammation of subcutaneous lymphatic channels, is usually caused by the spread of group A streptococcal infection from puncture wounds or other skin infections. This gram positive infection is characterized by fever, chills, malaise, headache, and leukocytosis. Treatment includes initial therapy with IV penicillin G for 3 days followed by oral penicillin VK to complete 10 days of antibiotics (Danziger et al., 2002; Stevens et al., 2005).

Cellulitis

Cellulitis is an infection of the epidermis and dermis that may spread to the superficial fascia. Cellulitis does not involve necrosis or formation of pustules. The affected area is hot, painful, and not elevated and has poorly defined margins; tenderness and lymphadenopathy at the infected site can also occur. Cellulitis is usually caused by trauma, abrasion, ulceration, or surgery. Because the lymphatic system is involved, cellulitis can spread to the blood and result in bacteremia. Bacteremia occurs in 30% of cases of cellulitis. Cellulitis can also cause local abscess, osteomyelitis (infection of the bone), or septic arthritis. Cellulitis of the lower extremities can cause thrombophlebitis (painful inflammation of the blood vessels). The most common causes of cellulitis are gram positive pathogens such as group A *Streptococcus* (*Streptococcus pyogenes*) and *Staphylococcus. aureus*. Obtaining cultures of the surface of intact skin associated with cellulitis is not helpful and may lead to inappropriate treatment of colonizing bacteria that are not the cause of the infection. Diabetics and other immunocompromised patients frequently are colonized with more pathogenic bacteria on the skin, such as gram-negative bacteria, and may develop cellulitis with a mixture of aerobic and anaerobic bacteria that can include gram-negative organisms. Infection that involves a mixture of types of bacteria (e.g., diabetic foot infection) may require treatment with antibiotics that are broader in spectrum than those used to treat most cases of cellulitis caused by the skin bacteria *Staphylococcus* and *Streptococcus* (Danziger et al., 2002; Stevens et al., 2005).

Necrotizing Skin Infections

Necrotizing soft-tissue infections include necrotizing fasciitis and clostridial myonecrosis (gas gangrene). Type I necrotizing fasciitis most often occurs in patients who recently underwent surgery that involved cutting through the bowel. Anaerobic bacteria may be involved in cellulitis in these patients, who may develop gas formation under the skin (termed crepitus) that may progress to gangrene. This type of infection is usually caused by a mixture of anaerobes such as *Bacteroides* or *Peptostreptococcus* and facultative bacteria (*Streptococcus* and other Enterobacteriaceae) that act synergistically to damage the fat and fascia of the skin. Common sites of this type of infection include the perineum, abdomen, and lower extremities. Expeditious surgical drainage, excision of necrotic tissue, and administration of appropriate IV antibiotics and supportive care is required for healing and preserving the surrounding tissue (Danziger et al., 2002; Stevens et al., 2005).

Type II necrotizing **fasciitis**, which is caused by virulent strains of *Streptococcus pyogenes*, is a rapidly progressing necrosis of the subcutaneous tissue and skin accompanied by **gangrene** and severe pain at the site. The infection spreads to the blood, resulting in shock and organ failure that can be fatal. Type II necrotizing fasciitis has symptoms that are similar to those of cellulitis but is also accompanied by bullae filled with clear liquid, fever, chills, and leukocytosis. The skin becomes maroon or violet after several days. Rapid diagnosis and intervention are required to prevent serious complications that can include death in 20% to 50% of patients affected. The rehabilitation specialist can help by rapidly referring to the emergency room any patient with skin lesions that are consistent with necrotizing fasciitis. Antibiotics used to treat necrotizing fasciitis can include high-dose IV penicillin, which can be combined with IV clindamycin to cover (kill) the Clostridia (Danziger et al., 2002; Stevens et al., 2005).

Stages of Wound Healing

Wounds occur when the integrity of the skin is compromised. Wound healing consists of four phases: the inflammatory phase, the proliferative phase, the epithelial resurfacing phase, and the maturation phase. The inflammatory phase lasts from the time of injury to day 4 to 6 after the injury. In this phase, vascular and cell responses include vasoconstriction at the site of injury along with deposition of fibrin–platelet clots and dilation of small venules. Antibodies, proteins, fluids, white blood cells, and red blood cells leave the microcirculation to permeate the affected area, which causes edema, redness, warmth, and pain, and neutrophils and monocytes enter for **phagocytosis**. The proliferative phase lasts for 2 to 21 days. Fibroblasts (connective tissue cells) multiply and migrate along fibrin strands that may serve as a matrix. New capillaries form and penetrate and nourish the injured tissue. Granulation tissue, which is the combination of budding capillaries and proliferating fibroblasts, forms during this phase. Active collagen synthesis by fibroblasts begins by day 5 to 7, and the wound gains tensile strength. Epithelial resurfacing occurs within 72 h of injury. During this phase the skin is impenetrable to bacteria but tensile strength is limited. The maturation phase begins on day 21 and lasts for months or years. During this phase, collagen fiber undergoes lysis and regeneration and becomes more organized, aligns more closely, and increases the tensile strength. Initially the scar is red, raised, hard and immature, and molds into a flat, soft, and pale mature scar. Scar tissue never achieves greater than 80% of preinjury strength (Bennett & Schultz, 1993; Bryant, 2003; Eaglstein, 1990).

Healthy wound healing is indicated by the presence of a healing ridge in which collagen deposition begins in the inflammatory phase (at time of injury) and peaks in the proliferative phase. If no ridge forms, the risk of wound dehiscence is increased. Induration (hardness) is noted beneath skin extending out 1 cm to each side of the wound and can be noted directly below the suture line on day 5 to 9 postoperatively (Bennett & Schultz, 1993; Bryant, 2003; Eaglstein, 1990).

Wound Care

The goal of wound care is to maintain a clean, moist wound bed. Meticulous care of a wound can prevent complications such as wound infections, osteomyelitis, and reduce the need for surgical removal of infected tissue. Complications can be prevented by debriding tissues via mechanical methods such as wet-to-dry dressings and wound irrigation, surgically removing dead tissue, using chemical enzymes, or **autolysis** using bio-occlusive dressings. Dressings protect the wound from trauma, maintain moisture, and act as a barrier against microorganisms and foreign matter and can help relieve pain and control odor. Dressings can be used to fill any dead space in the wound, control exudate, and prevent skin **maceration**. Gauze dressings are absorbent and can aid in the removal of necrotic tissue. Occlusive dressings can provide a moist wound bed, which facilitates proliferation and migration of epithelial cells, but can contribute to maceration. Hydrocolloid dressings adhere to dry and moist surfaces and form a gel, are waterproof, and stay in place for several days. Hydrogel dressings can be more than 90% water, are cooling, and maintain a moist wound bed. Absorptive dressing, which can include gels, powders, beads, granules, and pastes, should be used with heavy **exudates** (Bennett & Schultz, 1993; Bryant, 2003; Ciccone, 2007).

Factors that impair wound healing include poor nutrition and reduced supply of oxygen to the wound. Malnourished patients are at greater risk of postoperative morbidity and mortality. Members of the health care team should assess the patient's nutrition status and enlist the assistance of a clinical dietitian to develop a nutrition plan before and after surgery. Inadequate food intake over the week before surgery can impair wound healing response. Stress response can increase levels of epinephrine, glucagon, cortisol, and growth hormone. This can lead to decreases in circulating insulin, increases in circulating glucose, and vasoconstriction along with decreased perfusion of tissues, which can all impair wound healing. Inadequate oxygenation, which can be caused by pain, cold, fear, stress response with vasoconstriction, or the use of vasoconstricting medications such a intravenous epinephrine or dopamine or narcotics can also impair wound healing. Decreased tissue oxygenation causes decreases in collagen formation, new vessel formation, and epithelial formation by fibroblasts, resulting in decreased tissue tensile strength and increased potential for infection (Bennett & Schultz, 1993; Bryant, 2003).

Rehabilitation Considerations

The rehabilitation specialist commonly encounters wound infections in patients receiving care. Wounds can be classified as acute (occurring within the past month) or chronic (lasting for more than 30 days). Common types of wounds are arterial wounds, venous wounds, surgical wounds, pressure ulcers, and wounds associated with diabetic nephropathy (e.g., diabetic foot wounds). Wound contamination is defined as the presence of bacteria in a wound without an accompanying host reaction. Microorganisms can gain access to a wound through direct contact (e.g., transfer from equipment or the hands of caregivers), airborne dispersal, and self-contamination (i.e., the bacteria physically migrates from the patient's skin or gastrointestinal tract to another area). The classic signs of infection include localized erythema, pain, heat, cellulitis, and edema (Cameron, 2003).

Other symptoms of infection include abscess, discharge (may be viscous, discolored, and purulent), delayed healing, discoloration of tissues both in and at the wound margins, friability and bleeding of granulation tissue despite gentle handling, and unexpected pain or tenderness either at the time of dressing change or as reported by the patient. Infection can also be suspected when the wound smells abnormal or when wound breakdown associated with wound pocketing or bridging at base of wound (i.e., the wound develops strips of granulation tissue instead of a uniform spread across the whole of the wound bed) occurs.

The prescriber chooses an antibiotic treatment for surgical wound infections based on cultures from deep in the wound, wound biopsy or exudates, and sensitivity results that indicate which antibiotics effectively treat the causative organism. Swabbing the surface of a wound may provide unreliable cultures that may lead to inappropriately treating the organisms colonizing the wound surface rather than the causative bacteria. Common types of wound infections include infections of surgical, vascular, and arterial wounds and diabetic foot infections. The following sections discuss treatment of these wound infections.

Medication Therapy

Appropriate wound care may be limited to cleaning and dressing the wound as outlined in the previous sections and ensuring appropriate nutritional support. If the wound becomes infected, the site of the infection generally determines which antibiotic is used. Empiric treatment of wound infections of the skin includes an antibiotic that covers **Staphylococcus** and **Streptococcus**. More complex wounds that involve mucous membranes or abscess necessitate the addition of antibiotics that cover anaerobes, whereas wounds in proximity to the bowel necessitate the coverage of gram-negative bacteria. Once appropriate culture results are known, antibiotic therapy is geared toward treating the bacteria causing the infection. Table 16.4 summarizes antibiotics commonly used to treat skin and soft-tissue infections (Danziger et al., 2002; Stevens et al., 2005).

Surgical Wound Infections

The rehabilitation therapist will provide therapy for many patients who develop wound infections after surgery. Centers for Medicare and Medicaid Services (CMS) has developed guidelines, known as the Surgical Care Improvement Project, to help minimize

See table 16.4 in the web resource for a full list of medication-specific indications, dosing recommendations, and side effects.

Table 16.4   Antibiotic Treatment of Skin and Soft-Tissue Infections as Recommended by Infectious Diseases Society of America

Medication	Side effects affecting rehab							Other side effects or considerations
Penicillins: Penicillin is the drug of choice for *Streptococcus pyogenes* infection. Amoxicillin–clavulanate is an extended-spectrum aminopenicillin that covers *Staphylococcus* (not MRSA), *Streptococcus*, and anaerobes. Ampicillin–sulbactam is a broad-spectrum aminopenicillin that has activity against gram-positive, gram-negative, and anaerobic bacteria except MRSA and *Pseudomonas*.								
Penicillin	Cog +	S +	A +	Motor ++	D ++	Com +	F ++	Drug fever, rash, increased liver enzymes, nausea, vomiting, diarrhea, allergic reaction, *Clostridium difficile* colitis, bone marrow depression, dizziness, insomnia, confusion, agitation, convulsions, behavioral changes, serum sickness reactions, Stevens-Johnson skin reactions, tooth discoloration.
Amoxicillin–clavulanate (Augmentin)	Cog +	S +	A +	Motor ++	D ++	Com +	F +	
Ampicillin–sulbactam (Unasyn)	Cog +	S +	A +	Motor ++	D ++	Com +	F +	Probenecid increases levels. Increased rash when used with allopurinol.
First-generation cephalosporins: Cover *Staphylococcus, Streptococcus*, and some *Escherichia coli*.								
Cefazolin (Ancef)	Cog +	S +	A +	Motor ++	D ++	Com +	F +	Drug fever, rash, dyspepsia, gastritis, abdominal pain, allergic reactions, skin reactions, dizziness, hallucinations, fatigue, confusion, agitation, diarrhea, interstitial nephritis, bone marrow suppression.
Cephalexin (Keflex)	Cog +	S +	A +	Motor ++	D ++	Com +	F +	Additional side effect of cephalexin: Seizures when dose is not adjusted for renal insufficiency. No identified drug interactions.
Second-generation cephalosporin: Covers anaerobic bacteria, including *Bacteroides fragilis*, and many enteric gram-negative bacteria (not *Pseudomonas*).								
Cefoxitin (Mefoxin)	Cog +	S +	A +	Motor ++	D ++	Com +	F +	Thrombophlebitis at injection site, rash, allergic reaction, diarrhea, *Clostridium difficile* colitis, hypotension, exacerbation of myasthenia gravis, bone marrow suppression, hepatotoxicity, seizures when dose is not adjusted for renal insufficiency. No identified drug interactions.
Third-generation cephalosporins: Third-generation parenteral cephalosporin used to treat gram-negative bacteria other than the more resistant *Klebsiella* and *Pseudomonas acinetobacter*. Ceftriaxone is injectable; other agents are oral.								
Ceftriaxone (Rocephin)	Cog +	S +	A +	Motor ++	D ++	Com +	F +	Thrombophlebitis at injection site, rash, allergic reaction, diarrhea, *Clostridium difficile* colitis, hypotension, bone marrow suppression, nausea, vomiting, stomatitis, glossitis, hepatotoxicity, seizures when dose is not adjusted for renal insufficiency. Ceftriaxone does not need to be adjusted for renal insufficiency; it is eliminated in the bile and can cause biliary sludging leading to obstruction.
Cefpodoxime (Vantin)	Cog +	S +	A +	Motor ++	D ++	Com +	F +	
Cefprozil (Cefzil)	Cog +	S +	A +	Motor ++	D ++	Com +	F +	
Ceftibuten (Cedax)	Cog +	S +	A +	Motor ++	D ++	Com +	F +	No identified drug interactions.

Medication	Side effects affecting rehab							Other side effects or considerations
Third- and fourth-generation cephalosporins effective against *Pseudomonas*: Used to treat all gram-negative bacteria such as *Escherichia coli*, *Proteus*, *Klebsiella*, *Haemophilus*, and *Moraxella*; excellent coverage of *Pseudomonas*. Azactam is safe to use in most patients with penicillin allergy.								
Ceftazidime (Fortaz)	Cog +	S +	A +	Motor ++	D ++	Com +	F +	Thrombophlebitis at injection site, rash, allergic reaction, diarrhea, *Clostridium difficile* colitis, hypotension, bone marrow suppression, nausea hepatotoxicity, seizures when dose is not adjusted for renal insufficiency.
Aztreonam (Azactam)	Cog +	S +	A +	Motor ++	D ++	Com +	F +	
Cefepime (Maxipime)	Cog +	S +	A +	Motor ++	D ++	Com +	F +	No identified drug interactions.
Carbapenems without activity against *Pseudomonas*: Active against gram-positive bacteria (not MRSA), anaerobes, and gram-negative bacteria (not *Pseudomonas*).								
Ertapenem (Invanz)	Cog +	S +	A +	Motor ++	D +	Com +	F +	Thrombophlebitis at injection site, rash, allergic reaction, diarrhea, *Clostridium difficile* colitis, hypotension, bone marrow suppression, nausea, headache, hepatotoxicity, tremors, stiff muscles, seizures. Increases levels of antibiotic when combined with probenecid. Useful in outpatient treatment of diabetic foot and other polymicrobial infections with once/day dosing.
Carbapenems with activity against *Pseudomonas*: Active against gram-positive bacteria (not MRSA), anaerobes, and gram-negative bacteria, including *Pseudomonas*. Carbapenems are the agents of choice against *Acinetobacter* and resistant *Klebsiella*.								
Imipenem–cilastatin (Primaxin)	Cog +	S +	A +	Motor +++	D ++	Com +	F ++	Increased risk of seizures especially if dose not decreased with renal insufficiency (imipenem–cilastatin has the highest risk of seizures), somnolence, confusion, dizziness, abdominal pain, glossitis, tremor, paresthesias, heartburn, pharyngeal pain, bone marrow suppression.
Meropenem (Merrem)	Cog +	S +	A +	Motor ++	D +	Com +	F ++	Increases cyclosporine levels.
Doripenem (Doribax)	Cog +	S +	A +	Motor ++	D +	Com +	F ++	Ganciclovir increases risk of seizures. Probenecid increases levels.
Agents with anaerobic activity: Clindamycin is used to treat gram-positive organisms (not MRSA), anaerobes, and gram-negative bacteria such as *Escherichia coli*. Metronidazole, which is the most effective agent against anaerobic infection, works in an anaerobic environment; oral and IV therapies provide similar blood levels and effects.								
Clindamycin (Cleocin)	Cog 0	S 0	A 0	Motor ++	D +++	Com +	F ++	Diarrhea (occurs in 20% of treated patients), nausea, vomiting, esophagitis, dry mouth, taste perversion, rash, heart block with rapid IV administration, hypotension, hepatotoxicity, neuromuscular blockade, rash that can be severe (Stevens-Johnson) in rare instances. Increases muscle paralysis and apnea when used with neuromuscular relaxant and neuromuscular blockers. Kaolin decreases oral absorption of clindamycin.

› continued

Table 16.4 › *continued*

Medication	Side effects affecting rehab							Other side effects or considerations
Clindamycin (Cleocin) *(continued)*								Clindamycin increases theophylline levels and risk of seizures. *Clostridium difficile* diarrhea more common with oral administration than with IV administration.
Metronidazole (Flagyl)	Cog +	S +	A 0	Motor ++	D +++	Com +	F +	Nausea, vomiting, gastrointestinal upset, metallic taste, aseptic meningitis, encephalitis, seizures, brown discoloration of urine. Disulfiram (Antabuse) reaction occurs when used with alcohol. Increases INR when used with warfarin (Coumadin). Phenobarbital and phenytoin increase metabolism and decrease levels and effects.

Aminoglycosides: Bactericidal antibiotics that are highly effective against serious gram-negative pathogens, including *Pseudomonas.*

Medication								Other side effects or considerations
Gentamicin (Garamycin)	Cog 0	S 0	A 0	Motor ++	D 0	Com +	F ++	Neuromuscular blockade with rapid administration, nephrotoxicity, ototoxicity, vestibular toxicity, dizziness, vertigo, ataxia, peripheral neuropathy, encephalopathy, lethargy, confusion, worsened myasthenia gravis, hypomagnesemia, hypocalcemia, hypokalemia that can result in muscle weakness, tetany, respiratory depression, joint pain, hypotension, bone marrow suppression, rash, pyrogenic reaction to initial high-dose therapy with fever, shaking, chills, rigors, tachycardia.
Tobramycin (Nebcin, Tobi)	Cog 0	S 0	A 0	Motor ++	D 0	Com +	F ++	
Amikacin	Cog 0	S 0	A 0	Motor ++	D 0	Com +	F ++	Increased nephrotoxicity when used with amphotericin B, cyclosporine (Sandimmune), NSAIDs such as ibuprofen (Motrin), polymyxin B, radiographic contrast dye, vancomycin, or cisplatin (Platinol). Increased ototoxicity when used with loop diuretics such as furosemide (Lasix). Increases neuromuscular blockade with neuromuscular blockers used in anesthesia.

Agents active against MRSA: Used to treat infections caused by MRSA or MRSE. Linezolid and daptomycin are also effective against vancomycin-resistant *Enterococcus.* Tigecycline, a bacteriostatic synthetic derivative of tetracycline, is indicated for complicated infections of the skin and soft tissue.

Medication								Other side effects or considerations
Vancomycin	Cog 0	S 0	A 0	Motor +	D +	Com 0	F +	Red man syndrome (wheezing, dyspnea, upper-body rash, hypotension) with rapid infusion, thrombophlebitis, leukopenia, thrombocytopenia, hypotension, nephrotoxicity (especially when dose is not adjusted in patients with renal impairment or when used with other nephrotoxins), ototoxicity (hearing loss, vertigo, tinnitus) associated with high doses or concurrent use of other ototoxic medications, phlebitis at the site of the infusion, rare instances of rash with exfoliative dermatitis (Stevens-Johnson reaction or TENS).

Medication	Side effects affecting rehab							Other side effects or considerations
								Increased nephrotoxicity when used with amphotericin B, aminoglycosides (e.g., gentamicin, tobramycin or amikacin), polymyxin B, cisplatin (Platinol), or radiographic contrast dye.
Daptomycin (Cubicin)	Cog ++	S ++	A +	Motor ++	D ++	Com +	F ++	Constipation, somnolence, nausea, headache, diarrhea, vomiting, abdominal pain, dry mouth, stomatitis, jitteriness, rigors, taste disturbances, fatigue, eosinophilic pneumonia, dyspnea, rash, pruritus, paresthesias, peripheral neuropathy, hallucinations, anxiety, insomnia, confusion, worsening of renal function, decreases in electrolyte levels of potassium, phosphorus, and magnesium. Increased CPK; monitor for muscle pain and weakness; check CPK weekly. Suspend use of statins during use. False positive increase in INR when used with warfarin (Coumadin).
Linezolid (Zyvox)	Cog ++	S ++	A +	Motor ++	D ++	Com +	F ++	Serotonin syndrome, seizures, drowsiness, confusion, lactic acidosis, thrombocytopenia, anemia, leukopenia, peripheral neuropathy, diarrhea, headache, nausea, optic neuropathy that can progress to blindness, myelosuppression, tooth and tongue discoloration. Pseudoephedrine, foods containing tyramine, and serotonergic agents (selective serotonin reuptake inhibitors and tricyclic antidepressants) can increase risk of serotonin syndrome. Monitor visual function and CBC if taken for more than 2 wk.
Telavancin (Vibativ)	Cog +	S 0	A 0	Motor ++	D ++	Com 0	F ++	Nausea, vomiting, diarrhea, taste disturbances, dizziness, foamy urine, renal impairment, cardiac events, respiratory events, arrhythmias associated with QT prolongation. Avoid using with other medications known to prolong QT interval; causes cardiac arrhythmias.
Tigecycline (Tygacil)	Cog +	S +	A +	Motor +	D ++	Com +	F +	Nausea (35%), vomiting (20%), dyspepsia, pancreatitis, anorexia, diarrhea, taste disturbance, headache, dizziness, insomnia, somnolence, rash, hepatotoxicity (rare). May decrease effectiveness of oral contraceptives.

Cog = cognition; S = sedation; A = agitation or mania; Motor = discoordination; D = dysphagia; Com = communication; F = falls; IV = intravenous; MRSA = methicillin-resistant *Staphylococcus aureus*; NSAID = nonsteroidal anti-inflammatory drug; INR = international normalized ratio; TENS = toxic epidermal necrolysis; CPK = creatine phosphokinase; CBC = complete blood count; MRSE = methicillin–resistant *Staphylococcus epidermidis*.

The likelihood rating scale for encountering the side effects is as follows: 0 = Almost no probability of encountering side effects. + = Little likelihood of encountering side effects. +/++ = Low probability of encountering side effects; however, probability increases with increased dosage. ++ = Medium likelihood of encountering side effects. +++ = High likelihood of encountering side effects, particularly with high doses. ++++ = Highest likelihood of encountering side effects; best to avoid in at-risk patients.

infections, thrombus formation, and cardiac complications after surgery (Centers for Medicare and Medicaid Services, 2011).

Incidence

The incidence of surgical sites infections (SSIs) varies widely among countries. One Peruvian hospital reported an SSI incidence of 26.7%. The same study noted an SSI incidence of 9.7% in Mexico, 8.7% in Brazil, and 12% in Bolivia. Statistics show an SSI incidence of 21% in Spain and 22% in Vietnam (Hernandez et al., 2005). In the United States, SSIs occur in 2% to 5% of patients undergoing inpatient surgery, or approximately 500,000 patients/yr. Each patient with an SSI is hospitalized for an average of approximately 7 to 10 days post-surgery (Shuman et al., 2012).

Etiology and Pathophysiology

An estimated 40% to 60% of SSIs are preventable and many are associated with improper use of antibiotics (i.e., overuse, underuse, misuse, and improper timing) that occurs in 25% to 50% of surgeries. Risk factors for infection associated with surgery include failure to use appropriate aseptic technique during preparation for surgery or during surgery, shaving the surgical site, and failing to maintain adequate glucose control, warmth, and oxygenation in the patient during surgery. Patients with cardiac disease should receive beta blockers to control heart rate and insulin therapy to control glucose during surgery (Bratzler et al., 2005; Estrada et al., 2003; Stevens et al., 2005).

Rehabilitation Considerations

The rehabilitation therapist should ensure that appropriate wound care and an appropriate nutritional plan are initiated. The therapist may need to alter therapy sessions to prevent disrupting or damaging the wound dressings and to ensure the correct positioning of the patient is maintained to prevent further damage to the wound. At the beginning of each therapy session, the rehabilitation therapist should assess any wounds and determine whether healing is progressing appropriately. The therapist should promptly communicate to the patient's wound care practitioner any identified concerns. This valuable intervention may prevent associated complications such as wound infection, bacteremia, osteomyelitis, and amputation (Cameron, 2003).

Medication Therapy: Antibiotics Used to Prevent Surgical Wound Infections

Preoperative use of appropriate antibiotics within 1 h of incision protects the patient from postoperative infection by providing antibiotic levels that are adequate to reduce bacterial contamination of the blood and operative tissue. Surgeries are classified by their associated risk of infection. Table 16.5 summarizes the classification of surgeries based on infection risk as developed by the Centers for Disease Control and Prevention.

Guidelines have also been developed for appropriately selecting antibiotics based on the type of bacteria likely to be encountered during the surgery. Because all surgeries involve cutting through the skin, all antibiotics must cover Staphylococcus and Streptococcus. Surgeries that breach the bowel may require coverage of gram-negative bacteria and anaerobes, surgery of the mouth may require coverage of anaerobic bacteria, and vaginal surgery may require coverage of anaerobic bacteria. Surgeries are classified by their associated risk for bacterial contamination during surgery. Table 16.6 summarizes Surgical Care Improvement Project guidelines for the use of prophylactic antibiotics to prevent surgical infection.

Guidelines regarding the timing of the preoperative dose of antibiotics are based on providing peak antibiotic levels during the surgery. Guidelines regarding the length of the post surgery treatment are provided to reduce the risk of developed resistance and the risk to the patient of side effects associated with unnecessary antibiotic use. Prolonged use of antibiotics after surgery is not recommended because it does not provide added protection against infection and can increase the development of antibiotic resistance and adds unnecessary cost (Bratzler et al., 2005; Estrada et al., 2003; Latham et al., 2001; Stevens et al., 2005). Table 16.7 summarizes common causes of surgical wound infections as well as appro-

Table 16.5   Centers for Disease Control and Prevention Classification of Surgery By Infection Risk

Classification of surgery	Description of surgery	Expected risk of infection (%)
Clean (Class I)	Uninfected operative wound; no acute inflammation; primarily closed. Respiratory, gastrointestinal, biliary, and urinary tracts not entered. No break in aseptic technique; closed drainage used if necessary.	<2
Clean–contaminated (Class II)	Elective entry into respiratory, biliary, gastrointestinal, or urinary tract and minimal spillage. No evidence of infection or major break in aseptic technique. Example: appendectomy.	<10
Contaminated (Class III)	Nonpurulent inflammation present; gross spillage from gastrointestinal tract. Penetrating traumatic wounds <4 h prior to surgery; major break in aseptic technique during surgery.	~20
Dirty–infected (Class IV)	Purulent inflammation present; preoperative perforation of viscera; penetrating traumatic wounds >4 h before surgery.	~40

Table 16.6   Surgical Care Improvement Project Guidelines for Prophylactic Use of Antibiotics Based on Surgery Type

Surgery type	Prophylactic antibiotics recommended. Preoperative dose to be given within 60 min of incision (within 2 h of incision when using vancomycin and Levaquin). Last antibiotic dose to be given within 24 h of surgery completion (or within 48 h for cardiovascular surgery).
Cardiac, vascular, or orthopedic, surgery; abdominal hysterectomy	Cover gram-positive skin organisms. First-or second-generation cephalosporins cefazolin (Ancef) or cefuroxime (Zinacef). For patients with beta-lactam (penicillin) allergy: vancomycin or clindamycin (Cleocin).
Vaginal hysterectomy	Cover gram-positive skin organisms and anaerobes. First-generation cephalosporin cefazolin (Ancef) plus metronidazole (Flagyl) to cover anaerobes. For patients with beta-lactam (penicillin) allergy: clindamycin (Cleocin) to cover anaerobes.
Colon surgery	Cover gram-negative aerobes and anaerobes. First-generation cephalosporin cefazolin (Ancef) plus metronidazole (Flagyl) to cover anaerobes *or* use single agent that covers gram-negative aerobes and anaerobes: ertapenem (Invanz) or cefotetan (Cefotan). For patients with beta-lactam (penicillin) allergy: clindamycin (Cleocin) to cover anaerobes plus one of the following to cover gram-negative aerobes: gentamicin, tobramycin, levofloxacin (Levaquin), ciprofloxacin (Cipro), or aztreonam (Azactam) *or* metronidazole (Flagyl) to cover anaerobes plus one of the following to cover gram-negative aerobes: gentamicin, tobramycin, levofloxacin (Levaquin), ciprofloxacin (Cipro), or aztreonam (Azactam).

Table 16.7   Common Organisms Associated With Surgical Wound Infections

Bacterial class	Bacteria	Antibiotic treatment
Gram-positive cocci (Cause 50% of surgical wound infections)	Beta-hemolytic streptococci (*Streptococcus pyogenes*)	Penicillin
	Enterococci (*Enterococcus faecalis*)	Ampicillin
	Staphylococci sensitive to methicillin	First-generation cephalosporin: cefazolin (Ancef)
	Staphylococci resistant to methicillin: MRSE (methicillin-resistant *Staphylococcus epidermidis*), or MRSA (methicillin-resistant *Staphylococcus aureus*)	Vancomycin
Gram-negative facultative rods (Cause 15%-20% of surgical wound infections)	*Escherichia coli*	First-generation cephalosporin: cefazolin (Ancef)
	Enterobacter sp.	Third-generation cephalosporin ceftriaxone (Rocephin) or carbapenem ertapenem (Invanz)
	Klebsiella sp.	Third-generation cephalosporin ceftriaxone (Rocephin) or carbapenem ertapenem (Invanz)
	Proteus sp.	Third-generation cephalosporin ceftriaxone (Rocephin) or carbapenem ertapenem (Invanz)
Gram-negative aerobic rods (Cause 10% of surgical wound infections)	*Pseudomonas aeruginosa*	Antipseudomonal third-generation cephalosporin ceftazidime (Fortaz) or fourth-generation cephalosporin cefepime (Maxipime). For patients with beta-lactam allergy: aztreonam or aminoglycosides (gentamicin or tobramycin) plus an antipseudomonal quinolone antibiotic (levofloxacin or ciprofloxacin).
	Acinetobacter sp.	Carbapenem: imipenem (Primaxin), meropenem (Merrem), or doripenem (Doribax)
Anaerobes (Cause 5% of surgical wound infections)	*Bacteroides*, *Clostridium*	Agent of choice: metronidazole (Flagyl). Other options: cefoxitin (Mefoxin), clindamycin (Cleocin), cefotetan (Cefotan), ampicillin–sulbactam (Unasyn).

priate prophylactic use of antibiotics to prevent infections associated with surgery.

PATIENT CASE 2

R.M. is a 75-yr-old female who is 5 ft 3 in. (1.6 m) tall and weighs 210 lb (95.3 kg). R.M. has a history of diabetes, hypertension, and hyperlipidemia. She is also a smoker with chronic obstructive pulmonary disease (COPD). R.M. has chronic back pain associated with several herniated discs, and corrective spinal surgery is planned. Laboratory test results indicate the following: HbA1C (glycosylated hemoglobin) = 10; blood glucose = 169; blood pressure = 160/85; cholesterol = 240; HDL = 25;

LDL = 140; TG = 240; temperature = 98.6 °F; ABG (arterial blood gases): pO2 = 75, pCO2 = 47, pH = 7.35; albumin = 2.6, and Cr (serum creatinine) = 1.8. R.M.'s home medications include Glucophage 500 mg twice/day, Lasix 40 mg/day, Tenormin 50 mg/day, Zocor 10 mg by mouth/day, Advair inhaler twice/day, and prednisone 10 mg/day. Her current pain medications include Oxycontin 40 mg every 12 h and Percocet 2 tablets every 4 h as needed for breakthrough pain.

Question

What risk factors does R.M. have for developing an SSI while in the hospital?

Answer

Risk factors that predispose R.M. to developing a surgical wound include her histories of smoking, COPD, and diabetes. Her use of narcotics can also contribute to decreased oxygenation after surgery. Prednisone has immunosuppressive effects that can increase her risk of postoperative infection (Bratzler et al., 2005; Estrada et al., 2003).

Question

What steps can the health care team take to minimize R.M.'s risk of SSI? What cardiac risk factors should be considered to reduce surgical risk?

Answer

Health care team members should follow the guidelines outlined by the Surgical Care Improvement Project. These include ensuring that R.M. is given an appropriate antibiotic within 1 h of surgical incision and that the antibiotic is continued for less than 24 h postoperatively. Because R.M. is undergoing a clean surgery, the prophylactic antibiotic needs to cover only *Staphylococcus* and *Streptococcus*. Cefazolin (Ancef) is a first-generation cephalosporin and is an excellent choice. Other important measures include maintaining adequate oxygenation and normal temperature and controlling pain and blood glucose before, during, and after surgery. In addition, because R.M. is on a beta blocker for her

hypertension, team members should ensure that beta blockers are ordered and administered before and after surgery to prevent cardiac complications such as arrhythmia or myocardial infarction from occurring during or after her surgery (Bratzler et al. 2005; Estrada et al., 2003; Kjonniksen et al., 2002; Shammash et al., 2001).

Vascular Ulcers and Pressure Ulcers

The rehabilitation therapist commonly encounters vascular ulcers and pressure ulcers in the care of the patient undergoing rehabilitation therapy. The therapist can provide the patient and family with valuable information on properly caring for the wound and preventing wound infections.

Incidence

Worldwide, 8.5 million patients experience pressure ulcers and 12.5 million experience vascular ulcers (Driscoll, 2009). Vascular ulcers occur in about 1% of the population and up to 2.5% of patients admitted to long-term facilities. Of these, the majority (80%) are venous ulcers and the remainder are arterial ulcers (Gabriel et al., 2010). Pressure ulcers occur in up to 23% of individuals in skilled-care and nursing home facilities. Risk of forming pressure sores is increased in patients with quadriplegia (up to 60% incidence), elderly with femoral fracture (66% incidence), and patients with poor mobility, poor nutritional status, fecal or urinary incontinence, altered mental status, or loss of sensation associated with stroke or other neurologic disease (Cleveland Clinic, 2009; Eaglstein, 1990; Holloway, 1996; Wound Source, 2011).

Etiology and Pathophysiology

Arterial wounds are caused by **atherosclerosis**. The arteries and arterioles become narrowed and sclerotic with age, which results in decreased blood flow to tissues and increased incidence of breakdown. Risk factors for developing arterial wounds include diabetes, smoking, hyperlipidemia, hypertension, and sedentary lifestyle. Signs and symptoms of arterial disease include intermittent **claudication** (exercise pain); resting, positional, or nocturnal pain; diminished or absent peripheral pulses; cool skin; pallor on elevation; shiny, taut, and dry skin; hair loss; and thick, coarse toenails. Arterial wounds are commonly located on toe tips, phalangeal heads, the lateral malleolus, and locations associated with repetitive trauma or rubbing of footwear. The wound appearance is characterized by sharp edges; punched out, pale, or necrotic base; minimal or no granulation tissue; extension into deeper tissue; and minimal exudates. Wound infection with gangrene or necrosis is common. The wound periphery is erythematous, indurated with cellulitis and pain. Treatment involves treating the underlying cause by implementing smoking cessation and exercise, avoiding cold, and controlling edema. These wounds may require revascularization to heal. The wound should be protected and use of occlusive dressings should be avoided in these patients (Dosick, 1996; Holloway, 1996; Wound Source, 2011).

Venous wounds are associated with cardiac valvular disease or obstruction of the deep veins. Risk factors for venous ulcers include trauma, immobility, deep venous thrombosis, postphlebitic syndrome, congestive heart failure, and muscle weakness secondary to paralysis or arthritis (Gabriel et al., 2010). Venous ulcers are usually located on the medial aspect of the lower leg and ankle or superior to the medial malleolus. The appearance of the ulcer is characterized by irregular wound edges and a ruddy-colored base, and granulation tissue is often present. The wound is usually shallow and superficial with moderate to heavy exudates and erythema, induration, and cellulitis at the periphery. The wound is usually painless unless infected. Occlusive dressings should be used to protect the wound from the external environment, maintain a moist environment, encourage debridement, promote granulation, and decrease pain. Dressings should be changed every 3 to 7 days. This type of wound may require skin grafts to heal. Treatment includes leg elevation, therapeutic stockings, exercise, and treatment of underlying condition. Nonsteroidal anti-inflammatory

drugs (NSAIDs) and steroids should be avoided because they can delay healing. Complications of venous ulcers can include chronic ulceration and osteomyelitis (Dosick, 1996; Cleveland Clinic, 2009).

A pressure ulcer is defined as any lesion caused by unrelieved pressure that results in damage of underlying tissue. The most common sites of pressure ulcers include the ischial tuberosity (28%), the greater trochanter (9%), the sacrum and coccyx (17%), and the heels (9%). Table 16.8 describes the classifications and treatment of pressure ulcers. Braden or Norton scales are commonly used to stage the severity of the ulcer. Table 16.8 provides a description of the different wound types based on a stage classification and provides recommendations for treatment of wounds and associated precautions based on the wound's stage.

Offloading is a term used to describe providing mechanical support to lift the affected area and reduce pressure on the wound. This is accomplished by repositioning the patient and using pillows, boots, walkers, and other devices. It is an important intervention that assists in the healing of pressure ulcers. Table 16.9 summarizes recommended offloading interventions based on the site of the wound (Dosick, 1996; Krasner et al., 1996; Mulder et al., 1992; Stotts et al., 1998; Wound Source, 2011; Cleveland Clinic, 2009).

Rehabilitation Considerations

The rehabilitation therapist should be alert to any new wounds and ensure that appropriate wound care is initiated and that patients are referred to wound care specialists as necessary. The therapist should also implement infection-control measures to prevent the spread of infections to other patients. The therapist may need to alter therapy sessions to prevent disrupting or damaging the wound dressings. At the beginning of each therapy session, the therapist should inquire about the presence of any wounds and determine whether healing is progressing appropriately. The therapist should promptly communicate to the patient's wound care practitioner any identified concerns. This valuable intervention may prevent associated complications (Cameron, 2003).

Table 16.8   Classification and Treatment of Pressure Ulcers

Stage	Description of the wound	Recommended treatments and precautions
I	Nonblanchable erythema of intact skin. Redness remains 30 min after pressure is relieved. Usually reversible.	Offload, turn, prevent or reduce friction. Protect with transparent dressing. Ischial: Keep head of bed position at <30° if possible; limit sitting. Keep linens dry and wrinkle free.
II	Partial thickness involves epidermis or dermis. Superficial. Shallow crater, blister. Usually painful. Base is pink. May or may not have necrotic tissue or infection.	Offload, turn, draw sheet, limit time up, protect from moisture. Keep linens dry and wrinkle free. Protect with hydrocolloid or bio-occlusive dressing. Mechanical debridement as needed.
III	Full thickness involving damage or necrosis of subcutaneous tissue to, but not through, fascia with or without undermining tissue damage. Must be removed before staging if eschar is present.	Offload, bed rest. Protect with saline dressings or absorptive (Ca-alginate) dressings. Mechanical or surgical debridement.
IV	Deep-tissue destruction through subcutaneous tissue to fascia, muscle, tendon, joint, bone, and ligament. Often not painful. May be associated with gangrene or osteomyelitis.	Debride necrotic tissue by surgical, plastic, or mechanical (whirlpool) treatments. Cleanse with saline using minimal mechanical force. Do not use skin cleansers or antiseptics (cytotoxic to wound tissue).

Table 16.9   Offloading Tips

Anatomic location	Interventions
Feet	Special shoes (front or back of shoe adjusted to reduce or relieve pressure). Contact casts that disperse weight. Dorsal foot wounds: Cast shoes, surgical shoes, podus boots. Use insoles to prevent plantar ulcers. Heel protectors do not reduce pressure.
Ankles	Podus boots, E-Z Boot, waffle boots, rings, pillows, braces, controlled ankle motion walkers. Wheelchair: Assess arm strength and ability to manipulate the wheelchair. Crutches: Assess arm strength and level of coordination. Cane: Assess arm strength; for pronged or standard therapy.
Ischial	Air cushions: Watch inflation level. Foam pads: Check for bottoming out (ensure that pad provides adequate support under the patient's weight). Gels: Provides comfort but may not provide adequate pressure relief.
Trochanter or sacral	Beds: Low air loss, fluidized air therapy—indicated for flaps. Overlays: Alternate air overlays, foam overlays, and gel overlays.

Medication Therapy

Appropriate antibiotic treatment of wound infections usually includes antibiotics that cover *Staphylococcus* and *Streptococcus* such as cephalosporins or penicillins such as amoxicillin–clavulanate (Augmentin). Oral agents such as clindamycin or metronidazole (Flagyl) plus a quinolone antibiotic that covers *Pseudomonas* can be used in patients who are allergic to penicillin. IV therapy can include a cephalosporin such as cefazolin (Ancef) to cover gram-positive organisms or vancomycin to cover MRSA and sensitive *Staphylococcus* and *Streptococcus* plus an agent that covers gram-negative bacteria including *Pseudomonas* such as the third-generation cephalosporins ceftazidime (Fortaz), cefepime (Maxipime), or azactam (Aztreonam) which is used in patients with penicillin allergy. Alternatively, second-generation cephalosporins such as cefoxitin (Mefoxin) or ceftriaxone (Rocephin) or the penicillin ampicillin–sulbactam (Unasyn) may be used as monotherapy providing activity against most gram-positive (except MRSA or VRE) and most gram-negative organisms (except *Pseudomonas aeruginosa)*. Cefoxitin (Mefoxin) and ampicillin–sulbactam (Unasyn) are also active against anaerobic bacteria (Chambers, 2004). The **nephrotoxicity** and **ototoxicity** of IV vancomycin and the aminoglycoside antibiotics such as gentamicin or tobramycin necessitate careful dosing using monitoring of serum drug levels and serum creatinine and the pharmacokinetic dosing assistance of the clinical pharmacist to minimize toxicity (Ciccone, 2007; Katzung, 2004). The aminoglycosides carry a much higher risk of these effects than vancomycin and are usually avoided when at all possible in the diabetic who already is at risk for nephrotoxicity (Brill et al., 1994; Cuna, 2007; Safrin, 2004).

Diabetic Foot Infections

The rehabilitation specialist will commonly care for patients with diabetic foot infection, which is a common complication of diabetes. One of the most important ways that the patient can promote healing of this type of infection is to maintain their blood glucose levels lower than 200 mg/dl. One of the methods of monitoring a patient's long term blood glucose control is the HbA1C (glycosylated hemoglobin). Current recommendations are to keep the HbA1C less than 7% or lower to reduce many of the complications of diabetes such as impaired wound healing. Elevated glucose decreases the effectiveness of neutrophils as phagocytes and alters the deposition of

collagen by fibroblasts, resulting in decreased wound strength and impaired healing. Other methods of managing these types of infections are outlined in the sections below.

Incidence

The global incidence of diabetic foot infection ranges from 1.4% to 5.9%. Ulceration and amputation of the foot is a common complication seen in patients with diabetes. Worldwide, amputation of a lower limb secondary to diabetes occurs every 30 s (Papanas & Maltezos, 2009). Up to 25% of the 24 million diabetics in the United States will develop a diabetic foot infection at some point in life. Diabetic foot infections cause 20% of hospital admissions in diabetic patients and cause 55,000 amputations/yr. Amputations in the diabetic account for 85% of non-traumatic amputations/yr. After amputation, the diabetic patient's risk for developing a postoperative infection is up to 40%. Repeat amputations occur in up to 20% of these patients, and 39% to 60% of diabetics die within 5 yr of the initial amputation (Brill et al., 1995; Lipsky et al., 2004; Sherman, 2010).

Etiology and Pathophysiology

Diabetics are at increased risk for foot infections because of several factors, including associated neuropathy along with decreased perception of initial tissue injury, decreased tissue perfusion due to atherosclerotic changes in the blood vessels, and immunosuppression associated with the effects of prolonged hyperglycemia and tissue ischemia. Neuropathic changes seen in the diabetic can also result in autonomic nerve dysfunction and lead to neuromuscular imbalance, repetitive injury, and reduction of sweating, thus leading to dry, cracked skin that is more vulnerable to infection. Risk factors for developing a foot infection in the diabetic patient include having diabetes for more than 10 yr, previous history of foot ulcer, peripheral neuropathy, peripheral vascular disease, having a HbAIC (glycosylated hemoglobin) level of greater than 9%, nicotine use, visual impairment, and kidney disease associated with diabetes (Brill et al., 1995; Lipsky et al., 2004; Sherman, 2010).

Members of the health care team such as physicians, surgeons, diabetic specialists, wound care nurses, or rehabilitation specialists evaluate diabetic foot ulcers using a system called PEDIS (*p*erfusion, *e*xtent, and size of the ulcer; *d*epth of tissue loss; *i*nfection; and *s*ensation), which classifies diabetic foot infections as grade 1 through 4. Symptoms of infection include purulence accompanied by warmth, pain, tenderness, induration, erythema, or swelling. Patients with a wound without infection or inflammation symptoms are classified as grade 1. Patients with wounds with less than 2 cm of inflammation or infection around the ulcer are classified as grade 2. Any patient with ulcers of grade 2 or higher should be referred to a diabetes specialist. Patients with grade 1 foot ulcers that fail to heal after 4 wk should also see a diabetes specialist. Patients classified as grade 3 or 4 have systemic infections that are life threatening or more severe infections that threaten the limb and require hospitalization (Lipsky et al., 2004; Sherman, 2010).

Rehabilitation Considerations

Rehabilitation specialists and other members of the health care team should reinforce to patient and family the importance of regularly inspecting the feet and carefully maintaining the nails and feet. Patients with diabetes should not try to maintain their toenails themselves because damage to surrounding tissue caused by reduced visual perception and motor skills can increase risk of infection (Brill et al., 1995; Lipsky et al., 2004).

Medication Therapy

Diabetic foot infections are polymicrobial. *Staphylococcus* and *Streptococcus*, the normal bacteria on the skin, are the most common bacteria isolated from these wounds. Other bacteria that can contribute to these infections include gram-negative organisms (found 24% of the time) and anaerobes (found 31% of the time). Treatment includes wound care and antibiotic therapy. If the diabetic foot infection is caught early, using oral antibiotics for 7 to 10 days and proper wound care can successfully manage the infection. Radiologic exams may

be required to rule out spreading of the infection into the adjoining bone (osteomyelitis). If present, osteomyelitis requires prolonged IV antibiotic therapy for a minimum of 6 to 12 wk along with documented eradication of infection from the bone. Table 16.4 provides additional information on antibiotic use.

Pneumonia

Pneumonia is a serious infection involving the lower respiratory tract. In practice, the rehabilitation specialist will encounter patients with new-onset pneumonia who need to be referred for care, as well as patients who are recovering from pneumonia and are experiencing weakness or reduced respiratory capacity as they participate in rehabilitation therapy. Pneumonia is generally classified as community acquired or hospital acquired depending on where the patient developed the infection. A subtype of hospital-acquired pneumonia is ventilator-associated pneumonia. Signs and symptoms associated with pneumonia include cough, dyspnea, sputum production, pleuritic chest pain, fever or hypothermia, sweats or rigors, fatigue, myalgia, headache, anorexia, altered breath sounds, and localized rales. Elderly patients generally have fewer or less-severe symptoms. The physician makes the diagnosis based on the patient's physical exam with definitive diagnosis made based on the presence of an associated infiltrate on the chest X-ray (Lutfiyya et al., 2006; Mandell et al., 2007).

Incidence

Community-acquired pneumonia is one of the major causes of mortality and morbidity worldwide. Incidence ranges from 3 to 10/1,000 adults/yr (Welte & Kohnlein, 2009). Pneumonia is the seventh leading cause of death in the United States. Community-acquired pneumonia affects 5.6 million patients/yr and is the most deadly infectious disease in the United States, causing more than 50,000 deaths/yr. Community-acquired pneumonia costs the U.S. health care system an estimated $98.4 billion/yr (Lutfiyya et al., 2006; Mandell et al., 2007).

Etiology and Pathophysiology

The body has several protective mechanisms that prevent bacteria from causing infection in the lungs. One such mechanism is the immune system, which comprises humoral immunity (including the antibodies that tag invading microorganisms) and cellular immunity (including the lymphocytes and white blood cells that phagocytize invading organisms). Other protective mechanisms include the epiglottis, which physically prevents aspiration of bacteria from the mouth cavity into the lungs, and the cilia, which brush organisms up and out of the upper respiratory tract. Coughing and expectorating sputum (a composite of white blood cells and dead bacteria) are other methods of protecting the lower respiratory tract and preserving the vital exchange of oxygen and carbon dioxide needed for all the body's metabolic processes (Lutifiyya et al., 2006; Mandell et al., 2007).

Despite these effective mechanisms, bacteria can invade the lower respiratory tract and cause infection by several methods: inhalation of infectious particles such as *Legionella* delivered via air conditioning ducts and *Mycobacterium tuberculosis* delivered via the cough of an infected person; aspiration of oropharyngeal or gastric contents (risk of this is increased in patients with stroke, seizures, neuromuscular disease, or enteral feeding tubes and in patients who use antacids, which prevent stomach acid from killing bacteria in the stomach); hematogenous spread from an extrapulmonary organ infection such as bacteremia or sepsis; direct inoculation and contiguous spread associated with surgery, mechanical ventilation, or bronchoscopy; and reactivation of infection in an immunocompromised patient (e.g., *Pneumocystis carinii* or cytomegalovirus in a patient with human immunodeficiency virus infection or reactivation of tuberculosis in a patient being treated by tumor necrosis factor-alpha antagonist therapies for rheumatoid arthritis) (Lutifiyya et al., 2006; Mandell et al., 2007).

Rehabilitation Considerations

Patients with a history of smoking or chronic respiratory disease are at higher risk of developing respiratory infections and pneumonia. Respiratory infections can reduce oxygen exchange and severely compromise therapy progress. The therapist should be alert to symptoms of pneumonia such as coughing, shortness of breath, increased sputum production, fever, and weakness, which can increase fall risk. It is difficult to differentiate between chronic bronchitis exacerbation and pneumonia. In any case, patients with symptoms of respiratory infection should be promptly referred to their physician for evaluation and appropriate treatment. In addition, the therapist should implement infection-control measures, including hand washing and educating the patient on cough etiquette, to reduce the chance of transmitting infection to others.

Medication Therapy

The antibiotic therapy used depends on the causative organism. The causative organism may be isolated with blood cultures or sputum cultures, but much of the time these results are not available when therapy begins. In addition, sputum cultures can be contaminated from contact with the bacteria colonizing the upper respiratory tract when the sputum culture is expectorated (coughed up). Many times these cultures do not identify the causative organism, and the physician begins empiric antibiotic treatment based on the best guess regarding the causative bacteria. *Streptococcus pneumoniae* is the most common cause of pneumonia. Most strains of this pathogen have become resistant to ampicillin, which used to be the agent of choice (American Thoracic Society and Infectious Diseases Society of America, 2005; Mandell et al., 2007).

The rehabilitation therapist should adjust the patient's therapy once culture and sensitivity results of the sputum or blood cultures are obtained. Patients who are immunocompromised, on steroids, or on multiple courses of antibiotics are at risk for pneumonia caused by more resistant organisms. Patients on ventilators or in intensive care frequently are colonized with more pathogenic-resistant gram-negative bacteria that may be resistant to standard antibiotic therapy. For instance, *Acinetobacter baumannii* is a resistant gram-negative bacterium that can colonize tracheostomy tubes and cause pneumonia. It can survive on surfaces for days and many strains are resistant to all available antibiotics (Knox, 2009). Table 16.10 summarizes common causes of pneumonia (American Thoracic Society and Infectious Diseases Society of America, 2005; CMS Guidelines, 2010; Lutifiyya et al., 2006; Mandell et al., 2007). Table 16.11 summarizes antibiotics commonly used to treat pneumonia (American Thoracic Society and Infectious Diseases Society of America, 2005; Centers for Medicare and Medicaid Services, 2010; Lutifiyya et al., 2006; Mandell et al., 2007).

PATIENT CASE 3

M.T. is a 67-yr-old male who participates in respiratory rehabilitation sessions twice/wk for his severe chronic obstructive pulmonary disease (COPD). His medical history includes congestive heart failure, COPD, and hypertension. M.T. has cut back on his smoking to half a pack/day. His current medications include Advair inhaler, albuterol inhaler, prednisone, lisinopril (Prinivil), atenolol (Tenormin), and furosemide (Lasix). During this therapy session he is particularly winded after walking from the car. He seems confused and is coughing up purulent sputum. His rehabilitation specialist suspects that M.T.'s pulmonary condition is worsening and calls emergency medical services to transport him to the hospital. M.T. remains confused during transport and his vital signs in the emergency room include respiratory rate = 29, heart rate = 120, blood pressure = 185/98, and temperature = 101 °F.

Question
What risk factors for pneumonia does M.T. have?

Answer
M.T.'s risk factors include smoking and severe COPD.

Question
What tests should the emergency room staff perform to determine whether M.T. has pneumonia?

Answer
A chest X-ray should be done to determine whether infiltrates are present (infiltrates are also seen with congestive heart failure, so this should be ruled out as a cause), and oxygen should be administered if needed. The first dose of an appropriate antibiotic should be given as soon as possible; this will improve therapeutic outcomes tremendously. For patients who are sick enough to be admitted to the hospital, additional tests should include two sets of blood cultures obtained from different sites before the initiation of antibiotics, a complete blood count, and a complete metabolic profile. The emergency room physician should select an appropriate antibiotic based the severity of M.T.'s illness, history of antibiotic use, and medical history.

PATIENT CASE 3, continued

The recommended tests were performed on M.T. and his chest X-ray showed bilateral infiltrates. Additional findings included the following: BUN (blood urea nitrogen) = 56, Na = 135, glucose = 95, H/H (hemoglobin/hematocrit = 8.5/32.0, BNP (brain natriuretic peptide) = 212, and arterial blood gases are as follows: pH= 7.28, pCO_2 = 45, and pO_2 = 55. Blood and sputum cultures are taken but results are pending. The emergency room physician determines that M.T. is severely ill with community-acquired pneumonia and admits him to the intensive care unit. More resistant bacteria such as *Pseudomonas* may be the cause of M.T.'s pneumonia because his use of prednisone can compromise the function of his immune system. Therefore, he is placed on Levaquin 750 mg IV with Maxipime 1 g IV every 12 h and given tobramycin 5 mg/kg IV for one dose to cover more resistant pathogens. The clinical pharmacist is consulted to manage further dosing of the aminoglycoside based on pharmacokinetic dosing. M.T. improves with the therapy provided over the next 7 days in the hospital and is now ready for discharge.

Question
What therapies can reduce M.T.'s risk of recurrent pneumonia?

Answer
M.T. should receive influenza and pneumococcal vaccines. The influenza vaccine (inactivated) is recommended for persons over age 50 yr, patients with comorbid conditions, household contacts of high-risk patients, and health care providers. The influenza vaccine (live, attenuated) is recommended for healthy persons aged 5 to 49 yr. The pneumococcal vaccine is recommended for persons over age 65 yr and for select high-risk populations such as patients that have had their spleen removed. Smoking cessation should be addressed and encouraged in all patients with community-acquired pneumonia. A speech–language pathologist should be consulted in cases of suspected dysphagia. The rehabilitation specialist can assist patients and families by providing education about smoking cessation, causes of pneumonia, and important ways to prevent pneumonia.

Antibiotic-Associated Diarrhea

Patients undergoing rehabilitation therapy may be treated with antibiotics for various ailments. The therapist should be aware of antibiotic-associated diarrhea, which can be a life threatening complication of antibiotic therapy. Most cases of antibiotic-associated diarrhea are mild and respond to supportive measures such as increasing fluids, altering diet, and using over-the-counter **antidiarrheal** agents. Antibiotic-associated diarrhea can occur during treatment with antibiotics or up to 8 wk after antibiotic discontinuance. Symptoms include increased frequency of unformed stools accompanied by cramping, abdominal pain, and weakness. The prescriber should rule out other reasons for diarrhea, such as newly initiated enteral nutrition (especially if the nutrition was started at a high rate or after a prolonged time without oral intake) or initiation of medications that can cause osmotic diuresis. The prescriber should also review the patient's current drug list and ensure that the patient is not on laxative therapy such as lactulose that is causing the diarrhea (Halsey, 2008; O'Connor et al., 2004).

Incidence

C. difficile is responsible for almost all cases of pseudomembranous colitis and approximately 25% of antibiotic-associated diarrhea. *C. difficile*-associated disease (CDAD) is increasing in severity and frequency secondary to the emergence of more virulent strains of *Clostridia difficile*. Severe cases of toxic megacolon have been associated with *C. difficile* diarrhea and are associated with mortality rates of approximately 40%. Although CDAD is prevalent globally, its incidence varies considerably. For example, a study reviewing *C. difficile* diarrhea in Québec reported a 300% increase in CDAD along with increased cases of megacolon, colectomy, and death. Risk factors identified included use of antibiotics, immunosuppressants, and proton pump inhibitors (Vaishnavi, 2009).

C. difficile causes up to 25% of diarrhea associated with antibiotics. Symptoms of *C. difficile* diarrhea include profuse, mucus, foul-smelling diarrhea associated with cramps and tenesmus (painful defecation), and blood may be seen in the stool. Diarrhea is accompanied by nausea, vomiting, dehydration, and low-grade fever. White blood cell count is often elevated. The physician diagnoses *C. difficile* diarrhea based on these symptoms and a laboratory test of the stool for toxins A and B. This disease is also called pseudomembranous colitis because in severe cases endoscopic exam shows pseudomembranes over lesions in the bowel. The disease itself can cause severe illness and has been associated with dehydration, electrolyte disturbances, and even death, particularly in the older patient. Mortality associated with *C. difficile* infection increases dramatically with the age of the patient. The mortality rate of patients over 90 yr of age with antibiotic-associated diarrhea is 14%. *C. difficile* infection is associated with increased length of stay in the hospital (2.8 extra days) along with increased hospital

Table 16.10 Bacterial Causes of Community-Acquired Pneumonia and Antibiotic Treatments Recommended by Infectious Diseases Society of America

Pathogen	Cases (%)	Antibiotics commonly used
Streptococcus pneumoniae	20-60	Penicillin-susceptible strep: (e.g., amoxicillin or amoxicillin clavulanate [Augmentin]). Penicillin-resistant strep: third-generation cephalosporin (e.g., ceftriaxone [Rocephin]) plus an extended-spectrum quinolone (e.g., levofloxacin [Levaquin] or moxifloxacin [Avelox]) or vancomycin alone or extended-spectrum an quinolones (e.g., levofloxacin [Levaquin] or moxifloxacin [Avelox]) alone.
Haemophilus influenzae	3-10	Third-generation cephalosporin (e.g., ceftriaxone [Rocephin]) plus either doxycycline (Vibramycin) or a macrolide (e.g., azithromycin [Zithromax], clarithromycin [Biaxin]).
Staphylococcus aureus	3-5	Methicillin-sensitive *Staphylococcus aureus*: oxacillin. Methicillin-resistant *Staphylococcus aureus*: vancomycin.
Gram-negative bacilli	3-10	Antipseudomonal beta-lactam: (e.g., piperacillin–tazobactam [Zosyn], ceftazidime [Fortaz], cefepime [Maxipime]), with or without an aminoglycoside (e.g., gentamicin [Garamycin], tobramycin [Nebcin], or amikacin [Amikin]) or a carbapenem: (e.g., imipenem [Primaxin], meropenem [Merrem], doripenem [Doribax]) with or without an aminoglycoside (e.g., gentamicin [Garamycin], tobramycin [Nebcin], or amikacin [Amikin]).
Legionella sp.	2-8	Doxycycline (Vibramycin) or a macrolide: (e.g. azithromycin [Zithromax], clarithromycin [Biaxin]) or an extended-spectrum quinolone: (e.g., levofloxacin [Levaquin], moxifloxacin [Avelox]).
Mycoplasma pneumoniae	1-6	Doxycycline (Vibramycin) or a macrolide: (e.g., azithromycin [Zithromax], clarithromycin [Biaxin]) or an extended-spectrum quinolone: (e.g., levofloxacin [Levaquin], moxifloxacin [Avelox]).
Chlamydia pneumoniae	4-6	Doxycycline (Vibramycin) or a macrolide: (e.g., azithromycin [Zithromax], clarithromycin [Biaxin]) or an extended-spectrum quinolone: (e.g., levofloxacin [Levaquin], moxifloxacin [Avelox]).
Aspiration pneumonia	6-10	Agents with activity against anaerobes: (e.g., ampicillin–sulbactam [Unasyn], piperacillin–tazobactam [Zosyn], clindamycin [Cleocin]) or add metronidazole (Flagyl) to other agents covering the gram positive and gram negative pathogens listed above.
Viruses	2-15	Influenza A or B: oseltamivir (Tamiflu), zanamivir (Relenza).

See table 16.11 in the web resource for a full list of medication-specific indications, dosing recommendations, and side effects.

Table 16.11   Treatment of Pneumonia as Recommended by Infectious Diseases Society of America

Medication	Side effects affecting rehab							Other side effects or considerations
Beta-lactam antibiotics: Penicillins, cephalosporins, and carbapenems								
Penicillins: Amoxicillin is used to treat sensitive *Streptococcus pneumoniae* in ambulatory community-acquired pneumonia. Oxacillin, the agent of choice penicillin, is used to treat methicillin-sensitive staphylococcal pneumonia. Ampicillin–sulbactam, an extended-spectrum penicillin, is used to treat methicillin-sensitive *Staphylococcus* and *Streptococcus* and has good anaerobic activity for treating suspected aspiration pneumonia. Piperacillin–tazobactam, a broad spectrum antipseudomonal penicillin, is active against gram-positive bacteria, gram-negative bacteria, anaerobes, and *Pseudomonas*; it does not cover MRSA.								
Amoxicillin	Cog +	S +	A +	Motor ++	D ++	Com +	F ++	Drug fever, rash, increased liver enzymes, nausea, vomiting, diarrhea, allergic reaction, *Clostridium difficile* colitis, bone marrow depression, dizziness, insomnia, confusion, agitation, convulsions, behavior changes, serum sickness reactions, Stevens-Johnson skin reactions, tooth discoloration in pediatric patients. Increased rash when used with allopurinol.
Oxacillin	Cog +	S +	A +	Motor ++	D ++	Com +	F ++	Nausea, vomiting, diarrhea, stomatitis, *Clostridium difficile* colitis, bone marrow suppression, jaundice, hepatotoxicity, renal failure, interstitial nephritis, thrombophlebitis at infusion site, seizures when dose is not adjusted for renal insufficiency, hypokalemia with high doses, rash. Increases levels and effects when combined with probenecid.
Ampicillin–sulbactam (Unasyn)	Cog +	S +	A +	Motor ++	D ++	Com +	F ++	Gastrointestinal upset, diarrhea, drug fever, rash, increased liver enzymes, nausea, vomiting, allergic reaction, *Clostridium difficile* colitis, bone marrow depression, dizziness, insomnia, confusion, agitation, convulsions, behavioral changes, serum sickness reactions, Stevens-Johnson skin reactions, tooth discoloration. Increased rash when used with allopurinol.
Piperacillin–tazobactam (Zosyn)	Cog +	S +	A +	Motor ++	D ++	Com +	F ++	
Cephalosporins								
Third-generation cephalosporins without activity against *Pseudomonas*: Empiric use combined with a second agent such as quinolone, doxycycline, or macrolide in treatment of community-acquired pneumonia in patients who are not critically ill.								
Ceftriaxone (Rocephin) IV or IM	Cog +	S +	A +	Motor ++	D ++	Com +	F ++	Rash, allergic reaction, diarrhea, *Clostridium difficile* colitis, hypotension, bone marrow suppression, nausea, vomiting, stomatitis, glossitis, hepatotoxicity. Ceftriaxone only: Eliminated in the bile, no need to adjust dose for renal insufficiency; can cause biliary sludging leading to obstruction, thrombophlebitis.

Medication	Side effects affecting rehab							Other side effects or considerations
Cefpodoxime (Vantin) Oral	Cog +	S +	A +	Motor ++	D ++	Com +	F ++	No identified drug interactions.
Cefprozil (Cefzil) Oral	Cog +	S +	A +	Motor ++	D ++	Com +	F ++	
Ceftibuten (Cedax) Oral	Cog +	S +	A +	Motor ++	D ++	Com +	F ++	

Third- and fourth-generation cephalosporins with activity against *Pseudomonas*: Used to treat pneumonia in critically ill patients and patients with history of antibiotic or steroid use or bronchiectasis. Aztreonam is used in patients with penicillin allergy. Cefepime is a fourth-generation agent that also covers gram-positive bacteria.

Medication	Side effects affecting rehab							Other side effects or considerations
Aztreonam (Azactam)	Cog +	S +	A +	Motor ++	D ++	Com +	F ++	Thrombophlebitis at injection site, rash, allergic reaction, diarrhea, *Clostridium difficile* colitis, hypotension, bone marrow suppression, nausea, hepatotoxicity, seizures when dose is not adjusted for renal insufficiency.
Ceftazidime (Fortaz)	Cog +	S +	A +	Motor ++	D ++	Com +	F ++	
Cefepime (Maxipime)	Cog +	S +	A +	Motor ++	D ++	Com +	F ++	No identified drug interactions.

Carbapenems without activity against *Pseudomonas*: Active against gram-positive bacteria (not MRSA), anaerobes, and gram-negative bacteria.

Medication	Side effects affecting rehab							Other side effects or considerations
Ertapenem (Invanz)	Cog +	S +	A +	Motor ++	D +	Com +	F ++	Thrombophlebitis at injection site, rash, allergic reaction, diarrhea, *Clostridium difficile* colitis, hypotension, bone marrow suppression, nausea, headache, hepatotoxicity, tremors, stiff muscles, seizures. Increases levels of antibiotic when combined with probenecid.

Carbapenems with activity against *Pseudomonas*: Active against gram-positive bacteria (not MRSA), anaerobes, and gram-negative bacteria including *Pseudomonas*. Agent of choice against *Acinetobacter* and resistant *Klebsiella*.

Medication	Side effects affecting rehab							Other side effects or considerations
Imipenem–cilastatin (Primaxin)	Cog ++	S ++	A +	Motor +++	D +	Com +	F +++	Thrombophlebitis at injection site, rash, allergic reaction, diarrhea, *Clostridium difficile* colitis, hypotension, bone marrow suppression, nausea, headache, hepatotoxicity, tremors, stiff muscles, seizures, sedation, confusion, dizziness, abdominal pain, glossitis, tremor, paresthesias, heartburn, pharyngeal pain.
Meropenem (Merrem)	Cog +	S +	A +	Motor ++	D +	Com +	F ++	Increased risk of seizures, especially if dose not decreased with renal insufficiency. Imipenem has highest risk of seizures with renal impairment. Probenecid increases levels of carbapenem. Carbapenems increase cyclosporine levels.
Doripenem (Doribax)	Cog +	S +	A +	Motor ++	D +	Com +	F ++	

› continued

Table 16.11 › *continued*

Medication	Side effects affecting rehab							Other side effects or considerations
Macrolides: First-line therapy for outpatient community-acquired pneumonia and when combined with an antipneumococccal agent in hospitalized patients with pneumonia.								

Medication	Cog	S	A	Motor	D	Com	F	Other side effects or considerations
Azithromycin (Zithromax)	+	+	+	+	+	+	+	Nausea, gastrointestinal upset, diarrhea, rash which can rarely progress to an exfoliative rash such as Stevens-Johnson or TEN, hepatotoxicity, headache, somnolence, vertigo, interstitial nephritis, renal insufficiency, rare psychiatric disturbances. May increase QT interval. Increases cyclosporine and digoxin levels. Pimozide may increase QT interval.
Clarithromycin (Biaxin)	+	+	+	+	+	+	+	Nausea, gastrointestinal upset, abdominal pain, diarrhea, rash which rarely can progress to an exfoliative rash such as Stevens-Johnson or TEN, hepatotoxicity, headache, somnolence, vertigo, interstitial nephritis, renal insufficiency, rare psychiatric disturbances. May increase QT interval. Amiodarone, procainamide, sotalol, astemizole, terfenadine, cisapride, and pimozide increase QT interval. Increases levels and toxicity of carbamazepine and theophylline. Increases levels and effects of cimetidine, digoxin, ergot alkaloids, midazolam, triazolam, phenytoin, ritonavir, tacrolimus, and valproic acid. Decreases levels of zidovudine. Efavirenz, rifabutin, and rifampin decrease clarithromycin levels and effects. Increases INR when used with warfarin (Coumadin). Increases risk of rhabdomyolysis when used with statins.

| **Tetracycline:** Doxycycline is a first-line therapy combined with a second agent active against *Streptococcus* such as a beta-lactam; preferred agent in pneumonia suspected to be associated with *Chlamydia*. | | | | | | | | |

Medication	Cog	S	A	Motor	D	Com	F	Other side effects or considerations
Doxycycline (Vibramycin)	0	0	0	0	++	+	0	Nausea if not taken with food, anorexia, vomiting, glossitis, rash, increase in BUN, bone marrow suppression, phlebitis if given IV in inadequate volume. Avoid use in children or pregnant women; stains teeth of children. Decreased oral absorption occurs when used with iron, antacids containing calcium, magnesium, aluminum, sucralfate, or zinc. Bicarbonate decreases absorption, phenytoin, carbamazepine. Phenobarbital increases rate of doxycycline elimination and decreases doxycycline levels and effects. Increases INR when used with warfarin (Coumadin).

Medication	Side effects affecting rehab							Other side effects or considerations
Quinolones: First-line treatment of pneumonia as single agent in outpatient or inpatient therapy in patients who are not critically ill. Levaquin is active against *Pseudomonas*; moxifloxacin is not.								
Levofloxacin (Levaquin)	Cog +++	S 0	A ++	Motor +++	D +++	Com ++	F +++	Increases effects of warfarin (Coumadin). Absorption is decreased when taken with aluminum, magnesium, antacids containing calcium, or iron or zinc supplements. Increases effects on the central nervous system when taken with NSAIDs. Probenecid increases levofloxacin levels. Effective treatment for gram-negative bacteria, including *Pseudomonas aeruginosa*. Avoid use in pregnant women; can interfere with cartilage formation in children.
Moxifloxacin (Avelox)	Cog +++	S 0	A ++	Motor +++	D +++	Com ++	F +++	Taste perversion, abnormal dreams, vision changes, confusion, behavior changes, hallucinations, speech disorders, arthralgias, myalgias, bone marrow suppression, dysphagia, glossitis, gastritis, nausea, vomiting, stomatitis, *Clostridium difficile* colitis, altered coordination and gait, worsened myasthenia gravis, allergic reactions, liver dysfunction, tendon rupture, renal dysfunction, Stevens-Johnson reaction. Increases risk for QT prolongation with increased risk of arrhythmia and cardiac arrest. Increases effects of warfarin (Coumadin). Absorption is decreased when taken with aluminum, magnesium, antacids containing calcium, or iron or zinc supplements. Increases effects on the central nervous system when taken with NSAIDs. Probenecid increases levofloxacin levels. Avoid use in children and pregnant women; causes tooth discoloration and cartilage abnormalities.
Agents active against MRSA								
Vancomycin	Cog 0	S 0	A 0	Motor +	D +	Com 0	F +	Increased nephrotoxicity with amphotericin B and aminoglycosides, polymyxin B, cisplatin, or radiographic contrast dye. Central line needed for long-term therapy.
Linezolid (Zyvox)	Cog ++	S ++	A +	Motor ++	D ++	Com +	F ++	Serotonin syndrome, seizures, drowsiness, confusion, lactic acidosis, thrombocytopenia, anemia, leukopenia, optic neuropathy, peripheral neuropathy, diarrhea, headache, nausea, optic neuropathy that can progress to blindness, myelosuppression, tooth and tongue discoloration. Monitor visual function and CBC if taken for more than 2 wk. Pseudoephedrine, foods containing tyramine, and serotonergic agents (selective serotonin reuptake inhibitors and tricyclic antidepressants) can increase risk of serotonin syndrome.

› continued

Table 16.11 › *continued*

Medication	Side effects affecting rehab							Other side effects or considerations
Aminoglycosides: Used to treat pneumonia in critically ill patients or patients with history of antibiotic or steroid use, chronic obstructive pulmonary disease, and bronchiectasis.								
Gentamicin	Cog	S	A	Motor	D	Com	F	Neuromuscular blockade with rapid administration, nephrotoxicity, ototoxicity, vestibular toxicity, dizziness, vertigo, ataxia, peripheral neuropathy, encephalopathy, lethargy, confusion, worsened myasthenia gravis, hypomagnesemia, hypocalcemia, hypokalemia that can result in muscle weakness, tetany, respiratory depression, joint pain, hypotension, bone marrow suppression, rash, pyrogenic reaction to initial high-dose therapy with fever, shaking, chills, rigors, tachycardia.
	0	0	0	++	0	+	++	
Tobramycin (Nebcin, Tobi)	Cog	S	A	Motor	D	Com	F	
	0	0	0	++	0	+	++	
Amikacin	Cog	S	A	Motor	D	Com	F	Increases nephrotoxicity when used with amphotericin B, cyclosporine (Sandimmune), nonsteroidal anti-inflammatory drugs such as ibuprofen (Motrin), polymyxin B, radiographic contrast dye, vancomycin, or cisplatin (Platinol).
	0	0	0	++	0	+	++	Increased ototoxicity when used with loop diuretics such as furosemide (Lasix).
								Increased neuromuscular blockade when used with neuromuscular blockers used in anesthesia.
Antibiotics with activity against anaerobes: Agents with anaerobic activity that include the carbapenems and broad-spectrum penicillins.								
Metronidazole (Flagyl)	Cog	S	A	Motor	D	Com	F	Nausea, vomiting, gastrointestinal upset, metallic taste, aseptic meningitis, encephalitis, seizures, brown discoloration of urine.
	0	0	0	++	+++	+	++	Disulfiram (Antabuse) reaction occurs when used with alcohol.
								Increases INR when used with warfarin (Coumadin). Phenobarbital and phenytoin decrease levels and effects.
Clindamycin (Cleocin)	Cog	S	A	Motor	D	Com	F	Diarrhea (occurs in 20% of treated patients), nausea, vomiting, esophagitis, dry mouth, taste perversion, rash, heart block with rapid IV administration, hypotension, hepatotoxicity, neuromuscular blockade, rash that can be severe (Stevens-Johnson) in rare instances.
	+	+	0	+	++	+	+	Increases muscle paralysis and apnea when used with neuromuscular relaxant and neuromuscular blockers.
								Kaolin decreases oral absorption of clindamycin; clindamycin increases theophylline levels and risk of seizures.
								Clostridium difficile diarrhea more common with oral administration than with IV administration.

Cog = cognition; S = sedation; A = agitation or mania; Motor = discoordination; D = dysphagia; Com = communication; F = falls; MRSA = methicillin-resistant *Staphylococcus aureus*; IV = intravenously; BUN = blood urea nitrogen; INR = international normalized ratio; CBG = complete blood count; NSAID = nonsteroidal anti-inflammatory drug; TEN = toxic epidermal necrolysis.

The likelihood rating scale for encountering the side effects is as follows: 0 = Almost no probability of encountering side effects. + = Little likelihood of encountering side effects. +/++ = Low probability of encountering side effects; however, probability increases with increased dosage. ++ = Medium likelihood of encountering side effects. +++ = High likelihood of encountering side effects, particularly with high doses. ++++ = Highest likelihood of encountering side effects; best to avoid in at-risk patients.

costs. In addition, 20% of patients who have *C. difficile* colitis infection in the hospital require readmission (Cleveland Clinic, 2010; Cohen et al., 2010; Cuna, 2007; O'Connor et al., 2004).

Etiology and Pathophysiology

New epidemic strains of *C. difficile*, the causative organism, have emerged with increased virulence. The incidence of *C. difficile* diarrhea is associated with increased use of broad-spectrum antibiotics that eradicate the protective bacterial flora of the gastrointestinal tract. The risk of developing *C. difficile* diarrhea doubles after only 3 days of antibiotic therapy. Risk factors for colonization with disease-causing *C. difficile* include use of proton pump inhibitor antacids such as omeprazole (Prilosec) or histamine-2 blocker antacids such as cimetidine (Tagamet), use of more than three antibiotics, and use of second- or third-generation cephalosporins or fluoroquinolone antibiotics. Other risk factors for the development of *C. difficile* colitis include nutritional deficits denoted by serum albumin concentrations less than 3 g/dl, recent admission to a hospital or long term facility, and being female or of advanced age (Cleveland Clinic, 2010; Cohen et al., 2010; Halsey, 2008; O'Connor et al., 2004).

PATIENT CASE 4

L.A. is a 45-yr-old female who is participating in rehabilitation therapy after a recent hospitalization in which she underwent a colon resection. She is now receiving wound care for a surgical wound infection. She has a past medical history of diabetes, morbid obesity, and coronary artery disease (CAD). While in the hospital, L.A. received Zosyn 4.5 g IV every 8 h for 18 days. She is now taking a combination of Augmentin and ciprofloxacin as an outpatient. During this treatment session, L.A. looks flushed and she interrupts her therapy for an emergency trip to the bathroom. L.A. confides that she is having very smelly diarrhea and severe abdominal cramping and she thinks she has a fever. The therapist takes her temperature, which is 101 °F.

Question
What is the likely cause of L.A.'s fever?

Answer
Because L.A. has been on broad-spectrum antibiotics for an extended time, it is likely that she has antibiotic-associated (*C. difficile*) diarrhea. The therapist reviewed the patient's current medication list which does not include a laxative and asked L.A. about any recent changes to her diet. He then contacted L.A.'s physician, who scheduled her for immediate evaluation and stool testing. After evaluation and testing L.A. was diagnosed with *C. difficile* colitis.

Rehabilitation Considerations

Patients with antibiotic-associated *C. difficile* diarrhea can infect other patients or staff members if appropriate infection-control measures are not taken. Infection-control measures include using gloves and gowns when caring for patients with *C. difficile* diarrhea and frequently and meticulously washing the hands after patient contact using an antibacterial soap. One must create friction by rubbing while washing the hands because the *C. difficile* spores are difficult to remove (Knox, 2009). All health care professionals coming in contact with patients with *C. difficile* diarrhea should continue using contact precautions until symptoms resolve for at least 2 days and repeat stool cultures are found to be negative for *C. difficile* toxin. Patients should use equipment dedicated for their use when possible to reduce the risk of cross-infection of other patients. Because routine cleaning techniques do not kill *C. difficile* spores, meticulous infection-control measures are required to eradicate the spores and bacteria from the patient's living environment and prevent cross-infection of other persons. All high-touch areas (e.g., toilet seat, flush handle, bathroom door knob, bathroom handhold, bathroom light switch, bedpan cleaner, tray table, bedside rail, bedside table, nurse-call device, chair, telephone, and room door knobs) should be disinfected with 1:10 hypochlorite (diluted bleach solutions) (Cohen et al., 2010; O'Connor et al., 2004).

Medication Therapy

Treatment goals for managing *C. difficile* colitis include inhibiting the growth of *C. difficile* by using antibiotics active against *C. difficile* and preserving or re-establishing the protective bacteria in the bowel. The initial offending antibiotic that resulted in *C. difficile* overgrowth should be discontinued. Antibiotics used to inhibit growth of *C. difficile* and treat *C. difficile* colitis include oral or IV metronidazole and oral or rectal vancomycin. Initial therapy for mild colitis includes oral metronidazole (Flagyl) 500 mg every 8 h for 10 days. Therapy for restoring the bacterial flora in the gastrointestinal tract involves administering probiotics containing *Lactobacillus* or *Saccharomyces*. These products can be administered as a supplement and are available in enriched dairy products. Probiotics should be spaced at least 2 h from administration from any antibiotics to prevent the antibiotic from killing the good bacteria the probiotic provides (Cohen et al., 2010; O'Connor et al., 2004).

In the case of severe colitis or if the patient does not respond to metronidazole (Flagyl) treatment, oral vancomycin 125 mg every 6 h should be given for 10 days (intravenous vancomycin is ineffective for treating this infection). In patients who develop rare complications such as toxic megacolon or ileus, hospitalization is indicated and a combination of intracolonic vancomycin 500 mg in 500 ml of normal saline (NS) every 6 h via retention enemas plus metronidazole (Flagyl) 500 mg IV every 6 h for 10 days is administered. Other products that can be tried in patients not responsive to first-line therapies include rifaximin (Xifaxan) 400 mg by mouth twice/day or 200 mg by mouth every 8 h for 14 days or nitazoxanide (Alinia) 500 mg by mouth twice/day for 10 days. Anion-binding resins such as colestipol (Colestid) or cholestyramine (Questran) have also been used as adjunctive therapy to bind the *C. difficile* toxin, but care should be taken when using these agents because they can bind with and reduce the absorption and effects of other oral medications. Oral vancomycin is bound by these resins and inactivated. Because these resins also prevent oral absorption of many medications such as digoxin and thyroid supplements, they should be administered at least 6 h from all other oral medications. Use of intravenous immunoglobulin in doses of 200 to 300 mg/kg has been studied in small, non-controlled trials and been reported to be effective in case reports of patients not responsive to other therapies. However, intravenous immunoglobulin, a costly therapy that is in short supply, is not recommended or approved for this use (Cohen et al., 2010; Halsey, 2008).

Control of Infection in the Rehabilitation Center

The most important infection-control procedure is hand washing. Infection-control measures for reducing patient infection include sterilizing equipment and cleaning the rehabilitation area with disinfectant. *Pseudomonas*, a bacterium commonly found in water and soil, can cause infection in patients who come in contact with equipment contaminated by untreated water such as whirlpool tubs or respiratory equipment. Infection can be spread through direct contact with wounds or skin and accidental ingestion of water, aerosols, and sprays. Bacterial contamination can potentially occur with hydrotherapy and aquatics, thermal pharyngeal stimulation, intermittent urinary catheterization, and wound care. The whirlpool should be thoroughly disinfected between each patient use. In addition, equipment such as parallel bars, Hoyer lifts, and wheelchairs should be cleaned after each use (Friedman & Petersen, 2004; Flaherty, et.al., 1984; Mylotte, et al., 2000b).

The rehabilitation area may be contaminated by patients with undiagnosed infections. As such, it is important for referring physicians or nurses to inform the rehabilitation staff of any patient infection requiring precautions. The rehabilitation staff should look for signs of communicable infection such as skin lesions, productive cough, or rash. Patients exhibiting wounds and lesions of the skin, skin eruptions, exposed sub-epidermal blisters or tissue, or unmanaged bowel, bladder, or other infections should not use pool therapy. Personnel should use protective equipment such as gloves, masks, and goggles when caring for patients with infections, depending on the route through which the infecting pathogen is spread. The rehabilitation center must establish a system of infections surveillance and train the staff on methods of protecting themselves and other patients from the spread of infection (Friedman & Petersen, 2004).

Each rehabilitation unit should have a procedures manual that details the aspects of infection control specific to that unit. The manual should include procedures for reducing exposure of pathogens by reducing exposure to blood and other secretions, inhalation exposure, and direct contact. The program should have a hazardous material notebook that lists hazardous substances such as cleaning supplies and recommended methods of treating accidental toxic exposures. The program should also have a plan to educate staff, patients, and family and visitors to infection control procedures and methods to communicate this information appropriately so that these procedures can be meticulously followed. These infection control procedures should provide guidelines for hand washing, housekeeping, laundry handling, equipment maintenance, and cleaning and maintenance

of therapeutic equipment. Each unit should also have guidelines for safe storage and disposal of medications, care of patients with latex allergy, and establishment of a safety and infection-control committee. Each rehabilitation unit must conduct documented in-service training of all staff members regarding infection-control policy and procedures at least annually. Rehabilitation staff should also undergo an annual tuberculin skin test to detect tuberculosis infection associated with patient contact (Select Medical Corporation, 2010; Flaherty, et.al., 1984).

Summary

This chapter reviews basic principles of commonly encountered infections and the medications used to treat them. The rehabilitation specialist will commonly see patients with pneumonia, skin infections, and UTI. Rehabilitation specialists should be aware of any infections or antibiotic use in patients they care for and monitor for side effects associated with these therapies. In addition, the rehabilitation specialist should be cognizant of conditions that can exacerbate the spread of infections. This chapter reviews important infection-control procedures that should be part of providing a safe environment for patient care.

17

Medications Used to Treat Osteoarthritis, Gout, and Rheumatoid Arthritis

The rehabilitation specialist commonly cares for patients with various forms of arthritis. This chapter introduces various arthritic conditions such as osteoarthritis, gout, and rheumatoid arthritis and other forms of arthritis. This chapter describes how these disease states affect the rehabilitative process and methods the rehabilitation therapist can use to adjust sessions when caring for patients with arthritic conditions. Finally, this chapter presents medications commonly used to treat these conditions as well as the effects of these medications on rehabilitation.

Osteoarthritis

Osteoarthritis (also known as degenerative arthritis or degenerative joint disease) is defined as joint inflammation. Persistent, ongoing inflammation and **synovitis** can result in permanent joint damage (Altman et al., 2000). Osteoarthritis is characterized by joint disease that results in loss and erosion of **articular** cartilage, subchondral sclerosis, and the development of osteophytes (Altman et al., 2000). One of the most troubling features of osteoarthritis is the associated pain. The joint may have flare-ups of inflammation and effusion (swelling and collection of fluid in a joint).

Incidence

The incidence of osteoarthritis varies slightly among countries depending on factors such as obesity and inactivity. The prevalence of osteo-

arthritis in Canadians (approximately 17% of the overall population) is similar among Canadian provinces such as British Columbia, Alberta, and Ontario. The prevalence of osteoarthritis in the United States is approximately 21.6%. The difference in prevalence between Canada and the United States is attributable to the higher level of obesity and inactivity in the United States. The prevalence in the United Kingdom is 13%, whereas the prevalence in Australia and New Zealand ranges from 15% to 24%. The prevalence in countries in South America and the Caribbean ranges from 23% to more than 50%. In all instances, osteoarthritis is more prevalent in females and in patients of advanced age (Wong et al., 2010).

Osteoarthritis is the most prevalent form of arthritis in the United States. It affects more than 70% of adults between 55 and 78 yr of age (Brooks, 2003), and affects women more often than men. More than 26.9 million adults in the United States have been diagnosed with osteoarthritis (Lawrence et al., 2008). The prevalence of osteoarthritis is projected to increase to approximately 67 million individuals (25% of the population) by 2030 (Centers for Disease Control and Prevention, 2001).

Etiology and Pathophysiology

Osteoarthritis most often affects the weight-bearing joints of the hips, knees, and feet but also commonly affects the fingers and the spine. Unlike other systemic forms of arthritis, osteoarthritis does not affect the other organs of the body. The primary complaint associated with osteoarthritis is pain in the affected joint(s). The pain usually worsens with prolonged overuse and is relieved by rest and moderate therapeutic exercise that does not overload the joint. In addition to pain, many osteoarthritis sufferers experience stiffness that is relieved by moving the joint. Joint stiffness is especially prominent in the morning.

Orthopedic physicians often classify osteoarthritis as either primary or secondary osteoarthritis. Arthritis that is the result of wear and tear associated with the aging of hyaline articular cartilage (HAC) is often referred to as primary osteoarthritis. Arthritis that is caused by another disease or condition (e.g., obesity, repeated joint trauma, gout, diabetes, and **Lyme disease**) is often referred to as secondary osteoarthritis. Obesity puts excessive pressure on the weight-bearing joints and causes the production of enzymes that cause cartilage damage. Hence, weight reduction is commonly recommended for both preventing and relieving the pain and stiffness associated with osteoarthritis (Cooper et al., 2000).

As the pain and disability associated with osteoarthritis worsen, the ligaments and muscles supporting the joints weaken. This reduces the static stabilization of the joint by ligaments and the dynamic stabilization of the joint by the surrounding muscles. The pain often inhibits muscle function and results in significant atrophy due to disuse. Histologically, HAC comprises chondrocytes and their extracellular matrices. The HAC undergoes damage and degradation in osteoarthritis. The ongoing inflammation and synovitis associated with osteoarthritis progressively erode the HAC, resulting in permanent joint damage (Altman et al., 2000). HAC is aneural and avascular (Walker, 1998). It is separated from bone marrow cells by the subchondral bone layer (Jackson et al., 2001) and cannot depend on bloodborne mediators to assist with the healing process.

Classic symptoms of osteoarthritis include stiffness, joint pain, and swelling that worsen with activity or weight bearing and are relieved by rest. As osteoarthritis progresses, extensive bone changes, muscle weakness, and loss of joint integrity may lead to dramatic joint deformity and disability. The physical exam findings typically include joint-line point tenderness and painful, limited range of motion along with bony crepitus. In some instances varying degrees of joint effusion may be noted, especially during flare-ups of the condition. As the condition progresses, joint deformity, contracture, and osteophyte formation lead to severe pain and loss of joint function. The patient avoids using the painful joint, which ultimately leads to increased muscle tightness, joint contracture, loss of motion, and further disuse atrophy.

Synovial fluid analyses and blood tests are not used to diagnose osteoarthritis but typically are used to rule out other causes of the patient's symptoms or other common forms of arthritis (Sturmer et al., 2004). Radiographic studies are of value in patients who complain of osteoarthritis symptoms and are particularly useful in excluding other causes of the patient's symptoms and evaluating the extent of joint pathology. Radiographs typically show joint-space narrowing, effusions, bone cysts, and osteophyte formation. Computed tomography, magnetic resonance imaging (MRI), and diagnostic ultrasound can be used to rule out other conditions that may be causing joint pain.

Rehabilitation Considerations

The Osteoarthritis Research Society International (OARSI, 2010) provided evidence-based, expert-consensus guidelines for managing hip and knee osteoarthritis. These guidelines are incorporated into the text of this chapter.

Patient education is an important consideration in the treatment of osteoarthritis. Maintaining and improving function while managing the pain associated with osteoarthritis is typically achieved through a combination of nonpharmacologic and pharmacologic measures. Each patient will likely try a number of management options before finding the options that work best. The rehabilitation therapist should educate the patient on joint conservation and the use of joint-sparing exercise. For example, individuals with significant osteoarthritis of the hips or knees would benefit from minimizing running as a means of aerobic training and from increasing participation in non-weight-bearing or low-impact activities such as aquatic exercise (especially for patients with arthritic hips), cycling, using an elliptical machine, and walking.

Individuals with lower-extremity osteoarthritis should also chose joint-sparing exercises during strength training. For example, rather than performing weighted squats in the closed kinetic chain (i.e., weight bearing) position, the patient should perform strengthening exercises in an open kinetic chain (i.e., not weight bearing) position. The patient should especially perform quadriceps-strengthening exercises because the quadriceps muscles are known to atrophy as a result of prolonged knee pain and disuse (Zhang et al., 2008). Exercises such as seated knee extensions allow the patient to train the quadriceps without overburdening the already-compressed ankle, knee, and hip joints with excessive compressive loading. As osteoarthritis progresses, braces and assistive devices (e.g., cane or crutch on the contralateral side) can be used to further modify loading forces on the joint (Zhang et al., 2008). Diet and exercise geared toward weight reduction are also important in reducing the forces on the affected joint (Zhang et al., 2008).

OARSI recommends considering joint-replacement surgery (arthroplasty) in patients who do not achieve adequate pain relief and functional improvement using nonpharmacologic and pharmacologic modalities (Zhang et al., 2008). This surgical procedure involves removing the diseased or damaged joint and replacing it with a prosthetic joint made of a combination of metal, plastic, or ceramic materials. The primary indication for joint replacement is to relieve pain associated with severe arthritis. Joint-replacement surgery is reserved for those patients who have exhausted all conservative treatment methods and whose pain is severe and disabling.

Medication Therapy

No specific pharmacologic therapies can currently prevent the progression of joint damage due to osteoarthritis. Because osteoarthritis is progressive and degenerative, clinicians must take into consideration the adverse side effects that can result from long-term pharmacologic management and should make an effort to choose the most benign medications and use the lowest possible effective dose (Grosser et al., 2011). Pharmacotherapy should be initiated after nonpharmacologic interventions (e.g., rest, physical therapy, diet modification, assistive devices, and patient education) are employed. Table 17.1 summarizes medications used to treat osteoarthritis (Grosser et al., 2011).

Acetaminophen

Acetaminophen, a centrally acting analgesic, is recommended as first-line pharmacologic therapy in the treatment of osteoarthritis (Zhang et al., 2008). Acetaminophen is useful for relieving mild pain associated with osteoarthritis; it is also helpful when used before activities that may cause pain (e.g., exercise). Studies have shown that acetaminophen is more effective than a placebo for reducing pain in individuals with osteoarthritis (Towheed et al., 2006). Because it does not block prostaglandin, it does not reduce inflammation or carry the adverse effects of gastrointestinal bleeding or ulceration that can be associated with the use of aspirin or nonsteroidal anti-inflammatory drugs (NSAIDs). It also does not affect platelet function and therefore does not increase bleeding risk. It is the safest agent for treating mild pain in elderly patients and patients on oral anticoagulants such as warfarin (Coumadin). Acetaminophen is a relatively safe treatment and carries significantly lower risk of complications such as renal toxicity, confusion, fluid retention, and worsening of congestive heart failure compared with NSAIDs. Acetaminophen can provide substantial pain relief when taken on a regular basis in doses of 500 to 650 mg 3 or 4 times/day. Patients should try treating mild to moderate joint pain with acetaminophen before considering NSAIDs or other analgesic medications. If response to the use of acetaminophen is inadequate, the patient can try topical capsaicin or glucosamine chondroitin. Chapter 13 of this text provides additional information on acetaminophen

See table 17.1 in the web resource for a full list of medication-specific indications, dosing recommendations, side effects, and drug interactions.

Table 17.1 Medications Used to Treat Osteoarthritis

Medication	Side effects affecting rehab							Other side effects or considerations
Acetaminophen: Used to reduce fever and relieve pain.								
Acetaminophen (Tylenol)	Cog 0	S 0	A 0	Motor 0	D 0	Com 0	F 0	Hepatotoxicity with daily doses >3000 mg. Avoid use in patients with hepatic disease. Do not take with combination products containing acetaminophen (Percocet, Lortab, Norco, Ultracet).
NSAID nonselective inhibitors of cyclooxygenase 1 and 2: Used to reduce fever and inflammation and relieve pain.								
Diclofenac (Voltaren) Enteric coated (Cataflam EC) (Voltaren-XR) Combined with misoprostol to protect gastro-intestinal tract (Arthrotec; 50/200 mg, 75/200 mg)	Cog +	S 0	A 0	Motor 0	D ++	Com +	F +	Gastrointestinal upset, dyspepsia, xerostomia, oral ulceration, glossitis, gastrointestinal mucosal hemorrhage, abrupt acute renal insufficiency, fluid retention, worsening of congestive heart failure, memory loss, confusion, dizziness, headache. Reversible inhibition of platelet aggregation with NSAID lasts 1-3 days. Increased risk of bleeding with used with oral anticoagulant warfarin (Coumadin). Do not combine with aspirin. Antagonize effects of antihypertensives.
Diflunisal (Dolobid)	Cog +	S 0	A 0	Motor 0	D ++	Com +	F +	
Etodolac (Lodine, Lodine XR)	Cog +	S 0	A 0	Motor 0	D ++	Com +	F +	
Fenoprofen (Nalfon)	Cog +	S 0	A 0	Motor 0	D ++	Com +	F +	
Flurbiprofen (Ansaid)	Cog +	S 0	A 0	Motor 0	D ++	Com +	F +	
Ibuprofen (Motrin, Advil)	Cog +	S 0	A 0	Motor 0	D ++	Com +	F +	
Indomethacin (Indocin, Indocin SR)	Cog ++	S 0	A 0	Motor 0	D ++	Com +	F ++	
Ketoprofen (Orudis)	Cog +	S 0	A 0	Motor 0	D ++	Com +	F +	
Ketorolac (Toradol)	Cog +	S 0	A 0	Motor 0	D ++	Com +	F +	
Meclofenamate (Meclomen)	Cog +	S 0	A 0	Motor 0	D ++	Com +	F +	

› continued

Table 17.1   › continued

Medication	Side effects affecting rehab							Other side effects or considerations
Mefenamic acid (Ponstel)	Cog +	S 0	A 0	Motor 0	D ++	Com +	F +	Gastrointestinal upset, dyspepsia, xerostomia, oral ulceration, glossitis, gastrointestinal mucosal hemorrhage, abrupt acute renal insufficiency, fluid retention, worsening of congestive heart failure, memory loss, confusion, dizziness, headache.
Meloxicam (Mobic)	Cog +	S 0	A 0	Motor 0	D +	Com +	F +	
Nabumetone (Relafen)	Cog +	S 0	A 0	Motor 0	D ++	Com +	F +	Reversible inhibition of platelet aggregation with NSAID lasts 1-3 days.
Naproxen (Aleve, Naprosyn) Naproxen sodium (Anaprox) Naprelan sustained release	Cog +	S 0	A 0	Motor 0	D ++	Com +	F +	Increased risk of bleeding with used with oral anticoagulant warfarin (Coumadin). Do not combine with aspirin. Antagonize effects of antihypertensives.
Oxaprozin (Daypro)	Cog +	S 0	A 0	Motor 0	D ++	Com +	F +	
Piroxicam (Feldene)	Cog +	S 0	A 0	Motor 0	D ++	Com +	F +	
Sulindac (Clinoril)	Cog +	S 0	A 0	Motor 0	D ++	Com +	F +	
Tolmetin (Tolectin)	Cog +	S 0	A 0	Motor 0	D ++	Com +	F +	

Cog = cognition; S = sedation; A = agitation or mania; Motor = discoordination; D = dysphagia; Com = communication; F = falls; NSAID = nonsteroidal anti-inflammatory drug; XR = extended release; SR = sustained release.

The likelihood rating scale for encountering the side effects is as follows: 0 = Almost no probability of encountering side effects. + = Little likelihood of encountering side effects. +/++ = Low probability of encountering side effects; however, probability increases with increased dosage. ++ = Medium likelihood of encountering side effects. +++ = High likelihood of encountering side effects, particularly with high doses. ++++ = Highest likelihood of encountering side effects; best to avoid in at-risk patients.

(Boh & Elliott, 2002; Carl & Johnson, 2006; Grosser et al., 2011).

NSAIDs

NSAIDs inhibit the central and peripheral synthesis of **prostaglandins**, thus reducing inflammation and fever. Prostaglandins act as messengers in the process of inflammation and fever. They block the inflammatory action of prostaglandins peripherally at the site of injury, block leukocyte migration, and inhibit the release of lysosomal enzymes associated with inflammation.

NSAIDs can provide significant acute relief in patients with osteoarthritis (Zhang et al., 2008). However, because osteoarthritis occurs more commonly in older patients who often have other comorbidities, the use of NSAIDs is limited by their potential or actual side effects. A variety of NSAIDs have both analgesic and anti-inflammatory properties that can be helpful in the treatment of osteoarthritis. Over-the-counter NSAIDs such as aspirin, ibuprofen (Motrin), ketoprofen (Orudis), and naproxen (Aleve) may be used to control pain and inflammation. Even though these medications can be obtained without a prescription, their use is not without risk (Boh & Elliott, 2002; Carl & Johnson, 2006; Grosser et al., 2011).

NSAIDs are recommended by OARSI for short-term relief during inflammatory flare-ups that acetaminophen does not alleviate because NSAIDs can be more effective in reducing symptoms. According to OARSI, the lowest effective dose of NSAIDs should be used and NSAIDs should not be considered a long-term option. Chapters 13 and 14 contain additional information on NSAIDs (Zhang et al., 2008; Phillips & Brasington, 2010).

Topical Agents

The OARSI guidelines call for the use of topical agents, such as topical NSAIDs and capsaicin, for relief of symptoms on an as-needed basis (Zhang et al., 2008). Topical capsaicin relieves pain by depleting **substance P** in the peripheral sensory neurons. Substance P is thought to be one of the principal chemical mediators of pain impulses form the periphery to the central nervous system. Products containing capsaicin include Zostrix, Zostrix HP, Capzasin P, R-Gel, Capsin, and No Pain HP. This product should be applied to the affected area no more than 3 to 4 times/day, and contact with the eyes, contact lenses, and broken or irritated skin should be avoided. Use of gloves or an applicator during application is recommended. The person administering this agent should wash their hands immediately and thoroughly after each application. Adverse effects include transient burning, stinging, and erythema of area of application. Cough and respiratory irritation associated with exposure can also occur (Carl & Johnson, 2006; Grosser et al., 2011).

Other topical therapies include a transdermal lidocaine 5% (Lidoderm) patch applied for 12 h/day; and the topical NSAID diclofenac (Voltaren) in 1% gel or topical patch 1.3% (Flector). Topical NSAIDs such as diclofenac have been shown to provide small but clinically meaningful benefit in patients with osteoarthritis of the knee or hand (Roth & Shainhouse, 2004). An advantage of topical NSAIDs and other topical analgesics is that they cause less gastrointestinal upset than do oral medications. Dosing cards for measuring the dose and applying the gel to the treatment area are provided with the gel. The patches, which are applied directly to the area of pain, should be worn for up to 12 h and then removed. Medication patches should not be worn while bathing, showering, or swimming and can be secured using medical tape if they fall off. The used patch or dose should be folded in half and thrown away in an area that children or pets cannot access. Topical NSAIDs provide blood levels similar to those seen with oral agents. A recent FDA warning states that liver-function tests of patients receiving topical NSAIDs should be checked periodically during the first 6 wk of initiation and throughout therapy to identify hepatotoxic effects (Boh & Elliott, 2002; Grosser et al., 2011).

Intra-Articular Corticosteroid Injections

Use of systemic steroids is not recommended in patients with osteoarthritis due to lack of proven benefit and adverse effects of long-term use. Corticosteroid injections can be used to treat moderate to severe pain related to acute inflammatory flare-ups in the joint. They are best reserved for when oral medications are not effective in reducing flare-ups of joint inflammation. Aspiration of the effusion and injection of the steroid are carried out using aseptic technique. The physician should examine the aspirate to rule out infection. After injection the patient should minimize activity and stress on the joint for several days. Injection in the knee shows short-term (4 wk) improvement in pain relief and joint function (Arroll & Goodyear-Smith, 2004). Although corticosteroid injections are used in other joints, the benefits have not been as clearly established in the literature. It is widely recommended that a single joint not be injected more than 4 times/yr (Boh & Elliott, 2002; Grosser et al., 2011).

Intra-Articular Hyaluronic Acid Injections

High-molecular-weight hyaluronic acid is an important constituent of normal cartilage. It has viscoelastic properties that provide lubrication and assist with shock absorbency. Endogenous hyaluronic acid may also have anti-inflammatory effects. This product is injected once/wk for 3 to 5 wk. Viscosupplementation with hyaluronic acid does not reverse osteoarthritis but some studies have shown that it provides short-term relief that lasts 1 to 3 mo (Bellamy et al., 2006). However, results from a meta-analysis on the topic indicate that the efficacy data on hyaluronic acid injections are mixed and that some of the studies that showed positive benefits were methodologically flawed (Arrich et al., 2005). Because a significant improvement is seen with injection of placebo in studies, the efficacy of hyaluronic acid injections has not been well established. Despite the discrepancy in the literature, hyaluronic acid supplementation continues to be used to promote short-term relief of osteoarthritis symptoms in patients who note improved symptoms with this treatment (Boh & Elliott, 2002; Grosser et al., 2011).

Glucosamine

The most widely studied supplement in the treatment of osteoarthritis is glucosamine. Glucosamine is an amino-monosaccharide comprising glucose with a bound amino group. The sulfate salt is incorporated into keratin sulfate and hyaluronic acid, found in the synovial fluid and cartilage. The sulfate salt form is preferred over the hydrochloride salt because it is better absorbed from the gastrointestinal tract. The amount of glucosamine found in products in the United States can vary from 53% to more than 100% of what is listed on the label because it is considered a food supplement and manufacturing requirements are not as strict as those for medications, which are regulated by the FDA. A note of caution: Although glucosamine and chondroitin are safe, herbal products and food supplements may contain substances that are not proven to be safe. No governmental agency controls or regulates the practices for manufacturing these supplements (Miller & Bartels, 2009).

Opinion in the medical community is mixed regarding the effectiveness of glucosamine in reducing symptoms in patients with osteoarthritis. A Cochrane review of 25 studies involving 4,963 patients reported that glucosamine produces a moderate reduction in pain and increase in function compared with a placebo (Vlad et al., 2007). A recent 6 mo study of glucosamine supplementation in the treatment of osteoarthritis reported that glucosamine supplementation did not prevent joint damage from worsening in individuals with mild to moderate knee pain (Kwoh et al., 2009). Despite the conflicting studies, glucosamine supplementation is still commonly recommended on a trial basis to determine whether it will help reduce a patient's symptoms. Because the side effect profile for glucosamine is similar to that of a placebo, a 6 to 8 wk trial of glucosamine (1200-1500 mg/d) is often recommended for symptomatic patients. If no benefit is evident in 6 to 8 wk, discontinuation of the supplement is commonly recommended (Boh & Elliott, 2002; Miller & Bartels, 2009).

Narcotic Analgesics

Tramadol is available as Ultram, as a combination product with acetaminophen (Ultracet), and as an extended-release product (Ultram ER). It binds to mu receptors and is used to treat neuropathic pain because it inhibits norepinephrine and serotonin reuptake. It should be titrated slowly over several weeks in order to minimize the side effects of nausea and vomiting; therefore, it is less useful in managing acute pain. Its use has been associated with seizures and it should not be combined with monoamine oxidase inhibitors or tricyclic antidepressants, which can enhance the risk of this toxicity. The FDA recently advised prescribers to use this agent with caution in patients with history of substance abuse or psychiatric illness because of the increased risk for suicide and overdose in this patient population (Grosser et al., 2011).

Opioids

Short-term use of opioids can be considered in patients with continued pain despite the use of acetaminophen, NSAIDs, topical therapies, and glucosamine. Use of narcotic analgesics should be reserved for patients with severe joint disease and intolerable suffering who are not candidates for other therapeutic interventions or for whom other therapeutic interventions have failed. Chapters 14 and 15 contain additional information on the use of opioid pain products (Carl & Johnson, 2006; Grosser et al., 2011).

Gout

Gout is a form of arthritis characterized by acute gouty attacks, an inflammatory response caused by the precipitation of uric acid in the joints. Gout affects 0.5% to 1% of the population in Western countries. The most commonly affected joint is the big toe (metatarsal phalangeal joint), but it is not the only joint that can be afflicted. Uric acid is a waste product that is created via the metabolism of the purine components of protein and is removed by the kidneys. The body's overproduction of uric acid or the kidney's inability to eliminate it efficiently can cause an excessive buildup, known as hyperuricemia. Over time this excess uric acid can deposit in joints, where it forms into sharp uric acid crystals that lead to pain and swelling in the affected joint. Uric acid levels can be elevated because of decreased excretion, increased production, or increased purine intake. Purine-rich foods (e.g., liver, kidney, anchovies, asparagus, herring, meat gravies and broths, mushrooms, mussels, sardines, and sweetbreads) can contribute to hyperuricemia (Klippel, 2008).

Incidence

The incidence of gout is increasing worldwide. Factors that account for this increase include new classes of pharmacologic agents, metabolic syndrome, and increased longevity. Some ethnic populations do not demonstrate any of these factors but exhibit increased incidence of gout. This increase suggests that a genetic factor for gout exists (Zaka & Williams, 2006).

A gout attack occurs suddenly, and intensity may increase and decrease over a period of several days. Gout is the most common cause of inflammatory arthritis in men; the estimated prevalence among men aged 18 yr and older is 1.5% (Lawrence et al., 1989). It typically affects 6% to 7% of older men, although women become increasingly susceptible to gout after menopause. Gout is strongly associated with obesity, hypertension, hyperlipidemia, and diabetes. Other reported risk factors for gout include renal insufficiency, use of thiazide diuretics (which inhibit excretion of uric acid), alcohol intake, acidosis, physiological stress, and lead exposure (Klippel, 2008; Roubenoff et al., 1991).

PATIENT CASE 1

R.J. is a 45-yr-old male who weighs more than 310 lb (140.6 kg). R.J. works hard as a certified public accountant and normally does not have time to exercise. He loves having beer at the end of the work day and normally consumes four bottles of beer with dinner. R.J. has begun having pain in his left big toe. He makes an appointment with his primary physician, who informs him that he has gout.

Question
Would a change in diet help R.J.?

Answer
R.J.'s primary physician states that R.J. may improve his symptoms by changing his diet. He recommends limiting intake of alcohol and fat, choosing more complex carbohydrate, and choosing more low-fat or nonfat dairy products. R.J.'s primary care physician should also monitor for the development of kidney stones, which may develop if urate crystals collect in the urinary tract.

Etiology and Pathophysiology

With acute gout, onset of pain is usually sudden and often occurs at night. A common complaint is that the toe becomes so painful during the night that even the weight of the sheet against it becomes intolerable. The metatarsal phalangeal joint of the great toe is usually involved, but the instep, ankle, wrist, and elbows can also be affected. The joint becomes progressively more painful and inflamed, and the skin surrounding the joint becomes shiny and red or purple (Klippel, 2008). In some cases, fever, tachycardia, and malaise are possible. Gout is suspected when a patient experiences joint swelling and intense pain followed, at first, by pain-free periods between attacks (Klippel, 2008; Roubenoff et al., 1991).

A correct diagnosis of gout may depend on finding the characteristic monosodium uric acid crystals in synovial fluid of the joint. In this test, fluid is aspirated from the joint and examined for uric acid crystals under a microscope. Crystals can also be found in deposits that occur under the skin (called tophi) that occur in patients with advanced gout. Levels of uric acid in the blood can be misleading because they may be temporarily normal or even low during attacks. Furthermore, uric acid levels are often elevated in people who do not have gout. Joint involvement is commonly limited to one joint (usually the big toe) in the first several episodes of gout. Later attacks may affect several joints simultaneously or sequentially and persist for up to 3 wk if untreated (Porter & Kaplan, 2006). Subsequent attacks develop after progressively shorter symptom-free intervals. Eventually, several attacks may occur each year. Patient education typically involves lifestyle modifications such as gradually losing weight, avoiding alcohol, and reducing consumption of foods high in purines (Klippel, 2008; Roubenoff et al., 1991).

Rehabilitation Considerations

Rehabilitation for patients with gout is similar to that for patients with arthritis. Patients with gout usually benefit from outpatient physical and occupational therapy for controlling inflammation and pain and increasing flexibility and range of motion. During the acute phase of gout the therapist applies ice while the patient rests the joint. The application of ice diminishes pain in the joint by numbing the area and blocking nerve impulses. After the acute phase, the therapist instructs the patient to engage in strengthening exercises and gentle stretching. Patients who exhibit gait abnormalities may receive training in the use of a cane. Orthotics may also be useful in some cases. The patient may also require the services of an occupational therapist to address activities of daily living such as bathing and dressing. Joint protection and energy conservation may also be part of the therapy regimen (Medical Disability Advisor, 2010).

Medication Therapy

Acute gouty arthritis resolves spontaneously within a few days to several weeks. Medications are used to decrease the symptoms of an acute attack, decrease the risk of recurrent attacks, and lower levels of uric acid. The acute inflammation and pain associated with an acute gouty attack is treated with NSAIDs, colchicine, or corticosteroids given systemically or by **intra-articular** injection. Glucocorticoids, which provide relief within hours of administration, include prednisone, which is administered as 30 to 60 mg/day for 3 days and gradually tapered over the next 10 to 24 days. Intra-articular steroids are useful if the gouty attacks are limited to only a few joints, as long as septic arthritis has been ruled out. NSAIDs also provide relief within hours of initiation and are generally started at higher doses for 3 to 4 days and tapered over 7 to 10 days. Colchicine starts to relieve symptoms within 12 h, and symptoms are totally resolved within 2 to 3 days (Grosser et al., 2011; Hawkins & Rahn, 2002).

Colchicine and NSAIDs are also used to prevent inflammation associated with uric acid crystals. (Aspirin is not used because it can inhibit secretion of uric acid, which increases the risk of renal stone formation, and inhibits the uricosuric action of probenecid.) Medications that are used to prevent increases in uric acid levels include allopurinol (Zyloprim) and febuxostat (Uloric). Probenecid (Benemid) is a uricosuric agent that is used in patients with gout to increase excretion of uric acid (Grosser et al., 2011; Hawkins & Rahn, 2002).

Colchicine

Colchicine has been used since the sixth century to treat acute gouty attacks. It is now considered second-line therapy because it has a narrow therapeutic window and high incidence of side effects. Colchicine inhibits the release of histamine-containing granules from mast cells and may decrease inflammatory response by activated neutrophils. Colchicine dramatically relieves acute attacks of gout and provides relief in two thirds of patients if initiated within 24 h of the attack. Pain, swelling, and redness improve within 12 h and completely resolve within 2 to 3 d. Dosing is two 0.6 mg tablets at first sign of gout flare-up followed by a single 0.6 mg tablet 1 h later. Onset of action occurs 0.5 to 2 h after oral dosing and the half-life is

9 h. Because colchicine binds with many body tissues it has a large volume of distribution (drug compartment) and can be detected in the urine for up to 9 days after a single dose. Side effects include frequent gastrointestinal symptoms; bone marrow depression can also occur. Risk of side effects is increased in the elderly (Grosser et al., 2011; Hawkins & Rahn, 2002).

Colchicine is metabolized by CYP3A4 enzymes in the liver, and 10% to 20% of the drug is excreted in the urine. Dosage should be reduced in patients with renal or hepatic impairment or in patients who also take medications that inhibit CYP3A4 enzymes such as cimetidine (Tagamet) or that inhibit p-glycoprotein such as cyclosporine and verapamil. Colchicine also lowers body temperature, depresses the respiratory center, and induces vasoconstriction, which leads to increases in blood pressure. It can also affect gastrointestinal activity and alter neuromuscular function (Grosser et al., 2011; Hawkins & Rahn, 2002).

Colchicine enhances the effects of sympathomimetic medications and central nervous system depressants. Colchicine is also used off label to prevent recurrent gout. Dosing is 0.6 mg/day 3 to 4 times/wk for patients who have less than 1 attack/yr and 0.6 mg/day for patients who have more than 1 attack/yr. Doses of 0.6 mg 2 to 3 times/day have been used in patients who have severe attacks (Grosser et al., 2011; Hawkins & Rahn, 2002).

Xanthine Oxidase Inhibitors

The breakdown of protein involves the oxidation of xanthine and hypoxanthine by the enzyme xanthine oxidase and the resultant production of uric acid. Xanthine oxidase inhibitors inhibit this production of uric acid and relieve symptoms of gout.

Allopurinol Allopurinol (Zyloprim), a xanthine oxidase inhibitor that inhibits the breakdown of purine nucleosides in protein, is used to treat primary and secondary gout, hyperuricemia associated with malignancy, and renal stones caused by calcium oxalate. Allopurinol facilitates the dissolution of trophi and prevents the progression of gouty arthritis by lowering uric acid concentrations in the plasma. It is also used in higher doses to prevent complications associated with high levels of uric acid, which are associated with tumor lysis syndrome in patients undergoing high-dose chemotherapy regimens. Allopurinol should not be initiated during a gouty attack; colchicine is used instead. Gouty attacks may increase upon initiation of allopurinol as uric acid stored in the tissues is mobilized. Concurrent therapy with colchicine can minimize this adverse effect. Adequate fluid intake and alkalinization of the urine with sodium bicarbonate or modified Shohl's solution can minimize the risk of forming xanthine urinary stones when using allopurinol (Grosser et al., 2011; Hawkins & Rahn, 2002).

Allopurinol also has an active metabolite, oxypurinol, which contributes to its pharmacological effects. The half-life of allopurinol is 1 to 2 h, but the active metabolite oxypurinol has a longer half-life of 18 to 30 h, thus allowing this medication to be administered once/day. Allopurinol achieves peak concentration within 60 to 90 min of oral ingestion and can be given intravenously in patients who cannot take the oral form. Twenty percent is eliminated in the feces and 10% to 30% is eliminated unchanged in the urine. The remainder is metabolized by oxidation. Allopurinol is initiated at doses of 100 mg/day and titrated weekly in increments of 100 mg to an effective dose of 300 mg/day. Doses of up to 600 mg may be required to lower levels of uric acid to the desired range of less than 6 mg/dl. When used to prevent complications associated with chemotherapy treatment of hematologic malignancy, doses of up to 800 mg/day are used starting 2 to 3 days before chemotherapy. Doses greater than 300 mg/day should be given in 2 or 3 divided doses. Dosage should be reduced in patients with renal insufficiency: 200 mg/day for patients with creatinine clearance less than 60 ml/min and 100 mg/day in patients with creatinine clearance less than 30 ml/min (Grosser et al., 2011; Hawkins & Rahn, 2002).

Serious side effects of allopurinol include a maculopapular rash that is pruritic and erythematous. Patients who develop rash should discontinue therapy because the rash may progress to Stevens-Johnson syndrome or may precede the development of a hypersensitivity reaction. Hypersensitivity reactions can develop after months or years of therapy. Other side effects include fever, malaise, and myalgias. Transient leukopenia or eosinophilia occur rarely but require cessation of allopurinol therapy. Liver dysfunction and renal insufficiency can also occur (Grosser et al., 2011; Hawkins & Rahn, 2002).

Allopurinol increases the half-life of probenecid and enhances its uricosuric effects, and probenecid increases the rate of excretion of allopurinol, thus decreasing its length of action. Allopurinol inhibits the metabolism of 6-mercaptopurine (6-MP); when these two agents are used together the dose of the 6-MP should be decreased to 25% of the normal dose. Allopurinol also increases bone marrow suppression associated with cyclophosphamide (Cytoxan). Allopurinol inhibits the inactivation of warfarin (Coumadin) and may be associated with increased effects such as bleeding. It increases the half-life and effects of the active metabolite of theophylline and can contribute to theophylline toxicity. It has also been associated with an increased incidence of rash when used in patients taking ampicillin (Grosser et al., 2011; Hawkins & Rahn, 2002).

Febuxostat Febuxostat (Uloric), also a xanthine oxidase inhibitor, was recently approved for treatment of gout. It forms a stable complex with both reduced and oxidized forms of xanthine oxidase. A 40 mg dose of febuxostat provides action equivalent to 300 mg of allopurinol. Peak effects occur 1 to 1.5 h after administration. Antacids containing magnesium and aluminum delay absorption by 1 h. Febuxostat has a half-life of 5 to 8 h and is eliminated by both the liver and kidneys. It is metabolized by liver enzymes CYP1A2, CYP2C8, and CYP2C9 and by conjugation. Dosing should be initiated at 40 mg/day and increased after 2 wk to 80 mg/day if target uric acid levels are not achieved. Side effects include liver function abnormalities, nausea, joint pain, and rash. Increased gouty flares occur with initiation due to mobilization of uric acid from the tissues. An increase in myocardial infarction and stroke in patients taking this agent compared with those taking allopurinol prompted the FDA to require an additional study to assess cardiovascular risk associated with the use of febuxostat. Because this drug increases levels of medications that are metabolized by xanthine oxidase (e.g., theophylline, 6-mercaptopurine, and azathioprine) and can contribute to their toxicity, it should not be used with these agents (Grosser et al., 2011; Hawkins & Rahn, 2002).

Uricosuric Agents

Uricosuric agents increase the excretion of uric acid through the kidneys. Probenecid (Benemid) promotes uric acid excretion by inhibiting its reabsorption in the renal tubules. This action is blunted by the administration of salicylates. Probenecid is initiated at doses of 250 mg twice/day and increased over 1 to 2 wk to doses of 500 to 1000 mg twice/day. Patients taking probenecid should drink fluids liberally in order to prevent urate stones in the kidneys. Because gouty attacks occur in up to 20% of patients who are initiated on probenecid, concurrent use of colchicine or NSAIDs is indicated. Benemid also interferes with the excretion of methotrexate, ketorolac, the active metabolite of clofibrate, inactive metabolites of the NSAID naproxen, and indomethacin. The concurrent use of methotrexate or ketorolac with probenecid is contraindicated. Probenecid is used to increase penicillin levels in the treatment of gonorrhea or neurosyphilis. It may also interfere with the transport of penicillin into the cerebrospinal fluid (CSF). Common side effects include dyspepsia, hypersensitivity reactions (<4% of patients), and rash. This agent should not be used in patients with creatinine clearance less than 50 ml/min (Grosser et al., 2011; Hawkins & Rahn, 2002).

Rheumatoid Arthritis

Rheumatoid arthritis (RA) is a chronic, systemic, inflammatory autoimmune disorder of unknown etiology. It can affect many tissues in the body, but its most predominant characteristic is the inflammation and destruction of the synovium, which leads to articular cartilage destruction in synovial joints (Issa &

Ruderman, 2004). The disease causes pain, stiffness, symmetrical swelling, and limited motion in multiple joints (polyarthritis) (Harris, 1990). RA is further characterized by periods of exacerbation and remission. RA differs from osteoarthritis in that RA is a systemic autoimmune disorder that affects multiple joints and involves the **synovial membrane** of joints. Both RA and osteoarthritis can cause destruction of the HAC and may necessitate joint-replacement surgery. RA results in more than 9 million physician visits and more than 250,000 hospitalizations/yr (Cooper, 2000; Matsumoto et al., 2010).

Incidence

The global prevalence of RA is 0.3% to 1.2%. All populations except rural African populations report some instances of RA. Prevalence of RA is highest in American Indians and Alaskan Indians and lowest in Africans and Asians. European countries report intermediate prevalence rates (Carmona et al., 2002).

RA affects 1% of the adult population in the United States and affects women three times more often than men (Cooper, 2000). The onset of RA most frequently occurs between the ages of 40 and 50 yr, but RA can affect individuals of any age, including children (juvenile rheumatoid arthritis). RA can develop into a disabling and painful condition. Clinicians should make every effort to recognize and treat this condition early because RA is a systemic disease that may affect other organs of the body, including the skin, lungs, heart, and kidneys.

Etiology and Pathophysiology

The pathophysiology of RA is related to malfunction of cells in the immune system in which inflammation attacks healthy synovial joints in genetically susceptible individuals (Statsny, 1978). The trigger that initiates the autoimmune response in RA is not fully understood. One possible cause includes contact with a virus or other infectious agent. The inflammation occurs primarily in the synovium (the inner lining of the joint capsule). The inflammatory chemicals released by the immune

cells also cause swelling and damage to the synovium, articular cartilage, and bone. These arthritogenic chemical mediators include cytokines, prostaglandins, leukotrienes, and destructive enzymes such as proteases and collagenases (Firestein & Corr, 2005). The chemical mediators produced by the cells of the immune system are inflammatory and destructive to the synovium and cause an overgrowth of the synovium, called pannus. The **pannus** produces more enzymes that destroy nearby cartilage, aggravating the area and attracting more inflammatory white cells and thereby perpetuating the process (Klippel, 2008). Most patients experience a chronic fluctuating course of disease that, despite therapy, may result in progressive joint destruction, deformity, and varying levels of disability.

Due to the systemic nature of RA, patients with the disease have a higher incidence of cardiac disease and are at increased risk for diabetes (Hochberg, 1981; Klippel, 2008). RA can affect any joint, but tends to affect the small joints in the hands and feet more frequently. The stiffness seen in RA is typically worse in the morning and may last anywhere from 1 to 2 h to the entire day. Early identification of the disease is important in promoting a better treatment outcome and preventing as much damage to the synovium, articular cartilage, and joint (e.g., joint deformity) as possible. Important early signs include three or more swollen joints, involvement of the metatarsal or metacarpal phalangeal joints, and stiffness that lasts 30 min or more after waking (Emery et al., 2002).

Joint erosions occur early in RA. Up to 93% of patients with RA are likely to show radiographic abnormities less than 2 yr from onset of the disease. MRI can detect joint erosions within 4 mo of RA onset. Joint erosions progress much more rapidly in the first year than in the second or third years (Fuchs et al., 1989).

RA patients typically complain of morning stiffness in and around multiple joints that lasts at least 1 h. Physical examination typically reveals warmth, swelling, and pain in three or more joints. RA symptoms are often observed in the hand, including at least one swollen area in the wrist, metacarpal phalangeal joint, or proximal interphalangeal joint. Further findings include symmetrical arthritis, meaning that the same joint(s) are inflamed and symptomatic bilaterally. The clinician should also be alert to the presence of rheumatoid nodules, which can form in other areas of the body, often distant from the arthritic joints. Diagnostic testing of RA can be challenging, especially in early stages, because no test is 100% sensitive or specific. A positive serum rheumatoid factor is eventually found in approximately 80% of patients with RA but is found in only 30% in the early stage of RA (Klippel, 2008). X-rays are helpful in diagnosing RA but may not show any abnormalities in the first 3 to 6 mo of the disease process. X-rays that show erosions and bony decalcifications that correlate with the symptomatic joints support the diagnosis of RA (Arnett at al., 1988).

Rehabilitation Considerations

Patient education is an essential component in the management of rheumatoid diseases. Established patient-education programs such as the Arthritis Self-Management Program have been shown to reduce pain by 20% and reduce physician visits by 43% (Lorig et al., 1993). Programs such as this teach patients proactive approaches for managing their RA that include cognitive–behavioral techniques and joint-conservation techniques. The rehabilitation specialist is of great value to this patient population. Rehabilitation interventions include the implementation of appropriate devices to assist with mobility, activities of daily living, and functional activities. Therapeutic exercise focuses on range-of-motion and flexibility exercises that improve joint motion and prevent contracture. Strength-training programs should focus on joint-sparing exercises that strengthen the dynamic stabilizers (muscles) surrounding the joint. Educating patients about the importance of performing therapy exercises on a regular basis is essential to preventing disuse atrophy and contracture. The RA patient population responds especially well to aquatic exercise in a heated therapy pool.

Because pain is often a limiting factor that inhibits range of motion and muscle strength, the use of interventions such as transcutaneous electrical nerve stimulation (TENS) treatment can be of great benefit as a nonpharmacologic method of managing pain. Cold therapy and heat therapy are also commonly used in this population because both modalities have analgesic properties. Although most patients with RA prefer heat therapy (heat packs, paraffin bath, thermal short-wave diathermy, thermal ultrasound, warm-water immersion) over cold therapy, heat therapy should not be used during acute flare-ups of RA because it can increase local inflammation and exacerbate symptoms (Feibel & Fast, 1976).

Use of cold therapy (cold pack) 3 times/day for 1 mo was shown to decrease pain, improve mobility, improve sleep, and decrease the need for pain medication (Kagilaski, 1981). Low-level laser therapy has also been shown to reduce morning pain and stiffness and increase range of motion more than a placebo treatment (Brosseau et al., 2000). Splinting and bracing techniques can also be used to prevent or halt joint contracture and deformity.

Although RA is generally an inflammatory process of the synovium, structural or mechanical derangement is a frequent cause of pain or loss of joint function that may benefit from a surgical approach. Synovectomy of the wrist is recommended for patients with persistent, intense synovitis not responding to medical treatment; this surgery helps prevent extensor tendon sheath rupture that results in severe disability of hand function. Total joint arthroplasty of the knee, hip, wrist, knuckle, or elbow can be beneficial. Other surgeries that can be helpful include surgeries to release entrapped nerves (e.g., carpal tunnel syndrome), arthroscopic procedures, and, occasionally, removal of a symptomatic rheumatoid nodule (Boh & Elliott, 2002; Harris, 1990).

Medication Therapy

Medication therapy used to treat RA includes NSAIDs to relieve symptoms and disease-modifying antirheumatic drugs (DMARD) to reduce the activity of the disease and therefore reduce the progressive destruction of the affected parts of the body. Because cartilage damage and bony erosions frequently occur within the first 2 yr of disease, rheumatologists now move more aggressively to a DMARD agent early in the course of disease—usually as soon as a diagnosis is confirmed. The use of a single DMARD medication can achieve remission of the disease or significantly reduce disease activity in a large number of patients with RA. Combination therapy with two or three nonbiological DMARDs may be needed to treat moderate to severe disease or with failure of single-agent therapy. NSAIDs are commonly used in combination with the DMARD. Glucocorticoids are often used to bring the level of inflammation down quickly but are not used as long-term therapy due to their side effect profile. As in osteoarthritis, corticosteroids such as prednisone may be given orally at low doses or corticosteroids such as dexamethasone (Decadron) can be administered by injection into the joints (Grosser et al., 2011).

The first DMARDs available were gold therapy (Auralgan) and penicillamine (Cuprimine). These agents are now reserved for use in patients who have failed other therapies because of their reduced efficacy and significant side effect profile compared with the newer agents. DMARD include agents such as methotrexate, hydroxychloroquine (Plaquenil), azathioprine (Imuran), cyclosporine (Neoral, Sandimmune), and sulfasalazine (Azulfidine). The most commonly used **cytotoxic** drugs are azathioprine (Imuran), cyclosporine (Sandimmune, Neoral), cyclophosphamide (Cytoxan), and D-penicillamine. Because of their side effects, these agents are typically used to treat extra-articular manifestations of RA such as systemic vasculitis or severe articular disease that is refractory to other therapy (Grosser et al., 2011).

Biologic-response modifiers or biologic agents may target **tumor necrosis factor (TNF)-alpha**, **T-cell** function, **B-cell** function, or **interleukin** and can dramatically slow down the progression of the disease. FDA-approved treatments that target TNF-alpha include adalimumab (Humira), etanercept (Enbrel), golimumab (Simponi), certolizumab (Cimzia), and infliximab (Remicade). In addition, agents that deplete B-cell function such as rituximab (Rituxan), agents that interfere with

T-cell function such as abatacept (Orencia), and agents that block the actions of interleukin-1 such as anakinra (Kineret) are also used as biological DMARD in the treatment of RA. Biological DMARD are reserved for use in patients with persistent moderate or high disease activity; those with functional impairment, extra-articular disease, or radiographic bony erosions; and those who are positive for rheumatoid factor. Table 17.1 summarizes NSAIDs and table 17.2 summarizes DMARD agents used to treat RA (Grosser et al., 2011).

TNF Inhibitors

TNF is a proinflammatory **cytokine** produced by macrophages and lymphocytes. It is found in large quantities in the rheumatoid joint and is produced locally in the joint when synovial macrophages and lymphocytes infiltrate the joint synovium. TNF is one of the critical cytokines that mediate joint damage and destruction because it is active against many cells in the joint and has effects on other organs and body systems. TNF inhibitors such as adalimumab (Humira), golimumab (Simponi), and etanercept (Enbrel) are equally effective when used to treat patients with moderate to severe RA and are now approved for the treatment of other forms of inflammatory arthritis, including psoriatic arthritis and ankylosing spondylitis. Table 17.2 lists agent-specific dosing, adverse effects affecting rehabilitation, and monitoring considerations for patients receiving TNF inhibitors (Grosser et al., 2011).

T-Cell Blockers

Abatacept (Orencia) is the first of a class of agents known as T-cell blockers. T-cells recognize antigens as foreign and become active, proliferate, travel to inflamed sites, and secrete proinflammatory cytokines, including TNF. T-cell blockers interfere with the interactions between antigen-presenting cells and T-lymphocytes and affect early stages of inflammatory changes in RA (Grosser et al., 2011).

B-Cell Depletion

B-cells are important inflammatory cells with multiple functions in the immune response. They serve as antigen-presenting cells, secrete

See table 17.2 in the web resource for a full list of medication-specific indications, dosing recommendations, and side effects.

Table 17.2 Disease-Modifying Antirheumatic Drugs Used to Treat Rheumatic Disease

Medication	Side effects affecting rehab							Other side effects or considerations
Nonbiological DMARD								
Methotrexate Antifolate.	Cog 0	S 0	A 0	Motor 0	D ++	Com 0	F 0	Stomatitis in 3%-10%; diarrhea, nausea, and vomiting in up to 10%; thrombocytopenia in 1%-3%; elevated liver function tests (LFTs) in up to 15%, discontinue methotrexate if LFTs are sustained at more than 2 times normal. Rarer toxicities are leukopenia, pulmonary fibrosis, and pneumonitis. Teratogenic. DMARD of choice for initiation. Onset is 6-8 wk; patient should be supplemented with folic acid. Obtain baseline UA, CBC, and liver-function tests (AST/ALT, bilirubin, albumin); hepatitis B and C testing; repeat CBC, AST, and albumin every 1-2 mo to monitor for hepatotoxic side effects.
Leflunomide (Arava) Inhibits pyrimidine synthesis.	Cog 0	S 0	A 0	Motor 0	D ++	Com 0	F 0	Liver toxicity; contraindicated in patients with liver impairment. Teratogenic; takes months to clear but cholestyramine can enhance clearance. High incidence of gastrointestinal side effects. Onset of response in 1-2 mo; half-life is 14-16 days. Obtain baseline ALT and then repeat monthly to monitor for hepatotoxic side effects.
Hydroxy-chloroquine (Plaquenil) Antimalarial.	Cog 0	S 0	A 0	Motor ++	D ++	Com 0	F ++	Taking with food can reduce nausea, vomiting, and diarrhea. Ocular toxicity (accommodation defects, corneal deposits, blurred vision, scotomas, night blindness); patient should contact physician immediately if visual changes occur. Dermatologic rash, alopecia, increased skin pigmentation, mild neurologic side effects of headache, vertigo, and insomnia. Metabolized by liver and excreted by kidneys. Onset of effects is 2-4 mo; if no response occurs by 6 mo, drug should be discontinued. Baseline ophthalmologic exam and repeat every 9-12 mo. Conduct Amsler grid testing at home every 2 wk. Can be used in combination with methotrexate and sulfasalazine.

Medication	Side effects affecting rehab							Other side effects or considerations
Sulfasalazine (Azulfidine) Salicylate.	Cog	S	A	Motor	D	Com	F	Nausea, vomiting, diarrhea, and anorexia are minimized with low dose initiation and slow titration.
	0	0	0	0	+++	0	0	Rash, urticaria, and serum sickness reactions can be treated with antihistamines or steroids. Hypersensitivity reactions require discontinuance. Leukopenia, alopecia, stomatitis, elevated liver enzymes, yellow–orange skin discoloration; may cause photosensitivity.
								Baseline CBC, then repeat weekly for 1 mo and recheck every 1-2 mo.
								Onset is 6 wk-3 mo.
								Can be combined with methotrexate and hydroxychloroquine as triple therapy.

Nonbiological DMARD that are cytotoxic agents

Medication								
Azathioprine (Imuran)	Cog	S	A	Motor	D	Com	F	Reversible dose-related bone marrow suppression (leukopenia, macrocytic anemia, pancytopenia, thrombocytopenia), gastrointestinal intolerance, stomatitis, infection, drug fever, hepatotoxicity, hypertension, increased risk of infection, hyperglycemia, nephrotoxicity, tremor, hirsutism, gingival hyperplasia; may cause malignancies.
	0	0	0	0	+++	0	0	Hypertension and nephrotoxicity are reversed upon discontinuance.
								Baseline CBC and AST; repeat every 2 wk for first 2 mo, then every 1-2 mo. Eliminated by kidneys; adjust dose for renal insufficiency.
								If given with allopurinol, must reduce dose to 25% of original dose.
Cyclosporine (Neoral, Sandimmune)	Cog	S	A	Motor	D	Com	F	Hypertension, increased risk for infection, hyperglycemia, nephrotoxicity, tremor, gastrointestinal intolerances, hirsutism, gingival hyperplasia. Hypertension and nephrotoxicity are reversed upon discontinuance.
	0	0	0	+	+++	0	0	Measure serum creatinine and blood pressure at baseline and monthly.
								Onset of activity is 1-3 mo.
								Metabolized by liver (active metabolites) and excreted in bile.
								Interacts with anticonvulsants, ketoconazole, fluconazole, trimethoprim, erythromycin, verapamil, diltiazem, nonsteroidal anti-inflammatory drugs, and cyclophosphamide. Reserved for patients who fail more conventional therapies.
Cyclophosphamide (Cytoxan)	Cog	S	A	Motor	D	Com	F	Bone marrow suppression, hemorrhagic cystitis, premature ovarian failure, infection, secondary malignancy (particularly an increased risk of bladder cancer).
	0	0	0	0	+	0	0	Measure baseline UA and CBC; repeat weekly for first mo, then repeat every 2-4 wk.

› continued

Table 17.2 › *continued*

Medication	Side effects affecting rehab							Other side effects or considerations
Nonbiological DMARD that is a heavy metal-chelating agent								
Penicillamine (Cuprimine)	Cog 0	S 0	A 0	Motor +++	D +++	Com 0	F 0	Hypogeusia (lasts 2-3 mo and then resolves), stomatitis, nausea, vomiting, anorexia. Autoimmune complications that require discontinuance include glomerular nephritis with symptoms of proteinuria and hematuria, polymyositis, Goodpasture's syndrome, myasthenia gravis, systemic lupus erythematosus, and pemphigus. Dyspepsia improves by decreasing dose. Rash of metallic taste occurring after 6 mo of therapy requires decrease in dose. Food, antacids, and iron decrease absorption. Measure baseline UA with CBC and repeat weekly for 1 mo and then monthly, or after 2 wk if dose is adjusted.
Nonbiological DMARD: Gold salts								
Auranofin	Cog 0	S 0	A 0	Motor 0	D +++	Com 0	F 0	Metallic taste, proteinuria, hematuria, anemia, leukopenia, thrombocytopenia; gastrointestinal side effects of nausea, vomiting, or diarrhea resolve with time; skin rash or stomatitis require discontinuance. Onset delayed for 4-6 mo. Baseline UA and CBC every 1-2 mo. 35% of patients have side effects that require discontinuance. Reserved for patients who fail other therapies.
Aurothioglucose or gold sodium thiomalate (Solganal, Myochrysine) Injection	Cog 0	S 0	A 0	Motor ++	D ++	Com 0	F 0	Same side effects as oral gold; flushing, palpitations, hypotension, headache, and blurred vision can occur with injectable gold. Severe postinjection flare with increased joint symptoms requires discontinuance.
Biological DMARD								
Adalimumab (Humira)	Cog 0	S 0	A 0	Motor +	D ++	Com 0	F 0	Reactions at injection site, increased upper respiratory tract infections, bronchitis, urinary tract infection. Positive antinuclear antibody titers with lupus-like disease. Usual time to effect is 1-4 wk. Half-life is approximately 2 wk (ranging 10-20 days) after a standard 40 mg dose. Can reactivate latent infections such as tuberculosis or hepatitis B. Not recommended for patients with concurrent demyelinating disease or congestive heart failure.

Medication	Side effects affecting rehab							Other side effects or considerations
Etanercept (Enbrel)	Cog 0	S 0	A 0	Motor +	D ++	Com 0	F 0	Increased risk of infection, respiratory infection, positive antinuclear antibodies with lupus-like symptoms, transient neutropenia, mild reactions at injection site.
								1% of patients develop antietanercept antibodies. May increase risk of lymphoma.
								Onset of action is 1-4 wk; additional improvements seen over 3-6 mo.
								Half-life of 70 h after 25 mg dose.
								Can reactivate latent infections such as tuberculosis or hepatitis B.
								Not recommended for patients with concurrent demyelinating disease or congestive heart failure.
Golimumab (Simponi)	Cog 0	S 0	A 0	Motor 0	D +	Com 0	F 0	Headache, rash, cough, abdominal pain, nasopharyngitis, urinary tract infection, upper respiratory tract infection.
								Onset is days to weeks.
								Can reactivate latent infections such as tuberculosis or hepatitis B.
Infliximab (Remicade)	Cog 0	S 0	A 0	Motor ++	D ++	Com 0	F 0	Infusion reaction with fever, chills, body aches, headache.
								Symptoms can be reduced by slowing the infusion rate and administrating diphenhydramine, acetaminophen, and sometimes corticosteroids before infusion.
								Anti-infliximab antibodies occur in 10%-30% of patients; clinical systemic lupus erythematosus-like syndromes.
								Onset is days to weeks. Can reactivate latent infections such as tuberculosis or hepatitis B.
								Not recommended for patients with concurrent demyelinating disease or congestive heart failure. Should be given in combination with methotrexate.
Certolizumab (Cimzia)	Cog 0	S 0	A 0	Motor ++	D ++	Com 0	F 0	Headache, rash, cough, abdominal pain, nasopharyngitis, urinary tract infection, upper respiratory tract infection.
								Can reactivate latent infections such as tuberculosis or hepatitis B.
Abatacept (Orencia)	Cog 0	S 0	A 0	Motor +	D +	Com 0	F 0	Increased risk of infection. Respiratory infections, including pneumonia, especially in patients with chronic obstructive pulmonary disease.
								May increase risk of malignancy.
								Response occurs within 3 mo.
								Can reactivate latent infections such as tuberculosis or hepatitis B.

› continued

Table 17.2 › *continued*

Medication	Side effects affecting rehab							Other side effects or considerations
	Cog	S	A	Motor	D	Com	F	
Rituximab (Rituxan)	0	0	0	+	+	0	0	Infusion reactions with hives, itching, swelling, difficulty breathing, fever, chills, and changes in blood pressure are most common with the first infusion and are decreased with slowing the rate of the infusion.
								Increased infection risk. Can reactivate viral infections such as hepatitis B.
								Complete immunizations before starting therapy with rituximab; avoid live virus vaccinations.
								Effects are not seen for up to 3 mo after an infusion; however, effects may last 6 mo and up to 2 yr after a single infusion course.
Anakinra (Kineret)	Cog	S	A	Motor	D	Com	F	Reactions at injection site (erythema, itching, and discomfort) occur in 66% and resolve in 1-2 mo. Increased risk of serious infection.
	0	0	0	+	+	0	0	Opportunistic infections, including tuberculosis, are less common than with tumor necrosis factor antagonists.
								Neutropenia.
								Time to effect is 2-4 wk. Do not combine with tumor necrosis factor inhibitors.

Cog = cognition; S = sedation; A = agitation or mania; Motor = discoordination; D = dysphagia; Com = communication; F = falls; DMARD = disease-modifying antirheumatic drug; UA = urinalysis; CBC = complete blood count; ALT = alanine aminotransferase; AST = aspartate aminotransferase.

The likelihood rating scale for encountering the side effects is as follows: 0 = Almost no probability of encountering side effects. + = Little likelihood of encountering side effects. +/++ = Low probability of encountering side effects; however, probability increases with increased dosage. ++ = Medium likelihood of encountering side effects. +++ = High likelihood of encountering side effects, particularly with high doses. ++++ = Highest likelihood of encountering side effects; best to avoid in at-risk patients.

cytokines, and differentiate into antibody-forming plasma cells. The depletion of B-cells has been shown to be effective in reducing signs and symptoms of RA and in slowing radiographic progression of arthritis. One agent that depletes B-cells, rituximab (Rituxan), is currently available for the treatment of RA. Rituximab is effective in treating patients with RA who have failed other DMARD therapies. A single course of rituximab rapidly depletes B-lymphocytes; this depletion is sustained for 6 mo to 1 yr (Grosser et al., 2011).

Interleukin-1

Interleukin-1 (IL-1) is another proinflammatory cytokine implicated in the pathogenesis of RA. IL-1 receptor antagonist is an endogenous blocker of the cytokine IL-1, leads to cartilage degradation and inhibits repair, and potently stimulates osteoclasts, leading to bone erosion. One IL-1 antagonist, anakinra (Kineret), is approved for the treatment of RA and can be used alone or in combination with DMARD other than TNF-blocking agents. Anakinra is not recommended for use in combination with TNF inhibitors because studies have shown increased infections without additive clinical benefit (Grosser et al., 2011).

Narcotics

Chronic narcotic therapy is not used routinely due to side effects such as diminished mental status, hypersomnolence, constipation, and dependency. Furthermore, narcotics have no anti-inflammatory activity. Use of narcotics may be necessary in patients with severe joint destruction who are not candidates for surgery.

Related Rheumatic Diseases

Rheumatic diseases include more than 100 chronic systemic inflammatory diseases with autoimmune etiology (Klippel, 2008). The incidence of rheumatic diseases is increasing. Centers for Disease Control and Prevention (1990) predicts that approximately 11.6 million individuals in the United States will be affected by rheumatic diseases by 2020. The following sections describe several of the more common rheumatic diseases.

Juvenile Rheumatoid Arthritis

Juvenile rheumatoid arthritis (JRA) is the most common connective-tissue disease in children. This chronic inflammatory disease begins in patients under age 16 yr. The etiology is unknown, but researchers suggest that environmental factors may trigger the disease in genetically predisposed individuals. The pathophysiology of JRA is similar to that of adult RA. At onset the child may complain of joint pain or begin to limp without any previous injury or trauma. JRA commonly affects the knees or the small joints of the hands or feet. JRA typically affects multiple joints, which are painful, swollen, warm to the touch, point tender, and stiff. Like adult RA, JRA is often characterized by periods of exacerbation and remittance. JRA is classified into three main categories.

- *Pauciarticular JRA.* This is the most common form of JRA. It affects four or fewer joints and typically consists of milder joint inflammation and fewer extra-articular signs and symptoms compared with the other two forms of JRA. This variety is most likely to feature eye inflammation, which can cause blindness in rare cases (Porter & Kaplan, 2006).
- *Polyarticular JRA.* This is the second most common form of JRA. It affects 5 or more joints in a symmetrical presentation and may affect as many as 20 joints. This variety is more common in girls. The prognosis for polyarticular JRA is not as good as that for pauciarticular JRA, especially if the patient has a positive rheumatoid factor test (Porter & Kaplan, 2006).
- *Systemic onset.* This is the least common form of JRA and was previously known as Still's disease. Clinical features include swollen lymph nodes, rash, and high-spiking fever. Fevers may persist for up to 2 wk and are

typically worse in the afternoon and evening hours. Systemic JRA can also cause inflammation of internal organs. Splenomegaly, generalized adenopathy, and serositis with pericarditis or pleuritis are common. This form occurs in about 10% to 20% of patients with JRA (Porter & Kaplan, 2006).

NSAID are the agents of choice in treating JRA and are often used in combination with DMARD to relieve pain and swelling. Steroids such as prednisone and methylprednisolone (Solu-Medrol) are used on a short-term basis in acute management of flares. Pediatric dosing for prednisone is 0.05 to 2 mg/kg by mouth in 2 to 4 divided doses. Doses should be tapered over 2 wk as symptoms resolve and other antirheumatic drugs take effect. Pediatric dosing for methylprednisolone (Solu-Medrol) is 15 to 30 mg/kg by intravenous infusion/day given in 4 divided doses that are administered over 30 to 60 min for 2 to 3 days (Rabinovich, 2010).

DMARD used to treat JRA include methotrexate and sulfasalazine. The FDA issued a black-box warning regarding the use of the TNF-alpha antagonists due to the increased risk of malignancy when these agents are used in children. Table 17.2 provides additional information related to methotrexate and sulfasalazine (Rabinovich, 2010).

Systematic Lupus Erythematosus

Systemic lupus erythematosus (SLE) is a chronic inflammatory disease that can range from affecting only the skin to affecting multiple organ systems. Patients with SLE typically present with complaints of arthralgias (joint pain), fever, fatigue, and weight loss. Episodes of arthritis involving multiple joints that last for several weeks are common. A butterfly-shaped skin rash that appears over the cheeks and the bridge of the nose is present in 35% of patients with SLE (Stevens, 1983). Other skin rashes may also be present, especially on areas that are exposed to the sun. The patient may also experience sores in the mouth or nose that persist for more than 1 mo. Fatigue that interferes with quality of life, personal responsibilities, and functional activities is a primary complaint in 80% to 100% of patients with SLE (Schur, 1993).

Early treatment is important because SLE can cause blood clots, strokes, seizures, mental disorders, and miscarriages in some patients. Within 5 yr of diagnosis one half of patients develop organ damage, most often involving the skin, kidneys, joints, nervous system, and hematopoietic system. The most common symptoms (~75% of patients) include skin rashes and arthritis that are often accompanied by fatigue and fever. Other symptoms include sensitivity to light, headaches, depression, anxiety, heart complications, changes in weight, alopecia, swelling of the hands and feet, and anemia. SLE may cause Raynaud's syndrome, an exaggerated vascular response to cold temperatures and stress that can affect the fingers, toes, nose, and ears. SLE can also progress to seizures, psychosis, renal failure, pulmonary hemorrhage, or sepsis. The clinical course of SLE varies from mild to severe and typically involves alternating periods of remission and exacerbation. The associated mortality rate of patients with SLE is 4 times that of patients without the disease (Helms & Darbishire, 2010).

The Lupus Foundation of America estimates that between 1.5 and 2 million Americans have a form of lupus. Ninety percent of patients who develop SLE are females in their childbearing years (Schur, 1993). SLE is an autoimmune disorder that develops when the patient's immune system begins to attack the patient's own tissues. This first occurs through the production of autoantibodies (Schur, 1993). The disease leads to inflammation, blood vessel abnormalities (vasculitis), and deposition of inflammatory cells in organs, which causes tissue damage. This inflammatory reaction likely occurs as a result of some combination of hereditary predispositions and environmental factors (e.g., viruses, ultraviolet rays, silica dust, and allergies to medications). Recent research suggests that people affected by SLE may have a defect in the normal biological process of clearing old and damaged cells from the body; this defect causes abnormal stimulation of the immune system (Mattje & Turato, 2006). The Antinuclear Antibody (ANA) Test is used to detect and diagnose lupus. Antinuclear antibodies are present in virtually all patients with lupus, so these patients will have a positive ANA result. The patient must also present with 4 of the 11 diagnostic criteria for SLE (Helms & Darbishire, 2010; Tan et al., 1982).

Because the finding of histone antibodies can indicate possible medication-induced lupus, a thorough review of the patient's medications is essential. Medications that carry a high risk of causing lupus include procainamide (Pronestyl) and hydralazine (Apresoline). Quinidine carries a moderate risk of causing Lupus. Medications that infrequently have this effect include methyldopa (Aldomet), captopril (Capoten), acebutolol, chlorpromazine (Thorazine), isoniazid, minocycline (Minocin), propylthiouracil, D-penicillamine (Cuprimine), and sulfasalazine (Azulfidine) (Helms & Darbishire, 2010).

NSAID and DMARD are used as maintenance therapy when treating SLE. Hydroxychloroquine (Plaquenil) is a DMARD found to be particularly effective for SLE patients with fatigue, skin involvement, and joint disease. More aggressive therapy such as high-dose corticosteroids and immunosuppressive DMARD such as methotrexate (Rheumatrex, Trexall), azathioprine (Imuran), cyclophosphamide (Cytoxan), and cyclosporine (Sandimmune) are used for more serious manifestations such as kidney inflammation, lung or heart involvement, and central nervous system symptoms. Mycophenolate mofetil (CellCept) and rituximab (Rituxan) have been used to treat severe lupus kidney disease (Helms & Darbishire, 2010; Johnson & Heim-Duthey, 2002; Krenty et al., 2011).

Ankylosing Spondylitis

Ankylosing spondylitis is a chronic systemic inflammatory disease that affects the spine and almost always involves the sacroiliac joint. The classic symptoms include low-back pain, stiffness, fatigue, malaise, weight loss, and low-grade fever (Porter & Kaplan, 2006). Onset usually occurs in late adolescence or early adulthood, typically around 26 yr of age. It affects men more often than women. Low-back pain is the first complaint in 75% of individuals with ankylosing spondylitis (Khan, 1998). The disease is referred to as ankylosing spondylitis because the chronic inflammation of the spinal ligaments and joint capsule causes fibrosis and calcification that can, in some instances, lead to ankylosing (fusion) of the affected regions of the spine. The disease typically progresses from the sacroiliac joint up toward the cervical spine. It can progress in severity to the point that normal intervertebral disc spaces are eliminated due to calcification (called the "bamboo spine" on X-rays). The spine becomes exceedingly stiff, especially with inactivity. Ankylosing spondylitis can cause arthritis in the peripheral joints. It may also cause acute iritis, which occurs in up to 30% of patients with ankylosing spondylitis. Symptoms include eye pain, increased tearing, photophobia, and blurred vision, which is typically unilateral (Khan, 1998).

Psoriatic Arthritis

Psoriasis is the most prevalent autoimmune disease in the United States (National Psoriasis Foundation, 2010). More than 7.5 million Americans, or approximately 2.2% of the population, have psoriasis. Between 10% and 30% of people with psoriasis of the skin also develop **psoriatic arthritis** (PA; National Psoriasis Foundation, 2010). PA is an inflammatory autoimmune disorder of unknown etiology that likely involves a combination of genetic, immune, and environmental factors (Gottlieb et al., 2008). It is known that PA has risk factors associated with human leukocyte antigen and that T-cells and various cytokines play a role in both the initiation and perpetuation of the disease (Klippel, 2008).

Psoriatic arthritis (PA) primarily affects the skin and joints, but because it is a systemic rheumatic disease it can also cause inflammation in body tissues such as the eyes, heart, lungs, and kidneys. Some type of eye inflammation is seen in one third of patients (Veale et al., 1994). In 75% of PA cases, skin lesions appear before joint involvement begins. Skin lesions can precede joint involvement by as little as months or as long as many years. Onset of PA typically occurs between ages 30 and 50 yr, and the disease affects men and women with equal frequency. Common symptoms of PA include pain in multiple joints, swelling,

stiffness, and inflammation at the calcaneal insertion of the Achilles tendon and the plantar fascia. The joint symptoms commonly present in a symmetrical fashion, and pain and stiffness are greater in the morning, which can make it difficult to differentiate PA from RA. PA can also affect the spine and cause spondylitis and fusion of the spine, as in AS. PA is diagnosed largely based on clinical findings; no one laboratory test can diagnose PA (Gottlieb et al., 2008).

The European League Against Rheumatism (EULAR) Task Force proposed the following recommendations for managing PA. NSAID can be used as first-line treatment for musculoskeletal signs and symptoms in PA patients with joint involvement. DMARD, such as methotrexate, sulfasalazine, and leflunomide, should be considered early-stage treatment in patients with active disease and manifestations of structural damage plus inflammation. For patients with active PA and clinically relevant psoriasis, a DMARD that also improves psoriasis, such as methotrexate, should be considered. Patients with active PA and an inadequate response to at least one systemic DMARD, such as methotrexate, should be treated with a TNF-alpha inhibitor. TNF-alpha inhibitors should be considered first-line treatment for the following: patients with active enthesitis or dactylitis; patients with predominant axial disease who have had an insufficient response to NSAID or local steroids; and patients with very active PA who are naive to DMARD treatment, particularly those with swollen joints, structural damage in the presence of inflammation, or clinically relevant extra-articular manifestations, especially extensive skin involvement. Failure to respond to one TNF-alpha inhibitor warrants consideration of a switch to another TNF inhibitor. When adjusting therapy, the physician should consider disease activity, comorbidities, and concurrent drug therapy (European Conference Against Rheumatism, 2010).

Scleroderma

Scleroderma is an autoimmune disorder of the connective tissue that causes fibrosis of the skin, joints, and internal organs (especially the esophagus, lower gastrointestinal tract, lungs, heart, and kidneys). Scleroderma affects women four times as often as men. Onset typically occurs between ages 35 and 65 yr. Researchers believe that the etiology is related to immunologic mechanisms, heredity, and environmental exposure to various chemicals such as vinyl chloride. The term *scleroderma* literally means "hardening of the skin." Two types of scleroderma exist. Limited cutaneous scleroderma, the less severe of the two, affects mainly the skin distal to the knees and elbows and the lungs. It also may affect the face and neck. Fatigue and Raynaud's disease are also likely in this population (Porter & Kaplan, 2006).

Systemic scleroderma is a more aggressive form of the disease that is characterized by fibrosis of the internal organs, blood vessels, gastrointestinal tract, lungs, heart, and kidneys. It also causes fibrosis in tendons, muscles, joints, and the synovium, leading to polyarthralgia. Thickening of the skin occurs within months of onset of the disease and progresses over the course of 2 to 3 yr. About 50% of patients with systemic scleroderma have gastrointestinal and pulmonary disease. Many also have cardiopulmonary disease that can be life threatening.

PATIENT CASE 2

B.J. is a 40-yr-old female who sought medical help because she has constant heartburn. Her physician diagnoses the heartburn as gastroesophageal reflux disease (GERD), and after further workup also diagnoses B.J. with scleroderma.

Question
What is the connection between B.J.'s gastric symptoms and scleroderma?

Answer
Scleroderma is a disease of the smooth muscle. As a result, peristalsis in the esophagus may not occur. However, the lower esophageal sphincter may be open, resulting in gastroesophageal reflux disease. Heartburn is the primary symptom of gas-

troesophageal reflux disease. The heartburn typically occurs on the left side of the chest and may be confused with chest pain. The scleroderma can also lead to scarring of the esophagus and subsequently narrow the esophagus, resulting in dysphagia (Groher, 1997; Mayers, 2005). Scleroderma can also affect other parts of the body. For example, if scleroderma affects the skin, symptoms of itching, swelling, and pain may be evident. Scleroderma may also affect blood vessels, which will have a tendency to spasm when cold. This may result in Raynaud's disease, in which the fingers become discolored when the patient is chilled. Scleroderma in the lungs is usually characterized by shortness of breath and may lead to pulmonary hypertension. Scleroderma may also affect the bowels, resulting in constipation and eventually fecal impaction. The 10 yr survival rate in patients with systemic scleroderma is about 65%. Involvement of the lungs, heart, and kidneys accounts for most deaths (Porter & Kaplan, 2006).

Medications used to treat scleroderma include NSAID and corticosteroids, which are used to treat arthritis, myositis, or serositis (pericarditis or pleuritis). Anti-inflammatory agents that are used to control the inflammatory phase of this disease include methotrexate, cyclosporine (Neoral, Sandimmune), mycophenolate mofetil (CellCept), and cyclophosphamide (Cytoxan). Mycophenolate mofetil (CellCept) inhibits the function of the enzyme inosine monophosphate dehydrogenase, which is involved in guanine synthesis. Guanine synthesis is needed for B- and T-cell lymphocyte proliferation. Mycophenolate mofetil (CellCept) also inhibits antibody formation, cellular adhesion, and migration of white blood cells. Side effects include bone marrow depression, gastrointestinal side effects, and increased risk of infection. It is indicated for preventing transplant rejection but is also used as a DMARD in refractory arthritic disease and SLE kidney disease (Hummer & Wigley, 2010).

Three major features of scleroderma vascular disease potentially need treatment: vasospasm, proliferative thickening of blood vessels, and thrombosis. Vasospasm is best treated with vasodilator therapy that includes calcium channel blockers such as nifedipine. Calcium channel blockers can reduce the frequency of **Raynaud's disease** attacks and reduce the occurrence of digital ulcers. Angiotensin-converting enzyme inhibitors such as lisinopril can reverse the vasospasm of the scleroderma renal crisis. Bosentan (Tracleer) is an endothelin-1 (ET-1) receptor inhibitor that can improve blood flow in the lungs by reducing pulmonary vasoconstriction and decreasing pulmonary vascular resistance. Under normal conditions, endothelin-1 binding to endothelin-A (ET-A) or endothelin-B (ET-B) receptors causes pulmonary vasoconstriction. By blocking the endothelin's binding to these receptors, bosentan (Tracleer) decreases pulmonary vascular resistance. Prostacyclin is produced by healthy endothelial cells and, when activated, signals production of cyclic adenosine monophosphate. Cyclic adenosine monophosphate inhibits platelet activation and activates protein kinase-A, which inhibits myosin, leading to smooth muscle relaxation and vasodilation. The medications epoprostenol (Flolan) and iloprost (Ventavis) are synthetic prostacyclins that reduce pulmonary vascular resistance and can improve blood flow in the lungs (Hummer & Wigley, 2010).

In scleroderma, excess collagen is produced in the skin and other organs. Despite the lack of controlled studies to document its effectiveness, D-penicillamine (Cuprimine) is often used to reduce collagen production or destabilize tissue collagen. No medication has been documented to be effective in reversing the initial proliferation (thickening of the inner layer of the blood vessel) that is part of scleroderma vascular disease. Drugs that reverse vasospasm may also directly affect tissue fibrosis. For example, bosentan may be of benefit because it inhibits endothelin-1, a molecule produced by blood vessels that can directly activate tissue fibroblasts to make collagen (Hummer & Wigley, 2010).

Untreated scleroderma vascular disease can result in occlusion of the vessels by either thrombus formation or advanced fibrosis of the intima. Use of antiplatelet therapy in the form of low-dose aspirin is recommended in patients with scleroderma vascular disease in order to reduce platelet aggregation and to prevent thrombus formation. Acute digital ischemia associated with thrombus formation is treated short term with anticoagulants such as heparin, enoxaparin (Lovenox), or warfarin (Coumadin) (Hummer & Wigley, 2010).

Summary

Osteoarthritis, gout, RA, and related rheumatic conditions are prevalent in patients undergoing rehabilitation. This chapter introduces the different forms of arthritis and describes the effects these diseases have on rehabilitation. Medications used to treat these conditions and side effects that can impact rehabilitation are also discussed. The rehabilitation specialist must be well informed about the pathophysiology, medications, and rehabilitation considerations related to these conditions in order to optimize a patient's rehabilitative care.

18 Medications Used to Treat Cancer

In clinical practice, the rehabilitation therapist will often care for patients with cancer. This chapter introduces concepts in the diagnosis and care of the patient with cancer, medications commonly used to treat cancer, and the side effects and therapeutic effects of these medications. It also discusses the effect on rehabilitation of medication therapy used in the treatment of patients with cancer.

Definition of Cancer

Cancer is a group of diseases characterized by uncontrolled growth and spread of abnormal cells. This unregulated growth injures and compromises organ systems that are functioning normally and can result in death. Early tumor growth is exponential, which means that tumor growth rate is not limited and that the tumor continues to grow at a constant rate per unit time. During the early stages of tumor growth, a larger portion of the tumor cells are actively dividing. Tumors are most sensitive to the effects of chemotherapy medication during this stage. As the size of the tumor increases, the rate of growth slows. Tumor growth is often measured in doubling time, or the amount of time it takes for the size of the tumor to double. The doubling time of most solid tumors is about 2 to 3 mo, but the doubling time of some tumors, such as lymphomas, is only days (Balmer & Valley, 2002; Chabner et al., 2001; Chu & DeVita, 2010).

Incidence

Globally, cancer accounts for 1 out of every 8 deaths and causes more deaths than malaria, tuberculosis, and acquired immune deficiency syndrome combined. Cancer is the leading cause of death in developed countries and the second leading cause of death in developing countries. By 2030, new cancer cases will grow to more than 21 million/yr. The growth is attributable to the westernization of the world (e.g., smoking, diet, physical inactivity) as well as reductions in infections and childhood mortality and increased longevity (Center et al., 2011).

Each year in the United States, 1.5 million new cases of cancer (excluding noninvasive cancer and skin cancer) are diagnosed and 500,000 people die of cancer. Of these deaths, 170,000 are due to tobacco use; one third are due to obesity, physical inactivity, or poor nutrition; and one half could be prevented by screening, early detection, and treatment. Two million cases of skin cancer are diagnosed each year; one half of these could be prevented by using protection from the sun and avoiding indoor tanning. Cancer costs the U.S. health care system around $264 billion/yr. The most common causes of cancer-related deaths are lung, colon and rectum, and prostate cancers in males and breast, colon and rectum, and lung cancers in females. Today, 11.4 million living Americans have a history of cancer, and 68% of patients diagnosed with cancer survive 5 yr after diagnosis compared with 50% of patients diagnosed in the 1970s (American Cancer Society, 2011).

Etiology and Pathophysiology

Cancer is caused by both external factors (e.g., chemicals, radiation, viruses) and internal factors (e.g., hormones, immune conditions, inherited mutations). Cancer can develop in virtually any organ system. Tumor cells reproduce in a series of steps known as the cell cycle. The first phase is the mitosis phase, in which cell division occurs. This phase lasts for about 30 to 60 min. After mitosis the cell enters a dormant phase, also called the resting phase. Next is the gap phase in which the cell prepares for deoxyribonucleic acid (DNA) synthesis by making necessary enzymes. The next phase, called the DNA synthesis phase, usually lasts for 10 to 20 h. After the DNA synthesis phase, a second gap phase occurs as the cell prepares for mitosis by producing ribonucleic acid and the mitotic spindle apparatus. The cell then re-enters the mitosis phase and the cell cycle repeats. A certain percentage of cancer cells are killed with each course of chemotherapy, similar to the way each dose of antibiotic kills a certain percentage of bacteria. For example, the initial course of chemotherapy may kill 90% of the cells and leave 10% of the cells, the second administration of chemotherapy administration may kill another 90% and leave 10%, and so on. Tumors consisting of fewer than 10,000 cells are believed to be small enough for the immune system of the patient to eliminate (Balmer & Valley, 2002; Chabner et al., 2001; Chu & DeVita, 2010).

Cancer can be treated with surgery, radiation, chemotherapy, hormones, or immunotherapy. The prognosis and treatment of the patient and the likelihood of cancer cure are determined by the type of cancer, the size of the tumor, and whether the tumor has spread to distant sites. Such spreading of cancer cells is termed **metastasis**. Prognosis and treatment are determined by a process called staging. Stage 0 indicates that the disease is in an early stage, and stage IV indicates that tumor size and metastasis are significant. The stage of cancer is often classified by the T, N, and M system. T denotes the size of the tumor and is staged from T1 to T4, N denotes the degree of spread to regional lymph nodes and is classified as N0 (absent) to N3 (significant), and M denotes the amount of metastasis and is denoted M0 (none) or M1 (presence beyond regional lymph nodes). In addition, tumors that more closely resemble normal cells are termed low grade and carry a better prognosis whereas tumor cells with more distorted physiology are termed high grade and carry a poorer prognosis (Balmer & Valley, 2002; Chu & DeVita, 2010).

Depending on the type and stage of the cancer, a patient may require radiation therapy, chemotherapy, or surgical resection of the tumor. The selection of the form of therapy is tumor and patient specific and is guided by recommendations from cancer guidelines developed by experts in the field on the basis of published patient trials. Chemotherapy can be primary induction therapy for patients with advanced disease or cancer with no other effective treatment, **neoadjuvant** therapy for patients with localized disease that is not effectively treated with surgery or radiation alone, or adjuvant therapy to surgery or radiation. Chemotherapy can be directly instilled into the area of the body in which the cancer resides. Palliative therapy with chemotherapy is used to reduce tumor size to provide comfort or maintain function in the patient who is not expected to survive the disease (Balmer & Valley, 2002; Chu & DeVita, 2010).

Rehabilitation Considerations

The rehabilitation therapist should be aware of the many complications in the cancer patient that can affect rehabilitation, including fluid and electrolyte disorders that can cause weakness, altered mental status, and increase risk of falls. Chemotherapy medications can cause myelosuppression, which can reduce white blood cells, red blood cells, or platelets, which can in turn increase the risk of infection, anemia, and bleeding. The risk is greatest when cell counts are at the lowest point, termed the **nadir**. Patients with cancer who have an infection may not exhibit inflammatory symptoms commonly seen with infection due to their immunosuppression and low white blood cell counts, termed **neutropenia**. Febrile neutropenia is a life-threatening emergency and often is accompanied only by the single symptoms of fever. Because of this, patients who are neutropenic require special precautions (neutropenic precautions) to reduce their risk of exposure to pathogens and encountering infection. Neutropenic precautions can include isolation, dietary restrictions, and careful cleaning of their environment. Neutropenic patients should have their temperature carefully monitored while their white blood cell count is reduced. The therapist should also be aware that cancer patients often experience overwhelming fatigue known as cancer fatigue. Medications that may assist in the management of cancer fatigue are discussed later in the chapter.

The health care team should take special steps in caring for the cancer patient to prevent complications associated with immobility (e.g., pneumonia, urinary tract infections, decreased wound healing, and increased skin breakdown) and should implement special measures for reducing thrombotic complications such as deep venous thrombosis (DVT) and pulmonary embolism. Cancer patients are at higher risk for thrombosis because of their disease, as well as the debility that can accompany cancer. Patients should be encouraged to ambulate in order to prevent weakness and orthostasis associated with prolonged inactivity. Balance, coordination, and cognition also decline in the non-ambulatory patient. Reduction in cardiac output can reduce cerebral perfusion and produce lightheadedness and syncope, thus increasing patient risk for falls. The therapist should always ensure that an appropriate nutritional plan is in place for the patient, particularly if the patient is undergoing medication therapy or radiation therapy to treat the cancer. Finally, the therapist should be aware that many chemotherapy medications can induce neuropathy, which can negatively affect therapy participation and progress and increase the risk of falls.

Fluid and Electrolyte Disorders

Hyponatremia, which is common in cancer patients, is caused by the tumor, metastasis, or medications. **Hypovolemic** hyponatremia is associated with dehydration and can be caused by nausea, vomiting, and diarrhea induced by chemotherapy administration. Dehydration is associated with decreased skin turgor, dry mucous membranes, hypotension, and tachycardia. Hypovolemic hyponatremia is treated with sodium and fluid replacement. **Euvolemic** hyponatremia in cancer patients is usually caused by syndrome of inappropriate antidiuretic hormone (SIADH), steroids, hypothyroidism, stress, medications, and psychogenic polydipsia. SIADH occurs in 1% to 2% of all cancer patients and 10% of patients with small-cell lung cancer. Medications that can cause SIADH include vincristine (Oncovin), cyclophosphamide (Cytoxan), vinblastine (Velban), and cisplatin (Platinol). Treatment of SIADH includes identifying and discontinuing the causative agent, restricting salt and water, or administering demeclocycline if initial measures are not successful (Douglass, 1984; Finley & LaCivitia, 1992; Grunwald, 2003).

Tumor lysis syndrome is a life-threatening fluid and electrolyte disorder seen on days 1 through 5 of chemotherapy treatment of tumors such as Burkitt lymphoma, acute lymphoblastic leukemia, and solid tumors that have a high growth fraction and high sensitivity to chemotherapy. Chemotherapy-induced lysis of tumor cells results in rapid release of potassium, uric acid, phosphorus, and hypocalcemia associated with the hyperphosphatemia. Such electrolyte derangements can cause crystallization of uric acid or calcium and phosphate precipitation in the renal tubules, resulting in obstructive uropathy and acute renal failure. These electrolyte disorders can also cause cardiac arrhythmias and seizures. Calcium is often used to treat arrhythmias associated with high levels of potassium, and the combination of insulin, glucose, and bicarbonate is used to shift potassium from the serum into the cells to reduce toxic effects. Medications that bind potassium and phosphate may also be administered and hemodialysis may be used to rapidly correct electrolyte and metabolic disturbances associated with tumor lysis syndrome. Preventative therapy for reducing uric acid formation and uropathy is initiated with high-dose allopurinol (Zyloprim) along with aggressive hydration with intravenous fluids containing bicarbonate. Rasburicase (recombinant urate oxidase; Elitek) is a newer therapy that can be used if allopurinol (Zyloprim) is ineffective. Table 18.1 provides additional details on these medications (Bubalo, 2009; Krishnan & Hammad, 2009).

Infections in the Cancer Patient

Infections occur more frequently in the cancer patient as a result of impaired immune function associated with the disease or with cancer treatments. Prolonged bed rest or decreased ambulation can also result in infections in the cancer patient. Respiratory infections resulting from immobility can impair respiratory function by weakening the diaphragm and other muscles used in respiration and may lead to hypoxia and reduced ability to cough. Tumor in the lungs and adverse effects from both chemotherapy and radiation may impair the patient's ability to clear lung passages, increasing the risk of aspiration and pneumonia. The rehabilitation therapist should encourage the non-ambulatory patient to practice deep-breathing exercises, incentive spirometry, exercises that increase productive coughing, and exercises that promote stretching and strengthening of the trunk and abdominal muscles (Kaplan & Zandt, 2010).

Patients who remain supine often experience incomplete voiding, which can increase the risk of urinary tract infections. Removing unnecessary catheters, using condom catheters in males, using a bedside commode, and progressing the patient to bathroom privileges reduces the risk of urinary tract infections (Kaplan & Zandt, 2010).

Chemotherapy can cause significant decreases in neutrophils (myelosuppression) and can impair the patient's ability to fight off infection. Patients are at greatest risk when the neutrophil count reaches the lowest point, termed the nadir. Nadirs are usually predictable for each chemotherapy medication and are usually described as the number of days after a dose of chemotherapy. When the white count is very low the patient is termed neutropenic, and fever in these patients is usually the first and sometimes only symptom of life-threatening infection. Febrile neutropenia is a medical emergency that requires prompt hospitalization and the immediate initiation of intravenous antibiotics that are effective against the most common pathogenic bacteria seen in cancer patients (Balmer & Valley, 2002; Grunwald, 2003).

Bacterial infections, the infections most commonly encountered in the cancer patient, are often caused by the bacteria normally found on the skin or in the gastrointestinal tract. Initial treatment consists of intravenous administration of an antibiotic that is active against gram-negative bacteria such as *Escherichia coli* (the bacteria most commonly found in the lower gastrointestinal tract) combined with an agent that covers bacteria most often found on the skin (*Staphylococcus* and *Streptococcus*). Examples of such a regimen include a combination of cefepime (Maxipime) and vancomycin or the use of a broad-spectrum agent such as imipenem–cilastatin (Primaxin) that covers both gram-positive and gram-negative bacteria. If the fever does not improve after 4 days of antibiotics, fungal infection is suspected and **antifungal** agents are added to the antibacterial regimen (Balmer & Valley, 2002; Grunwald, 2003).

Oral fluconazole (Diflucan) is used to treat or prevent fungal infections of the mouth and esophagus (oral thrush or candida esophagitis). Intravenous fluconazole (Diflucan) is used in empiric treatment of suspected fungal infections or in treatment of documented fungal infections caused by *Candida albicans*. Intravenous echinocandin antifungal agents are used if the patient does not improve with Diflucan or if the fungus identified is a more resistant variety. Herpes simplex viral infections of the mucous membranes of the mouth and lips are treated with antiviral agents such as topical, oral, or intravenous acyclovir (Zovirax), oral famciclovir (Famvir), and oral valacyclovir (Valtrex) (Balmer & Valley, 2002; Grunwald, 2003).

Complications Associated With Immobility

Cancer patients are at increased risk of complications associated with immobility that is associated with frequent hospitalization, fatigue and weakness, and the effects of cancer treatments such as chemotherapy, radiation, and surgery. Reduced ambulation associated with bed rest can significantly decrease muscle strength. Strength in the lower extremities may decrease by about 10%/wk and up to 25% after 5 wk. Lack of use can also result in muscle shortening, which can lead to joint contractures (Bubalo, 2009; Kaplan & Zandt, 2010).

Prolonged inactivity can result in orthostatic hypotension. Balance, coordination, and cognition also decline in the non-ambulatory patient. Reduced cardiac output can reduce cerebral perfusion and produce lightheadedness and syncope, thus increasing the patient's risk of falls. Patients should be encouraged to sit up as soon as possible after periods of bed rest or surgery to reduce these adverse effects. Early ambulation helps prevent respiratory complications associated with inactivity, minimizes urinary tract infections, promotes bowel function, and reduces the risk of DVT associated with inactivity (Bubalo, 2009; Kaplan & Zandt, 2010).

Cancer-Associated Thrombosis

Thrombosis is a common complication of cancer and its treatment. Risk of DVT in patients receiving chemotherapy is 6.5 times that seen in the general population. Risk of DVT appears to be highest within 3 to 6 mo of diagnosis and is very common in patients diagnosed with cancer of the pancreas, stomach, brain, kidney, ovary, or lung and in patients with lymphoma and metastatic cancers. The survival rate of cancer patients who develop thrombosis decreases to one third of the survival rate of cancer patients who do not develop thrombosis. Prophylactic use of anticoagulant therapy that includes low-molecular-weight heparin, such as enoxaparin (Lovenox) or fondaparinux (Arixtra), is recommended in patients who are hospitalized with cancer. Documented DVT should be treated with low-molecular-weight heparin such as enoxaparin (Lovenox) for a minimum of 6 mo. Patients with bleeding risk that cannot be safely treated with an anticoagulant should receive an inferior vena cava filter to reduce the risk of pulmonary embolus and should use nonpharmacologic methods of DVT prevention such as elastic stockings and increased ambulation (Bubalo, 2009).

Skin Care

Wound healing can be impeded by poor nutrition, vitamin deficiencies, smoking, and reduced oxygenation of the tissues. **Vasoconstrictors** (e.g., dopamine) used to treat hypotension in the critical care setting can decrease perfusion of tissues and reduce tissue oxygenation. In addition, medications such as chemotherapy and steroids can increase skin breakdown and impede wound healing. Early ambulation reduces the patient's risk of developing skin breakdown and pressure ulcers. Interventions that reduce formation of pressure ulcers in patients that cannot ambulate include frequent repositioning, uploading to reduce pressure, minimizing skin exposure to moisture, and nutritional support (Bubalo, 2009; Kaplan & Zandt, 2010).

Nutrition in the Cancer Patient

Providing adequate nutrition is an important supportive measure in the cancer patient and can significantly affect the patient's ability to participate in rehabilitation therapies. Patients with cancer may have significant problems with dysphagia due to surgical resection, radiation therapy, and chemotherapy-related toxicities such as mucositis, xerostomia, peripheral neuropathy, nausea, and vomiting. Initiation of a bowel regimen that includes adequate hydration, fiber in the diet, laxative use, and exercise can prevent or minimize constipation and impaction. Cancer patients receiving opiate therapy require a stool softener as well as a stimulant laxative such as Senokot-S to counter the severe constipation that can result from the effects of the opiate on the mu receptors in the gastrointestinal tract (Berger & Kilroy, 1997; Carl & Johnson, 2006).

Chemotherapy-Induced Neuropathy

Chemotherapy-induced neuropathy can significantly impair the rehabilitation progress. A patient may complain of symptoms such as cramps in the muscles or reduced feeling in the hands or feet. Chemotherapy-induced autonomic neuropathies can affect balance and impair gastrointestinal motility, which may contribute to gastrointestinal symptoms. The patient may complain of dizziness when standing up or bending over and may experience repeated falls. Chemotherapy-induced neuropathy may cause weight loss, vomiting, or symptoms of gastroesophageal reflux after eating. Table 18.1 summarizes chemotherapy agents that commonly cause neuropathy.

Table 18.1 Chemotherapy Agents That Commonly Induce Neuropathy

Medication	Neuropathy	Symptoms	Comments
Vinca alkaloids			
Vincristine (Oncovin) Vinblastine (Velban)	Damage to small C-fibers and damage to the autonomic nervous system, resulting in orthostasis, impaired gastrointestinal motility, impotence, and urinary retention	Early symptoms are gradual in onset and include myalgias and distal paresthesias. Cranial neuropathies are rapid in onset and are seen with toxic levels of vincristine. These include ptosis and ophthalmoplegia that cause visual disturbance and laryngeal neurotoxicity that can result in stridor.	Vincristine is the most neurotoxic of the Vinca alkaloids. Maximum individual dose of 2 mg and maximum total dose of 12 mg. Recovery from vincristine neuropathy may take 3-4 yr.
Taxane			
Paclitaxel (Taxol)	Sensory-motor neuropathy	The most common initial symptoms include numbness, tingling, and burning pain in a stocking-and-glove distribution. Symptoms are typically symmetric, severe neuropathy accompanied by significant weakness may occur after exposure to large cumulative doses of 200-600 mg/m^2.	Severe orthostasis seen with higher doses.
Platinols			
Cisplatin (Platinol)	High-dose cisplatin commonly causes peripheral neuropathy at cumulative doses of 300 mg/m^2 and in all patients who receive doses >500 mg/m^2. Administering as smaller, more frequent doses or continuous infusions is less toxic than high-bolus dosing.	Early symptoms include cramps, distal paresthesias, and a decrease in ankle jerk and ability to sense vibration. Delayed autonomic dysfunction may also occur.	Risk factors for toxicity include preexisting neuropathy, increased age, ethanol use, and diabetes. Amifostine has shown benefit in the prevention of cisplatin-induced neurotoxicity.
Oxaliplatin (Eloxatin)	Acute sensory neuropathy associated with the infusion that is transient and completely reversible (occurs in 85%-95% of patients), chronic sensory neuropathy	Acute toxicity symptoms include distal or perioral paresthesias, pharyngolaryngeal dysesthesias that affect swallowing and breathing, and muscle contractions of distal extremities (less frequent). Patient should avoid cold, which increases acute symptoms. Dose-limiting chronic neuropathy is associated with cumulative dose and causes pronounced distal dysesthesias and persistent paresthesias of the extremities.	Oxaliplatin causes significant neurotoxicity with an incidence similar to cisplatin. Carboplatin is the platinol product that poses the least risk of neurotoxicity, but can also cause neurotoxicity when used in higher dose regimens or when combined with other neurotoxins.
Individual agents			
Thalidomide	Progressive distal sensory neuropathy	Predominant in the distal limbs. Sensory symptoms include tingling, numbness, and an extreme sensitivity (burning, freezing, or electric-like) to touch.	Occurs with cumulative doses >20 g.
Etoposide (VP-16)	Moderate to severe distal axonal sensorimotor polyneuropathy	Associated with severe autonomic dysfunction (orthostatic hypotension and gastroparesis).	Reversible neuropathy occurs in 4%-10% of patients.
Bortezomib (Velcade)	Peripheral and sensory neuropathy	Sensory symptoms include tingling, numbness, and an extreme sensitivity (burning, freezing, or electric-like) to touch.	Risk of neuropathy increases with increased doses or long-term therapy.

Medication Therapy: Cancer Treatment

The two major classes of medications that are used to kill cancer cells and induce remission in the cancer patient are chemotherapy medications and biologic-response modifiers. Each type of chemotherapy medication targets different stages of tumor growth. Some chemotherapy medications are not cell cycle specific, meaning that they kill cancer cells in all phases of growth. Examples include classic alkylating agents, anthracycline antibiotics, products containing platinum, and nitrosoureas. Other medications target a specific phase of cell replication. For example, chemotherapy medications that target the gap phase include steroids and asparaginase (Elspar). Medications that target the mitotic phase include vinca alkaloids and taxanes. Chemotherapy medications that target the DNA synthesis phase include **antimetabolites** and lymphokines. Finally, bleomycin and podophyllotoxins target the second gap phase. Table 18.2 provides additional information on chemotherapy medications (Balmer & Valley, 2002; Chabner et al., 2001; Chu & DeVita, 2010).

Biologic-response modifiers that help the body fight cancer by altering the response of the immune system are increasingly being used in the treatment of cancer. These agents include monoclonal antibody therapies and cytokines such as interleukin and interferon. Table 18.3 provides information on these medications.

Chemotherapy

Chemotherapy medication is usually administered in 4 to 6 cycles of 3 to 4 wk. Specific dosing is based on the pharmacokinetics of each medication and the growth pattern of the tumor. A combination of several types of chemotherapy medications is used in many regimens to target different stages of tumor growth. Combination therapy can be more effective than a single agent and can reduce overall toxicity and minimize development of tumor resistance. Medications in combination chemotherapy regimens are also chosen based on the side effect profile of each medication in order to minimize additive effects of the same toxicity (Balmer & Valley, 2002; Chabner et al., 2001; Chu & DeVita, 2010; Finley & LaCivitia, 1992; Grunwald, 2003).

Side effects that occur frequently with chemotherapy and that can necessitate suspending the administration of the chemotherapy are called dose-limiting toxicities (designated as DLT in the chapter tables). Examples of dose-limiting toxicities include myelosuppression, severe nausea and vomiting, stomatitis, and cardiotoxicity. Chemotherapy can cause fatigue, myelosuppression, and impaired immune function and can increase risk of infection in patients with cancer (Balmer & Valley, 2002; Chabner et al., 2001; Chu & DeVita, 2010; Finley & LaCivitia, 1992; Grunwald, 2003).

When chemotherapy agents are administered with other medications, the health care provider must monitor for possible drug interactions as well as additive toxicities from the other agents. Numerous drug interactions exist with these agents. These interactions can result in altered rates of metabolism or elimination and contribute to increased toxicity or reduced efficacy. An important potential drug interaction involves competitive antagonism of antimetabolite chemotherapy agents cytotoxic action by nutritional or vitamin products. For example, the action of methotrexate can be reduced by folic acid supplementation. Monitoring for side effects and drug interactions is an important component of patient care. Several herbal products can reduce the effects of chemotherapy or harm patients with impaired immune systems such as cancer patients. Some can impair nutrient absorption, contribute to bleeding risk, and even cause depression. Patients with cancer should avoid black cohosh and chamomile (can interfere with absorption of vitamins and nutrients), valerian (can cause depression), aristolochia (contains carcinogens and can contribute to cancer), bioflavonoids and echinacea (can decrease the effectiveness of chemotherapy agents), flaxseed (can increase growth of hormone-dependent cancers), and sweet clover and ginkgo (can increase bleeding risk, especially in patients with low platelet counts due to chemotherapy

See table 18.2 in the web resource for a full list of medication-specific indications, dosing recommendations, and side effects.

Table 18.2 Chemotherapy Medications

Medication and indication	Side effects affecting rehab							Dose-limiting toxicities and other side effects or considerations
Antimetabolites: Inhibit DNA action or replication.								
Cytarabine (Cytosine, Cytosine arabinoside, Ara-C) Acute myelogenous leukemia, acute lymphocytic leukemia, chronic myelogenous leukemia, leptomeningeal carcinomatosis, non-Hodgkin's lymphoma	Cog +++	S +	A +	Motor +++	D +++	Com +++	F +++	Side effects: DLT: Myelosuppression. Mild nausea with lower-dose regimens, alopecia (common). With high doses >1 g/m²: Severe nausea, neurotoxicity, dysarthria, nystagmus, ataxia, encephalopathy, seizures, chemical conjunctivitis, and CNS, ocular, hepatic, dermatologic, and pulmonary toxicity. Other: Use steroid eye drops and saline eye drops to prevent ocular toxicity. Drug interactions: Antagonizes activity of gentamicin and 5-FU; decreases levels and activity of digoxin. Enhances cytotoxicity of alkylating agents. Pretreatment with methotrexate, fludarabine, and hydroxyurea enhances activity. Granulocyte- and monocyte-stimulating factors and interleukin-3 potentiate cytotoxic effects. Increased risk of pancreatitis when L-asparaginase is given before cytarabine.
Gemcitabine (Gemzar) Pancreatic cancer, non-small-cell lung cancer, breast cancer, ovarian cancer, bladder cancer, soft-tissue sarcoma	Cog ++	S ++	A 0	Motor 0	D +	Com +	F ++	Side effects: DLT: Myelosuppression, with WBCs affected to a greater extent than platelets; nadir on days 10-14; recovery by day 21. Others: Infusion reactions are related to infusion rate and include flushing, facial swelling, headache, dyspnea, hypotension, elevated LFTs, proteinuria, mild hematuria (50%). Flu-like syndrome 6-12 h after dose (20%), rash 2-3 days after administration (25%), mild to moderate nausea and vomiting (70%), diarrhea or mucositis (15%-20%), pulmonary toxicity, dyspnea, pneumonitis, maculopapular skin rash (trunk and extremities with pruritus). Potent radiosensitizer. Drug interactions: Enhances cytotoxicity of cisplatin. Etoposide may enhance cytotoxicity.
6-Mercaptopurine Acute lymphoblastic leukemia	Cog +	S +	A 0	Motor 0	D ++	Com +	F +	Side effects: Mild bone marrow suppression with WBC nadir days 10-14; recovery by day 21; mucositis or diarrhea with higher doses; elevated serum bilirubin, liver enzymes, jaundice (onset occurs 2-3 mo after therapy).

› continued

Table 18.2 › *continued*

Medication and indication	Side effects affecting rehab							Dose-limiting toxicities and other side effects or considerations
6-Mercaptopurine Acute lympho-blastic leukemia (continued)								Other: Elevated serum bilirubin and liver enzymes, mild nausea and vomiting (dose-related). Drug interactions: Reduce dose by 50% when combined with allopurinol. Inhibits anticoagulant effects of warfarin (Coumadin). Bactrim DS may enhance myelosuppressive effects.
6-Thioguanine (6-TG) Acute and chronic myelog-enous leukemia, acute lympho-blastic leukemia	Cog ++	S ++	A 0	Motor 0	D +++	Com +	F ++	Side effects: DLT: Myelosuppression where leukopenia precedes thrombocytopenia; nadir is 10-14 days; recovery by day 21; severe mucositis and diarrhea. Other: Elevated serum bilirubin and liver enzymes, mild nausea and vomiting (dose-related). Drug interactions: None known.
5-Fluorouracil (5-FU) (Efudex) Cell cycle spe-cific, active in S phase. Used in colorec-tal, breast, GI, head and neck, liver, ovarian, skin cancers	Cog +++	S +++	A +++	Motor +++	D +++	Com ++	F +++	Side effects: DLT: Myelosuppression, mucositis, diarrhea, neu-rotoxicity (head-foot syndrome, ataxia, seizures). Use pyridoxine 50 mg bid prophylaxis to reduce neurotoxic effects. Others: Ischemia in patients with cardiac dis-ease, conjunctivitis, blepharitis, skin discolor-ation, metallic taste. Drug interactions: Leucovorin enhances activity, toxicity. Methotrexate pretreatment increases 5-FU metabolite formation and effects. Thymidine or vistonuridine rescue patient from toxic effects of 5-FU.
Fludarabine monophosphate (F-ara-A, Fludara) Chronic lymphocytic leukemia, non-Hodgkin's lymphoma	Cog +++	S +++	A +++	Motor +++	D +++	Com ++	F +++	Side effects: DLT: Myelosuppression with WBC nadir is 10-13 days; recovery by days 14-21. Immunosuppression common with decreased CD4+ and CD8+ T-cells. Recovery of CD4+ count is slow and may take more than 1 yr to return to normal. With high dose: Weakness, agitation, confusion, progressive encephalopathy, cortical blindness, seizures, coma. Other: Tumor lysis syndrome (1%-2%), hyper-sensitivity reaction (maculopapular skin rash, erythema, pruritus), reversible interstitial pneumonitis after several courses of therapy, neurotoxicity (somnolence, mild peripheral neu-ropathy, paresthesias, visual disturbances), auto-immune hemolytic anemia (rare), drug-induced aplastic anemia (rare).

Medication and indication	Side effects affecting rehab							Dose-limiting toxicities and other side effects or considerations
								Fever, fatigue, malaise, myalgias, arthralgias, and chills (20%-30%) 5-7 days after dose due to release of pyrogens from tumor cells.
								Drug interactions: Enhances the antitumor activity of cytarabine, cyclophosphamide, cisplatin, and mitoxantrone.
								Increases incidence of fatal pulmonary toxicity when used with pentostatin. Use of this combination is absolutely contraindicated.
Cladribine (Leustatin) Hairy cell leukemia, chronic lymphocytic leukemia, non-Hodgkin's lymphoma	Cog ++	S ++	A +	Motor ++	D +	Com ++	F ++	Side effects: DLT: Myelosuppression with WBC nadir is 7-14 days; recovery in 3-4 wks. Immunosuppression with decrease in CD4+ and CD8+ cells and increased risk of opportunistic infections. Recovery of CD4+ takes up to 40 months. Other: Erythema, pain, pruritus, swelling at injection site, neurotoxicity (headache, insomnia, dizziness). Fever, fatigue, malaise, myalgias, arthralgias, and chills occur in 40%-50% of patients on days 5-7 of therapy. Drug interactions: None known.
Methotrexate (MTX, Trexall, Rheumatrex) Breast cancer, head and neck cancer, osteogenic sarcoma, acute lymphoblastic leukemia, non-Hodgkin's lymphoma, meningeal leukemia, bladder cancer, colorectal cancer, gestational cancer, trophoblastic cancer	Cog ++	S ++	A +	Motor ++	D +++	Com ++	F ++	Side effects: DLT: Myelosuppression and mucositis. Mucositis occurs 3-7 days after dose. Mucosal ulceration can be life threatening and can require dose interruption. Renal toxicity is prevented with vigorous hydration and IV administration of bicarbonate and leucovorin rescue to prevent crystallization in the renal tubules. Leucovorin rescues the host toxic effects of methotrexate but may impair antitumor activity. Other: Mild nausea and vomiting, photosensitivity, eye discomfort, allergic reactions; hepatic, renal, neurologic, and pulmonary toxicities (can be fatal). Symptoms of pulmonary toxicity are fever, dry cough, dyspnea, and chest pain. Irreversible chronic demyelinating encephalopathy with dementia, spasticity, and coma can occur months or years after treatment (usually occurs with cranial irradiation). Drug interactions: Cisplatin decreases elimination. Aspirin, penicillins, probenecid, nonsteroidal anti-inflammatory drugs, cephalosporins, and phenytoin inhibit renal excretion, increasing toxicity. Increases anticoagulant effect of warfarin (Coumadin).

› continued

Table 18.2 › *continued*

Medication and indication	Side effects affecting rehab							Dose-limiting toxicities and other side effects or considerations
Methotrexate (MTX, Trexall, Rheumatrex) Breast cancer, head and neck cancer, osteogenic sarcoma, acute lymphoblastic leukemia, non-Hodgkin's lymphoma, meningeal leukemia, bladder cancer, colorectal cancer, gestational cancer, trophoblastic cancer *(continued)*								Enhances antitumor activity of 5-fluorouracil when given 24 h before fluoropyrimidine treatment. Thymidine rescues the host toxic effects of methotrexate, causing impaired antitumor activity. Folic acid supplements may counteract the antitumor effects. Omeprazole increases serum methotrexate levels, leading to enhanced antitumor activity and host toxicity. L-asparaginase antagonizes the antitumor activity of MTX.

Vinca alkaloids: Mitotic inhibitors that reduce cell replication and cause apoptosis.

Medication and indication	Cog	S	A	Motor	D	Com	F	Dose-limiting toxicities and other side effects or considerations
Vincristine (Oncovin) Acute lymphoblastic leukemia, Hodgkin's and non-Hodgkin's lymphoma, multiple myeloma, rhabdomyosarcoma, neuroblastoma, Ewing's sarcoma, Wilms' tumor, chronic leukemias, thyroid cancer, brain tumors, trophoblastic neoplasm	++	++	+	++++	++++	++	++++	Side effects: DLT: Dose-limiting toxicity is neurotoxicity (distal, symmetric). Affects sensation and motor function; earliest symptoms are depressed deep-tendon reflexes, paresthesias of the fingers and toes, and cranial nerve toxicities of hoarseness, facial palsies, and jaw pain. Autonomic neuropathy, constipation, colicky abdominal pain, orthostasis, paralytic ileus, cranial nerve palsies (ataxia, cortical blindness, seizures, coma), and pain in the bone, back, limb, jaw, and parotid gland. Alopecia, skin rash, fever, a prophylactic bowel regimen for neurotoxicity associated constipation is recommended. Other: SIADH form of hyponatremia. Vesicant; treat with warm compresses if extravasation occurs. Drug interactions: Occur with medications metabolized by the CYP3A liver enzymes. Reduces the blood levels of phenytoin and digoxin. Concurrent administration with other neurotoxins (cisplatin, paclitaxel) increases neurotoxicity. Should be administered 12-24 hrs before L-asparaginase when used in combination; L-asparaginase inhibits vincristine clearance and increases its toxicity. Increases the cellular uptake of methotrexate, resulting in enhanced antitumor activity and host toxicity. Concurrent use with filgrastim may result in severe atypical neuropathy.

Medication and indication	Side effects affecting rehab							Dose-limiting toxicities and other side effects or considerations
Vinblastine (Velban) Vinorelbine (Navelbine) Hodgkin's and non-Hodgkin's lymphomas, testicular cancer, breast cancer, Kaposi's sarcoma, renal cell carcinoma	Cog	S	A	Motor	D	Com	F	Side effects:
	++	++	+	++++	++++	++	++++	DLT: Myelosuppression with WBC nadir at days 4-6.
								Neurotoxicity presents with the same manifestations as seen with vincristine: Peripheral neuropathy (paresthesias, paralysis, loss of deep-tendon reflexes, constipation) and dysfunction of the autonomic nervous system (orthostatic hypotension, paralytic ileus, urinary retention).
								Other: Mucositis, stomatitis, nausea, vomiting, anorexia, diarrhea, alopecia (common, mild, and reversible), SIADH, headache, depression, and vascular events (stroke, myocardial infarction, Raynaud's syndrome).
								Less common: Cranial nerve paralysis, ataxia, cortical blindness, seizures, coma.
								Vesicant; treat with warm compresses if extravasation occurs.
								Drug interactions: Occur with medications that are metabolized by CYP3A liver enzymes, such as the calcium channel blockers, cimetidine, cyclosporine, erythromycin, metoclopramide, and ketoconazole.
								Reduces blood levels of phenytoin through either reduced absorption of phenytoin or an increase in the rate of its metabolism and elimination.
								Risk of Raynaud's syndrome increases when combined with bleomycin.

Taxane alkaloids: Have antimitotic effects by microtubule polymerization in the mitotic phase of cell replication that prevents tumor cell replication, induces angiogenesis, and promotes cell death.

Medication and indication	Side effects affecting rehab							Dose-limiting toxicities and other side effects or considerations
Paclitaxel (Taxol) Ovarian cancer, breast cancer, non-small-cell and small-cell lung cancer, head and neck cancer, esophageal cancer, prostate cancer, bladder cancer, Kaposi's sarcoma related to acquired immune deficiency syndrome	Cog	S	A	Motor	D	Com	F	Side effects:
	++	++	0	+++	+++	++	+++	DLT: Myelosuppression with WBC nadir at days 8-10; recovery by day 15-21; nadir is decreased with shortened infusion.
								Cumulative and dose-dependent neurotoxicity (sensory neuropathy with numbness and paresthesias, motor and autonomic neuropathy); more frequent with longer infusions and at doses >175 mg/m^2.
								Other: Bradycardia (30% of patients), alopecia (all patients; total loss of hair), mucositis or diarrhea (30%-40%).
								Hypersensitivity (skin rash, flushing, erythema, hypotension, dyspnea, bronchospasm) occurs in first 2-10 min of an infusion in 30%-60% of patients due to the Camphor-EL vehicle. Pretreatment reduces hypersensitivity reaction incidence to 2%-4%.

› continued

Table 18.2 › *continued*

Medication and indication	Side effects affecting rehab							Dose-limiting toxicities and other side effects or considerations
Paclitaxel (Taxol) Ovarian cancer, breast cancer, non-small-cell and small-cell lung cancer, head and neck cancer, esophageal cancer, prostate cancer, bladder cancer, Kaposi's sarcoma related to acquired immune deficiency syndrome *(continued)*								Pretreatment regimen: Decadron 20 mg given by mouth or by IV at 12 hrs and at 6 hrs prior to the dose h plus Benadryl 50 mg IV and oral cimetidine 300 mg given 30-60 min before the chemo dose. Radiosensitizing agent. Drug interactions: Concomitant use of inhibitors or activators of CYP3A4 liver enzymes may affect metabolism, levels, and toxicity. Phenytoin and phenobarbital increase metabolism. Myelosuppression increases when a platinum compound or cyclophosphamide is administered before paclitaxel. Must be given first when administered with platinum analog. Decreases clearance of doxorubicin by 30%-35%; administer after doxorubicin to reduce severity of neutropenia.
Docetaxel (Taxotere) Breast cancer, locally advanced or metastatic breast cancer, non-small-cell lung cancer, small-cell lung cancer, head and neck cancer, gastric cancer, refractory ovarian cancer, bladder cancer	**Cog** +++	**S** +++	**A** 0	**Motor** ++++	**D** ++++	**Com** ++	**F** +++	Side effects: DLT: Myelosuppression with WBC nadir at days 7-10 and recovery by day 14. Cumulative peripheral neuropathy (sensory, motor neuropathy, autonomic neuropathy, and CNS effects). Others: Hypersensitivity reactions associated with the Camphor-EL vehicle (severe <5%), skin rash, erythema, hypotension, dyspnea, bronchospasm. Usually occurs in first 2-10 min of an infusion with first 2 treatments; reduced with weekly dosing regimens. Pretreat with dexamethasone (Decadron) 80 mg by mouth every 12 h starting 24 h before dose and continued every 12 h after dose for 3 more days. Fluid-retention syndrome (50%): Weight gain, peripheral or generalized edema, pleural effusion, ascites. Incidence increases with total doses >400 mg/m². Pretreat with steroid to prevent edema and allergic reactions. Phlebitis, swelling at the injection site, maculopapular skin rash (50% in first wk), alopecia (up to 80% of patients), mucositis or diarrhea (40% of patients), generalized fatigue, arthralgias, myalgias and asthenia (60-70%), reversible elevations in liver enzymes and bilirubin, fever (30%), vesicant. Radiosensitizing agent. Drug interactions: Medications metabolized by CYP3A4 liver enzymes such as cyclosporine, ketoconazole, and erythromycin alter metabolism, blood levels, and toxicity of the taxanes.

Medication and indication	Side effects affecting rehab							Dose-limiting toxicities and other side effects or considerations
Podophyllotoxin derivatives: Cause breakage of DNA strands by inhibiting double-stranded DNA repair enzyme topoisomerase II.								
Etoposide (Toposar, Vepesid) Germ cell tumors, small-cell lung cancer, non-small-cell lung cancer, non-Hodgkin's lymphoma, gastric cancer	Cog +	S +	A 0	Motor +	D +	Com ++	F +	Side effects: DLT: Infusion reactions; propylene glycol vehicle contributes to infusion reaction. Orthostasis can be prevented with slowed infusion over 30-60 min. Others: Metallic taste during infusion, reaction at local injection site, radiation recall skin changes. Drug interactions: Prolongs INR with warfarin (Coumadin) therapy.
Teniposide (Vumon) Acute lymphoblastic leukemia	Cog ++	S ++	A 0	Motor 0	D ++	Com +	F ++	Side effects: DLT: Myelosuppression is dose-limiting toxicity. Neutrophil nadir is 7-10 days; recovery by day 21. Severe, life-threatening hypersensitivity reactions (tachycardia, bronchospasm, facial and tongue swelling, hypotension, chills, fever, flushing, urticaria) can occur. Camphor-EL vehicle contributes to allergic reactions. Mucositis may be dose limiting with high-dose regimens. Other: Diarrhea; prevent dose-associated diarrhea with atropine. Treat delayed-onset diarrhea with loperamide (Imodium) 4 mg at symptom onset, then 2 mg every 2 h until no bowel movement for 12 h. Reaction at local injection site, mild nausea and vomiting (30%; pretreat for nausea and vomiting), alopecia (10%-30%). Drug interactions: Incompatible with heparin; precipitates can form.
Camptothecin alkaloids: Causes breakage of DNA strands by inhibiting single-stranded DNA repair enzyme topoisomerase I.								
Irinotecan (Camptosar) Colorectal cancer, non-small-cell lung cancer, small-cell lung cancer	Cog ++	S ++	A 0	Motor 0	D ++++	Com +	F ++	Side effects: DLT: Myelosuppression with WBC nadir is 7-10 days; recovery by days 21-28. Dose-limiting diarrhea: Early and late forms. Early form occurs within 24 h with flushing, diaphoresis, abdominal pain, and diarrhea. Late form occurs 3-10 days after treatment (severe and prolonged with dehydration and electrolyte imbalance in 20%). 80%-90% of patients experience late diarrhea. Other: Mild alopecia, rash, low-grade fevers, malaise, elevated liver enzymes, eosinophilia (20%), severe nausea, and vomiting. Drug interactions: None known.

› continued

Table 18.2 › *continued*

Medication and indication	Side effects affecting rehab							Dose-limiting toxicities and other side effects or considerations
	Cog	S	A	Motor	D	Com	F	
Topotecan (Hycamtin)	+	+	0	++	+++	+	++	**Side effects:**
Ovarian cancer, small-cell lung cancer, acute myelogenous leukemia								DLT: Myelosuppression is dose limiting with WBC nadir at days 7-10; recovery by days 21-28.
								Others: Headache, fever, malaise, arthralgias, myalgias, alopecia, mild to moderate nausea, and vomiting (60-80%; dose related).
								Drug interactions: None known.

Anthracycline antibiotics and anthracenediones: Cause breakage of DNA strands by inhibiting double-stranded DNA repair enzyme topoisomerase II; bind with iron to form free radicals that cleave DNA.

Medication and indication	Side effects affecting rehab							Dose-limiting toxicities and other side effects or considerations
	Cog	S	A	Motor	D	Com	F	
Anthracycline antibiotic: Doxorubicin (Adriamycin)	++	++	0	0	+++	+	++	**Side effects:**
Breast cancer, Hodgkin's and non-Hodgkin's lymphomas, soft tissue sarcoma, ovarian cancer, non-small-cell and small-cell lung cancers, bladder cancer, thyroid cancer, hepatoma, gastric cancer, Wilms' tumor, neuroblastoma, acute lymphoblastic leukemia								DLT: Cardiotoxicity; acute, chronic, and late onset. Acute: ST wave changes, tachycardia, and PVC can occur with dose. Chronic: Cardiomyopathy limits cumulative dose to >550 mg/m²; 50% incidence with doses >1000 mg/m². Liposomal forms produce less cardiotoxicity. Cardiac monitoring of ejection fraction is recommended. Cardiotoxic effects inhibited by dexrazoxane (Zinecard). Small weekly doses or continuous infusion for 2-4 days markedly decrease cardiotoxicity. Late onset (5-20 yr after treatment): Progressive left ventricular dysfunction, arrhythmias, sudden death.
								Myelosuppression with WBC nadir at days 10-14; recovery by day 21.
								Mucositis and diarrhea (dose limiting with infusion protocols).
								Others: Red–orange discoloration of urine within 1-2 days after dose, mild nausea and vomiting (50% in first 1-2 h of dose; premedicate for nausea and vomiting), alopecia in all (reverses in 3 mo), dermatologic flare at site during infusion, radiation recall skin reaction, acute myeloid leukemia.
								Extravasation is associated with significant tissue damage; application of ice is recommended.
								Drug interactions: Incompatible with dexamethasone, 5-fluorouracil, and heparin; leads to precipitate formation.
								Increased risk of hemorrhagic cystitis and cardiotoxicity when combined with cyclophosphamide.
								Levels decreased when used with barbiturates and phenytoin.
								Increased cardiotoxicity when used with herceptin or mitomycin C.
								Decreases oral bioavailability of digoxin.
								Increased risk of hepatotoxicity when used with 6-mercaptopurine.

Medication and indication	Side effects affecting rehab							Dose-limiting toxicities and other side effects or considerations
Anthracycline antibiotic: Daunorubicin (Cerubidine) Acute myelogenous leukemia (remission induction and relapse), acute lymphoblastic leukemia (remission induction and relapse)	Cog ++	S ++	A 0	Motor 0	D +++	Com +	F ++	Side effects: DLT: Myelosuppression with WBC nadir at 10-14 days; recovery by day 21. Cardiotoxicity: Acute, chronic, and delayed. Acute occurs within the first 2-3 days as arrhythmias and electrocardiography changes; transient and asymptomatic. Chronic: cardiomyopathy and CHF can limit cumulative dose to >550 mg/m^2; 50% incidence with doses >1000 mg/m^2. Delayed (5-20 yr after treatment): Progressive left ventricular dysfunction, arrhythmias, and sudden death. Mucositis can be dose limiting in infusion protocols. Others: Nausea and vomiting (usually mild; 50% in first 1-2 h of dose; premedicate for nausea and vomiting), photosensitivity, hyperpigmentation of nails, skin rash (rare), urticaria, alopecia (occurs in all; reverses 5-7 wk after treatment), red–orange discoloration of urine (lasts 1-2 days after administration), radiation recall skin reaction. Drug interactions: Incompatible with dexamethasone and heparin; precipitate will form.
Anthracycline antibiotic: Idarubicin (Idamycin) Acute myelogenous leukemia, acute lymphoblastic leukemia, chronic myelogenous leukemia in blast crisis, myelodysplastic syndrome (MDS)	Cog ++	S ++	A 0	Motor 0	D +++	Com +	F ++	Side effects: DLT: Cardiotoxicity; acute, chronic, and late onset. Acute: ST wave changes, tachycardia, and PVC can occur with dose. Chronic: Cardiomyopathy can limit cumulative doses >550 mg/m^2; 50% incidence with doses >1000 mg/m^2. Late onset (5-20 yr after treatment): Progressive left ventricular dysfunction, arrhythmias, and sudden death. Preventative IV administration of dexrazoxane reduces cardiotoxicity. Monitoring of ejection fraction is recommended. Small weekly doses or continuous infusion for 2-4 days markedly decrease cardiotoxicity. Myelosuppression with WBC nadir at 10-14 days; recovery by day 21. Mucositis and diarrhea may be dose limiting in infusion protocols. Others: Moderate to severe nausea and vomiting (80-90%; premedicate for nausea and vomiting), alopecia (occurs in all; reversible), photosensitivity, mucositis, and diarrhea (common but not severe), reversible effects on liver enzymes, red discoloration of urine in first 1-2 days of dose, radiation recall skin reaction. Drug interactions: Avoid combining with probenecid or sulfinpyrazone to avoid uric acid nephropathy. Incompatible with heparin; precipitates can form.

› continued

Table 18.2 › *continued*

Medication and indication	Side effects affecting rehab							Dose-limiting toxicities and other side effects or considerations
Anthracycline antibiotic: Epirubicin (Ellence) Breast cancer, metastatic breast cancer, gastric cancer	Cog	S	A	Motor	D	Com	F	Side effects:
	++	++	0	0	++	+	++	DLT: Myelosuppression with WBC nadir at 8-14 days; recovery by day 21.
								Cardiotoxicity: acute, chronic, and late onset. Acute: ST wave changes, tachycardia, PVC, chest pain, and myopericarditis can occur within 24-48 h of dose. Chronic can limit cumulative dose >550 mg/m^2; 50% incidence with doses >1000 mg/m^2. Chronic: Cardiotoxicity presents as a dilated cardiomyopathy with congestive heart failure. Risk increases significantly with cumulative doses >900 mg/m^2. Late onset (5-20 yr after treatment): Progressive left ventricular dysfunction, arrhythmias, and sudden death. Preventative IV administration of dexrazoxane reduces cardiotoxicity. Monitoring of ejection fraction is recommended. Continuous infusion and weekly schedules decrease risk of cardiotoxicity.
								Others: Mild nausea and vomiting (premedicate for nausea and vomiting), mild mucositis and diarrhea (common and dose dependent), alopecia (25%-50%; occurs within 10 days of dose; reverses with discontinuance), red–orange discoloration of urine for 24 h after dose, radiation recall skin reaction.
								Potent vesicant. Extravasation is associated with significant tissue damage. Apply ice.
								Drug interactions: Incompatible with heparin; precipitates can form.
								Increased myelosuppression when used with 5-FU or cyclophosphamide.
								Cimetidine reduces levels and effects by 50%.
Anthracenedione: Mitoxantrone (Novantrone) Hodgkin's disease, non-Hodgkin's lymphoma	Cog	S	A	Motor	D	Com	F	Side effects:
	++	++	0	0	+	+	+	DLT: Myelosuppression with WBC and platelet nadirs at day 7-10; recovery by day 21.
								Severe nausea and vomiting can be dose limiting in first 3 h after drug administration and last 4-24 h. Premedicate for nausea and vomiting.
								Others: Pain, inflammation, and necrosis at injection site.
								Reduced cardiotoxicity and less ulceration with extravasation. Nausea, vomiting, alopecia, and mucositis are less severe than with the anthracycline antibiotics.
								Powerful vesicant.

Medication and indication	Side effects affecting rehab							Dose-limiting toxicities and other side effects or considerations
Alkylating agents: Highly reactive alkyl groups; covalently bind with nucleic acids in proteins, causing cross-linking of DNA and inhibition of DNA synthesis. Nitrogen mustard derivatives and nitrosoureas which transform into alkylating agents.								
Alkylating agent: Cyclophosphamide (Cytoxan) Breast cancer, non-Hodgkin's lymphoma, chronic lymphocytic leukemia, ovarian cancer, bone and soft-tissue sarcoma, rhabdomyosarcoma, neuroblastoma, Wilms' tumor	Cog +	S +	A 0	Motor 0	D +	Com +	F +	Side effects: DLT: Myelosuppression with WBC leukopenia nadir at 7-14 days; recovery by day 21. Dose-limiting hemorrhagic cystitis (5%-10% of patients). Time of onset is variable and may begin within 24 h of therapy or may be delayed for up to several weeks. Usually reversible upon discontinuation of drug. Minimized with prehydration with at least 3 L of fluid before the dose (low-dose regimens) or with prehydration and Mesna administration (high-dose regimens; mandatory to prevent bladder toxicity). Continuous bladder irrigations may also be useful. Others: Dose-related nausea and vomiting (severe with high-dose regimens; onset is within 2-4 h of dose and lasts up to 24 h; premedicate for nausea and vomiting), dose-related alopecia (severe with high-dose regimens; occurs 2-3 wk after dose), hyperpigmentation of skin and nails, anorexia, cardiotoxicity (observed with high-dose therapy), immunosuppression, SIADH, hypersensitivity reaction (rhinitis, irritation of the nose and throat), thrombocytopenia (usually with high-dose therapy), nephrotoxicity (may occur with high-dose regimens). Drug interactions: Phenobarbital, phenytoin, and other drugs that stimulate the liver P450 system increase the rate of metabolic activation of cyclophosphamide to its toxic metabolites. Increases the effect of anticoagulants; may need to decrease dose of anticoagulants depending on coagulation parameters. Decreases plasma levels of digoxin by activating its metabolism in the liver. May increase risk of doxorubicin-induced cardiotoxicity.

› *continued*

Table 18.2 › *continued*

Medication and indication	Side effects affecting rehab							Dose-limiting toxicities and other side effects or considerations
Nitrogen mustard alkylating agent: Ifosfamide (Mitoxana, Ifex) Recurrent germ cell tumors, soft-tissue sarcoma, osteogenic sarcoma, non-Hodgkin's lymphoma, Hodgkin's disease, non-small cell and small-cell lung cancers, bladder cancer, head and neck cancer, cervical cancer, Ewing's sarcoma	Cog +++	S +++	A ++	Motor +++	D +++	Com ++	F +++	Side effects: DLT: Myelosuppression with WBC nadir at 10-14 days; recovery in 21 days. Dose-limiting toxicity is hemorrhagic cystitis; prehydrate and administer Mesna. Minimize dose-limiting side effect of hemorrhagic cystitis. Continuous bladder irrigations may also be useful. Others: Dose-related nausea and vomiting (severe with high-dose regimens; occurs within 3-6 h of dose and may last up to 3 days; premedicate for nausea and vomiting); CNS toxicity (lethargy, confusion, seizure, cerebellar ataxia, weakness, hallucinations, cranial nerve dysfunction, and, rarely, stupor and coma; risk increased with high-dose therapy and renal impairment), alopecia (>80% of patients; dose related and severe with high-dose regimens), SIADH. Drug interactions: Phenobarbital, phenytoin, and other drugs that induce CYP450 enzymes increase the rate of metabolic activation of ifosfamide to its toxic metabolites and increase its toxicity. Cimetidine and allopurinol increase the formation of ifosfamide metabolites and its toxicity. Cisplatin increases renal toxicity. Increases anticoagulant effects and toxicity of warfarin (Coumadin).
Nitrosourea: Carmustine (BiCNU—IV) Brain tumors, Hodgkin's disease, non-Hodgkin's lymphoma, multiple myeloma	Cog ++	S ++	A 0	Motor +	D ++	Com ++	F ++	Side effects: DLT: Dose-limiting interstitial lung disease and pulmonary fibrosis (cough, dyspnea, pulmonary infiltrates, respiratory failure) with cumulative doses >1400 mg/m². Pulmonary symptoms treated with steroids. Myelosuppression is dose limiting; involves all blood elements; delayed, prolonged, and cumulative. Lasts 6-8 wks. Affects WBCs and platelets. Platelet nadir is 4-6 wk after dose and lasts 1-3 wk. Others: Severe nausea and vomiting (occurs within 2 h of dose and lasts 4-6 h; premedicate for nausea and vomiting), facial flushing, burning sensation at injection site with faster rates of administration, hepatotoxicity with elevated liver enzymes (90%) within 1 wk of therapy, hepatic veno-occlusive disease with high doses (5%-20%). Skin contact with drug may cause brownish discoloration and pain. Drug interactions: Cimetidine increases toxicity.

Medication and indication	Side effects affecting rehab							Dose-limiting toxicities and other side effects or considerations
								Amphotericin B increases cellular levels of carmustine, increasing toxicity (including renal toxicity).
								Decreases digoxin and phenytoin levels.
Nitrosourea: Lomustine (CeeNU—oral) Brain tumors, Hodgkin's disease, non-Hodgkin's lymphoma	Cog ++++	S ++++	A ++	Motor +++	D +++	Com ++	F +++	Side effects: DLT: Myelosuppression is dose-limiting toxicity; delayed, cumulative, and prolonged; lasts 6-8 wk; affects all elements. Platelet nadir is 4-6 wks after dose and lasts 1-3 wks. Renal toxicity with cumulative doses >1,000 mg/m² (azotemia, decreased kidney size, renal failure, glomerulosclerosis, severe tubular loss, interstitial fibrosis). Others: Nausea and vomiting (occurs 2-6 hrs after dose and lasts up to 24 hrs; premedicate for nausea and vomiting), neurotoxicity (confusion, lethargy, dysarthria, ataxia). Drug interactions: Cimetidine increases levels and toxicity. Avoid alcohol for at least 1 h before and after dose.
Nitrosourea: Dacarbazine (DTIC—IV) Metastatic malignant melanoma, Hodgkin's disease, soft-tissue sarcomas, neuroblastoma	Cog ++++	S +++	A +	Motor ++++	D +++	Com ++	F ++++	Side effects: DLT: Myelosuppression with WBC and platelet nadir at 21-25 days. CNS toxicity (paresthesias, neuropathies, ataxia, lethargy, headache, confusion, seizures). Others: Pain or burning at injection site, severe nausea and vomiting (occurs within 1-3 h and lasts up to 12 h; pretreat with antiemetic therapy), anorexia, flu-like syndrome (fever, chills, malaise, myalgias, arthralgias) for several days after therapy, increased risk of photosensitivity. Drug interactions: Incompatible with heparin, lidocaine, and hydrocortisone. Phenytoin and phenobarbital decrease levels by increasing CYP450 metabolism.
Nitrosourea: Temozolomide (Temodar—oral) Brain tumors, metastatic melanoma	Cog ++	S ++	A 0	Motor ++++	D +	Com +	F ++	Side effects: DLT: Myelosuppression affecting WBC and platelets. Mild to moderate nausea and vomiting (occurs 1-3 h after dose and lasts up to 12 h); headache (25%; can be severe), fatigue, flu-like symptoms (occur several days after dose administration), constipation, photosensitivity. Drug interactions: None known.

› continued

Table 18.2 ›*continued*

Medication and indication	Side effects affecting rehab							Dose-limiting toxicities and other side effects or considerations
Busulfan (Myleran—oral) Drug of choice for palliative treatment of chronic myelogenous leukemia (CML). Remission rate ~90% after one dose. Used in bone marrow ablation prior to bone marrow transplant.	Cog ++	S ++	A 0	Motor +	D +++	Com +	F +	Side effects: DLT: Severe myelosuppression. Others: Nausea and vomiting is mild with standard doses, but can be severe with high dose regimens; pretreat for nausea and vomiting. Associated with hyperpigmentation and pulmonary fibrosis. Use prophylactic anticonvulsants to prevent seizures with high-dose regimens. Use allopurinol to prevent hyperuricemia.
Procarbazine (Matulane—oral) Hodgkin's lymphoma, non-Hodgkin's lymphoma, brain tumors, cutaneous T-cell lymphoma	Cog ++	S ++	A 0	Motor +	D +++	Com +	F +	Side effects: DLT: Myelosuppression, nausea, and vomiting is mild with standard doses but can be severe with high dose regimens; pretreat for nausea and vomiting. Others: Disulfiram reaction when combined with alcohol, CNS effects (depression, headache, mania, insomnia, hallucinations).
Chlorambucil (Leukeran—oral) Leukemia's drug of choice for CLL and lymphomas	Cog ++	S ++	A 0	Motor +	D +++	Com +	F +	Side effects: DLT: Severe myelosuppression; conduct weekly blood counts. Others: Nausea and vomiting is mild with standard doses, but can be severe with high dose regimens; pretreat for nausea and vomiting. Known carcinogen in humans, mutagenic and teratogenic; use contraception!
Nitrogen mustard: Melphalan (Oral: Alkeran) (IV: L-PAM, L-phenylalanine mustard) Multiple myeloma, breast cancer, ovarian cancer, polycythemia vera, and in transplant setting	Cog +	S +	A 0	Motor +	D +++	Com +	F +	Side effects: DLT: Myelosuppression with WBC and platelet nadir at 4-6 wks; delayed and prolonged nadir. Nausea and vomiting may be severe and dose limiting with high dose therapy. Others: Hypersensitivity reactions with IV form (rare), alopecia (uncommon), skin reactions at injection site (uncommon), secondary malignancies, teratogenic. Drug interactions: Cimetidine decreases levels and effects by 30%; steroids enhance antitumor effects; Cyclosporine enhances renal toxicity secondary to melphalan.

Medication and indication	Side effects affecting rehab							Dose-limiting toxicities and other side effects or considerations
Mechloretha-mine (Mustargen, nitrogen mustard)

Hodgkin's lymphoma, non-Hodgkin's lymphoma, cutaneous T-cell lymphoma (topical use), treatment of pleural effusions caused by metastatic disease | Cog ++ | S ++ | A 0 | Motor + | D +++ | Com + | F + | Side effects:

DLT: Myelosuppression with WBC and platelet nadir at 7-10 days; recovery by day 21.

Nausea and vomiting within first 3 hrs, lasts for 4-8 hrs and up to 24 hrs.

Others: Potent vesicant, use central line and running IV to administer; alopecia; amenorrhea; azoospermia; hyperuricemia; weakness; sleepiness; headache; hypersensitivity reactions (rare); secondary malignancies.

Drug interactions: Sodium thiosulfate inactivates effects of Mechlorethamine. |
| Thiotepa (IV: Triethylene-thiophosphora-mide, Thioplex)

Breast cancer, ovarian cancer, superficial bladder cancer, Hodgkin's and non-Hodgkin's lymphoma, transplant setting for ovarian and breast cancer | Cog ++ | S ++ | A 0 | Motor + | D +++ | Com + | F + | Side effects:

DLT: Myelosuppression; WBC nadir at 7-10 days, recovery by day 21. Platelet nadir at day 21 with recovery by day 28-35.

Mucositis may be dose limiting, allergic reactions (rare), nausea and vomiting is mild with standard doses but can be severe with high dose regimens (pretreat for nausea and vomiting), chemical or hemorrhagic cystitis after bladder instillation, skin reactions, teratogenic, carcinogenic with secondary malignancies. |
| **Heavy metal compounds:** Platinum products bind to tumor DNA and forms cross-links and bending of DNA resulting in impaired tumor cell synthesis. | | | | | | | | |
| Cisplatin (Platinol)

Testicular cancer, ovarian cancer, bladder cancer, head and neck cancer, esophageal cancer, small-cell and non-small-cell lung cancers, non-Hodgkin's lymphoma, trophoblastic neoplasms | Cog ++ | S ++ | A 0 | Motor ++++ | D ++++ | Com ++ | F ++++ | Side effects:

DLT: Severe dose-limiting nausea and vomiting; acute and delayed. Acute occurs within 1 h of dose and lasts 8-12 h; delayed can last 3-5 days and cause severe dehydration and electrolyte losses. Pretreat nausea and vomiting with corticosteroids and serotonin-receptor agents such as ondansetron (Zofran).

Dose-related electrolyte disturbances associated with starting first dose; wasting of potassium and magnesium and reduction of creatinine clearance, hypomagnesemia, hypocalcemia, and hypokalemia common.

Myelosuppression in 25-30%. White blood cells, platelets, and red blood cells equally affected (dose related). Anemia can be severe; manage with erythropoietin and iron supplementation. Hemolytic anemia can also occur. Nephrotoxicity is dose-limiting toxicity; progressive (35%-40%). Incidence of nephrotoxicity is decreased by careful diuresis with mannitol and aggressive hydration with saline. |

› continued

Table 18.2 › *continued*

Medication and indication	Side effects affecting rehab							Dose-limiting toxicities and other side effects or considerations
Cisplatin (Platinol)

Testicular cancer, ovarian cancer, bladder cancer, head and neck cancer, esophageal cancer, small-cell and non-small-cell lung cancers, non-Hodgkin's lymphoma, trophoblastic neoplasms

(continued) | | | | | | | | Neurotoxicity is dose limiting; cumulative toxicity, irreversible ototoxicity, vestibular damage. Peripheral neuropathy (distal stocking glove distribution) post dose pain and paresthesias reverse within 1 yr. Ototoxicity: High-frequency hearing, tinnitus.

Ocular toxicity: Optic neuritis, papilledema, cerebral blindness, disturbances in color perception.

Others: Raynaud's phenomenon, SIADH, hypersensitivity reactions with dose (facial edema, wheezing, bronchospasm, hypotension), myelosuppression (25%-30%), metallic taste of food, loss of appetite.

Drug interactions: Decreases effect of phenytoin. Directly inactivated by Amifostine and Mesna.

Increases nephrotoxicity from aminoglycosides and amphotericin B.

Increases levels and toxicity of etoposide, methotrexate, ifosfamide, and bleomycin, increasing accumulation of each drug.

May enhance antitumor activity of etoposide. |
| Carboplatin (Paraplatin)

Ovarian cancer, germ cell tumors, head and neck cancer, small-cell and non-small-cell lung cancer, bladder cancer, relapsed and refractory acute leukemia, endometrial cancer | Cog
+ | S
+ | A
0 | Motor
++ | D
++ | Com
+ | F
++ | Side effects:

DLT: Myelosuppression is dose limiting; dose-dependent; cumulative toxicity. Platelet nadir at day 21.

Others: Significantly less nausea and vomiting and renal toxicity than seen with cisplatin; hypocalcemia, hypokalemia, hypomagnesemia, hyponatremia, peripheral neuropathy (<10%), allergic reaction (25%; skin rash, urticaria, pruritus).

Skin testing may be helpful in identifying patients at risk for allergic reactions; mild and reversible elevation of LFT's. |
| Oxaliplatin (Eloxatin, Iproplatin, Ormaplatin)

Metastatic colorectal cancer | Cog
+ | S
+ | A
0 | Motor
+++ | D
+++ | Com
+ | F
+++ | Side effects:

DLT: Neurotoxicity is dose limiting; peripheral sensory neuropathy with distal paresthesias; worsened by cold, usually reversible after 3-4 months.

Laryngopharyngeal dysesthesias can cause difficulty breathing or swallowing immediately or 1-3 days after dose. >50% risk of neurotoxicity with cumulative doses of 1200 mg/m^2. |

Medication and indication	Side effects affecting rehab							Dose-limiting toxicities and other side effects or considerations
								Others: Nausea and vomiting (65% with oxaliplatin, 90% when combined with 5-FU/LV; well controlled with antiemetic therapy), diarrhea (30% with oxaliplatin, 80%-90% when combined with 5-FU/LV), myelosuppression (mild thrombocytopenia, anemia).
								Drug interactions: None known.

Antitumor antibiotic: From *Streptomyces* fungus; causes breakage of tumor cell DNA strands and formation of free radicals after binding with iron; active against cells in the second gap phase of the cell cycle.

Medication and indication	Cog	S	A	Motor	D	Com	F	Dose-limiting toxicities and other side effects or considerations
Bleomycin (Blenoxane) Hodgkin's disease and non-Hodgkin's lymphoma, germ cell tumors, head and neck cancer, squamous cell carcinomas	+	+	0	+	++	+	+	Side effects:
								DLT: Pulmonary toxicity is dose limiting (10%). Increased risk with patients >70 yr of age and with cumulative doses >450 units. Presents with cough, dyspnea, dry inspiratory crackles, and infiltrates on chest X-ray. Risk of pulmonary side effects increased with previous lung disease, advanced age, chest irradiation, and renal dysfunction. Radiation therapy enhances pulmonary toxicity.
								Pulmonary function tests (PFTs) with specific focus on diffusing capacity (DL_{CO}) and vital capacity is the most sensitive approach for detecting pulmonary toxicity. A decrease of 15% or more in PFT mandates immediately stopping the drug.
								Fatal fibrosis (1%).
								Others: Hypersensitivity reactions (25%; fever and chills), fever (25%-50%) within 1 h up to 2 days after dose, mild nausea and vomiting, common **mucocutaneous** reactions (mild stomatitis; hyperpigmentation of the elbows, knees, hand joints; thickened nail beds; alopecia; skin erythema and edema).
								Drug interactions: Oxygen therapy at high concentrations may enhance pulmonary toxicity. Fraction of inspired oxygen (FIO_2) should be maintained at <25%.
								Phenothiazines increase levels and toxicity by reducing metabolism of liver P450 enzymes.
								Cisplatin decreases renal clearance, increasing levels and toxicity.

Enzyme produced by *Escherichia coli* bacteria: Degrades the nonessential amino acid L-asparagine, reducing protein synthesis.

Medication and indication	Cog	S	A	Motor	D	Com	F	Dose-limiting toxicities and other side effects or considerations
L-asparaginase (Elspar, Oncaspar long acting) Acute lymphocytic leukemia	+++	+++	++	+++	+++	++	+++	Side effects:
								DLT: Liver toxicity (common, dose limiting), mild elevation in LFTs (including serum bilirubin and liver enzymes), hemorrhage and thrombosis due to impaired synthesis of clotting factors and anticoagulants with risk of bleeding and clotting (50%), decreased production of lipoproteins and albumin.

› continued

Table 18.2 › *continued*

Medication and indication	Side effects affecting rehab							Dose-limiting toxicities and other side effects or considerations
L-asparaginase (Elspar, Oncospar) Acute lymphocytic leukemia *(continued)*								Life-threatening allergic reactions (bronchospasm, respiratory distress, hypotension; resuscitation drugs and equipment required at bedside), fever, chills, nausea, vomiting (50%). Skin testing is helpful for identifying patients with increased risk of allergy. Neurologic toxicity (25%; lethargy, confusion, agitation, hallucinations; coma requires discontinuance).
								Others: Mild hypersensitivity (25%; skin rash, urticaria), pancreatitis (up to 10% of patients; reverses with discontinuance), hyperglycemia (decreased insulin production).
								Drug interactions: Reduces effects of methotrexate; administer these drugs 24 hrs apart.
								Increases effects of vincristine; administer vincristine 12-24 hrs before L-asparaginase.

Tyrosine kinase inhibitors: Decreases production of cancer cells.

Medication and indication	Cog	S	A	Motor	D	Com	F	Dose-limiting toxicities and other side effects or considerations
Imatinib mesylate (Gleevec—oral) Chronic myelogenous leukemia, acute lymphoblastic leukemia, gastrointestinal stromal tumors	+	+	0	++	++	+	++	Side effects: Well tolerated due to selectivity for cancer cells. Myelosuppression with neutropenia and thrombocytopenia.
								Nausea and vomiting (50%; reduced by taking with meal), diarrhea, pleural effusion, ascites, pulmonary edema (5%), muscle cramps, rash, diarrhea, fluid retention (dose related; pleural effusion, ascites, pulmonary edema, weight gain), transient ankle and periorbital edema, mild elevation of liver enzymes; skin reactions which can be severe (Stevens-Johnson syndrome).
								Drug interactions: Dilantin, carbamazepine, rifampicin, phenobarbital, and St. John's wort increase rate of metabolism and decrease effects.
								Ketoconazole, itraconazole, erythromycin, and clarithromycin inhibit CYP3A4 metabolism, increasing levels and toxicity.
								Reduces metabolism of warfarin (Coumadin), increasing levels and toxicity.

Cog = cognition; S = sedation; A = agitation or mania; Motor = discoordination; D = dysphagia; Com = communication; F = falls; CNS = central nervous system; DNA = deoxyribonucleic acid; IV = intravenous; LV = left ventricular; SIADH = syndrome of inappropriate antidiuretic hormone; INR= international normalized ratio; PVCs= premature ventricular contractions; ST= ST portions of the electrocardiogram reflecting cardiac contraction; CHF = congestive heart failure; WBC = white blood cells; DLT = dose-limiting toxicities; LFT = liver function test; CLL = chronic lymphocytic leukemia.

The likelihood rating scale for encountering the side effects is as follows: 0 = Almost no probability of encountering side effects. + = Little likelihood of encountering side effects. +/++ = Low probability of encountering side effects; however, probability increases with increased dosage. ++ = Medium likelihood of encountering side effects. +++ = High likelihood of encountering side effects, particularly with high doses. ++++ = Highest likelihood of encountering side effects; best to avoid in at-risk patients.

See table 18.3 in the web resource for a full list of medication-specific indications, dosing recommendations, and side effects.

Table 18.3 Biologic-Response Therapies Used in Cancer Patients

Medication and indication	Side effects affecting rehab							Dose-limiting toxicities and other side effects or considerations
Monoclonal antibodies								
Alemtuzumab (Campath) Chronic lymphocytic leukemia, relapsed or refractory B-cell chronic lymphocytic leukemia, T-cell prolymphocytic leukemia	Cog ++	S ++	A 0	Motor ++	D +++	Com ++	F ++	Side effects: DLT: Severe prolonged myelosuppression of white cells, red cells, and platelets (pancytopenia with marrow hypoplasia, which can be fatal, occurs in rare instances); immunosuppression (recovery of CD4 and CD8 counts may take >1 yr). Severe infusion-related fever, chills, nausea, vomiting, urticaria, skin rash, fatigue, headache, diarrhea, dyspnea, hypotension, mucositis, edema; premedicate with diphenhydramine and acetaminophen. Start with a low dose and gradually increase to full dose. Infuse over 2 h to reduce infusion reactions. Patient should receive prophylaxis therapy for *Pneumocystis carinii*, cytomegalovirus, herpes zoster, *Candida*, *Cryptococcus*, and *Listeria* meningitis infection until CD4 counts are >200. Drug interactions: None known.
Bortezomib (Velcade) Relapsing or refractory multiple myeloma, non-Hodgkin's lymphoma	Cog ++	S ++	A 0	Motor ++++	D ++	Com ++	F ++++	Side effects: DLT: Nausea, vomiting, and diarrhea; myelosuppression with thrombocytopenia and neutropenia; peripheral sensory neuropathy or sensorimotor neuropathy (improves with discontinuation). Others: Orthostatic hypotension (12%), fever (40%), fatigue, malaise, and generalized weakness (onset during the first and second cycles of therapy). Drug interactions: None known.
Gemtuzumab (Mylotarg) Acute myelogenous leukemia	Cog ++	S ++	A 0	Motor 0	D ++	Com ++	F ++	Side effects: DLT: Myelosuppression is dose-limiting toxicity; neutropenia and thrombocytopenia. Patients frequently require red blood cell and platelet transfusions. Infusion-related symptoms within 2 h of infusion (fever, chills, nausea, vomiting, urticaria, skin rash, fatigue, headache, diarrhea, dyspnea, hypotension; incidence decreases with second dose); premedicate with diphenhydramine and acetaminophen.

› continued

Table 18.3 › *continued*

Medication and indication	Side effects affecting rehab							Dose-limiting toxicities and other side effects or considerations
Gemtuzumab (Mylotarg) Acute myelogenous leukemia (continued)								Others: Hepatotoxicity (20%), increased bilirubin and liver enzymes, nausea, vomiting, mucositis, rare cases of veno-occlusive disease. Drug interactions: None known.
Rituximab (Rituxan) Non-Hodgkin's lymphoma	Cog 0	S 0	A 0	Motor 0	D +	Com 0	F 0	Side effects: DLT: Infusion-related symptoms within 30 min-2 h of dose (fever, chills, urticaria, flushing, fatigue, headache, bronchospasm, rhinitis, dyspnea, angioedema, nausea, hypotension). Tumor lysis syndrome within first 12-24 hrs of treatment, mucocutaneous reactions (pemphigus, Stevens-Johnson syndrome, lichenoid dermatitis, toxic epidermal neurolysis; usual onset from 1-13 wk after dose; requires drug discontinuation). Others: Arrhythmias, chest pain, mild nausea, vomiting, rare myelosuppression, respiratory symptoms in 40%, cough, rhinitis, dyspnea, sinusitis. Drug interactions: None known.
Tositumomab (Bexxar) Relapsed or refractory CD20-positive, follicular non-Hodgkin's lymphoma	Cog +	S +	A 0	Motor 0	D +	Com 0	F 0	Side effects: DLT: Myelosuppression is most common side effect; all elements affected. Nadir at 4-7 wks; recovery is 30 days, but cytopenias may persist for 12 weeks in 5-7% of patients. Others: Infusion-related symptoms (fever, chills, urticaria, flushing, fatigue, headache, bronchospasm, rhinitis, dyspnea, angioedema, nausea, hypotension; usually resolve upon slowing or interrupting infusion), mild nausea, vomiting, mild asthenia and fatigue (40%), infections (45%), hypothyroidism. Drug interactions: None known.
Trastuzumab (Herceptin) Metastatic breast cancer	Cog +	S +	A 0	Motor +	D +	Com 0	F 0	Side effects: DLT: Infusion-related symptoms in 40%-50% with initial dose, fever, chills, urticaria, flushing, fatigue, headache, bronchospasm, dyspnea, angioedema, hypotension. Infusion-related reactions can also include anaphylaxis and pulmonary toxicity (dyspnea, pulmonary infiltrates, effusions, pulmonary edema, ARDS).

Medication and indication	Side effects affecting rehab	Dose-limiting toxicities and other side effects or considerations
		Cardiotoxicity (dyspnea, peripheral edema, reduced left ventricular function which is reversible). Patients should undergo baseline and periodic evaluation of cardiac function. Risk is increased with past or concurrent use of anthracyclines or cyclophosphamide (Cytoxan). Others: Generalized pain, asthenia, headache, mild nausea, vomiting, diarrhea. Drug interactions: Additive immunosuppression with other chemotherapy agents, avoid administration of live vaccines as these may result in disseminated infections, immunize patient prior to treatment.

Interferon: Makes the cancer cells more easily recognized by the cells of the immune system.

Medication and indication	Side effects affecting rehab							Dose-limiting toxicities and other side effects or considerations
Interferon-alpha (Roferon, Intron-A) Malignant melanoma, chronic myelogenous leukemia, hairy cell leukemia, Kaposi's sarcoma related to acquired immune deficiency syndrome, cutaneous T-cell lymphoma, multiple myeloma, non-Hodgkin's lymphoma, renal cell cancer, hemangioma	Cog +++	S +++	A ++	Motor ++	D ++	Com +	F ++	Side effects: DLT: Fatigue and anorexia are dose-limiting toxicities. Others: Flu-like syndrome (fever, chills, malaise, myalgias, headache; develops over 1-2 wk; manage with acetaminophen), mild myelosuppression, dose-related gastrointestinal side effects, elevated liver enzymes. Depression, mental slowing, and memory loss increase with chronic use. Rare instances of mania, severe depression, and suicidal behaviors. Antidepressants may manage depression side effects. Drug interactions: Increases effects of phenytoin and phenobarbital due to inhibition of their CYP450 metabolism.

Interleukins: Promotes B- and T-cell proliferation; initiates a cytokine cascade that increases levels of natural killer cells; increases tumor cell death without damaging normal cells.

Medication and indication	Side effects affecting rehab							Dose-limiting toxicities and other side effects or considerations
Interleukin-2 (Aldesleukin) Renal cell cancer, malignant melanoma	Cog +++	S +++	A ++	Motor +++	D ++	Com ++	F +++	Side effects: DLT: Vascular leak syndrome is dose-limiting toxicity (weight gain, arrhythmias, hypotension, edema, oliguria, renal insufficiency, pleural effusion, pulmonary congestion). Others: Delirium, confusion, somnolence, memory impairment, flu-like symptoms (fever, chills, malaise, myalgias, arthralgias; 100%), elevated hepatic enzymes (bilirubin reverses 4-6 days after dose), changes in thyroid function, skin rash, itching, myelosuppression with neutropenia, thrombocytopenia, and anemia.

› continued

Table 18.3 › *continued*

Medication and indication	Side effects affecting rehab							Dose-limiting toxicities and other side effects or considerations
Interleukin-2 (Aldesleukin) Renal cell cancer, malignant melanoma *(continued)*								Drug interactions: Steroids can decrease dose-limiting toxicities but can also decrease antitumor effects of interleukin-2. Nonsteroidal anti-inflammatory drugs may increase capillary leak syndrome. Potentiates effects of hypotensive agents; administration requires holding these agents for 12-24 hrs prior to dose.
Denileukin diftitox (Ontak) T-cell lymphoma	Cog +	S +	A +	Motor +++	D +++	Com +	F +++	Side effects: DLT: Hypersensitivity reactions (hypotension, back pain, dyspnea, chest pain; 70% of patients) within 24 h of infusion, anaphylaxis occurs in 1%-2% of patients. Prevent infusion-related reactions by using antihistamines and acetaminophen; avoid steroid pretreatment. Vascular leak syndrome (hypotension, edema). Delayed and prolonged diarrhea, anorexia, nausea, vomiting; pretreat. Others: Elevated liver enzymes (resolve within 2 wk of dosing). Drug interactions: None known.
Immodulator and antiangiogenic agent: Thalidomide (Thalomid) Multiple myeloma, erythema nodosum leprosum, myelodysplastic disease, solid tumors	Cog ++	S ++	A 0	Motor ++++	D ++	Com ++	F ++	Side effects: DLT: Neurotoxic effects (orthostatic hypotension, dizziness, peripheral neuropathy in the form of numbness, tingling, and pain in the feet or hands), constipation (common). Serious dermatologic reactions including Stevens-Johnson syndrome (development of skin rash during therapy requires discontinuance). Others: Milder maculopapular skin rash, urticaria, dry skin, sedation or fatigue following an evening dose (occurs with larger initial doses; manage with dose reduction), increased risk of deep venous thrombosis and pulmonary embolism. Teratogenic. Drug interactions: Sedative effect is enhanced with concurrent use of barbiturates, chlorpromazine, reserpine, or alcohol.

Medication and indication	Side effects affecting rehab							Dose-limiting toxicities and other side effects or considerations
Hormone therapies								
Antiestrogen: Tamoxifen (Nolvadex) Used to prevent osteoporosis and recurrence of breast cancer in premenopausal and hormone receptor-positive patients	Cog 0	S 0	A 0	Motor 0	D ++	Com 0	F 0	Side effects: Menopausal symptoms (hot flashes, nausea, vomiting, vaginal bleeding, menstrual irregularities), vaginal discharge, vaginal dryness, skin rash, pruritus, hair thinning, elevations in serum triglycerides, fluid retention and peripheral edema (30%), tumor flare (usually occurs within first 2 wk of starting therapy), anorexia, increased risk of endometrial cancer, ocular toxicity with cataract formation and xerophthalmia. Deep vein thrombosis, pulmonary embolism, and superficial phlebitis are rare but may be increased when administered concomitantly with chemotherapy. Drug interactions: Can increase anticoagulant effect of warfarin (Coumadin). Bromocriptine increases levels and effects. Inhibits CYP P450 metabolism and increases levels and effects of cyclophosphamide, erythromycin, calcium channel blockers, and cyclosporine.
Antiestrogen: Raloxifene (Evista) Used to prevent osteoporosis and recurrence of breast cancer in postmenopausal women	Cog 0	S 0	A 0	Motor 0	D ++	Com 0	F 0	Side effects: DLT: Deep vein thrombosis, pulmonary embolism, and superficial phlebitis are rare but may be increased when given concomitantly with chemotherapy; ocular toxicity with cataract formation and xerophthalmia. Others: Menopausal symptoms (hot flashes, nausea, vomiting, vaginal bleeding, menstrual irregularities), vaginal discharge, vaginal dryness, skin rash, pruritus, hair thinning, elevations in serum triglycerides, fluid retention and peripheral edema (30%), tumor flare (usually occurs within the first 2 wk of starting therapy), anorexia, increased risk of endometrial cancer.

› continued

Table 18.3 › *continued*

Medication and indication	Side effects affecting rehab							Dose-limiting toxicities and other side effects or considerations
Antiestrogen:	Cog	S	A	Motor	D	Com	F	Side effects:
Toremifene	0	0	0	0	++	0	0	DLT: Deep vein thrombosis, pulmonary embolism, and superficial phlebitis are rare but may be increased when given concomitantly with chemotherapy; ocular toxicity with cataract formation and xerophthalmia.
(Fareston)								
Used to prevent osteoporosis and recurrence of breast cancer in hormone receptor-positive and negative patients								Others: Menopausal symptoms (hot flashes, nausea, vomiting, vaginal bleeding, menstrual irregularities), vaginal discharge, vaginal dryness, skin rash, pruritus, hair thinning, elevations in serum triglycerides, fluid retention and peripheral edema (30%), tumor flare (usually occurs within the first 2 wk of starting therapy), anorexia, increased risk of endometrial cancer.
								Drug interactions: Thiazide diuretics decrease the renal clearance of calcium and increases the risk of hypercalcemia associated with toremifene.
								Increases anticoagulant effect of warfarin (Coumadin).
								Phenobarbital, carbamazepine, and phenytoin increase metabolism, decreasing levels and effects.
								Ketoconazole and erythromycin inhibit metabolism, increasing levels and effects.
Progestin:	Cog	S	A	Motor	D	Com	F	Side effects: Weight gain, hot flashes, vaginal bleeding, edema, increased risk of thrombus formation.
Medroxyprogesterone acetate	0	0	0	+	0	0	0	
Used as second-line therapy with tamoxifen for prevention of osteoporosis and breast cancer recurrence in breast cancer patients								Drug interactions: None identified.
Progestin:	Cog	S	A	Motor	D	Com	F	
Megestrol acetate	0	0	0	+	0	0	0	
Used as second-line therapy with tamoxifen for prevention of osteoporosis and breast cancer recurrence in breast cancer patients								

Medication and indication	Side effects affecting rehab							Dose-limiting toxicities and other side effects or considerations
LHRH analogs: Leuprolide (Lupron) Used in prostate and breast cancers to induce medical castration by decreasing gonadotropin-releasing hormone activity (agonist), decreasing hormone production	Cog 0	S 0	A 0	Motor 0	D +	Com 0	F 0	Side effects: Amenorrhea, hot flashes, occasional nausea. Drug interactions: None identified.
LHRH analogs: (Zoladex) Goserelin Used in prostate and breast cancers to induce medical castration by decreasing gonadotropin-releasing hormone activity (agonist), decreasing hormone production	Cog 0	S 0	A 0	Motor 0	D +	Com 0	F 0	
Antiestrogen: Anastrozole (Arimidex) Aromatase inhibitor that blocks the effects of estrogen on estrogen receptors in patients with early breast cancer and metastatic breast cancer	Cog +	S +	A 0	Motor +	D +	Com 0	F +	Side effects: Profile of aromatase inhibitors is more favorable than that of aminoglutethimide; nausea, hot flashes, mild fatigue. Increases in cholesterol may occur; lipid profile monitoring recommended. Drug interactions: None identified.
Antiestrogen: Letrozole (Femara) Aromatase inhibitor that blocks the effects of estrogen on estrogen receptors in patients with early breast cancer and metastatic breast cancer	Cog +	S +	A 0	Motor +	D +	Com 0	F +	
Antiestrogen: Exemestane (Aromasin) Aromatase inhibitor that blocks the effects of estrogen on estrogen receptors in patients with early breast cancer and metastatic breast cancer	Cog +	S +	A 0	Motor +	D +	Com 0	F +	

› continued

Table 18.3 › *continued*

Medication and indication	Side effects affecting rehab							Dose-limiting toxicities and other side effects or considerations
Antiestrogen: Aminoglutethimide (Cytadren) Blocks the effects of estrogen on estrogen receptors in patients with early breast cancer and metastatic breast cancer	Cog ++	S ++	A 0	Motor +++	D +	Com +	F +++	Side effects: Lethargy, rash, orthostasis, ataxia, nystagmus, nausea. Drug interactions: Decreases conversion of cholesterol to glucocorticoids; must be administered with hydrocortisone.
Dexamethasone (Decadron) Steroid used to manage hematologic malignancies due to cytotoxic effects; used in supportive care of patients	Cog +	S 0	A +	Motor +	D +	Com 0	F +	Side effects: Immunosuppression, hyperglycemia, mental status changes, edema, weight gain. Preferred (minimal mineralocorticoid effect and fewer psychiatric side effects) in treatment of cerebral edema associated with brain metastases or cranial irradiation; spinal cord treatment of nausea and vomiting, hypercalcemia, transfusion reactions, appetite stimulation, pneumonitis associated with chemotherapy or radiation, preventing allergic reactions, fluid retention from chemotherapy agents, treatment of graft-versus-host disease, and compression-associated pain. Drug interactions: Increased immunosuppression and infection risk with other immunosuppressives, antagonizes hypoglycemic effects of diabetic agents.

Cog = cognition; S = sedation; A = agitation or mania; Motor = discoordination; D = dysphagia; Com = communication; F = falls; DLT = dose-limiting toxicities; LHRH = luteinizing hormone releasing hormone; ARDS = acute respiratory distress syndrome.

The likelihood rating scale for encountering the side effects is as follows: 0 = Almost no probability of encountering side effects. + = Little likelihood of encountering side effects. +/++ = Low probability of encountering side effects; however, probability increases with increased dosage. ++ = Medium likelihood of encountering side effects. +++ = High likelihood of encountering side effects, particularly with high doses. ++++ = Highest likelihood of encountering side effects; best to avoid in at-risk patients.

treatments). Finally, cancer patients should avoid St. John's wort, which is metabolized by CYP3A4 liver enzymes. Use of St. John's wort can increase or decrease the effects of medications metabolized by the same pathway. This is significant because the majority of medications that are metabolized are cleared by this pathway. Table 18.2 summarizes the classes of chemotherapy medications as well as common side effects, drug interactions, and pertinent information regarding administration of each agent (Balmer & Valley, 2002; Chabner et al., 2001; Chu & DeVita, 2010; Finley & LaCivitia, 1992; Grunwald, 2003).

PATIENT CASE 1

E.O. is an 85-yr-old male with lung cancer who was referred for physical rehabilitation. He developed postoperative respiratory failure and pneumonia during a prolonged hospitalization for his lung resection and as a result lost significant weight and muscle strength. E.O. is to begin a chemotherapy combination of cisplatin (Platinol) and etoposide (VP-16) plus radiation therapy for his non-small-cell lung cancer.

Question

What side effects should be monitored for with the initiation of his chemotherapy? What preventative therapies should be used to minimize side effects associated with his chemotherapy regimen?

Answer

Cisplatin (Platinol) is a product containing platinum. Its use is associated with severe nausea and vomiting that requires pretreatment with corticosteroids and ondansetron (Zofran). His nutritional status may be affected by the nausea and vomiting and associated dehydration as well as an associated metallic taste and anorexia. Cisplatin (Platinol) may cause neurotoxicity that can include ototoxicity, vestibular damage, peripheral neuropathy, and even ocular toxicity. Such neurotoxicity may affect E.O.'s balance and ability to participate in ambulation and exercise. Nephrotoxicity associated with cisplatin (Platinol) requires pretreatment with intravenous fluid hydration and diuretics. E.O. will require careful monitoring and replacement of potassium, magnesium, and calcium because these can affect muscle function. Cisplatin (Platinol) can cause myelosuppression and associated decrease in white blood cells, platelets, and red blood cells, which can impair E.O.'s ability to fight infection and may contribute to bleeding and anemia. His anemia will need to be managed with erythropoietin and iron supplementation and may contribute to increased cancer-related fatigue, which can reduce his ability to participate in rehabilitation.

Etoposide (VP-16) is a topoisomerase-targeting chemotherapy agent that can cause severe myelosuppression and low white cell counts from days 10-14 through day 21 after each chemotherapy dose. This neutropenia will reduce E.O.'s ability to fight infection and will require administration of a medication such as filgrastim (Neupogen) to stimulate production of white blood cells. Nausea and vomiting are mild with this medication. Loss of hair (alopecia) is expected with etoposide administration. The combination of mucositis, nausea, vomiting, metallic taste, and diarrhea associated with this medication can interfere with maintaining oral intake and nutrition. The clinical dietitian should be consulted to provide nutrition support for E.O. as he undergoes his cancer treatments and tries to gain muscle strength. The rehabilitation therapist should adjust scheduled sessions with these expected side effects in mind.

Biologic-Response Modifiers

Biologic-response modifiers help the body fight cancer by altering the response of the immune system. These agents are increasingly being used in the treatment of cancer. These agents include monoclonal antibody therapies and cytokines such as interleukin and interferon. Table 18.3 provides information on these medications. Antibodies or immuno-globulins are part of the immune system and circulate in the blood and lymphatic system. They help the body eliminate foreign materials such as tumors by binding to antigens on foreign cells, marking them for destruction by macrophages and complement. Monoclonal antibodies are made by injecting cells or protein from human cancer cells into mice whose immune systems create antibodies against the cancer cells. Monoclonal antibodies recognize a particular protein associated with a certain cancer cell and assist with destruction of the cancer cell through direct killing effects or indirect effects. Direct effects produce apoptosis or programmed cell death or block growth factor receptors, resulting in tumor cell death. Indirect effects include the recruitment of cells that have cytotoxicity, such as monocytes and macrophages. This type of antibody-mediated cell killing is called antibody-dependent cell-mediated cytotoxicity. Monoclonal antibodies can also bind to complement, leading to direct cell toxicity, known as complement-dependent cytotoxicity (Bishop, 2010).

The two types of monoclonal antibodies are naked or unconjugated monoclonal antibodies and conjugated monoclonal antibodies. No drugs or radiation attach to naked or unconjugated monoclonal antibodies. Typically, these antibodies attach to antigens on the cancer cell, which signals for the body's immune system to destroy them. Conjugated monoclonal antibodies act as a carrier to deliver drugs, toxins, or radioactive isotopes directly to the cancer cell. When the antibodies bind with antigen-bearing cells, they deliver their load of toxin directly to the tumor. Monoclonal antibodies cause infusion-related reactions that can range from mild fever, chills, nausea, and rash to severe, life-threatening anaphylaxis and cardiopulmonary collapse. Patients must be monitored closely during the infusion and should be premedicated with antihistamines and acetaminophen before the dose to minimize infusion-related reactions (Bishop, 2010).

Cytokines, which are proteins or glycoproteins secreted by immune cells, act as the messengers of the immune system. They regulate natural killer cells, macrophages, and neutrophils as well as T-cell and B-cell response. Interleukin-2 and interferon alpha-2b are two cytokines used in the treatment of cancer. Interleukin-2 has demonstrated activity against renal cell carcinoma, melanoma, lymphoma, and leukemia. Interferon is active against Kaposi's sarcoma, chronic myelogenous leukemia, and hairy cell leukemia (Weber, 2010).

Medication Therapy: Supportive Medication Therapies

Supportive therapies used in the cancer patient include medication therapies that treat myelosuppression and cancer fatigue and medications that treat and prevent nausea and vomiting. Tumor spread to the bone can be particularly painful; the bisphosphonates pamidronate (Aredia) and zoledronate (Zometa, Aclasta) are used to prevent fracture, treat hypercalcemia, and inhibit formation of osteoclasts in order to reduce metastatic bone pain. High-dose allopurinol (Zyloprim) and rasburicase (recombinant urate oxidase; Elitek) are medications that are used to reduce uric acid levels in a life-threatening fluid and electrolyte disorder associated with the lysis of a large burden of cancer cells at once. Table 18.4 provides information on supportive therapies.

Medication Treatment of Myelosuppression

Chemotherapy medications may cause **myelosuppression** along with reduced production of white blood cells (neutropenia), platelet cells (thrombocytopenia), and red blood cells (anemia). Myelosuppression is a dose-limiting toxicity associated with many chemotherapy agents. Neutropenia can result in significant immunosuppression and interfere with the patient's ability to survive an infection during the period of myelosuppression (Chu & DeVita, 2010; Finley & LaCivitia, 1992; Grunwald, 2003).

Colony-stimulating growth factors are cytokines that stimulate the proliferation, differentiation, and activation of progenitor cells for neutrophils in the bone marrow and the

See table 18.4 in the web resource for a full list of medication-specific indications, dosing recommendations, and side effects.

Table 18.4 Supportive Therapies Used in the Cancer Patient

Medication	Side effects affecting rehab							Other side effects or considerations
Granulocyte and macrophage colony-stimulating factors: Increase production of granulocytes or macrophages in bone marrow; increase phagocytic activity of mature granulocytes and macrophages.								
Filgrastim (Neupogen) Pegfilgrastim (Neulasta)	Cog 0	S 0	A 0	Motor +	D 0	Com 0	F +	Side effects: Bone pain, rupture of the spleen. Avoid administration during period 24 h before chemotherapy through 24 h after completion of chemotherapy. Drug interactions: None identified.
Sargramostim (Leukine)	Cog +	S +	A 0	Motor ++	D +	Com 0	F +	Side effects: Flu-like syndrome (fever, chills, lethargy, malaise, headache), transient bone pain (may be prevented by acetaminophen), fluid-retention syndrome, injection reaction, transient elevation in serum bilirubin and liver transaminases. Hold for at least 24 hrs after last dose of chemotherapy and 12 hrs after radiation therapy. Monitor complete blood counts at least twice/wk during treatment. Therapy should be terminated once total white blood cells >10000/mm^3 or ANC > 1000/mm^3 for 3 days. Drug interactions: None identified.
Erythropoietin-stimulating factor: Increases production of erythropoietin, a hormone manufactured in the kidney that stimulates the formation of red blood cells.								
Erythropoietin (Procrit, Epogen) Darbepoetin (Aranesp)	Cog 0	S 0	A 0	Motor +	D 0	Com 0	F 0	Side effects: DLT: Increased risk of tumor progression, increased risk of thrombus in patients with cancer. Indicated only in patients not expected to attain cancer cure; Food and Drug Administration restrictions for use (Risk Evaluation and Mitigation Strategy program) apply. Not indicated for treating anemia in cancer patients due to other factors such as iron or folate deficiencies, hemolysis, or gastrointestinal bleeding. Drug interactions: Administration requires concurrent monitoring of iron levels and stores and the administration of iron supplementation.
Substance P inhibitor antiemetic therapy: Highly effective in preventing acute and delayed nausea and vomiting with highly emetogenic chemotherapy.								
Aprepitant (oral) Fosaprepitant (IV) (Emend)	Cog ++	S ++	A 0	Motor ++	D +	Com +	F ++	Side effects: Fatigue, nausea, weakness, hiccups. Expensive therapy. Drug interactions: Induces CYP2C9; decreases effects of warfarin (Coumadin), dexamethasone, methylprednisolone, ethinyl estradiol, and norgestimate contraceptives. Avoid concurrent ingestion of grapefruit juice as it can increase levels and toxicity.

› continued

Table 18.4 › *continued*

Medication	Side effects affecting rehab							Other side effects or considerations
Serotonin receptor antagonist antiemetics: Highly effective in treating nausea and vomiting associated with chemotherapy and upper-abdominal irradiation and other causes of nausea and vomiting. Oral doses are the same as the IV doses.								
	Cog	S	A	Motor	D	Com	F	Side effects: Constipation, insomnia, diarrhea, dizziness, headache, arrhythmia with QT pro-
Ondansetron (Zofran)	+	+	0	++	+	+	++	longation, dystonia, extrapyramidal symptoms, arthralgias, depression.
	Cog	S	A	Motor	D	Com	F	
Granisetron (Kytril)	+	+	0	++	+	+	++	Drug interactions: Antiarrhythmics, tricyclic anti-
	Cog	S	A	Motor	D	Com	F	depressants (thioridazine, mesoridazine, and ziprasidone), and anesthetics can increase QT
Dolasetron (Anzemet)	+	+	0	++	+	+	++	interval and cause life threatening arrhythmias.
	Cog	S	A	Motor	D	Com	F	
Palonosetron (Aloxi)	+	+	0	++	+	+	++	
Benzodiazepine antiemetics: Effective for treating anticipatory nausea and vomiting.								
	Cog	S	A	Motor	D	Com	F	Side effects: Sedation, confusion, hypotension, ataxia.
Lorazepam (Ativan—IV or oral)	+++	+++	0	++	++	++	++	Drug interactions: Some antidepressants, anti-
	Cog	S	A	Motor	D	Com	F	epileptic drugs (e.g., phenobarbital, phenytoin, carbamazepine), sedative antihistamines, opiates,
Alprazolam (Xanax—oral)	+++	+++	0	++	++	++	++	antipsychotics, and alcohol may enhance seda-tive effects of these agents.
Glucocorticoid: Used in combination with a serotonin antagonist before each dose of chemotherapy. May be useful in treating delayed and refractory nausea and vomiting. Treats nausea in patients with disseminated cancer by suppression of inflammation and prostaglandin production caused by tumor encroachment.								
	Cog	S	A	Motor	D	Com	F	Side effects: Gastrointestinal upset, hyperglyce-mia, altered mental status.
Dexametha-sone (Decadron) Prednisone	+	0	+	+	+	0	+	Drug interactions: Increased immunosuppression and infection risk with other immunosuppres-sives, antagonizes hypoglycemic effects of dia-betic agents.
Cannabinoid antiemetic: Derivative of marijuana that is used in treatment of nausea in cancer patients in which other agents have failed.								
	Cog	S	A	Motor	D	Com	F	Side effects: Sedation, altered mental status.
Dronabinol (Marinol)	+++	+++	0	++	0	++	++	Most effective in patients with previous positive experiences with marijuana.
								Drug interactions: Can increase sedation and CNS depression when combined with other CNS depressants such as alcohol, sedatives, antipsy-chotics.

Medication	Side effects affecting rehab							Other side effects or considerations
Dopamine antagonist antiemetic: Rescue antiemetic in chemotherapy patients; used postoperative and in other causes of nausea and vomiting. Metoclopramide has additional prokinetic activity associated with effects on muscarinic receptors.								
Metoclo-pramide (Reglan)	Cog +++	S +++	A ++	Motor +++	D +	Com +++	F +++	Side effects: Restlessness, drowsiness, dizziness, lassitude, dystonia, headache, changes in blood pressure, extrapyramidal effects, hyperprolactinemia, constipation, depression. Drug interactions: Additive sedation when used with other central nervous system depressants. Antagonizes dopamine-enhancer therapy used in treatment of Parkinson's disease.
Phenothiazine antiemetics: Anticholinergic and antihistaminic properties make them useful in treating motion sickness, postoperative nausea, and other types of nausea.								
Promethazine (Phenergan)	Cog +++	S +++	A ++	Motor +++	D +	Com +++	F +++	Side effects: Strong sedative and anticholinergic effects, dry mouth and throat, increased heart rate, pupil dilation, urinary retention, constipation. At high doses: Hallucinations or delirium, motor impairment (ataxia), flushed skin, blurred vision, abnormal sensitivity to bright light, difficulty concentrating, short-term memory loss, visual disturbances, irregular breathing, dizziness, irritability, itchy skin, confusion, decreased body temperature (generally in the hands or feet), erectile dysfunction, additive sedation when used with other central nervous system depressants. Drug interactions: Additive sedation when used with other central nervous system depressants. Additive confusion and anticholinergic side effects when combined with other anticholinergic agents. Antagonizes dopamine-enhancer therapy used in treatment of Parkinson's disease.
Prochlorpera-zine (Compazine)	Cog +++	S +++	A ++	Motor +++	D +	Com +++	F +++	
Histamine-1 receptor antagonist (antihistamine) antiemetics: Used as rescue antiemetics and in treating delayed nausea and vomiting associated with chemotherapy; used in treating postoperative nausea and vomiting and other causes of nausea and vomiting, especially with vestibular effects. These agents are useful in treating postoperative nausea and motion sickness due to additional effects on the muscarinic receptors. Diphenhydramine is often used to treat allergic reactions.								
Hydroxyzine (Vistaril)	Cog +++	S +++	A ++	Motor +++	D +	Com +++	F +++	Side effects: Strong sedative and anticholinergic effects, dry mouth and throat, increased heart rate, pupil dilation, urinary retention, constipation. At high doses: Hallucinations or delirium, motor impairment (ataxia), flushed skin, blurred vision, abnormal sensitivity to bright light, difficulty concentrating, short-term memory loss, visual disturbances, irregular breathing, dizziness, irritability, itchy skin, confusion, decreased body temperature (generally in the hands or feet), erectile dysfunction. Drug interactions: Additive sedation when used with other central nervous system depressants. Additive confusion and anticholinergic side effects when combined with other anticholinergic agents. Antagonizes dopamine-enhancer therapy used in treatment of Parkinson's disease.
Diphenhydr-amine (Benadryl)	Cog +++	S +++	A ++	Motor +++	D +	Com +++	F +++	
Meclizine (Dramamine)	Cog +++	S +++	A ++	Motor +++	D +	Com +++	F +++	
Scopolamine (Hyoscine, Transderm Scop patch)	Cog +++	S +++	A ++	Motor +++	D +	Com +++	F +++	

› continued

Table 18.4 › *continued*

Medication	Side effects affecting rehab							Other side effects or considerations
Bisphosphonates: Used to prevent fracture and to treat hypercalcemia; inhibits osteoclasts to reduce metastatic bone pain.								
Pamidronate (Aredia)	Cog 0	S 0	A 0	Motor 0	D ++	Com 0	F 0	Common side effects: Fatigue, anemia, muscle aches, fever, swelling in the feet or legs, flu-like symptoms with initial infusion. Uncommon side effects: Severe bone, joint, or musculoskeletal pain. Drug interactions: Increased nephrotoxicity when combined with other agents associated with nephrotoxicity (aminoglycosides; polypeptide, glycopeptide, and polymyxin antibiotics; amphotericin B; adefovir; cidofovir; foscarnet; cisplatin; deferasirox; gallium nitrate; lithium; mesalamine; certain immunosuppressants; intravenous pentamidine; high intravenous dosages of methotrexate; high dosages or chronic use of nonsteroidal anti-inflammatory drugs or immunoglobulin therapy).
Zoledronate (Zometa, Aclasta)	Cog 0	S 0	A 0	Motor 0	D ++	Com 0	F 0	
Xanthine oxidase inhibitors: Used to reduce uric acid levels in tumor lysis syndrome.								
Allopurinol (Zyloprim)	Cog 0	S 0	A 0	Motor 0	D +	Com 0	F 0	Side effects: Rash, kidney stones, acute interstitial nephritis, pneumopathy, fever, eosinophilia. Drug interactions: Reduce dose when used with 6-mercaptopurine, 6-thioguanine, or azathioprine.
Rasburicase (Elitek)	Cog 0	S 0	A 0	Motor 0	D +	Com 0	F 0	Converts uric acid to water-soluble metabolites. Effectively decreases plasma and urinary uric acid levels. Does not increase excretion of xanthine and is not associated with xanthine stone uropathy. Contraindicated in glucose-6-phosphate dehydrogenase deficiency and pregnancy. Very expensive.

Cog = cognition; S = sedation; A = agitation or mania; Motor = discoordination; D = dysphagia; Com = communication; F = falls; DLT = dose-limiting toxicities; IV = intravenous; CNS = central nervous system; ANC = absolute neutrophil count.

The likelihood rating scale for encountering the side effects is as follows: 0 = Almost no probability of encountering side effects. + = Little likelihood of encountering side effects. +/++ = Low probability of encountering side effects; however, probability increases with increased dosage. ++ = Medium likelihood of encountering side effects. +++ = High likelihood of encountering side effects, particularly with high doses. ++++ = Highest likelihood of encountering side effects; best to avoid in at-risk patients.

activity of mature granulocytes. These agents enhance neutrophil chemotaxis and phagocytosis, thus improving the immune function of patients with chemotherapy-induced neutropenia. Products used to treat myelosuppression include filgrastim (Neupogen) and a longer-acting product called pegfilgrastim (Neulasta). Administration of these products should be avoided in the period 24 h before through 24 h after completion of chemotherapy in order to avoid chemotherapy-induced destruction of newly formed neutrophils. A complete blood count should be performed twice/wk while the patient is receiving these agents. Increased bone pain due to increased activity in the bone marrow is associated with the use of these products. Splenic rupture associated with overproduction of white cells can occur with the use of these agents (Chu & DeVita, 2010; Finley & LaCivitia, 1992; Grunwald, 2003).

Erythropoietin is a natural hormone produced by the kidneys that stimulates production of red blood cells. Chemotherapy treatment can dramatically reduce the production of red blood cells and can result in severe anemia. Chemotherapy-induced **anemia** is treated with a combination of iron supplementation and erythropoiesis stimulating agents (ESAs) to stimulate red blood cell production. Failure to treat chemotherapy-induced anemia can reduce oxygen delivery to tissues and may necessitate transfusion of red blood cells. Chemotherapy-induced anemia can cause fatigue and reduce exercise tolerance, which can reduce the patient's ability to participate in rehabilitation (Bubalo, 2009; Grunwald, 2003).

In anemic patients, serum ferritin concentrations are less than 100 ng/ml and transferrin saturation is less than 20%. Individual patient laboratory values determine the appropriate dosage of iron therapy. Oral iron can cause constipation, nausea, and vomiting. Administering iron parenterally provides faster results and prevents gastrointestinal side effects but is more expensive and carries the risk of infusion-related hypersensitivity reactions. Parenteral iron products include iron dextran, iron sucrose, and sodium ferric gluconate. A small test dose of iron dextran is given before the first dose to identify patients with risk

of allergic reaction (Bubalo, 2009; Kaplan & Zandt, 2010).

Currently available erythropoiesis stimulating agents (ESAs) include darbepoetin (Aranesp) and epoetin alpha (Procrit, Epogen). Epoetin alpha (Procrit, Epogen) is human erythropoietin produced in cell culture using recombinant DNA technology. Another ESA is darbepoetin (Aranesp), which is also produced by DNA recombinant technology but has a longer half life and may be dosed as infrequently as once/mo. Because the use of these agents may increase the risk of thrombotic events, lower doses of erythropoiesis stimulating agents (ESAs) are now used to reach lower target hemoglobin levels of 11 to 12 g/dl. These agents may increase tumor progression; therefore, use in patients in which cancer cure is anticipated is not recommended. Because of these risks, in 2009 the FDA required a change in the prescribing information for these agents in oncology patients and in 2010 the FDA required that all ESA prescribed to cancer patients be monitored using an FDA-mandated Risk Evaluation and Mitigation Strategy (REMS). As part of the REMS, prescribers and pharmacists must provide to all patients receiving ESA a medication guide explaining the risks and benefits of ESA. Only hospitals and health care professionals who have enrolled and completed training in the program can prescribe and dispense ESA to patients with cancer (FDA, 2012).

Medications Used to Treat Cancer-Associated Fatigue

Cancer-related fatigue is a persistent sense of tiredness that interferes with daily activities. Cancer-related fatigue affects 70% to 100% of patients with cancer. Although factors that contribute to fatigue in cancer patients are multifactorial and the exact pathophysiology of cancer-related fatigue is not known, increased levels of interleukin-1, interleukin-6, and tumor necrosis factor have been noted in cancer patients. Insomnia, anxiety, and depression occur frequently in cancer patients and can cause fatigue. Chemotherapy-related fatigue is greatest at 2 to 3 days after therapy and gradually improves over the next 3 wk. Radiation can also cause fatigue that peaks at

4 wk after initial radiation treatment and then resolves within 1 to 3 mo after completion of radiation treatment (Bubalo, 2009; Kaplan & Zandt, 2010).

PATIENT CASE 2

R.P. is a 75-yr-old male patient receiving the PEB combination chemotherapy regimen along with radiation therapy for testicular cancer. The PEB regimen includes cisplatin, etoposide, and bleomycin given in a cycle every 28 days. He is referred for cancer rehabilitation therapy and to increase muscle strength and ability to ambulate after a recent hospitalization for febrile neutropenia. At his therapy session, he confides to his rehabilitation therapist that after completing his initial chemotherapy cycle he feels tired all the time and that getting out of bed each day is a real effort. He asks whether this is an emotional response that is all in his head or whether he feels so tired for another reason. He wonders whether he needs a vitamin or whether he should consult with someone at the health food store for help.

Question

What advice should the therapist give R.P. regarding his symptoms of fatigue?

Answer

The therapist is aware that several factors, including decreased white cell count, preexisting anemia, and anemia associated with his cancer or the chemotherapy treatment, may be contributing to R.P.'s fatigue. Depression can also contribute to fatigue. The therapist contacts R.P.'s oncologist's office and R.P. communicates his new symptoms to his oncologist's nurse, who asks the patient to come in later that day for additional evaluation. His oncologist performs an examination and orders appropriate laboratory studies. During his next therapy session R.P. notifies the therapist of three new medications that he needs to take after each cycle of chemotherapy: filgrastim (Neupogen), epoetin (Procrit),

and ferrous sulfate to treat the low white cell counts and anemia he was experiencing. He reports that his symptoms of fatigue have improved.

Medications Used to Treat Chemotherapy-Induced Nausea and Vomiting

The introduction and use of newer agents and the use of preventative combination antiemetic therapy regimens have improved control of nausea and vomiting. The amount of nausea and vomiting associated with chemotherapy agents differs by agent. In addition, chemotherapy agents that are not emetogenic on their own can cause emesis when combined with other chemotherapy agents in the chemotherapy regimen. Whether a patient experiences nausea and vomiting depends on the potential of each chemotherapy medication to cause nausea and vomiting, the dosage of the medications used, the patient's previous experience with chemotherapy, and the additive effect of all the agents used in the regimen. Even with preventative measures about 10% to 50% of patients receiving chemotherapy experience nausea and vomiting. Nausea and vomiting are usually classified as acute, delayed, anticipatory, breakthrough, or **refractory**. Acute nausea and vomiting are experienced at the time of the chemotherapy administration, and delayed nausea and vomiting occur several hours or days afterward. Anticipatory nausea and vomiting occur before chemotherapy administration when the patient anticipates the nausea and vomiting that occurred with a previous cycle of chemotherapy. Breakthrough nausea and vomiting occur when a patient has nausea and vomiting despite preventative measures; breakthrough nausea and vomiting are treated with rescue antiemetic agents. Refractory nausea and vomiting do not respond to antiemetics and can occur with administration of highly emetogenic chemotherapy. It is now standard practice for patients receiving chemotherapy to receive aggressive and preventative combinations of antiemetic therapy with the goal of preventing nausea and vomiting and reducing anticipatory nausea and vomiting that occurs when patients have experienced severe nausea and vomiting with previous regimens. Anticipatory nausea and vomiting are usually treated with preventative dosing of a benzodiazepine such as lorazepam (Ativan) before chemotherapy administration. A combination of antiemetics, such as a serotonin receptor antagonist (Zofran), dexamethasone (Decadron), and aprepitant (Emend), is administered before the chemotherapy dose to prevent acute and delayed nausea and vomiting in highly emetogenic regimens. Antiemetic therapy should be administered on a scheduled basis for a defined period to control the symptoms and then be tapered off as the patient starts to tolerate oral intake (Balmer & Valley, 2002; Bubalo, 2009; Kaplan & Zandt, 2010).

Medications that are used to treat nausea and vomiting fall into several classes. Antiemetics block dopamine receptors, histamine receptors, serotonin receptors, and cholinergic receptors in the chemotherapy receptor trigger zone. In addition, substance P is a neurokinin-1 receptor agonist that can trigger emesis. Agents that block substance P such as aprepitant can prevent chemotherapy-induced nausea and vomiting in both the acute and delayed phases. Rescue agents include phenothiazines such as promethazine (Phenergan), dopamine antagonists such as metoclopramide (Reglan), antihistamines such as hydroxyzine (Vistaril), **cannabinoids** such as Marinol, corticosteroids such as dexamethasone (Decadron), and benzodiazepines such as lorazepam (Ativan). Serotonin antagonists such as ondansetron (Zofran) are not usually effective as rescue agents. Table 18.4 summarizes medications used to treat nausea and vomiting and other supportive therapies (Bubalo, 2009; Grunwald, 2003).

PATIENT CASE 2, continued

R.P. is quite anxious about receiving his second cycle of chemotherapy. He complains that he has lost weight and has no interest in eating. He wants to stop his chemotherapy treatments because he does not want to experience the severe, prolonged nausea and vomiting that occurred with his first cycle.

Question
What type of nausea and vomiting is R.P. likely to experience? What should the rehabilitation therapist tell R.P. about nausea and vomiting associated with chemotherapy administration?

Answer
Because R.P. is receiving a highly emetogenic chemotherapy regimen, he likely will experience acute, delayed, and even breakthrough and refractory nausea and vomiting. Because of his experience with his previous chemotherapy, anticipatory nausea and vomiting is also likely. The therapist should advise R.P. to discuss his concerns with his oncologist and request that a combination antiemetic regimen that includes a serotonin receptor antagonist, dexamethasone, and aprepitant be administered before the chemotherapy dose to prevent acute and delayed nausea and vomiting. In addition, R.P. should receive lorazepam (Ativan) to reduce anticipatory nausea and vomiting before the second course of chemotherapy. R.P. can also reduce his nausea by drinking plenty of liquids, eating cold food to reduce cooking smells that can trigger nausea, avoiding strong fragrances that can trigger nausea, and eating small, frequent meals instead of larger meals three times a day.

Summary

This chapter discusses important concepts of cancer, medications used to treat cancer, and supportive therapies (e.g., medications used to treat nausea and vomiting, anemia, cancer-related fatigue, and chemotherapy induced neutropenia) used in the cancer patient. This chapter also addresses considerations regarding rehabilitation therapy in the cancer patient such as chemotherapy and immunotherapy-induced immunosuppression with increased infection risk, cancer fatigue, complications associated with immobility in the cancer patient, and chemotherapy-induced neuropathy.

PART VI

Medications Used to Treat Chronic Disease

The chapters in part VI summarize chronic diseases commonly encountered in rehabilitation, including diabetes, cardiac disease, thyroid and parathyroid disease, respiratory disease, and gastrointestinal disease, as well as dysphagia associated with these disease states. Patients may not be referred to rehabilitation for assistance in management of these diseases in all instances. However, because these diseases and the associated medications can affect rehabilitation, the rehabilitation therapist must consider them when developing a rehabilitative treatment plan.

Chapter 19, the first of two chapters dealing with various cardiac diseases, discusses hypertension, congestive heart failure, and cardiac arrhythmias such as atrial fibrillation or premature ventricular contraction. Chapter 20 reviews disease states associated with atherosclerosis, including peripheral artery disease, stroke, and coronary heart disease. Atherosclerosis is responsible for the pathogenesis of these cardiovascular diseases and is associated with dyslipidemia that can be inherited or associated with lifestyle decisions such as diet and exercise. Atherosclerosis can lead

to accumulation of fat deposits in the lining of blood vessels, which results in inflammation and obstruction of the pathway of the blood vessel. Eventual rupture of the blood vessel wall can lead to acute cardiovascular events such as claudication, stroke, or heart attack. Chapters 19 and 20 review how these disease states can affect rehabilitation, and how medications used to treat them can also require alteration of planned rehabilitation activities to optimize results while maintaining a safe patient environment.

Chapter 21 provides an overview of diabetes. It explains the difference between insulin-dependent diabetes and non-insulin-dependent diabetes and how treatment of the two types differs. The complications associated with diabetes can lead to disabilities such as blindness, amputation, and kidney failure. Other clinical conditions that can result from diabetes, such as heart disease, hyperlipidemia, and hypertension, can lead to complications of stroke, peripheral neuropathy, and diabetic foot infections that can negatively affect the patient's rehabilitation plan. This chapter reviews medication therapies used to treat diabetes and discusses how the different outcomes and side effects of these therapies can affect the patient's ability to participate in exercise and rehabilitation.

Chapter 22 discusses common respiratory diseases such as asthma and chronic obstructive pulmonary disease, which includes chronic bronchitis and emphysema. This chapter reviews the medications and other therapies used to treat respiratory disease and provides practical methods for appropriately adjusting therapy sessions to meet patient rehabilitation needs and ensure patient safety during exercise.

Chapter 23 reviews thyroid disease, parathyroid disease, and osteoporosis. Thyroid disease can affect all metabolic processes in the body as well as cognition and learning, which are essential for successful rehabilitation. Disease associated with parathyroid function can significantly affect calcium levels, muscle function, bone formation, and maintenance of a healthy skeletal structure. Osteoporosis, or bone loss that can occur as a result of parathyroid disease or postmenopausal hormone loss, can significantly affect a patient's ability to participate in exercise and rehabilitation. This chapter discusses current treatments for hypothyroidism, hyperthyroidism, hypoparathyroidism, and hyperparathyroidism as well as the prevention and treatment of osteoporosis.

Finally, chapter 24 reviews some of the gastrointestinal disorders a therapist may encounter in caring for patients in a rehabilitation setting. Gastrointestinal disorders can significantly affect nutritional status, and failure to manage them can result in fatigue, muscle weakness, and impaired immune function and healing. In addition, conditions such as gastrointestinal reflux disease often make patient participation in exercises that involve bending difficult. This chapter discusses commonly seen disorders (i.e., nausea, vomiting, and constipation) that often result from side effects of medications or the patient's clinical condition (i.e., diabetic gastroparesis, achalasia, gastroesophageal reflux disease, and inflammatory bowel diseases such as Crohn's disease or irritable bowel syndrome). Finally, the chapter discusses medication-induced dysphagia as well as methods for identifying, preventing, and treating this common cause of dysphagia.

19

Medications Used to Treat Hypertension, Congestive Heart Failure, and Cardiac Arrhythmias

In clinical practice, the rehabilitation therapist will encounter many patients who require cardiac rehabilitation or who have concurrent cardiac disorders such as **hypertension**, arrhythmias, and **congestive heart failure** (CHF). This chapter reviews important concepts pertaining to the effect of heart disease on the patient undergoing rehabilitation therapy and reviews how medication therapies used to treat heart disease change the approach to designing a rehabilitation plan. This chapter also serves as an introduction to chapter 20, which discusses concepts associated with atherosclerosis, ischemic heart disease, and stroke and provides information on acute treatment and prevention of these disorders.

Cardiovascular Disease

Cardiovascular disease is another name for heart disease. Heart diseases include congenital defects to the heart, arrhythmias, acquired inflammatory heart diseases, heart valve problems, degenerative cardiovascular disorders, and heart failure (American Heart Association, 2012). Many cardiovascular problems are related to atherosclerosis. Atherosclerosis occurs when plaque builds up in the artery walls, causing the arteries to narrow and thus making it more difficult for blood to flow through the arteries. Blood flow may be blocked, and a heart attack or stroke may result. Atherosclerosis is discussed in detail in chapter 20.

Incidence

Heart disease is the leading cause of death in the United States. The U.S. ranks 135th in the world for prevalence of coronary heart disease; the death rate is 80.5 per 100,000 deaths. The statistics are similar in many European countries. African and Middle Eastern countries have the highest rates of death from coronary heart disease. Turkmenistan ranks first in the world (405.1/100,000) and Ukraine is second (399/100,000 deaths). Japan and France have the lowest rates of death from cardiac disease (World Health Organization, 2012).

According to American Heart Association statistics for 2006, 81 million people in the United States had one or more forms of cardiovascular disease. Of those, more than 74.5 million had high blood pressure and 17.6 million had coronary heart disease. In addition, 8.5 million Americans experienced an associated heart attack and 10.2 million experienced associated angina. Diabetes is considered to be a risk factor for coronary heart disease because it is highly associated with atherosclerosis. Most strokes are ischemic and are associated with atherosclerosis. Stroke affected an estimated 6.4 million Americans in 2006. Finally, heart failure affected an estimated 5.8 million Americans in 2006.

Cardiovascular disease is the leading cause of death in the United States. In 2006 it claimed 831,272 lives and caused 34.3% of all deaths, or 1 of every 2.9 deaths in the United States.

More than 151,000 of these deaths occurred in Americans under 65 yr of age (American Heart Association, 2006).

Etiology and Pathophysiology

Cardiac disease is also related to obesity and weight gain. Approximately 66% of Americans over the age of 20 yr are overweight or obese, and about 32% of children aged 2 to 19 yr are overweight or obese. Obesity is clearly associated with increased lipid levels, high blood pressure, and increased risk for developing adult-onset diabetes. Obesity is also associated with increased risk of heart disease, heart failure, cancer, degenerative joint disease, asthma, stroke, and diabetes in children (Jones et al., 2010).

Rehabilitation Considerations

Cardiac disease is associated with atrophy of neural tissue, an overall reduction in whole-brain volume, and enlarged ventricles. Certain brain regions, such as the basal ganglia and hippocampus (subcortical structures known to contribute to cognitive functioning), appear to be particularly vulnerable to atrophy related to cardiovascular disease. Patients with cardiovascular disease can exhibit problems with sensory memory and, as a result, have difficulty with processing speed and attention span, which can include problems with sustained attention and alternating attention. Patients may also exhibit difficulties with executive functions such as reasoning, inhibition, and planning. They may have problems with immediate and delayed verbal recall, difficulty learning, and problems with visual memory. Cardiac patients may have language difficulties, such as difficulties with word retrieval or with higher-level lexical–semantic processing (e.g., identifying synonyms) (Murray, 2006).

Cognitive dysfunction that results from reduced cardiac output associated with heart failure is called cardiogenic dementia. Heart failure is associated with cognitive difficulties. More than 50% of patients with mild to moderate heart failure exhibit signs of mild cognitive impairment in multiple cognitive realms (most frequently memory, attentional deficits,

and verbal learning) (Almeida & Flicker, 2001; Trojano et al., 2003). Patients with heart failure generally exhibit increased cognitive difficulties when ventricular **ejection fraction** is less than 30% (Almeida & Tamai, 2001b; Zuccala et al., 1997).

Attention deficits are associated with impaired sensory memory and, as a result, psychomotor speed. The resulting problems include slow motor-response times and problem-solving difficulties. Most cognitive impairments are classified as mild; however, at least 25% of patients with heart failure have moderate to severe cognitive difficulties (Bennett & Sauve, 2003). Because sensory memory and attention respond to rehabilitation efforts, cognitive rehabilitation can reverse the attention problems of the patient with heart failure (Almeida & Tamai, 2001a). Improvements in attention problems can potentially increase the patient's motor response and problem-solving abilities.

A number of studies have examined cognitive impairments (i.e., psychomotor slowing, difficulties with executive functioning, and loss of short- and long-term memory) that occur after coronary artery bypass grafting (CABG) surgery. In a study by McKhann and colleagues (1997), 10% of patients undergoing CABG reported a persistent decline in attention, verbal memory, visual memory, and visuoconstruction whereas 24% reported a late decline in visuoconstruction. The visuoconstruction difficulties are a result of a problem coordinating visuospacial abilities and fine motor skills. The patient may have difficulty writing, doing arithmetic, or driving. Short-term and long-term changes in cognition occur after CABG. Short-term deficits appear to be directly related to the cardiopulmonary bypass (Seines & McKhann, 2005). Moller and colleagues (1998) investigated short- and long-term cognitive deficits post surgery. Their results indicate that the risk factors for early (short-term) cognitive difficulties include the duration of anesthesia, advanced age, low educational level of the patient, history of multiple surgeries, postoperative respiratory complications, and postoperative infection. Long-term changes in cognition after surgery may result from factors such as ischemic injury from microemboli and hypoperfusion after major surgery, and occur more often in patients with a history of cerebrovascular disease or hypertension (Newman et al., 1994; Seines & McKhann, 2005). In a study by Selnes and colleagues (2003), patients who underwent CABG surgery experienced short-term memory loss 5 times more often than the controls with coronary artery disease that did not undergo CABG surgery.

Cardiac rehabilitation is an important component of managing patients with heart disease. Rehabilitation promotes recovery, improves quality of life, and instructs the patient in preventive practices. Rehabilitation can take place before or after hospital admission and can be provided in a rehabilitation hospital, skilled-nursing facility, outpatient center, or home health care setting. Rehabilitation is multidisciplinary and includes medical, psychological, social, and emotional support and patient and family education (Evans et al., 2009). The goals of a cardiac-rehabilitation program are to reduce negative emotions and effects of heart disease, provide a safe exercise program that increases exercise tolerance and fitness, and improve patient compliance with lifestyle changes such as smoking cessation, improving diet, exercising, and reducing stress. Patients with most forms of heart disease (including high-risk patients) participate in multidisciplinary programs (Taylor et al., 2001).

For treatment to be effective and specific to each patient, the rehabilitation specialist must use tests and measurements that provide a detailed analysis of the patient's communication or cognitive functioning and use the results of this analysis to accurately target specific deficits for remediation. General communication-assessment tools may fail to properly identify the patient's specific problems (Murray, 2006). The rehabilitation therapist should break down cognitive functions into component parts to better identify the patient's deficit(s). For example, memory deficits can be categorized as affecting sensory memory, working memory, declarative memory, and nondeclarative memory. The rehabilitation therapist should also educate other health care

professionals about the relationship between cognitive or communication deficits and cardiovascular disease and should work with these professionals to ensure that the materials and instructions (verbal and nonverbal), equipment, exercises, compensatory devices, and strategies used for a patient are compatible with the patient's cognitive and communication abilities (Murray, 2006). The rehabilitation therapist should also work with the patient to encourage patient compliance with the treatment plan and patient adherence in taking prescribed medications.

A physician should supervise the patient's treatment program, and the exercises should be prescribed based on the findings of the physical examination and the information obtained from exercise testing. Exercise testing is typically performed using a treadmill or a stationary bicycle ergometer. During exercise testing, the intensity of exercise is progressively increased until the workload is maximal, symptom limited, or submaximal. The patient's heart rate, blood pressure, and electrocardiography are monitored throughout the test. The specific test parameters used are based on the individual patient's history and clinical presentation. The clinician should terminate the exercise test if the patient exhibits any of the signs or symptoms listed in table 19.1.

Once exercise testing is completed and the results are analyzed, the physician and rehabilitation therapist can develop an individualized exercise prescription. The rehabilitation therapist assesses the patient's functional capacity, psychosocial and educational status, and concurrent cardiac disease states (i.e., arrhythmias, ventricular dysfunction, or myocardial ischemia) and uses this information to individualize the patient's exercise-training prescription and identify the amount of supervision the patient will require. Adequate supervision and monitoring is important since noncompliance with exercise programs, pharmacological regimens, dietary or nutritional changes, or smoking cessation are common. Noncompliance can exacerbate a patient's cardiac difficulties and can play a role in hospital recidivism. Readmission rates for patients with CHF over 65 yr of age approach 50% (Quinn, 2006; Taylor et al., 2001).

Exercise training offers numerous benefits such as increased maximal cardiac output, increased maximal oxygen uptake (Taylor et al., 2001), and improved capacity for exercise. The exercise program includes a warm-up period, cardiovascular conditioning, resistance training, and a cool-down period. The gradual warm-up and cool-down periods are particularly important in cardiac rehabilitation. A gradual warm-up (typically 5-10 min) at low intensity is believed to reduce the risk of myocardial ischemia by allowing the collateral vessels to open and preventing vascular spasm. The cool-down (typically 5-10 min) allows the heart rate and blood pressure to gradually return to resting levels. This enhances venous return and limits post-exercise hypotension.

Cardiac rehabilitation programs often include the judicious use of resistance training. The rehabilitation therapist must be familiar with the medical contraindications to resistance training, including ischemic changes during exercise, poor left ventricular function, uncontrolled arrhythmias and hypertension, and abnormal hemodynamic responses to exercise (Taylor et al., 2001). The American College of Sports Medicine lists additional medical contraindications to resistance training, including unstable angina, untreated severe left main coronary artery disease, angina, hypotension, arrhythmias provoked by resistance training, end-stage CHF, and severe valvular disease (Coe & Fiatarone-Singh, 2010).

Resistance training is often added to cardiac rehabilitation programs as an adjunct to aerobic training after the patient has successfully undergone regular aerobic training for a period of time (this time period depends on the patient's specific cardiac condition and response to aerobic training). The resistance-training program is often a circuit-training program in which the patient alternates upper- and lower-body resistance-training exercises with brief (15-30 s) rest periods. Intensive upper-body exercises are more taxing than lower-body exercises on the cardiovascular system. The prescribed resistance is of lower intensity and usually begins with loads that approximate 40% to 60% of the patient's 1 repetition maximum. The prescribed number of repetitions is usually 10 to 15. This type of low-weight, high-repetition training allows for both improvement of strength and cardiovascular benefit. It also better prepares the patient to perform activities of daily living using the muscle groups they are training. The therapist must instruct the patient in proper breathing technique and the importance of not performing a valsalva maneuver during training. If the load and repetitions are prescribed appropriately, the patient will not need to use a valsalva maneuver to complete the exercise.

Exercise may increase heart rate and may trigger arrhythmia, especially in patients who become dehydrated or who have electrolyte disorders associated with concurrent diuretic therapy. Electrocardiogram recording can identify arrhythmias in the clinic or hospital setting. The therapist should monitor for dizziness, fainting, or altered pulse rate or rhythm in patients with arrhythmia and notify the patient's physician as soon as these symptoms occur (Ciccone, 2007). The rehabilitation therapist should be aware of whether the patient is taking medications that can influence the patient's ability to communicate, learn, and exercise and should consider how these medications may impact the patient's ability to participate in the exercise routine (Youse, 2008). Exercise testing or training should be discontinued if the patient exhibits any of the signs or symptoms listed in table 19.1.

Exercise prescription for patients with cardiovascular disease varies depending on the patient's cardiac pathology, exercise test results, and coexisting medical conditions and the clinical discretion of the physician and rehabilitation specialist. The American College of Sports Medicine provides research-based guidelines for modes of exercise, training intensities, frequency of training, and monitoring the patient based on the specific cardiac condition (Cuccurullo, 2004). The guidelines for exercise prescription in patients with cardiovascular disease recommend training intensities as low as 40% of heart rate reserve and as high as 85% of heart rate reserve, depending on the patient's specific cardiac pathology and response to exercise (Schairer et al., 2010).

Exercise intensity should ideally be determined based on the results of exercise testing. In the absence of an exercise test, one can use

Table 19.1   Indications for Terminating an Exercise Test or Training Session in Cardiac Patients

- Decrease in systolic blood pressure >10 mm Hg from baseline
- Ventricular tachycardia
- Moderate to severe angina
- ST elevation >1 mm in leads without diagnostic Q waves
- Ataxia, dizziness, or near syncope
- Technical difficulties in obtaining electrocardiography or blood pressure readings
- Cyanosis or pallor
- Patient requests to terminate the test or training session

the resting heart rate plus 10 beats/min as the baseline for exercise intensity once the patient has physician clearance to begin exercising. From this level, exercise intensity can progressively increase depending on the patient's symptoms and rating of perceived exertion on the Borg scale. Patients are then provided a target heart rate range (based on their resting heart rate plus 15-25 beats/min) which they maintain during exercise. Use of the Borg scale is especially important in patients taking cardiac medications that blunt exercising heart rate (e.g., beta blockers). In this instance, therapists should not use maximum heart rate and target heart rate as predicted from equations in developing an exercise plan (Brawner, 2010; Brawner et al., 2004).

The American College of Cardiology and the American Heart Association recommend that all patients entering a cardiac rehabilitation program undergo a symptom-limited exercise test. In patients with myocardial ischemia, exercise should be modified so that maximal heart rate is 10 beats/min lower than the heart rate that produces ischemia. Patients with myocardial ischemia, arrhythmia, and CHF require a modified exercise program and electrocardiographic monitoring (Singh et al., 2008).

Medication Therapy

Numerous types of medications are used to control cardiac disease and include medications to control blood pressure and cardiac arrhythmia, as well as to modify and prevent disability associated with heart failure. In all cases, these medications should be combined with lifestyle modifications such as appropriate diet, exercise, weight management, smoking cessation, moderation in alcohol intake, and employment of stress management techniques to help manage their cardiac disease. Later sections in this chapter describe the different categories of medications used to manage heart disease and to improve quality of life in these patients. Special attention is given to mechanism of action, therapeutic effects, side effects, and drug interactions that the therapist should be aware of in providing rehabilitation therapy to patients treated with these medications.

Hypertension

High blood pressure, or hypertension, is frequently called the silent killer because the disease is asymptomatic and many people are unaware that their blood pressure is high. Of those with high blood pressure in the United States in 2006, only 77.6% were aware of their condition. Of all people with high blood pressure, 67.9% were under current treatment, 44.1% had well controlled hypertension, and 55.9% had been treated but their blood pressure remained uncontrolled.

Incidence

One in three adults worldwide has hypertension (World Health Organization, 2012). More than 30% of Americans suffer from hypertension, which becomes more prevalent with increased age (Carter & Saseen, 2002; Ciccone, 2007; Colbert & Mason, 2002; Dobesch & Stacy, 2011; Michel & Hoffman, 2011). High blood pressure (hypertension) was responsible for 56,500 deaths in the United States in 2006. From 1996 to 2006, the rate of death from high blood pressure increased 19.5% and the number of deaths increased 48.1%. In 2006, the rate of death from hypertension was 15.6/100,000 people for white males, 51.1/100,000 for black males, 14.3/100,000 for white females, and 37.7/100,000 for black females (American Heart Association, 2012). Non-Hispanic blacks are more likely to suffer from high blood pressure than are non-Hispanic whites. In the African American community, those with the highest rates of hypertension are more likely to be middle aged or older, less educated, overweight or obese, and physically inactive and are more likely to have diabetes. Complications associated with high blood pressure include acute myocardial infarction, stroke, aneurysm, heart failure, renal failure, blindness, and memory disorders. Direct and indirect costs associated with treatment of essential hypertension exceeded $74 billion in 2009 (American Heart Association, 2012; Mayo Clinic, 2010).

Etiology and Pathophysiology

The cardiovascular system works with the pulmonary system and, via the arterial system, delivers oxygenated blood from the lungs to all parts of the body. Every metabolic process in the body requires oxygen. The cardiovascular system also carries venous blood containing carbon dioxide, a waste product generated by the body's metabolic processes, to the lungs for elimination from the body. Adequate blood pressure is needed to pump oxygenated blood from the heart and to provide adequate perfusion and delivery to all the organs and the brain. If blood pressure is too high, serious consequences such as kidney failure, blindness, heart attack (MI), and stroke can result.

High blood pressure is one of the leading causes of heart attack or stroke. High blood pressure can cause the arteries to harden and thicken, which can lead to a heart attack, stroke, or other complication. People with high blood pressure are more likely to develop coronary artery disease because high blood pressure puts added force against the artery walls. Over time, this extra pressure can damage the arteries, making them more vulnerable to the narrowing and plaque buildup associated with atherosclerosis. High blood pressure can cause blood vessels to weaken and bulge, forming an **aneurysm**, which carries a high risk of rupture and death. High blood pressure can also increase the risk of heart failure. The force of heart contraction must increase in order for the heart to pump blood through blood vessels that are thickened; this can lead to hypertrophy (thickening of the heart muscle). Heart failure occurs when the enlarged heart cannot maintain the work needed to pump enough blood to oxygenate all the body tissues. High blood pressure can also affect blood vessels in the eyes and kidneys, leading to vision loss and kidney failure, and can decrease memory and impair cognition (Mayo Clinic, 2010).

Hypertension is classified as either essential (primary) or secondary. Essential hypertension exists if the hypertension has no specific cause. Most individuals (95%) with hypertension have essential hypertension (Jennings & Cook, 2010). Secondary hypertension exists if the elevation in blood pressure is caused by another disorder. Common causes of secondary hypertension include renal failure, pheochromocytoma (adrenal tumor), **Cushing's syndrome**, hyperthyroidism, hyperparathyroidism, primary **aldosteronism**, pregnancy, and medication use. Medications associated with hypertension include corticosteroids, alcohol, amphetamines, medications or herbals that promote weight loss, antidepressants, cyclosporine, estrogens and oral contraceptives, nonsteroidal anti-inflammatory drugs, decongestants, and thyroid supplements. Treatment of secondary hypertension is straightforward and involves treating the underlying cause (Ciccone, 2007; Colbert & Mason, 2002).

Arterial blood pressure is determined by two major factors: cardiac output (the force of the heart's contraction) and total peripheral resistance (the force from the blood vessels through which the heart must push blood). Arterial blood pressure has two components: systolic blood pressure (the pressure reached during cardiac contraction and the highest blood pressure) and diastolic blood pressure (the pressure reached at the end of the heart's contraction and the lowest blood pressure). Hypertension is defined as blood pressure greater than 140 systolic or 89 diastolic. Elderly patients frequently have elevated systolic blood pressure and normal diastolic blood pressure. This type of hypertension has only recently been recognized as an important risk factor for cardiac death (Carter & Saseen, 2002; Dobesch & Stacy, 2011; Michel & Hoffman, 2011).

Cardiac output is determined by stroke volume (how much blood is pushed out through the heart) and heart rate. Cardiac output is a major determinant of systolic blood pressure. Factors that increase stroke volume or heart rate increase cardiac output and therefore can increase systolic blood pressure (Carter & Saseen, 2002; Dobesch & Stacy, 2011; Michel & Hoffman, 2011).

Total peripheral resistance, which is the amount of pressure exerted by the blood vessels, is determined by the elasticity of the blood vessels and the viscosity of the blood. Elasticity of the blood vessels varies with the amount of constriction by smooth muscle in the blood vessel (vasoconstriction or vasodilation) and the thickness of the blood vessel wall itself. Increased accumulation of fatty deposits in the blood vessel wall, as seen with hyperlipidemia, can lead to thickening of the blood vessel wall (atherosclerosis) and a resultant increase in total peripheral resistance. The narrowed artery limits or blocks the flow of blood to the heart muscle, depriving the heart of oxygen. The hardened surface of the artery can also encourage the formation of small blood clots.

Venous capacitance (the amount of volume held in the venous system) affects the volume of blood that returns to the heart through the central venous circulation (called preload). A decrease in total peripheral resistance (vasodilation) results in increased flow to tissues and increased venous flow back to the heart. Vasoconstriction is associated with an increase in total peripheral resistance and increased diastolic blood pressure. An increase in total peripheral resistance results in decreased flow to tissues and decreased venous flow back to the heart.

Blood pressure is measured in millimeters of mercury. The difference between diastolic and systolic blood pressures is called the pulse pressure. This pressure reflects the tension from the arterial wall. Mean arterial pressure, which is a measure of pressure throughout the entire contraction of the heart, takes into account the systolic and diastolic pressures as well as the time in systole and diastole (Carter & Saseen; 2002, Dobesch & Stacy, 2011; Michel & Hoffman, 2011).

The central and autonomic nervous systems regulate blood pressure. Sympathetic neuronal fibers are located on the surface of the blood vessels. Stimulation of alpha receptors results in vasoconstriction. Stimulation of cardiac beta-1 receptors results in increased heart rate and contractility, whereas stimulation of beta-2 receptors in blood vessels causes vasodilation. Alpha-2 adrenergic stimulation in the central nervous system decreases blood pressure by inhibiting the vasomotor center, whereas increased **angiotensin** II increases sympathetic outflow from the vasomotor center and increases blood pressure (Carter & Saseen, 2002; Dobesch & Stacy, 2011; Michel & Hoffman, 2011).

The baroreceptor reflex system is a negative-feedback mechanism that transmits impulses to the brainstem through the ninth cranial and vagus nerves to control sympathetic activity. An acute elevation in blood pressure results in vasodilation and a decrease in heart rate and myocardial contractility. An acute decrease in arterial blood pressure has the opposite effect and causes vasoconstriction. The kidney helps maintain normal blood pressure by altering excretion of sodium and water. When blood pressure drops the kidneys respond by increasing retention of sodium and water. On the other hand, when blood pressure increases the kidneys respond by increasing the excretion of sodium and water (Carter & Saseen, 2002; Dobesch & Stacy, 2011; Michel & Hoffman, 2011).

The renin–angiotensin–aldosterone system also regulates sodium, potassium, and fluid balance. It significantly affects vascular tone and sympathetic nervous system activity and contributes to the regulation of blood pressure. Renin is an enzyme stored in the juxtaglomerular apparatus in the kidneys. When renal perfusion decreases, the juxtaglomerular apparatus stimulates the release of renin, which converts angiotensin I to angiotensin II. Angiotensin II causes vasoconstriction, the release of catecholamines, and a centrally mediated increase in activity of the sympathetic nervous system. The result is an increase in retention of sodium and water and an increase in heart rate and blood pressure (Carter & Saseen, 2002; Dobesch & Stacy, 2011; Michel & Hoffman, 2011).

Rehabilitation Considerations

The rehabilitation therapist will undoubtedly interact with patients exhibiting either high or low blood pressure. The specialist working with patients who are being treated with antihypertensives that cause orthostasis must be aware that rapidly changing positions can increase the risk of falls. The therapist should carefully consider therapeutic modalities that cause vasodilation if the patient is on vasodilation medications. For example, the use of heat (e.g., whirlpools) may result in an inappropriate reduction in blood pressure if used with patients taking vasodilation medication, calcium channel blockers, or alpha blockers. Exercise may also facilitate skeletal muscle perfusion by vasodilation. In addition, exercising patients who take beta blockers may experience blunted cardiac output and heart rate. Patients who are receiving diuretic therapy should have their sessions later in the day in order to prevent urinary urgency during rehabilitation sessions.

The rehabilitation therapist should also encourage the patient to control blood pressure through nonpharmacological methods when at all possible. The specialist may play a key role in educating the patient about smoking cessation, weight reduction, heart-healthy diet, and regular cardiovascular exercise as part of the overall plan for managing hypertension. Including stress-management techniques in patient-education sessions can also be valuable (Ciccone, 2007).

Medication Therapy

Treatment of essential hypertension includes nonpharmacologic measures such as losing weight, instituting a heart-healthy diet, restricting salt intake, restricting alcohol intake, smoking cessation, and exercise. These measures should always be included in a plan of care in addition to pharmacologic interventions. Antihypertensive drugs can be divided into nine classes: diuretics, beta blockers, angiotensin-converting enzyme (ACE) inhibitors, calcium channel blockers, angiotensin II receptor blockers (ARB), alpha blockers, central alpha-2 agonists, adrenergic inhibitors, and vasodilators. Medications used to treat hypertension target one of several mechanisms associated with blood pressure elevation. Medications that decrease cardiac output, such as the beta adrenergic blockers and the calcium channel blockers, reduce heart rate and the force of myocardial contraction. These agents are useful in patients with ischemic heart disease because they reduce oxygen demand by the heart and help prevent chest pain associated with cardiac ischemia. Medications that reduce blood volume include the diuretics. These agents promote excretion of sodium and water through the kidneys. Medications that reduce vascular resistance include the vasodilators. Angiotensin-converting enzyme (ACE) inhibitors and angiotensin II receptor blockers (ARBs) alter sodium and fluid retention as well as sympathetic responses that affect heart rate and blood pressure via the renin–angiotensin–aldosterone system (Carter & Saseen, 2002; Dobesch & Stacy, 2011; Michel & Hoffman, 2011).

The choice of medication for treating hypertension depends on concurrent disease states, and the recommended choices for initiation continue to change based on evidence in the literature. Table 19.2 summarizes the most current recommendations from the American Heart Association and the American College of Cardiology (ACC), published in 2007 and 2008, for choice of antihypertensives based on patient risk factors. The age, sex, and nationality of the patient can also be used to predict response of different medication classes. If blood pressure does not lower to the target goal after a medication is initiated, these guidelines recommend adding a second agent rather than using high doses of a single agent, as high dose

Table 19.2   Initial Antihypertensive Therapy Choices and Target Blood Pressures Based on Patient Risk Factors

Patient category	Target blood pressure	Initial therapy choices
Primary treatment in patients without other risk factors	<130/80	ACE inhibitor or ARB, calcium channel blocker, thiazide diuretic, or combination
Patients with high risk of coronary heart disease (e.g., patients with diabetes and kidney disease)	<130/80	First choice: ACE inhibitor or ARB Second choice: thiazide diuretic Third choice: calcium channel blocker
Patients with coronary heart disease (e.g., high cholesterol, history of acute myocardial infarction or angina)	<130/80	First choice: beta blocker, ACE inhibitor, or ARB Second choice: thiazide diuretic Third choice: calcium channel blocker
Patients with carotid artery disease (previous stroke or transient ischemic attack [TIA])	<130/80	First choice: ACE inhibitor or ARB Second choice: calcium channel blocker
Patients with left ventricular dysfunction and no symptoms of heart failure	<120/80	ACE inhibitor or ARB and beta blocker
Patients with left ventricular dysfunction and current or previous symptoms of heart failure	<120/80	ACE inhibitor or ARB, beta blocker, diuretic, aldosterone antagonist, and hydralazine plus isosorbide dinitrate

ACE = angiotensin-converting enzyme; ARB = angiotensin receptor-blocking agent.

single agent therapy is associated with more side effects and toxicity than is combination low dose therapy. Some patients require several types of antihypertensive therapy to meet their blood pressure goals. Table 19.2 summarizes recommendations for initial therapy and target goals for blood pressure (Carter & Saseen, 2002; Dobesch & Stacy, 2011; Michel & Hoffman, 2011).

Several evidence-based guidelines provide recommendations for choosing an initial antihypertensive agent based on the patient's concurrent disease state and other characteristics. These guidelines include the Joint National Committee on Prevention, Detection, Evaluation and Treatment of High Blood Pressure (JNC7); the joint scientific statements from the American Heart Association (AHA) and the American Society of Hypertension; the Canadian Hypertension Education Program; and the European Society of Cardiology and the European Society of Hypertension practice guidelines. The JNC7 guidelines, published in 2003, provide a simplified classification structure for patients and staged goals for treatment. They

also establish more aggressive blood pressure targets for patients with diabetes and kidney disease. The JNC7 guidelines recommend thiazide diuretics as the preferred first-line therapy and combination therapy for patients with higher blood pressure. They also recommend the use of ACE inhibitors or angiotensin receptor blockers in patients with diabetes or kidney disease because these agents have protective effects on kidney function (Carter & Saseen, 2002; Dobesch & Stacy, 2011; Michel & Hoffman, 2011; Jennings & Cook, 2010).

The AHA and ACC guidelines were published in 2007 and 2008, respectively. These guidelines recommend thiazide diuretics, ACE inhibitors (or ARBs), or calcium channel blockers as first-line treatment of hypertension and recommend reserving beta blockers for patients with a history of coronary artery disease. They still recommend the use of ACE inhibitors (or ARBs) in patients with diabetes because these agents have renal-protective effects. Patients receiving thiazide diuretics should take these medications in low doses and be carefully monitored for potassium and magnesium loss (which can be associated with new-onset diabetes), cardiac arrhythmia, and muscle weakness. The European guidelines, published in 2007, still recommend the use of beta blockers for initial therapy. The Canadian guidelines still recommend using beta blockers as first-line therapy in patients under 60 yr of age and using thiazide diuretics as first-line therapy in patients without diabetes or coronary artery disease. Table 19.3 summarizes recommendations for selecting antihypertensive therapies based on the individual patient's concurrent disease states (Carter & Sassen, 2002; Dobesch & Stacy, 2011; Michel & Hoffman, 2011; Jennings & Cook, 2010).

Table 19.4 summarizes medications used to treat hypertension and CHF and includes information on dosing and associated side effects that can affect the patient's ability to participate in rehabilitation.

Diuretics are used to treat hypertension as well as edema. Three types of diuretics are used in the management of hypertension: thiazide diuretics, loop diuretics, and potassium-sparing diuretics. Diuretics increase the excretion of water and sodium. When administered acutely, diuretics lower blood pressure by causing diuresis and reducing plasma volume and cardiac output. However, after chronic use, diuretics reduce blood pressure by lowering peripheral

Table 19.3 Antihypertensives Recommended or Contraindicated Based on Concurrent Disease of the Patient

Condition	Antihypertensive medications recommended	Antihypertensive medications to avoid
Heart failure	ACE inhibitors, diuretics, carvedilol or metoprolol, spironolactone	Calcium channel blockers, alpha blockers, beta blockers other than carvedilol or metoprolol
Diabetes	ACE inhibitors	Beta blockers, high-dose diuretics, calcium channel blockers as monotherapy
Elderly age	Diuretics	Alpha agonists or alpha blockers
Myocardial infarction	Non-ISA beta blockers	Hydralazine, minoxidil, dihydropyridine calcium channel blockers (except amlodipine and felodipine)
Angina	Non-ISA beta blockers	Hydralazine, minoxidil
Bronchospasm	Calcium channel blockers	Beta blockers, ACE inhibitors
Pregnancy	Methyldopa, hydralazine, labetalol	ACE inhibitors, ARB, diuretics
Gout	Beta blockers, ACE inhibitors	Diuretics
Renal insufficiency	ACE inhibitors, loop diuretics, diltiazem, hydralazine, minoxidil	Thiazide diuretics, potassium-sparing diuretics
African American descent	Choice 1: diuretics Choice 2: calcium channel blockers	Beta blockers or ACE inhibitors may be tried after diuretics or calcium channel blockers
Left ventricular hypertrophy	Choice 1: ACE inhibitors Diuretics are also effective	—
Coronary artery disease	Choice 1: non-ISA beta blockers	Calcium channel blockers are third-line treatment
Sexual dysfunction	ACE inhibitors, calcium channel blockers, and cardioselective beta blockers when a beta blocker is needed	Alpha-1 blockers, central alpha-2 agonists

ACE = angiotensin-converting enzyme; ARB = angiotensin receptor-blocking agent; ISA = intrinsic sympathomimetic activity.

See table 19.4 in the web resource for a full list of medication-specific indications, dosing recommendations, and side effects.

Table 19.4 Medications Used to Treat Hypertension and Congestive Heart Failure

Medication	Side effects affecting rehab							Other side effects or considerations
Thiazide diuretics: Used to treat hypertension. Useful for reducing edema and blood volume in patients with normal renal function; helpful in elderly patients with systolic hypertension; more effective than loop diuretics except in patients with creatinine clearance <30 ml/min.								
Chlorthalidone (Hygroton)	Cog 0	S 0	A 0	Motor ++	D +	Com 0	F ++	Side effects: Dizziness, orthostatic hypotension, increased risk of falls, cardiac arrhythmia, weakness, muscle fatigue, cramps, orthostasis.
Hydrochloro-thiazide (Hydrodiuril)	Cog 0	S 0	A 0	Motor ++	D +	Com 0	F ++	Carefully monitor for electrolyte imbalances, hypokalemia, hypomagnesemia, hypercalcemia, hyperuricemia, hyperglycemia, hyperlipidemia, sexual dysfunction.
Indapamide (Lozol)	Cog 0	S 0	A 0	Motor ++	D +	Com 0	F ++	Drug interactions: Toxic effects of digoxin are increased if potassium loss occurs.
Metolazone (Mykrox)	Cog 0	S 0	A 0	Motor ++	D +	Com 0	F ++	Diuretics increase levels of lithium and toxicity.
Metolazone (Zaroxolyn)	Cog 0	S 0	A 0	Motor ++	D +	Com 0	F ++	Nonsteroidal anti-inflammatory drugs may reduce diuretic effects. Corticosteroids, amphotericin B, or aminoglycosides may further increase potassium loss.
Loop diuretics: Used to treat hypertension or CHF. Useful in patients with creatinine clearance <30 ml/min; agents of choice in patients with CHF; higher doses needed for patients with renal impairment or CHF.								
Bumetanide (Bumex)	Cog 0	S 0	A 0	Motor ++	D +	Com 0	F ++	Side effects: Dizziness, orthostatic hypotension, increased risk of falls, cardiac arrhythmia, weakness, muscle fatigue, cramps, orthostasis.
Furosemide (Lasix)	Cog 0	S 0	A 0	Motor ++	D +	Com 0	F ++	Carefully monitor for electrolyte imbalances, hypokalemia, hypomagnesemia, hypercalcemia, hyperuricemia, hyperglycemia, hyperlipidemia, sexual dysfunction.
Torsemide (Demadex)	Cog 0	S 0	A 0	Motor ++	D +	Com 0	F ++	Drug interactions: Toxic effects of digoxin are increased if potassium loss occurs.
								Diuretics increase levels of lithium and toxicity.
								Nonsteroidal anti-inflammatory drugs may reduce diuretic effects.
								Corticosteroids, amphotericin B, or aminoglycosides may further increase potassium loss.

Medication	Side effects affecting rehab							Other side effects or considerations
Potassium-sparing diuretics: Used to treat hypertension or CHF. Use in combination with another diuretic.								
Amiloride (Midamor) Amiloride–hydrochlorothiazide (Moduretic)	Cog 0	S 0	A 0	Motor ++	D +	Com 0	F ++	Side effects: Hyperkalemia (symptoms include irregular heartbeat, confusion, numbness, unusual tiredness, weakness or a heavy feeling in the legs, confusion, nervousness, breathing problems). Drug interactions: ACE inhibitors may increase the risk of hyperkalemia in patients with renal dysfunction or those taking potassium supplements.
Spironolactone (Aldactone) Spironolactone–hydrochlorothiazide (Aldactazide)	Cog +	S 0	A 0	Motor ++	D +	Com 0	F ++	
Triamterene (Dyrenium) Triamterene–hydrochlorothiazide (Dyazide, Maxzide)	Cog +	S 0	A 0	Motor ++	D +	Com 0	F ++	
Beta blockers: Reduce sympathetic tone, myocardial oxygen demand, and ischemia. Indicated in patients with ischemic heart disease or history of acute myocardial infarction; cardioselective in low doses.								
Propranolol (Inderal; Inderal LA [long acting])	Cog +++	S +++	A ++	Motor ++	D ++	Com +	F +++	Side effects: As listed below with other beta blockers. In addition, because it is highly lipophilic it crosses into the CNS more readily and has higher incidence of CNS side effects (hallucinations, decreased concentration, insomnia, nightmares, depression). Drug interactions: Avoid using with medications that increase sympathetic tone (e.g., cocaine, amphetamines, decongestants such as pseudoephedrine); increase in heart rate and arrhythmia may occur.
Atenolol (Tenormin)	Cog ++	S ++	A 0	Motor ++	D ++	Com +	F ++	Cardioselective in low doses. Precautions: Beta blockers prevent an increase in heart rate with exercise. Avoid abrupt discontinuation, as this may result in acute myocardial infarction or arrhythmia. Side effects: Nausea, diarrhea, bronchospasm, cold extremities, exacerbation of Raynaud's syndrome, bradycardia, heart block, orthostasis, fatigue, dizziness, alopecia, abnormal vision, hyperglycemia, hyperlipidemia, sexual dysfunction. Drug interactions: Avoid using with medications that increase sympathetic tone (e.g., cocaine, amphetamines, decongestants such as pseudoephedrine); increase in heart rate and arrhythmia may occur.
Betaxolol (Kerlone)	Cog ++	S ++	A 0	Motor ++	D ++	Com +	F ++	
Bisoprolol (Zebeta)	Cog ++	S ++	A 0	Motor ++	D ++	Com +	F ++	
Metoprolol (Lopressor, Toprol XL)	Cog ++	S ++	A 0	Motor ++	D ++	Com +	F ++	
Nadolol (Corgard)	Cog ++	S ++	A 0	Motor ++	D ++	Com +	F ++	
Timolol (Blocadren)	Cog ++	S ++	A 0	Motor ++	D ++	Com +	F ++	

› continued

Table 19.4 › *continued*

Medication	Side effects affecting rehab	Other side effects or considerations
Beta blockers with intrinsic sympathomimetic activity: Used to treat hypertension or CHF. Act as partial agonists on the beta receptors; may be useful in patients with CHF or sinus bradycardia. Cardioselective in low doses.		
Acebutolol (Sectral)	Cog ++ S ++ A + Motor ++ D ++ Com + F ++	Intrinsic sympathomimetic activity beta blockers have fewer metabolic side effects than other beta blockers. Cardioselective in low doses.
Carteolol (Cartrol)	Cog ++ S ++ A + Motor ++ D ++ Com + F ++	Side effects: Nausea, diarrhea, broncho-spasm, cold extremities, exacerbation of Raynaud's syndrome, orthostasis, fatigue, dizziness, alopecia, abnormal vision, sexual dysfunction.
Nebivolol (Bystolic)	Cog ++ S ++ A + Motor ++ D ++ Com + F ++	
Penbutolol (Levatol)	Cog ++ S ++ A + Motor ++ D ++ Com + F ++	Drug interactions: Avoid using with medications that increase sympathetic tone (e.g., cocaine, amphetamines, decongestants such as pseudoephedrine); increase in heart rate and arrhythmia may occur.
Pindolol (Visken)	Cog ++ S ++ A + Motor ++ D ++ Com + F ++	
Beta blockers with alpha-blocking activity: Carvedilol is indicated in treatment of CHF and after myocardial infarction. Labetalol is frequently used in managing acute hypertension in stroke patients. Increased risk of orthostasis.		
Carvedilol (Coreg)	Cog ++ S ++ A + Motor ++ D ++ Com + F ++	Side effects: Higher risk of orthostasis due to vasodilating effects, nausea, diarrhea, bronchospasm, cold extremities, exacerbation of Raynaud's syndrome, orthostasis, fatigue, dizziness, alopecia, abnormal vision, sexual dysfunction.
Labetalol (Normodyne, Trandate)	Cog ++ S ++ A + Motor +++ D ++ Com + F +++	Drug interactions: Avoid using with medications that increase sympathetic tone (e.g., cocaine, amphetamines, decongestants such as pseudoephedrine); increase in heart rate and arrhythmia may occur.
Calcium channel blockers: Used to treat hypertension. Control heart rate and increase vasodilation. Fewer side effects than with beta blockers.		
Diltiazem (Cardizem, Cardizem CD, Dilator SR)	Cog 0 S 0 A 0 Motor + D + Com 0 F +	Side effects: Bradycardia, nausea, peripheral edema, hypotension. Increased risk of falls from orthostasis. Verapamil is associated with severe constipation; use laxative with this medication.
Verapamil (Calan, Calan SR, Isoptin, Isoptin SR, Covera-HS)	Cog 0 S 0 A 0 Motor + D +++ Com 0 F +	Food interactions: Grapefruit juice (>200 ml) can increase levels of these medications and should not be consumed within 2 hrs before or 4 hrs after administration.
		Drug interactions: Decreases liver metabolism of carbamazepine (Tegretol), simvastatin (Zocor), atorvastatin (Lipitor), and lovastatin (Mevacor) that can result in rhabdomyolysis or liver toxicity.

Medication	Side effects affecting rehab							Other side effects or considerations
Calcium antagonists (dihydropyridines): Cause vasodilation without controlling heart rate; should be combined with another agent that controls heart rate. Grapefruit juice (>200 ml) can increase levels of these medications and should not be consumed within 2 h before or 4 h after administration.								
Amlodipine (Norvasc)	Cog +	S 0	A +	Motor +	D ++	Com +	F ++	Side effects: Dizziness, orthostasis with increased risk of falls, flushing, headache, gingival hyperplasia, peripheral edema, mood changes, gastrointestinal side effects.
Felodipine (Plendil)	Cog +	S 0	A +	Motor +	D ++	Com +	F ++	Side effects: Dizziness, orthostasis with increased risk of falls, flushing, headache, gingival hyperplasia, peripheral edema, mood changes, gastrointestinal side effects.
Isradipine (Dynacirc)	Cog +	S 0	A +	Motor +	D ++	Com +	F ++	Drug interactions: Decreases liver metabolism of carbamazepine (Tegretol), simvastatin (Zocor), atorvastatin (Lipitor), and lovastatin (Mevacor) that can result in rhabdomyolysis or liver toxicity,
Nicardipine sustained release (Cardene SR)	Cog +	S 0	A +	Motor +	D ++	Com +	F ++	
Nifedipine long acting (Adalat CC, Procardia XL)	Cog +	S 0	A +	Motor +	D ++	Com +	F ++	
Nisoldipine (Sular)	Cog +	S 0	A +	Motor +	D ++	Com +	F ++	
ACE inhibitors: Improve exercise tolerance in patients with CHF; reduce ventricular hypertrophy; prevent diabetic nephropathy in diabetics with hypertension. Well tolerated with few side effects.								
Benazepril (Lotensin)	Cog +	S +	A 0	Motor +	D +	Com 0	F +	Precautions: Reduce dose with renal impairment; may cause acute renal failure with renal artery stenosis.
Captopril (Capoten)	Cog +	S +	A 0	Motor +	D ++	Com 0	F +	Hold diuretics for several days before initiating these agents to avoid acute hypotension.
Enalapril (Vasotec)	Cog +	S +	A 0	Motor +	D +	Com 0	F +	Diuretics can increase the risk of acute renal failure when used with ACE inhibitors.
Fosinopril (Monopril)	Cog +	S +	A 0	Motor +	D +	Com 0	F +	Side effects: Hypotension, cough, hyperkalemia, headache, dizziness, fatigue, nausea, angioedema, renal impairment.
Lisinopril (Prinivil, Zestril)	Cog +	S +	A 0	Motor +	D +	Com 0	F +	Drug interactions: Use of potassium-sparing diuretics or potassium supplements increases risk of hyperkalemia, especially in patients with renal impairment.
Moexipril (Univasc)	Cog +	S +	A 0	Motor +	D +	Com 0	F +	
Quinapril (Accupril)	Cog +	S +	A 0	Motor +	D +	Com 0	F +	
Ramipril (Altace)	Cog +	S +	A 0	Motor +	D +	Com 0	F +	
Trandolapril (Mavik)	Cog +	S +	A 0	Motor +	D +	Com 0	F +	

› continued

Table 19.4 › continued

Medication	Side effects affecting rehab							Other side effects or considerations

<table>
<tr><td colspan="9">Angiotensin II receptor blockers: Used to treat hypertension and CHF and to prevent diabetic nephropathy in patients with CHF or diabetics who cannot tolerate ACE inhibitors and ACE inhibitor-associated cough; well tolerated with few side effects.</td></tr>
<tr>
<td>Candesartan
(Atacand)</td>
<td>Cog
+</td><td>S
+</td><td>A
0</td><td>Motor
+</td><td>D
+</td><td>Com
0</td><td>F
+</td>
<td rowspan="5">Side effects: Hypotension, hyperkalemia, headache, dizziness, fatigue, nausea, angioedema, renal impairment.

Drug interactions: Diuretics can increase the risk of acute renal failure when used with angiotensin II receptor blockers.

Use of potassium-sparing diuretics or potassium supplements increases risk of hyperkalemia, especially in patients with renal impairment.</td>
</tr>
<tr>
<td>Irbesartan
(Avapro)</td>
<td>Cog
+</td><td>S
+</td><td>A
0</td><td>Motor
+</td><td>D
+</td><td>Com
0</td><td>F
+</td>
</tr>
<tr>
<td>Losartan
(Cozaar)</td>
<td>Cog
+</td><td>S
+</td><td>A
0</td><td>Motor
+</td><td>D
+</td><td>Com
0</td><td>F
+</td>
</tr>
<tr>
<td>Telmisartan
(Micardis)</td>
<td>Cog
+</td><td>S
+</td><td>A
0</td><td>Motor
+</td><td>D
+</td><td>Com
0</td><td>F
+</td>
</tr>
<tr>
<td>Valsartan
(Diovan)</td>
<td>Cog
+</td><td>S
+</td><td>A
0</td><td>Motor
+</td><td>D
+</td><td>Com
0</td><td>F
+</td>
</tr>
<tr><td colspan="9">Alpha-1 adrenergic blockers: Used to treat hypertension or BPH (benign prostatic hypertrophy). Can improve urinary flow in patients with prostatic hypertrophy; high risk of orthostasis and falls.</td></tr>
<tr>
<td>Doxazosin
(Cardura)</td>
<td>Cog
++</td><td>S
++</td><td>A
+</td><td>Motor
+++</td><td>D
0</td><td>Com
++</td><td>F
+++</td>
<td rowspan="3">Side effects: Headache, asthenia, hypotension, lassitude, vivid dreams, depression.

Initial doses can cause acute dizziness, faintness, syncope; orthostasis can persist in some patients.

Drug interactions: Increased hypotension when used with vardenafil (Levitra) or sildenafil (Viagra).

Increased hypotension when doxazosin is concurrently used with CYP3A4 inhibitors: clarithromycin (Biaxin), indinavir (Crixivan), itraconazole (Sporanox), ketoconazole (Nizoral), nefazodone (Serzone), nelfinavir (Viracept), ritonavir (Norvir), saquinavir (Invirase), or voriconazole (Vfend).</td>
</tr>
<tr>
<td>Prazosin
(Minipress)</td>
<td>Cog
++</td><td>S
++</td><td>A
+</td><td>Motor
+++</td><td>D
0</td><td>Com
++</td><td>F
+++</td>
</tr>
<tr>
<td>Terazosin
(Hytrin)</td>
<td>Cog
++</td><td>S
++</td><td>A
+</td><td>Motor
+++</td><td>D
0</td><td>Com
++</td><td>F
+++</td>
</tr>
<tr><td colspan="9">Central alpha-2 agonist: Used to treat hypertension not responsive to other agents. Avoid abrupt discontinuance; high risk of orthostasis and falls.</td></tr>
<tr>
<td>Clonidine
(Catapres)</td>
<td>Cog
++</td><td>S
++</td><td>A
0</td><td>Motor
+++</td><td>D
++</td><td>Com
++</td><td>F
+++</td>
<td rowspan="3">Side effects: Dry mouth, sedation, orthostasis, dizziness, fluid retention (usually requires addition of diuretic).

Drug interactions: Potentiates the depressive effects of alcohol, barbiturates, and other sedating drugs on the central nervous system.

Tricyclic antidepressants may reduce effects of clonidine.

Increased bradycardia when combined with digitalis, calcium channel blockers, and beta blockers.

Methyldopa is safe to use in pregnancy.</td>
</tr>
<tr>
<td>Clonidine patch
(Catapres-TTS)</td>
<td>Cog
++</td><td>S
++</td><td>A
0</td><td>Motor
+++</td><td>D
++</td><td>Com
++</td><td>F
+++</td>
</tr>
<tr>
<td>Methyldopa
(Aldomet)</td>
<td>Cog
++</td><td>S
++</td><td>A
0</td><td>Motor
+++</td><td>D
++</td><td>Com
++</td><td>F
+++</td>
</tr>
</table>

Medication	Side effects affecting rehab	Other side effects or considerations
Peripheral adrenergic antagonist: Used to treat hypertension not controlled by other agents. High risk of orthostasis and falls.		
Reserpine	Cog S A Motor D Com F ++ ++ 0 +++ +++ ++ +++	Side effects: Dry mouth, nausea, vomiting, diarrhea, anorexia, arrhythmia, dizziness, nasal congestion, extrapyramidal symptoms (rare), nightmares, depression, drowsiness, muscle aches, sexual dysfunction, gynecomastia, optic atrophy, deafness. Drug interactions: Avoid using with digitalis or quinidine; can increase arrhythmia. Avoid combining with catecholamines, monoamine oxidase inhibitors, or medications that are sedating.
Direct vasodilators: Minoxidil is used as an adjunctive treatment of hypertension not responsive to other agents; high risk of orthostasis and falls. Hydralazine is used to treat life-threatening hypertension or as an adjunctive treatment of hypertension not responsive to other agents.		
Minoxidil (Loniten)	Cog S A Motor D Com F 0 + 0 +++ ++ + +++	Pretreat with beta blocker and diuretic to reduce fluid retention and reflex tachycardia. Side effects: Reflex tachycardia, weakness, postural hypotension, dizziness, headache, nausea, fluid retention (requires addition of diuretic), hirsutism. Drug interactions: Avoid concurrent use of guanethidine; causes profound hypotension.
Hydralazine (Apresoline)	Cog S A Motor D Com F 0 + 0 +++ ++ + +++	Pretreat with beta blocker and diuretic to reduce fluid retention and reflex tachycardia. Side effects: Reflex tachycardia, weakness, postural hypotension, dizziness, headache, nausea, fluid retention (requires addition of diuretic). Drug interactions: Avoid concurrent use of monoamine oxidase inhibitors. Additive hypotensive effects when used with other antihypertensives.

Cog = cognition; S = sedation; A = agitation or mania; Motor = discoordination; D = dysphagia; Com = communication; F = falls; ACE = angiotensin-converting enzyme; CHF = congestive heart failure; CNS = central nervous system.

The likelihood rating scale for encountering the side effects is as follows: 0 = Almost no probability of encountering side effects. + = Little likelihood of encountering side effects. +/++ = Low probability of encountering side effects; however, probability increases with increased dosage. ++ = Medium likelihood of encountering side effects. +++ = High likelihood of encountering side effects, particularly with high doses. ++++ = Highest likelihood of encountering side effects; best to avoid in at-risk patients.

resistance (i.e., vasodilation). The mechanism of this effect is unclear, but it may involve either direct vasodilator actions or effects on whole-body or renal autoregulation. Thiazide diuretics provide a gentler diuresis over a longer period of time than do loop diuretics and are more effective in treating hypertension in patients with normal renal function than are other diuretics. Loop diuretics have a shorter duration of action but are effective in patients with renal insufficiency and provide significant diuresis that is consistent with the size of the dose. They are particularly helpful in managing acute edema and in CHF. Potassium-sparing diuretics are weak and are usually used with thiazide diuretics to minimize potassium loss associated with the thiazide diuretics (Carter & Saseen, 2002).

Use of thiazide diuretics is associated with side effects of hypokalemia, hypomagnesemia, hypercalcemia, hyperuricemia, hyperglycemia, hyperlipidemia, and sexual dysfunction. Loss of potassium and magnesium can result in cardiac arrhythmias, muscle weakness, fatigue, and muscle cramps. Therefore, therapists should carefully monitor for these symptoms in patients taking diuretics and notify the prescriber if they occur so that these electrolytes can be checked and replacement therapy can be administered to maintain the electrolytes within therapeutic range. Dizziness and orthostasis can occur, especially with initiation of therapy, so appropriate fall prevention measures must be implemented in the therapy plan. The metabolic effects on glucose and lipids are most pronounced when these agents are used in higher doses and can increase the risk for diabetes and coronary heart disease (Carter & Saseen, 2002; Dobesch & Stacy, 2011; Michel & Hoffman, 2011).

The side effects of loop diuretics are similar to those of thiazide diuretics except that use of loop diuretics usually decrease calcium levels, and resultant hypocalcemia can result in muscle weakness and reduced bone strength. Patients should understand that all diuretics cause the urgent need to pass a large volume of urine, which may require the patient to make regular trips to the restroom. This effect may be felt within 1 h of taking the diuretic and may last several hours. Patients may experience dizziness or lightheadedness, especially when getting up from a sitting or lying position. Urgency to go to the restroom paired with dizziness and lightheadedness can increase the risk for falls in patients taking diuretics. Patients should be instructed to take diuretics in the morning to avoid sleep interference. The potassium-sparing diuretics are less potent but may be associated with hyperkalemia (especially when combined with ACE inhibitors or potassium supplements) or with acute changes in renal function. Patients should understand the symptoms of high levels of potassium in the body (i.e., irregular heartbeat, confusion, numbness, unusual tiredness, weakness or a heavy feeling in the legs, nervousness, and breathing problems) and contact their physician if these symptoms occur. The therapist should monitor the patient for any of these symptoms as well, contacting the prescriber when identified so that electrolytes can be tested and medication dosage adjusted as needed (Carter & Saseen, 2002).

For many years, beta-blocking agents, which have been documented to reduce morbidity and mortality in patients with hypertension, were considered first-line therapy for treating hypertension. However, because of their side effect profile, they are now used as first-line agents only in treating hypertension in patients with angina or a history of myocardial infarction. In these patients, the beta blockers carvedilol (Coreg) and metoprolol (Toprol XL) are still recommended as first-line therapy. The negative **chronotropic** and **inotropic** effects of beta blockers on the heart reduce cardiac output, thus reducing myocardial ischemia in these patients. Physicians must be cautious about using beta blockers in patients with insulin-dependent diabetes or peripheral vascular disease. Because the adrenergic nervous system mediates insulin secretion and glycogenolysis, blockage of the beta-2 receptors can reduce these processes and blunt the peripheral side effects of hypoglycemia (shakiness). Beta blockers can also reduce blood flow to the peripheral tissues and worsen symptoms of peripheral vascular disease (Carter & Saseen, 2002; Dobesch & Stacy, 2011; Michel & Hoffman, 2011).

Beta blockers are subdivided into categories based on their selectivity for different beta receptors in the body. Use of beta blockers can cause the unwanted effects of bronchospasm, increased glucose levels, and increased lipid levels. Beta-1 selective (also called cardioselective) agents are more selective for blocking beta-1 receptors located in the heart and kidneys and have less blocking action of the beta-2 receptors which are primarily located in the peripheral tissues (lungs, pancreas, and arteriolar smooth muscle). This selective blockade results in decreased heart rate, contractility, and renin release and a decreased tendency to cause bronchospasm and vasoconstriction. Beta blockers that are cardioselective include bisoprolol (Zebeta), metoprolol (Toprol XL), atenolol (Tenormin), and acebutolol (Sectral). When used in low doses, these agents are safer to use in patients with respiratory disease or peripheral ischemia. Beta blockers that have intrinsic sympathomimetic activity are safer to use in patients with bradycardia and are less likely to increase glucose and lipid levels. Beta blockers that have alpha- and beta-blocking effects, such as labetalol (Normodyne) or carvedilol (Coreg), carry a higher risk of producing orthostatic hypotension and therefore carry an increased risk of falls. Many of the side effects of beta blockers, including bradycardia, reduced exercise capacity, heart failure, hypotension, and blockage of atrioventricular (AV) nodal conduction, are related to their cardiac mechanisms. These side effects result from excessive blockage of normal sympathetic influences on the heart. Beta blockers should not be used in patients with sinus bradycardia and partial AV block. Table 19.4 summarizes the dosing, side effects, and drug interactions of beta blockers (Carter & Saseen, 2002; Ciccone, 2007; Colbert & Mason, 2002; Dobesch & Stacy, 2011; Michel & Hoffman, 2011).

Contraction of cardiac and smooth muscle cells requires increased levels of intracellular calcium, resulting in activation of myosin and contraction. Calcium channel blockers inhibit the influx of calcium into the cell and cause relaxation of cardiac muscle, resulting in decreased contractility, or relaxation of smooth muscle in the blood vessels, resulting in vasodilation. Both of these effects lower blood pressure. Two calcium channel blockers that relax heart muscle and slow AV nodal conduction, diltiazem and verapamil, can be used to treat cardiac arrhythmias (supraventricular tachycardia). These agents have negative inotropic and chronotropic effects on heart function. The dihydropyridine group of calcium channel blockers relaxes vascular smooth muscle, resulting in vasodilation, but does not affect heart conduction or heart rate. These agents can cause a compensatory increase in heart rate and can worsen angina by increasing cardiac output and oxygen demand in patients with angina or CHF (Dobesch & Stacy, 2011; Michel & Hoffman, 2011).

Angiotensin-converting enzyme (ACE) inhibitors reduce peripheral arterial resistance without influencing cardiac output and heart rate. ACE is found primarily in endothelial cells of the blood vessels. It converts angiotensin I to angiotensin II. Angiotensin II, a potent vasoconstrictor, stimulates aldosterone production and antidiuretic hormone. Aldosterone and antidiuretic hormone promote retention of sodium and water in the kidneys. The ACE inhibitors block the conversion of angiotensin I to angiotensin II, resulting in vasodilation, lowered blood pressure, and blocking of aldosterone, resulting in decreased fluid and sodium retention. The ACE inhibitors also block metabolism of bradykinin, a substance that lowers blood pressure. ACE inhibitors stimulate the synthesis of other vasodilating substances, including prostacyclin and prostaglandins. ACE inhibitors can prevent or reverse left ventricular hypertrophy, prevent proteinuria, and help preserve kidney function. These agents are preferred in patients with kidney disease, diabetics, and patients with CHF. ACE inhibitors can increase potassium retention, resulting in hyperkalemia (a higher-than-normal level of potassium), especially when concurrently used with potassium supplements or potassium-sparing diuretics. In addition, these agents can precipitate acute renal failure in patients with renal artery stenosis; they should be initiated cautiously in low doses in patients with renal insufficiency. Angioedema can also occur with the use of ACE inhibitors (Carter & Saseen, 2002; Dobesch & Stacy, 2011; Michel & Hoffman, 2011).

One side effect of ACE inhibitors is the "Captopril cough", which is attributed to elevated bradykinin levels. The cough occurs in approximately 30% of patients. Patients who have cough associated with ACE inhibitors are usually treated with an angiotensin II receptor blocker (ARB) and still receive many of the positive therapeutic effects of ACE inhibitors without the cough. These agents block angiotensin II at the receptor site and are not associated with elevated bradykinin levels. Although it causes cough in some patients, bradykinin also causes regression of myocyte hypertrophy and regression of fibrosis; these beneficial effects improve cardiac function in patients with heart failure. The ARBs block angiotensin II action at the angiotensin II receptor site; this blocks vasoconstriction, aldosterone release, sympathetic activation, antidiuretic hormone release, and constriction of the efferent arterioles of the **glomerulus**. The ARBs do not block angiotensin I, which allows the beneficial effects of angiotensin I (i.e., vasoconstriction, tissue repair, and inhibition of cell growth) on the angiotensin I receptor to continue. Side effects of the ARBs include hyperkalemia, renal insufficiency, and angioedema. Angioedema occurs less frequently with these agents than with ACE inhibitors, but patients with allergic reactions to ACE inhibitors may also have an allergic response to ARBs (Dobesch & Stacy, 2011; Michel & Hoffman, 2011).

Peripheral alpha-1 adrenergic receptor blockers block vasoconstriction in the blood vessels and reduce blood pressure by causing vasodilation. These medications can cross the blood–brain barrier and can cause **lassitude**, vivid dreams, and depression. Initial doses can cause acute dizziness, faintness, and syncope within the first 1 to 3 h of the dose, so the patient should take the initial dose at bedtime. Orthostasis can persist with chronic administration in some patients. The rehabilitation therapist should teach patients to change positions slowly to avoid falls (Colbert & Mason, 2002).

Central alpha-2 receptor agonists lower blood pressure by stimulating alpha-2 receptors in the brain, thus increasing vagal tone and reducing sympathetic tone at peripheral alpha sites. Resultant effects include reduced heart rate, reduced cardiac output, reduced peripheral resistance, reduced renin, and blunted baroreceptor response. Chronic use of these agents causes fluid retention and usually requires addition of a diuretic to the regimen. Side effects include dry mouth, sedation, orthostasis, and dizziness. These side effects can significantly affect a patient's participation in rehabilitative exercise, decrease cognition, and increase risk for falls. Because of these side effects, these agents are usually avoided in the elderly (Carter & Saseen, 2002; Ciccone, 2007; Dobesch & Stacy, 2011; Michel & Hoffman, 2011).

Direct vasodilators, including minoxidil (Loniten) and hydralazine (Apresoline), are typically not the first medications used in the treatment of hypertension. They are generally used as add-on therapy when other agents fail to control blood pressure. Because hirsutism is common with minoxidil, this agent is also used topically to treat baldness (Carter & Saseen, 2002; Ciccone, 2007; Dobesch & Stacy, 2011; Michel & Hoffman, 2011).

PATIENT CASE 1

S.D. is a 38-yr-old male college professor who has participated in a regular jogging program for the past 5 yr. He was recently diagnosed with hypertension and was put on beta blockers. This medication, which is the only medication he is taking, controls his hypertension well. S.D. uses a heart-rate monitor while jogging and is concerned that he is unable to elevate his exercising heart rate above 135 beats/min when jogging at the same pace and for the same distance as in the past. Despite not being able to reach his previous age-adjusted target heart rate, he feels like he is working as hard as he used to during his jogs.

Question

What can contribute to S.D.'s inability to meet his target heart rate?

Answer

S.D. is experiencing a lower exercising heart rate because beta blockers decrease heart rate and the contraction force of the heart. This decreases resting heart rate and maximum exercise capacity. Therefore, S.D.'s resting heart rate and exercising heart rate goals should be adjusted to compensate for the effects of the beta blocker. The rehabilitation therapist should counsel S.D. about the effects of beta blockers on resting and exercising heart rates and should encourage him to consult his physician to determine whether an exercise stress test is indicated. The exercise stress test allows the physician to check the blood flow through the heart while the patient is exercising and to measure how hard the heart pumps while the patient is on beta blockers. S.D.'s physician can use this information to adjust his target heart rate to an appropriate level. The rehabilitation therapist should also advise S.D. to use the Borg scale of perceived exertion during exercise. In the absence of a stress test, S.D. could try lowering his target heart rate by the amount that the beta blocker lowers his resting heart rate. For example, if his resting heart rate has decreased from 70 to 50, he could try working at a target heart rate 20 beats/min lower than that at which he used to train. (Note: This method of calculating adjusted target heart rate is not precise and sometimes the peak exercise heart rate is affected much more than is the resting heart rate. An exercise stress test is the best way to establish a new target heart rate on beta blockers.)

Congestive Heart Failure

The terms *heart failure* and *congestive heart failure* have been used interchangeably in the past. However, *heart failure* is now the preferred term because patients can have heart failure without having symptoms of congestion.

Incidence

Heart failure affects almost 6 million Americans. It is the leading cause of hospital admission in patients receiving Medicare benefits and incurs Medicare costs of $2.9 billion annually. More than 550,000 patients are newly diagnosed with heart failure each year, and heart failure is responsible for 15 million office visits and 16.5 million hospital days each year. Heart failure is most prevalent in the elderly. Approximately 1% of 50-yr-old individuals have CHF, whereas 5% of individuals over 75 yr of age have CHF. More men than women have CHF between 40 and 75 yr of age. After age 75 yr, however, little difference in incidence exists between the sexes. African Americans are twice as likely as Caucasians to experience CHF. Approximately 50% of patients diagnosed with CHF die within 5 yr of the diagnosis. The most common causes of heart failure are hypertension, coronary artery disease, and dilated cardiomyopathy (Ciccone, 2007; Quinn, 2006).

Etiology and Pathophysiology

Heart failure occurs when the contractility of the heart decreases or ventricular filling is restricted and the heart is no longer able to pump oxygenated blood to the tissues in adequate amounts. Decreased contractility is associated with a reduction in cardiac muscle mass due to ischemia or myocardial infarction, alcoholic or viral cardiomyopathy, ventricular hypertrophy due to pressure overload (systemic or pulmonary hypertension), or volume overload caused by cardiac valve dysfunction. Pressure or volume overload over a long period of time can cause ventricular hypertrophy, or enlargement of the heart muscle. This hypertrophy at first improves muscle function and cardiac output. However, over time, this hypertrophied muscle becomes fibrotic and contractility decreases. Ventricular hypertrophy increases ventricular stiffness and slows relaxation of the heart, resulting in impaired cardiac filling and decreased cardiac output. Restricted ventricular filling can result from increased ventricular stiffness due to hypertrophy, myocardial ischemia or infarction, valvular stenosis, or pericardial disease (Johnson et al., 2002; Maron & Rocco, 2011).

Heart failure occurs when the body's compensatory mechanisms for improving perfusion are no longer adequate and cardiac output and tissue oxygenation are subsequently reduced. Decreased tissue perfusion results in weakness and fatigue and triggers 1) activation of the neuroendocrine systems of the sympathetic nervous system in an attempt to increase myocardial contractility and venous return by vasoconstriction and 2) activation of the renin–angiotensin–aldosterone system in an attempt to increase blood volume and myocardial filling by retaining sodium and water. Increased venous pressure and volume result in symptoms of congestion, edema, dyspnea, and **orthopnea**. Vasodilators and diuretics are used to treat these symptoms. Beta blockers are used to reduce activation of the sympathetic system (i.e., increased heart rate and vasoconstriction), and ACE inhibitors are used to reverse vasoconstriction and retention of sodium and water. Beta blockers and ACE inhibitors also limit cardiac remodeling (fibrotic changes) and can reduce cardiac hypertrophy associated with the prolonged increase in cardiac work (Johnson et al., 2002; Maron & Rocco, 2011).

Symptoms of heart failure include **tachypnea**, fatigue, weakness, exercise intolerance, pallor, **cyanosis**, and **nocturia**. Right sided heart failure is associated with systemic venous congestion and occurs when the right ventricle cannot accept or eject blood presented to it. Such heart failure is associated with hepatic congestion, jugular venous distention, peripheral edema, abdominal pain, anorexia, and nausea. Left sided heart failure occurs when the left ventricle cannot accept or eject blood delivered to it. Such heart failure is associated with symptoms of respiratory congestion along with pulmonary edema, tachypnea, dyspnea on exertion, orthopnea, cough, and rales (crackling sounds on auscultation) (Colbert & Mason, 2002; Johnson et al., 2002; Maron & Rocco, 2011; Young & Mills, 2004).

The treatment of heart failure includes both nonpharmacologic and pharmacologic therapies. Which therapeutic interventions are employed depends on the symptoms and severity of the disease. Two major methods are used to classify heart failure. The New York Heart Association's functional classification system for heart failure, summarized in table 19.5, is widely used. The system divides heart failure into four classes based on the patient's ability to function. Class I is the mildest form of the disease and class IV is the most severe (Quinn, 2006; Young & Mills, 2004). The American College of Cardiology and American Heart Association heart failure staging tool, summarized in table 19.6, classifies disease into stages based on symptoms and recommends interventions for each stage of disease (American College of Cardiology & American Heart Association, 2005).

Rehabilitation Considerations

The rehabilitation therapist should be aware of the medications the patient is taking and the role these medications play in reducing symptoms of CHF. Symptoms of CHF include shortness of breath, frothy sputum, rales, and increased cough. The therapist should

Table 19.5   New York Heart Association Classification System for Heart Failure

Class	Symptoms	Therapy recommended
Class I	No symptoms and no limitation in ordinary physical activity (e.g., shortness of breath when walking or climbing stairs); ejection fraction <40%	Initiate ACE inhibitor and consider a beta blocker
Class II	Mild symptoms (e.g., mild shortness of breath or angina) and slight limitation during ordinary activity	Initiate a diuretic for volume overload or an ACE inhibitor and beta blocker if no volume overload
Class III	Marked limitation in activity due to symptoms, even during less-than-ordinary activity (e.g., walking short distances of 20-100 m); comfortable only at rest	Add digoxin and a diuretic
Class IV	Severe limitations and symptoms even while at rest; mostly bedbound	Add aldosterone antagonist, ARB, and intravenous inotrope
Classes I-IV	Fluid overload	Add diuretics; restrict sodium and fluid
	Persistent hypertension	Add ARB, calcium channel blockers (amlodipine or felodipine), or hydralazine
	Concomitant angina	Add nitrates or calcium channel blockers (amlodipine or felodipine)

ACE = angiotensin-converting enzyme; ARB = angiotensin receptor-blocking agent.

Table 19.6   American College of Cardiology and American Heart Association Stages of Heart Failure

	Stage A	Stage B	Stage C	Stage D
Description of heart failure	Patients at risk for heart failure without structural disease	Structural heart disease without heart failure symptoms	Structural heart disease with previous or current heart failure symptoms	Refractory heart failure
Examples of disease states and symptoms	Hypertension, atherosclerosis, diabetes, obesity, metabolic syndrome	Previous myocardial infarction, asymptomatic valvular heart disease, LV remodeling (LV hypertrophy or low ejection fraction)	Symptoms: Shortness of breath, fatigue, exercise intolerance	Marked symptoms despite medication therapy
Treatment goals and nonpharmacologic treatments	Goals: Treat hypertension, lipid disorders, and metabolic syndrome; encourage exercise, healthy diet, and smoking cessation; discourage use of alcohol or illicit drugs	Goals outlined in stage A	Goals outlined in stage A plus dietary salt restriction	Goals outlines in stages A, B, and C; decisions regarding level of care
Medication treatments	Medications: ACE inhibitor or ARB in diabetics or patients with valvular heart disease	Medications: ACE inhibitors or ARB, beta blockers	Medications: Diuretics, ACE inhibitors or ARB, beta blockers. For advanced symptoms: Aldosterone antagonists, digitalis, hydralazine with nitrates.	Compassionate end-of-life care or hospice, chronic inotropes
Surgical therapies	N/A	N/A	Devices: Pacemakers or implanted defibrillators	Cardiac transplant

ACE = angiotensin-converting enzyme; ARB = angiotensin II receptor-blocking agent; N/A = not applicable; LV= left ventricular.

also be aware of side effects and toxicity of medications used to treat cardiac disease. For example, symptoms of digitalis toxicity include confusion, nausea, and dizziness. Symptoms of excessive weakness, hypotension, and fatigue in patients taking diuretics may indicate depletion of fluid and electrolytes. Patients on vasodilators may have symptoms of hypotension and postural hypotension; the rehabilitation therapist should be cautious when asking these patients to stand up quickly. In addition, certain exercises and whirlpools that create systemic vasodilation may cause hypotension in patients using vasodilators. The rehabilitation therapist should contact the physician upon identifying side effects associated with medications (Ciccone, 2007).

Medication Therapy

Table 19.4 summarizes the medications used to treat CHF and provides information on side effects that can affect the patient's ability to participate in rehabilitation. The text that follows includes additional information on these therapies.

ACE Inhibitors

ACE inhibitors are the cornerstone of medication therapy for patients with heart failure. These agents cause arterial and venous vasodilatation and reduce both preload and afterload by reducing formation of angiotensin II and reducing breakdown of bradykinin. ACE inhibitors significantly increase cardiac index and stroke work index and reduce left ventricular filling pressure, systemic vascular resistance, mean arterial pressure, and heart rate. The use of these agents significantly improves clinical status, functional class, exercise tolerance, and left ventricular size and reduces mortality by 20% to 30%. These agents also help prevent heart failure in patients who have had a myocardial infarction, especially those with a reduced ejection fraction. Any patient with left ventricular dysfunction should receive an ACE inhibitor unless contraindicated (Johnson et al., 2002; Maron & Rocco, 2011).

Typical side effects of ACE inhibitors include angioedema (swelling of the lips, tongue, or throat), cough, loss of taste or metallic taste, loss of appetite, dizziness, fainting, and fatigue (Quinn, 2006). A number of these side effects can affect the patient's ability to eat or swallow. ARBs function like ACE inhibitors and result in vasodilation and elimination of salt and water. Use of an ARB is considered for patients who have cough associated with use of ACE inhibitors. ARBs are generally well tolerated and have few side effects. More information on ACE inhibitors and ARBs can be found in table 19.4 and in the "Hypertension" section found earlier in this chapter (Quinn, 2006; Young & Mills, 2004).

Beta Blockers

Beta blockers reduce compensatory sympathetic activation, thus reducing cardiac rate and the vasoconstriction that is responsible for cardiac remodeling and the progression of heart failure. The two beta blockers documented to improve outcomes are metoprolol and carvedilol; these are the agents of choice in patients with heart failure. These agents increase ejection fraction, decrease ventricular mass, improve the shape and function of the ventricle, and reduce left ventricular end systolic and diastolic volumes. These changes improve quality of life in many patients. Despite the negative inotropic effects of beta blockers, they can reduce the number of hospi-

talizations and mortality in patients with heart failure if they are initiated at low doses and slowly titrated up. They may not be tolerated in stage 4 heart failure. Additional information on beta blockers can be found in table 19.3 and earlier in this chapter (Ciccone, 2007; Colbert & Mason, 2002; Quinn, 2006).

Diuretics

Diuretics counteract the compensatory retention of fluid and sodium mediated by the angiotensin–renin–aldosterone system and antidiuretic hormone in patients with heart failure. Additional detail on diuretics can be found in table 19.3 and in the "Hypertension" section found earlier in this chapter (Carter & Saseen, 2002; Quinn, 2006; Young & Mills, 2004).

Diuretics carry numerous side effects because they affect the balance of fluid and electrolytes. Excessive use of diuretics may result in dehydration, weakness, and cardiac arrhythmias. Excessive diuresis can result in fatigue, postural hypotension, and an increase in the patient's blood urea nitrogen. Excessive dehydration induced by the use of diuretics can result in decreased perfusion of the kidneys and can cause acute renal failure. The rehabilitation therapist should teach the patient signs and symptoms associated with dehydration and depletion of electrolytes such as potassium, magnesium, and calcium and should monitor for these symptoms during rehabilitation sessions. If such symptoms are noted, the prescriber should be notified to check the patient's blood work in order to detect electrolyte depletion and replenish electrolytes when necessary. Patients taking diuretics should be taught to weigh themselves daily in order to detect fluid accumulation or excessive losses of fluid. A loss of more than 2 lb (0.9 kg) may indicate excessive loss of fluids and risk of dehydration with accompanying electrolyte depletion. Patients who are using diuretics and exercising should ensure adequate hydration but avoid electrolyte drinks (e.g., Gatorade) that contain high amounts of sugar and sodium. Diuretic-associated dehydration can increase the risk of orthostatic hypotension and thereby increase the risk of falls.

In contrast, an increase of more than 2 lb (0.9 kg) over a few days indicates excessive intake of sodium or water in the diet or the need to increase the diuretic dose. Patients should be taught to monitor for fluid accumulation in their extremities (peripheral edema) as signs that they are accumulating fluid. Most of the time, this edema is due to dietary intake of a high sodium food or from exceeding prescribed fluid intake. In many instances, it is the result of over-the-counter medication intake, such as a NSAID (e.g. ibuprofen). Some patients demonstrate resistance to diuretics, and review of the patient's medications by the pharmacist may help identify a medication cause of the resistance. Altering the dose, changing the type of diuretic, or adding a second diuretic may help prevent or correct diuretic resistance. The rehabilitation therapist should keep these cautions in mind when developing a patient-specific program (Ciccone, 2007; Quinn, 2006).

Vasodilator Therapies

Nitrates and hydralazine were frequently used as vasodilatory therapy in patients with heart failure before ACE inhibitors were available; they are still used in patients with heart failure and symptoms of angina. For patients who cannot tolerate ACE inhibitors or ARB, the combination of nitrates and hydralazine is still recommended (Johnson et al., 2002; Maron & Rocco, 2011).

Nitrates such as nitroglycerin increase cyclic GMP in vascular smooth muscle and cause vasodilation of the venous system, thus reducing preload. Hydralazine, on the other hand, is a direct vasodilator that causes vasodilation of arterial smooth muscle, thus decreasing systemic vascular resistance and increasing stroke volume and cardiac output. When used together, nitrates inhibit ventricular remodeling and hydralazine prevents nitrate tolerance. Nitrates can be administered in a number of forms, including oral, topical, intravenous, and sublingual. Nitrate therapy can improve the patient's exercise tolerance. Use of nitrate–hydralazine therapy has been associated with reduced mortality but not to the extent that use of ACE inhibitors has been associated with reduced mortality (Quinn, 2006). Sublingual

nitroglycerin is frequently used to treat acute chest pain associated with angina, whereas intravenous nitroglycerin is used to manage acute decompensated CHF associated with CHF exacerbations that require hospitalization. Continuous administration of nitrates can result in patient tolerance and, subsequently, reduced drug effectiveness. A daily drug-free interval may be prescribed in order to maintain medication effectiveness. Typical nitrates are nitroglycerin (Nitro-Dur, Nitrostat) and isosorbide dinitrate (Imdur, Isordil). Nitrates have few side effects regardless of the administration route. Typical side effects include headache, bradycardia (low heartbeat), hypotension, skin reactions, and nausea. Headache is associated with vasodilation of blood vessels in the head (Johnson et al., 2002; Maron & Rocco, 2011; Quinn, 2006).

Hydralazine has been used as an antihypertensive medication for more than 40 yr. Hydralazine has been shown to increase resting cardiac performance and increase the patient's exercise ability. Patients with severe chronic CHF and African American patients can achieve improved control of their hypertension with the addition of hydralazine to their antihypertensive regimen. The side effects of hydralazine (Apresoline) include joint pain, rapid heartbeat, and headache (Elkayam et al., 2007; Quinn, 2006).

Brain natriuretic peptide (BNP) is released when the left ventricle experiences an increase in pressure, usually as a result of cardiomyopathy associated with long standing heart failure. This BNP causes a compensatory vasodilation as the body attempts to reduce the increased pressure. Emergency room physicians often use the measurement of BNP in the blood to quantify the degree of decompensation associated with an acute exacerbation of CHF. Nesiritide (Natrecor) is a recombinant form of B-type natriuretic peptide that counteracts the angiotensin–renin–aldosterone system and causes vasodilation and excretion of sodium and water by the kidney. It is used in patients who are admitted to the hospital with acute decompensated heart failure that does not respond to first-line vasodilator therapies such as intravenous nitroglycerin. Its use has declined with evidence in the literature that it may be associated with a decline in renal function. Side effects of Nesiritide (Natrecor) include lightheadedness, low blood pressure, and dizziness (Johnson et al., 2002; Maron & Rocco, 2011; Quinn, 2006).

Digitalis

Digitalis has been used to treat cardiac patients for more than 200 yr. Digitalis is primarily used to treat arrhythmias and CHF. This medication increases the force of the heart's contractions, thus allowing the heart to beat more efficiently and less frequently. CHF symptoms and cardiac output during rest and exercise improve when the ability of the heart to pump efficiently improves. Little evidence shows that digitalis decreases patient mortality, but it can decrease hospitalizations and morbidity. Digitalis is usually introduced if additional symptomatic improvement is needed with the use of standard therapy (e.g., ACE inhibitors and diuretics). Patients with severe left ventricular dysfunction appear to benefit the most from digitalis. Digitalis should not be discontinued abruptly. This medication is dosed to therapeutic digoxin levels of 0.5 to 1.0 ng/ml. It is eliminated renally; therefore, dose should be adjusted down in patients with renal insufficiency and in older patients (Carter & Saseen, 2002; Ciccone, 2007; Quinn, 2006).

Aldosterone Antagonists

Aldosterone is a neurohormone that increases collagen deposition of the cardiac cell matrix, thus promoting fibrotic changes in the heart. Spironolactone is an aldosterone antagonist that produces a weak potassium-sparing diuretic effect. A new agent that also antagonizes aldosterone is eplerenone. In the Randomized Aldactone Evaluation Study involving 1,600 patients with class III and IV heart failure, the use of spironolactone was associated with a 30% reduction in total mortality, a 36% reduction in death due to progressive heart failure, and a 29% reduction in sudden death in patients with heart failure. Symptoms in patients receiving spironolactone also improved (Marcy & Ripley, 2006).

Spironolactone is a nonselective aldosterone antagonist, and eplerenone is selective to the aldosterone receptor. Both agents have been shown to improve morbidity and mortality in patients with advanced heart failure. A side effect of both spironolactone and eplerenone is potentially life-threatening hyperkalemia, which can be caused by acute renal insufficiency or concurrent drug therapy. Patients at risk for acute renal insufficiency with resultant hyperkalemia include those with diabetes mellitus, advanced heart failure, and those of advanced age. The Randomized Aldactone Evaluation Study and the Eplerenone Post-Acute Myocardial Infarction Heart Failure Efficacy and Survival Study have established aldosterone antagonists as life-saving additions in the treatment of heart failure. Prescribers should consider use of these agents in patients with class III or IV heart failure (Marcy & Ripley, 2006).

Surgical Interventions

Patients with heart failure may experience arrhythmias that do not respond to medication alone and may require surgical placement of pacemakers or implanted cardioversion defibrillators. Pacemakers can control the beating rhythm of each chamber or can shock the heart to normal rhythm during a dangerous arrhythmia. Another frequent intervention is surgical ablation of an area of the heart precipitating a recurrent arrhythmia (Quinn, 2006). Cardiac transplant is considered in stage 4 heart failure.

PATIENT CASE 2

K.B. is a 65-yr-old female with a history of congestive heart failure. She is being seen in home care 1 wk after a recent right total knee replacement. During the physical therapy evaluation K.B.'s chief complaint is right knee pain and decreased mobility. She also reports that she has been experiencing significantly more bilateral ankle edema than usual and slightly more shortness of breath than usual. Prior to being discharged from the hospital her cardiologist examined her and performed additional testing to rule out other cardiac and respiratory conditions. Because of her increased symptoms of heart failure, the cardiologist increased her digitalis from 0.125 mg/d to 0.25 mg/d.

Question

Heart failure of which side of the heart is most typically involved when ankle edema is a prevailing feature?

Answer

Right sided heart failure results in peripheral edema including swollen ankles and enlarged organs. Left sided heart failure results mainly in pulmonary edema.

Question

During the next physical therapy session K.B. demonstrates increased lethargy and apathy toward her therapy program. She is also confused and states that she thinks she has a stomach bug because she is experiencing nausea. What is the likely cause of K.B.'s new symptoms?

Answer

It is likely that K.B. is exhibiting symptoms of digitalis toxicity, as her current digoxin dose is higher than most elderly patients can tolerate. Symptoms of digitalis toxicity include lethargy, confusion, nausea, dizziness, fatigue, and arrhythmias. These side effects can result after a recent increase in the dosage of digitalis or if the patient has a sudden decline in kidney function, resulting in less efficient elimination of the medication. A sudden decline in kidney function can result from dehydration or the addition of a medication such as a diuretic or an over-the-counter NSAID (e.g. ibuprofen) in an older patient.

Question

If the physical therapist suspects digitalis toxicity, what is the next immediate action?

Answer

The physical therapist should immediately contact K.B.'s cardiologist to communicate this change in K.B.'s status. Blood tests are used to confirm the diagnosis of digitalis toxicity.

Question

Blood tests confirmed that K.B. was indeed experiencing digitalis toxicity. K.B.'s cardiologist decreased her dose of digitalis. What other category of medication may K.B.'s cardiologist consider to reduce K.B.'s fluid retention?

Answer

K.B.'s cardiologist may give strong consideration to adding a low dose diuretic to gradually reduce fluid retention and avoid acute dehydration. The therapist educates K.B. on the importance of following her physician's restrictions of sodium, fluid intake, and monitoring her weight on a daily basis to detect rapid changes in fluid status. Any changes of greater than 2 lbs (0.9 kg) over a few days should be reported to her physician.

Cardiac Arrhythmias

In clinical practice, the rehabilitation therapist will care for patients with cardiac arrhythmias. An **arrhythmia** occurs when the heart contracts as a response to electrical impulses caused by any portion of the heart other than the normal pacemaker of the heart, the sinoatrial (SA) node resulting in an abnormal heart rate or rhythm. The abnormal heart rate or rhythm may lead to incomplete or inefficient cardiac contraction, inefficient movement of blood through the heart, and inefficient delivery of oxygenated blood to the body's tissues. Cardiac arrhythmias can result from damage to the heart that interferes with the normal circuitry of the heart, from electrolyte imbalances that result in impaired nerve transmission to the muscle, or from medication use. Signs and symptoms associated with cardiac arrhythmia include palpitations, chest pain, lightheadedness, weakness, fatigue, dizziness, and syncope. The electrocardiogram measures the electrical activity of the heart throughout the cardiac contraction cycle. Some arrhythmias are asymptomatic and are diagnosed only after diagnostic use of the electrocardiogram or other radiologic studies (Berrios-Colon & Cha, 2010).

Arrhythmias are classified by where in the heart they originate and the resultant heart rate and rhythm shown on the electrocardiogram. Supraventricular arrhythmias originate above the ventricle in the atria, and ventricular arrhythmias originate in the lower chambers of the heart, or ventricles. Tachycardia is defined as a heart rate that is faster than normal, and bradycardia is a heart rate that is slower than normal. Fibrillation is a rapid partial contraction of the heart that occurs so quickly that all chambers do not contract and pump efficiently. Arrhythmias may vary in severity, and the outcome can range from mild irritation to death (Berrios-Colon & Cha, 2010).

Supraventricular arrhythmias include **atrial fibrillation**, autonomic atrial tachycardia, and paroxysmal supraventricular tachycardia. Patients with atrial fibrillation are at risk for inefficient pumping of blood from the atria to the ventricles, which can result in pooling of the blood in the atria and the formation of clots in the atria; these clots can travel to the brain and cause a stroke. Because of this, patients with atrial fibrillation are frequently placed on anticoagulants such as warfarin (Coumadin) to help prevent the formation of these clots. Atrial fibrillation doubles the risk of mortality and causes one out of every six strokes. Causes of atrial fibrillation include hypertension, heart failure, valvular heart disease, and ischemic heart disease. Treatment includes converting the patient's heart rhythm to normal sinus rhythm and maintaining the patient's sinus rhythm by reducing AV node conduction with medications such as amiodarone, dofetilide, flecainide, propafenone, sotalol, or dronedarone. Nonpharmacologic interventions that are frequently used to convert the patient to sinus rhythm include radiofrequency **ablation** and pacemaker insertion (Berrios-Colon & Cha, 2010; Draskovich & O'Dell, 2010). Common ventricular arrhythmias include premature ventricular contractions, ventricular tachycardia, ventricular fibrillation, and torsades de pointes. Uncontrolled ventricular arrhythmias commonly lead to cardiac arrest and sudden cardiac death (Bauman & Scoen, 2002; Berrios-Colon & Cha, 2010; Colbert & Mason, 2002; Sampson & Kass, 2011; Sanoski, 2011).

Incidence

Cardiac arrhythmias are common. Atrial fibrillation is the most common form of arrhythmia. It accounts for one third of the cardiac arrhythmias diagnosed in the United States and affects 2.2 million Americans. It is a common cause of stroke (Draskovich & O'Dell, 2010). The Centers for Disease Control and Prevention estimates that more than 600,000 sudden cardiac deaths occur each year. Sudden death is the first manifestation of cardiac disease in up to 50% of patients with arrhythmia (Zheng et al., 2002; Bauman & Scoen, 2002; Berrios-Colon & Cha, 2010; Colbert & Mason, 2002; Sampson & Kass, 2011; Sanoski, 2011).

Etiology and Pathophysiology

The heart comprises four chambers. The upper chambers include the right and left atria, and the lower chambers include the right and left ventricles. These chambers contract in response to electrical signals that originate in specialized cardiac cells in the heart, called pacemakers. The pacemakers include the SA node in the upper atrial chamber, the AV node located between the atria and the ventricles, and the Purkinje fibers that run down the center and to the outer edges of the ventricles. The heart's natural pacemaker is the SA node; it spreads electrical activity across the right and left atria, the top chambers of the heart. The electrical signal is slightly delayed by the AV node and then travels down the center of the ventricles along the electrical pathway called the bundle of His and on to the Purkinje fibers, resulting in contraction of the ventricles. If the SA node stops firing, the AV node takes over the pacemaker function; if the AV node fails, the Purkinje fibers pick up the pacemaker function. Heart rate is set by the frequency of the heart's contractions, which are usually set by the heart's normal pacemaker, the SA, which provides sinus rhythm (usually 60-80 beats/min).

Rehabilitation Considerations

The rehabilitation therapist should be aware of medications the patient is taking and the role these medications play in reducing symptoms of arrhythmia. Symptoms of arrhythmia, which include heart palpitations, dizziness, fatigue, and shortness of breath, can lead to increased risk of falls in rehabilitation sessions, particularly sessions that include exercise. The therapist should also be aware of the side effects of medications used to treat arrhythmia. For example, symptoms of digitalis toxicity include confusion, nausea, dizziness, fatigue, and arrhythmias. Many antiarrhythmic therapies can affect heart rate achievable during exercise. The rehabilitation therapist must consider the effects of these therapies when designing a patient-specific rehabilitation plan and should contact the physician upon identifying side effects associated with medications. Table 19.1 summarizes symptoms that warrant the discontinuation of exercise (Ciccone, 2007).

Medication Therapy

The decision to treat arrhythmias with pharmacology is usually based on a number of variables such as the patient's heart rate and blood pressure, medication side effects, and quality-of-life issues. Because antiarrhyth-

mic medications frequently have serious side effects, nonpharmacologic antiarrhythmic interventions are also used. Implantable devices such as defibrillators and procedures such as electrode catheter ablation have also been used to control arrhythmias.

Antiarrhythmic medications establish and maintain normal sinus rhythm, suppress excitable cardiac activity (**ectopic foci**), and control ventricular rate (Colbert & Mason, 2002). Chronotropic medications influence the rate of the heart, inotropic medications influence the force of the contraction, and dromotropic medications influence the electrical conduction of the heart. Antiarrhythmic medications fall into four categories; the first class is subdivided into three sections. The different drug classes affect different phases of the action potential or ionic channels and affect calcium and sodium channels, prolong the repolarization phase of the cardiac contraction, or block beta-adrenergic activity. The properties of some medications fall into more than one class. Table 19.7 summarizes

 See table 19.7 in the web resource for a full list of medication-specific indications, dosing recommendations, and side effects.

Table 19.7   Classes of Antiarrhythmic Medications

Medication	Side effects affecting rehab	Other side effects or considerations
Type 1a: Sodium channel blockers. Used to maintain sinus rhythm in patients with supraventricular tachycardia and prevent recurrence of ventricular arrhythmia.		
Quinidine (Quinaglute)	Cog S A Motor D Com F ++ 0 ++ + ++ ++ ++	Side effects: Diarrhea in up to 50%, cinchonism (headache and tinnitus seen with elevated levels), confusion, blurred vision. Drug interactions: Quinidine is a CYP2D6 inhibitor; it reduces clearance of digoxin and propafenone and decreases metabolism and therapeutic levels and effects of codeine. Phenytoin, rifampin, and phenobarbital may decrease quinidine levels and effects. Quinidine toxicity is increased when taken with ritonavir, beta blockers, amiodarone, verapamil, cimetidine, alkalinizing agents, or nondepolarizing or depolarizing muscle relaxants. Quindine may enhance effect of warfarin (Coumadin).

› *continued*

Table 19.7 › *continued*

Medication	Side effects affecting rehab							Other side effects or considerations
Procainamide (Pronestyl— long acting)	Cog ++	S 0	A ++	Motor ++	D ++	Com ++	F ++	Side effects: Lupus-like syndrome, anemia, neutropenia, agranulocytosis, allergy, rash, nausea, vomiting, diarrhea, taste changes, elevated liver enzyme, hepatomegaly (rare), dizziness, giddiness, mental depression, psychosis (rare), hypotension, cardiac arrhythmia, and heart block after IV administration. Drug interactions: Increased levels of the active metabolite NAPA in patients taking cimetidine, ranitidine, beta blockers, amiodarone, trimethoprim, or quinidine. May increase effect of skeletal muscle relaxants (e.g., quinidine, lidocaine) and neuromuscular blockers. Ofloxacin inhibits tubular secretion and may increase levels and effects of procainamide.
Disopyramide (Norpace)	Cog ++	S ++	A 0	Motor +++	D ++	Com ++	F +++	Side effects: Dry mouth, urinary hesitancy, constipation, blurred vision, urinary retention, nausea, bloating, flatulence, dizziness, fatigue, muscle weakness, headache, malaise, muscle pain. Drug interactions: Do not administer within 48 h before or 24 h after verapamil. Cases of life-threatening interactions have been reported when given with clarithromycin and erythromycin; administering disopyramide with cytochrome 3A4 inhibitors could result in a potentially fatal interaction.

Type 1b: Sodium channel blockers. Used to treat ventricular arrhythmias (premature ventricular contractions, ventricular tachycardia).

Medication	Side effects affecting rehab							Other side effects or considerations
Lidocaine (Xylocaine)	Cog ++	S ++	A 0	Motor ++	D +	Com ++	F ++	Side effects: Disorientation, confusion, dizziness, respiratory depression. Drug interactions: Coadministration with cimetidine or beta blockers increases toxicity. Coadministration with procainamide and tocainide may result in additive cardiodepressant action. May increase effects of succinylcholine.
	Not used in rehab.							
Mexiletine (Mexitil)	Cog ++	S +	A +	Motor +++	D ++	Com +	F ++	Side effects: Blurred vision, clumsiness, constipation, diarrhea, dizziness or lightheadedness, headache, heartburn, incoordination, nausea, nervousness, tremor, vomiting. Drug interactions: Decreased levels when used with aluminum–magnesium hydroxide compounds, atropine, narcotics, hydantoins, rifampin, or urinary acidifiers. Metoclopramide and urinary alkalinizers increase levels. Cimetidine can either increase or decrease levels. Increases levels of caffeine and theophylline.

Medication	Side effects affecting rehab							Other side effects or considerations
Tocainide (Tonocard)	Cog	S	A	Motor	D	Com	F	Side effects: Nausea, vomiting, dizziness, vertigo, paresthesias, tremor, confusion, arrhythmia, agranulocytosis (rare), pulmonary fibrosis, respiratory arrest, skin rash. No drug interactions identified.
	++	+	+	+++	++	+	++	

Type 1c: Sodium channel blockers. Used to maintain sinus rhythm in patients with supraventricular tachycardia.

Medication	Side effects affecting rehab							Other side effects or considerations
Flecainide (Tambocor)	Cog	S	A	Motor	D	Com	F	Side effects: Dizziness, visual disturbances, dyspnea, headache, nausea, fatigue, palpitations, chest pain, asthenia, tremor, constipation, edema, abdominal pain. Drug interactions: May increase toxicity of digoxin. Beta-adrenergic blockers, verapamil, and disopyramide may have additive inotropic effects when administered with flecainide. CYP4502D6 inhibitors (e.g., ritonavir, cimetidine, amiodarone) may increase flecainide levels and cardiotoxicity.
	++	+	+	+++	++	+	++	
Propafenone (Rythmol)	Cog	S	A	Motor	D	Com	F	Side effects: Hypotension, bradycardia, torsades de pointes. Drug interactions: Rifampin may decrease plasma levels. Quinidine may increase Rythmol's effects. May increase levels of beta blockers, cyclosporine, warfarin, and digoxin. CYP2D6 inhibitors (e.g., ritonavir, cimetidine, amiodarone) may increase Rythmol's levels and toxicity.
	+	0	0	++	0	0	++	

Type II: Beta blockers. Reduce sympathetic tone, myocardial oxygen demand, ischemia, heart rate, and blood pressure. See table 19.2.

Type III: Potassium channel blockers. Used to treat ventricular arrhythmia. Maintains sinus rhythm in patients with atrial fibrillation.

Medication	Side effects affecting rehab							Other side effects or considerations
Amiodarone (Cordarone, Pacerone)	Cog	S	A	Motor	D	Com	F	Side effects: Pulmonary fibrosis, hypothyroidism, corneal microdeposits, elevated liver enzymes, hepatitis (rare), jaundice, blue–gray discoloration of skin. Increases effect and blood levels of theophylline, quinidine, procainamide, phenytoin, methotrexate, flecainide, digoxin, cyclosporine, beta blockers, and anticoagulants. Ritonavir and disopyramide increase cardiotoxicity. Coadministration with calcium channel blockers may cause an additive effect and further decrease myocardial contractility. Cimetidine may increase levels. Protease inhibitors (e.g., indinavir, ritonavir, amprenavir, nelfinavir) inhibit metabolism, resulting in increased serum levels and possible prolongation of QT interval.
	+	0	0	+	0	0	+	

› continued

Table 19.7 › *continued*

Medication	Side effects affecting rehab							Other side effects or considerations
Bretylium (Bretylol)	Cog	S	A	Motor	D	Com	F	Side effects: Hypertension followed by hypotension, ventricular ectopy.
	+	0	0	++	0	0	++	Drug interactions: Digitalis toxicity may be aggravated by the initial release of norepinephrine caused by bretylium.
								Enhances the pressor effects of catecholamines (e.g., dopamine, norepinephrine).
Dofetilide (Tikosyn)	Cog	S	A	Motor	D	Com	F	Side effects: Bradycardia, headache, chest pain, dizziness, torsades de pointes.
	0	0	0	++	0	0	++	Drug interactions: Avoid concurrent use of thiazide diuretics verapamil, cimetidine, trimethoprim (alone or in combination with sulfamethoxazole), or ketoconazole; each of these drugs causes a substantial increase in Tikosyn levels.
								Do not use with other known inhibitors of renal cation transport (e.g., prochlorperazine, megestrol).
Dronedarone (Multaq)	Cog	S	A	Motor	D	Com	F	Side effects: Diarrhea, nausea, bradycardia, torsades de pointes.
	+	0	0	++	+	0	++	Drug interactions: Increased risk of torsades de pointes when used with drugs that prolong QT interval (e.g., certain phenothiazines, tricyclic antidepressants, macrolide antibiotics, class I and III antiarrhythmics).
								Concurrent use of digoxin, verapamil, diltiazem, or beta blockers potentiates Multaq's effects.
								Avoid concurrent use of ketoconazole as well as other potent CYP3A inhibitors (e.g., itraconazole, voriconazole, ritonavir, clarithromycin, and nefazodone).
								Grapefruit juice is contraindicated.
								Rifampin or other CYP3A inducers (e.g., phenobarbital, carbamazepine, phenytoin, St. John's wort) decrease levels and effects of Multaq.
								Verapamil and diltiazem are moderate CYP3A inhibitors and increase Multaq levels 1.4- to 1.7-fold.
								Multaq increases simvastatin levels 2- to 3-fold; increases verapamil, diltiazem, or nifedipine levels by 50%; and increases digoxin levels 2.5-fold.
								Can increase plasma concentrations of tacrolimus, sirolimus, beta blockers, tricyclic antidepressants, and selective serotonin reuptake inhibitors.

Medication	Side effects affecting rehab							Other side effects or considerations
Sotalol (Betapace)	Cog	S	A	Motor	D	Com	F	Side effects: Fatigue, dizziness, bradycardia, asthenia.
	++	++	0	++	+	++	++	Drug interactions: Aluminum salts, barbiturates, nonsteroidal anti-inflammatory drugs, penicillins, calcium salts, cholestyramine, and rifampin may decrease bioavailability and plasma levels, possibly resulting in decreased pharmacologic effect.
								May increase cardiotoxicity when used with calcium channel blockers, quinidine, flecainide, or contraceptives.
								Increased toxicity when used with digoxin, flecainide, acetaminophen, clonidine, epinephrine, nifedipine, prazosin, haloperidol, phenothiazines, or catecholamine-depleting agents.
Ibutilide (Corvert)	Cog	S	A	Motor	D	Com	F	Side effects: Arrhythmia, nausea.
	+	0	0	+	+	0	+	Drug interactions: No drug interactions identified.

Type IV: Calcium channel blockers

Medication	Side effects affecting rehab							Other side effects or considerations
Verapamil (Calan, Calan SR, Isoptin, Isoptin SR, Covera-HS)	Cog	S	A	Motor	D	Com	F	Side effects: Bradycardia, nausea, peripheral edema, hypotension. Increased risk of falls from orthostasis. Verapamil is associated with severe constipation; use laxative with this medication.
	+	0	0	++	+	0	++	
Diltiazem (Cardizem, Cardizem CD, Dilator SR)	Cog	S	A	Motor	D	Com	F	Food interactions: Grapefruit juice (>200 ml) can increase levels of these medications and should not be consumed within 2 hrs before or 4 hrs after administration.
	+	0	0	++	+	0	++	Drug interactions: Decreases liver metabolism of carbamazepine (Tegretol), digoxin, and cyclosporine levels. May decrease metabolism and increase levels of simvastatin (Zocor), atorvastatin, (Lipitor), and lovastatin (Mevacor) that can result in rhabdomyolysis or liver toxicity.
								Coadministration with amiodarone can cause bradycardia and decrease cardiac output.
								May increase cardiac depression when used with beta blockers.
								Cimetidine may increase levels.
								May increase theophylline levels.

Cog = cognition; S = sedation; A = agitation or mania; Motor = discoordination; D = dysphagia; Com = communication; F = falls; IV = intravenously; NAPA = N-acetylprocainamide.

The likelihood rating scale for encountering the side effects is as follows: 0 = Almost no probability of encountering side effects. + = Little likelihood of encountering side effects. +/++ = Low probability of encountering side effects; however, probability increases with increased dosage. ++ = Medium likelihood of encountering side effects. +++ = High likelihood of encountering side effects, particularly with high doses. ++++ = Highest likelihood of encountering side effects; best to avoid in at-risk patients.

the medications used to treat cardiac arrhythmias and lists dosing, side effects, and precautions the rehabilitation therapist should keep in mind when caring for patients taking these medications (Bauman & Scoen, 2002; Colbert & Mason, 2002; Sampson & Kass, 2011; Sanoski, 2011).

Class I antiarrhythmic medications are used to treat ventricular tachycardia and supraventricular arrhythmias (atrial fibrillation and paroxysmal atrial tachycardia). They block the cardiac sodium channel in the muscle cell, thus preventing depolarization. Class IA medications, such as quinidine (Quinaglute) and procainamide (Pronestyl), are used to treat arrhythmias that originate in the atria or ventricles. Class IB arrhythmic medications, such as lidocaine (Xylocaine), are used to treat ventricular arrhythmias (premature ventricular contractions and ventricular tachycardia). Class IC antiarrhythmic medications are usually used to treat ventricular arrhythmias (ventricular tachycardia and premature ventricular contractions) (Bauman & Scoen, 2002; Ciccone, 2007; Colbert & Mason, 2002; Sampson & Kass, 2011; Sanoski, 2011).

Class II antiarrhythmic medications are beta blockers that slow heart rate. Beta blockers decrease the probability of sudden death secondary to arrhythmias after a myocardial infarction (MI). Class II antiarrhythmics should be used with caution in patients with chronic obstructive pulmonary disease or asthma. Class III antiarrhythmics are potassium channel blockers. These medications, which prolong repolarization of the heart, are used to treat ventricular arrhythmias (ventricular tachycardia and ventricular fibrillation) (Ciccone, 2007; Colbert & Mason, 2002).

Class IV antiarrhythmic medications are calcium channel blockers. These medications, which reduce heart rate, are used to treat supraventricular tachycardia as well as hypertension and angina (Bauman & Scoen, 2002; Ciccone, 2007; Colbert & Mason, 2002; Sampson & Kass, 2011; Sanoski, 2011). The main calcium channel blockers used to treat arrhythmia are verapamil (Calan) and diltiazem (Cardizem).

Summary

This chapter reviews the pathophysiology of hypertension, cardiac arrhythmia, and CHF and provides an overview of medication therapy. It also discusses considerations for adjusting rehabilitation and monitoring cardiac patients and introduces cardiac rehabilitation.

Medications Used to Treat Peripheral Artery Disease, Stroke, and Coronary Heart Disease

20

The rehabilitation specialist commonly treats patients with **coronary heart disease**, **peripheral artery disease**, and **stroke**. This chapter describes these conditions, the relevant medications used to treat and prevent these conditions, and rehabilitation considerations in developing rehabilitation treatment plans for these patients. Coronary heart disease, peripheral artery disease, and stroke are all associated with atherosclerosis and are highly associated with **hyperlipidemia**, obesity, and weight gain. Diabetes is considered to be a risk factor for coronary heart disease and stroke and is highly associated with hyperlipidemia and coronary heart disease (American Heart Association, 2012a).

Atherosclerosis

New (primary) and recurrent (secondary) strokes occur approximately 800,000 times/yr in the United States. Of these strokes, more than 600,000 are primary strokes. Someone in the United States has a stroke approximately every 40 s. Most are ischemic stroke associated with atherosclerosis (American Heart Association, 2012b).

Atherosclerosis is the thickening and hardening of arteries due to the formation of plaque (inflammatory lipid deposits) along the inner walls of arteries that leads to reduced or blocked blood flow (Tamparo & Lewis, 2000). Atherosclerosis is facilitated by repeated microtrauma to the walls of arteries, often as a result of high blood pressure. Once the inner wall of an artery begins to take on damage, platelets accumulate at the injury site in an effort to repair the artery. This process leads to inflammation and the formation of plaque. Over time this pathologic process leads to loss of flexibility of the artery, stenosis, calcification, and compromised blood flow through the lesion portions of the blood vessel. Total occlusion of blood flow can occur if plaque accumulation is large enough. Rupture of a plaque formation can result in dislodgement of the plaque and formation of an **embolus** (Tamparo & Lewis, 2000).

Atherosclerosis can affect arteries of the brain, heart, kidneys, and other vital organs. Many factors contribute to the development of atherosclerosis, including high blood pressure, smoking, diabetes, obesity, and high levels of cholesterol in the blood (Beers & Porter, 2006). Preventing and treating atherosclerosis is essential in preventing heart attack and stroke. No symptoms may be present in early stages of atherosclerosis. The first recognizable symptoms are often pain or cramps in tissue when that tissue's need for oxygen cannot be met due to compromised blood flow (Beers & Porter, 2006; Tamparo & Lewis, 2000).

Atherosclerosis is related to obesity and weight gain. Approximately 66% of Americans over age 20 yr are overweight or obese. About 32% of American children aged 2 to 19 yr are overweight or obese. Research has shown that obesity is clearly associated with increased lipid levels, high blood pressure, increased risk for developing diabetes, and increased risk of heart disease, heart failure, cancer, degenerative joint disease, asthma, and stroke (American Heart Association, 2010).

Peripheral Artery Disease

Peripheral artery disease (PAD) is a narrowing of peripheral arteries as a result of buildup of atherosclerotic plaque on the inner walls of the artery. The condition compromises the flow of blood to the tissues supplied by the affected artery and leads to **ischemia**.

Incidence

More than 27 million individuals in North America and Europe have PAD. In the United States, more than 413,000 people are discharged from the hospital with chronic PAD. More than 88,000 of these hospitalizations involve arteriography of the lower extremity, and 28,000 discharges indicate embolectomy or thrombectomy of the lower limb per year (Harris, 2008). PAD affects approximately 12% of people in the United States, or more than 8 million Americans. PAD is more prevalent in men than in women. In 2005, atherosclerosis was the leading cause of morbidity and mortality in the United States. It is expected to be the leading cause of death worldwide by 2020 (Beers & Porter, 2006).

Etiology and Pathophysiology

The rehabilitation specialist should be alert to signs and symptoms of arterial insufficiency associated with atherosclerosis, including intermittent claudication, changes in skin temperature and color, bruits over the involved artery, headache, dizziness, and memory deficits (Tamparo & Lewis, 2000). PAD and intermittent claudication symptoms are a result of arterial insufficiency due to the buildup of atherosclerotic plaque in the affected arteries. Claudication symptoms often begin to appear after the disease progresses to the point the vessel diameter narrows to approximately 50% (Goodman et al., 2008).

Intermittent claudication commonly occurs in the vasculature supplying the lower extremities. The condition and related symptoms can be unilateral or bilateral and can affect the calves, feet, thighs, hips, or buttocks depending on where the PAD causes narrowing of the vasculature. Because the **popliteal** artery is frequently affected, symptoms are most common in the calf muscles. In the classic presentation of intermittent claudication, calf pain, muscle cramping, and limping due to ischemia limit the distance a patient is able to walk. More subtle symptoms of intermittent claudication include a sense of weakness or tiredness in the affected lower extremity. A hallmark sign of intermittent claudication is that rest from walking often provides relief. With a more severe occlusion, the patient may experience no relief with rest due to the extent of arterial insufficiency (Rowe, 2009).

Rehabilitation Considerations

The rehabilitation specialist should be aware that elevating the legs can aggravate symptoms and that positioning the feet below heart level lessens symptoms (Beers & Porter, 2006). For this reason, patients often complain of experiencing ischemic pain in the lower extremities at night while in bed. Moderate to severe PAD can diminish popliteal, tibialis posterior, and dorsal pedal pulses (Beers & Porter, 2006). Recognizing intermittent claudication and referring the patient for treatment is essential in preventing complications and adverse events associated with this condition. Intermittent claudication affects more than 5 million individuals in the United States (Murabito et al., 2005). Diagnosis of intermittent claudication is made based on the patient's history, physical examination, ankle–brachial blood pressure index, ultrasonography, and angiography. Accurately diagnosing and treating PAD or intermittent claudication is important because PAD increases an individual's risk for coronary artery disease, heart attack, stroke, and transient ischemic attack six- to sevenfold (Beers & Porter, 2006).

Reducing modifiable risk factors through smoking cessation, following a heart-healthy diet, and exercising is an important part of treatment. Patients with concurrent hypertension (Mehler et al., 2003) or diabetes (Collins et al., 2004) should maintain blood pressure and blood glucose levels in their target range.

Smoking is the most important risk factor for PAD. If a patient smokes, the quickest way to reduce the symptoms and progress of PAD is to stop smoking. Extensive evidence shows that smoking cessation improves the prognosis of patients with PAD. Patients with PAD have a tendency to walk less due to claudication pain. Reduction of walking increases progression of the disease and symptoms, whereas a regular walking program leads to substantial improvement in most patients with claudication by conditioning muscles to work more efficiently and increasing the formation of collateral vessels. A daily walking program of 45 to 60 min is recommended. The rehabilitation therapist should instruct the patient to walk until claudication pain occurs, rest until the pain subsides, and repeat the cycle (Rowe, 2009).

The rehabilitation specialist plays an important role in designing therapeutic exercise programs for patients with intermittent claudication. Patients who are able should participate in carefully prescribed and supervised interval-training programs that alternate periods of walking and rest. The program may start out with an interval of as little as 1 min of walking followed by rest and repeated as tolerated. The intensity and duration of exercise should be gradually progressed based on the patient's exercise tolerance and onset of symptoms. Rehabilitation therapists recommend treating intermittent claudication by building exercise tolerance and increasing circulation through treadmill-walking programs and other forms of aerobic exercise that increase blood flow (Hiatt et al., 1991). Additional exercise routines for this patient population include the use of muscle-pumping exercises that promote increased circulation. Activities such as ankle pumps, ankle circles, and various active range-of-motion exercises for the lower extremities along with alternating periods of rest are commonly used.

Medication Therapy

Because atherosclerosis is a systemic disease that occurs throughout the blood vessels of the body, lipid-lowering therapy combined with antiplatelet therapy is the mainstay of treatment in the patient with PAD. Platelet aggregation results in the formation of the initial hemostatic plug when a blood vessel is injured. Platelet aggregation and the inflammatory response associated with injury can then lead to thrombus, which results in acute events associated with myocardial infarction (MI), stroke, and acute claudication. Medications that inhibit platelet aggregation can decrease the occurrence of these acute events and reduce morbidity and mortality. Although antiplatelet drug therapies effectively reduce fatal ischemic events in patients with PAD, these therapies as well as other secondary prevention efforts appear to be underused in patients with the disease (Murabito et al., 2005). Pentoxifylline (Trental) and cilostazol (Pletal) are antiplatelet therapies that are specifically used to treat claudication. Table 20.1 summarizes dosing and side effects associated with these agents.

Pentoxifylline

Pentoxifylline (Trental) is a methylxanthine derivative that is used to improve blood flow in patients with circulation problems in order to reduce aching, cramping, and tiredness in the hands and feet. It decreases the thickness (viscosity) of blood and allows blood to flow more easily, especially in the small blood vessels of the hands and feet. It is dosed at 400 mg 3 times/day. Side effects include belching, bloating, blurred vision, diarrhea, dizziness, flushing, nausea, and dyspepsia (Michel & Hoffman, 2011).

Cilostazol

Cilostazol (Pletal) increases cyclic adenosine monophosphate, thus inhibiting platelet aggregation and producing vasodilation. Pletal is dosed at 100 mg twice/day and is taken at least 0.5 h before or 2 h after breakfast and dinner. It is metabolized by CYP3A4 and CYP2C19 and can interact with other medications metabolized by these pathways. Prescribers should consider a dose of 50 mg twice/day when coprescribing CYP3A4 inhibitors (e.g., ketoconazole, itraconazole, erythromycin, and diltiazem) or CYP2C19 inhibitors (e.g., omeprazole). Side effects include diarrhea, back pain, bloating, dizziness, gas, headache,

See table 20.1 in the web resource for a full list of medication-specific indications, dosing recommendations, side effects, and drug interactions.

Table 20.1   Medications Used to Treat Claudication

Medication	Side effects affecting rehab							Other side effects or drug interactions
Antiplatelet therapies: Used to prevent clot formation and reduce symptoms of claudication.								
Cilostazol (Pletal)	Cog 0	S 0	A 0	Motor ++	D ++	Com 0	F ++	Side effects: Diarrhea, back pain, bloating, dizziness, gas, headache, cough, dyspepsia, muscle aches, cold symptoms, swelling of feet, ankles, or hands. Drug interactions: Increased levels and effects with concurrent use of CYP3A4 inhibitors (e.g., ketoconazole, itraconazole, erythromycin, and diltiazem) and coadministration of CYP2C19 inhibitors (e.g., omeprazole); reduce dose to 50 mg twice/day.
Pentoxifylline (Trental)	Cog 0	S 0	A 0	Motor ++	D ++	Com 0	F ++	Side effects: Belching, bloating, blurred vision, diarrhea, dizziness, flushing, nausea, dyspepsia. Drug interactions: May increase risk of bleeding in patients on warfarin (Coumadin). May increase theophylline levels and toxicity.
Aspirin therapy	Cog 0	S 0	A 0	Motor 0	D +	Com 0	F 0	Side effects: Headache, nausea, dyspepsia, tinnitus with high doses. Drug interactions: Increases risk of bleeding when combined with anticoagulants and other antiplatelet medications.
Statin therapy: Used to reduce atherosclerosis and obstruction of blood flow. See table 20.2.								

Cog = cognition; S = sedation; A = agitation or mania; Motor = discoordination; D = dysphagia; Com = communication; F = falls.

The likelihood rating scale for encountering the side effects is as follows: 0 = Almost no probability of encountering side effects. + = Little likelihood of encountering side effects. +/++ = Low probability of encountering side effects; however, probability increases with increased dosage. ++ = Medium likelihood of encountering side effects. +++ = High likelihood of encountering side effects, particularly with high doses. ++++ = Highest likelihood of encountering side effects; best to avoid in at-risk patients.

cough, dyspepsia, muscle aches, cold symptoms, and swelling of feet, ankles, or hands, (Michel & Hoffman, 2011).

Cilostazol improves claudication symptoms but does not improve cardiovascular mortality. Side effects include headache and cardiac arrhythmia. Its use is contraindicated in patients with heart failure. Trials have documented modest improvements in walking distance in patients using this agent, and full effects have been seen after 2 to 3 mo of therapy. Several randomized studies have shown that the use of cilostazol (Pletal) has increased both the distance walked before the onset of claudication pain and the distance walked before exercise-limiting symptoms became intolerable (i.e., maximal walking distance) (Michel & Hoffman, 2011; O'Donnell et al., 2009).

Statin Therapy

Lipid-lowering agents reduce the accumulation of atherosclerotic plaque and help reduce occlusion as well as ischemic events in patients with PAD. The Heart Protection Study documented that the use of simvastatin lowered by 25% the risk of major vascular events in patients with PAD. The next section deals with stroke and provides additional information on the use of statins (Bersot, 2011; Rowe, 2009).

Stroke

The term *stroke* is commonly used to describe a cerebrovascular accident. Stroke is a sudden focal interruption in cerebral blood flow that results in neurologic deficit (Beers & Porter, 2006). The two broad categories of stroke include ischemic stroke, which accounts for roughly 80% of all strokes, and hemorrhagic stroke, which account for about 20% of all strokes (Beers & Porter, 2006). Ischemic strokes typically result from a thrombosis or an embolism. Hemorrhagic strokes are the result of a vascular rupture that leads to bleeding.

Incidence

More than 15 million people in the world suffer a stroke annually; of these, 5 million die and 5 million are permanently disabled. Hypertension and tobacco use are the major risk factors for stroke globally. Other risk factors include heart attack, heart failure, and atrial fibrillation. The incidence of stroke has declined in developed countries; however, the actual number of patients with stroke in the world is increasing because the population is aging (World Health Organization, 2012).

Stroke is the third leading cause of death in the United States. Each year, 780,000 strokes occur; 180,000 of these are recurrent strokes. About 25% of these strokes occur in persons who are aged 45 to 65 yr. Approximately 900,000 patients are discharged from medical facilities with the diagnosis of stroke each year. Two million to three million stroke survivors are either partially or totally disabled. Direct and indirect costs associated with stroke in the United States are approximately $73.3 billion (ATP III pocket guideline, 2004; Furie et al., 2011; Goodman et al., 2008; Summers et al., 2009).

Etiology and Pathophysiology

The etiology and pathophysiology of stroke varies depending on the type of stroke a patient experiences. Accurately diagnosing the type of stroke is essential in determining the most effective medical management for the condition (Fonarow et al., 2010).

General risk factors for stroke include older age, family history of stroke, alcoholism, male sex, hypertension, smoking, hypercholesterolemia, diabetes, previous stroke or **transient ischemic attack** (TIA), and abuse of stimulants such as cocaine and amphetamines (Beers & Porter, 2006). Certain risk factors predispose individuals to a particular type of stroke. Those at risk for arterial ischemic stroke include Native Americans (6.7%), persons of multiple races (4.6%), African American men and women (4%), Hispanic men (3.1%), Hispanic women (2.7%), and Caucasian men and women (2.3%). Those with hypercoagulability are predisposed to thrombotic stroke, and those with atrial fibrillation are at greater risk for embolic stroke. Risk also increases with advancing age (Summers et al., 2009). Individuals at greater risk for intracranial hemorrhage (hemorrhagic stroke) include African Americans and those with hypertension, high cholesterol, high consumption of alcohol, and liver disease. Greater risk for subarachnoid hemorrhages is present in individuals who develop a cerebral aneurysm in the brain that can lead to rupture or those with arteriovenous malformation (Furie et al., 2011; Summers et al., 2009).

Atherosclerosis is responsible for most cerebral infarctions and MI (Schell Frazier & Wist Drzymkowski, 2004). An early study by Friedman and colleagues (1968) found that coronary or arteriosclerotic heart disease was diagnosed before the stroke date in 41.9% of the stroke cases. Both atherosclerosis and hypertension are predominant factors that contribute to stroke (Schell Frazier & Wist Drzymkowski, 2004).

In instances where atherosclerotic plaque is built up in the arteries leading to the brain, early signs of pathology may include episodes of TIA. Some signs and symptoms of TIA include sudden numbness or weakness in the arms or legs, difficulty speaking or slurred speech, and facial droop. Up to 40% of individuals who experience a TIA go on to experience a stroke; 5% of patients who experience a TIA experience a stroke within 7 days and 15% experience a stroke within 30 days (National Stroke Association, 2010). Because of this, in

2009 the definition of TIA was changed from experiencing stroke symptoms for less than 24 h to "any transient episode of neurologic dysfunction, focal ischemia of the brain, spinal cord or retina not associated with infarction" (Easton et al., 2009). Symptoms include sudden but transient loss of vision, weakness, changes in brain function, or changes in motor function that improve spontaneously and do not qualify as a stroke. This change in definition is extremely important, because it focuses less on the length of time symptoms are present and instead identifies warning signs that should lead a person to seek an immediate medical evaluation and perhaps prevent a stroke. Scoring systems such as the ABCD2 scoring system for assessing the severity of TIA have been developed. Current guidelines recommend that those who experience a TIA undergo evaluation and neuroimaging within 24 h of symptom onset and that those with an ABCD2 score of 3 or greater be admitted for further evaluation (Easton et al., 2009; Goldstein et al., 2011). Patients who experience a TIA should be educated on the condition and recommended changes in lifestyle in order to lower their risk factors for stroke. Antiplatelet therapy should be initiated in all patients who experience a TIA, and lipid-lowering agents should be initiated in patients with low-density lipoprotein levels greater than 100 mg/dl (>70 mg/dl in patients with other cardiac risk factors) (Furie et al., 2011).

Because a patient may have a TIA or stroke at any time, the rehabilitation specialist must be proficient in recognizing the symptoms of a TIA or stroke. Signs and symptoms include a sudden change in speech, facial drop, loss of vision, diplopia, paralysis, hemiparesis, dizziness, loss of balance, and numbness or weakness in the face, arm, or leg (especially on one side of the body). Patients may also experience difficulty understanding what others are saying (Goldstein & Simel, 2005). In some instances a sudden headache with no known cause may be present and is often associated with hemorrhagic stroke. Dysphagia commonly occurs after stroke. To avoid aspiration and associated complications, patients with symptoms of stroke should not take food,

drink, or medications by mouth and should remain nothing per oral (NPO) until a health care provider determines that they can swallow safely (Summers et al., 2009).

Ischemic Stroke

Ischemic stroke, sometimes referred to as occlusive stroke, accounts for up to 87% of all strokes. The most common cause of ischemic stroke is the development of a thrombus or embolus that occludes a blood vessel. Most embolic strokes occur when a cholesterol-filled plaque ruptures and part of the plaque travels and lodges in an artery occluding blood flow to a portion of the brain, resulting in brain ischemia. Approximately 50% of adults in the United States have elevated total cholesterol; 26% have cholesterol levels greater than 240 mg/dl. Poorly controlled cholesterol that leads to plaque formation is considered a modifiable risk factor that can increase one's risk for ischemic stroke (Beers & Porter, 2006; Summers et al., 2009). Hypertension is another modifiable risk factor that the rehabilitation specialist should be aware of and diligently monitor for in patients. A transient and dramatic increase in blood pressure is common during an acute ischemic stroke as the body attempts to compensate for the reduction in blood flow to the brain (Adams et al., 2007; Furie et al., 2011; Goldstein et al., 2011; Sacco et al., 2006; Semplicini et al., 2003; Summers et al., 2009).

Cardiogenic embolism accounts for approximately 20% of ischemic strokes/yr. Cardioembolic strokes are associated with atrial fibrillation and valvular disease in which cardiac pumping is less efficient, which contributes to pooling of blood in the cardiac chambers and resultant clot formation. Atrial fibrillation is associated with between 75,000 and 95,000 strokes/yr in the United States (Hart & Halperin, 2001). Hart and colleagues (1983) reported a 20% rate of recurrence of cerebral embolism within 11 days of the initial embolus in patients who had not started anticoagulant therapy. Approximately 2.5% of patients with acute MI experience a stroke within 2 to 4 wk of the MI. Most emboli occur within 1 to 2 wk of the cardiac event. An estimated 38,000 strokes/yr in the United States are directly related to acute MI (Cerebral Embolism Study Group, 1989).

Intracranial Hemorrhage

Intracranial hemorrhage (ICH), also sometimes referred to as a cerebral hemorrhage or a hemorrhagic stroke, is bleeding that occurs within the brain tissue. ICH accounts for approximately 10% of all strokes. In this type of stroke, bleeding from an arterial source into the brain occurs (Goodman et al., 2008). The likelihood of death or major disability is greater in patients experiencing ICH than in those experiencing ischemic stroke or subarachnoid hemorrhage. Secondary cell death occurs in the central nervous system (CNS) tissue supplied by the ruptured artery because the tissue no longer receives oxygen and nutrients, resulting in brain ischemia. Additional CNS tissue damage and disruption of brain function occur as a result of the ruptured artery clots and the swelling that pushes on healthy brain tissue. A contributing factor to ICH is persistent, long-term hypertension, which decreases the integrity of the arteries in the brain and increases their risk of rupture (Furie et al., 2011; Summers et al., 2009).

Subarachnoid Hemorrhage

Subarachnoid hemorrhage, in which bleeding into the subarachnoid space between the pia mater and arachnoid mater membranes occurs, accounts for 3% of all strokes. A common cause of subarachnoid hemorrhagic stroke is a burst aneurysm or the rupture of an arteriovenous malformation (a congenitally malformed tangle of thin-walled blood vessels) (Furie et al., 2011; Summers et al., 2009).

Physiology of Clot Formation

Clot formation is a protective mechanism for preventing blood loss associated with injury, but clot formation is also involved with the formation of thrombus or embolus associated with acute cardiovascular events such as cardioembolic stroke, hemorrhagic stroke, and myocardial infarction. Clot formation also can occur in areas where blood pools as a result of stasis, such as in cardioembolic stroke due to inefficient cardiac pumping. Clot formation begins when platelets adhere to the injured blood vessel, where they become activated. They then release inflammatory substances that recruit more platelets to the site of injury, forming the primary hemostatic plug. The injured vessel wall also releases tissue factor, which activates the coagulation system. This activation triggers a complex series of steps known as the coagulation cascade, which ultimately results in the formation of thrombin, which converts fibrinogen to fibrin. Fibrin reinforces the platelet clot and anchors it to the vessel wall. Thrombin also recruits additional platelets to the area of injury, contributing to clot formation (Colbert & Mason, 2002).

The coagulation cascade involves a series of activation reactions in which enzymatic processes systematically convert clotting factors to activated clotting factors. The tissue factor pathway (formerly the extrinsic pathway), which initiates clot formation, involves tissue factor and factor VII. This pathway activates the contact activation pathway (formerly called the intrinsic pathway), which activates factors IX and VIII. Both pathways meet at the final common pathway involving factors X, V, and II, which results in the final activation of prothrombin (factor II) to thrombin (activated factor IIa). Activated thrombin then converts fibrinogen (factor I) to fibrin (factor Ia) and clot formation results. Anticoagulants block clot formation by interfering during one or more of these enzymatic steps needed for clot formation (Colbert & Mason, 2002).

After the wound heals the clot is dissolved and removed by fibrinolytic agents (clot busters) in the body such as tissue plasminogen activator. Tissue plasminogen activator promotes the conversion of plasminogen to plasmin, which digests fibrin, the glue that holds the clot together. Medications such as antiplatelet therapy prevent clot formation by preventing the initial step of platelet aggregation, whereas anticoagulants interfere with clot formation by interfering with the formation of the fibrin clots at one or more of the steps in the coagulation cascade. Finally, the fibrinolytics (also known as clot busters) work in a manner similar to the body's natural tissue plasminogen activator to degrade fibrin holding clots together. The fibrinolytic most commonly used to treat clots that cause stroke is tissue plasminogen activator (TPA) (Activase), which is a recombinant form of tissue plasminogen activator. Other recombinant variants of TPA that are used as clot busters in treating MI include reteplase (Retavase) and tenecteplase (TNKase) (Colbert & Mason, 2002).

Rehabilitation Considerations

The impairments associated with a stroke depend on the anatomic location of the stroke and the type and severity of the stroke. CNS tissue does not regenerate, but cortical reorganization does occur. Cortical reorganization is the basis for many rehabilitation techniques, including constraint-induced movement therapy. This therapy approach involves discouraging the use of the noninvolved extremity and encouraging the use of the involved limb. For example, in a patient with a hemiplegic right upper extremity, the rehabilitation therapist may place a mitt on the patient's nonaffected hand to encourage the patient to use the affected limb during therapeutic interventions and daily activities. Therapy involves using the affected upper extremity to do activities such as picking and stacking small objects (e.g., cone stacking) and practicing other tasks that are necessary for activities of daily living.

Patients with stroke commonly present with a variety of motor control impairments, including hemiplegia or hemiparesis, hemiparetic shoulder, wrist drop, foot drop, and difficulty with motor control of the trunk. Clinical presentations vary considerably based on the location, type, and severity of the stroke. The rehabilitation therapist designs a rehabilitation program that addresses the specific impairments and functional limitations that are identified during the initial examination. For example, therapeutic activities that restore proximal stability and good neuromuscular control of the trunk serve as a base to help the patient develop better neuromuscular control of the affected limbs. Using functional electrical stimulation to treat hemiparetic shoulder, drop foot, and wrist drop is recommended because the final common pathway is intact

and can be retrained in upper motor neuron lesions. Recovery depends on many factors, including anatomical location of the stroke, how quickly the initial diagnosis was made, and how soon treatment was initiated. Rehabilitation programs that employ principles of motor control and include constraint-induced movement therapy show good carryover to functional activities and promote improved outcomes. Dromerick (2003) found that use of constraint-induced movement therapy resulted in a marked improvement in motor impairment.

The rehabilitation specialist must also focus on protecting and rehabilitating the hemiparetic shoulder in afflicted patients. The specialist should ensure that the glenohumeral joint capsule is not overstretched and that the dynamic stabilizers of the shoulder (muscles) are trained to stabilize the shoulder joint to prevent or correct shoulder subluxation in this population. Upper-extremity weight-bearing exercises that apply compression to the joint help promote stability and activate the shoulder muscles. The use of functional electrical stimulation can enhance many therapeutic interventions and functional activities for the upper extremity. Electromyography (EMG) and EMG-triggered electrical stimulation can also be used to treat weak, inhibited muscles in this patient population. With both functional electrical stimulation and EMG-triggered electrical stimulation, the patient must volitionally participate in the task while muscles are being electrically stimulated. The combination of volitional participation and electrical stimulation is believed to stimulate cortical reorganization. Individuals who have recalcitrant functional deficits that do not respond to treatment should be taught compensatory techniques for performing functional tasks (Goodman et al., 2008).

Falls are common in this patient population. The rehabilitation specialist should focus on fall prevention through functional training, using appropriate assistive devices, and modifying the patient's environment to eliminate fall risks. Falls are common during the transition from sitting to standing because the patient overcompensates by shifting their weight toward the noninvolved side in an effort to gain more stability. The entire movement from sit to stand is also significantly slower in this patient population, which can negatively influence motor control, especially if the patient has deficits in trunk control and balance (Goodman et al., 2008).

Gait training in this patient population can be challenging due to unequal weight distribution through the affected lower extremity, drop foot in the affected lower extremity, deficits in trunk control, and impaired arm swing in the affected upper extremity. Partially weighted treadmill walking and aquatic gait training can promote improved gait. The use of functional electrical stimulation is advocated to restore functional dorsiflexion during gait in patients with drop foot. An orthosis, such as the molded ankle–foot orthosis, is commonly used to passively maintain the ankle in a neutral position during gait and prevent falls associated with the inability to clear the affected foot over the ground during gait (Goodman et al., 2008).

Because stoke is an upper motor neuron lesion, the common symptoms of hyperreflexia, hypertonicity (spasticity), and spastic paralysis are often present. The rehabilitation specialist can use antispastic pattern positioning, range-of-motion exercise, stretching, and splinting to prevent or treat contracture. The rehabilitation therapist should also be alert to signs of angina, PVD, and deep vein thrombosis (DVT) that can develop after stroke (Rodgers et al., 1999).

PATIENT CASE 1

P.T. is a 75-yr-old woman who is receiving rehabilitation therapy for muscle strengthening and gait training after a prolonged hospitalization for pneumonia with respiratory failure. P.T.'s medical history includes diabetes, chronic obstructive pulmonary disease (COPD), hypertension, and hyperlipidemia. Her current medications include Glucophage for diabetes, Advair and albuterol rescue inhalers for COPD, diltiazem (Cardizem CD) for hypertension, and atorvastatin (Zocor) for hyperlipidemia. While exercising, P.T. loses her balance.

The rehabilitation specialist notices that P.T. is now confused and exhibits weakness on the right side, muscle twitching, and a facial droop. The rehabilitation specialist suspects a stroke and calls 911 to summon emergency medical services.

Question

What symptoms are consistent with stroke in P.T.?

Answer

Symptoms in P.T. consistent with stroke (also called a brain attack) include sudden onset of altered mental status, weakness on the right side, muscle twitching, and a facial droop.

The main stroke symptoms can be remembered using the acronym FAST (face, arms, speech, time), which was developed to assist the public and first responders in early identification of stroke. The FAST test is able to identify nearly 9 out of 10 strokes (Wall et al., 2008).

- Face: The person's face may be drooped on one side, the person may be unable to smile, or the mouth or eye may have drooped.

- Arm weakness: The person with suspected stroke may not be able to lift one or both arms and keep them there due to arm weakness or numbness. Ask the patient to hold both arms out in front of them (90° shoulder flexion). The test is positive if one arm drifts down (i.e., they cannot hold it up).

- Speech impairment: The person's speech may be slurred or garbled or the person may not be able to talk at all despite appearing to be awake.

- Time: It is time to activate emergency medical services (EMS) if any of these three signs are present. Note the time of onset and report it to the EMS personnel who will immediately communicate this while in transit to the treating emergency room physician.

Once it is identified that a patient is experiencing a stroke or TIA, the patient should be transported without delay via EMS for prompt treatment. In the past, only supportive treatment was available when a person experienced a stroke. Now, patient outcome can be markedly improved by use of the clot buster TPA (Activase), which can break up the obstructing clot and provide rapid reperfusion to the obstructed site in the brain. The longer the delay in treatment, the more likely that the patient will experience residual neuromuscular damage associated with prolonged brain ischemia. Prompt referral and initiation of thrombolytic therapy in patients eligible for TPA can reverse brain ischemia and reduce residual disability associated with stroke (Furie et al., 2011).

Once the patient arrives in the emergency department, emergency practitioners will ask important questions about the timing of symptom onset, the patient's medical history, and the patient's current medications. This important information can help the emergency room physician determine whether the symptoms were caused by a stroke or other conditions with similar symptoms. This information also helps determine whether the patient is a candidate for thrombolytic therapy to reverse the occlusion in the brain and re-establish perfusion of the brain tissue. Sample questions include the following: What time was the patient last known to be well? When were symptoms first observed? Was anyone with the patient when symptoms began? If yes, who? Does the patient have a history of diabetes, hypertension, seizure, or trauma related to current event? Does the patient have a history of MI, angina, cardiac arrhythmias, or atrial fibrillation? Does the patient have a history of stroke or TIA? What medications is the patient currently taking? Is the patient receiving anticoagulation therapy with warfarin? The rehabilitation therapist can help the patient and family by ensuring that the patient's medical information and list of medications accompany the patient to the emergency department (Summers et al., 2009).

PATIENT CASE 1, *continued*

Based on the case history for P.T., answer the following questions.

Question
What pertinent facts about P.T.'s history and symptoms need to be shared with the emergency room staff?

Answer
The emergency room staff should be informed about P.T.'s risk factors (diabetes, hypertension, hyperlipidemia, COPD), her recent hospitalization, and her current medications.

In the emergency department, emergency practitioners can use more comprehensive stroke scales such as the National Institutes of Health Stroke Scale to classify the severity of the stroke. The patient's level of orientation, memory, emotional control, motor control and balance, sensation, hearing, vision, and ability to read and write are tested using these scales. A review of the patient's medical history, medications, and a thorough physical examination are essential in establishing an accurate diagnosis. A working diagnosis of the type and location of the stroke can usually be established based on the patient's history and the results of the physical examination. Accompanying laboratory tests and imaging studies can help rule out differential diagnoses, identify concurrent conditions that require emergency treatment, confirm stroke diagnosis, and assist in developing the best emergency treatment for the patient (Furie et al., 2011).

Diagnostic testing performed on all patients presenting with symptoms of a stroke includes an emergent brain computed tomography (CT) scan or magnetic resonance imaging to determine whether the patient is having a hemorrhagic or embolic stroke, an electrocardiogram to rule out MI or arrhythmia (some patients present with both acute cardiac and stroke events), serum blood tests for electrolytes, blood glucose (symptoms of hypoglycemia can mimic stroke symptoms), complete blood count, prothrombin time/international normalized ratio (PT/INR) and PTT tests to determine the patient's level of anticoagulation, and assessment of oxygenation level. Additional tests that may be performed based on the patient's history include liver function tests, toxicology screen, blood alcohol levels, pregnancy test, lumbar puncture for suspected subarachnoid hemorrhage, and electroencephalogram to confirm suspected seizure (Furie et al., 2011). These tests need to be performed with expert efficiency to allow the medical team to treat the patient's urgent symptoms and decide whether the patient is a candidate for thrombolytic therapy.

Medication Therapy

Tissue plasminogen activator (TPA), a thrombolytic, has significantly improved outcomes in the acute management of the stroke patient. In patients who are candidates for TPA, adjunctive medications that can optimize the effects of TPA therapy include hyperglycemic agents, antipyretic agents, and analgesics.

PATIENT CASE 1, *continued*

The following are the results of P.T.'s diagnostic tests:

Brain CT: nonhemorrhagic stroke

Electrocardiogram: no arrhythmia or MI

Blood glucose: 252

Serum electrolytes: within normal limits

Renal-function tests: creatinine = 1.2

Complete blood count (CBC) including, WBC: 8.0; Hemoglobin/hematocrit (H/H): 12.0/34.3; Platelets: 150,000

Coagulation tests including, Prothrombin time/international normalized ratio (PT/INR): normal; Partial thromboplastin time (PTT): normal

Electroencephalogram (EEG): no seizure activity noted

Blood pressure (BP): 195/122

Temperature: 98.6 °F

Chest film: no infiltrates

O_2 saturation: 85%

Question

What therapeutic interventions are needed at this time?

Answer

P.T. is exhibiting acute hypoxemia, which should be addressed with emergent administration of ventilatory support including oxygen therapy. Because the emergency room physician and consulting neurologist have determined that P.T. is a candidate for thrombolytic therapy, interventions must be made to control blood pressure, temperature, pain, and blood sugar in order to provide the best outcome for the TPA treatment.

After emergency diagnosis and treatment of acute stroke symptoms, medications used to prevent complications from a stroke include antiplatelet therapy initiated after 24 h and within 48 h, and anticoagulants initiated at least 24 h after a stroke, which prevent deep vein thrombosis and pulmonary embolism. In order to avoid complications of pneumonia, deep vein thrombosis, pulmonary embolism, contractures, and pressure sores, the physical therapist should initiate range-of-motion exercises in the patient within the first 24 h, turn the patient frequently, and initiate mobilization when the patient is stable (Summers et al., 2009).

Medication therapies are also used to prevent a second stroke. Such therapies include antiplatelet therapies, anticoagulants, and medications used to control preventable risk factors for stroke (e.g., antihypertensives, hypoglycemic agents, and lipid-lowering agents).

Thrombolytic Therapy

Thrombolytic therapy is used to dissolve or break up blood clots. Thrombolytic therapy is most effective when given within 3 h of onset of symptoms but can also cause bleeding. The longer administration is delayed, the higher the risk of bleeding associated with the stroke. Recent guidelines permit expanding the window of treatment to up to 4.5 h in low-risk populations but not in elderly patients or patients with history of stroke, diabetes, or anticoagulant use (Del Zoppo et al., 2009). Minimum times have been established by the National Institute of Neurologic Disorders and Stroke (NINDS) for accomplishing steps of emergent care of stroke patients. The physician should see the patient within 10 min of arrival, the CT should be completed within 25 min of arrival, and the CT should be read within 45 min of arrival. Patients are considered to be candidates for TPA if they are of adult age, the CT shows no hemorrhage, and they have stroke symptoms (Furie et al., 2011).

Patients with extensive thrombus (more than one third occlusion of middle cerebral artery or with clearly identifiable hypodensity on initial CT), or patients with minor or rapidly improving stroke symptoms should not receive TPA because the risk of hemorrhage outweighs possible benefits of TPA in these patients. Factors that increase the risk of bleeding, such as a history of bleeding, recent surgery, head trauma, or use of anticoagulant therapy with associated high levels of anticoagulation, also rule out the use of TPA. Patients who present with seizures, have pericarditis after a MI, or patients who are pregnant are not candidates for TPA. Intra-arterial TPA, a treatment option that is available in comprehensive stroke centers, can be administered by specially trained interventional neurologists in appropriate patients who are not eligible for intravenous TPA. Embolectomy (mechanical removal of the clot) by the interventional neurologist is another therapy that may be available in the comprehensive stroke center (Furie et al., 2011).

Antihypertensive Therapy

Embolic stroke can evolve into a hemorrhagic stroke in patients whose blood pressure is too high. Eighty percent of patients with stroke present with markedly elevated blood pressure that spontaneously improves within 24 h and declines to baseline levels over the next 7 to 10 days. However, excessively high blood pressure can worsen a stroke and increases the risk that an embolic stroke will evolve into a hemorrhagic stroke. In addition, patients must have systolic blood pressure less than 185 and diastolic blood pressure less than 110 to receive TPA. The use of intravenous beta blockers such as labetalol or esmolol (Brevibloc) or the intravenous infusion of the calcium channel blocker nicardipine (Cardene) can emergently reduce blood pressure to a safe level in patients who are otherwise eligible for TPA and allow administration of this thrombolytic therapy (Bath et al., 2001; Harrington, 2003; Summers et al., 2009).

Ten percent of the total TPA dose is given as a bolus over 1 min, the rest is infused over 1 h. If the patient develops severe headache, acute hypertension, nausea, or vomiting during TPA administration, the TPA infusion should be discontinued and an emergent repeat CT scan should be obtained. A repeat CT should be done after the completion of TPA therapy. Symptoms worsen within 24 to 48 h after the stroke in one fourth of patients who experience a stroke. Therefore, patients should be admitted to the ICU or stroke unit and closely monitored during this period of time. Neurological assessments should be done every 15 min during infusion of TPA, every 30 min for next 6 h, and then hourly for the remainder of the initial 24 h. Patients require bed rest, hydration with intravenous saline, and close monitoring and control of blood pressure, oxygenation, temperature, fluid intake and urine output, and glucose levels. Automatic blood pressure cuffs, toothbrushes, and venipuncture should be avoided after TPA administration to minimize hematoma and bleeding (Furie et al., 2011; Summers et al., 2009).

Blood Glucose Control

Patients with high blood sugar do not receive maximum benefit from thrombolytic therapy. Short-acting insulin should be used to maintain blood sugar levels less than 150 mg/dl after a stroke (Summers et al., 2009).

Temperature

Temperature should be checked every 4 h. To minimize bleeding risk associated with TPA administration, temperature should be maintained below 99.6 through administration of acetaminophen after a stroke (Summers et al., 2009).

Antibiotic Therapy

Concurrent infection should be identified and treated with appropriate antibiotic therapy. Patients experiencing a stroke may be admitted with concurrent urinary tract infection, pneumonia, chronic obstructive pulmonary disease, or bacteremia. Aspiration pneumonia resulting from dysphagia is a common infection seen early after a stroke (Summers et al., 2009).

Analgesics

Managing the patient's acute pain and taking appropriate physical therapy measures can minimize chronic pain after a stroke. Risk factors for pain in the stroke patient include central pain associated with ischemia and nerve damage in the brain, immobility, and subluxation of the shoulder with improper movement of the patient's affected arm. Frequent repositioning also helps manage pain in these patients. Stroke patients are at high risk for experiencing pain but may not be able to communicate their pain effectively due to altered cognition, aphasia, and sensory loss. Patient caregivers should use nonverbal pain scales to detect pain in stroke patients, and parenteral pain medications should be used until it is determined that the patient can safely take oral medications.

Antiplatelet and Anticoagulant Therapy

Antiplatelet therapy (aspirin 325 mg once daily) should be implemented 24 h after the administration of TPA. Aspirin is used in acute treatment of stroke and also as preventative therapy for stroke recurrence. In platelets the inflammatory response is mediated by thromboxane A2, a cyclooxygenase product that induces platelet aggregation and vasoconstriction. Aspirin blocks the production of thromboxane A2 by acting on cyclooxygenase 1, an enzyme that produces the precursor for thromboxane A2. This inhibitory effect lasts for the life of the platelet (usually 7-10 days). Because blocking platelet aggregation increases bleeding risk, aspirin should be held for 7 to 10 days before any surgery. Complete inactivation of cyclooxygenase 1 occurs at doses of 75 mg/day; higher doses can interfere with production of prostacyclin, the body's natural anticoagulant. Higher doses are also associated with increased bleeding. For this reason, low-dose (81 mg) aspirin is used as chronic therapy to prevent thrombosis and secondary stroke. Other nonsteroidal anti-inflammatory drugs (NSAIDs) such as ibuprofen do not have antithrombotic activity and can actually interfere with the antithrombotic effects of aspirin. Therefore, patients receiving aspirin for thrombus prevention should not be placed on concurrent NSAID therapy.

Anticoagulants

Health care practitioners should also implement measures to prevent pulmonary embolism (PE), which causes 10% of all stroke-related deaths, and to prevent deep vein thrombosis (DVT). Intermittent pneumatic compression or elastic stockings should be used when anticoagulants are contraindicated. Anticoagulants such as low-dose subcutaneous heparin 5000 U every 8 h or enoxaparin (Lovenox) 30 mg every 12 h should be used to prevent DVT or PE. Use of full-dose anticoagulants should be avoided in patients with acute ischemic stroke except in the case of cerebral venous sinus thrombosis, when treatment-dose anticoagulants are used in the acute phase, even in patients with hemorrhage, and followed with oral anticoagulants for 3 to 6 mo. Patients with a history of atrial fibrillation who experience cardioembolic stroke should be started on a combination of full-dose heparin or enoxaparin (Lovenox) and oral warfarin (Coumadin) 24 h after TPA administration. Cardioembolic stroke is caused by a clot that is formed in the heart due to inefficient ejection of blood from the heart caused by arrhythmia (usually atrial fibrillation) or valvular disease.

Medications and Interventions Used to Prevent Stroke Recurrence (Secondary Stroke)

An estimated 180,000 patients in the United States experience a second stroke. Much research has been conducted to identify methods of preventing secondary stroke, and specific guidelines for preventing secondary stroke have been developed. A number of medications can decrease modifiable risk in the stroke patient, including antiplatelet therapy, anticoagulants, lipid-lowering therapy, antihypertensive therapy, and diabetes therapy. The patient should also initiate lifestyle changes such as smoking cessation, weight reduction, diet therapy, and exercise to prevent stroke recurrence. The following sections summarize medications useful in preventing secondary stroke.

PATIENT CASE 1, continued

P.T. is ready for discharge. Because her treatment with TPA was successful and because she received expert care from the hospital team, she is leaving the hospital with minimal residual effects from her stroke.

Question

What medications should P.T. receive on discharge for prevention of secondary stroke? What education regarding needed lifestyle interventions should be provided to P.T. and her family before her discharge?

Answer

Patients who have an ischemic stroke should be initiated on lifelong therapy to prevent another stroke. Therapy includes antiplatelet medications for a noncardioembolic stroke or anticoagulant therapy for a cardioembolic stroke. Statin therapy for reducing formation of atherosclerotic plaque should also be initiated if the patient's cholesterol levels are elevated. Therapy for hypertension or diabetes should be optimized in order to reduce these risk factors for repeat stroke. In addition, patients should begin a program of exercise, stop smoking, reduce weight when appropriate, and follow a heart-healthy diet.

Antiplatelet Therapy   All patients who have had a noncardioembolic ischemic stroke or a TIA should receive lifelong antiplatelet therapy. The Antithrombotic Trialists did a meta-analysis of studies that included a total of 144,051 patients and found that the use of antiplatelet therapy after stoke reduced the risk of a second stroke, MI, and vascular death by 25%. The use of aspirin 50 to 325 mg /day after stroke reduced recurrent stroke, MI, and vascular deaths by 23%; the use of clopidogrel (Plavix) 75 mg/day reduced recurrent stroke, MI, and vascular death by 30%; and the use of Aggrenox ER (aspirin 25 mg with dipyridamole 200 mg) twice/day reduced recurrent stroke, MI, and vascular death by 38%. Carotid endarterectomy is a surgical intervention in which plaque is removed from inside the carotid arteries. Patients who have a carotid endarterectomy should be given aspirin 81 to 325 mg/ day before and chronically after the procedure. Combination therapy of aspirin and clopidogrel (Plavix) is not routinely recommended for patients with ischemic stroke or TIA unless they have a specific cardiac indication for this therapy (e.g., coronary stent or acute coronary syndrome) because dual therapy is no more effective than a single agent and increases bleeding risk (Colbert & Mason, 2002; Weitz, 2011).

Dipyridamole (Persantine) interferes with platelet function by inhibiting phosphodiesterase, which causes an accumulation of adenosine, adenosine nucleotides, and cyclic adenosine monophosphate. It has vasodilatory properties and is used in a long-acting combination product with 25 mg of aspirin to prevent stroke recurrence in patients who have had a stroke. Because the aspirin component is only 25 mg, many practitioners add a baby aspirin to Aggrenox therapy so that the patient receives full cardioprotective effects (Colbert & Mason, 2002; Weitz, 2011).

Thienopyridine antiplatelet agents irreversibly inhibit platelet purinergic receptors and reduce adenosine diphosphate-induced platelet aggregation. The thienopyridines are prodrugs and require activation by metabolism to the final active medication. The thienopyridines include clopidogrel (Plavix), ticlopidine (Ticlid), and prasugrel (Effient). These agents continue to have antiplatelet effects for at least 5 days after discontinuance. Ticlopidine is seldom used as first-line therapy because serious neutropenia and agranulocytosis with thrombocytopenia can occur within the first 3 mo of therapy. Several trials have documented the effectiveness of clopidogrel (Plavix) therapy in reducing secondary stroke. It is used as an alternative to aspirin in patients who do not tolerate aspirin therapy. Prasugrel (Effient) is an alternative to clopidogrel in patients with coronary heart disease. It has a faster onset of action than clopidogrel but increases the risk of bleeding in the elderly patient. It is not used in the treatment of stroke (Colbert & Mason, 2002; Weitz, 2011).

Anticoagulants Anticoagulants (blood thinners) interfere with clot formation, thus decreasing the risk of stroke, heart attack, DVT, and PE. Anticoagulants such as low-dose subcutaneous heparin, fondaparinux (Arixtra), and low-dose enoxaparin (Lovenox) can be used in low doses to prevent clot formation, particularly in patients who are immobile after surgery or stroke or with acute medical illness or patients in the intensive care unit who are critically ill. These agents bind to antithrombin, which inhibits activated clotting factors in the intrinsic and common pathways of the anticoagulation cascade, thus interfering with factors IXa and Xa. Patients with a history of DVT, PE, atrial fibrillation, or stroke may be prescribed anticoagulants to prevent recurrence. Intravenous heparin or subcutaneous low-molecular-weight heparins such as enoxaparin (Lovenox) in higher doses may be administered when the patient requires immediate anticoagulation, as in the treatment of a clot. Low-molecular-weight heparins such as enoxaparin provide anticoagulant results that are uniform and consistent with the dosage used (based on patient weight and renal function), so frequent laboratory tests to assure adequate anticoagulation is achieved are generally unnecessary. Conversely, the results of heparin infusion vary widely from patient to patient and infusion rates must be adjusted based on frequent laboratory monitoring of the anticoagulation level via testing of activated partial thromboplastin time (aPTT). Patients treated with heparin products with DVT or PE require long-term anticoagulation therapy as outpatients and may be treated with oral warfarin (Coumadin) dosed based on regular PT/INR testing or by subcutaneously administered anticoagulants such as enoxaparin (Lovenox) dosed based on patient weight and renal function (Colbert & Mason, 2002; Weitz, 2011).

Cardioembolic stroke results when the heart fails to pump blood out of the cardiac chambers efficiently due to cardiac arrhythmia (usually atrial fibrillation) or valvular disease. When this occurs, some of the blood may remain in the chambers of the heart resulting in blood stasis and clot formation. Cardioembolic stroke results when the clot dislodges, becomes an embolus which lodges in the cerebral arteries and obstructs blood flow to the brain. In patients who have atrial fibrillation, oral anticoagulants such as warfarin (Coumadin) are used to prevent any pooled blood in the heart from forming a clot and causing cardioembolic stroke. Warfarin (Coumadin) interferes with the formation of vitamin K–dependent clotting factors in the liver (factors II, V, VII, and IX). Warfarin effects vary highly from patient to patient, and dosing must be adjusted based on laboratory measurement of the degree of anticoagulation via prothrombin time or the international normalized ratio (INR), a more accurate assessment of the degree of anticoagulation. Degree of anticoagulation should be checked at least monthly in patients using warfarin (Coumadin), or more frequently after dosage changes or changes in the patient's medication regimen. The amount of vitamin K ingested in the diet can change the anticoagulant effect of Coumadin. High amounts of green leafy vegetables and fats with high amounts of vitamin K can antagonize the effects of warfarin. In addition, many medications can change the metabolism of warfarin and alter its anticoagulation effects. Medications that inhibit the CYP2C9 pathways can increase warfarin effects and increase bleeding risk in patients taking warfarin. These include amiodarone (Cordarone), the fluoroquinolone antibiotics levofloxacin (Levaquin) and ciprofloxacin (Cipro), the macrolide antibiotics azithromycin (Zithromax) and clarithromycin (Biaxin), and the antibiotic sulfamethoxazole/trimethoprim (Septra Bactrim). The desired range for INR is 2.0 to 3.0 for most patients and 2.5 to 3.5 for patients with mechanical heart valves. In patients with atrial fibrillation or a history of cardioembolic stroke, the use of oral warfarin (Coumadin) in doses to achieve target INR of 2.0 to 3.0 is recommended. Aspirin is recommended in patients who cannot use warfarin, but aspirin is far less effective than warfarin in preventing stroke recurrence (Colbert & Mason, 2002; Weitz, 2011).

Dabigatran (Pradaxa), a new oral anticoagulant that directly interferes with thrombin in the coagulation cascade, has recently been approved for reducing stroke in patients with atrial fibrillation. This agent is dosed at 150 mg twice/day, and the frequent blood tests required with the use of warfarin (Coumadin) are not necessary. This agent has a peak onset of 2 h and a half-life of 12 to 14 h. It should not be given with other medications that increase the risk of bleeding (i.e., NSAIDs and anticoagulants). Rifampin should not be given with dabigatran because it decreases levels and therapeutic effects of dabigatran. Patients should watch for signs or symptoms of bleeding and notify their physician immediately if unexplained bruising or bleeding occurs (Colbert & Mason, 2002; Pradaxa, 2012; Weitz, 2011).

Unintended bleeding can be a side effect of anticoagulants. Patients receiving heparin or enoxaparin should be monitored for symptoms of bleeding and should routinely have blood work done to monitor platelet counts and monitor for anemia associated with undetected blood loss. An unusual side effect called heparin-induced thrombocytopenia, which can occur within the first 5 to 7 days of therapy, is associated with rapid decline in platelet counts and can be life threatening. Additional side effects of anticoagulant use include loss of appetite, upset stomach, vomiting, diarrhea, and bloating. Patients on anticoagulants should be taught to monitor for unusual or unexplained bruising, blood in the stool or urine, nosebleeds, and gum bleeding and to contact their physician if any of these are noted (Colbert & Mason, 2002; Weitz, 2011).

Lipid-Lowering Therapy   High-density lipoproteins (HDLs), also called the good cholesterol, are considered to be protective against stroke or cardiovascular events. Low-density lipoproteins (LDLs), also called the bad cholesterol, are associated with increased risk of stroke or other cardiovascular events such as MI. Elevated triglycerides (TG) can also increase stroke risk. Dyslipidemia is defined as an imbalance of lipids that includes one or more of the following: LDL greater than 100 mg/dl, HDL less than 40 mg/dl, or TG greater than 240 mg/dl. Statins, also known as HMG-CoA reductase inhibitors, are the first-line therapy for lowering lipids. HMG-CoA reductase is an enzyme that catalyzes an early rate-limiting step in cholesterol synthesis by the liver. These agents lower levels of LDL, total cholesterol, and TG. Some statins also increase HDL levels. They are the most effective and best-tolerated agents for lowering cholesterol and treating dyslipidemia. Table 20.2 lists dosing and common side effects associated with statins.

The most serious adverse reaction associated with statins is rhabdomyolysis, which is associated with breakdown of skeletal muscle and leads to release of intracellular content (e.g., myoglobin, potassium, and creatine kinase) into the bloodstream. **Myoglobin** can cause serious kidney damage and hyperkalemia can cause fatal arrhythmia. Presentation of rhabdomyolysis can range from **myopathy** to acute liver or renal dysfunction. Laboratory test findings usually include elevated creatine kinase; increased liver enzymes such as aspartate aminotransferase (AST), alanine transaminase (ALT), bilirubin, and INR denoting liver toxicity; and increased serum creatinine and blood urea nitrogen with renal failure (Bersot, 2011; Sanoski, 2011; Sisson & Van Tassell, 2011).

Other therapies that are used to decrease triglycerides or increase HDL include nicotinic acid (Niacin, Niaspan), which increases HDL by inhibiting lipid breakdown in the tissues, and fibrates such as gemfibrozil (Lopid), which increases HDL and decreases triglyceride levels by increasing lipid metabolism. Combining statin with medications that inhibit CYP3A4 or CYP2C9 can result in increased levels of statins and associated toxicity. Table 20.3 lists important drug interactions with medications that decrease lipids (Bersot, 2011; Sanoski, 2011).

See table 20.2 in the web resource for a full list of medication-specific indications, dosing recommendations, and side effects.

Table 20.2 Medications Used to Decrease Lipids

Medication	Side effects affecting rehab							Other side effects or considerations
High-potency statins: Decrease lipids by 35%-55%.								
Atorvastatin (Lipitor)	Cog +	S +	A 0	Motor +	D +	Com 0	F +	Available in generic form. Side effects: Headache, gastrointestinal intolerance, flu-like symptoms, myalgia (5%), myopathy (0.2%-0.4%), fatigue. Liver effects: Increased liver enzyme (AST/ALT). Dose dependent (0.5%-2.5%); managed by reducing dose. Rare events of liver damage, hepatitis, or jaundice can occur. Drug interactions: Metabolized by CYP3A4. When used with medications metabolized by the same pathway can increase risk of rhabdomyolysis. This drug interaction is managed by avoiding these interacting medications whenever possible and by using lowest effective statin dose.
Rosuvastatin (Crestor)	Cog +	S +	A 0	Motor +	D +	Com 0	F +	Side effects: Headache, gastrointestinal intolerance, flu-like symptoms, myalgia (5%), myopathy (0.2%-0.4%), fatigue. Liver effects: Increased liver enzymes (AST/ ALT); managed by reducing dose. Rare liver damage, hepatitis, or jaundice can occur. Drug interactions: Metabolized by CYP2C9. When used with medications metabolized by the same pathway can increase risk of rhabdomyolysis. This drug interaction is managed by avoiding these interacting medications whenever possible and by using lowest effective statin dose. Can potentiate effects of warfarin (Coumadin); may require Coumadin dose adjustment.
Intermediate-potency statin: Decreases lipids by 30%-45%.								
Simvastatin (Zocor)	Cog +	S +	A 0	Motor +	D +	Com 0	F +	Available in generic form; 30% eliminated by kidneys. Side effects: Headache, gastrointestinal intolerance, flu-like symptoms, myalgia (5%), myopathy (0.2%-0.4%), fatigue. Liver effects: Increased liver enzyme (AST/ALT). Dose dependent (0.5%-2.5%); managed by reducing dose. Rare events of liver damage, hepatitis, or jaundice can occur. Drug interactions: Metabolized by CYP3A4. When used with medications metabolized by the same pathway can increase risk of rhabdomyolysis. This drug interaction is managed by avoiding these interacting medications whenever possible and by using lowest effective statin dose.

› continued

Table 20.2 › *continued*

Medication	Side effects affecting rehab							Other side effects or considerations
Low-potency statins: Decrease lipids by 20%-40%.								
Lovastatin (Mevacor)	Cog	S	A	Motor	D	Com	F	Available in generic form; 30% eliminated by kidneys.
	+	+	0	+	+	0	+	Side effects: Headache, gastrointestinal intolerance, flu-like symptoms, myalgia (5%), myopathy (0.2%-0.4%), fatigue.
								Liver effects: Increased liver enzyme (AST/ALT). Dose dependent (0.5%-2.5%); managed by reducing dose. Rare events of liver damage, hepatitis, or jaundice can occur.
								Can lead to rhabdomyolysis in rare cases. Managed by avoiding interactions and using lowest effective dose.
								Drug interactions: Metabolized by CYP3A4. When used with medications metabolized by the same pathway can increase risk of rhabdomyolysis. This drug interaction is managed by avoiding these interacting medications whenever possible and by using lowest effective statin dose.
Pravastatin (Pravachol)	Cog	S	A	Motor	D	Com	F	Available in generic form. 60% eliminated by kidneys; avoid in patients with renal insufficiency.
	+	+	0	+	+	0	+	Side effects: Headache, gastrointestinal intolerance, flu-like symptoms, myalgia (5%), myopathy (0.2%-0.4%), fatigue.
								Drug interactions: None.
								Metabolized by sulfonation.
								Safest to use with warfarin (Coumadin).
Fluvastatin (Lescol)	Cog	S	A	Motor	D	Com	F	Available in generic form.
	+	+	0	+	+	0	+	Side effects: Headache, gastrointestinal intolerance, flu-like symptoms, myalgia (5%), myopathy (0.2%-0.4%), fatigue.
								Liver effects: Increased liver enzyme (AST/ALT). Dose dependent (0.5%-2.5%); managed by reducing dose. Rare events of liver damage, hepatitis, or jaundice can occur.
								Can lead to rhabdomyolysis in rare cases.
								Drug interactions: Potentiates warfarin (Coumadin) effects. Managed by avoiding interactions and using lowest effective dose. Metabolized by CYP2C9. When used with medications metabolized by the same pathway can increase risk of rhabdomyolysis. This drug interaction is managed by avoiding these interacting medications whenever possible and by using lowest effective statin dose.

Medication	Side effects affecting rehab							Other side effects or considerations
Agents that increase HDL: Nicotinic acid increases HDL by 15%-35%, decreases LDL by 5%-25% and TG by 20%-50%, and inhibits lipid breakdown from adipose tissue. Gemfibrozil increases HDL by 10%-30% and decreases TG by 20%-50%.								
Nicotinic acid (Niaspan, Niacin)	Cog 0	S 0	A 0	Motor +	D 0	Com 0	F 0	Achieves better results in elderly—less hepatotoxic than fibrates. Must titrate dose; increase by 500 mg every 4 wk. Long acting prescription form preferred, less hepatotoxic than short acting over-the-counter forms. Side effects: Flushing (use aspirin to prevent it), itching, headache, reduced insulin sensitivity.
Gemfibrozil (Lopid)	Cog 0	S 0	A 0	Motor ++	D ++	Com 0	F ++	Available in generic form. Side effects: Diarrhea, myopathy, cholelithiasis, abdominal pain. Drug interactions: Can increase international normalized ratio when used with warfarin (Coumadin).

Cog = cognition; S = sedation; A = agitation or mania; Motor = discoordination; D = dysphagia; Com = communication; F = falls; HDL = high-density lipoprotein; LDL = low-density lipoprotein; TG = triglyceride; AST = aspartate aminotransferase; ALT = alanine transaminase.

The likelihood rating scale for encountering the side effects is as follows: 0 = Almost no probability of encountering side effects. + = Little likelihood of encountering side effects. +/++ = Low probability of encountering side effects; however, probability increases with increased dosage. ++ = Medium likelihood of encountering side effects. +++ = High likelihood of encountering side effects, particularly with high doses. ++++ = Highest likelihood of encountering side effects; best to avoid in at-risk patients.

Table 20.3   Drug Interactions With Medications That Decrease Lipids

Statin medication	Interacting medication	Effects of interaction
All statins	Red yeast rice, Niacin, fibrates (gemfibrozil, fenofibrate), daptomycin (Cubicin), danazol (Danocrine)	Increased statin levels and toxicity. Hold statins while receiving daptomycin. Increased risk of myopathy and rhabdomyolysis; requires dose adjustment of statin or interacting agent.
Lovastatin (Mevacor) Simvastatin (Zocor)	HIV antivirals: indinavir (Crixivan), nelfinavir (Viracept), ritonavir (Norvir), saquinavir (Invirase) Azole antifungals: ketoconazole (Nizoral), fluconazole (Diflucan), itraconazole (Sporanox) Macrolides: erythromycin, clarithromycin (Biaxin) Calcium channel blockers: verapamil (Isoptin, Calan), diltiazem (Cardizem) Antiarrhythmic: amiodarone (Cordarone) Proton pump inhibitor: omeprazole (Prilosec) Cyclosporine (Sandimmune) Other: nefazodone (Serzone), aprepitant (Emend), imatinib (Gleevec), grapefruit juice	Increased statin levels and toxicity. Increased risk of myopathy and rhabdomyolysis; requires dose adjustment of statin or interacting agent.

› continued

Table 20.3 › *continued*

Statin medication	Interacting medication	Effects of interaction
Lovastatin (Mevacor) Fluvastatin (Lescol)	HIV antivirals: efavirenz (Sustiva), nevirapine (Viramune) Barbiturates: phenobarbital (Luminal), butabarbital (Butisol) Antidiabetic: pioglitazone (Actos) Anticonvulsants: phenytoin (Dilantin), carbamazepine (Tegretol) Other: rifampin, St. John's wort	Decreased statin levels and effects. Increased risk of high lipid levels, cardiac event, or stroke; requires increase of statin dose.
Simvastatin (Zocor) Lovastatin (Mevacor) Gemfibrozil (Lopid)	Anticoagulant: warfarin (Coumadin)	Decreased metabolism and increased effects of warfarin (Coumadin). Increased risk of bleeding; requires dose decrease of warfarin (Coumadin).
Fibrate: Gemfibrozil (Lopid)	All statins	Increased levels, effects, and toxicity of statins. Increased risk of myopathy and rhabdomyolysis; requires dose adjustment of statin or interacting agent.
	Anticoagulant: warfarin (Coumadin)	Increased effects, international normalized ratio, and toxicity of warfarin (Coumadin). Increased risk of bleeding; requires 50% decrease of warfarin (Coumadin) dose.

HIV = human immunodeficiency virus.

The Stroke Prevention by Aggressive Reduction in Cholesterol Levels (SPARCL) Trial, published in 2006, studied the effects of initiating statin therapy in almost 5,000 patients with no known cardiovascular disease who had recently experienced a stroke or TIA. Of these patients, 2,365 patients were placed on atorvastatin 80 mg/day and an additional 2,366 patients were treated with a placebo to see whether statin therapy had an effect on the incidence of secondary stroke. Compared with the patients who were treated with a placebo, the group placed on atorvastatin had an 18% reduction in the risk of stroke, a 35% reduction in the risk of major coronary events, a 42% reduction in coronary heart disease events, and a 45% reduction in revascularization procedures such as coronary artery bypass grafting (CABG). This landmark trial prompted a change in stroke-prevention guidelines (SPARCL Investigators, 2006).

The American Heart Association (AHA) and American Stroke Association (ASA) guidelines recommend that patients with elevated cholesterol who experience an ischemic stroke or TIA be initiated on statin therapy to reach target LDL levels of less than 70 mg/dl (Liu-DeRyke & Bladwin, 2012). In addition, patients with ischemic stroke or TIA with low HDL levels should be considered candidates for niacin or gemfibrozil. The 2011 AHA/ASA Guidelines for Treatment of Patients with Stroke or TIA were revised to also recommend that all patients who experience stroke or TIA (even without diagnosed cardiovascular artery disease) be started on lipid-lowering therapy (Furie et al., 2011; Goldstein et al., 2011).

PATIENT CASE 2

H.B. is an 82-yr-old male who was admitted to the emergency room after 2 wk of unexplained muscle stiffness and soreness. His medical history includes prostate carcinoma, coronary artery disease with coronary artery bypass grafting (CABG), hyperlipidemia, atrial fibrillation, and cardioembolic cerebrovascular accident. He is married, retired, and uses no tobacco, alcohol, or illicit drugs. His home medications include the anticoagulant Coumadin for atrial fibrillation; Cordarone for cardiac arrhythmia; aspirin; potassium; and Zocor (simvastatin), which he recently started at 80 mg/day. His laboratory results on admission included the following:

Creatine kinase: 6670

Aspartate aminotransferase (AST): 1508

Alanine transaminase (ALT): 601

Blood urea nitrogen (BUN): 110

Creatinine: 3.5

INR: >5.0

K: >6.0

Question

What adverse drug reaction may explain these findings? What drug interactions may have been involved?

Answer

He was recently started on simvastatin (Zocor) 80 mg, which is metabolized by CYP3A4 liver enzyme systems. H.B. was already taking amiodarone (Cordarone), which is a known CYP3A4 inhibitor. This drug interaction resulted in increased levels of simvastatin, thus causing myopathy, elevated liver function, and rhabdomyolysis. In addition, both simvastatin and amiodarone can increase the INR in patients taking Coumadin, resulting in increased anticoagulation and increased bleeding risk in H.B.

In patients who are older or who are on medications that interact with a medication to be added, one must remember the following rule of thumb: Start low and go slow (especially with the elderly). Always consider possible drug interactions of the new medication with concurrent drug therapy, and always consider the effects of concurrent disease states.

Coronary Artery Disease

Coronary artery disease (CAD), also known as ischemic heart disease, is the leading cause of death in the United States. Ischemic heart disease may present as stable angina, unstable angina, or acute MI. CAD is associated with hyperlipidemia and atherosclerosis of the coronary vessels. Hyperlipidemia causes progressive development of plaques (deposits of lipids accompanied by inflammatory products) in the coronary vessel wall. This process begins early in life and continues throughout the lifespan. By middle age enough fatty deposits have accumulated to cause episodes of acute obstruction of blood flow to the heart, resulting in ischemia and chest pain. Risk factors for CAD include diabetes, smoking, hypertension, hyperlipidemia, obesity, sedentary lifestyle, high uric acid levels, type A personality, and the use of corticosteroids and progestins (Dobesch & Stacy, 2011; Michel & Hoffman, 2011).

Incidence

CAD is one of the leading causes of death globally, and it appears that this high incidence will persist for at least the next two decades. In Europe, one in five males and one in seven females die from CAD. The high incidence of CAD globally has turned this disorder into an epidemic (Clarify, 2009). CAD is the leading cause of death in both sexes and accounts for one third of all deaths in developed countries. CAD is more common in males earlier in life. After age 75 yr the incidence in females is equal to or exceeds that in males.

Etiology and Pathophysiology

The rehabilitation therapist needs to be acutely aware of symptoms of ischemic heart disease because of the high incidence of the disease in the United States and the severe complications associated with it. The therapist also needs to understand how exercise affects ischemic heart disease and how medications used to treat this disease may affect the rehabilitation process (Colbert & Mason, 2002; Ciccone, 2007).

Stable angina is also known as effort angina. Stable angina pain occurs when myocardial oxygen demand exceeds what the heart can deliver. The typical underlying cause of stable angina is a fixed coronary stenosis along with compromised blood flow and slow, progressive plaque growth that allows for the occasional development of collateral flow. Stable angina typically presents as chest discomfort and associated symptoms precipitated by some activity (e.g., running, walking). Symptoms are minimal or nonexistent at rest. Symptoms typically abate several minutes after cessation of precipitating activities and resume when activity resumes (Carter & Saseen, 2002; Dobesch & Stacy, 2011; Michel & Hoffman, 2011).

Angina associated with ischemic heart disease is described as pressure, crushing, burning, or tightness associated with anterior chest pain (96%), left arm pain (84%), left lower arm pain (30%), and neck pain (22%). Some patients have angina without any pain; this is termed silent ischemia. Diabetics tend to have silent ischemia, and women tend to have atypical chest pain or silent ischemia. Ischemic chest pain may resemble pain arising from other sources, such as gastric pain associated with gastroesophageal reflux disease. Classic stable angina has symptoms of chest pain of a characteristic quality and duration that is provoked by exertion or emotional stress. This pain is relieved with nitroglycerin administration (Carter & Saseen, 2002; Dobesch & Stacy, 2011; Michel & Hoffman, 2011).

Acute coronary syndrome includes unstable angina as well as acute MI. Acute coronary syndrome is most often associated with a rupture of lipid plaque along with an inflammatory cascade of platelet migration and aggregation at the site, activation of thrombin and the formation of a thrombus, and coronary artery vasoconstriction. This results in complete or partial obstruction of the coronary artery and reduced blood flow to the heart. Goals of treatment of acute coronary syndrome

are to relieve chest pain and restore coronary blood flow. Additional goals are to prevent progression of unstable angina to MI, minimize cardiac tissue damage associated with an MI, and prevent event-associated heart failure or death (Carter & Saseen, 2002; Dobesch & Stacy, 2011; Michel & Hoffman, 2011).

Unstable angina is a reversible event that involves acute obstruction of coronary flow due to partial obstruction of the coronary artery with or without spasm. Unstable angina is defined as angina pectoris that worsens, occurs at rest, and is more severe than stable angina. Attacks of unstable angina last longer and occur more frequently than attacks of stable angina. Unstable angina may occur unpredictably at rest; this may be a serious indicator of an impending heart attack. What differentiates stable angina from unstable angina (other than symptoms) is the pathophysiology of the atherosclerosis. In unstable angina, the reduction of coronary flow is due to transient platelet aggregation on apparently normal endothelium, coronary artery spasm, or coronary thrombosis (Dobesch & Stacy, 2011; Michel & Hoffman, 2011).

Acute coronary syndrome differs from stable angina in that the initial event is thought to be a reduction in coronary blood flow associated with plaque rupture rather than an increase in myocardial oxygen demand associated with inadequate blood flow due to stable obstruction. Treatment of unstable angina includes addressing the pain, supplemental oxygen, nitroglycerin, and aspirin. Anticoagulant therapy such as intravenous heparin is used to prevent clot formation; intravenous beta blockers, followed by oral beta blockers, are used to reduce oxygen demand by the heart; and intravenous morphine is commonly used to treat pain. An angiotensin-converting enzyme inhibitor is added if left ventricular dysfunction is present. Anyone with acute coronary syndrome should be emergently treated with chew-and-swallow aspirin (two baby aspirin or one full-strength aspirin). This should be followed by an anticoagulant such as low-molecular-weight heparin or intravenous heparin because platelet aggregation and development of thrombosis plays a major role in acute coronary syndrome. Clopidogrel (Plavix) is given before percutaneous coronary intervention (PCI), and a combination of aspirin and clopidogrel should be continued as long-term therapy after PCI to prevent platelet aggregation and reocclusion of the coronary arteries. A new agent called prasugrel (Effient), which is similar in efficacy to clopidogrel, is used as an alternative in patients who are undergoing PCI or with acute coronary syndrome. Its onset is more rapid, its metabolic process has fewer steps, and it is less prone to drug interactions than clopidogrel (Dobesch & Stacy, 2011; Michel & Hoffman, 2011). However, prasugrel also increases the risk of bleeding, especially in the elderly patient compared to clopidogrel.

In 2006, 1.57 million patients were admitted to the hospital for acute coronary syndrome, 1.47 million were admitted for unstable angina or acute MI not associated with ST elevation, and 0.33 million were admitted for acute MI associated with ST elevation. Survivors of MI continue to have a poor prognosis, and their risk of mortality and morbidity is up to 15 times greater than that of the rest of the population. A 30% reduction in mortality from CAD has occurred in the past 30 yr. Factors that have reduced mortality include the introduction of coronary care units, coronary artery bypass grafting, thrombolytic therapy, percutaneous coronary intervention, and a renewed emphasis on lifestyle modification (Dobesch & Stacy, 2011; Michel & Hoffman, 2011).

Acute MI associated with ST elevation on the electrocardiogram, called STEMI, is associated with complete obstruction by a fibrin-rich thrombus. Acute MI not associated with ST elevation, called non-STEMI, is associated with incomplete obstruction of a dynamic clot composed of platelets without fibrin (white clots). Both ST-elevated and non-ST-elevated MI can be treated with percutaneous coronary interventions (PCI), which is the mechanical opening of the coronary artery obstruction conducted in the cardiac catheterization laboratory. Percutaneous transluminal coronary angioplasty (PTCA) involves inflating a balloon in the coronary artery to compress the plaque in the walls of the artery and increase the size of the lumen to facilitate blood flow. Another procedure that is done during a percutaneous coronary intervention (PCI) is implantation of

a stent (a small mesh tube) into the artery to prop it open. The stent may be impregnated with medication to help prevent reocclusion of the vessel. Plaque formation may also be mechanically removed with rotational or laser atherectomy (Dobesch & Stacy, 2011; Michel & Hoffman, 2011). After an acute MI, patients should be on lifelong therapy of aspirin, a beta blocker, and a medication to lower lipid levels such as a statin. An angiotensin-converting enzyme inhibitor should also be added if the MI is associated with left ventricular dysfunction and associated decrease in ejection fraction (EF) by the heart are present. The addition of an antiplatelet medication such as clopidogrel (Plavix) is recommended in all patients who have PCI, especially with stent placement, to help to prevent stent or coronary artery reocclusion by thrombus formation associated with vascular trauma of the PCA and stent insertion (Dobesch & Stacy, 2011; Michel & Hoffman, 2011).

STEMI can also be treated with thrombolytic (clot buster) medication such as tissue plasminogen activator to break up the occluding thrombus and provide coronary reperfusion in the event that cardiac catheterization is not readily available. Time is of the essence in re-establishing coronary flow and minimizing the extent of cardiac necrosis and residual cardiac damage associated with acute MI. Non-STEMI is not treated with thrombolytic therapy but is treated with emergent interventional cardiac catheterization. In the event that cardiac catheterization is delayed, potent antiplatelet therapy such as the intravenous glycoprotein IIb/IIIa inhibitors can be used short term until the cardiac catheterization can take place.

Rehabilitation Considerations

The rehabilitation specialist should be cognizant of whether patients are taking medications for coronary artery (ischemic heart) disease and should ensure that the patient taking sublingual nitroglycerin to manage angina pain has the drug within reach during rehabilitation sessions. Angina attacks may occur during rehabilitation because exercise increases oxygen demand. The rehabilitation specialist should be acutely aware of the limitations of each patient treated in therapy and should consider whether the rehabilitation activities can increase myocardial oxygen demand and precipitate angina pain. The specialist should also be aware of the effects of the patient's medications on exercise. For example, some calcium blockers and beta blockers slow down heart rate and decrease contractility. The therapist needs to take this into account when designing an exercise program for the patient taking these medications. The rehabilitation specialist should also be aware of the side effects of medications. For example, calcium channel blockers and nitrates can cause orthostatic or postural hypotension; this may place the patient at risk for falls when bending or changing positions rapidly (Ciccone, 2007).

Medication Therapy

Ischemic pain is associated with oxygen delivery that is inadequate to meet the demands of the heart. Therapy for angina is focused on either increasing oxygen delivery or decreasing oxygen demand by the heart. The amount of oxygen required by the heart is determined by the rate of heart contraction, heart wall tension, and heart contractility. Calcium channel blockers, nitrates, and beta blockers are effective in increasing oxygen delivery or reducing myocardial oxygen demand and can be used as chronic therapy in the management of angina. Table 20.4 summarizes medications used to treat ischemic heart disease (Colbert & Mason, 2002; Dobesch & Stacy, 2011; Michel & Hoffman, 2011).

 See table 20.4 in the web resource for a full list of medication-specific indications, dosing recommendations, side effects, and other considerations.

Table 20.4   Medications Used to Treat Ischemic Heart Disease

Medication	Side effects affecting rehab							Other side effects or considerations
Beta blockers: Reduce sympathetic tone, myocardial oxygen demand, and ischemia.								
Atenolol* (Tenormin)	Cog ++	S ++	A 0	Motor ++	D ++	Com +	F ++	Indicated in ischemic heart disease. Avoid abrupt discontinuation.
Betaxolol* (Kerlone)	Cog ++	S ++	A 0	Motor ++	D ++	Com +	F ++	Do not allow heart rate to increase with exercise.
Bisoprolol* (Zebeta)	Cog ++	S ++	A 0	Motor ++	D ++	Com +	F ++	Side effects: Nausea, diarrhea, bronchospasm, cold extremities, exacerbation of Raynaud's syndrome, bradycardia, heart block, orthostasis, fatigue, dizziness, alopecia, abnormal vision, hyperglycemia, hyperlipidemia, sexual dysfunction.
Metoprolol* (Lopressor, Toprol XL— extended release)	Cog ++	S ++	A 0	Motor ++	D ++	Com +	F ++	
Nadolol* (Corgard)	Cog ++	S ++	A 0	Motor ++	D ++	Com +	F ++	Drug interactions: Avoid administering with medications that increase sympathetic tone (e.g., cocaine, amphetamines, decongestants such as pseudoephedrine); increased heart rate and arrhythmia may occur.
Propranolol (Inderal, Inderal LA— long acting)	Cog +++	S +++	A ++	Motor ++	D ++	Com +	F +++	Propranolol is lipophilic and has higher incidence of effects on central nervous system (i.e., hallucinations, decreased concentration, insomnia, nightmares, and depression).
Timolol (Blocadren)	Cog ++	S ++	A 0	Motor ++	D ++	Com +	F ++	

Medication	Side effects affecting rehab							Other side effects or considerations
Calcium channel blockers: Used to treat angina; control heart rate and increase vasodilation, increasing risk of bradycardia and orthostasis.								
Diltiazem (Cardizem, Cardizem CD—extended release, Dilacor SR—extended release)	Cog 0	S 0	A 0	Motor +	D +	Com 0	F +	Side effects: Bradycardia, nausea, peripheral edema, hypotension. Verapamil is associated with severe constipation; administer laxative with this medication. Food and drug interactions: Grapefruit juice (>200 ml) can increase levels of this medication and should not be consumed within 2 h before or 4 h after administration.
Verapamil (Calan, Isoptin, Calan SR, Isoptin SR, Covera-HS)	Cog 0	S 0	A 0	Motor +	D +++	Com 0	F +	Decreases liver metabolism of carbamazepine (Tegretol), simvastatin (Zocor), atorvastatin (Lipitor), and lovastatin (Mevacor). This can lead to toxicity from these drugs.
Calcium antagonists (dihydropyridines): Used to treat angina; cause vasodilation without controlling heart rate. Should be combined with another agent that controls heart rate. Vasodilatory effects increase the risk of orthostasis.								
Amlodipine (Norvasc)	Cog +	S 0	A +	Motor +	D ++	Com +	F ++	Side effects: Dizziness, flushing, headache, gingival hyperplasia, peripheral edema, mood changes, gastrointestinal side effects. Food interactions: Grapefruit juice (>200 ml) can increase levels of this medication and should not be consumed within 2 h before or 4 h after administration.
Felodipine (Plendil)	Cog +	S 0	A +	Motor +	D ++	Com +	F ++	Side effects: Dizziness, flushing, headache, gingival hyperplasia, peripheral edema, mood changes, gastrointestinal side effects. Food interactions: Grapefruit juice (>200 ml) can increase levels of this medication and should not be consumed within 2 h before or 4 h after administration. Drug interactions: Decreases liver metabolism of carbamazepine (Tegretol), simvastatin (Zocor), atorvastatin (Lipitor), and lovastatin (Mevacor). This can lead to toxicity from these drugs.
Isradipine (Dynacirc)	Cog +	S 0	A +	Motor +	D ++	Com +	F ++	
Nicardipine (Cardene SR)	Cog +	S 0	A +	Motor +	D ++	Com +	F ++	
Nifedipine (Adalat CC, Procardia XL)	Cog +	S 0	A +	Motor +	D ++	Com +	F ++	
Nisoldipine (Sular)	Cog +	S 0	A +	Motor +	D ++	Com +	F ++	

› *continued*

Table 20.4 › *continued*

Medication	Side effects affecting rehab							Other side effects or considerations

ACE inhibitors: Used to improve exercise tolerance in patients with congestive heart failure and ventricular hypertrophy and to prevent diabetic nephropathy in diabetics with hypertension. Well tolerated with few side effects.

Medication	Cog	S	A	Motor	D	Com	F	Other
Benazepril (Lotensin)	+	+	0	+	+	0	+	May cause acute renal failure with renal artery stenosis.
Captopril (Capoten)	+	+	0	+	++	0	+	Reduce dose with renal impairment.
Enalapril (Vasotec)	+	+	0	+	+	0	+	Side effects: Hypotension, cough, hyperkalemia, headache, dizziness, fatigue, nausea, angioedema, renal impairment, allergic reactions, taste loss, and taste disturbances are more common with captopril and are believed to be associated with its sulfhydryl group.
Fosinopril (Monopril)	+	+	0	+	+	0	+	
Lisinopril (Prinivil, Zestril)	+	+	0	+	+	0	+	Drug interactions: Diuretics can increase the risk of acute renal failure with ACE inhibitors. Hold diuretics for several days before initiating these agents to avoid acute hypotension.
Moexipril (Univasc)	+	+	0	+	+	0	+	
Quinapril (Accupril)	+	+	0	+	+	0	+	Use of potassium-sparing diuretics or potassium supplements increases risk of hyperkalemia, especially in patients with renal impairment.
Ramipril (Altace)	+	+	0	+	+	0	+	
Trandolapril (Mavik)	+	+	0	+	+	0	+	

Angiotensin II receptor blockers: Used in patients with congestive heart failure or diabetics who cannot tolerate ACE inhibitor-associated cough. Well tolerated with few side effects.

Medication	Cog	S	A	Motor	D	Com	F	Other
Candesartan (Atacand)	+	+	0	+	+	0	+	Side effects: Hypotension, hyperkalemia, headache, dizziness, fatigue, nausea, angioedema, renal impairment.
Irbesartan (Avapro)	+	+	0	+	+	0	+	Drug interactions: Diuretics can increase the risk of acute renal failure with angiotensin II receptor blockers.
Losartan (Cozaar)	+	+	0	+	+	0	+	
Telmisartan (Micardis)	+	+	0	+	+	0	+	Use of potassium-sparing diuretics or potassium supplements increases risk of hyperkalemia, especially in patients with renal impairment.
Valsartan (Diovan)	+	+	0	+	+	0	+	

Nitrates used in angina

Medication	Cog	S	A	Motor	D	Com	F	Other
Nitroglycerin Sublingual intravenous, topical paste, and patch	+	0	+	+	++	+	++	Dizziness, flushing, headache, gingival hyperplasia, peripheral edema; tolerance develops with continuous use. Allow a nitrate free interval (8-12 h) to reduce tolerance with chronic use.

Medication	Side effects affecting rehab							Other side effects or considerations
Isosorbide dinitrate (Isordil) Isosorbide mononitrate (Ismo)	Cog	S	A	Motor	D	Com	F	Dizziness, flushing, headache, gingival hyperplasia, peripheral edema; tolerance develops with continuous use.
	+	0	+	+	++	+	++	

*Cardioselective in low doses.

Cog = cognition; S = sedation; A = agitation or mania; Motor = discoordination; D = dysphagia; Com = communication; F = falls; ACE = angiotensin-converting enzyme; MI = myocardial infarction.

The likelihood rating scale for encountering the side effects is as follows: 0 = Almost no probability of encountering side effects. + = Little likelihood of encountering side effects. +/++ = Low probability of encountering side effects; however, probability increases with increased dosage. ++ = Medium likelihood of encountering side effects. +++ = High likelihood of encountering side effects, particularly with high doses. ++++ = Highest likelihood of encountering side effects; best to avoid in at-risk patients.

Beta Blockers

Beta blockers decrease heart rate, blood pressure, contractility, and afterload, resulting in decreased myocardial oxygen consumption. This can be beneficial during exercise. Exercise may also facilitate skeletal muscle vasodilation. Exercising patients on beta blockers may experience blunted cardiac output and heart rate. Several rehabilitation concerns are related to the side effects of beta blockers. The reduction in blood pressure can result in orthostatic hypotension, putting the patient at risk for an episode of syncope and a related fall. The decrease in heart rate and contraction force, although helpful in minimizing tachycardia and exertion on the heart, decreases the patient's maximal exercise capacity. This means that the patient's resting heart rate and exercising heart rate will not be as high as they would be if the patient was unmedicated. The rehabilitation specialist must be cognizant of this and not overtax the heart by trying to reach maximal age-adjusted target heart rates for unmedicated individuals (Peel & Mossberg, 1995).

Beta blockers are effective for treating chronic exertional angina as monotherapy and in combination with nitrates or calcium channel blockers. Beta blockers should be first-line drug therapy for chronic angina because they are more effective in reducing episodes of silent ischemia, reducing early morning ischemic activity, and improving mortality after a non-Q-wave MI than are nitrates or calcium channel blockers. Beta blockers are used in the treatment of all patients with acute coronary events because they reduce the extent of cardiac tissue necrosis and permanent damage to the heart after an acute event. Patients with severe asthma, rest angina, or angina associated with coronary vasospasm may be better treated with calcium channel blockers or long-acting nitrates. One of the most common reasons for discontinuing beta blocker therapy is related to side effects of fatigue, malaise, and depression. Beta blockers should be tapered over about 2 days to minimize risk of withdrawal reactions in patients who are discontinuing therapy (Ciccone, 2007; Colbert & Mason, 2002; Dobesch & Stacy, 2011; Michel & Hoffman, 2011).

Nitrates

Nitrates increase cyclic guanosine monophosphate (GMP) in vascular smooth muscle and cause vasodilation of the venous system, thus reducing preload. Nitroglycerin also alleviates angina attacks by causing vasodilation of the coronary arteries. It is administered sublingually or by spray in the outpatient setting and is provided by intravenous administration in the hospital setting in the management of acute angina or MI. Nitrates can also be used routinely by oral or topical (paste or patch) routes to prevent angina attacks. Isosorbide dinitrate and isosorbide mononitrate are administered orally. Chronic nitrate administration over a 24 h period can be associated with reduced effectiveness, called tolerance. Therefore, nitroglycerin patches are placed in the morning for 12 h and then removed for 12 h during sleep and oral products are administered during waking hours. Side effects of nitrates include headache, orthostatic hypotension, dizziness, and nausea. The orthostatic hypotension and headache are due to venodilation. Nitrates can also cause reflex tachycardia (compensatory increase in heart rate) because they cause vasodilation. This is why beta blockers (slow heart rate) and nitrates may be combined in angina treatment (Ciccone, 2007; Colbert & Mason, 2002).

Calcium Channel Blockers

Calcium channel blockers inhibit the initiation of contraction and function as vasodilators by influencing the vascular smooth muscle. Calcium channel blockers block voltage gated calcium channels in cardiac muscle and blood vessels resulting in decreased contractility, automaticity, and AV conduction. Cardiac relaxation and vasodilatation is caused by the decreased influx of calcium into cardiac muscle and into vascular smooth muscle cells. Resultant vasodilation increases blood and oxygen supply into the myocardial muscle and reduced cardiac contraction reduces the myocardial oxygen demand. Calcium channel blockers are also effective in preventing angina attacks because of their vasodilatory properties. They are more effective than beta blockers in preventing angina associated with spasm of the coronary arteries but are not as effective as beta blockers in preventing acute coronary events. Beta blockers are the preferred agents in patients with ischemic heart disease after an acute MI. Patients who do not tolerate beta blockers are good candidates for calcium

channel blocker therapy. Table 20.4 provides additional information on beta blockers and calcium channel blockers (Dobesch & Stacy, 2011; Michel & Hoffman, 2011).

An appropriate regular exercise program is an important component in the treatment of angina. Exercise increases production of nitric oxide (a vasodilator), improves exercise tolerance, can reduce fatigue, and improves the patient's ability to accomplish daily activities. Chronic prophylactic therapy should be instituted for patients who have more than one angina episode per day. Beta-adrenergic blocking agents are the agents of choice for managing angina but are associated with fatigue and limit heart rate. Calcium channel blockers, which can also be used, provide better skeletal muscle oxygenation, resulting in decreased fatigue and better exercise tolerance. Diltiazem (Cardizem) or verapamil (Isoptin, Calan) are preferred agents when a calcium channel is needed because they control heart rate and increase vasodilation. The dihydropyridine calcium channel blockers do not control heart rate and can excessively elevate heart rate with exercise, which can contribute to angina pain. The dihydropyridine calcium channel blockers should only be used when the patient is receiving concurrent medications to control the heart rate.

Antiplatelet Therapies

Because acute coronary syndrome is associated with platelet aggregation and thrombus formation, antiplatelet therapy such as aspirin and clopidogrel (Plavix) is used in primary and secondary prevention of acute coronary events. Patients who are undergoing PCI are usually given a loading dose of clopidogrel to prevent platelet aggregation during and after the procedure and reduce the chances of reocclusion of the coronary arteries. A newer therapy, prasugrel (Effient), is similar to clopidogrel (Plavix) in efficacy but increases the risk of bleeding, particularly in the older patient. Because the metabolic processes involved in converting prasugrel (Effient) to its active form differ from those associated with activating clopidogrel (Plavix), prasugrel may have less potential for reduced activity when combined with the proton pump inhibitors such as omeprazole (Prilosec) (Dobesch & Stacy, 2011; Michel & Hoffman, 2011).

Side effects to monitor for in patients taking antiplatelet therapy include bleeding and gastrointestinal upset. Enteric-coated aspirin can be used to reduce gastrointestinal upset. After PCI, patients are placed on a combination of aspirin and clopidogrel; this combination increases bleeding risk, particularly in the elderly patient. Health care professionals must counsel these patients to avoid self-medicating with over-the-counter NSAIDs such as ibuprofen (Motrin) or naproxen (Aleve) or combination products containing aspirin when they are on these medications in order to avoid increasing risk of gastrointestinal bleeding as well as reducing the cardioprotective effects of the antiplatelet therapy (Dobesch & Stacy, 2011; Michel & Hoffman, 2011).

Lipid-Lowering Agents

Medications used to lower lipid levels, such as the statins, are essential in managing coronary heart disease. Fifty percent of Americans have elevated cholesterol and 25% have hypercholesterolemia (cholesterol levels >240 mg/dl). In addition to heart-healthy diet, exercise, and weight reduction, these use of lipid-lowering medications can reduce cardiac risk. Treatment of hyperlipidemia slows, stops, and may even reverse atherosclerotic plaque buildup in the blood vessels. Treatment improves endothelial structure and results in more stable plaques and less risk of rupture with an acute coronary event (Bersot, 2011; Grundy, 2001; Knopp, 1999; Sanoski, 2011; Talbert, 2005).

HDL, the good cholesterol, is cardioprotective and decreases acute coronary risk. LDL, the bad cholesterol, increases cardiac risk. Elevated triglycerides (TG) also increase cardiac risk. Dyslipidemia is defined as an imbalance of lipids that includes one or more of the following: LDL >100 mg/dl, HDL <40 mg/dl, and TG >240 mg/dl. Goals for patients with cardiac risk factors are to reduce LDL to <70 mg/dl, increase HDL to >60 mg/dl, and maintain total cholesterol <200 mg/dl and triglycerides <150 mg/dl. Statins are the first-line therapy for lowering lipids. Other therapies include nicotinic acid (Niacin, Niaspan), bile acid sequestrants such as cholestyramine (Questran) and colestipol (Colestid), and fibrates such as gemfibrozil (Lopid) and fenofibrate (Tricor). Combining statin with medications that inhibit CYP3A4 or CYP 2C9 can result in increased levels of statins and associated toxicity. Table 20.2 summarizes medications used to lower lipids, and table 20.3 summarizes important drug interactions (Bersot, 2011; Grundy, 2001; Heart Protection Study Collaborative Group, 2002; Knopp, 1999; Muls et al., 2001; Sanoski, 2011; Talbert, 2005).

Summary

This chapter introduces atherosclerosis and explains how ischemic heart disease and stroke can result from this disorder. This chapter also reviews medications used to treat these disorders acutely, those used as chronic medication therapy, and medications used to prevent the recurrence of acute ischemic events. Finally, the chapter discusses the therapeutic effects and side effects of these medications and how the rehabilitation therapist should tailor therapy sessions to minimize problems associated with these disease states and with associated side effects of these medications.

21

Medications Used to Treat Diabetes

In clinical practice, the rehabilitation therapist will care for many patients who have diabetes. This chapter introduces diabetes and outlines how the disease can affect patients undergoing rehabilitation. It also discusses medications used to treat the diabetic patient and provides recommendations for adjusting the rehabilitation therapy session based on the effects of these medications.

Diabetes Mellitus

Diabetes mellitus is a chronic metabolic disorder caused by an absolute or relative deficiency of insulin, which is a peptide hormone. Insulin is essential in the regulation of carbohydrate fat and protein metabolism in the body. Insulin decreases levels of blood glucose by facilitating the entry of glucose into muscle cells and stimulating the conversion of glucose to glycogen as a storage unit of carbohydrate by a process called glycogenesis. Insulin also inhibits the release of stored glucose from the liver glycogen (**glycogenolysis**) and slows the breakdown of protein and fat for glucose production (**gluconeogenesis**) in both the liver and kidneys. Glucose is the sole energy source for red blood cells, the kidneys, and provides energy for the metabolic processes of the brain and central nervous system. Insulin is produced by the beta cells of the islets of Langerhans, located in the pancreas. Maintenance of blood glucose requires a balance between the actions of insulin and **glucagon**. Incretin hormones, which are released in response to

food ingestion, help stimulate insulin secretion and inhibit glucagon secretion.

Incidence

Globally, 1 in 10 adults has diabetes (World Health Organization, 2012). Diabetes mellitus is expected to affect 380 million people worldwide by 2025. In the United States alone, 24 million adults, or 7% of the population, are diabetics. Diabetes is the leading cause of blindness in adults under 75 yr of age, the leading cause of non-traumatic amputation of the lower extremity (60% of all amputations), and the leading cause of end-stage renal disease. In 2006, diabetes was the seventh leading cause of death (Marquess, 2010; Sherman, 2010).

Etiology and Pathophysiology

Type 1 (insulin-dependent) diabetes occurs when the islets of Langerhans are destroyed and can no longer make insulin. Type 1 diabetes usually develops in childhood and occurs 50% more often in Caucasian Americans than in African Americans or Hispanics. Type 1 diabetes is characterized by uncontrolled hyperglycemia due to the absence of insulin and the associated symptoms which can be fatal if left untreated by insulin replacement. The most easily recognized symptoms of type 1 diabetes are associated with hyperglycemia, Hyperglycemia, defined as fasting blood glucose levels greater than 200 mg/dl, occurs when insulin deficiency allows production of uninhibited amounts of glucose and prevents the use and storage of this circulating glucose. Symptoms associated with hyperglycemia include general malaise, irritability, headache, and weakness. Hyperglycemia can lead to polydipsia (increased thirst) and polyuria (increased frequency and volume of urine). Because the kidneys cannot reabsorb the excess glucose load, glucose spills into the urine (**glucosuria**), resulting in osmotic **diuresis**. Osmotic diuresis results in thirst, dehydration, and severe electrolyte imbalance because the water loss is accompanied by loss of electrolytes. Inability of tissues to use glucose causes breakdown of fat and protein to meet energy needs, leading to ketone production and weight loss. Failure to thrive and wasting may be the first symptom of diabetes in the infant or child (Lamb, 2011; Marquess, 2010; Sherman, 2010).

Many diabetics are initially diagnosed with diabetes after presenting to the emergency room with diabetic ketoacidosis. **Diabetic ketoacidosis** is a life-threatening syndrome of extremely high glucose levels, severe dehydration, and electrolyte imbalance. It is accompanied by ketones in the blood, respiratory distress, hypotension, tachycardia, vomiting, and altered mental status that may present as diabetic coma. Treatment requires hospitalization, replacement of fluids and electrolytes, and administration of an insulin drip to stabilize the patient (Marquess, 2010; Sherman, 2010).

Type 2 diabetes (non-insulin-dependent) is characterized by peripheral insulin resistance and an insulin secretory defect (as opposed to insulin deficiency in type 1 diabetes). Most diabetics (90%-95%) are type 2 diabetics, and most are obese. All overweight persons have insulin resistance, but diabetes develops in those who are not able to increase beta-cell production to compensate for the insulin resistance. Weight loss can normalize blood glucose in these patients. More children are being diagnosed with type 2 diabetes, and most of those diagnosed have associated childhood obesity.

Rehabilitation Considerations

When working with the diabetic patient, the rehabilitation therapist should check whether the patient's medications have changed since the last therapy session and should consider the scheduling of medications and meals when designing sessions. Many patients with diabetes require a snack before exercise to prevent hypoglycemia. Hypoglycemia, which can occur in both type 1 and type 2 diabetics, is characterized by nausea, extreme hunger, jitteriness, cold or clammy skin, excessive perspiration, tachycardia, numbness of fingertips or lips, and trembling. If blood glucose falls below 55 mg/dl, altered mental status, along with irritability, anxiety, restlessness, confusion, and difficulty thinking or concentrating can occur. Difficulty in ambulation, blurred vision, lethargy, and slurred speech can also occur. If blood glucose decreases below 40 mg/dl, seizures, loss of consciousness, and coma can occur (Marquess, 2010; Sherman, 2010).

The therapist should monitor the patient for symptoms of hyperglycemia or hypoglycemia during the session and make appropriate interventions to reduce fall risk associated with fluctuations in glucose levels in the diabetic patient. The therapist should ensure that the patient receives education regarding appropriate diet, exercise, smoking cessation, and foot care. The patient should be assisted by a clinical dietitian in developing an appropriate diet plan and should receive education about how diet and exercise affects the control of glucose and cholesterol levels. The clinical pharmacist can provide additional education about the appropriate use of blood glucose monitoring and use of medications to control diabetes, hypertension, and high cholesterol in order to reduce risk of diabetic complications (DeHart & Worthington, 2005).

In addition to diet and medication therapy, other forms of therapy in diabetic neuropathy are useful. Physical therapy may be a useful when the patient's neuropathy manifests in muscle pain and weakness. The physical therapist can instruct the patient in general exercise techniques for maintaining mobility and strength and in pain-management and relaxation strategies. The physical therapist can also provide transcutaneous electrical nerve stimulation treatment for neuropathic pain and assist with wound care of diabetic foot ulcers using modalities of whirlpool treatment and debridement. Patients with autonomic neuropathy need balance training and fall-prevention education. The therapist also determines whether the patient requires braces, orthotics, prosthetics, or assistive devices to promote safe and efficient gait and functional performance (Brock, 2010; Montfort et al., 2010; Sherman, 2010; Votey & Peters, 2010; White, 2010).

Patients with severe loss of function may need occupational therapy. When only the lower limbs are involved, patients may need home modifications and equipment. When the upper limbs are involved, patients may need more extensive functional restoration and adaptive equipment. When a person loses a limb, even more intensive functional retraining is required. Involvement of a speech–language pathologist can help patients affected by gastroparesis or dysphagia (Brock, 2010; Montfort et al., 2010; Sherman, 2010; Votey & Peters, 2010; White, 2010).

Surgical intervention is indicated in the case of aggressive debridement or an amputation for necrosis or infection of a diabetic foot ulcer, insertion of a jejunostomy tube in order to feed the patient with intractable gastroparesis by bypassing the paralytic stomach, or penile prosthesis for impotence not responsive to alternative therapy. Treatment of Charcot joint (denervated joint deformity associated with osteoporosis) may include surgery to correct the deformity along with bracing and placing the joint in a boot (Brock, 2010; Montfort et al., 2010; Sherman, 2010; Votey & Peters, 2010; White, 2010).

PATIENT CASE 1

J.K. is a 23-yr-old female college volleyball player with a history of diabetes who was referred to her athletic trainer for help developing a regimen of strength-training exercises. She is 5 ft 8 in. (1.72 m) tall and weighs 125 lb (56.7 kg). She reports difficulty finishing a game due to weakness, extreme thirst, and headaches despite carbohydrate loading and drinking sport drinks before the game.

Question

What actions should the athletic trainer take at this time?

Answer

J.K. is exhibiting symptoms of hyperglycemia, probably due to consumption of inappropriate carbohydrate drinks before the game. The patient is most likely a type 1 (insulin-dependent) diabetic. J.K.'s blood glucose should be checked and insulin should be administered as prescribed by her physician. J.K. should be instructed to have a snack of complex carbohydrates rather than a high-sugar drink before exercise. The athletic trainer should ask about J.K.'s medications, her diet regimen, and how often she monitors her glucose levels and provide follow-up education and referral as needed.

Long-term complications associated with type 1 and type 2 diabetes include increased risk of infections; microvascular complications of retinopathy, cataracts, **nephropathy**, or progressive renal failure; neuropathic complications; and macrovascular disease leading to coronary artery disease, hypertension, myocardial infarction, or stroke. Macrovascular complications such as stroke or myocardial infarction is the leading cause of death in patients with diabetes. They cause up to 75% of deaths in diabetics compared with 35% of deaths in patients without diabetes. Diabetes increases the risk of myocardial infarction twofold in men and fourfold in women. Because atherosclerosis occurs earlier in the diabetic and is more severe in patients with this disease, aggressive treatment of **dyslipidemia** with medications such as statins is required to avoid these complications in patients with diabetes. The risk of hypertension in the diabetic is twice that in the nondiabetic. Medications that reduce hypertension to control glucose levels should be initiated early and used to aggressively control blood pressure and blood glucose in order to reduce complications associated with macrovascular disease. An angiotensin-converting enzyme inhibitor should be used in the diabetic patient to reduce blood pressure and protect against diabetic nephropathy.

Infections can cause considerable morbidity and mortality in the diabetic. Diabetics can have poor tissue perfusion, decreased sensation due to peripheral neuropathy, and impaired immunity that increases the risk of developing infections. Neuropathy associated with diabetes includes peripheral and autonomic neuropathy, and a symmetric distal sensorimotor neuropathy in a stocking-and-glove distribution is commonly seen. Loss of peripheral sensation allows foot injury to go undetected and can result in diabetic foot ulcers (Sherman, 2010).

Prolonged hyperglycemia causes several biological changes, including an increase in the attachment of glucose to tissues producing glycosylated products. Glycosylated hemoglobin (hemoglobin A1C) is used as a laboratory marker for tracking long-term glycemic control over a period of several months. For every point decrease in hemoglobin A1C, patients can reduce their risk of microvascular complications by 40%. The American Diabetes Association recommends a target hemoglobin A1C level of 7%, the American Association of Clinical Endocrinologists recommends a hemoglobin A1C level of 6.5% or lower. The Diabetes Control and Complications Trial, which studied outcomes in patients with type 1 diabetes, and the United Kingdom Prospective Diabetes Study, which studied outcomes in patients with type 2 diabetes, both showed that lowering glucose levels and associated hemoglobin A1C levels resulted in lowered risk for microvascular and macrovascular disease (Marquess, 2010; Sherman, 2010).

PATIENT CASE 1, *continued*

When speaking with J.K., the athletic trainer learns that J.K. has had diabetes since she was 8 yr old. J.K. takes long-acting insulin each morning and checks her blood sugar every morning before taking her insulin. Her physician has asked her to check her blood sugar more often, but she finds it inconvenient.

Question
What can the athletic trainer tell J.K. about the importance of checking her blood sugar more often and maintaining normal glucose throughout the day?

Answer
The athletic trainer should tell J.K. that checking blood glucose levels more frequently (usually before each meal and at bedtime) and maintaining normal blood glucose levels throughout the day (hemoglobin A1C level <7.0 mg/dl) are important in preventing or postponing diabetes-associated complications (e.g., nerve impairment, damage to circulation, and impaired ability to fight infections) and reducing her risk for developing infections of the urinary tract, bloodstream, and skin, which can lead to diabetic ulcers. It will also help her reduce the risk of damage to the small blood vessels (microvascular disease) in the eyes that can lead to blindness and damage to the blood vessels in the kidneys that can lead to kidney failure that may require dialysis. Keeping her blood sugars in normal range also can reduce her risk for disease of the larger blood vessels (macrovascular disease) and the accompanying complications such as heart attack and stroke. The athletic trainer should tell J.K. that appropriate and scheduled meal intake is an important part of maintaining euglycemia and that she should eat appropriate snacks before exercise to prevent hypoglycemia (Sherman, 2010).

PATIENT CASE 1, *continued*

At her next rehabilitation session, J.K. mentions that she does not feel well when she exercises. She wonders whether she is better off not exercising at all.

Question
How should the athletic trainer advise J.K.?

Answer
The athletic trainer should explain that exercise is an important aspect of managing diabetes and that patients should exercise regularly with an exercise plan approved by their physician. Exercise can improve blood pressure and cholesterol levels and help maintain normal glucose levels (euglycemia). The therapist should

advise J.K. that exercising vigorously for more than 30 min lowers glucose levels and can cause symptoms of **hypoglycemia**. To prevent hypoglycemia, the physician may advise J.K. to decrease her insulin by 10% to 20% or consume an extra snack before exercise. The therapist should also stress the importance of maintaining hydration status during exercise with water rather than sport drinks that contain caffeine and sugar (Sherman, 2010).

Medication Therapy

In the past two decades, only two classes of medications were used to treat diabetes: insulin and sulfonylureas. However, the complex mechanisms involved in glucose and glucagon control are now better understood and the number of classes of medications used to treat diabetes has increased dramatically. The patient must self-monitor blood glucose levels in order to maintain optimal control. Both the American Diabetes Association and the American Association of Clinical Endocrinologists stress the importance of achieving and maintaining glycemic levels as near to normal as possible in order to delay or prevent diabetes-related complications. New types of drugs allow for the combination of more than one type of oral therapy or the combination of oral and insulin therapies, which often improves glycemic control. Table 21.1 summarizes the therapies used to treat diabetes (Joffe et al., 2010; Quinn, 2006; Rochester et al., 2010; Sherman, 2010).

Insulin

Subcutaneously injected insulin is the first-line therapy in the treatment of type 1 diabetes. Insulins are categorized based on time of onset and duration of action. Rapid onset, short-, intermediate-, and long-acting insulins are available. Regular, lispro, and aspart insulins are the only types that can be administered intravenously. The term *basal insulin* describes the insulin levels that maintain metabolic processes during periods of fasting. In healthy adults, basal insulin concentrations of 5 to 15 µU/ml help maintain normal fasting plasma glucose concentrations. Long-acting insulin analogs provide insulin coverage that mimics normal fasting insulin levels. Long-acting insulin analogs include insulin glargine (Lantus) and insulin detemir (Levemir). The onset of action of these products is about 1 h. Because these products provide stable blood levels of insulin for up to 24 h, they are usually dosed once or twice per day. These products have taken the place of the older intermediate-acting products called neutral protamine hagedorn (NPH) insulin (Humulin N, Novolin N). The onset of action of NPH insulin is 2 to 4 h, effects peak at 4 to 10 h, and effects last for 10 to 16 h. NPH insulin is usually dosed twice/day (before breakfast and before dinner) (Quinn, 2006; Rochester et al., 2010).

Insulin concentration peaks at 60 to 80 µU/ml immediately after meal is ingested and returns to basal levels 1 to 3 h later. Several types of insulin help provide insulin coverage after a meal. These insulin products are classified as rapid acting or short acting. Examples of rapid-acting insulin include insulin glulisine (Apidra), insulin lispro (Humalog), and insulin aspart (NovoLog). The onset of action of these products is less than 15 min, effects peak at 1 to 2 h, and effects lasts for 3 to 4 h. These products may be given after the meal has been ingested and still provide good coverage of the glucose spikes associated with the meal. Regular insulin is short acting and is available as Humulin R and Novolin R. The onset of action is 0.5 to 1 h, effects peak at 2 to 3 h, and effects last for 3 to 6 h. Use of this product to cover meals is more problematic because the medication must be administered before meals and hypoglycemia can occur if the meal is not ingested or delayed (Quinn, 2006; Rochester et al., 2010).

Use of treatment regimens that include a combination of rapid- and long-acting insulins has resulted in improved hemoglobin A1C levels, better glycemic control, and reduced hypoglycemia compared with use of treatment regimens that include regular insulin along with NPH insulin. An example of this is a basal-bolus insulin regimen that includes 0.2-0.4 U/kg of long-acting product combined with 0.1 U/kg of rapid-acting product after each meal. Glucose levels are also checked before meals and at bedtime and out of range glucose

Table 21.1 Medications Used to Treat Diabetes

Medication	Side effects affecting rehab							Other side effects or considerations
Biguanide: Increases sensitivity of insulin by decreasing hepatic gluconeogenesis (primary effect) and increasing peripheral insulin sensitivity (secondary effect).								
Metformin (Glucophage)	Cog 0	S 0	A 0	Motor 0	D ++	Com 0	F 0	Used as monotherapy or with sulfonylurea, thiazolidinedione, or insulin. Decreases A1C by 1%-2% and decreases FPG by 60-80 mg/dl. Decreases levels of vitamin B$_{12}$; provide B-12 supplementation. Avoid in patients with creatinine >1.5 due to increased risk of lactic acidosis. Advantages: When used as monotherapy Glucophage rarely causes hypoglycemia and it does not increase insulin levels. Glucophage improves cardiovascular health by lowering lipid levels and by not causing weight gain; most effective in patients who are overweight or who have dyslipidemia or high fasting plasma glucose. Disadvantages: Side effects of nausea, vomiting, diarrhea, and metallic taste; take with food to minimize adverse gastrointestinal side effects.
Sulfonylureas: Secretagogues; increase production of insulin by the beta cells in the pancreas in patients with residual beta-cell function.								
Glipizide (Glucotrol, Glucotrol XL)	Cog +	S 0	A 0	Motor +	D 0	Com 0	F +	Achieves A1C decreases of 1%-2%. Advantages: Inexpensive. More effective in newly diagnosed patients (diagnosed within the previous 5 yrs) who are close to ideal body weight and who have fasting plasma glucose levels of <200 mg/dl. Disadvantages: Weight gain, allergy, photosensitivity, beta-cell burnout with decreased efficacy, hypoglycemia. May increase cardiovascular risk (increased weight gain and lipid levels).
Glyburide (Diabeta, Glycron, Glynase, Micronase)	Cog +	S 0	A 0	Motor +	D 0	Com 0	F +	
Glimepiride (Amaryl)	Cog +	S 0	A 0	Motor +	D 0	Com 0	F +	
Meglitinides: Short-acting insulin secretagogues; act on the adenosine triphosphate-dependent potassium channels in pancreatic beta cells, allowing calcium channels to open and increasing insulin release.								
Repaglinide (Prandin)	Cog 0	S 0	A 0	Motor 0	D 0	Com 0	F 0	Advantages: Low risk of hypoglycemia, minimizes hyperglycemia after meals, needs glucose to work (food dependent); give only with meals. Stimulates pancreatic insulin secretion within 20 min of oral administration.
Nateglinide (Starlix)	Cog 0	S 0	A 0	Motor 0	D 0	Com 0	F 0	

› continued

Table 21.1 › *continued*

Medication	Side effects affecting rehab							Other side effects or considerations
Insulins: Exogenous replacement of natural hormone insulin used to prevent and treat hyperglycemia in type 1 and type 2 diabetics; decreases A1C 1-2%.								
Glargine (Lantus) Long-acting insulin: Onset is 1 h, peak is 1 h, and duration is 24 h. Usually dosed once/day (twice/day in brittle diabetics).	Cog +	S 0	A +	Motor +	D +	Com +	F +	Side effects: Weight gain, hypoglycemia. Loses effectiveness after time. Patients with type 2 diabetes need relatively large doses. Rotate site of injection to prevent lipodystrophy. Glargine: Longer effects than detemir (Levemir) allows once/day dosing in more patients.
Detemir (Levemir) Long-acting insulin: Onset is 1 h, peak is 1 h, and duration is 24 h. Usually dosed once/day (twice/day in brittle diabetics).	Cog +	S 0	A +	Motor +	D +	Com +	F +	Used with short-acting insulin given with meals. Detemir may need to be dosed twice/day.
NPH insulin (Humulin N, Novolin N) Intermediate-acting insulin: Onset is 2-4 h, peak is 4-10 h, and duration is 10-16 h. Usually dosed twice/day before breakfast and before dinner.	Cog +	S 0	A +	Motor +	D +	Com +	F +	May be used with short-acting insulin administered with meals. Side effects: Weight gain, hypoglycemia. Loses effectiveness after time. Patients with type 2 diabetes need relatively large doses. Rotate site of injection to prevent lipodystrophy.
Regular insulin (Novolin R, Humulin R) Short-acting insulin: Onset is 2-4 h, peak is 2-3 h, and duration is 3-6 h. Can be given as IV infusion.	Cog +	S 0	A +	Motor +	D +	Com +	F +	Side effects: Weight gain, hypoglycemia. Loses effectiveness after time. Patients with type 2 diabetes need relatively large doses. Rotate site of injection to prevent lipodystrophy. Multiple daily injections: Before meals 3 times/day along with basal insulin at bedtime.

Medication	Side effects affecting rehab							Other side effects or considerations
Glulisine (Apidra) Lispro (Humalog) Aspart (NovoLog) Rapid-acting insulin: Onset is <15 min, peak is 1-2 h, and duration is 3-4 h.	Cog +	S 0	A +	Motor +	D +	Com +	F +	Commonly given with meals; may be administered immediately after meal. Side effects: Weight gain, hypoglycemia. Loses effectiveness after time. Patients with type 2 diabetes need relatively large doses. Rotate site of injection to prevent lipodystrophy.

Thiazolidinediones: Act as insulin sensitizers; reduce glucose production in the liver and increase glucose utilization in skeletal muscle. Onset of action is 12-16 wk; may preserve beta function and slow progression of diabetes.

Medication	Side effects affecting rehab							Other side effects or considerations
Rosiglitazone (Avandia)	Cog 0	S 0	A 0	Motor +	D +	Com 0	F +	These agents are used as monotherapy or with sulfonylurea, metformin, meglitinide, DPP-4 inhibitors, exenatide, or insulin. Decreases A1C by 0.6%-1.9%; decreases fasting plasma glucose by 50-80 mg/dl.
Pioglitazone (Actos)	Cog 0	S 0	A 0	Motor +	D +	Com 0	F +	Side effects: Liver failure (rare), plasma volume expansion, edematous weight gain increasing the risk of congestive heart failure exacerbations. Osteoporosis; increased rates of upper and distal lower limb fracture in both men and women. Do not use while pregnant or breastfeeding or in children. Rosiglitazone is now available only via a restricted-access program by the Food and Drug Administration due to increased cardiovascular risk. Actos may be associated with increased risk of bladder cancer.

Alpha-glycosidase inhibitors: Inhibit carbohydrate digestion in the gastrointestinal tract, delaying postmeal glucose spikes.

Medication	Side effects affecting rehab							Other side effects or considerations
Acarbose (Precose)	Cog 0	S 0	A 0	Motor 0	D ++	Com 0	F 0	Decreases A1C by 0.5%-1%; decreases fasting plasma glucose by 40-50 mg/dl.
Miglitol (Glyset)	Cog 0	S 0	A 0	Motor 0	D ++	Com 0	F 0	Used as monotherapy or with sulfonylurea, thiazolidinedione, metformin, or insulin therapy. Useful in treatment of patients with significant PPG blood glucose, obese patients, or those with a high risk of hypoglycemia. Dose should be increased slowly. Dose is taken with the first bite of a meal of at least 300 cal. If the patient does not eat, the medicine should not be taken. Advantages: Does not cause hypoglycemia when used as monotherapy. Side effects: Gastrointestinal upset, take with food to minimize gastrointestinal upset. Elevated liver enzyme levels.

› continued

Table 21.1 › *continued*

Medication	Side effects affecting rehab							Other side effects or considerations
Dipeptidyl peptidase-4 (DPP-4) inhibitors: Prevent degradation of GIP and GLP-1, increasing their effects and slowing insulin response to meals; improve insulin secretion and inhibit glucagon production.								
Sitagliptin (Januvia)	Cog +	S 0	A 0	Motor 0	D +	Com 0	F +	Decrease A1C by 0.5%-0.8%; decrease fasting plasma glucose by 15-30 mg/dl; decrease postprandial glucose by 35-50 mg/dl.
Saxagliptin (Onglyza)	Cog +	S 0	A 0	Motor 0	D +	Com 0	F +	Advantages: Generally well tolerated; possible hypoglycemia when used in combination with insulin or secretagogues, but does not cause hypoglycemia when used alone.
								Modest antihyperglycemic effects useful in the elderly. Reduce dosage for renal impairment or concurrent use of other medications that inhibit liver metabolism via the 3A4/5 pathway. May increase risk for acute pancreatitis.
GLP-1 agonists: Incretin analogs that enhance glucose-dependent insulin secretion, suppress glucagon, delay gastric emptying, and promote satiety and weight loss.								
Exenatide (Byetta) 5 mcg and 10 mcg fixed-dose prefilled pens	Cog 0	S 0	A 0	Motor 0	D ++	Com 0	F +	Decreases A1C by 1%-2%; decreases FPG by 25-60 mg/dl; decreases PPG glucose by 35-50 mg/dl. Advantages: Improved glucose levels with reduced risk of hypoglycemia; modest improvements in blood pressure and lipids.
Liraglutide (Victoza) 6 mg/ml pre-filled cartridge pen	Cog +	S 0	A 0	Motor 0	D ++	Com 0	F +	Promote satiety and weight loss. Side effects: Transient nausea and vomiting. Initial dose of 0.6 mg/day is intended to reduce gastrointestinal symptoms during initial titration and does not result in adequate glycemic control.
								During initiation, reduce dose of concomitantly administered insulin secretagogues (i.e., sulfonylureas, meglitinides) to reduce risk of hypoglycemia.
								FDA approved REMS in place due to possible link to thyroid C-cell cancer; prescriber to determine whether benefits outweigh risk.
								Drug interactions: Delayed gastric emptying and decreased acid secretion may affect absorption of other medications.

Medication	Side effects affecting rehab							Other side effects or considerations
Amylin derivative: Synthetic analog of human amylin, a naturally occurring hormone made in pancreatic beta cells; used in patients who have not achieved desired glucose control despite optimal insulin therapy.								
Pramlintide acetate (Symlin) 60 prefilled pen injector for lower doses of 15-60 mcg and 120 prefilled pen injector for doses of 60-120 mcg	Cog 0	S 0	A 0	Motor 0	D +	Com 0	F 0	Indicated to treat type 1 or type 2 diabetes in combination with insulin. Advantages: Improves long-term control (A1C) compared with insulin alone. Reduces spikes in PPG, glucagon secretion, and regulates food intake by centrally mediated appetite modulation. Reduces needed dose of insulin and promotes weight loss. May need to adjust dose of insulin to maintain euglycemia. Side effects: Nausea. Drug interactions: Slows gastric emptying, which can affect absorption of other medications.

Cog = cognition; S = sedation; A = agitation or mania; Motor = discoordination; D = dysphagia; Com = communication; F = falls; A1C = glycosylated hemoglobin; GIP = glucose-dependent insulinotropic polypeptide; GLP-1 = glucagon-like peptide-1; IV = intravenously; FPG = fasting plasma glucose; PPG = postprandial glucose; mcg = microgram (1/1000 of a milligram); NPH = neutral protamine hagedorn; FDA = U.S. Food and Drug Administration; REMS = risk evaluation and mitigation strategy.

The likelihood rating scale for encountering the side effects is as follows: 0 = Almost no probability of encountering side effects. + = Little likelihood of encountering side effects. +/++ = Low probability of encountering side effects; however, probability increases with increased dosage. ++ = Medium likelihood of encountering side effects. +++ = High likelihood of encountering side effects, particularly with high doses. ++++ = Highest likelihood of encountering side effects; best to avoid in at-risk patients.

levels are corrected with a rapid-acting product using a sliding scale dosage column with doses determined by the patient's blood glucose and weight (Quinn, 2006; Rochester et al., 2010; Sherman, 2010).

Mixtures of insulin preparations with different time to onset and duration of action can usually be administered in a single injection by drawing measured doses of two preparations into the same syringe immediately before use. The exception is insulin glargine (Lantus), which should not be mixed with any other form of insulin. Preparations that contain a mixture of 70% NPH and 30% regular human insulin (i.e., Novolin 70/30, Humulin 70/30) are available, as is Humulin 50/50 and a 75%/25% mixture of NPH and lispro insulin. The fixed ratios of intermediate-acting to rapid-acting insulin are convenient for patients on stable insulin regimens, but use of these agents may be restricted if dosing must be adjusted. Insulin is routinely provided in preparations containing 100 U/ml (U-100 insulin). However, concentrations of up to 500 U/ml

are available for people with marked insulin resistance. A multiple-dose insulin-injection device, commonly referred to as an insulin pen, uses a cartridge that contains enough doses for several days. Unopened insulin should be refrigerated but never frozen. For ease of use, insulin preparations can be stored at room temperature after they are opened (Quinn, 2006; Rochester et al., 2010; Sherman, 2010).

Insulin therapy is used to treat both type 1 and type 2 diabetes. Type 1 diabetics do not produce insulin and require insulin therapy. Type 2 diabetics produce some insulin, but tissues do not efficiently utilize insulin. Levels of normal insulin secretion are often reduced by 50% in patients at initial diagnosis of type 2 diabetes and six years after diagnosis levels are often reduced by 75%. Consequently, the majority of patients with type 2 diabetes will eventually require insulin supplementation. Treatment of type 2 diabetes aims to lower insulin resistance (i.e., increase the ability of the peripheral tissues to use insulin) and to increase release of insulin by the beta cells in the pancreas. Because patients with type 2 diabetes have insulin resistance and beta-cell dysfunction, oral medications that increase insulin sensitivity at the peripheral tissue site may be given along with daily administration of long-acting insulin. Medications that increase the secretion of insulin, termed insulin secretagogues, include the sulfonylureas. The goal of using combination therapy of insulin with oral therapy is to lower the fasting glucose level to 100 mg/dl by titration of the long-acting insulin dose. When this target is achieved, the oral agents can effectively maintain preprandial and postprandial blood glucose levels throughout the day. If a regimen of combined oral agents and long-acting insulin fails to maintain glucose levels within normal range, the patient's regimen should be changed to an intensive insulin regimen which combines daily injections of long-acting insulin combined with injections of rapid-acting insulin immediately before each meal to control postprandial increases in blood glucose (Drabb, 2009a; Grossman, 2009; Marquess, 2010; Montfort et al., 2010). The most commonly reported adverse effect associated with insulin is hypoglycemia. Hyperthyroidism may increase renal clearance of insulin (more insulin may be needed to treat hyperglycemia). Hypothyroidism may delay insulin turnover (less insulin may be needed to treat hyperglycemia). Dose adjustments may be necessary in patients with renal or hepatic dysfunction. Table 21.2 summarizes current recommendations from the American Diabetes Association and the European Association for the Study of Diabetes for the use of combination medication therapies in managing patients with type 2 diabetes.

PATIENT CASE 1, continued

Three months later, J.K. reports she has consulted with her physician and she is now able to participate in volleyball without hypoglycemic symptoms. She eats a high-fiber protein bar before games. She has adjusted her diet and is eating appropriate meals on a scheduled basis and is now

checking her blood glucose before and after each meal and at bedtime. She reports that her hemoglobin A1C has decreased from 8.0 to 7.5 mg/dl.

When reviewing J.K.'s medication list, the therapist notices that she is now taking Lantus insulin 40 U subcutaneously/day in the morning along with NovoLog insulin 8 U subcutaneously before each meal. Her blood glucose level before meals is 90 to 100 mg/dl, but her glucose level after meals is more than 200 mg/dl. Her physician wants her to start taking a new medication called Symlin. She asks why the doctor cannot just increase her insulin dose and why another injection is necessary. She also wonders why she cannot take a pill to improve her glucose control like one of her coworkers does.

Question

What information can the therapist provide to J.K.?

Answer

The therapist can tell J.K. that she may have a different form of diabetes than her coworker. In patients with type 1 diabetes, damage to the beta cells in the pancreas prevents the pancreas from producing insulin. Therefore, the patients require insulin injections to control their blood glucose. Most oral medications (pill formulations) are designed for type 2 diabetics. These pills help the type 2 diabetic use the insulin produced by the pancreas more efficiently and help the pancreas produce more insulin. Symlin is a new medication that the type 1 diabetic can take with insulin to reduce the amount of insulin taken and to help better control glucose spikes seen after consumption of meals.

New Medication Therapies

Many new types of medications for the diabetic patient are available. A new group of medications targets the incretin system, a group of hormones that the gastrointestinal tract produces when stimulated by meal ingestion.

Table 21.2   The 2012 ADA/EASD Consensus Algorithm for Management of Hyperglycemia in Patients With Type 2 Diabetes

Step 1: Initiate lifestyle changes and add metformin (Glucophage).

Step 2: Medication choices to be added to metformin:

Choice 1: To avoid weight gain, add DPP-4 inhibitor or GLP-1 agonist.

Choice 2: To avoid hypoglycemia, add DPP-4 inhibitor or GLP-1 agonist or TZD.

Choice 3: To minimize costs, add sulfonylurea or insulin.

Step 3: Medication choices to be added to drug regimen chosen from step 2:

Choice 1: To avoid weight gain, add DPP-4 inhibitor or GLP-1 agonist.

Choice 2: To avoid hypoglycemia, add DPP-4 inhibitor or GLP-1 agonist or TZD.

Choice 3: To minimize costs, add sulfonylurea or insulin.

Alternative to above: Initiate intensive insulin therapy with long-acting and short-acting insulin in patients not well controlled or those with medication contraindications.

Note: Check A1C every 3 months until <7%, change therapy if A1C is >7%.

DPP-4 inhibitor = sitagliptin (Januvia) or saxagliptin (Onglyza); GLP-1 agonist = liraglutide (Victoza) or exenatide (Byetta); TZD = pioglitazone (Actos); sulfonylurea = glipizide (Glucotrol), glyburide (Diabeta), or glimepiride (Amaryl).

Based on Inaucchi et al. 2012.

The incretin system includes two hormones: glucose-dependent insulinotropic polypeptide (GIP) and glucagon-like peptide-1 (GLP-1) (Drabb, 2009a,b). These hormones improve survival of beta cells. GLP-1 improves defective glucose-stimulated insulin secretion, slows insulin secretory response to meals, inhibits the secretion of glucagon, and increases the production of proinsulin in the beta cells of the pancreas. Two new medication classes that affect the incretin system are GLP-1 agonists and (dipeptidyl peptidase-4) DPP-4 inhibitors. The action of these medications is regulated by the body's glucose levels and therefore their use is not associated with the side effects of hypoglycemia seen with the use of many oral hypoglycemic agents or insulin. GLP-1 agonists act on the same receptor site as GLP-1, resulting in actions similar to those of endogenous GLP-1. DPP-4 inhibitors include sitagliptin (Januvia) and saxagliptin (Onglyza) and are oral agents that decrease the deactivation of, and promote the actions of, GLP-1 and GIP. GLP-1 agonists include exenatide (Byetta) and liraglutide (Victoza) and are given by injection. These agents have been linked to an increased risk of acute pancreatitis and may be associated with an increased risk of thyroid cancer. Pramlintide (Symlin) is a synthetic analog of human amylin, a naturally occurring hormone made in pancreatic beta cells. This medication elicits endogenous amylin effects, resulting in delayed gastric emptying, decreased postprandial glucagon release, and modulated appetite (Grossman, 2009; Joffe et al., 2010; Leahy & Marquess, 2010; Montfort et al., 2010; Quinn et al., 2006; Rochester et al., 2010; Zaharowitz & Conner, 2009).

Diabetic Neuropathy

Neuropathies, the most common complication of diabetes mellitus, affect 28% to 55% of patients with diabetes. Patients at greatest risk of developing neuropathy include those with prolonged hyperglycemia as well as those with concurrent dyslipidemia, hypertension, and cardiovascular disease. Diabetic neuropathy is more common in smokers, people older than 40 yr of age, and those who have uncontrolled diabetes mellitus. More severe symptoms are seen in patients with poor glycemic control, advanced age, hypertension, a long history of diabetes, dyslipidemia, smoking, or heavy alcohol intake. Members of minority groups (e.g., Hispanics, African Americans) experience more secondary complications from diabetic neuropathy, such as lower-extremity amputations, than Caucasians and are hospitalized for neuropathic complications more often. Neuropathy can result in severe pain, impotence, ileus, diarrhea, cardiac arrhythmia (often associated with death), dizziness with resultant falls and fractures, and foot ulcers that often lead to amputation and associated disability (Brock, 2010; Montfort et al., 2010; Sherman, 2010; Votey & Peters, 2010; White, 2010).

Pathogenic factors associated with diabetic neuropathy include derangement of glucose metabolism, vascular insufficiency, loss of growth factor tropism, and autoimmune destruction of small unmyelinated nerves (C-fibers) found in visceral organs and in skin and soft tissue. Symptoms and complications of diabetic neuropathy are associated with degeneration of nerve fibers and grossly diseased blood vessels that supply those nerve fibers. Proper circulation determines whether nerve fibers repair themselves or proceed to permanent nerve damage. Glycosylation of nerve and blood vessel proteins causes nerve ischemia and nerve hypoxia and increases oxidative stress in the nerve. Ischemia also induces oxidative stress, resulting in nerve injury. Sensory neuropathy involves the smallest nerve fibers (i.e., C-fibers). These small nerve fibers are supported by neurotrophic factor and nerve growth factor. Levels of these factors are reduced significantly in diabetic neuropathy. Autoimmune damage may also be associated with diabetic nerve damage (Brock, 2010; Montfort et al., 2010; Sherman, 2010; Votey & Peters, 2010; White, 2010).

Peripheral neuropathies may be associated with pathology associated with one or a combination of sensory, motor, or autonomic neurons. The most common type of diabetic neuropathy is generalized sensory–motor neuropathy, which involves both sensory and motor nerves. Sensory symptoms include pain, numbness, and a feeling of pins and needles related to altered sensation in the distal feet or hands, and motor symptoms include decreased strength and atrophy in the muscles of the lower limbs. The distribution of symptoms, termed a stocking-and-glove distribution, is stronger distally and less strong proximally. Symptoms include dysesthesias, **paresthesias**, and muscle pain. Patients with diabetic autonomic neuropathies may report ataxia, gait instability, or near syncope. Manifestation of autonomic neuropathies varies with the anatomic site of nerve damage and can result in gastrointestinal neuropathy, cardiovascular blood vessel neuropathy, and sex organ and bladder neuropathy. Associated symptoms with gastrointestinal neuropathy can include bloating, diarrhea, constipation, nausea, vomiting, and early satiety. Blood vessel neuropathy can result in orthostasis, tachycardia, and hypotension. Urogenital neuropathy can result in sexual dysfunction, incontinence, and inability to empty bladder (Brock, 2010; Montfort et al., 2010; Sherman, 2010; Votey & Peters, 2010; White, 2010). Table 21.3 summarizes medications used to treat diabetic neuropathic pain (Brock, 2010; Montfort et al., 2010; Sherman, 2010; Votey & Peters, 2010; White, 2010).

PATIENT CASE 2

A.T. is a 65-yr-old man with a diabetic foot wound who is referred for whirlpool therapy and gait training. He is 5 ft 10 in. (1.78 m) tall and weighs 230 lb (104.3 kg). He has a history of elevated cholesterol, hypertension, and diabetic kidney disease. During gait training he complains of dizziness, weakness, nausea, and shakiness.

Question
What actions should the therapist take at this time?

Answer
A.T.'s symptoms are consistent with hypoglycemia. Hypoglycemia can be treated with 4 oz (118.3 ml) of orange juice, 6 oz (177.4 ml) of regular soda, or 8 oz (236.6 ml) of nonfat milk. Patients with renal disease should be treated with 4 oz (118.3 ml) of apple juice or 6 oz (177.4 ml) of ginger ale.

The therapist should review A.T.'s medication list and ask when A.T. last took these medications. In addition, the therapist should ask when A.T. ate his most recent meal. Diabetics should take medications and eat at scheduled times. Failure to maintain therapeutic glucose levels can interfere with A.T.'s ability to participate in physical exercise and rehabilitation. In addition, the therapist should ask A.T. about his current methods of monitoring blood glucose levels at home; this monitoring is vital to keeping the diabetic patient's glucose levels in the appropriate range and preventing diabetic complications (Marquess, 2010; Sherman, 2010).

Individuals with diabetes who keep their blood glucose in the normal range throughout the day have a decreased risk of developing complications such as poor circulation and decreased ability to feel foot pain, and injury to the feet. These complications can lead to diabetic foot injury and infection. Patients should be counseled about foot care, including wearing only comfortable, well-fitting athletic shoes (not open-toed shoes or sandals) and never going barefoot, even indoors. Patients should not wear the same shoes for more than 5 h at a time or new shoes for more than 2 h at a time. When purchasing new shoes patients should shop at the end of the day when the feet are enlarged. Patients should be advised to wear cotton socks with shoes and to change the socks frequently. The feet should be inspected and washed daily, paying attention to the spaces between the toes, and the feet should be lubricated (except between the toes) daily with lotion. Patients should avoid exposing the feet to extreme temperatures and use sunscreen on them before exposing them to the sun. Toenails should be trimmed straight across, and a medical professional should be consulted for removal of corns or calluses. Pumice stones should not be used because they can introduce bacteria into skin abrasions and promote infection. Patients should have the feet inspected by a physician at least once/yr or sooner if a blister, sore, or puncture on the foot occurs.

PATIENT CASE 2, *continued*

When reviewing A.T.'s medication list further, the therapist notices that he is taking the following medications: simvastatin 40 mg/day for high cholesterol, lisinopril 20 mg/day for high blood pressure, and a baby aspirin each morning and Toprol XL 25 mg/day for high blood pressure. A.T. complains that 20 yr ago he was healthy and wonders why the doctor thinks he needs all of these medications now. He wonders if the therapist can explain what has caused all of his health problems.

Question
What insight can the therapist provide to A.T. about the link between diabetes and cardiovascular disease?

Answer
The therapist explains that diabetes increases the risk of high cholesterol, high blood pressure, myocardial infarction, and stroke. High levels of cholesterol can also cause circulation problems in the legs, called peripheral artery disease (PAD). A.T. can minimize these complications by working to improve his health through weight loss, maintaining a healthy diet, and using medications to control his diabetes, blood pressure, and cholesterol levels. Taking the baby aspirin each day can help prevent stroke and heart attack. High blood pressure also increases cholesterol levels, so managing his blood pressure reduces his risk of complications. Lisinopril is an angiotensin-converting enzyme inhibitor that lowers blood pressure and also helps prevent kidney damage in patients with diabetes. Simvastatin, along with a healthy diet and weight loss, can help lower cholesterol levels. The therapist should encourage A.T. to purchase blood pressure- and glucose-monitoring devices and maintain a daily log of his blood pressure and blood glucose levels. He should bring the log with him to each physician visit. For best results, A.T. should maintain his blood pressure at less than 120/80, his low-density lipoprotein (LDL) at less than 70 mg/dl, and his blood glucose at less than 120 mg/dl.

One of the first steps in managing diabetes is diet control. The rehabilitation therapist should ensure that the patient is assisted by a clinical dietitian to create an individualized diet plan. Clinical dietitians should teach patients about the timing, size, frequency, and composition of

See table 21.3 in the web resource for a full list of medications, dosing recommendations, and side effects.

Table 21.3 Medications Used to Treat Pain Associated With Diabetic Neuropathy

Medication	Side effects affecting rehab							Other side effects or considerations
NSAIDs: Used in acute treatment of neuropathy to relieve mild to moderate pain. Antipyretic, analgesic, anti-inflammatory. Reversible inhibition of platelet aggregation with NSAIDs lasts for 1-3 days.								
Ibuprofen (Motrin)	Cog +	S 0	A 0	Motor 0	D ++	Com +	F +	Side effects: Gastrointestinal upset, dyspepsia, xerostomia, oral ulceration, glossitis, gastrointestinal mucosal hemorrhage, abrupt acute renal insufficiency, fluid retention, worsening of congestive heart failure, memory loss, confusion (especially in the elderly), dizziness, headache.
Naproxen (Naprosyn, Anaprox, Naprelan)	Cog +	S 0	A 0	Motor 0	D ++	Com +	F +	Drug interactions: Increased risk of bleeding with oral anticoagulant warfarin (Coumadin). Do not combine with aspirin. Antagonizes effects of antihypertensives.
Skeletal muscle relaxants: Helpful in initial 2 wk of treatment of diabetic neuropathy.								
Carisoprodol (Soma)	Cog ++	S +++	A 0	Motor +++	D ++	Com ++	F ++	Abuse potential. Metabolized by CYP2C19 to meprobamate. Side effects: Headache, dizziness, drowsiness, facial flushing, insomnia, coordination problems, dependence. Drug interactions: Potentiates effects of opiates, allowing reduction of opiate dosage.
Cyclobenzaprine (Flexeril)	Cog ++++	S ++++	A 0	Motor +++	D ++	Com ++	F ++++	Limit use to no more than 3 wk. Side effects: Somnolence, confusion, dizziness, paresthesias, seizures, arrhythmias. Drug interactions: Chemically related to tricyclic antidepressants. Avoid with monoamine oxidase inhibitors, selective serotonin reuptake inhibitors, guanethidine, and concurrent central nervous system depressants.
Methocarbamol (Robaxin, Skelex)	Cog ++++	S ++++	A ++	Motor +++	D ++	Com ++	F +++	Side effects: Somnolence, dizziness, vertigo, syncope, muscular incoordination, stomach upset, flushing, blurred vision, fever, skin rash, pruritus, bradycardia, jaundice, mood changes, slow heart rate, fainting, clumsiness, difficulty urinating; may cause discoloration of urine (black, blue, or green). Drug interactions: Additive sedation when used with other central nervous system depressants. Metabolized by demethylation; no significant drug interactions.

Medication	Side effects affecting rehab							Other side effects or considerations
Tricyclic antidepressants: Inhibit reuptake of serotonin and norepinephrine; should be used as first-line therapy in patients with underlying insomnia or depression; are effective for paresthesic pain (e.g., the feeling of pins and needles, electricity, numbness, or achy, knifelike shooting).								
Amitriptyline (Elavil)	Cog ++++	S ++++	A 0	Motor ++	D ++++	Com ++++	F ++++	Weight gain +++ Seizure +++ Cardiac +++ Sexual ++ Not recommended in elderly due to high sedative and anticholinergic effects that increase risk of falls.
Desipramine (Norpramin)	Cog ++	S ++	A +	Motor ++	D ++	Com ++	F ++	Weight gain + Seizure ++ Cardiac ++ Sexual ++ Prolongs QT interval.
Nortriptyline (Pamelor)	Cog ++	S ++	A 0	Motor ++	D ++	Com ++	F +	Weight gain + Seizure ++ Cardiac ++ Sexual ++ Preferred tricyclic antidepressant in elderly due to low anticholinergic and sedative effects.
Norepinephrine serotonin reuptake inhibitor antidepressant: Enhances norepinephrine and serotonin; used to treat depression, anxiety disorder, diabetic peripheral pain, neuropathic pain, chronic skeletal muscle pain, and fibromyalgia.								
Duloxetine (Cymbalta)	Cog +	S 0	A +	Motor 0	D ++	Com 0	F +	Weight gain 0/+ Seizure 0 Cardiac 0 Sexual + Drug interactions: Metabolized by CYP1A2 and CYP2D6; potential interactions with other medications metabolized by the same pathways.
Anesthetic patch: Can be used for both dysesthetic and paresthesic pain as adjunct to oral therapy; may relieve intractable pain not relieved by other agents.								
Lidocaine 5% topical patch (Lidoderm)	Cog +	S +	A +	Motor +	D +	Com +	F +	Side effects: Confusion, nervousness, light-headedness, euphoria, tremors, blurred vision, vomiting, hypotension.
Anticonvulsants: Used to treat pain by blocking sodium, potassium, calcium channels, and neurotransmitters such as gamma amino butyric acid to relieve neuropathic pain.								
Gabapentin (Neurontin)	Cog ++	S ++	A +	Motor +++	D 0	Com ++	F +++	Side effects: Peripheral edema, tremor, dizziness, fatigue, ataxia, drowsiness, weight gain, behavior changes.
Pregabalin (Lyrica)	Cog ++	S ++	A +	Motor +++	D 0	Com ++	F +++	Side effects: Dizziness, somnolence, dry mouth, edema, blurred vision, weight gain, difficulty with concentration and attention.
Substance P enhancer: Topical agent used as an adjunct to oral therapy. Can relieve dysesthetic pain when applied to affected area.								
Capsaicin cream	Cog 0	S 0	A 0	Motor 0	D 0	Com 0	F 0	May cause stinging and burning pain during the initial applications; use gloves and applicator to apply and wash hands after application; avoid contact with the eyes.

› *continued*

Table 21.3 › *continued*

Medication	Side effects affecting rehab							Other side effects or considerations
Opiate analgesics: Used for severe pain that is not relieved with other agents.								
Oxycodone (Oxycontin)	Cog ++	S ++	A +	Motor +++	D ++	Com ++	F +++	Side effects: Constipation, somnolence, dizziness, nausea, vomiting, itching, sedation, respiratory depression.
Morphine (MS Contin)	Cog ++	S ++	A +	Motor +++	D ++	Com ++	F +++	Drug interactions: Additive sedation with other CNS depressants.
Tramadol (Ultram)	Cog ++	S ++	A +	Motor +++	D ++	Com ++	F +++	Side effects: Constipation, somnolence, dizziness, nausea, vomiting, itching. Risk of addiction, physical dependence, and tolerance. Contraindications: Avoid use in those with seizure disorder or alcohol or drug abuse. Drug interactions: Reduce risk for serotonin syndrome by avoiding concurrent use of selective serotonin reuptake inhibitors (SSRIs).

Cog = cognition; S = sedation; A = agitation or mania; Motor = discoordination; D = dysphagia; Com = communication; F = falls; NSAID = nonsteroidal anti-inflammatory drug; CNS = central nervous system.

The likelihood rating scale for encountering the side effects is as follows: 0 = Almost no probability of encountering side effects. 0/+ = Very low probability of encountering side effects but increased with higher dosages. + = Little likelihood of encountering side effects. +/++ = Low probability of encountering side effects; however, probability increases with increased dosage. ++ = Medium likelihood of encountering side effects. +++ = High likelihood of encountering side effects, particularly with high doses. ++++ = Highest likelihood of encountering side effects; best to avoid in at-risk patients.

meals to prevent hypoglycemia or **postprandial** hyperglycemia. Patients should receive a comprehensive diet plan that includes a prescription for daily caloric intake; recommendations for amounts of dietary carbohydrate, fat, and protein; and instructions for dividing calories among meals and snacks. As a rule of thumb, patients should consume 20% of daily calories at breakfast, 35% at lunch, 30% at dinner, and 15% as a late-evening snack. The minimum protein requirement for good nutrition is 0.9 g/kg/day (range = 1-1.5 g/kg/day), but a reduced protein intake is indicated in cases of nephropathy. Patients should limit fat intake to 30% or less of the total calories, and a low-cholesterol diet is recommended. Patients should consume sucrose in moderation and increase dietary intake of whole grains, fresh fruits and vegetables, and fiber. In some individuals, healthy midmorning and midafternoon snacks are important for avoiding hypoglycemia. Chapter 3 discusses additional considerations in providing nutritional support for diabetic patients (Sherman, 2010).

PATIENT CASE 2, *continued*

A.T. returns for additional therapy several months later. He is experiencing numbness along with tingling in his feet and burning and shooting pain in his legs. In addition, he is experiencing dizziness when he stands up and gait abnormalities. He has fallen three times in the past month. He is referred to therapy for help with ambulation. He wants to know whether the medications he is taking are causing his symptoms of dizziness. The therapist reviews his list of medications and finds that he is now taking amitriptyline (Elavil) 150 mg at bedtime for neuropathic pain and oxycodone 5 mg tablets as needed up to 4 times/day for breakthrough pain. He has been taking the amitriptyline (Elavil) for 4 wk and the oxycodone for 2 wk. His other medications remain unchanged.

Question

How should the therapist advise A.T.?

Answer

The therapist consults with the patient's physician, reporting these new symptoms. A.T. is exhibiting significant neuropathic symptoms. His paresthesias and dysesthesias are symptoms of peripheral sensory–motor neuropathy. Amitriptyline is effective for treating this type of pain but also has significant anticholinergic effects such as orthostasis that increase A.T.'s fall risk. Use of amitriptyline is not recommended in the older patient because of the associated side effects. In addition, the onset of falls and symptoms occurred when A.T. started taking amitriptyline. The therapist should ask whether A.T.'s neuropathic pain can be treated with another agent such as the anticonvulsants pregabalin (Lyrica) or gabapentin (Neurontin). These agents can also cause dizziness and gait abnormalities, so the prescriber should start at a low dose and slowly titrate the dose up. In addition, the prescriber may need to adjust the dose down if A.T. has renal insufficiency, as many diabetics do. The therapist could also suggest that the prescriber consider discontinuing the oxycodone to reduce symptoms of sedation and dizziness. Opiates are generally not as effective as anticonvulsants or antidepressants in managing neuropathic pain. Other products that could be considered would be topical products such as Lidoderm or Capsaicin.

Pain is transmitted through the peripheral nerves, the brain, and the spinal cord. Tissue injury can trigger pain and result in changes in levels and activity of neurotransmitters and the sodium-, potassium-, and calcium-mediated pathways involved in neurotransmission. Nerve injury can cause an increase in calcium and sodium channel activity and a decrease in potassium channel activity, resulting in a release of the neurotransmitters substance P and glutamate, and can lead to allodynia. In addition, nerve damage can increase the release of interleukin-1 and tumor necrosis factor, which can exacerbate and prolong transmitted pain. Medications used to treat neuropathic pain often affect pain transmission by altering the levels of neurotransmitters (glutamate, serotonin, and norepinephrine) via antidepressants or the activity of sodium, potassium, or calcium pathways involved in neurotransmission via anticonvulsants.

Neuropathies associated with diabetes can be categorized as acute or chronic. Acute neuropathy, which is self-limited, has an acute onset and lasts less than 12 mo. This type of neuropathy is treated with tight glucose control and analgesics. Chronic neuropathy persists beyond acute neuropathy, and analgesics cannot effectively control the pain. Medications used to treat diabetic neuropathy target sensory–motor neuropathy, cardiovascular autonomic neuropathy resulting in orthostatic hypotension, and diabetic autonomic neuropathy resulting in sexual or bladder dysfunction. Table 21.4 lists medications used to treat diabetic autonomic neuropathies (Brock, 2010; Montfort et al., 2010; Sherman, 2010; Votey & Peters, 2010; White, 2010).

Based on the symptoms and type of neuropathy, the physician can implement an appropriate treatment regimen. Dysesthesias can be treated with capsaicin cream, pregabalin, or gabapentin therapy. Paresthesias can be treated with tricyclic antidepressants, lidocaine patch, tramadol, opiates, anticonvulsants, and selective serotonin and norepinephrine reuptake inhibitors. Simple stretching exercises and proper footwear can help relieve muscle pain. Occasionally, muscle relaxants such as carisoprodol (Soma) or cyclobenzaprine (Flexeril) may be of benefit in the first 2 wk of therapy. Table 21.5 summarizes medications used to treat diabetic enteropathy (Brock, 2010; Montfort et al., 2010; Sherman, 2010; Votey & Peters, 2010; White, 2010).

Summary

This chapter introduces important concepts in the pathophysiology of diabetes and the complications associated with the disease. It also reviews the use of insulin and other hypoglycemic agents and the medications used to

See table 21.4 in the web resource for a full list of medication-specific indications, dosing recommendations, and side effects.

Table 21.4   Medications Used to Treat Diabetic Autonomic Neuropathy

Medication	Side effects affecting rehab							Other side effects or considerations
Treatment of orthostatic hypotension								
Fludrocortisone acetate (Florinef)	Cog +	S 0	A +	Motor ++	D ++	Com +	F ++	Used if salt tablets and pressure stockings fail to alleviate hypotension. Used to increase standing blood pressure; increases sodium retention and expands plasma volume. Side effects: Fluid retention, insomnia, dizziness, lightheadedness, increased sweating, hyperglycemia, indigestion, psychosis.
Treatment of diabetic impotence								
Sildenafil (Viagra)	Cog +	S 0	A +	Motor ++	D ++	Com +	F ++	All other causes of impotence must be excluded. Older methods such as vacuum devices or intracavernosal papaverine injections may also be tried. Side effects: Headache, flushing, dyspepsia, dizziness, diarrhea, rash, vision changes. Avoid nitrate therapy.
Treatment of neurogenic bladder								
Bethanechol (Urecholine)	Cog +	S 0	A +	Motor +++	D +++	Com +	F +++	In cases of neurogenic bladder, encourage voiding every 3-4 h. Side effects: Malaise, belching, abdominal cramps, colicky pain, diarrhea, increased salivation, urinary urgency, flushing, lacrimation, miosis, hypotension with reflex tachycardia.

Cog = cognition; S = sedation; A = agitation or mania; Motor = discoordination; D = dysphagia; Com = communication; F = falls.

The likelihood rating scale for encountering the side effects is as follows: 0 = Almost no probability of encountering side effects. + = Little likelihood of encountering side effects. +/++ = Low probability of encountering side effects; however, probability increases with increased dosage. ++ = Medium likelihood of encountering side effects. +++ = High likelihood of encountering side effects, particularly with high doses. ++++ = Highest likelihood of encountering side effects; best to avoid in at-risk patients.

treat diabetic neuropathy and outlines how to appropriately adjust the patient's therapy session based on the side effects of these medications. Finally, the chapter discusses diabetic neuropathy and nonpharmacologic treatments of type 1 and type 2 diabetes.

See table 21.5 in the web resource for a full list of medications, dosing recommendations, and side effects.

Table 21.5 Medications Used to Treat Diabetic Enteropathy

Medication	Side effects affecting rehab							Other side effects or considerations
Antidiarrheal medications for diabetic diarrhea: Patients with autonomic dysfunction of the gastrointestinal tract are taught to eat very small meals several times a day. In severe cases, reducing the dietary fiber to near zero may improve symptoms. Diabetic diarrhea is a diagnosis of exclusion and can be difficult to control. A high-fiber diet, along with diphenoxylate, loperamide, or clonidine, can be helpful. Should not be used to treat diarrhea associated with bacterial infections.								
Atropine–diphenoxylate (Lomotil)	Cog +	S +	A ++	Motor ++	D ++	Com +	F ++	Maximum of 8 tablets per day to reduce chance of development of tolerance. Side effects: Blurred vision, constipation, insomnia, dizziness, drowsiness, nausea, loss of taste, xerostomia, tachycardia.
Loperamide (Imodium)	Cog +	S +	A ++	Motor ++	D ++	Com +	F ++	Maximum of 8 capsules daily to reduce chance of development of tolerance. Side effects: Tightness in chest, constipation, nausea, vomiting, abdominal cramps, decreased urination, skin reactions, bloating, drowsiness, dizziness.
Antibiotics for bacterial overgrowth: Small bowel stasis results in bacterial overgrowth, causing diarrhea.								
Amoxicillin	Cog +	S 0	A +	Motor +	D ++	Com +	F +	Take before meals on an empty stomach to ensure adequate absorption. Side effects: Nausea, vomiting, diarrhea, colitis, allergic reactions, agitation, insomnia, confusion, dizziness.
Metronidazole (Flagyl)	Cog +	S 0	A +	Motor ++	D ++	Com +	F ++	Side effects: Seizures, peripheral neuropathy with prolonged use, nausea, anorexia, diarrhea, vomiting, abdominal cramping, dizziness, vertigo, ataxia, depression, weakness, insomnia, bone marrow suppression, confusion, urinary incontinence. Drug interactions: Avoid alcohol; can result in severe nausea and vomiting (Antabuse effect).
Ciprofloxacin (Cipro)	Cog +	S 0	A +	Motor ++	D ++	Com +	F ++	Space by 2 h from calcium, iron supplements, vitamins, antacids containing magnesium or aluminum, dairy products, and sucralfate to ensure adequate absorption. Side effects: Nausea, vomiting, rash, restlessness, dizziness, tremor, ataxia, hallucinations, insomnia, depression, dysphagia, arthralgias, foot pain, pain in the extremities.
Doxycycline (Vibramycin)	Cog 0	S 0	A 0	Motor 0	D ++	Com +	F 0	Space by 2 h from calcium, iron supplements, vitamins, antacids containing magnesium or aluminum, dairy products, and sucralfate to ensure adequate absorption. Side effects: Photosensitivity, nausea, vomiting, loss of appetite, glossitis, dysphagia, esophageal ulceration, rash, bone marrow suppression.

› continued

Table 21.5 › *continued*

Medication	Side effects affecting rehab							Other side effects or considerations
Macrolide antibiotic used for diabetic gastroparesis: Binds to and activates motilin receptors; duplicates the action of motilin.								
Erythromycin (E-Mycin, Erythrocin, Ery-Tab, EES)	Cog 0	S 0	A +	Motor 0	D ++	Com 0	F 0	Intravenous administration enhances the emptying rate of both liquids and solids. Effect can be seen with oral erythromycin. Substitution of the enteric-coated form may be tolerated better by the patient. Side effects: Nausea, vomiting, abdominal pain, diarrhea, hepatotoxicity (rare), rash, ototoxicity with high doses or renal dysfunction, QT prolongation with intravenous form, nightmares.
Serotonin receptor agonist: Used to treat diabetic gastroparesis; available via a limited-access treatment program through the manufacturer, IND treatment protocol was removed from the market because treatment resulted in serious cardiac arrhythmias.								
Cisapride (Propulsid)	Cog ++	S ++	A ++	Motor ++	D +	Com +	F ++	Side effects: Arrhythmias, headache, somnolence, dizziness, fatigue, extrapyramidal symptoms, insomnia, anxiety, depression, urinary frequency, bone marrow suppression. Drug interactions: Risk of QT prolongation and arrhythmia increases when cisapride is combined with clarithromycin, erythromycin, nefazodone, fluconazole, itraconazole, ketoconazole, indinavir, or ritonavir.
Dopamine agonist that acts as a prokinetic agent: Stimulates acetylcholine release in the **myenteric plexus**; acts centrally on chemoreceptor triggers in the floor of the fourth ventricle, which provides important antiemetic activity.								
Metoclopramide (Reglan)	Cog ++	S 0	A ++	Motor +++	D ++	Com +	F +++	Side effects: Tardive dyskinesia, dystonias, neuroleptic malignant syndrome, extrapyramidal symptoms, galactorrhea, impotence, changes in heart rate and blood pressure, nausea, diarrhea, urinary frequency or retention. Contraindications: Avoid use in patients with Parkinson's disease. Precautions: Monitor for extrapyramidal side effects in elderly or patients with creatinine clearance <30 ml/min.
Serotonin agonist used for chronic ileus: Temporarily withdrawn from the U.S. market in March 2007; now available under manufacturer IND treatment protocol.								
Tegaserod (Zelnorm)	Cog ++	S ++	A 0	Motor ++	D ++	Com ++	F ++	Side effects: Abdominal pain, diarrhea, flatulence, headache, dizziness, fatigue, migraine, leg pain, back pain, arthropathy, rash.

Cog = cognition; S = sedation; A = agitation or mania; Motor = discoordination; D = dysphagia; Com = communication; F = falls; IND = investigational new drug application.

The likelihood rating scale for encountering the side effects is as follows: 0 = Almost no probability of encountering side effects. + = Little likelihood of encountering side effects. +/++ = Low probability of encountering side effects; however, probability increases with increased dosage. ++ = Medium likelihood of encountering side effects. +++ = High likelihood of encountering side effects, particularly with high doses. ++++ = Highest likelihood of encountering side effects; best to avoid in at-risk patients.

Medications Used to Treat Respiratory Disease

The rehabilitation therapist will care for many patients with respiratory disease. This chapter introduces the pathophysiology and treatment of the chronic pulmonary diseases **emphysema**, **chronic bronchitis**, and **asthma**, outlines the effect of these diseases on the patient's ability to participate in the rehabilitation session, and provides methods for adjusting the therapy session to assist these patients. This chapter also reviews the most common medications used to treat respiratory disease, outlines their effects and side effects, and provides the rehabilitation specialist with guidelines for monitoring these patients during their rehabilitative sessions.

Respiratory System

The role of the respiratory system is to exchange respiratory gases between the outside environment and the bloodstream. The respiratory gases consist of oxygen and carbon dioxide. Anatomically, the respiratory system comprises the trachea, bronchi, **bronchioles**, and alveolar ducts that transmit air containing oxygen and carbon dioxide through the alveoli in the lungs. A series of capillaries surrounds the alveoli. Oxygen and carbon dioxide are diffused through this single cell layer of the capillaries and alveoli, resulting in oxygenation of the blood and removal of carbon dioxide waste from the blood. Smooth muscle and cartilage compose the pathways of the respiratory system. This smooth muscle, which is controlled by the autonomic nervous system, regulates the size of the passages. The

autonomic nervous system also innervates the involuntary smooth muscles in blood vessels and the heart, the visceral organs, and the endocrine and exocrine glands. Respiration is regulated by the autonomic nervous system, although conscious control can also be initiated. Respiratory disorders can reduce this gas exchange and result in decreased oxygen delivery to the tissues, thus interfering with normal metabolic processes throughout the body (Brenner, 2010; Raissy & Kelly, 2008).

Chronic Obstructive Pulmonary Disease

The Global Initiative for Chronic Obstructive Lung Disease (GOLD, 2013) guidelines define chronic obstructive pulmonary disease (COPD) as a pulmonary disease characterized by airflow limitation that is not fully reversible, is usually progressive, and is associated with abnormal inflammatory response to exposure to noxious particles or gases. Patients with COPD may have a mixture of symptoms associated with emphysema, chronic bronchitis, or asthma (Beers & Porter, 2006; Brenner, 2010).

Incidence

COPD is associated with a high rate morbidity and mortality globally. The incidence of COPD in the elderly is 9.2/1000 person-years. The incidence of COPD is 14.4/1000 person-years in males and 6.2/1000 person-years in women. Between 1990 and 2020, COPD will move from the sixth leading to the third leading cause of death worldwide (van Durme et al., 2009). In the United States, COPD affects approximately 12 million individuals, is the fourth leading cause of death, and results in 5% of all deaths each year. Ten to fifteen percent of patients with COPD also have asthma (Kamanger & Nikhani, 2010; World Health Organization, 2004).

Etiology and Pathophysiology

Cigarette smoking is the predominant COPD risk factor, but pipe and cigar smoking also increase the risk of developing COPD. COPD occurs in 15% of all cigarette smokers. COPD can also be caused by secondhand smoke, environmental pollutants, or routine inhalation of chemicals, fumes, or dust. An inherited form of COPD that is associated with alpha-1 antitrypsin deficiency can also occur and affects 1-3% of COPD patients and can be associated with development of cirrhosis in adults and children.

PATIENT CASE 1

K.L. is a 76-yr-old female who was recently discharged after a prolonged hospitalization with COPD and pneumonia. She lives in an assisted living facility, has a 300 pack/yr history of smoking, and has cut back to one half pack/day. Her forced expiratory volume (**FEV1**) is 50% and she has continuous symptoms of shortness of breath. Since her admission to the assisted living facility, she has lost 15 lb and has fallen twice. She was referred to the rehabilitation therapist for assistance with pulmonary rehabilitation.

Question
Which risk factors for pneumonia and COPD are associated with K.L.'s medical history? What are some initial symptoms associated with COPD?

Answer
K.L.'s history of smoking increases her risk for COPD, and her COPD increases her risk for developing pneumonia. Between 4% and 10% of the population globally

has COPD. The main risk factor for COPD is cigarette smoking. The inhalation of secondhand smoke may contribute to the onset of COPD in nonsmokers. Air pollution, occupational chemicals, and conditions such as tuberculosis and human immunodeficiency virus can also contribute to COPD. The initial symptom of COPD is cough, which the patient may overlook. The symptoms of shortness of breath and fatigue usually encourage the patient to seek medical help.

Emphysema

Emphysema and chronic bronchitis are the two most common conditions that make up COPD. With emphysema, oxidative stress from phagocytes and exposure to free radicals in cigarette smoke cause cell death in the central airways, peripheral bronchioles, and lung parenchyma. With emphysema, the alveoli become enlarged and alveolar cell walls are destroyed, resulting in collapsed airways and air becoming trapped in the airways, which results in an enlarged pulmonary air space. This enlargement decreases the elasticity of the lungs and reduces the patient's ability to exchange gases (oxygen and carbon dioxide) in and out of the lungs. The reduction of gas exchange results in shortness of breath and decreased exercise capacity, along with an expanded (barrel) chest, tachypnea, use of accessory muscles for breathing, and forward leaning while breathing. Bronchoconstriction associated with inflammation may be partially reversible with medication therapy in emphysema (Kamanger & Nikhani, 2010; Prosser & Bollmeier, 2008). Patients with emphysema may be treated with medications, exercises to enhance respiratory efficiency, and oxygen therapy. Bronchodilators and **mucolytic agents** are often prescribed for bronchial dilatation and secretion expectoration (Hitner & Nagle, 2001a).

Incidence

The Burden of Obstructive Lung Disease Study shows that the worldwide prevalence of COPD is around 10%. Prevalence varies by geographic location (Buist et al., 2007). The National Health Interview Survey reports the prevalence of emphysema at 18/1000 persons and chronic bronchitis at 34/1000 persons. The rate of emphysema has stayed largely unchanged since 2000, and the rate of chronic bronchitis has decreased (Adams et al., 2008).

Etiology and Pathophysiology

Smoking is the primary cause of emphysema. The inflammatory response from the exposure to toxins results in infiltration of the lung tissue by activated white blood cells and monocytes, which release destructive proteases. Emphysema occurs if an imbalance exists between the destructive proteases and the protective antiproteases in the lungs. Cigarette smoke inactivates alpha-1 antitrypsin and impairs other antiproteases such as secretory leukoprotease inhibitor. Secretory leukoprotease inhibitor also down regulates tissue necrosis factor. These proteases destroy alveoli and collagen, resulting in decreased lung elasticity, increased airway obstruction, and alveolar collapse. Cigarette smoke and tar contain high concentrations of reactive oxidants and overwhelm the lung's protective factors of mucin, glutathione, catalases, superoxide dismutases, and ascorbic acid, resulting in damage to lung cells and elastin (Kamanger & Nikhani, 2010; Prosser & Bollmeier, 2008).

Chronic Bronchitis

Chronic bronchitis is characterized by enlargement of the mucous glands and chronic inflammation of the medium airways of the lungs (bronchioles). Chronic bronchitis is defined by chronic cough accompanied by persistent production of sputum for at least 3 mo/yr for at least 2 yr. Airway obstruction in chronic bronchitis results from narrowing of the airways, increased airway resistance associated with inflammation, and increased production of sputum. Symptoms include shortness of breath, expectorating cough, and wheezing. Tobacco smoking is the most common cause of chronic bronchitis (Kamanger & Nikhani, 2010; Prosser & Bollmeier, 2008).

Incidence

The global prevalence of chronic bronchitis is estimated to be about 2.6%; prevalence varies from country to country. In comparison, prevalence of smoking is estimated to be 20% to 57%. Only 30% of the geographical variability in prevalence is explained by differences in smoking habits, suggesting that factors such as genetics or environmental exposure to toxins may also play an important role. According to estimates from national interviews conducted by the National Center for Health Statistics in 2006, approximately 9.5 million people, or 4% of the U.S. population, were diagnosed with chronic bronchitis. Many believe that this is an underestimate of true incidence because many patients with chronic bronchitis go undiagnosed. Chronic bronchitis is more prevalent in people over 50 yr of age (Cerveri et al., 2001).

Etiology and Pathophysiology

Chronic bronchitis is viewed as progressive in nature and is caused by pulmonary inflammation after exposure to noxious gases or particles. Cigarette smoking causes 85% to 90% of cases of chronic bronchitis. Studies indicate that smoking pipes, cigars, and marijuana cause similar damage. Air pollution has been associated with increased respiratory health problems among people living in affected areas. Occupational exposures that can cause chronic bronchitis include coal, manufactured vitreous fibers, oil mist, cement, silica, silicates, osmium, vanadium, welding fumes, organic dusts, engine exhaust, fire smoke, and secondhand cigarette smoke.

Chronic inflammation impairs ciliary movement, inhibits the function of alveolar macrophages, and leads to hypertrophy and hyperplasia of mucous-secreting glands. This results in increased and thickened mucous secretions in the pulmonary passages. These mucous secretions affect the exchange of pulmonary gas, and fibrotic alterations in the lining of the respiratory system can result. Subsequently, the patient exhibits a chronic cough along with production of sputum. The copious amount of mucus causes breathing difficulty, increases susceptibility to respiratory infections, and reduces the patient's ability to engage in physical activity (Fischer et al., 2007; Hitner & Nagle, 2001a).

Asthma

In contrast to COPD, asthma is a chronic lung condition of reversible bronchospasm. It is characterized by episodes of intermittent, acute narrowing of the bronchioles (bronchospasm) accompanied by diffuse airway inflammation, termed an asthma attack. This inflammation is accompanied by increased mucosal edema, production of bronchial mucus, and impaired ciliary clearance of mucus from the lower respiratory airways. Symptoms of asthma include cough, dyspnea, and wheezing. Patients experiencing an asthma attack may have difficulty speaking, exhibit stridor (harsh, high-pitched wheezing), use the accessory muscles to breathe, have decreased level of alertness, and have difficulty in maintaining a reclining position due to their shortness of breath (Brenner, 2010; Raissy & Kelly, 2008).

Incidence

The prevalence of asthma and the associated mortality and morbidity have dramatically increased over the past 4 decades. The prevalence of asthma increases 50% every 10 yr. Worldwide, it is estimated that more than 300 million people have asthma and that more than 180,000 deaths are attributable to asthma (Braman, 2006).

Asthma affects approximately 6% to 10% of the U.S. population, or 20 million to 25 million people; half of these are children. Onset of asthma usually occurs in childhood. Childhood asthma affects 8% to 20% of all children; asthma persists into adulthood in about 50% of these children. Asthma accounts for 2% of all visits to the emergency room. The incidence of asthma is higher in African Americans and Hispanics than in Caucasians. About 4,500 Americans die from asthma each year (Brenner, 2010).

Etiology and Pathophysiology

Triggers of asthma attacks include respiratory tract infections, emotional upset, exercise, and exposure to allergens (e.g., dust mites, cold) or respiratory irritants (e.g., tobacco smoke). Exposure to allergens or irritants causes membrane phospholipases to produce arachidonic acid, and activation of the arachidonic cascade of inflammation. Arachidonic acid is metabolized by cyclooxygenase to vasoactive prostaglandins (thromboxane and prostacyclin) and to leukotrienes that cause vasoconstriction of the bronchial smooth muscles and bronchoconstriction. Bronchoconstriction from other triggers is mediated through the neurotransmitters of the autonomic nervous system. Asthmatic attacks can be relieved through the use of bronchodilators and medications that reduce the inflammatory response of the respiratory airways (Brenner, 2010; Hitner & Nagle, 2001a; Raissy & Kelly, 2008).

Rehabilitation Considerations for Respiratory Disease

The rehabilitation therapist treating patients with respiratory disease is likely to encounter individuals with a variety of diagnoses such as COPD, asthma, chronic bronchitis, and emphysema. These patients present with numerous difficulties with nutrition, dysphagia, breathing, posture, behavior, or cognition that directly or indirectly affect their respiratory ability and ability to participate in rehabilitation. The rehabilitation specialist needs to be sensitive to and aware of these difficulties and should be cognizant of the medications that the patient is taking and be aware of these medications' therapeutic effects, as well as potential side effects and drug interactions that can affect rehabilitation.

Nutritional Assessment and Therapy

Nutritional difficulties frequently occur in patients with pulmonary disease. Some patients are so weak that their inability to self-feed jeopardizes their nutritional status. This reduced nutritional intake coupled with an increase in nutritional needs seen in the patient with chronic pulmonary disease can make maintaining a good nutritional status especially challenging. Counseling that addresses planning and preparing nutritionally adequate meals, the adequacy of the patient's food supply, and the use of nutritional supplements is essential in helping patients meet their nutritional needs. Patients should also be evaluated for possible dysphagia, which commonly occurs in the respiratory patient. Approximately 50% of hospitalized patients with COPD reportedly suffer from protein and calorie malnutrition. The onset of weight loss in a patient with chronic respiratory disease is a poor prognostic indicator. Inadequate dietary intake, increased resting energy expenditure, and failure of the normal adaptive response to malnutrition lead to energy imbalance and progressive weight loss. With an adequate provision of calories, the usual intervention for a malnourished patient with chronic respiratory disorder results in weight gain. A calorie intake of 1.7 times the resting energy expenditure is recommended, and provision of adequate nitrogen to maintain body stores, replace structural tissue, and spare calories is required. Based on trials, it appears that protein supplementation of at least 1.7 g/kg of body weight/day is associated with nitrogen retention and physiologic improvement (DeHart & Worthington, 2005; Drive et al., 1982).

Dysphagia

Dysphagia can occur in the patient with pulmonary disease and can adversely affect nutritional status. Skeletal muscle wasting and dysfunction seen in respiratory disease can result in a decreased ability to move the bolus posterior. In addition, the COPD patient may fail to exhibit adequate oral sensation and perception, and anterior–posterior bolus movements in the oral cavity may decrease as a result. The COPD patient may exhibit swallowing that is discoordinated with the phases of respiration (Harding, 2002). Disrupted coordination of breathing and swallowing can increase the risk of aspiration (Gross et al., 2009). Oral pharyngeal dysphagia, commonly seen in COPD patients, may lead to nutritional changes and weight loss. The speech–language pathologist (SLP) working with the COPD

patient needs to be cognizant of decreases in oral and pharyngeal musculature abilities in the patient. Common difficulties include reduced tongue control, reduced anterior–posterior tongue movement, delayed pharyngeal swallow, and dysfunctional swallow (Mokhlesi et al., 2002). The SLP also needs to be aware that the COPD patient will most likely exhibit rhonchi during thoracic auscultation. The rhonchi may or may not indicate aspiration. The SLP must be able to differentiate the lung sounds of aspiration from the lung sounds of COPD because both may produce rhonchi. Asking the patient to cough or change position may help the therapist differentiate the lung sounds (Carl & Johnson, 2006; Mokhlesi, 2003; Mokhlesi et al., 2001, 2002).

The SLP needs to provide patient education which helps the patient focus on oral sensation and perception and anterior–posterior movement of the bolus as well as decrease the patient's reliance on altered diets and thickened liquids by increasing oral and pharyngeal motor strength. Pulmonary rehabilitation programs that include nutritional counseling and dysphagia instruction improve the management of dysphagia and the patient's respiratory disease (McKinstry et al., 2010).

Secondary Effects of COPD

The effects of COPD are seen far beyond pulmonary dysfunction. This disease can lead to skeletal muscle dysfunction, systemic inflammation, nutritional changes, and weight loss. The COPD patient is also more likely to develop osteoporosis, resulting in an increased probability of fractures. Consequences of respiratory disease such as COPD include peripheral muscle dysfunction, respiratory muscle dysfunction, nutritional abnormalities, cardiac impairment, skeletal disease, sensory deficits, reduced cognition, and psychosocial dysfunction. These consequences occur because of deconditioning, malnutrition, persistent hypoxemia, steroid myopathy, hyperinflation, diaphragmatic fatigue, frequent hospitalizations, and effects of various medications. Psychosocial dysfunction results from anxiety, depression, guilt, dependency, and sleep disturbance. COPD patients experience insomnia more frequently due to decreased gas exchange and depression-related sleep deprivation, hypoventilation, and cough. Patients with COPD should use medications to treat insomnia with care because hypnotics may influence the functioning of the respiratory system. Sleep apnea combined with hypoventilation may result in a lack of oxygen and premature mortality.

All of these factors contribute to increased risk of falls in individuals with COPD. Fractures are considered a secondary cause of mortality and morbidity among COPD patients. The occupational therapist and physical therapist should outline the therapeutic procedures for preventing and treating fractures in this population (Fischer et al., 2007). Clinical dietitians and pharmacists can assist with appropriate recommendations for diet and medication supplements to optimize bone health.

Patients with COPD tend to be more anxious than patients with normal respiratory function; 10% to 16% of patients with COPD experience anxiety compared with 5% of patients without respiratory disease. In addition, 8% to 37% of patients with COPD experience panic attacks (Brenes, 2003). Patients with COPD are at increased risk for depression, especially those who live alone. Depression and solitary living can reduce the chance of successful smoking cessation. The lack of social contact may also increase the patient's anxiety, depression, and feeling of isolation. Successful rehabilitation addresses both the physical and emotional issues seen in the patient with COPD. In some instances, collaboration with a social worker, psychologist, or psychiatrist may be necessary to provide an effective individualized rehabilitation plan (Fischer et al., 2007; Kim et al. 2000; Puhan et al., 2008; Sharma & Arneja, 2010).

The COPD patient also can exhibit cognitive dysfunction secondary to the systemic effects of reduced oxygen exchange. The COPD cognitive pattern generally consists of deficits in verbal memory due to difficulties with active recall as well as deficits in passive recognition of learned data. Sensory memory and attention span can be affected. COPD patients can also exhibit deficits in deductive thinking (Incalzi et al., 2003), working memory, and long-term memory. These cognitive dysfunctions are at least partially related to hypoxemia and can have an immediate effect on the patient's prognosis for rehabilitation and daily functioning. Oxygen therapy or physical activity can reduce cognitive deficits in this population (Derkacz et al., 2007). Therapies involving continuous oxygen and pulmonary rehabilitation have been shown to increase attention and verbal fluency and decrease anxiety and depression. Advanced age does not hamper the COPD patient's response to rehabilitation. In addition, one study reported that the most physically impaired patients received the most benefit from rehabilitation. Patients undergoing lung volume-reduction surgery to improve airflow and reduce hyperinflation have shown improvements in verbal memory, psychomotor speed, and naming (DiMeo et al., 2008; Emory et al., 2008; Kozora et al., 2008).

COPD can affect the patient's self-concept. Being dependent on medications and caregivers and being unable to perform certain functional abilities may negatively affect the patient's self-esteem and self-efficacy. The patient's feeling of shortness of breath in particular exacerbates the feeling of inadequacy in performing activities of daily living. Chronic systemic inflammation associated with COPD is a causative factor in the patient's increased risk for developing other chronic diseases. Patients with COPD are at higher risk for depression, cancer, heart disease, high blood pressure, sinusitis, ulcers, and migraines (Fischer et al., 2007; Incalzi et al., 1997).

Oxygen Therapy

COPD is commonly associated with progressive hypoxemia. Use of oxygen reduces mortality rates in patients with advanced COPD due to the favorable effects of oxygen on pulmonary hemodynamics. Long-term oxygen therapy improves survival twofold or more in hypoxemic patients with COPD. Hypoxemia is defined as having a partial pressure of oxygen (PaO_2) of less than 55 mm Hg or having an oxygen saturation of less than 90%. Specialists recommend long-term oxygen therapy in patients with PaO_2 less than 55 mm Hg or PaO_2 less than 59 mm Hg along with evidence of polycythemia or cor pulmonale. These patients should be re-evaluated in 1 to 3 mo to determine whether continued therapy is warranted. Oxygen supplementation during exercise can reduce dyspnea, improve exercise tolerance, and prevent increases in pulmonary artery pressure. When used as prescribed, oxygen therapy is generally safe. Oxygen toxicity from inspiring high concentrations (>60%) is well recognized and should be avoided. The continuous-flow nasal cannula is the standard means of oxygen delivery for the stable hypoxemic patient. This means of oxygen delivery is simple, reliable, and generally well tolerated. Each liter of oxygen flow adds 3% to 4% to the fractional inspired oxygen. Nasal oxygen delivery is also beneficial for most patients who breathe through the mouth. Oxygen-conserving devices deliver all of the oxygen during early inhalation. These devices improve the portability of oxygen therapy and reduce overall costs (Sharma & Arneja, 2010). The major physical hazards of oxygen therapy are fires and explosions. Patients, family members, and other caregivers must be warned not to smoke. However, major accidents are rare and can be prevented by good patient and family training (Garrod et al., 2000; Sharma & Arneja, 2010).

Pulmonary rehabilitation is an integral part of the clinical management and health maintenance of patients with chronic respiratory disease who remain symptomatic or continue to have decreased function despite standard medical treatment. Pulmonary rehabilitation aims to reduce symptoms, decrease disability, increase participation in physical and social activities, and improve the overall quality of life of patients with chronic respiratory disease. These goals are achieved through patient and family education, exercise training, psychosocial and behavioral intervention, and outcome assessment. The rehabilitation interventions are patient specific and implemented by a multidisciplinary team of health care professionals. The rehabilitation team is led by a physician rehabilitation specialist and includes a physical therapist, occupational therapist, SLP, rehabilitation nurse, pharmacist, social worker, respiratory therapist, vocational counselor, and psychologist. Outcomes of a comprehensive pulmonary rehabilitation program include increased independence and improved quality of life as well as fewer hospitalizations or shorter hospitalization time (Sergysels et al., 1979). Outcome measures to be evaluated after 6 to 12 mo include level of dyspnea, exercise ability, health status, and activity level (Boueri et al., 2001; Brown et al., 2000; Fischer et al., 2007; Sergysels et al., 1979; Sharma & Arneja, 2010).

Although COPD is the major disease involved in referral for pulmonary rehabilitation services, patients with other conditions may be appropriate candidates for pulmonary rehabilitation. The same principles of ameliorating secondary morbidity apply to conditions such as asthma, chest wall disease, cystic fibrosis, bronchiectasis, interstitial lung disease, lung cancer, selected neuromuscular diseases, post polio syndrome, and perioperative conditions (e.g., thoracic or abdominal surgery, lung transplantation, and lung volume-reduction surgery) (Sharma & Arneja, 2010).

Exercise Training

Exercise does not alter underlying respiratory impairment, but it does ameliorate dyspnea and improve other outcome measures. A closely monitored, gradual progression of physical exercise is the foundation of rehabilitation for the COPD patient. Rehabilitation also focuses on energy-conservation exercises, relaxation exercises, smoking cessation, nutrition, and cognitive rehabilitation (Fischer et al., 2007). Patients with COPD who participate in a medically supervised aerobic-training program demonstrate significant improvement in the 6 min walking distance test, maximal exercise performance test, peripheral and respiratory muscle strength tests, and quality of life scores (Koppers et al., 2006; Sharma & Arneja, 2010; Troosters et al., 2000).

In COPD patients, a major portion of oxygen consumption goes toward supporting the work of breathing. During exercise, this will likely reduce the overall workload that these patients are able to tolerate. The rehabilitation therapist should grade exercise intensity carefully and monitor the patient for signs of early fatigue or distress such as cyanosis and abnormal vital signs. The major components of physical training in the COPD patient are breathing exercises, strength training for respiratory muscles, and endurance training for the lower and upper extremities. Resistance-training programs should train each major muscle group 2 to 3 times/wk. Training the muscle groups of the lower extremity, such as the quadriceps and hip extensors, is especially important because these muscles have a predisposition to weakness and play an essential role in sit-to-stand transfers and gait. Functional multijoint resistance exercises such as the bodyweight squat are commonly used to target these muscle groups. Outcomes related to resistance-training programs in patients with COPD include increased muscle strength, endurance, and function; increased exercise tolerance; and reduced dyspnea. Flexibility exercises typically focus on stretching the thoracic and shoulder girdle areas to improve thoracic and shoulder girdle compliance and to reduce the workload involved in breathing (Fischer et al., 2007; Mueller et al., 1970; Sergysels et al., 1979).

The effects of training are reversible and are maintained only if the patient continues to exercise. Therefore, improving long-term adherence to exercise training at home is essential to the long-term effectiveness of pulmonary rehabilitation (Bourbeau et al., 2003; Finnerty et al., 2001; Hill, 2006; Reardon et al., 1994).

Breathing Techniques

The three major breathing techniques used in pulmonary rehabilitation include pursed-lip breathing, posture techniques, and diaphragmatic breathing. In pursed-lip breathing, the patient exhales slowly for 4 to 6 s through pursed lips that are held in a whistling position. This technique relieves dyspnea by increasing expiratory airway pressure, thereby inhibiting dynamic expiratory airway collapse. Patients also shift their breathing pattern from a rapid rate of respiration, which is under the control of the involuntary respiratory center, to a slower, more controlled pattern governed by voluntary cortical function. The overall work of breathing does not change and, in fact, may decrease slightly. The pursed-lip breathing shifts a major portion of the inspiratory work

of breathing from the diaphragm to the ribcage muscles, thus resting the diaphragm and reducing dyspnea.

Forward-leaning postures frequently relieve dyspnea in patients with COPD by reducing respiratory effort. The shifting of abdominal contents cranially elevates the depressed diaphragm, resulting in improved performance. The greatest benefit occurs in patients with severe hyperinflation who experience paradoxical inward movement of the upper abdomen.

In diaphragmatic breathing, the patient is taught to use only the diaphragm during inspiration and to maximize abdominal protrusion. During expiration, the patient may contract the muscles of the abdominal wall to displace the diaphragm more cephalic (Fischer et al., 2007; Mueller et al., 1970; Sergysels et al., 1979; Sharma & Arneja, 2010).

Chest Physical Therapy

Controlled-breathing techniques and chest physical therapy are the two major components of the multidisciplinary approach to rehabilitation in patients with COPD, bronchiectasis, and cystic fibrosis. Although only smoking cessation and long-term oxygen therapy prolong life in patients with COPD, chest physical therapy likely prolongs life in patients with cystic fibrosis and diffuse bronchiectasis (Fischer et al., 2007; Mueller et al., 1970; Sergysels et al., 1979).

Chest physical therapy, along with postural drainage, enhances clearance of mucus from the central and peripheral lung airways. The value of this therapy in stable patients with COPD and in acute COPD exacerbation is uncertain. Nonetheless, chest physical therapy combined with postural drainage and effective coughing techniques enhances sputum expectoration in patients who produce more than 30 ml of sputum/24 h or who have difficulty expectorating sputum.

Chest physical therapy and respiratory hygiene can help the patient maintain a clear airway. The clinician should also encourage the patient to cough and expectorate secretions. Rehabilitation treatments should be coordinated with respiratory therapy. For example, patients should participate in chest physical therapy after medications used in respiratory therapy have loosened secretions in the chest. Clinicians should know how to respond to a bronchospastic attack and should encourage patients to bring their portable aerosol bronchodilator to treatment sessions (Ciccone, 2007; Reardon et al., 1994). Chest physical therapy remains an essential component of therapy for patients with bronchiectasis and cystic fibrosis. The frequency of treatments must be individualized based on the severity of disease and the amount of airway secretion that must be cleared. Standard chest physical therapy with postural drainage, cough, and the forced expiratory technique is the cornerstone of such a treatment regimen. Chest physiotherapy is essential for managing atelectasis in postoperative or seriously ill patients with COPD who are hospitalized (Fischer et al., 2007; MacIntyre et al., 2001; Mueller et al., 1970; Sergysels et al., 1979).

The rehabilitation therapist should extensively educate the patient with COPD about their condition in order to engage the patient to actively participate in rehabilitation. Educational sessions should include information about the patient's disease state, nutrition, relaxation and stress-management training, coping-skills training, realistic goal setting, self-monitoring, energy conservation, and cognitive–behavioral therapy and should include physical exercise. In several studies, sessions that did not include physical exercise actually increased anxiety, whereas sessions that included a combination of physical exercise and education decreased anxiety among patients with COPD (Devine & Pearcy, 1996; Fischer et al., 2007).

Medication Therapy for Respiratory Disease

Impaired oxygen exchange that results in airway obstruction is common to asthma, bronchitis, and emphysema. This airway obstruction is a result of bronchoconstriction and inflammation. Medication therapy is directed at preventing or reducing bronchial constriction and inflammation. Bronchodilators are medications that reduce bronchoconstriction by inducing relaxation of smooth muscle in the lung tissues, which is controlled by the autonomic nervous system. The autonomic nervous system comprises sympathetic (adrenergic) and parasympathetic (cholinergic) nerves. Stimulation of the sympathetic nervous system results in "fight or flight" responses, including bronchodilation. Stimulation of the parasympathetic (cholinergic) nervous system results in bronchoconstriction mediated by the neurotransmitter acetylcholine. Anticholinergic medications counteract the effects of acetylcholine and can facilitate bronchodilation. Medications that are used to induce bronchodilation include beta-2 adrenergic agonists and inhaled anticholinergic agents (Brenner, 2010; Raissy & Kelly, 2008).

Medications are also used to reduce inflammation. These include inhaled and oral anti-inflammatory agents (corticosteroids) and inhaled and oral leukotriene inhibitors. Medications used to reduce congestion associated with increased production of sputum include inhaled and oral mucolytics, xanthine inhibitors, expectorants, and antitussives. Antibiotics are used to treat acute COPD exacerbations that are characterized by an increased amount of **purulent** sputum associated with bacterial infection. In addition, medication therapy is often used to assist in smoking cessation in the patient with respiratory disease. Finally, vaccine administration is important in preventing exacerbations and reducing the number of hospitalizations in the patient with respiratory disease.

Medication Therapy for COPD

Patients with COPD are staged by severity of illness; a patient's stage determines treatment. Stage I disease is defined by FEV1 values of greater than 80% with or without symptoms, stage II disease is defined by FEV1 values of 50% to 80% with or without symptoms, stage III disease is defined by FEV1 of 30% to 50% with or without symptoms, and stage IV disease is defined by FEV1 of 30% to 50% with chronic symptoms of respiratory failure. Mild disease is treated with a short-acting inhaled beta agonist when needed. The Global Initiative for Chronic

Obstructive Lung Disease guidelines recommend an inhaled long-acting beta agonist or an inhaled anticholinergic agent as first-line maintenance therapy for all patients with stage II disease. The addition of an inhaled corticosteroid to long-acting inhaled bronchodilators has been shown to reduce mortality by 27% in patients with stage III or stage IV disease. All patients should have a short-acting beta agonist on hand to treat intermittent symptoms of shortness of breath. Table 22.1 summarizes medication therapies used to treat asthma and COPD (Prosser & Bollmeier, 2008).

PATIENT CASE 1, *continued*

K.L. is the 76-yr-old female discussed earlier who was recently discharged after a prolonged hospitalization with COPD and pneumonia and is admitted to rehabilitation services for pulmonary rehabilitation after two recent falls. Her FEV1 is 50% and she has continuous symptoms of shortness of breath. In addition to exercise training and breathing exercises, what are some medication therapies that may help control K.L.'s respiratory symptoms?

Answer

K.L. should use a combination of a long-acting inhaled bronchodilator to open airway passages and to improve oxygen exchange and an inhaled corticosteroid to reduce respiratory airway inflammation as scheduled chronic therapy. She should also be taking a short-acting beta-2 agonist by inhalation to treat immediate symptoms of dyspnea as needed.

Medication Therapy for Asthma

Asthma is classified by frequency and severity of symptoms and the percentage of forced expiratory volume compared with normal values. A patient's classification determines which medications to use in treatment. Classifications include mild intermittent (symptoms <2 times/wk and FEV1 >80% of normal), mild persistent (symptoms 3-6 times/wk and FEV1 >80% of normal), moderate persistent (daily symptoms and FEV1 60%-80% of normal), and severe persistent (continual symptoms and FEV1 <60% of normal values). Intermittent

asthma is managed by the use of short-acting inhaled beta agonists taken on an as-needed (prn) basis. Symptoms consistent with mild persistent disease are controlled with low-dose inhaled corticosteroids, inhaled cromolyn, a leukotriene inhibitor, or theophylline taken on a scheduled chronic basis. Symptoms seen with moderate persistent disease are managed with an intermediate-dose inhaled corticosteroid in combination with a long-acting inhaled bronchodilator taken on a scheduled chronic basis. Symptoms associated with severe disease require high-dose inhaled corticosteroids in combination with a long-acting inhaled bronchodilator taken on a scheduled chronic basis. In all stages of disease, a short acting bronchodilator should be available for immediate treatment of acute bronchospasm. Acute exacerbations of asthma (severe asthma attacks) are managed with use of short-term systemic corticosteroids along with continuously nebulized beta agonists in the emergency room setting (Raissy & Kelly, 2008). Table 22.1 summarizes medications used to treat asthma and COPD (Springhouse, 2009).

Bronchodilators

Bronchodilators reverse the bronchospasm associated with COPD and asthma. Because the bronchospastic component of asthma is much more reversible than that of COPD, beta-2 agonists produce more bronchodilation and more dramatic symptom relief in patients with asthma than in patients with COPD. Inhaled beta-2 agonists are the initial treatment of choice for acute exacerbations of COPD and asthma. They increase muscle relaxation in the bronchioles, thus increasing the surface area available for oxygen and carbon dioxide exchange. This results in reduced carbon dioxide retention and improved delivery of oxygen to the organs via the bloodstream (Raissy & Kelly, 2008).

Inhaled beta-2 agonist bronchodilators activate specific beta-2 adrenergic receptors on the surface of smooth muscle cells. This increases levels of intracellular cyclic adenosine monophosphate and increases relaxation of smooth muscle. These medications can be administered orally, subcutaneously, or by inhalation. The inhalation route is preferred because it

See table 22.1 in the web resource for a full list of medication-specific indications, dosing recommendations, and side effects.

Table 22.1 Medications Used in Respiratory Rehabilitation

Medication	Side effects affecting rehab							Other side effects or considerations
Short-acting beta-2 agonists: Immediate-onset bronchodilator used as rescue therapy for acute symptoms of shortness of breath.								
Albuterol (Ventolin) Pirbuterol (Maxair) Levalbuterol (Xopenex)	Cog ++	S 0	A ++	Motor ++	D +	Com 0	F ++	May be helpful before physical exercise to control symptoms; keep on hand during exercise. Side effects: Tachycardia, arrhythmia, nervousness, anxiety, insomnia, hallucinations, dizziness, tremor, increased blood pressure, paradoxical bronchospasm, hypokalemia, muscle pain, cough. Drug interactions: Avoid combining with other sympathomimetics such as the decongestants pseudoephedrine and phenylpropanolamine; may potentiate side effects.
Long-acting beta-2 agonists: Delayed-onset bronchodilator used for continuous bronchodilation to prevent acute symptoms of shortness of breath.								
Formoterol (Foradil) Salmeterol (Serevent)	Cog ++	S 0	A ++	Motor ++	D +	Com 0	F ++	Side effects: Tachycardia, arrhythmia, nervousness, anxiety, insomnia, hallucinations, dizziness, tremor, increased blood pressure, paradoxical bronchospasm, hypokalemia, muscle pain, cough. Drug interactions: Avoid combining with other sympathomimetics such as the decongestants pseudoephedrine and phenylpropanolamine; may potentiate side effects.
Short-acting anticholinergics: Used as bronchodilator with beta-2 agonist to enhance bronchodilator effects.								
Ipratropium bromide (Atrovent)	Cog +	S 0	A ++	Motor +	D +	Com 0	F +	Side effects: Tachycardia, nervousness, paradoxical bronchospasm, dry mouth, nausea, vomiting, tremor, sinus irritation. Drug interactions: Avoid combining with other anticholinergics such as antihistamines that potentiate dry mouth and sympathomimetics that can potentiate tachycardia and nervousness.
Long-acting anticholinergic: Delayed-onset anticholinergic used for continuous bronchodilation to prevent acute symptoms of shortness of breath.								
Tiotropium (Spiriva)	Cog +	S 0	A ++	Motor +	D +	Com 0	F +	Side effects: Tachycardia, nervousness, paradoxical bronchospasm, dry mouth, nausea, vomiting. Drug interactions: Avoid combining with other anticholinergics such as antihistamines that potentiate dry mouth and sympathomimetics that can potentiate tachycardia and nervousness.

› continued

Table 22.1 › *continued*

Medication	Side effects affecting rehab							Other side effects or considerations

Corticosteroids: Inhaled corticosteroids reduce chronic inflammation in air passages and improve oxygen and carbon dioxide exchange; they are often combined with beta-2 agonist therapy. Oral and parenteral steroids are used for short-term treatment of acute exacerbations. Patients should use lowest effective dose of parenteral steroids.

Medication	Cog	S	A	Motor	D	Com	F	Other side effects or considerations
Combination inhaled: Fluticasone–salmeterol (Advair) Budesonide–formoterol (Symbicort)	+	0	+	+	+	0	+	Side effects seen with systemic corticosteroids are minimized with inhaled dosage forms. Always rinse out the mouth after medication administration to reduce the risk of mouth infections.
Oral steroids: Prednisone, methylprednisolone Parenteral steroids: Methylprednisolone dexamethasone	+	0	+	+	+	0	+	Side effects: Personality changes, insomnia, euphoria, muscle weakness or wasting, thinning of the skin, glaucoma, hyperglycemia, cataracts, depression of immune function, lipodystrophy (e.g., moon facies, truncal obesity). Precautions: Avoid abrupt discontinuation of long-term or high-dose oral therapy; may cause severe depression and acute adrenal insufficiency.

Leukotriene inhibitors: Reduce inflammation of air passages by inhibiting effects of leukotrienes, improving oxygen and carbon dioxide. Singulair is used on chronic basis to reduce inflammation associated with asthma, allergic rhinitis, and chronic obstructive pulmonary disease and can be used on an as-needed basis for acute symptoms of allergic rhinitis or as a preventative for bronchospasm when used 2 h before exercise in asthmatic patients.

Medication	Cog	S	A	Motor	D	Com	F	Other side effects or considerations
Zafirlukast (Accolate)	++	++	++	+	++	+	+	Side effects: Sleep disorders, behavioral changes.
Montelukast (Singulair)	++	++	++	+	++	+	+	Most common: Sinusitis, nausea, pharyngolaryngeal pain.
Zileuton (Zyflo; Zyflo CR—sustained release)	++	++	++	+	++	+	+	Common: Fever, headache, pharyngitis, cough, abdominal pain, diarrhea. Less common: Agitation, aggressive behavior or hostility, anxiousness, depression, disorientation, dream abnormalities, hallucinations, insomnia, irritability, restlessness, somnambulism, suicidal thinking and behavior, vasculitis paresthesias, swelling of the sinuses. With zafirlukast, observe liver enzymes to monitor for rare instances of hepatotoxicity and changes in behavior. Drug interactions: Zafirlukast may increase levels of theophylline, cimetidine (Tagamet), amiodarone (Cordarone), and fluconazole (Diflucan). No drug interactions with montelukast are known. Zileuton can increase levels of warfarin (Coumadin), propranolol (Inderal), and theophylline.

Medication	Side effects affecting rehab							Other side effects or considerations
Theophylline: Improves respiratory muscle function, stimulates the respiratory center, promotes bronchodilation, and reduces inflammation. May also improve contractility of the diaphragm muscle.								
Theophylline sustained release: (Theo-24, Theo-Dur) Immediate release: (Theophylline and aminophylline syrup liquid or theophylline intravenous infusion)	Cog ++	S ++	A ++	Motor ++	D +	Com +	F ++	Take product on consistent basis with meals or fasting. Not effective in treatment of acute bronchospasm. Adjust dosing to maintain levels of 5-10 mg/L; recheck blood levels with addition of new medications listed in table 22.2. Side effects seen with serum levels <20 mg/L: Diarrhea, irritability, tachycardia, restlessness, tremors of fine skeletal muscle, and transient diuresis may occur. Levels >20 mg/L: Life-threatening arrhythmias and seizures may occur. Drug interactions: Multiple drug interactions; see table 22.2.
Mucolytic: Used to break up mucus so it can be removed via coughing or suction.								
Acetylcysteine (Mucomyst) 10%-20% solution	Cog 0	S 0	A 0	Motor 0	D +	Com 0	F 0	Respiratory irritant that can result in bronchospasm; administer with bronchodilator to counter bronchospasm. Side effects: Stomatitis, rhinorrhea, nausea, bronchospasm.
Expectorant: Used to thin mucus in air passages to make it easier to cough up mucus and clear airways.								
Guaifenesin (Robitussin—immediate-acting liquid, tablets, dissolving granules, capsules; Mucinex—extended-release tablet)	Cog 0	S 0	A 0	Motor 0	D +	Com 0	F 0	Side effects: Headache, nausea, vomiting.

Cog = cognition; S = sedation; A = agitation or mania; Motor = discoordination; D = dysphagia; Com = communication; F = falls.

The likelihood rating scale for encountering the side effects is as follows: 0 = Almost no probability of encountering side effects. + = Little likelihood of encountering side effects. +/++ = Low probability of encountering side effects; however, probability increases with increased dosage. ++ = Medium likelihood of encountering side effects. +++ = High likelihood of encountering side effects, particularly with high doses. ++++ = Highest likelihood of encountering side effects; best to avoid in at-risk patients.

provides direct administration of the medication to the lungs and the onset of action is more rapid. Using this route also minimizes side effects such as increased heart rate, blood pressure, and jitteriness that can occur when medications are administered orally or subcutaneously. If a patient encounters these side effects, dose reduction may be necessary (Raissy & Kelly, 2008).

These medications are provided in short-acting or long-acting forms. Short-acting formulations, which are used to treat acute bronchospasm or shortness of breath, have immediate effects and are frequently used on an as-needed basis. Long-acting inhaled beta-2 agonist medications such as formoterol (Foradil) and salmeterol (Serevent) provide continuous bronchodilation and are used on a chronic basis to prevent or reduce frequency of acute symptoms. Because their onset is delayed, these products should not be administered to treat acute symptoms. In addition, continuous use of these long-acting products alone results in decreased effectiveness. A recent FDA alert warned that patients should never be treated with long-acting formulations alone and that these agents should always be prescribed in combination with other therapies such as inhaled corticosteroids along with short-acting beta-2 agonists for immediate relief of acute bronchospasm. One study found an increased risk of death in asthma patients who used long-acting formulations to treat acute bronchospasm (Springhouse, 2009).

Anticholinergic Agents

Anticholinergic drugs compete with acetylcholine for postganglionic muscarinic receptors and inhibit cholinergically mediated bronchomotor tone, resulting in bronchodilation. They also block vagally mediated reflex arcs that cause bronchoconstriction. The onset of action is slow (i.e., 30-60 min). Anticholinergic medications can produce bronchodilation and are useful in the treatment of COPD. Adverse reactions associated with anticholinergics include tachycardia, nervousness, paradoxical bronchospasm, dry mouth, nausea, and vomiting. These medications do not cause centralized anticholinergic effects because they are poorly absorbed by inhalation. Ipratropium nasal spray is also used to treat vasomotor rhinitis (runny nose) that results from excess cholinergic activity (Springhouse, 2009).

Ipratropium bromide (Atrovent) is an anticholinergic that is used as a bronchodilator. This medication is used to treat COPD and as an adjunct to beta-2 adrenergic agonists. Treatment with aerosolized anticholinergic agents (i.e., ipratropium bromide or tiotropium) may be more effective than treatment with a beta-2 agonist in patients with COPD. Ipratropium bromide has bronchodilatory activity and minimum adverse effects and is administered via a metered-dose inhaler. Studies in patients with stable COPD have shown that the activity of ipratropium bromide is equivalent or superior to that of a beta-2 agonist. In combination with a beta-2 agonist, ipratropium bromide produces an additional 20% to 40% bronchodilation. This medication has slower onset and a longer duration than a beta-2 agonist and is less suitable for as-needed use. Tiotropium (Spiriva) is also an anticholinergic bronchodilator (Ciccone, 2007; Hitner & Nagle, 2001b). Use of inhaled anticholinergic bronchodilators does not influence the long-term decline of FEV1. Therapy with ipratropium should be scheduled at 2 to 4 puffs 4 times/day and a beta-2 agonist should be added as needed. The effect of beta-2 agonists is additive when they are used with an anticholinergic agent. Combination products such as Combivent and Duonebs are commonly prescribed (Gardenhire, 2008b; Springhouse, 2009). The clinician may note cardiac side effects in patients taking beta-2 agonists and xanthine derivatives. Symptoms of nervousness and confusion may be side effects of bronchodilators and are more pronounced with higher doses or more frequent use. Such symptoms should be reported to the prescriber and may require dosage reduction.

Glucocorticoids

Glucocorticoids (corticosteroids) are potent anti-inflammatory agents that act on all stages of the inflammatory response. Use of these agents can reduce inflammatory response, thus increasing opening of airway passages and reducing mucus production and plugging associated with chronic bronchitis. Corticosteroids are often used in the treatment of asthma and COPD. Glucocorticoids are administered in oral, intravenous injection, intramuscular injection, aerosol inhalant, or intranasal spray formulations. When the medication is administered via the inhaled and intranasal routes, the steroid is delivered directly to the inflamed respiratory tissue and systemic absorption is limited, thus minimizing most of the adverse effects. Corticosteroids do not slow the decline in lung function but do decrease the frequency of exacerbations and improve quality of life. Combination products that combine steroids with bronchodilators are frequently prescribed to enhance control of symptoms and minimize acute exacerbations of COPD. Examples include Advair (fluticasone–salmeterol), Dulera (mometasone-formoterol), and Symbicort (budesonide–formoterol) (Ciccone, 2007; Gardenhire, 2008a; Hitner & Nagle, 2001c; Springhouse, 2009).

Adverse effects are more frequently seen with oral doses, high doses, and long-term use of steroids. High–dose, long–term use of steroids can suppress action of the adrenal gland, and abrupt discontinuation can result in acute adrenal insufficiency. Alternate-day oral administration minimizes this effect (Ciccone, 2007; Gardenhire, 2008c; Hitner & Nagle, 2001c).

The use of oral corticosteroids should be carefully evaluated in patients who develop an acute exacerbation or fail to improve sufficiently despite being on appropriate maintenance therapy. An increase in FEV1 of more than 20% has been used as a surrogate marker for steroid response. In acute exacerbation of COPD, oral or even injected steroids are used routinely to improve symptoms and lung function. Oral steroids can be used successfully to treat acute exacerbations and prevent hospitalization, but once stable these patients should be weaned off oral corticosteroids because of the adverse effects associated with long-term steroid use (Ciccone, 2007; Gardenhire, 2008c; Hitner & Nagle, 2001c; Springhouse, 2009). Use of corticosteroids (especially prolonged systemic administration) can cause thinning of the skin and may result in skin breakdown, reduced bone density and osteoporosis, as well as myopathy. Other side effects include hyperglycemia, acute changes in mental status or personality changes, and immunosuppression that can increase the risk of infection. Upon noting these side effects or evidence of infection, the clinician should immediately bring them to the attention of the physician and the rest of the team (Ciccone, 2007).

Leukotriene inhibitors, which are used to treat asthma, reduce inflammation by interfering with the formation of leukotrienes that act as mediators of inflammation (Springhouse, 2009). Theophylline improves respiratory muscle function, stimulates the respiratory center, promotes bronchodilation, and reduces inflammation. Theophylline may also improve contractility of diaphragm muscle. Theophylline (Theo-Dur, Theo-24) and the related product aminophylline are now used only if first-line agents are ineffective in controlling symptoms. Because of the potential for toxicity associated with theophylline, it is now recommended that physicians monitor patient serum levels and maintain levels between 5 and 10 mg/L rather than the formerly used range of 10 to 20 mg/L. Table 22.2 summarizes the many drug interactions associated with theophylline (Gardenhire, 2008d; Springhouse, 2009).

PATIENT CASE 1, *continued*

K.L. is the 76-yr-old female discussed earlier who was recently discharged after a prolonged hospitalization with COPD and pneumonia and was admitted to rehabilitation services for pulmonary rehabilitation after two recent falls. While taking K.L.'s history, the rehabilitation specialist reviews the list of K.L.'s prescription medications. The list includes the following: Advair 250/50 for COPD, albuterol inhaler 2 puffs every 6 h as needed for shortness of breath, atenolol 50 mg/day for blood pressure, simvastatin 40 mg/day for high cholesterol, and Paxil 20 mg/day for depression. K.L. states that she does not understand why she has to take all of these medications and that she was fine without them before she went into the hospital. She wonders why she needs two prescriptions for breathing, especially because the Advair is expensive and she does not have insurance. To reduce expenses, she has been taking Advair only when she needs it and takes the less expensive albuterol instead.

Question
How should the therapist respond to K.L.'s question regarding her COPD medications?

Answer
The therapist should alert the physician regarding K.L.'s concerns and ensure additional medication teaching is provided. The therapist should consult the pharmacist to provide additional teaching and should explain that her symptoms of shortness of breath are caused by inflammation and constriction of the air sacs in her lungs, which reduces the ability of the lungs to absorb oxygen and eliminate carbon dioxide. Her medication regimen contains Advair and albuterol (Ventolin). Advair is

a combination product containing a steroid to reduce inflammation and a long-acting bronchodilator (salmeterol) that keeps her air passages open. Advair works best if taken regularly to maintain a reduction in the chronic inflammation in her lungs and to help prevent episodes of shortness of breath. Her albuterol (Ventolin) is a fast acting bronchodilator that provides immediate relief of shortness of breath and works best when used to treat acute symptoms or to prevent shortness of breath immediately prior to exercise. K.L. is also instructed to exhale fully before taking the inhaled dose, then place the mouthpiece to her lips and breathe in quickly and deeply through the inhaler. She should hold her breath for about 10 s or for as long as is comfortable and then breathe out slowly. After each dose of Advair she should rinse her mouth with water and spit the water out to minimize the chance of developing a fungal infection in the mouth. Finally, K.L. is told that she should never take an extra dose, even if she did not taste or feel the medicine.

PATIENT CASE 1, *continued*

After hearing this information, K.L. states that she does not believe in taking steroids because she has heard they have dangerous side effects in athletes.

Question
How should the therapist respond to K.L.'s concerns?

Answer
The therapist should inform K.L. that Advair contains fluticasone, a corticosteroid similar to cortisol, a normal hormone in her body. Corticosteroids such as those in Advair are not anabolic steroids that athletes and bodybuilders have abused. Corticosteroids can reduce inflammatory response, which can increase the opening of airway passages and reduce mucus production and plugging associated with chronic bronchitis. When inhaled, the medication is delivered directly to the inflamed respira-

tory tissue, which limits systemic absorption and minimizes the risk of most side effects.

Antibiotics

Antibiotics are recommended only for treatment of acute exacerbations of COPD accompanied by symptoms of infection (i.e., production of increased amounts of sputum, more purulent sputum, dyspnea accompanied by fever, elevated white blood cell count, and infiltrates on the chest X-ray). Empiric antimicrobial therapy of such an acute exacerbation should cover the likely pathogens. The airways of patients with COPD are commonly colonized with *Streptococcus pneumoniae*, *Haemophilus influenzae*, and *Moraxella catarrhalis*. The goal of antibiotic therapy in COPD is not to completely eliminate the organisms from the air passages but rather to improve symptoms associated with the acute exacerbation. In patients with frequent infectious exacerbations (>3/yr), oral antibiotic therapy that is initiated promptly at the initial onset of symptoms can help rapidly resolve the symptoms and reduce the frequency of hospitalizations (Ciccone, 2007; Gardenhire, 2008a; Sharma & Arneja, 2010; Springhouse, 2009).

PATIENT CASE 1, *continued*

K.L. asks whether antibiotics would clear up her lungs and help improve her shortness of breath. She mentions that she has some Zithromax left over from before she was admitted to the hospital.

Question
What should the therapist tell K.L. about the appropriate use of antibiotics in COPD?

Answer
The therapist should explain that unnecessary use of antibiotics can do more harm than good. Antibiotics can kill susceptible bacteria that are present in the airway passages but not causing infection (termed colonization). More resistant bacteria can take their place, thus increasing the risk for developing more serious infections that require stronger and more expensive, or more toxic, antibiotics.

Table 22.2   Drug Interactions With Theophylline

Medication	Drug interaction	Effects produced
Adenosine	Theophylline blocks adenosine receptors.	Higher doses of adenosine may be required to achieve desired effect.
Alcohol	A single, large dose of alcohol (3 ml/kg of whiskey) decreases theophylline clearance for up to 24 h.	30% increase in theophylline levels and effects.
Allopurinol (Zyloprim)	Allopurinol doses ≥ 600 mg/day decrease theophylline clearance.	25% increase in theophylline levels and effects.
Aminoglutethimide (Cytadren)	Increases theophylline clearance by inducing microsomal enzyme activity.	25% decrease in theophylline levels and effects.
Carbamazepine (Tegretol)	Increases theophylline clearance by inducing microsomal enzyme activity.	30% decrease in theophylline levels and effects.
Cimetidine (Tagamet)	Decreases theophylline clearance by inhibiting cytochrome P4501A2.	70% increase in theophylline levels and effects.
Ciprofloxacin (Cipro)	Decreases theophylline clearance by inhibiting cytochrome P4501A2.	40% increase in theophylline levels and effects.
Clarithromycin (Biaxin)	Erythromycin metabolite decreases theophylline clearance by inhibiting cytochrome P4503A3.	25% increase in theophylline levels and effects.
Diazepam (Valium)	Benzodiazepines increase CNS concentrations of adenosine, a potent CNS depressant; theophylline blocks adenosine receptors.	Larger diazepam doses may be required to produce desired level of sedation. Discontinuing theophylline without reducing diazepam dose may result in respiratory depression.
Disulfiram (Antabuse)	Decreases theophylline clearance by inhibiting hydroxylation and demethylation.	50% increase in theophylline levels and effects.
Enoxacin (Penetrex)	Decreases theophylline clearance by inhibiting cytochrome P4501A2.	300% increase in theophylline levels and effects.
Ephedrine	Increased side effects of CNS stimulation.	Increased frequency of nausea, nervousness, and insomnia.
Erythromycin	Erythromycin metabolite decreases theophylline clearance by inhibiting cytochrome P4503A3.	35% increase in theophylline and 35% decrease in erythromycin levels.
Estrogen replacements	Oral contraceptives containing estrogen decrease theophylline clearance in a dose-dependent fashion. The effect of progesterone on theophylline clearance is unknown.	30% increase in theophylline levels and increased effects.
Flurazepam (Dalmane)	Benzodiazepines increase CNS concentrations of adenosine, a potent CNS depressant; theophylline blocks adenosine receptors.	Larger diazepam doses may be required to produce desired level of sedation. Discontinuing theophylline without reducing flurazepam dose may result in respiratory depression.
Fluvoxamine (Luvox)	Decreases theophylline clearance by inhibiting cytochrome P4501A2.	70% increase in theophylline levels and effects.
Halothane	Halothane sensitizes the **myocardium** to catecholamines; theophylline increases release of endogenous catecholamines.	Increased risk of ventricular arrhythmias.
Interferon, human recombinant alpha-A	Decreases theophylline clearance.	100% increase in theophylline levels and effects.
Isoproterenol (Isuprel—intravenous)	Increases theophylline clearance.	20% decrease in theophylline levels and effects.

› continued

Table 22.2 ›*continued*

Medication	Drug interaction	Effects produced
Ketamine	Increases CNS effects.	May lower theophylline seizure threshold.
Lithium (Eskalith)	Theophylline increases renal lithium clearance.	Lithium dose required to achieve a therapeutic serum concentration increases an average of 60%.
Lorazepam (Ativan)	Benzodiazepines increase CNS concentrations of adenosine, a potent CNS depressant; theophylline blocks adenosine receptors.	Larger diazepam doses may be required to produce desired level of sedation. Discontinuing theophylline without reducing lorazepam dose may result in respiratory depression.
Methotrexate	Decreases theophylline clearance.	20% increase in theophylline levels and effects after low dose of methotrexate. Higher dose of methotrexate may have greater increases in levels and effects.
Mexiletine (Mexitil)	Decreases theophylline clearance by inhibiting hydroxylation and demethylation.	80% increase in levels and effects of theophylline.
Midazolam (Versed)	Benzodiazepines increase CNS concentrations of adenosine, a potent CNS depressant; theophylline blocks adenosine receptors.	Larger midazolam doses may be required to produce desired level of sedation. Discontinuing theophylline without reducing midazolam dose may result in respiratory depression.
Pancuronium (Pavulon)	Theophylline may antagonize nondepolarizing neuromuscular-blocking effects, possibly due to phosphodiesterase inhibition.	Larger doses of pancuronium may be required to achieve neuromuscular blockade.
Pentoxifylline (Trental)	Decreases theophylline clearance.	30% increase in theophylline levels and effects.
Phenobarbital	Increases theophylline clearance by inducing microsomal enzyme activity.	25% decrease in theophylline and effects are seen after 2 wk of concurrent phenobarbital.
Phenytoin (Dilantin)	Increases theophylline clearance by increasing microsomal enzyme activity; theophylline decreases phenytoin absorption.	About 40% decrease in both theophylline and phenytoin levels and effects.
Propafenone (Rythmol)	Decreases theophylline clearance and pharmacologic interaction.	40% increase in theophylline levels and effects. Beta-2 blocking effect of propafenone may decrease efficacy of theophylline.
Propranolol (Inderal)	Decreases theophylline clearance by inhibiting CYP1A2 and pharmacologic interaction.	100% increase in theophylline levels and effects. Beta-2 blocking effect of propranolol may decrease efficacy of theophylline.
Rifampin	Increases theophylline clearance by increasing CYP1A2 and CYP3A3 activity.	20%-40% decrease in theophylline levels and effects.
St. John's wort	Decreases theophylline plasma concentrations.	Higher doses of theophylline may be required to achieve desired effect. Discontinuing use of St. John's wort may result in theophylline toxicity.
Sulfinpyrazone (Anturane)	Increases theophylline clearance by increasing demethylation and hydroxylation; decreases renal clearance of theophylline.	20% decrease in theophylline levels and effects.
Tacrine (Cognex)	Decreases theophylline clearance by inhibiting CYP1A2; increases renal clearance of theophylline.	90% increase in theophylline levels and effects.
Thiabendazole (Mintezol)	Decreases theophylline clearance.	190% increase in theophylline levels and effects.
Ticlopidine (Ticlid)	Decreases theophylline clearance.	60% increase in theophylline levels and effects.
Verapamil (Isoptin, Calan)	Decreases theophylline clearance by inhibiting hydroxylation and demethylation.	20% increase in theophylline levels and effects.

CNS = central nervous system.

Mucolytics and Expectorants

Mucolytics and expectorants are agents that assist in the removal of mucus from the lower respiratory airways. Mucolytic agents reduce sputum viscosity and improve clearance of secretions. Viscous lung secretions in patients with COPD consist of mucus-derived glycoproteins and leukocyte-derived deoxyribonucleic acid. Mucolytics are administered to break up the mucus so that it can be removed via coughing or suction. Acetylcysteine (Mucomyst), the primary mucolytic medication currently used, is usually administered via inhalation or intratracheal installation. Because it is a respiratory irritant that can cause bronchospasm, a bronchodilator is concurrently administered with acetylcysteine. Expectorants increase gastric and respiratory secretions by stimulating gastric reflexes and thus decrease irritation and cough (Gardenhire, 2008a).

Smoking Cessation

Smoking cessation continues to be the most important therapeutic intervention in the pulmonary patient. Many patients with COPD have a history of smoking, and many currently smoke. A smoking-cessation plan is an essential part of a comprehensive management strategy. Success rates associated with smoking cessation are low. Any smoking-cessation program must involve multiple interventions. According to the U.S. Preventative Services Task Force guidelines, clinicians should ask all adults about use of tobacco products and should provide interventions to encourage smoking cessation to smokers.

The guideline uses a "five A" approach to counseling:

- Ask about tobacco use.
- Advise to quit through personalized messages.
- Assess willingness to quit.
- Assist smoking cessation.
- Arrange for follow-up.

The transition from smoking to abstention from smoking consists of five stages: pre-contemplation, contemplation, preparation, action, and maintenance. Depression and anxiety can negatively affect the COPD patient's motivation to quit smoking. It is therefore important for health care providers to be aware of the signs of psychological problems when smoking cessation is advised (Fischer et al., 2007).

Physicians and other health care providers should help the patient set the target quit date and should follow up with respect to progress in following the plan for smoking cessation. Brief (<10 min) behavioral counseling and pharmacotherapy are each effective alone but are most effective when used together. The task force also advises clinicians to ask all pregnant women, regardless of age, about tobacco use. Those who currently smoke should receive pregnancy-tailored counseling supplemented with self-help materials. Successful cessation programs use tools such as patient education, a quit date, follow-up support, relapse prevention, advice for healthy lifestyle changes, social support systems, and adjuncts to treatment (e.g., pharmacologic agents) (U.S. Preventative Services Task Force, 2009).

Supervised use of pharmacologic agents is an important adjunct to self-help and group smoking-cessation programs. Medications used to help patients stop smoking include nicotine-replacement products such as nicotine patches and oral medications such as Chantix or Zyban. Table 22.3 summarizes medications used to assist with smoking cessation.

Nicotine is the ingredient in cigarettes that is primarily responsible for addiction. Withdrawal from nicotine may cause adverse effects including anxiety, irritability, difficulty concentrating, anger, fatigue, drowsiness, depression, and sleep disruption. These effects usually occur during the first several weeks of any attempt at smoking cessation. Nicotine-replacement therapies help reduce withdrawal symptoms. A smoker who requires a cigarette within 30 min of waking is likely to be highly addicted and could benefit from nicotine-replacement therapy.

Several nicotine-replacement therapies exist. Nicotine polacrilex is a chewing gum that leads to better quit rates than counseling alone. Nicotine-replacement chewing pieces are marketed in two strengths: 2 mg and 4 mg. An individual who smokes 1 pack/day should

See table 22.3 in the web resource for a full list of medication-specific indications, dosing recommendations, and side effects.

Table 22.3 Medications Used to Help Patients Quit Smoking

Medication	Side effects affecting rehab							Other side effects or considerations
Nicotine replacement: Used for smoking cessation. Provides increased quit rates of up to 22% compared to 2-35% rates with counseling alone.								
Nicotine gum	Cog	S	A	Motor	D	Com	F	Side effects: Increased heart rate and blood pressure, arrhythmias, sore throat, increased sweating, nausea, dry mouth, dyspepsia, diarrhea, abnormal dreams, irritability, dizziness, arthralgias, myalgias.
	+	0	++	+	++	0	+	
Nicotine patches (NicoDerm, Nicotrol, Habitrol)	Cog	S	A	Motor	D	Com	F	
	+	0	++	+	++	0	+	
Nicotine receptor partial agonist: Used for smoking cessation. Provides 44% quit rates compared to 23-30% with Zyban or 2-25% quit rates seen with counseling alone.								
Varenicline (Chantix)	Cog	S	A	Motor	D	Com	F	Side effects: Gastrointestinal upset, bad taste in mouth, changes in appetite, insomnia, unusual dreams or nightmares, headache, hostility, agitation, depression, suicidal thoughts.
	+	0	++	0	++	0	+	Contraindications: Depression, bipolar disorder, schizophrenia, or other mental illness.
Antidepressant: Used for smoking cessation. Provides 23-30% quit rates for cessation compared to 2-25% attained with counseling alone.								
Bupropion (Zyban)	Cog	S	A	Motor	D	Com	F	Side effects: Dry mouth, insomnia, dizziness, difficulty concentrating, nausea, anxiety, constipation, tremors, skin problems or rashes.
	0	++	++	++	++	0	0	Taking the evening dose in the afternoon at least 8 h after the morning dose may minimize difficulty with insomnia.
								Contraindications: Seizure disorders, eating disorders, or alcoholism.

Cog = cognition; S = sedation; A = agitation or mania; Motor = discoordination; D = dysphagia; Com = communication; F = falls.

The likelihood rating scale for encountering the side effects is as follows: 0 = Almost no probability of encountering side effects. + = Little likelihood of encountering side effects. +/++ = Low probability of encountering side effects; however, probability increases with increased dosage. ++ = Medium likelihood of encountering side effects. +++ = High likelihood of encountering side effects, particularly with high doses. ++++ = Highest likelihood of encountering side effects; best to avoid in at-risk patients.

use the 4 mg pieces, and an individual who smokes less than 1 pack/day should use the 2 mg pieces. For the first 2 wk, patients should chew a piece hourly as well as at the time of cravings. Patients should gradually reduce frequency of chewing over the next 3 mo. Transdermal nicotine patches are also readily available. Long-term success rates of patches range from 22% to 42% whereas those of a placebo range from 2% to 25%. These agents are well tolerated and the adverse effects are limited to localized skin reaction. Nicotine patches are sold under the trade names NicoDerm CQ, Nicotrol, and Habitrol. The usual dosing schedule is the same for all three brands. Individuals who smoke more than 1 pack/day should initially place the 21 mg patch on the skin each day for 30 days, then apply the 14 mg patch for 30 days, and then apply the 7 mg patch for 30 days. Those that smoke less than

1 pack/day should start with the 14 mg patch for 30 days and then apply the 7 mg patch for 30 days. There is no benefit to using nicotine replacement patches for more than 2 months.

Bupropion (Zyban) is an antidepressant that is effective in smoking cessation. Twenty-three percent of smokers using bupropion maintained cessation 1 yr after quitting whereas only 12% of smokers using a placebo maintained cessation. Bupropion was shown to be effective when used in patients who failed to quit smoking while using nicotine-replacement therapy.

Varenicline (Chantix) binds to nicotinic acetylcholine receptors and prevents nicotine from binding to these receptors. This product also provides 44% successful quit rates compared to 12% attained with counseling alone. The dose should be titrated up to 1 mg by mouth twice/day after meals at least 1 wk before the quit date. The dose should be decreased to 0.5 mg twice/day in patients with severe renal impairment or to 0.5 mg/day in patients with end-stage renal disease. Serious neuropsychiatric symptoms, reported during post-marketing surveillance, may include changes in behavior, agitation, depressed mood, suicidal ideation, and attempted and completed suicide (Sharma & Arneja, 2010; U.S. Preventative Services Task Force, 2009).

Preventative Medications

Pneumococcal vaccine (Pneumovax) is recommended for patients at risk of pneumococcal infection, including diabetics, alcoholics, patients living in chronic-care facilities, and patients older than 65 yr who have chronic cardiovascular, liver, or pulmonary disease. It is also recommended for patients who are immunocompromised (e.g., patients receiving immunosuppressants or chemotherapy, organ-transplant patients). The vaccine is administered intramuscularly as a single 0.5 ml dose. In rare cases, a second dose may be administered 5 yr later. Mild irritation at the site of injection may develop, and systemic reactions such as fever and muscle aches may occur in rare instances (Sharma & Arneja, 2010).

Worldwide outbreaks and epidemics of influenza, an acute respiratory illness caused by influenza A or B viruses, occur almost every year. In patients with chronic lung disease, administration of influenza vaccine substantially decreases mortality, hospitalization for influenza and pneumonia, exacerbation of chronic lung disease, and physician visits for respiratory complaints and annual immunization is recommended. Other patients who should receive the vaccine include those 65 yr or older, those in chronic-care facilities, and patients with chronic cardiac disease, respiratory disease, diabetes, renal dysfunction, or disease that impairs immune function. The influenza vaccine causes low-grade fever and mild systemic symptoms in 5% of patients and should not be administered to patients who are allergic to egg products. A small risk of Guillain-Barré syndrome (approximately 1/1 million vaccine recipients) may exist (Sharma & Arneja, 2010).

Other products used to prevent and treat influenza include zanamivir (Relenza), an inhaled compound, and oseltamivir (Tamiflu), an oral medication. If taken within 2 days of exposure to influenza, both decrease the duration and severity of influenza symptoms. Because resistance to Tamiflu (oseltamivir) emerged in the United States during the 2008 and 2009 influenza seasons, Relenza (zanamivir) is now the first choice for antiviral **prophylaxis** or treatment when influenza A infection or exposure is suspected (Sharma & Arneja, 2010).

Summary

This chapter reviews important concepts in respiratory disease and summarizes the medications used to treat respiratory disease. It also presents appropriate methods for monitoring patients with chronic respiratory disease participating in rehabilitation and provides interventions that the rehabilitation therapist can make to improve the care of patients with respiratory disease. The rehabilitation therapist needs to work with the pharmacist, respiratory therapist, physician, nurse, and patient in the management of pulmonary difficulties. All members of the team need to be aware of the side effects of medications used to manage respiratory disease.

23 Medications Used to Treat Thyroid Disease, Parathyroid Disease, and Osteoporosis

The rehabilitation therapist will provide care for patients with thyroid disease and patients with bone disorders such as osteoporosis associated with parathyroid disease. This chapter discusses the pathophysiology of thyroid disease, parathyroid disease, and osteoporosis, the medications used to treat these conditions, and the implications for rehabilitation.

Thyroid disorders profoundly affect all metabolic processes, cognition, energy, and organ function and can impact rehabilitation success. The rehabilitation therapist may be the first health professional to detect symptoms consistent with these diseases. In addition, bone health is tremendously important in fracture prevention. The rehabilitation therapist can educate the patient and family in dietary intake and medication use in order to help prevent or treat osteoporosis. Finally, the rehabilitation therapist should tailor sessions to minimize fall risk in patients with these disease states.

Thyroid Disease

The **thyroid gland** is a butterfly-shaped gland located in the anterior portion of the lower neck, below the larynx and anterior to the trachea. In the child, thyroid function is needed for growth and development. In the adult, thyroid function maintains metabolic stability of all organ systems of the body. The thyroid gland synthesizes, stores, and secretes thyroid hormone that regulates metabolism and protein synthesis. Inside the thyroid gland

are four parathyroid glands. Two are located on each side of the posterior surface of each lobe of the thyroid gland. The **parathyroid hormone** (PTH) that is secreted from these glands regulates calcium and phosphorus metabolism. PTH works along with calcitonin and vitamin D to regulate calcium levels in the body and bone health (Guyton & Hall, 2010; Mehta et al., 2010).

Incidence

Incidence of thyroid disease is high globally; approximately 200 million individuals worldwide have thyroid disease (Shomon, 2010). Thyroid disease affects women, especially those with a family history of thyroid disease, more than men; women have as much as a 1 in 7 chance of developing thyroid disease (McConnell, 2007). An estimated 27 million Americans have thyroid disease. Hyperthyroidism occurs in about 2% of the U.S. population; half of these individuals have subclinical hyperthyroidism and show no symptoms of the disease. Many individuals with thyroid dysfunction go undiagnosed because early symptoms of thyroid disease are often subtle and later symptoms can mimic various other medical conditions (McConnell, 2007; Mehta et al., 2010).

Etiology and Pathophysiology

The most common forms of thyroid disorder—thyroid nodules, **goiter**, and thyroid enlargement—are associated with normal amounts of circulating thyroid hormone. Pathology arises when hormone secretion from the thyroid gland is deficient (**hypothyroidism**) or excessive (**hyperthyroidism**). Altered thyroid hormone levels are accompanied by clinical symptoms. Because thyroid hormones act on nearly all body systems, abnormalities can negatively affect the rate of metabolism and can negatively influence the musculoskeletal, integumentary, nervous, gastrointestinal, and cardiovascular systems. In some areas of the world, goiter results from insufficient intake of iodine. Recommended daily allowances for iodine are 90 to 120 µg for children, 150 µg for adults, 220 µg for pregnant women, and 290 µg for lactating mothers. The most practical method for ensuring adequate intake is to use iodized table salt. Good dietary sources of iodine include dairy products and fish (Brent & Koenig, 2011; Reasner & Talbert, 2011).

Thyroid hormone is synthesized and stored as amino acid residues of thyroglobulin, a protein that makes up a large portion of the thyroid mass. This allows the thyroid gland to store a great deal of potential hormone. The thyroid gland takes up and oxidizes dietary iodine, thus incorporating it into the thyroglobulin. Iodine ingested in the diet reaches circulation in the form of iodide ion, which is transported by the thyroid gland via a transporter protein. This transporter protein is found in greater amounts in the salivary glands, gastric mucosa, midportion of the small intestine, choroid plexus, skin, mammary glands, and placenta. More iodide is found in these tissues than in the blood. Thyroid hormone is stored in the thyroid gland in the form of thyroglobulin and is secreted in the prohormone form **thyroxine** (T4), which must be metabolized to the active form **tri-iodothyronine** (T3) by the action of the enzyme 5-monodeiodinase in liver and other tissues. Thyroid hormone mediates most of its action by binding to the nuclear thyroid hormone receptors in tissues and by modulating transcription of specific genes (Brent & Koenig, 2011; Mehta et al., 2010; Reasner & Talbert, 2011).

Thyroid levels are regulated by the hypothalamic–pituitary–thyroid axis, which is extremely sensitive to changes in the level of thyroid in the bloodstream and maintains thyroid hormone in a very narrow therapeutic range. The growth and function of the thyroid gland are mediated by the regulating hormone **thyrotropin** (TSH), which is secreted by the pituitary gland. TSH stimulates the thyroid to release thyroid hormone. Levels of TSH, T3, and T4 are commonly used in the diagnosis of thyroid disorders. High TSH levels generally indicate that the body is trying to compensate for hypothyroidism, and low levels indicate that the body is trying to compensate for excessive levels of thyroid hormone. The release of TSH by the pituitary gland is regulated by thyroid-releasing hormone (TRH), which is released by the hypothalamus. Low TRH levels, which can cause thyroid disease, occur as a result of cranial cancer, irradiation, or trauma. Different medical conditions and medications can alter levels of these hormones and affect thyroid function. For instance, high levels of glucocorticoids, dopamine, and somatostatin can reduce TRH action, and metformin can decrease TSH levels (Brent & Koenig, 2011; Mehta et al., 2010; Reasner & Talbert, 2011).

Rehabilitation Considerations

Most thyroid remediation is accomplished through surgery and medication therapy. Rehabilitation efforts may also involve changes in diet and lifestyle as well as exercise. For example, a patient with an underactive thyroid may be instructed to avoid sugar and refined carbohydrates in drinks and food because these tend to contribute to adrenal stress. Refined and processed foods also contain chemicals that can deplete nutrients in the body that are necessary for thyroid function. The patient may be instructed to instead eat foods rich in iodine such as onions, garlic, and artichokes as well as poultry, whole grains, fruits, and vegetables.

The patient with hypothyroidism may also be encouraged to exercise because exercise increases thyroid secretions. Patients should engage in 20 min of light to moderate-intensity exercise 3 times/wk. Types of exercise include aerobics, swimming, cycling, jogging, and walking (Howard, 2009).

Medication Therapy

Thyroid hormones have long half-lives because they bind to plasma proteins, which protects them from metabolism and excretion. T4, which has a half-life of 6 to 8 days, is eliminated from the body slowly. The half-life is reduced to 3 to 4 days in patients with hyperthyroidism and is increased to 9 to 10 days in patients with hypothyroidism. The use of certain medications increases binding, resulting in higher levels of total thyroid hormone that can contribute to misdiagnosis if the laboratory measures total rather than free (active) thyroid hormone. Conversely, use of other medications can decrease binding. Also, certain medications and food can impair the absorption of thyroid supplements, thus increasing dose requirements. Other medications can increase the metabolic rate of thyroid supplements, thus increasing dose requirements. Amiodarone can affect thyroid function because it contains iodine that can reduce the conversion of T4 to the active form T3. Decreased doses of thyroid supplements may be needed in patients of advanced age and women receiving estrogen therapy (Guyton & Hall, 2010). Table 23.1 lists medications that can alter thyroid levels.

Table 23.1   Drug Interactions With Thyroid Hormone Replacement Therapy

Mechanism of drug interaction with thyroid hormone	Interacting medications	Result of interaction
Medications that increase protein binding of thyroid hormone	Estrogens (Premarin, oral contraceptives), tamoxifen (Nolvadex), estrogen receptor modulators, 5-fluoruracil, heroin, methadone	Decreased thyroid hormone availability to act at the thyroid hormone receptor with decreased effects of thyroid hormone
Medications that decrease protein binding of thyroid hormone	Glucocorticoids, androgens, L-asparaginase, salicylates furosemide (Lasix), anticonvulsants (phenytoin [Dilantin], carbamazepine [Tegretol])	Increased thyroid hormone availability to act at the thyroid hormone receptor; increased effects of thyroid hormone
Medications that impair absorption of thyroid supplements	Antacids containing aluminum (Maalox, Mylanta), sucralfate (Carafate), bile acid sequestrants (cholestyramine [Questran], colestipol [Colestid], colesevelam [Welchol]), calcium carbonate, chromium supplements, iron supplements, phosphate binders sevelamer [Renagel], raloxifene (Evista), proton pump inhibitors (Prevacid, Nexium, Protonix, Prilosec)	Decreased thyroid hormone availability to act at the receptor; decreased effects of thyroid hormone
Medications that increase metabolism of thyroxine	Bexarotene (Targretin), rifampin, sertraline (Zoloft), anticonvulsants (carbamazepine [Tegretol], phenytoin [Dilantin])	Decreased thyroid hormone availability to act at the thyroid hormone receptor; decreased effects of thyroid hormone
Medications that alter conversion of thyroxine to tri-iodothyronine	Amiodarone (Cordarone, Pacerone)	Decreased thyroid hormone availability to act at the thyroid hormone receptor; decreased effects of thyroid hormone
Medications that decrease secretion of tri-iodothyronine and thyroxine	Lithium (Eskalith)	Decreased thyroid hormone availability to act at the thyroid hormone receptor; decreased effects of thyroid hormone
Medications that lower thyrotropin levels	Glucocorticoids, dopamine, somatostatin	Decreased thyroid hormone availability to act at the thyroid hormone receptor; decreased effects of thyroid hormone
Medications that lower thyroid-releasing hormone	Metformin (Glucophage)	Decreased thyroid hormone availability to act at the thyroid hormone receptor; decreased effects of thyroid hormone

Hyperthyroidism

Approximately one third of the world's population lives in areas that are deficient in iodine. When iodine is low the thyroid compensates in an effort to maintain the production of thyroid hormone. This disequilibrium affects the body in many ways that are described in the coming sections.

Incidence

The global incidence of hyperthyroidism is reported to be 102.8/100,000 people per year, and onset typically occurs between 30 and 50 yr of age (Pederson et al., 2006; Tamparo & Lewis, 2000). Hyperthyroidism affects approximately 2% of women and 0.2% of men (Franklyn, 1994). McGrogan and colleagues (2008) report an incidence of hyperthyroidism of 80/100,000 women/yr and 8/100,000 men/yr. The most common form of hyperthyroidism is Graves' disease, which accounts for 70% to 85% of all cases of hyperthyroidism. Another cause of hyperthyroidism is toxic multinodular goiter, also known as Parry's disease or Plummer's disease, which accounts for about 5% of hyperthyroidism in the United States.

Etiology and Pathophysiology

Hyperthyroidism, also sometimes referred to as thyrotoxicosis, is defined as an overactive thyroid that excessively produces thyroid hormone. This overproduction increases the metabolic rate in the body. Pituitary disease can also cause hyperthyroidism and inappropriate production of TSH despite adequate levels of thyroid hormone (Goodman et al., 2003). Graves' disease is an autoimmune disorder that produces autoantibodies that stimulate TSH receptors on the thyroid gland, resulting in increased production and secretion of T4 (Goodman et al., 2003). The etiology of Graves' disease has been related to both immunologic and genetic factors. The immune system in individuals with Graves' disease produces autoantibodies that stimulate the thyroid gland and cause excessive production of thyroid hormone. With toxic multinodular goiter, which usually occurs in patients over 40 yr of age living in iodine-deficient regions, thyroid nodules are hyperfunctional and produce excess thyroid hormone. A short-term type of hyperthyroidism can occur 3 to 6 mo postpartum in 5% to 10% of women due to inflammation of the thyroid gland; this usually resolves over time. Finally, excessive intake of dietary iodine or medications containing iodine can induce hyperthyroidism. Medications that contain iodine include amiodarone (Cordarone, Pacerone), which can disrupt thyroid function in 14% to 18% of patients treated with this medication, and iodine-containing radiographic contrast used in diagnostic testing. Because amiodarone can induce hyper- or hypothyroidism, patients on this medication should have their thyroid function tested every 6 mo (Mehta et al., 2010; Reid & Wheeler, 2005).

The diagnosis of hyperthyroidism is made based on clinical history, physical examination, and laboratory testing, including radioimmunoassay for T4 and T3, testing TSH levels, thyroid scan (contraindicated during pregnancy), and ultrasonography. Common laboratory findings that support a diagnosis of hyperthyroidism include increased T3 and T4 levels and decreased TSH levels (Frazier & Drzymkowski, 2004).

The signs and symptoms of **Graves' disease** include enlargement of the thyroid gland (goiter), nervousness, tremor, sweating, heat intolerance, alopecia (hair loss), weight loss without calorie reduction, diarrhea, and possibly dysphagia. Hyperthyroidism is equally prevalent in the elderly and general populations. Additional signs and symptoms of hyperthyroidism include fatigue, anorexia, and skeletal muscle myopathy. The bulbar muscles may be involved, resulting in aspiration, nasal speech, and dysphagia, which may result from pharyngeal and esophageal dysmotility. More than 50% of patients complain of muscle weakness and 63% demonstrate evidence of proximal muscle weakness and wasting (Guildiken et al., 2006; Konstantitinos et al., 2011).

Cardiopulmonary symptoms of hyperthyroidism include palpitations, tachycardia, increased cardiac output, systolic hypertension, increased respiration rate, and **dyspnea**. Protrusion of the eyes (exophthalmos) is characteristic but not always present. The patient may experience cyclical mood changes (from feeling low to feeling euphoric), and excessive thyroid activity may be associated with fatigue. Older adults do not present with all of the classic symptoms. Seniors typically become more apathetic instead of hyperactive and have a higher incidence of cardiovascular abnormalities (Kennedy & Carlo, 1996). As a result, hyperthyroidism is more difficult to diagnose in this population.

Musculoskeletal abnormalities associated with hyperthyroidism include osteoporosis, periarthritis (inflammation of the tendons, ligaments, and joint capsules), and increased incidence of adhesive capsulitis, which most commonly affects the shoulder (i.e., frozen shoulder). Periarthritis involvement can be unilateral or bilateral and usually resolves with early intervention and medication. Proximal muscle weakness and atrophy in the pelvic girdle and thigh muscles are common impairments in this patient population (Kocabas et al., 2009). These strength impairments may cause difficulties with gait and transfers from sitting to standing positions. Musculoskeletal symptoms usually begin to resolve within 2 mo of initiating medication (Kocabas et al., 2009). The rehabilitation therapist should focus on strengthening the quadriceps, hamstrings, and hip musculature with the expectation that strength gains will occur as prescribed medication treatment normalizes thyroid hormone concentrations.

In individuals with hyperthyroidism, stress associated with surgery, infection, pregnancy, or diabetic acidosis may lead to thyroid storm, which is an acute exacerbation of thyrotoxicosis. Other precipitating factors include radioactive iodine therapy and withdrawal from antithyroid medications. Thyroid storm is a medical emergency that can lead to life-threatening cardiac, hepatic, or renal complications. It is characterized by extreme irritability, hypertension, tachycardia, vomiting, and fevers of up to 106 °F. The condition can lead to delirium and coma (Beers & Porter, 2006).

Treatment of thyroid storm includes prompt suppression of thyroid hormone formation and secretion, initiation of antiadrenergic therapy (i.e., beta blockers) to control heart rate, administration of corticosteroids, and treatment of the triggering incident. Table 23.2 summarizes therapies used to treat thyroid storm. If iodides are used, they should be given after propylthiouracil (PTU) or methimazole (MMI) to prevent the use of the iodide as substrate for hormone production. Acetaminophen (not aspirin or nonsteroidal anti-inflammatory drugs) should be used to treat fever to avoid displacement of thyroid hormone that is bound to protein (Brent & Koenig, 2011; Reasner & Talbert, 2011).

Rehabilitation Considerations

The rehabilitation therapist often is the first to recognize early signs and symptoms of hyperthyroidism in rehabilitation patients. The cli-

Table 23.2   Medications Used to Treat Thyroid Storm

Medication	Dosing
Propylthiouracil	900-1200 mg by mouth/day in 4-6 divided doses
Methimazole	90-120 mg by mouth/day in 4-6 divided doses
Sodium iodide	Up to 2 g by mouth/day in single or divided doses
Lugol's solution	5-10 drops by mouth in water or juice 3 times/day
Saturated solution of potassium iodide	1-2 drops by mouth in water or juice 3 times/day
Propranolol (Inderal)	40-80 mg by mouth every 6 h
Dexamethasone (Decadron)	5-20 mg by mouth or intravenously/day in divided doses
Prednisone	25-100 mg by mouth/day in divided doses
Methylprednisolone (Solu-Medrol)	20-80 mg intravenously/day in divided doses
Hydrocortisone (Solu-Cortef)	100-400 mg/day in divided doses

nician should be alert to these symptoms and be proficient in screening patients for possible hyperthyroidism. Key findings on physical assessment include swelling or enlargement of the neck in the area of the thyroid gland (with or without accompanying pain), point tenderness, vocal difficulties, dysphagia, and exophthalmos (protrusion of the eyes). Because the thyroid controls metabolism, hyperthyroidism increases the metabolism in the body. As a result, the patient may feel hot. In addition, the patient may lose weight without decreasing food intake due to increases in metabolism. On the other hand, the patient may rapidly gain weight due to increased appetite (Norman, 2010). During therapy sessions the clinician should monitor the patient's vital signs closely due to the cardiopulmonary effects of hyperthyroidism. Although patients generally tolerate warm therapy pools, hot full-body whirlpools may exacerbate the patient's heat intolerance and should be avoided. The clinician must carefully monitor the patient's exercise intensity and progression when prescribing therapeutic exercise because hyperthyroidism is often associated with exercise intolerance and increased heart rate with possible arrhythmia. Carefully monitoring vital signs and using

rating of perceived exertion scales (e.g., Borg scale) is recommended.

The rehabilitation therapist must also be aware that a small percentage of patients on thyroid medication will experience fever, rash, or arthralgias (joint pain). The therapist should report these occurrences to the patient's prescriber and pharmacist to assist in determining whether these symptoms are a result of a side effect or drug interaction and whether change of medication therapy is necessary.

Medication Therapy

The usual treatment of hyperthyroidism includes the use of antithyroid drugs, the administration of radioactive iodine, or surgical resection. Goals of medication therapy are to eliminate excess thyroid hormone and minimize symptoms and consequences of hyperthyroidism. Table 23.3 summarizes treatments for hyperthyroidism, including MMI, PTU, and radioactive iodine therapy, as well as medications that can affect thyroid function (Brent & Koenig, 2011; Mehta et al., 2010; Reasner & Talbert, 2011). PTU is the agent of choice in patients with hyperthyroidism during pregnancy.

 See table 23.3 in the web resource for a full list of medication-specific indications, dosing recommendations, and side effects.

Table 23.3   Medications Used to Treat Hyperthyroidism

Medication	Side effects affecting rehab	Other side effects
Thiourea medications: Used to inhibit thyroid hormone synthesis and peripheral conversion of thyroxine to iodothyronine. First-line therapy for Graves' disease; used short term before surgical thymectomy or radioactive iodine ablation of the thyroid.		
Propylthiouracil	Cog S A Motor D Com F ++ ++ + +++ ++ ++ +++	Common side effects: Skin rash, urticaria, nausea, vomiting, epigastric distress, arthralgias, paresthesias, loss or changes of taste, myalgias, drowsiness, vertigo. Less common side effects: Jaundice, liver failure, drug fever, interstitial pneumonitis, bone marrow suppression.
Methimazole (Tapazole)	Cog S A Motor D Com F ++ ++ 0 ++ ++ + ++	Side effects: Arthralgias, myalgias, paresthesias, nausea, vomiting, loss of taste perception, bone marrow suppression, hepatotoxicity, headache, drowsiness, vertigo, fever.

› continued

Table 23.3 › continued

Medication	Side effects affecting rehab							Other side effects
Beta-adrenergic blocking agents: Used as adjunctive therapy for managing symptoms such as tachycardia and hypertension. Ameliorate action of thyroid hormone in tissues.								
Propranolol (Inderal)	Cog +++	S +++	A ++	Motor ++	D ++	Com +	F +++	Highly lipophilic. Side effects: This beta blocker has a higher incidence of CNS side effects than other beta blockers, including hallucinations, decreased concentration, insomnia, nightmares, and depression. Other side effects include nausea, diarrhea, bronchospasm, cold extremities, exacerbation of Raynaud's syndrome, bradycardia, heart block, orthostasis, fatigue, dizziness, alopecia, abnormal vision, hyperglycemia, hyperlipidemia, sexual dysfunction.
Nadolol (Corgard)	Cog ++	S ++	A 0	Motor ++	D ++	Com +	F ++	Side effects: Nausea, diarrhea, bronchospasm, cold extremities, exacerbation of Raynaud's syndrome, bradycardia, heart block, orthostasis, fatigue, dizziness, alopecia, abnormal vision, hyperglycemia, hyperlipidemia, sexual dysfunction.
Compounds containing iodine: Used to inhibit thyroxine and tri-iodothyronine release in preparation for surgery or in treatment of thyrotoxic crisis.								
Lugol's solution	Cog ++	S +	A +	Motor ++	D ++	Com +	F ++	Side effects: Diarrhea, mild nausea, fever, vomiting, arrhythmia, confusion, tiredness, numbness, tingling, joint pain, weakness, metallic taste.
Potassium iodide	Cog ++	S +	A +	Motor ++	D ++	Com +	F ++	
Glucocorticoids: Used to treat severe subacute thyroiditis and thyrotoxic crisis. Ameliorates actions of thyroid hormone on tissues and exerts immunosuppression in treatment of Graves' disease.								
Glucocorticoids	Cog +	S 0	A +	Motor +	D +	Com 0	F +	Side effects: Personality changes, insomnia, euphoria, muscle weakness or wasting, thinning of the skin, glaucoma, hyperglycemia, cataracts, depression of immune function, lipodystrophy (e.g., moon facies, truncal obesity).
Ablation of thyroid gland: First-line therapy for Graves' disease. Treatment of choice for recurrent thyrotoxicosis.								
Radioactive iodine (Iodine-131)	Cog ++	S +	A +	Motor ++	D ++	Com +	F ++	Side effects: Diarrhea, mild nausea, fever, vomiting, arrhythmia, confusion, tiredness, numbness, tingling, joint pain, weakness, metallic taste. Contraindicated in children, pregnant women, and those with ophthalmic disease.
Surgical removal of thyroid gland								
Thyroidectomy	N/A							Patients should be euthyroid before surgery.

Cog = cognition; S = sedation; A = agitation or mania; Motor = discoordination; D = dysphagia; Com = communication; F = falls; CNS = central nervous system; N/A = not applicable.

The likelihood rating scale for encountering the side effects is as follows: 0 = Almost no probability of encountering side effects. + = Little likelihood of encountering side effects. +/++ = Low probability of encountering side effects; however, probability increases with increased dosage. ++ = Medium likelihood of encountering side effects. +++ = High likelihood of encountering side effects, particularly with high doses. ++++ = Highest likelihood of encountering side effects; best to avoid in at-risk patients.

Thyroidectomy

Thyroidectomy involves removal of the hyper-secreting gland. Before thyroidectomy, PTU or MMI are administered for about 6 to 8 wk until the patient is biochemically euthyroid. Then, iodides (500 mg/day) are administered for 10 to 14 days before surgery to decrease the vascularity of the thyroid gland and minimize the blood loss associated with the surgery. Levothyroxine may be added to maintain euthyroid levels while PTU or MMI is being administered. Propranolol is administered starting several weeks before surgery to maintain pulse less than 90 beats/min and is continued for 10 to 14 days postoperatively. Morbidity with this surgery is 2.7%. Complications can include postoperative hypothyroidism (49%), hypoparathyroidism (4%), and vocal cord abnormalities (5%) (Brent & Koenig, 2011; Reasner & Talbert, 2011).

Antithyroid Medication Therapy

Propylthiouracil (PTU) and methimazole (Tapazole, MMI) inhibit the synthesis of thyroid hormone by preventing the incorporation of iodine into thyroglobulin and inhibit coupling of monoiodothyronine and di-iodothyronine to form T3 and T4. Within 4 to 8 wk of initiation, symptoms are diminished and thyroid hormone levels return to normal. Once levels are normal, the medications are tapered once/mo to maintenance doses of PTU 50 to 300 mg/day or MMI 5 to 30 mg/day. Patients should remain on therapy for 12 to 24 mo. Forty to fifty percent of patients on these medications obtain long-term remission. If a relapse occurs, the patient is not retreated with these agents but instead receives radioactive iodine therapy. Side effects associated with PTU and MMI include pruritic maculopapular rash with or without **vasculitis**, arthralgias, and fever in 5% of patients. Administration of antihistamines may help relieve rash. **Leukopenia** can occur in up to 12% of patients and is usually benign. Leukopenia is the most serious adverse effect and is accompanied by fever, malaise, gingivitis, oropharyngeal infection, and granulocyte counts of less than 250 per cu mm and usually develops in the first 3 mo of therapy. Patients should discontinue their medications and contact their prescriber if symptoms of fever, malaise, or sore throat develop. Arthralgias and lupus-like symptoms can occur in 4% to 5% of patients; these usually occur after 6 mo of therapy. Hepatotoxicity develops in about 1% of patients (Brent & Koenig, 2011; Mehta, 2010; Reasner & Talbert, 2011).

Iodides

Iodide inhibits synthesis of thyroid hormone, blocks release of thyroid hormone, and decreases the size and vascularity of the thyroid gland, resulting in improved symptoms within 2 to 7 days after initiation. This effect lasts for 1 to 2 wk, after which the thyroid adapts by decreasing active transport of iodine into the gland. These agents are used to prepare patients for surgery, to acutely inhibit thyroid gland release, and to reduce thyroid levels in patients who are thyrotoxic and have cardiac decompensation. Potassium iodide or Lugol's solution is administered 7 to 14 days before thymectomy and as an adjunct to radioactive iodine therapy starting 3 to 7 days after the radioactive iodine is given. Side effects include hypersensitivity reactions (rash, fever, conjunctivitis, swelling in the salivary gland), iodism (metallic taste, burning of mouth and throat, sore teeth and gums), cold symptoms, and gynecomastia (Brent & Koenig, 2011; Reasner & Talbert, 2011).

Adrenergic Blocking Agents

Beta blockers are used as adjunctive therapy when treating Graves' disease or toxic nodules, in preparation for surgery, or in thyroid storm. Doses of propranolol (Inderal) 20 to 40 mg 4 times/day are usually effective. Beta blockers should not be used in patients with bradycardia or patients receiving monoamine oxidase inhibitors or tricyclic antidepressants. Beta blockers should be used with caution in patients with congestive heart failure, chronic obstructive pulmonary disease, asthma, and diabetes as they can worsen these clinical conditions. Side effects of beta blockers include nausea, vomiting, anxiety, insomnia, lightheadedness, bradycardia, and hematologic disturbances (Brent & Koenig, 2011; Reasner & Talbert, 2011).

Radioactive Iodine Therapy

An alternative procedure is the use of radioactive iodine to ablate the thyroid tissue. Sodium iodine-131 is the agent of choice for treating patients with Graves' disease, toxic autonomous nodules, and toxic multinodular goiters. This agent is colorless and tasteless and is incorporated into thyroid hormones and thyroglobulin, resulting in tissue necrosis, edema, and fibrosis of the interstitial tissue of the thyroid gland. This procedure results in hypothyroidism that may be seen months to years after treatment. A euthyroid state is achieved in 60% of patients after this procedure, and 100% become euthyroid within 1 yr after repeat dosing. Beta blockers can be given concurrently with radioactive iodine, but iodine therapy should be deferred until after the ablation to ensure that the radioactive material is adequately absorbed. Thionamides such as PTU and MMI should be discontinued 4 days before administration of radioactive iodine and restarted 4 days after administration. Repeat dosing of radioactive iodine should not occur sooner than 6 mo after the initial procedure. Patients are often advised to avoid contact with children for up to 3 wk after receiving radioactive iodine (Brent & Koenig, 2011; Reasner & Talbert, 2011).

PATIENT CASE 1

G.G. is a 44-yr-old female that is in rehabilitation for treatment of adhesive capsulitis in her right shoulder. She reports that there was no previous injury to the shoulder and that she simply noticed a gradual decrease in mobility of the shoulder. She went to her primary care physician after noticing that she was having difficulty putting her shirt on due to limited range of motion in the right shoulder. G.G.'s primary care physician diagnosed her with adhesive capsulitis and referred her to therapy.

During her therapy evaluation, G.G. describes several symptoms that are unrelated to her orthopedic condition. These symptoms include a recent weight loss of 12 pounds without dieting or increasing exercise, increased appetite, tachycardia, nervousness, anxiety, sweating, and fine, brittle hair. Lastly, she adds that she has been experiencing some swelling at the base of her neck. This finding is evident on both observation and palpation of the area.

Question
Based on the information provided, what would be your next action in regard to G.G.'s medical symptoms?

Answer
Communicate symptoms to the patient's primary care physician.

Question
What is the swelling at the base of the neck most likely related to?

Answer
An enlarged thyroid gland (goiter).

Question
What condition are G.G.'s symptoms consistent with?

Answer
Hyperthyroidism.

Question
G.G.'s primary care physician makes a diagnosis of hyperthyroidism and prescribes methimazole. What side effects should the rehabilitation specialist monitor G.G. for while taking methimazole?

Answer
Side effects include arthralgias, myalgia, paresthesia, nausea, vomiting, loss of taste perception, jaundice, headache, drowsiness, vertigo, and fever.

Question
Do you think that G.G.'s development of adhesive capsulitis could be related to the condition of hyperthyroidism?

Answer
Yes, musculoskeletal abnormalities associated with hyperthyroidism include osteoporosis, periarthritis (inflammation of the tendons, ligaments, and joint capsules), and increased incidence of adhesive capsulitis, which most commonly affects the shoulder.

Hypothyroidism

Hypothyroidism is an endocrine disorder that most commonly occurs when the thyroid gland produces insufficient amounts of thyroid hormone. In a smaller percentage of cases, it can result from a lack of secretion of thyroid hormone due to inadequate secretion of either TSH from the pituitary gland or thyrotropin-releasing hormone (TRH) from the hypothalamus (Guyton & Hall, 2010). Because hypothyroidism causes a decrease in the body's metabolism, symptoms of lethargy, weight gain, constipation, and bradycardia are typically seen after the onset of hypothyroidism. The disorder is more prevalent in females and in patients with a family history of this condition.

Incidence

The international incidence of hypothyroidism ranges between 2% and 5% and can increase up to 15% in patients that are age 75 yr or older (Bharaktiya et al., 2012). Hypothyroidism is currently the most common thyroid dysfunction in the United States. Epidemiologic studies on the incidence and prevalence of hypothyroidism are lacking, but a recent estimate indicates that the incidence of hypothyroidism is likely 350/100,000 women/yr and 80/100,000 men/yr (McGrogan et al., 2008). It is estimated that more than half of people with hypothyroidism go undiagnosed.

Hypothyroidism occurs at any age but is particularly common in the elderly. It occurs in 10% of women and 6% of men older than age 65 yr (Beers & Porter, 2006). It is typically easier to diagnose hypothyroidism in younger adults because the disorder may be subtle and present atypically in the elderly (Beers & Porter, 2006). In newborn and pediatric patients, early detection of congenital hypothyroidism is important because it can result in cretinism if left untreated. Congenital hypothyroidism affects 1/4,000 newborns (Delange, 1998).

Etiology and Pathophysiology

A variety of factors and conditions can lead to hypothyroidism. The most common cause of hypothyroidism in the United States is chronic autoimmune thyroiditis, also known as Hashimoto's disease (Blackwell, 2004). Hypothyroidism can also result from decreases in functional thyroid tissue, impaired hormonal synthesis or release, congenital defects in the thyroid gland, loss of thyroid tissue, radio iodine treatment for hyperthyroidism, surgical removal of part or all of the thyroid, radiation therapy for throat or neck cancer, and dietary iodine deficiency (Tamparo & Lewis, 2000). Dysfunction of the hypothalamus or pituitary contributes to hypothyroidism in 10% of cases. Hypothalamic disease contributes by resulting in a failure to produce TRH, while pituitary disease (e.g., pituitary tumor or insufficiency) results in failure to produce TSH (Boissonnault, 1995).

Early signs of hypothyroidism are often subtle and difficult to diagnose. Symptoms may include low energy, cold intolerance, constipation, forgetfulness, and personality changes. Unexplained weight gain is common due to fluid retention and decreased metabolism. Paresthesias of the hands and feet and carpal tunnel syndrome may be additional early signs of the condition. Women with hypothyroidism may develop menstrual disturbance (Brent & Koenig, 2011; Reasner & Talbert, 2011).

Cardiorespiratory effects of hypothyroidism include bradycardia, deceased cardiac output, and poor peripheral circulation (Goodman et al., 2003). The rehabilitation therapist must be careful to not overtax the patient's cardiovascular system during therapy sessions. Monitoring vital signs and using a perceived exertion scale can help determine intensity of exercise. Also, weakness in respiratory muscles can result in dyspnea on exertion (Goodman et al., 2003).

Gastrointestinal effects of hypothyroidism include decreased gastrointestinal tract motility, constipation, achlorhydria (absence of hydrochloric acid from gastric juice), and decreased lipid metabolism. Decreased lipid metabolism can lead to increased serum cholesterol and triglycerides, **arteriosclerosis**, and coronary disease (Goodman et al., 2003).

Neurologic effects include slowed neurologic function, depression, headache, forgetfulness, slurred speech, and hoarse voice. Lethargy, fatigue, and an increased requirement for sleep are common complaints. Hypothyroidism can affect the patient's thermoregulation, which can result in a decrease in production of body heat and cause the patient to report always feeling cold (Beers & Porter, 2006).

Effects on the musculoskeletal system include myalgia and proximal muscle weakness of the quadriceps and hamstrings (Kocabas et al., 2009). The patient may also experience chronic trigger points, edema, carpal tunnel syndrome, paresthesias, low-back pain, and joint pain.

The integumentary effects of hypothyroidism can be profound. In more severe cases, a condition known as myxedema may develop. It is characterized by a dry, waxy type of non-pitting edema along with abnormal deposits of mucin in the skin and other tissues. The condition results in distinctive physical changes: The face become bloated, the lips become swollen, and the nose thickens (Frazier & Drzymkowski, 2004). Additional skin changes that occur with hypothyroidism include the presence of dry, flaky, inelastic skin; coarse hair; hair loss; and general puffiness of the face along with periorbital edema. Hypothyroidism may also cause non-pitting edema in the hands and feet and poor wound healing.

A serious complication of hypothyroidism is **myxedema** coma. Myxedema coma is a severe form of hypothyroidism that results in altered mental status, hypothermia, bradycardia, hypercarbia (abnormally high level of carbon dioxide in the circulating blood), and hyponatremia. **Cardiomegaly**, pericardial effusion, cardiogenic shock, and ascites may be present. Myxedema coma most commonly occurs in individuals with undiagnosed or untreated hypothyroidism who are subjected to external stressors such as low temperature, infection, or medical interventions (e.g., surgery or hypnotic drugs).

The diagnosis of hypothyroidism is made based on clinical history, physical examination, and laboratory testing. History and physical examination findings vary based on the severity of the condition. In more severe cases, the patient often presents with facial myxedema (periorbital edema, dry skin, coarse hair, puffy face). Although enlargement of the thyroid gland (goiter) is usually associated with hyperthyroidism, it can be present in some forms of hypothyroidism, such as **Hashimoto's disease** (Tamparo & Lewis, 2000).

Diagnosis of hypothyroidism is normally made based on measurement of TSH levels and measurement of T3 and T4 levels by radioimmunoassay. Radioimmunoassay provides information on the unbound levels (active form) of thyroid hormone and is more accurate than measurement of total thyroid levels. Measurement of TSH levels is considered the most sensitive screening test for establishing the diagnosis of primary hypothyroidism. Common laboratory findings that support a diagnosis of hypothyroidism include low or normal T3 and T4 levels and increased TSH levels. The high TSH level is a result of the pituitary producing more TSH in an effort to stimulate the thyroid gland to produce more thyroid hormone. Because many patients with primary hypothyroidism have normal circulating levels of T4, measurement of the serum T3 or T4 levels alone is not enough to diagnose hypothyroidism (Beers & Porter, 2006). In subclinical hypothyroidism, also referred to as mild hypothyroidism, T4 levels are typically normal but TSH concentration is slightly elevated. Because thyroid hormone has a half-life of about 1 wk, thyroid levels should be reassessed 6 wk after making a dosage change. Other diagnostic laboratory tests can include thyroid scan (contraindicated during pregnancy) and ultrasonograpy (Brent & Koenig, 2011; Reasner & Talbert, 2011).

Rehabilitation Considerations

The rehabilitation specialist should prescribe and carefully monitor exercise in patients with hypothyroidism. This population often demonstrates exercise intolerance, bradycardia, reduced stroke volume, and dyspnea on exertion (Klein & Ojamaa, 1996). Exercise-induced myalgia and, in rare instances, rhabdomyolysis can occur with exercise in untreated patients. Apathy and depression, which are common in patients with untreated hypothyroidism, may affect the patient's participation in and compliance with an exercise program. The rehabilitation therapist may also see an increased prevalence of fibromyalgia and trigger points in individuals with hypothyroidism due to metabolic distress in the muscle tissue.

The rehabilitation therapist should monitor patients with cardiac disease closely after thyroid-replacement therapy and should watch for tachycardia, hypertension, and any exacerbation of their existing cardiac condition. Patients with existing cardiac conditions should be started at low doses of thyroid medication to prevent adverse cardiac effects. The rehabilitation therapist should also monitor all patients on thyroid-replacement therapy for signs of hyperthyroidism and should communicate such signs to the patient's prescriber and pharmacist, who may identify any possible side effects or drug interactions that may be involved and determine whether a medication dosage change is needed.

Medication Therapy

The goal of medication therapy in hypothyroidism is to restore normal levels of thyroid hormone in the body. Improvement of symptoms, such as restoration of left ventricular performance, can occur as early as 2 wk after supplement initiation. Treatment of hypothyroidism usually involves daily thyroid hormone replacement with synthetic forms of T4 (levothyroxine [Synthroid]) or T3 (liothyronine [Cytomel]). Liothyronine, which has a more rapid rate of onset, is used in the emergent treatment of low thyroid levels. Levothyroxine is preferred over liothyronine for chronic dosing because liothyronine requires more frequent dosing (3 times/day), costs more, and is associated with transient increases in T3. Peak levels of both occur 2 to 4 h after dosing. Liotrix (Euthroid, Thyrolar) is a synthetic supplement that combines T4 and T3 in a 4:1 ratio. The older Armour thyroid product (desiccated thyroid product from sheep, hogs, or beef) is still occasionally encountered. Thyroglobulin (Proloid) is a partially purified, pork-derived thyroid protein. A dose of 60 mg (or 1 grain) of either of these animal products is equivalent to 80 µg of T4. These animal-derived products are seldom used now due to possible development of antigens to the animal protein. When a patient cannot take oral levothyroxine, intravenous levothyroxine can be administered at 80% of the oral dose. Table 23.4 summarizes

Table 23.4 Thyroid Supplements Used to Treat Hypothyroidism

Medication	Content	Dose equivalent to 60 mg of levothyroxine	Comments
Thyroid (Armour Thyroid)	Desiccated beef, pork, or sheep thyroid gland	1 grain (65 mg)	Generic brands may not be equivalent. Unpredictable hormone activity.
Thyroglobulin	Partially purified pork thyroglobulin	1 grain (65 mg)	Standardized to give T4:T3 ratio of 2.5:1.
Levothyroxine (Synthroid, Levothroid, Levoxyl)	Synthetic T4	50-60 µg	Agent of choice due to stable levels and predictable potency. Generics are equivalent. Half-life = 7 days.
Liothyronine (Cytomel)	Synthetic T3	15-37.5 µg	Uniform absorption. Rapid onset. Half life = 1.5 days. Must be dosed 3 times/day.
Liotrix (Euthroid, Thyrolar)	Synthetic T4:T3 in ratio of 4:1	50-60 µg of T4 and 12.5-15 µg of T3	Predictable levels and effects. Expensive.

T3 = tri-iodothyronine; T4 = thyroxine.

medications used to treat hypothyroidism (Brent & Koenig, 2011).

Adverse effects from thyroid supplementation rarely occur as long as the dose is carefully initiated and titrated. Allergic reactions occasionally occur with administration of animal-derived products. The Synthroid 50 mcg tablet, which contains no dyes and very few additives, should be tried if allergic reaction to thyroid supplements is suspected. Excessive supplementation of thyroid hormone can result in heart failure, angina pectoris, and myocardial infarction. It can also cause excessive remodeling of bone along with decreased bone density and increased risk of fracture (Brent & Koenig, 2011; Reasner & Talbert, 2011).

Medications Used to Treat Goiter

Goiter, the leading thyroid disease throughout the world, affects more than 200 million people. Most goiters also contain thyroid nodules. The incidence of goiter has declined with the introduction of iodine supplementation into the diet in the form of iodized salt. Goiter results from inadequate thyroid hormone secretion, compensatory TSH secretion, and thyroid enlargement. In treating goiter, a trial of thyroid supplementation is first conducted in order to rule out elevated TSH levels as the cause of the hyperplasia. Large, long-standing goiters do not spontaneously decrease in size. Surgical resection is required when large goiters compress surrounding structures and cause symptoms of dysphagia or dyspnea (Brent & Koenig, 2011; Reasner & Talbert, 2011).

Osteoporosis

Osteoporosis is a condition of low bone mass and microarchitectural disruption in which fractures result from minimal trauma. Osteomalacia (deficient bone mineralization) can lead to skeletal muscle weakness and fracture as well. Bone mineral density (BMD), which describes the balance between bone resorption and reformation, is classified based on a T-scoring system. Each individual's T-score reflects the number of standard deviations away from the mean BMD for that individual's age. Normal bone mass is reflected in a T-score

greater than −1, osteopenia is reflected in a T-score of −1 to −2.5, and osteoporosis is reflected in a T-score at or below −2.5. BMD peaks between 20 and 35 yr of age (Friedman, 2011; O'Connell & Elliott, 2002).

Incidence

Osteoporosis is a major global problem that affects more than 200 million individuals (American Association of Orthopedic Surgeons, 2009). Osteoporosis affects 10 million Americans, and an additional 44 million Americans over 50 yr of age have low bone mass along with increased risk of developing osteoporosis. Approximately 1.5 million fractures associated with osteoporosis occur each year. Thirty to fifty percent of women and 15% to 30% of men worldwide suffer a fracture due to osteoporosis. Risk increases in women after menopause due to lower levels of estrogen, a female hormone that helps to maintain bone mass. In the first decade after menopause women lose 10% to 25% of bone mass; about 10% is lost in each subsequent decade. The incidence of osteoporosis in men is about 20%. Although women are at risk for osteoporosis during and immediately after menopause, both sexes lose bone mass at about the same rate after age 70 yr.

Etiology and Pathophysiology

Hyperparathyroidism (discussed later) can increase the risk for osteoporosis. Modifiable risk factors for osteoporosis include low intakes of calcium and vitamin D, estrogen deficiency, physical inactivity, excessive caffeine intake, cigarette smoking, corticosteroid use, and prolonged overuse of thyroid hormone. Table 23.5 lists mechanisms and treatments of metabolic bone disease.

The skeleton provides structural support for the body, acts as a reservoir of calcium and phosphorus, and protects vital organs and houses the hematopoietic system contained in the bone marrow. One fifth of bone is trabecular bone, comprising a meshwork of horizontal and vertical structures. Trabecular bone has a large surface area and is in close contact with cells in the marrow affecting bone turnover. Cortical bone is compact and is formed in

Table 23.5 Mechanisms and Treatment of Metabolic Bone Disorders

Disorder	Description	Primary treatment
Hyperparathyroidism	Increased parathyroid hormone and hypercalcemia can lead to bone demineralization, bone fractures, and kidney damage	Surgical removal of the hypersecreting parathyroid gland. Cinacalcet (Sensipar) is used to treat secondary hyperparathyroidism associated with chronic renal disease or parathyroid cancer.
Hypoparathyroidism	Decreased parathyroid hormone and hypocalcemia can lead to osteoporosis and bone fracture	Calcium supplements, vitamin D
Osteoporosis	Bone demineralization; effects of aging, metabolic disease, and hormonal changes in postmenopausal women	Calcium supplements, vitamin D, calcitonin (Miacalcin), raloxifene (Evista), bisphosphonates, parathyroid hormone fragment teriparatide (Forteo)
Rickets	Deficient bone mineralization in children caused by vitamin D deficiency	Calcium supplements, vitamin D
Osteomalacia	Softening of bone; adult form of rickets	Calcium supplements, vitamin D
Paget's disease	Chronic disorder of the skeleton in which areas of bone undergo abnormal turnover, resulting in areas of enlarged and softened bone; elevated alkaline phosphatase levels	Bisphosphonates, calcitonin
Renal osteodystrophy	Increased phosphate levels; reduced calcium and reduced renal activation of vitamin D	Phosphate binders: calcium acetate (Phoslo), lanthanum carbonate (Fosrenol), sevelamer (Renagel)

layers. The mature bone undergoes constant remodeling: 4% of cortical bone and 28% of trabecular bone is replaced each year.

Bone is a highly organized, three-dimensional structure comprising an organic matrix and crystalline minerals. The organic matrix comprises protein (90% collagen) and specialized cells involved in bone remodeling: the osteoblasts, osteoclasts, and osteocytes. Osteoblasts promote mineralization and rebuilding of bone, and osteoclasts break down bone in preparation for remodeling (resorption). Osteocytes are retired osteoblasts that identify fatigue damage in the bone structure and summon osteoclasts to initiate resorption. The mineral structure (apatite) is mainly calcium and phosphate. In fact, bone contains 99% of the body's calcium and 85% of its phosphorus. Constant balance of these ions within the body is essential for metabolic and muscle function. Bone resorption and loss are part of the process of maintaining balance of calcium and phosphorus levels.

Parathyroid hormone (PTH) is produced by the parathyroid glands and works along with calcitonin and vitamin D in maintaining bone health. PTH increases the release of calcium and phosphorus from bone and increases the absorption of calcium and excretion of phosphate by the kidneys. PTH also promotes calcium absorption in the gastrointestinal tract. The regulation of calcium is essential because calcium is vital in synaptic transmission for muscle contraction and in bone mineralization. The receptors in the **parathyroid gland** sense changes in calcium levels in the bloodstream and respond by increasing calcium release of PTH or decreasing PTH release as needed to maintain homeostasis. The release of PTH increases blood calcium levels by altering calcium metabolism in bone, the kidneys, and the gastrointestinal tract (Tfelt-Hansen & Brown, 2005).

PTH increases renal excretion of phosphate and decreases renal reabsorption of phosphate in the proximal tubules. Decreased phosphate levels promote production of calcitriol (the active form of vitamin D), whereas high phosphate levels suppress production of calcitriol. Vitamin D is not a vitamin; rather, it is a hormone that is synthesized and acts to regulate calcium levels. Active vitamin D requires two successive hydroxylation steps in the kidney to form the active form 1,25 dihydroxyvitamin D. Calcitriol augments absorption and retention of calcium and phosphorus. Newly synthesized calcitriol promotes intestinal reabsorption of calcium, thus increasing serum calcium levels (Friedman, 2011; O'Connell & Elliott, 2002). Calcitonin, another hormone that regulates calcium levels and promotes bone health, is synthesized in the parafollicular C-cells of the thyroid gland. The actions of calcitonin generally oppose those of PTH and produce hypocalcemia (Friedman, 2011; O'Connell & Elliott, 2002).

Parathyroid gland dysfunction can be classified as hyperparathyroidism or hypoparathyroidism. Associated alterations in PTH and calcium can profoundly affect central nervous system function, muscle function, and bone health. Several additional metabolic bone disorders, including osteoporosis, rickets, osteomalacia, and **Paget's disease**, are treated with medications. Table 23.5 summarizes the primary effects of these disorders and the associated medication therapies (Friedman, 2011; O'Connell & Elliott, 2002).

Rehabilitation Considerations

Fracture associated with postmenopausal osteoporosis usually involves trabecular bone. Common sites of fracture in the elderly are the hip, vertebra, and forearm. Fracture can also occur in the proximal femur and ribs. Fracture risk increases with age, and survival rates are reduced in patients who experience fractures of the hip or spine (Friedman, 2011; O'Connell & Elliott, 2002). Patients are commonly seen in rehabilitation after suffering a fall and resulting hip fracture. Many of these patients exhibit cognitive difficulties such as problems with attention, short-term memory impairment, and verbal memory problems. The physical therapist needs to work on the patient's cognitive problems using occupational therapy and speech–language pathology in order to enhance the probability that the patient will have a successful rehabilitation outcome. A large number of patients continue to experience cognitive difficulties 6 mo after the hip fracture and subsequent surgery, which can increase the probability that the patient will continue to fall and require additional surgery.

Preventative measures for osteoporosis include regular weight-bearing and muscle-strengthening exercise and adequate intakes of calcium and vitamin D, especially in the elderly adult. Smoking and excessive drinking are also risk factors and should be avoided. Table 23.6 lists factors and medications that can contribute to increased risk of falls and fracture (Friedman, 2011; O'Connell & Elliott, 2002).

Medication Therapy

The goals of treatment are to restore bone strength and prevent fracture. Adequate dietary intake of calcium and vitamin D is essential in maintaining healthy bone structure and reducing risk of osteoporosis and bone fracture. Daily requirements for calcium and vitamin D vary with age. Children under 1 yr of age require 210 to 270 mg of calcium/day. The requirement increases to 500 mg for children 1 to 3 yr of age, 800 mg for children 4 to 8 yr of age, and 1300 mg/day for children 9 to 18 yr of age. Adults require 1000 mg/day until age 51 yr, when the requirement increases to 1200 mg/day. A good rule of thumb to ensure adequate calcium intake is to count each serving of low-fat dairy products as 200 mg of calcium and to provide the balance for the day with calcium supplements. The requirement for vitamin D is 200 IU/day until age 51 yr, when the requirement increases to 400 IU/day. Patients over age 71 yr require 600 IU/day. Table 23.7 compares calcium supplements.

Agents that inhibit resorption of bone, including bisphosphonates, estrogen supplements, the selective estrogen receptor modulator (SERM) raloxifene (Evista), and calcitonin, are also used to treat patients with osteoporosis. A newer therapy is the biologically active PTH fragment teriparatide (Forteo). Hormone-

Table 23.6   Factors That Contribute to Bone Loss and Increased Fall Risk

Factors that contribute to bone loss	
Genetic factors	Caucasian or Asian ethnicity, family history of osteoporosis, small or thin body frame, older age
Lifestyle factors	Sedentary lifestyle, minimal exercise, smoking, excessive alcohol intake, minimal sun exposure
Dietary factors	Low calcium intake, lactose intolerance, high caffeine intake, high phosphorus intake, weight loss of >10% after 50 yr of age, anorexia nervosa, long-term parenteral nutrition
Hormonal factors	Late menarche, early menopause, oophorectomy without estrogen replacement, nulliparity, amenorrhea associated with anorexia nervosa, medication use, excessive exercise
Chronic illnesses	Hyperthyroidism, Cushing's disease, multiple myeloma, cancer of the bone, diabetes, gastrointestinal disease or surgery, arthritis, cognitive impairment, stroke, post transplantation
Medications that increase risk of osteoporosis	Glucocorticoids, excessive thyroid replacement, lithium, chemotherapy, anticonvulsants, gonadotropin-releasing hormone agonists or antagonists
Medications that increase risk of osteoporosis by impairing calcium absorption	Tetracyclines, phenothiazines, cyclosporine, antacids containing aluminum, phosphate binders used in renal failure
Medications that increase risk of osteoporosis by promoting renal elimination of calcium	Loop diuretics (furosemide, bumetanide)
Factors that contribute to falls	
Medications that increase fall risk	Antianxiety medications, insomnia medications (benzodiazepines), antidepressants, antihypertensives, antiarrhythmics, vasodilators, diuretics, antipsychotics, antiparkinson agents, skeletal muscle relaxants, antihistamines, use of 4 or more medications of any type
Non-medication risk factors	Physical disability, slow gait, orthostatic hypotension, difficult tandem walk, decreased visual acuity, decreased auditory acuity, poor depth perception, decreased quadriceps and grip strength, inability to rise from a chair, use of walking aids, presence of stairs or uneven footpaths, polished floors, thick mats or carpet in the living environment, poor footwear choices

replacement therapy (in which estrogen or progesterone is administrated in postmenopausal women to preserve bone mass and protect against fracture) was once endorsed. However, the increased risk of cardiac disease and breast cancer has limited the use of estrogen and progesterone to short-term use in managing vasomotor symptoms associated with menopause in females without cardiac risk factors. Table 23.8 summarizes medications that are used to treat osteoporosis and other metabolic bone disorders (Friedman, 2011; O'Connell & Elliott, 2002).

PATIENT CASE 2

P.G. is a 73-yr-old retired male who was referred to the outpatient physical therapy clinic after a recent visit to the metabolic bone clinic at the local hospital. He was referred with a diagnosis of osteoporosis, an old T1 fracture, and thoracic and low-back pain. P.G. has a notable thoracic kyphosis. He also has Crohn's disease and has been treated with the corticosteroid prednisone during repeated, uncontrolled periods of

Table 23.7   Comparison of Calcium Products

Product		Elemental calcium (%)	Calcium provided per dose
Calcium carbonate products	Titralac liquid	40	400 mg/5 ml (teaspoon)
	Titralac tablets		168 mg
	Titralac Extra Strength		300 mg
	Tums Chewable		200 mg
	Tums EX		300 mg
	Tums Ultra		500 mg
	Viactiv chews		500 mg
	Calcium carbonate with vitamin D		600 mg/125 IU of vitamin D
	Caltrate with vitamin D		600 mg/125 IU of vitamin D
	Oscal with vitamin D		500 mg/125 IU of vitamin D
Calcium citrate products	Citracal	24	200 mg
	Citracal Liquitab		500 mg
	Citracal with vitamin D		316 mg/200 IU of vitamin D
Calcium phosphate tribasic products	Posture	39	600 mg
	Posture-D		600 mg/125 IU of vitamin D
	Dical-D chewable wafers with vitamin D		232 mg/200 IU of vitamin D

exacerbation throughout his adult life. P.G. is approximately 30 lb (13.6 kg) overweight and does not participate in any type of regular physical activity. P.G.'s physician wants P.G. to receive therapy exercises to treat the musculoskeletal impairments associated with his back pain and receive recommendations for a general exercise program that will help prevent further bone demineralization and lower his risk for fractures. P.G.'s physician has prescribed calcium and vitamin D supplements as well as the bisphosphonate medication alendronate (Fosamax). P.G. also smokes 1 pack of cigarettes/day; his doctor has asked him to stop smoking. P.G. reports that since starting these medications he has noticed a change in bowel movements. P.G. reports that he previously had loose stools and that he is now experiencing constipation.

Question

Could the treatment that P.G. received for his Crohn's disease be associated with his development of osteoporosis?

Answer

One of the potential side effects of long-term use of corticosteroids is osteoporosis. Corticosteroids directly inhibit osteoblast function, directly enhance bone resorption, inhibit absorption of gastrointestinal calcium, increase loss of calcium via the kidney, and inhibit gonadal hormones.

Question

What are some possible causes of P.G.'s constipation?

Answer

One side effect of increasing calcium intake is constipation. A close look at P.G.'s diet and level of calcium supplementation is necessary. It is possible that P.G. has increased his calcium intake through recommended dietary changes and that he does not require as much calcium supplementation as previously thought. If P.G.'s constipation persists after his calcium intake is optimized through diet and supplementation, P.G.'s doctor may want to consider recommending a stool softener.

See table 23.8 in the web resource for a full list of medication-specific indications, dosing recommendations, and side effects.

Table 23.8 Medications Used to Treat Osteoporosis and Metabolic Bone Disorders

Medication	Side effects affecting rehab							Other side effects or considerations
Medications used to treat osteomalacia, osteoporosis, and hypoparathyroidism								
Calcium	Cog	S	A	Motor	D	Com	F	Side effects: Constipation, gas, kidney stones (rare).
	0	0	0	0	+	0	0	Drug interactions: Antacids decrease absorption. Take at least 2 h apart from antacids, sucralfate, iron products, laxatives, and tetracycline or quinolone antibiotics.
Vitamin D	Cog	S	A	Motor	D	Com	F	Side effects: Excessive dosing can cause hypercalcemia.
	0	0	0	0	+	0	0	Precautions: Must use activated form (calcitriol) in patients with renal impairment.
Bisphosphonates used to treat osteoporosis and Paget's disease: Pamidronate and zoledronate (Zometa) are also used to treat bone metastasis, multiple myeloma, and hypercalcemia associated with malignancy and Paget's disease.								
Oral: Alendronate (Fosamax) Risedronate (Actonel) Ibandronate (Boniva)	Cog	S	A	Motor	D	Com	F	To prevent esophageal complications, take in the morning with a full glass of water while sitting upright.
	0	0	0	0	++	0	0	Side effects: Heartburn, esophageal irritation or esophagitis, abdominal pain, diarrhea. Serious osteonecrosis of the jaw has been reported.
								Drug interactions: Calcium supplements, antacids, food, and iron supplements interfere with intestinal absorption.
								Contraindications: Avoid use in patients with renal impairment.
Parenteral: Pamidronate (Aredia) Zoledronate (Reclast, Zometa)	Cog	S	A	Motor	D	Com	F	Side effects: Bisphosphonates given intravenously have been associated with nephrotoxicity, which increases with higher doses and rapid intravenous administration. Longer administration times decrease risk of nephrotoxicity.
	0	0	0	0	++	0	0	Contraindications: Avoid in patients with renal impairment.
Selective estrogen receptor modulator (SERM) used to prevent and treat osteoporosis								
Raloxifene (Evista)	Cog	S	A	Motor	D	Com	F	Used in postmenopausal women; also used to reduce the risk of breast cancer.
	0	0	0	+	0	0	+	Side effects: Hot flashes, leg cramps, thromboembolic events.
Calcitonin: Hormone produced by the thyroid and used to treat osteoporosis, Paget's disease, hypercalcemia, and bone metastases.								
Calcitonin Intramuscular or subcutaneous injection or intranasal spray	Cog	S	A	Motor	D	Com	F	Side effects: Nasal formulation, runny nose, nausea, hand swelling, urticaria, intestinal cramping.
	0	0	0	0	+	0	0	Injection: Discomfort at injection site.
								Salmon derivative.
								Resistance associated with antigen development can occur.

› continued

Table 23.8 › continued

Medication	Side effects affecting rehab							Other side effects or considerations
Recombinant form of parathyroid hormone used to treat osteoporosis								
Teriparatide (Forteo) injection	Cog 0	S 0	A 0	Motor ++	D ++	Com 0	F ++	Increases formation of new bone; synthetic parathyroid hormone fragment. Side effects: Pain at injection site, nausea, leg cramps, headache, dizziness.
Agent used to treat secondary hyperparathyroidism in patients with chronic kidney disease on dialysis and hypercalcemia in patients with parathyroid cancer								
Cinacalcet (Sensipar)	Cog 0	S 0	A 0	Motor +	D 0	Com 0	F 0	Side effects: Monitor for seizures associated with rapid drops in calcium or adynamic bone disease with parathyroid levels <100 pg/ml. Drug interactions: CYP3A4 inhibitors such as ketoconazole (Nizoral), erythromycin, and itraconazole (Sporanox) and CYP2D6 inhibitors such as beta blockers, flecainide (Tambocor), vinblastine, and tricyclic antidepressants can increase levels and effects of cinacalcet. Phosphate binders, vitamin D, bisphosphonates, calcitonin, and glucocorticoids can interfere with the action of cinacalcet.

Cog = cognition; S = sedation; A = agitation or mania; Motor = discoordination; D = dysphagia; Com = communication; F = falls.

The likelihood rating scale for encountering the side effects is as follows: 0 = Almost no probability of encountering side effects. + = Little likelihood of encountering side effects. +/++ = Low probability of encountering side effects; however, probability increases with increased dosage. ++ = Medium likelihood of encountering side effects. +++ = High likelihood of encountering side effects, particularly with high doses. ++++ = Highest likelihood of encountering side effects; best to avoid in at-risk patients.

Question

What type of exercise program should the rehabilitation therapist recommend for P.G.?

Answer

The goals of the exercise program should be to increase bone mass, slow bone loss, and minimize risk for fractures and falls. Common recommendations include weight-bearing aerobic exercise (e.g., walking programs) or resistance training with an emphasis on weight-bearing exercises. The rehabilitation therapist must also assess and treat any impairment in the patient's balance that could increase the risk for falls. P.G. will also benefit from postural-awareness training and spine-stabilization exercises. The rehabilitation therapist should also reinforce the doctor's recommendation regarding smoking cessation. Addressing this modifiable risk factor will help improve P.G.'s bone health and his overall ability to tolerate physical exercise.

Paget's Disease

Paget's disease is a bone disorder characterized by single or multiple sites of disordered bone remodeling.

Incidence

Paget's disease occurs globally; however, it is more common in New Zealand, Australia, and Europe. In these locations this disease occurs in 5% of the elderly. The prevalence of this disease ranges from 1.5% to 8%, depending on the country and the age of the population (Cohen, 2008). Paget's disease affects 2% to 3% of patients over 60 yr of age in North America.

Etiology and Pathophysiology

Paget's disease is thought to be caused by infection with the measles virus. Patients experience increased bone resorption followed by rapid formation of bone that is disorganized and of poor quality, resulting in bowing of the bones, stress fractures, thickened bone, and arthritis of joints adjacent to poorly formed bone. Bone lesions contain abnormal multinucleated osteoclasts. Complications of this disease include deafness, spinal cord compression, high-output heart failure, and pain. In rare instances, this disease progresses to osteogenic sarcoma, which can be fatal (Friedman, 2011).

Rehabilitation Considerations

The rehabilitation therapist should emphasize that patients need to take prescribed amounts of calcium and vitamin D on a daily basis. In addition, the patient should exercise to maintain good skeletal health and increase joint mobility. The rehabilitation therapist plays a major role in helping the patient exercise without putting strain on the bones (Cleveland Clinic, 2009). The rehabilitation specialist also sees patients for therapy after surgical repair, such as total joint replacement and fracture repair. Pain management is part of the rehabilitative effort in these patients. Patients should receive gait and balance training as needed. Patients also may require correction for leg length with supportive devices and may require assistance in activities of daily living (ADL) in order to increase safety and independent mobility. The rehabilitation therapist may recommend adaptive equipment and provide patient instruction and training in the use of these devices and equipment (Chow, 2011).

Medication Therapy

Most patients with Paget's disease do not require medication therapy. Patients with symptoms of severe pain, neural compression, progressive deformity, hypercalcemia, high-output congestive heart failure, or repeated fractures should receive medication treatment (Friedman, 2011). **Bisphosphonate** therapy is standard therapy and is initiated for 6 mo. With treatment, patients experience a decrease in bone pain over several weeks. Single-dose infusions of pamidronate can induce long-term remission. Long-term response is also obtained with the administration of zoledronate (Reclast). Bisphosphonates inhibit bone resorption by concentrating in the sites of active remodeling and incorporating into

the bone's matrix. Table 23.8 summarizes the dosing of the bisphosphonates used in treatment of Paget's disease. Their side effects include heartburn, esophageal irritation or **esophagitis**, abdominal pain, and diarrhea. To prevent esophageal complications, patients should take these products with a full glass of water while sitting upright and should take them in the morning rather than at bedtime. Serious osteonecrosis of the jaw has also been reported with the use of these agents. Important drug interactions include calcium supplements, antacids, food, and iron supplements, which interfere with intestinal absorption of the oral bisphosphonates.

Calcitonin is also used to treat Paget's disease. Calcitonin is given by subcutaneous injection in a dose of 100 U/day initially and is then reduced to 50 U/day. Long-term use results in a decrease in serum alkaline phosphatase and improved symptoms. Side effects include nausea, hand swelling, urticaria, and intestinal cramping. Antigens to this product can develop and cause resistance to medication effects (Friedman, 2011; O'Connell & Elliott, 2002).

Hyperparathyroidism

Hyperparathyroidism is a disease caused by overactivity of one or more of the four parathyroid glands. This overactivity results in increased secretion of PTH, which causes hypercalcemia (Frazier & Drzymkowski, 2004). Hyperparathyroidism disrupts calcium and phosphate balance and disrupts bone metabolism, which can lead to osteoporosis.

Incidence

The incidence of primary hyperparathyroidism in the United States is estimated to be 1/1000 for men, 2-3/1,000 for women, and 21/1,000 in postmenopausal females (Clarke, 2008). Women are two to three times more likely to be affected than are men, and the disease is seen more frequently in women over 40 yr of age (Regina-Cammon et al., 2002). Onset typically occurs after age 60 yr. Hyperparathyroidism is characterized by excessive circulating PTH in the blood. This can lead to hypercalcemia, bone damage, and kidney damage (Vestergaard et al., 2000).

Etiology and Pathophysiology

Primary hyperparathyroidism is most often caused by a single **adenoma** or multiple endocrine neoplasms. Overproduction of PTH by a tumor increases intestinal calcium absorption, reduces renal calcium clearance, and increases bone calcium release. Secondary hyperparathyroidism can be seen with vitamin D deficiency or chronic renal failure.

The central nervous system symptoms of hyperparathyroidism include lethargy, drowsiness, paresthesias, slow mentation, memory difficulties, depression, and personality changes. The rehabilitation therapist should be aware that the patient is likely to fatigue easily. The musculoskeletal effects associated with hyperparathyroidism include muscle wasting and myopathy that is most notable in the proximal muscles. Myopathy related to parathyroid dysfunction appears to result from altered PTH levels and impaired action of vitamin D (Schapira & Griggs, 2000). Bone decalcification accompanied by bone pain, especially in the spine, can put the patient at risk for pathologic fractures (Goodman et al., 2003). Other musculoskeletal symptoms include gout, pseudo gout, arthralgias, and joint hypermobility. Gastrointestinal symptoms include peptic ulcers, pancreatitis, nausea, vomiting, constipation, and abdominal pain. Genitourinary effects include the development of kidney stones, hypercalcemia resulting in polyuria, polydipsia, constipation, kidney infections, and renal hypertension.

Hyperparathyroidism is the most common cause of hypercalcemia; other causes of hypercalcemia should be ruled out. Hypercalcemia can be caused by milk–alkali syndrome, which is caused by concurrent ingestion of large amounts of milk and antacids. Sustained use of antacids can also cause low phosphate levels and can result in osteomalacia characterized by an undermineralized bone matrix. Newly diagnosed hypercalcemia can also be caused by malignancy, with or without bony metastasis, due to a PTH-like protein produced by tumor cells. Excessive vitamin D intake (>50,000 U/day) can cause vitamin D toxicity and associated symptoms of hypercalcemia.

A diagnosis of hyperparathyroidism is made if the serum calcium level and the PTH level are high at the same time. In a small percentage of patients, the serum calcium level may be high but the PTH level may not.

Surgery, the most common treatment of primary hyperparathyroidism, provides a cure in at least 90% of all cases (Chen et al., 1998). The surgeon removes only the glands that are enlarged or have a tumor (adenoma). If all four glands are affected, the surgeon likely removes only three glands and perhaps a portion of the fourth in an attempt to leave some functioning parathyroid tissue (Chen et al., 1998). Surgery is the treatment of choice in patients with symptoms of primary hyperparathyroidism. Guidelines recommend that patients with asymptomatic primary hyperparathyroidism undergo surgery when concentration of serum calcium is high (>1 mg/dl above normal range), urine calcium output is high, and organs are involved (e.g., reduced kidney function or reduced BMD) (Bilezikian et al., 2002). Patients treated surgically for primary hyperparathyroidism have fewer fractures and gastric ulcers than patients treated conservatively (Vestergaard & Mosekilde, 2003).

Rehabilitation Considerations

The rehabilitation therapist should be aware that the patient with hyperparathyroidism is prone to fractures due to demineralization (Vestergaard et al., 2000) and should move the patient carefully during transfers and put fall precautions in place. Strengthening exercises that address weakness and atrophy in the proximal muscles and in the legs are often necessary (Goodman et al., 2003). Some patients develop inflammatory polyarthritis or tendinopathy (most commonly of the Achilles, triceps, and obturator tendons); these secondary conditions are less common now that recognition and treatment of hyperparathyroidism have improved. The rehabilitation therapist should carefully monitor patients who are taking digitalis for any toxic effects produced by elevated calcium levels. Patients with hypercalcemia, hypokalemia, or hypomagnesemia are hypersensitive to the effects of digitalis and may quickly develop toxic symptoms (arrhythmias, nausea, fatigue, and visual changes).

Medication Therapy

Calcimimetics are a new group of medications that mimic the action of calcium on tissue by activating the calcium-sensing receptors and inhibit production of PTH by the parathyroid glands. Cinacalcet (Sensipar) is indicated for treating secondary hyperparathyroidism in patients with chronic kidney disease on dialysis and treating hypercalcemia associated with parathyroid cancer. Sensipar is dosed at 30 mg by mouth/day for hypercalcemia in patients with kidney failure and can be titrated up to a maximum of 180 mg/day. Dosing for treatment of parathyroid cancer starts at 30 mg by mouth twice/day and the maximum dose is 90 mg 4 times/day. Dosing for treatment of secondary hyperparathyroidism or for normalizing calcium levels in patients with parathyroid cancer should be titrated up every 2 to 4 wk to maintain a PTH level between 150 and 300 pg/ml. Side effects can include seizures associated with rapid decreases in calcium or adynamic bone disease in patients whose PTH levels decrease below 100 pg/ml. Phosphate binders, vitamin D, bisphosphonates, calcitonin, and glucocorticoids can interfere with the action of cinacalcet. In addition, medications that inhibit CYP3A4 metabolism such as ketoconazole (Nizoral), erythromycin, and itraconazole (Sporanox) can increase levels and effects of cinacalcet. Medications that inhibit CYP2D6 such as beta blockers, flecainide (Tambocor), vinblastine, and tricyclic antidepressants can also increase levels and effects of cinacalcet.

Hypoparathyroidism

Hypoparathyroidism results when the parathyroid gland produces and secretes insufficient amounts of PTH. This disease is much rarer than hyperparathyroidism (Bringhurst et al., 2008). Hypoparathyroidism is characterized by abnormally low levels of parathyroid hormone.

This deficiency leads to low calcium levels in the blood and bones and to an increased amount of phosphorus. The goal of treatment is to normalize the levels of calcium and phosphorus.

Incidence

Hypoparathyroidism is classified as a rare disease. The incidence is 4/100,000 individuals (Medical Disability Advisor, 2010).

Etiology and Pathophysiology

The most common cause of hypoparathyroidism is injury to the parathyroid glands during surgery. The severity and nature of signs and symptoms of hypoparathyroidism usually depend on the degree of hypocalcemia (Tamparo & Lewis, 2000). Hypocalcemia is associated with neuromuscular irritability, which may result in tetany that can lead to painful spasms, laryngospasm, and arrhythmias (Bringhurst et al., 2008). The onset on tetany usually begins with tingling in the fingers, around the mouth, and occasionally in the feet. Central nervous system effects include irritability, agitation, anxiety, and depression; seizures are possible in severe cases (Tamparo & Lewis, 2000). Cardiovascular effects can be severe and include arrhythmias and eventual cardiac failure if left untreated. Integumentary effects include dry, scaly, coarse skin; increased likelihood of skin infections; thinning hair; and brittle fingernails and toenails (Beers & Porter, 2006). Gastrointestinal effects include nausea, vomiting, constipation, and abdominal pain.

The practitioner should rule out other causes of hypocalcemia when making the diagnosis of hypoparathyroidism. For example, vitamin D deficiency results in inadequate absorption of calcium and phosphate, thus impairing mineralization of newly formulated bone and cartilage. This can cause rickets in children and osteomalacia in adults. Blood tests that check serum calcium, phosphorus, magnesium, and PTH levels may be used to confirm a diagnosis of hypoparathyroidism. Electrocardiogram testing may reveal prolonged QT and ST intervals or other arrhythmias due to hypocalcemia.

A urine test may also be done to determine how much calcium is being renally eliminated (Tamparo & Lewis, 2000). Positive laboratory results that support a diagnosis of hypoparathyroidism include decreased PTH concentration, decreased serum calcium, and increased serum phosphorus (Springhouse, 2008).

Rehabilitation Considerations

The rehabilitation therapist should watch for signs of muscle **tetany** in patients with hypoparathyroidism during therapy sessions. Tetany may cause difficulties that make gait unsafe and inefficient and may negatively influence balance. Hyperventilation may worsen tetany; therefore, the use of breathing exercises is recommended. The clinician should monitor the patient's cardiac function; chronic hypoparathyroidism can lead to arrhythmia, heart block, and decreased cardiac output.

Medication Therapy

The goal of medication treatment is to restore calcium and mineral balance in the body. Treatment involves calcium carbonate and vitamin D supplements, which the patient usually must take for life (Wysolmerski & Insogna, 2008). In addition, a high-calcium, low-phosphorus diet is recommended. Patients with metabolic bone disease should be monitored with routine measurement of their serum electrolytes, vitamin D, and bone density to assure their vitamin D, calcium, magnesium, phosphorus, and potassium levels remain in therapeutic range to determine necessary adjustments in the dosage of supplements. This is especially important in patients treated with digoxin, diuretics, chemotherapy, and antibiotics such as aminoglycosides that can alter these electrolyte levels. Acute hypocalcemia can result from administration of multiple units of blood products due to the citrate preservative in these products (Tamparo & Lewis, 2000).

Patients who have life-threatening attacks of low calcium levels or prolonged muscle contractions are given intravenous calcium. Critical care practitioners take precautions to prevent seizures or laryngospasm and monitor the heart for abnormal rhythms until repletion is completed and the patient is stable. Once the life-threatening attack has been controlled, treatment continues with oral supplementation.

Summary

The rehabilitation professional commonly cares for patients with thyroid disease, parathyroid disease, and osteoporosis. This chapter introduces these disease states and the medication therapies used to treat them. The chapter also discusses methods the rehabilitation therapist can use to provide optimal care for these patients. The rehabilitation therapist must understand the functions of the thyroid and parathyroid glands, how thyroid and parathyroid disease can affect rehabilitation and the pharmacologic management of these disorders in order to develop and maintain safe and effective rehabilitation regimens for patients with these diseases.

Medications Used to Treat Gastrointestinal Disorders

24

The rehabilitation therapist commonly encounters patients with gastrointestinal (GI) disorders. Common disorders that can affect the patient's nutritional status and ability to participate in therapy include nausea and vomiting, constipation, irritable bowel syndrome, inflammatory bowel disease, dyspepsia, eosinophilic esophagitis, and dysphagia. This chapter summarizes these disorders and the medication therapies used to prevent and treat them. It also explains how these disorders can affect rehabilitation and provides guidance on adjusting the therapy session to enhance patient participation.

Nausea and Vomiting

Nausea and vomiting are protective mechanisms that remove potential toxins from the upper digestive tract. Nausea is an unpleasant sensation in the throat and epigastric area associated with the urge to vomit, whereas vomiting is the forceful expulsion of gastric contents. This process includes a pre-ejection phase (stomach relaxation and retroperistalsis), **retching** (rhythmic abdominal, intracostal, and diaphragmatic contraction against a closed glottis), and ejection (intense contraction of the abdominal muscle and relaxation of the upper esophageal sphincter). Retching is also known as the dry heaves. Nausea and vomiting are two of the most commonly encountered side effects associated with medication use and most often occur with initiation of therapy or with upward titration of dosage. Nausea and vomiting also commonly occur after surgical procedures, chemotherapy, or radiation therapy. Nausea and vomiting can affect the nutritional status of the patient, interfere with wound healing, and decrease the patient's ability to participate in the cognitive and motor training required in the rehabilitative session (Pasricha, 2001; Sharley & Wallace, 2011).

Incidence

Even with preventative medications about 10% to 50% of patients receiving chemotherapy experience nausea and vomiting. Postoperative nausea and vomiting occur in 25 million people annually and in one third of patients undergoing surgical procedures. Sixty-five percent of surgeries are now done in the outpatient setting; post discharge nausea and vomiting occurs in 30% of patients undergoing outpatient surgeries. **Emesis** (vomiting) is associated with increased risk of aspiration and has been associated with additional complications such as suture **dehiscence**, esophageal rupture, subcutaneous emphysema, and bilateral pneumothorax (Wender, 2009).

Etiology and Pathophysiology

Nausea and vomiting are regulated by the central emesis center, which processes neurotransmitter input from the chemoreceptor trigger zone (CTZ) and the nucleus tractus solitarius of the vagal nerve, as well as the cerebral cortex and the vestibular apparatus. The CTZ has a high concentration of serotonin receptors, dopamine receptors, and opioid receptors, whereas the nucleus tractus solitarius contains receptors for histamine, serotonin, and dopamine. Histamine and muscarinic receptors mediate the vestibular apparatus, and medications that block these central neuroreceptors are frequently used to treat patients with dizziness or balance difficulties (Eng & White, 2007; Wender, 2009).

Vomiting is controlled by the emetic center in the lateral reticular formation of the medulla. Efferent impulses from the emetic center communicate with the vagus, phrenic, and spinal nerves of the abdominal muscles. The emetic center is not exposed to blood or cerebral spinal fluid. The emetic center receives afferent nerve signals from the higher cortical centers and the optic, olfactory, vagal, glossopharyngeal, and trigeminal nerves. A major source of input to the emetic center is the CTZ located in the area postrema fourth ventricle. The CTZ is activated by direct chemical stimulation through the cerebrospinal fluid or blood. The CTZ is the major protective organ against toxic substances in the brain and is involved with the development of nausea and vomiting. The vestibular labyrinthian system of the middle ear can cause nausea and vomiting when stimulated with motion and vestibular toxicity. In addition, certain emotions, pain, sights, smells, and tastes can induce nausea and vomiting when mediated through the cerebral cortex. Memory, fear, and anticipation can provide input from the higher cortical centers to the vomiting center in the medulla to activate the vomiting reflex. Sensory information from the GI tract, mediastinum, testes, pharynx, and heart also provides input to the emetic center. The visceral afferents from the GI tract provide input to the emetic center when the GI tract is obstructed, is affected by medications, or is afflicted with gastroparesis (Eng & White, 2007; Wender, 2009).

Symptoms of nausea can interfere with the patient's ability to participate in the rehabilitative session and can reduce appetite and energy, thus interfering with physical, social, and psychological function. In the initial assessment, the rehabilitation therapist should ask the patient about the timing of meals, medication intake, and presence of symptoms such as nausea. Scheduling sessions for periods that are less likely to be associated with nausea and scheduling with consideration to the timing of patient meals and medication intake can contribute to successful rehabilitation. The therapist should also consider triggers associated with nausea and vomiting when designing sessions. Patients may be highly sensitive to strong smells and cooking smells, and such triggers should be avoided.

Medication Therapy

Central structures involved with the vomiting response are rich in dopamine, muscarinic, serotonergic, histamine, and opioid receptors. Many antiemetics work via their action at these receptors (Wender, 2009). Table 24.1 summarizes neurotransmitters that are involved with emesis and that are targeted by antiemetics (Eng & White, 2007; Wender, 2009).

PATIENT CASE 1

A.S. is a 43-yr-old female administrative assistant at a local university. She is currently 7 days status after open reduction internal fixation surgery on her right ankle for repair of a bimalleolar fracture. After surgery A.S. was given a prescription for oxycodone HCl–acetaminophen (Percocet) and instructed to take 2 tablets every 4 to 6 h as needed for postsurgical pain. Today is A.S.'s first visit to the outpatient rehabilitation clinic. During the history portion of her examination, A.S. reports that the Percocet controls the pain in her right ankle well (resulting in a pain level of 4 out of a pain score of 1-10 pain level at rest). However, she reports that since beginning the medication she has had intolerable nausea that is interfering with her ability to perform activities of daily living and therapy exercises. She states that she has vomited an average of 3 to 4 times each day since beginning the pain medication. She is strongly considering not using the pain medication despite pain scores of 8 to 10 when unmedicated. Her pain, untreated with this medication, does not allow her to fully participate in the session.

Table 24.1   Sites, Receptors, and Neurotransmitters that Mediate Nausea and Vomiting and the Appropriate Medication Treatments

Site	Receptor	Neurotransmitter	Antiemetic medication (receptor antagonist)
Vomiting center (medulla)	Serotonin-3 receptor	Serotonin	Serotonin antagonists: ondansetron (Zofran), granisetron (Kytril), dolasetron (Anzemet), palonosetron (Aloxi)
	Neurokinin-1 receptor	Substance P	Aprepitant (Emend)
	Dopamine receptor	Dopamine	Dopamine antagonists: metoclopramide (Reglan), droperidol (Inapsine)
Chemoreceptor trigger zone	Serotonin-3 receptor	Serotonin	Dopamine antagonists: metoclopramide (Reglan), droperidol (Inapsine)
	Neurokinin-1 receptor	Substance P	Aprepitant (Emend)
	Dopamine receptor	Dopamine	Dopamine antagonists: metoclopramide (Reglan), droperidol (Inapsine)
Gastrointestinal tract (sensory afferents)	Serotonin-3 receptor	Serotonin	Serotonin antagonists: ondansetron (Zofran), granisetron (Kytril), dolasetron (Anzemet), palonosetron (Aloxi)
Brain (higher cortical centers)	Benzodiazepine receptor	Gamma amino butyric acid	Benzodiazepine: lorazepam (Ativan)
Vestibular apparatus and nucleus tractus solitarius	Histamine receptor	Histamine	Anticholinergics: promethazine (Phenergan), hydroxyzine (Vistaril, Atarax)
Cerebral cortex and pons	Muscarinic cholinergic receptor	Acetylcholine	Scopolamine (Transderm Scop)

Question

What is an appropriate intervention for the rehabilitation therapist to make regarding A.S.'s pain medication?

Answer

The symptoms of nausea and vomiting A.S. described are frequent side effects of narcotic pain medication. Other frequent side effects of pain medication include dizziness, drowsiness, syncope, general weakness, hypotension, malaise, and constipation. The rehabilitation therapist notified A.S.'s orthopedic surgeon of the side effects that A.S. was experiencing. The surgeon prescribed promethazine 25 mg (Phenergan) tablets. Promethazine (Phenergan) is an antiemetic used to reduce nausea. The pharmacist instructed A.S. to take 1 promethazine (Phenergan) tablet with each oxycodone–acetaminophen (Percocet) dose for the next 2 wk. A.S.'s pain is now well controlled (achieving a pain level of ≤4 on a scale of 1-10) and she no longer experiences nausea or vomiting. Both the rehabilitation therapist and pharmacist told A.S. to watch for signs of constipation and sedation which, are common side effects of both oxycodone–acetaminophen (Percocet) and promethazine, and to avoid driving and drinking alcoholic beverages when taking these medications. The pharmacist recommended using a laxative with stool-softening and stimulant action such as senna–docusate (Senokot-S) to prevent opiate-induced constipation.

Chemotherapy-Induced Nausea and Vomiting

Treating nausea and vomiting in the oncology patient receiving chemotherapy or radiation therapy can be especially challenging. Nausea and vomiting in these patients are mediated by different mechanisms and usually require aggressive multidrug regimens to be given before and after treatment. Nausea and vomiting are usually classified as acute, delayed, anticipatory, breakthrough, or refractory. Acute nausea and vomiting are experienced at the time of chemotherapy administration, whereas delayed nausea and vomiting occur several hours or days after chemotherapy administration. Anticipatory nausea and vomiting occur before the chemotherapy dose as the patient anticipates the nausea and vomiting that occurred with a previous cycle of chemotherapy. Breakthrough nausea and vomiting occur when a patient has nausea and vomiting despite preventative measures. Breakthrough nausea and vomiting are treated with rescue antiemetic agents. Refractory nausea and vomiting do not respond to antiemetics and can occur with highly emetogenic chemotherapy (Bubalo, 2009).

Medication Therapy for Chemotherapy-Induced Nausea and Vomiting

It is now standard practice for patients receiving chemotherapy to receive aggressive and preventative combinations of antiemetics with the goal of preventing nausea and vomiting. Table 24.2 summarizes common antiemetic regimens used before and after chemotherapy administration. Anticipatory nausea and vomiting are usually treated with administration of a benzodiazepine before chemotherapy. A combination of antiemetics, that can include a serotonin receptor antagonist such as ondansetron (Zofran), a steroid medication such as dexamethasone (Decadron), and aprepitant (Emend), is administered before the chemotherapy dose to prevent acute and delayed nausea and vomiting with highly emetogenic regimens. Table 24.3 outlines the approach for managing nausea and vomiting based on the emetogenic potential of the chemotherapy regimen (Bubalo, 2009).

 See table 24.2 in the web resource for a full list of medication-specific indications, dosing recommendations, and side effects.

Table 24.2   Medications Used to Treat Nausea and Vomiting

Medication	Side effects affecting rehab							Other side effects and considerations
Substance P inhibitor: Highly effective in preventing acute and delayed nausea and vomiting with highly emetogenic chemotherapy when combined with serotonin antagonist and dexamethasone (Decadron).								
Aprepitant (Emend—oral; Fosaprepitant—IV)	Cog ++	S ++	A 0	Motor ++	D +	Com ++	F ++	Side effects: Fatigue (≤18%), nausea (≤13%), weakness (≤18%), hiccups (11%). Drug interactions: Emend induces CYP2C9; decreases warfarin (Coumadin) by 34% with a 14% decrease in INR and anticoagulant effects and decreases levels of dexamethasone (Decadron) and methylprednisolone (CYP3A4 substrates) by 50%. Decreases effectiveness of ethinyl estradiol and norgestimate contraceptives. Grapefruit juice (CYP3A4 inhibitor) can increase Emend levels. High-cost therapy.

Medication	Side effects affecting rehab							Other side effects and considerations
Serotonin receptor antagonists: Highly effective in treating nausea and vomiting associated with chemotherapy and upper-abdominal irradiation and other causes of nausea and vomiting.								
Ondansetron (Zofran)	Cog +	S +	A 0	Motor ++	D +	Com +	F ++	Side effects: Constipation, insomnia, diarrhea, dizziness, headache, arrhythmia with QT prolongation, dystonia, EPS arthralgias, depression. Drug interactions: Can increase QT prolongation and arrhythmias when combined with other agents that prolong the QT such as antiarrhythmics, tricyclic antidepressants, thioridazine (Mellaril), mesoridazine (Serentil), ziprasidone (Geodon), anesthetics, and medications that cause loss of potassium or magnesium.
Granisetron (Kytril)	Cog +	S +	A 0	Motor ++	D +	Com +	F ++	
Dolasetron (Anzemet)	Cog +	S +	A 0	Motor ++	D +	Com +	F ++	
Palonosetron (Aloxi)	Cog +	S +	A 0	Motor ++	D +	Com +	F ++	
Benzodiazepines: Provide effective preventative therapy for anticipatory nausea and vomiting.								
Lorazepam (Ativan)	Cog +++	S +++	A 0	Motor ++	D ++	Com ++	F ++	Side effects: Sedation, confusion, hypotension, ataxia, dysphagia, dry mouth. Drug interactions: Enhanced sedative effects when used with some antidepressants, antiepileptic drugs (e.g., phenobarbital, phenytoin, carbamazepine), sedative antihistamines, opiates, antipsychotics, or alcohol.
Alprazolam (Xanax)	Cog +	S +	A 0	Motor ++	D 0/+	Com +	F +	
Glucocorticoids: Steroids are used in combination with a serotonin antagonist before each dose of chemotherapy. May be useful in treating delayed and refractory nausea and vomiting; also used to treat nausea in patients with disseminated cancer by suppressing inflammation and prostaglandin production caused by tumor encroachment.								
Dexamethasone (Decadron) Prednisone	Cog +	S 0	A +	Motor +	D +	Com +	F +	Side effects: Personality changes, insomnia, euphoria, muscle weakness or wasting, thinning of the skin, glaucoma, hyperglycemia, cataracts, depressed immune function, lipodystrophy (moon facies, truncal obesity). Avoid abrupt discontinuation of long-term or high-dose oral therapy to avoid severe depression and acute adrenal insufficiency. Drug interactions: Can antagonize glycemic control of antidiabetic agents.
Cannabinoid: Derivative of marijuana used to treat nausea in cancer patients in which other agents have failed. It is most effective in patients with previous positive experiences with marijuana.								
Dronabinol (Marinol)	Cog ++	S ++	A 0	Motor ++	D +	Com ++	F ++	Side effects: Sedation, confusion, hypotension, ataxia, dry mouth. Drug interactions: Enhanced sedative effects when used with other central nervous system depressants or alcohol.
Dopamine antagonists antiemetic: Used as a rescue antiemetic in chemotherapy patients. Used to treat postoperative and other causes of nausea and vomiting. Metoclopramide (Reglan) has additional prokinetic activity associated with effects on muscarinic receptors.								
Metoclopramide (Reglan)	Cog +++	S +++	A ++	Motor +++	D +	Com +++	F +++	Common side effects: Restlessness, drowsiness, dizziness, lassitude, dystonia. Infrequent side effects: Headache, extrapyramidal effects such as **oculogyric** crisis, hypotension, hypertension, hyperprolactinemia leading to galactorrhea, constipation, depression.

› continued

Table 24.2 › *continued*

Medication	Side effects affecting rehab	Other side effects and considerations
Metoclo-pramide (Reglan) *(continued)*		Drug interactions: Additive sedation with other central nervous system depressants. Antagonizes dopamine-enhancer therapy used in treatment of Parkinson's disease.

Phenothiazine antiemetics: Phenothiazine agents that are dopamine antagonists; used as rescue antiemetics in chemotherapy patients. Useful in treating postoperative nausea and vomiting, motion sickness, and other causes of nausea and vomiting due to additional effects on the muscarinic receptors.

Medication	Side effects affecting rehab	Other side effects and considerations
Promethazine (Phenergan)	Cog S A Motor D Com F +++ +++ ++ +++ ++ +++ +++	Side effects: Strong sedative and anti-cholinergic effects, dry mouth and throat, increased heart rate, pupil dilation, urinary retention, constipation.
Prochlorpera-zine (Compazine)	Cog S A Motor D Com F +++ +++ ++ +++ ++ +++ +++	At high doses: Hallucinations or delirium, motor impairment (ataxia as well as extra-pyramidal side effects), flushed skin, blurred vision, abnormal sensitivity to bright light (photophobia), difficulty concentrating, short-term memory loss, visual disturbances, irregular breathing, dizziness, irritability, itchy skin, confusion, decreased body temperature (generally in the hands or feet), erectile dysfunction, excitability. Drug interactions: Additive sedation when used with other central nervous system depressants. Antagonizes dopamine-enhancer therapy used in treatment of Parkinson's disease.

Histamine-1 receptor antagonist (antihistamine) antiemetics: Used as rescue antiemetics and to treat delayed nausea and vomiting associated with chemotherapy. Useful in treating postoperative nausea and vomiting, motion sickness, and other causes of nausea and vomiting due to additional effects on the muscarinic receptors.

Medication	Side effects affecting rehab	Other side effects and considerations
Hydroxyzine (Vistaril)	Cog S A Motor D Com F ++ ++ + ++ ++ ++ ++	Side effects: Strong sedative and anti-cholinergic effects, dry mouth and throat, increased heart rate, pupil dilation, urinary retention, constipation.
Diphenhydr-amine (Benadryl)	Cog S A Motor D Com F +++ +++ + +++ +++ +++ +++	At high doses: Hallucinations or delirium, motor impairment (ataxia), flushed skin, blurred vision, abnormal sensitivity to bright light (photophobia), difficulty concentrating, short-term memory loss, visual disturbances, irregular breathing, dizziness, irritability, itchy skin, confusion, decreased body temperature (generally in the hands or feet), erectile dysfunction, excitability.
Meclizine (Antivert)	Cog S A Motor D Com F ++ ++ + ++ ++ ++ ++	Drug interactions: Additive sedation when used with other central nervous system depressants.
Scopolamine (Hyoscine, Transderm Scop patch)	Cog S A Motor D Com F ++ ++ + ++ ++ ++ ++	Antagonizes dopamine-enhancer therapy used in treatment of Parkinson's disease.

Cog = cognition; S = sedation; A = agitation or mania; Motor = discoordination; D = dysphagia; Com = communication; F = falls; IV = intravenous; INT = international normalized ratio; EPS = extrapyramidal symptoms.

The likelihood rating scale for encountering the side effects is as follows: 0 = Almost no probability of encountering side effects. 0/+ = Slightly higher probability of encountering side effects. + = Little likelihood of encountering side effects. +/++ = Low probability of encountering side effects; however, probability increases with increased dosage. ++ = Medium likelihood of encountering side effects. +++ = High likelihood of encountering side effects, particularly with high doses. ++++ = Highest likelihood of encountering side effects; best to avoid in at-risk patients.

Table 24.3   Antiemetic Regimens Based on Emetogenic Risk of Chemotherapy Regimen

Expected emesis	Prechemotherapy regimens	Postchemotherapy regimens
Mild emesis caused by chemotherapy	Prochlorperazine (Compazine) 10-25 mg by mouth, 5-25 mg IV, or 25 mg rectally (PR) before chemotherapy.	10-25 mg by mouth every 4-6 h as needed.
	Ondansetron (Zofran) 8 mg by mouth twice/day; first dose 30 min before chemotherapy.	8 mg 8 h after chemotherapy.
	Ondansetron (Zofran) 32 mg IV 30 min before chemotherapy.	None.
	Dexamethasone (Decadron) 4-8 mg by mouth or 10-20 mg IV.	Repeat every 4-6 h as needed.
	Prochlorperazine (Compazine) plus dexamethasone (Decadron) in doses listed previously.	Prochlorperazine (Compazine) 10-25 mg by mouth every 4-6 h as needed plus dexamethasone (Decadron) 4 mg by mouth every 6 h for total of 4 doses as needed.
	Metoclopramide (Reglan) 20-40 mg by mouth or IV and diphenhydramine (Benadryl) 25-50 mg by mouth or IV every 4-6 h as needed.	
Moderate emesis caused by chemotherapy	Ondansetron (Zofran) 32 mg IV and dexamethasone (Decadron) 4-8 mg by mouth or 10-20 mg IV 30 min before chemotherapy.	Ondansetron (Zofran) 16 mg by mouth and dexamethasone (Decadron) 8 mg by mouth each morning on days 2 and 3 plus prochlorperazine (Compazine) 10 mg by mouth every 6 h as needed.
	Aprepitant (Emend) 125 mg by mouth 60 min before chemotherapy plus dexamethasone (Decadron) 12 mg by mouth and ondansetron (Zofran) 32 mg IV 30 min before chemotherapy.	See regimens for breakthrough nausea and vomiting.
	Dexamethasone (Decadron) 4-8 mg by mouth or 10-20 mg IV 1 dose plus lorazepam (Ativan) 1.5 mg/m^2 and prochlorperazine (Compazine) 5-25 mg by mouth or IV 30 min before chemotherapy.	See regimens for breakthrough nausea and vomiting.
Severe emesis caused by chemotherapy	Ondansetron (Zofran) 32 mg IV and dexamethasone (Decadron) 10-20 mg IV plus lorazepam (Ativan) 1 mg by mouth or IV 30 min before chemotherapy.	Ondansetron (Zofran) 16 mg by mouth and dexamethasone (Decadron) 8 mg by mouth each morning on days 2 and 3 plus prochlorperazine (Compazine) 10 mg by mouth every 6 h as needed.
	Aprepitant (Emend) 125 mg by mouth 60 mins before chemotherapy on day 1 plus dexamethasone (Decadron) 12 mg by mouth and ondansetron (Zofran) 32 mg IV 30 min before chemotherapy.	Aprepitant (Emend) 80 mg by mouth on days 2 and 3.
	Metoclopramide (Reglan) 2-3 mg/kg IV, dexamethasone (Decadron) 10-20 mg IV, and diphenhydramine (Benadryl) 25-50 mg IV 60 min before chemotherapy and orally at same doses 30 min before chemotherapy.	Metoclopramide (Reglan) 20-40 mg by mouth and dexamethasone (Decadron) 8 mg by mouth in the morning on days 2 and 3 plus prochlorperazine (Compazine) 10 mg by mouth every 6 h as needed.
	Palonosetron (Aloxi) 0.25 mg IV 30 min before chemotherapy, aprepitant (Emend) 125 mg by mouth 60 min before chemotherapy on day 1, and dexamethasone (Decadron) 12 mg by mouth 30 min before chemotherapy.	Aprepitant (Emend) 80 mg by mouth on days 2 and 3 plus dexamethasone (Decadron) 8 mg by mouth on days 2 and 3.

› continued

Table 24.3 › *continued*

Expected emesis	Prechemotherapy regimens	Postchemotherapy regimens
Anticipatory nausea and vomiting	Lorazepam (Ativan) 0.5-2 mg by mouth 60 min before or IV 10 min before chemotherapy; repeat every 6 h as needed.	
	Alprazolam (Xanax) 0.25-0.5 mg 60 min before chemotherapy; repeat every 6 h as needed.	
Breakthrough nausea and vomiting	Metoclopramide (Reglan) 40 mg by mouth every 4-6 h and dexamethasone (Decadron) 4-8 mg every 4-6 h for 4 days.	
	Aprepitant (Emend) 80 mg by mouth and dexamethasone (Decadron) 8-12 mg by mouth once/day on days 2 and 3.	
	Aprepitant (Emend) 80 mg by mouth/day, dexamethasone (Decadron) 8-12 mg by mouth/day, and ondansetron (Zofran) 8 mg by mouth twice/day on days 2 and 3.	
	Metoclopramide (Reglan) 20-40 mg by mouth and diphenhydramine 50 mg by mouth every 3-4 h.	
	Dronabinol (Marinol) 5-10 mg by mouth every 4-6 h.	
	Prochlorperazine (Compazine) 25 mg rectally every 12 h.	

IV = intravenous.

Postoperative Nausea and Vomiting

Postoperative nausea and vomiting are associated with administration of opioids, nitrous oxide, and volatile anesthetics during surgery. Risk is increased with administration of high-dose anticholinesterase medications (e.g., neostigmine, edrophonium) postoperatively to reverse neuromuscular blockade. Measures for reducing postoperative nausea and vomiting include using prophylactic antiemetics and minimizing the administration of agents that increase emetic risk (Kloth, 2009). Pediatric patients have a higher incidence of postoperative nausea and vomiting, especially with strabismus surgery.

The antiemetic therapy regimen used depends on the type of surgery and the associated risk for nausea and vomiting. Patients undergoing surgeries that are associated with a low risk of emesis (i.e., emesis seen in <10% of patients) do not require prophylaxis, and postoperative nausea and vomiting can usually be controlled with rescue antiemetic therapy with a serotonin antagonist such as ondansetron (Zofran) 2 mg or dolasetron (Anzemet) 12.5 mg. Patients undergoing surgeries that cause nausea and vomiting 10% to 30% of the time should receive prophylactic dosing of intravenous droperidol 0.625 to 1.25 mg plus glucocorticoid therapy such as dexametha-

sone (Decadron) 4 to 8 mg and receive rescue therapy with a serotonin antagonist as needed after the procedure. Patients undergoing procedures that cause nausea and vomiting 30% to 60% of the time should receive preventative doses of droperidol (Inapsine) 0.625 to 1.25 mg plus a steroid plus a serotonin antagonist such as ondansetron (Zofran) 4 to 8 mg or aprepitant (Emend) and receive a serotonin antagonist after the procedure. Patients undergoing surgeries that cause nausea and vomiting more than 60% of the time should receive preventative propofol (Diprivan) 20 to 30 mg, plus droperidol (Inapsine) 0.625 to 1.25 mg, plus a glucocorticoid such as dexamethasone (Decadron), plus a serotonin antagonist such as ondansetron (Zofran) 4 to 8 mg or aprepitant (Emend) preoperatively; and postoperatively should receive rescue therapy with dopamine antagonist antiemetics such as the phenothiazine antiemetics or metoclopramide (Reglan) (Eng & White, 2007).

Constipation

Constipation may frequently affect patients undergoing rehabilitation. Constipation is defined as having one or more of the following symptoms: hard stools, infrequent stools, excessive straining with defecation, a sense of incomplete evacuation, or excessive time spent on the toilet with unsuccessful defecation.

Chronic constipation can reduce appetite and energy and can interfere with physical, social, and psychological function. Constipation can cause reduced food intake and compromise the nutritional status of the patient. Straining associated with attempting to have a bowel movement can result in transient cardiac ischemia, arrhythmia, and even myocardial infarction. Chronic constipation can lead to hemorrhoids, rectal fissures, rectal prolapse, fecal impaction, reduced blood supply to the colon, and even perforation of the bowel. Fecal impaction is usually associated with nausea, vomiting, and abdominal pain, and treatment may require hospitalization or surgery. When assessing the patient, the rehabilitation therapist should ask the patient about symptoms and frequency of constipation and timing of bowel movements. Constipation should be prevented and managed with a patient-specific bowel regimen that includes diet, exercise, fluid intake, and laxative use to maintain regular, formed stools that are achieved every 1 to 2 days without straining. Scheduling rehabilitation sessions for times that are less likely to interfere with bowel movements and scheduling sessions with consideration to the timing of patient meals can help enhance patient participation in the therapy session.

The Rome III criteria defines chronic constipation as having fewer than 3 bowel movements/wk and at having least 2 of the following occur during at least 25% of bowel movements: straining, lumpy or hard stools, sensation of incomplete evacuation, sensation of anorectal blockage or obstruction, and manual maneuvers that facilitate defecation (e.g., digital evacuation, use of the pelvic floor). The Bristol Stool Form Scale helps describe the stool. Descriptions range from type 1 (separate hard lumps that are associated with slow gut transit) to type 7 (watery stools with no solid pieces that are associated with rapid gut transit) (Cash, 2007).

Constipation is a common condition. Approximately 12% of the world's population suffers from constipation. The frequency of constipation varies in different parts of the world. Constipation occurs twice as often in individuals in the Americas and Pacific Asia as it does in individuals in Europe (17.3% vs. 8.75%) (Wald et al., 2006). In the United States, constipation affects 63 million Americans. Females suffer from constipation twice as often males. Americans spend $800 million/yr on over-the-counter laxatives, and constipation is responsible for 2.5 million physician office visits annually. People who are more prone to chronic constipation include those who are not Caucasian, those with lower incomes, those with lower levels of education, older people, people who are depressed, and those under psychological stress (Cash, 2007).

Etiology and Pathophysiology

Primary idiopathic constipation can be categorized as normal-transit constipation, slow-transit constipation, or constipation associated with defecatory disorders. Patients with normal-transit constipation complain of hard stools and difficulty evacuating stools. They may also have reduced rectal sensation, increased rectal compliance, or pelvic floor dysfunction. Slow-transit constipation is associated with colonic inertia and is most common in young women who have an infrequent urge to defecate, decreased stool frequency, bloating, and abdominal discomfort. Sleep, meals, and physical and emotional stressors can affect colonic transit time. Pelvic floor dyssynergia involves anal spasm during attempted defecation. Patients with this type of constipation have hard stools, impaction, feelings of blockage, and severe straining with defecation and require digital evacuation (Cash, 2007). Secondary causes of constipation can include medication-induced constipation; metabolic disorders such as hypothyroidism, diabetes, hypercalcemia, hypomagnesemia, and hypokalemia; neurologic disorders such as Parkinson's disease, multiple sclerosis, and muscular dystrophy; and psychiatric disorders.

Changes in the diet, adequate hydration, and addition of bulk in the form of fruits, vegetables, and whole grains may help prevent and alleviate constipation. The addition of prunes or prune juice is effective in many patients. The initial step in treating constipation should be making corrective changes in the diet or fluid intake and incorporating daily exercise rather than adding medication to the patient's regimen. Decreased fluid intake is associated with constipation in patients who are elderly, confused, or in long-term care. Making fluids accessible throughout the day for these patients and patients with limited mobility can help these patients maintain hydration and prevent constipation. Poor mobility is also associated with constipation. Regular exercise can improve symptoms of constipation in the patient with limited mobility (Carl & Johnson, 2006; Cassagnol et al., 2010).

The use of opioid pain medications or medications with anticholinergic effects (e.g., antiemetics, antihistamines, antidepressants, antipsychotics, bladder-control products) can cause constipation. Other medications that can cause constipation include calcium-containing antacids, iron supplements, antispasmodics, anticonvulsants, medications used to treat Parkinson's disease, calcium channel blockers, diuretics, and vinca alkaloid chemotherapy. Constipation may be reduced by reducing the dose of these agents or using a similar agent with less anticholinergic effects. For patients on chronic opioid pain medications, a scheduled bowel regimen is essential for preventing severe constipation and bowel obstruction. This bowel regimen should comprise adequate hydration and dietary fiber, a stool softener, and a stimulant laxative in doses adequate to maintain a bowel movement at least every 2 days (Carl & Johnson, 2006; Cassagnol et al., 2010).

Medication Therapy

Many types of laxatives are available. Laxatives can increase the frequency of bowel movements by increasing the bulk of the stools; increasing the osmotic gradient in the bowel and drawing water into the colonic **lumen**, resulting in increased motility and bowel transit time; acting as a surfactant, thus softening the feces; and stimulating propulsion of the feces by directly irritating the bowel (Carl & Johnson, 2006; Cash, 2007; Cassagnol et al., 2010; Wallace & Sharkey, 2011).

Methylnaltrexone (Relistor) is a new injectable opioid antagonist that reduces opioid-associated constipation in patients on long-term opioids for palliative care. The chemical structure of methylnaltrexone is similar to that of naltrexone (ReVia) and differs only by the addition of a methyl group that prevents the medication from crossing the blood–brain barrier. Therefore, opioid antagonism is limited to the mu receptors in the GI tract. This medication reverses opioid-induced constipation without reversing the centrally mediated opioid induced analgesia (Kraft, 2007). Table 24.4 summarizes the types of laxatives available (Carl & Johnson, 2006; Cash, 2007; Wallace & Sharkey, 2011).

Irritable Bowel Syndrome

The rehabilitation therapist will at some time provide care for patients with irritable bowel syndrome (IBS), and should be aware of the effect of medication use on these patients during rehabilitation sessions and of methods for minimizing symptoms during these sessions. IBS is characterized by symptoms associated with visceral hypersensitivity and hyperalgesia. Symptoms include chronic or intermittent abdominal discomfort accompanied by changes in stool consistency or frequency. IBS can cause reduced food intake and compromise the nutritional status of the patient. Symptoms of IBS can interfere with the patient's ability to participate in the rehabilitative session and can reduce appetite and energy, thus interfering with physical, social, and psychological function. When assessing the patient, the rehabilitation therapist should ask the patient about timing of symptoms. Scheduling rehabilitation sessions for periods that are less likely to be associated with bowel symptoms and scheduling sessions with consideration to the timing of patient meals can contribute to successful patient participation in therapy sessions.

IBS is classified as constipation predominant, diarrhea predominant, or pain predominant depending on the symptoms that predominate in the individual patient. Psychosocial disturbances such as anxiety, depression, panic disorder, inability to cope, and sleep disorders are also associated with IBS. The Rome III diagnostic criteria define IBS as having symptoms for at least 6 mo as well as having discomfort at least 3 days/mo for the past 3 mo. Other

See table 24.4 in the web resource for a full list of medication-specific indications, onset of action, side effects, and drug interactions and precautions.

Table 24.4 Medications Used to Treat Constipation

Medication	Side effects affecting rehab	Other side effects and considerations
Bulk-forming laxatives: Used on routine basis to prevent constipation by absorbing water from the bowel lumen to increase stool bulk. Onset of effects is up to 3 days.		
Bran: Psyllium preparations (Metamucil) Methylcellulose (Citrucel) Calcium polycarbophil (Fibercon)	Cog S A Motor D Com F 0 0 0 0 + 0 0	Side effects: Bloating, gas, stomach pain. These products absorb water from the bowel lumen to increase bulk and should be taken with adequate fluid to prevent impaction and bowel obstruction. Contraindicated in patients with bowel obstruction, megacolon, and **megarectum**. May be used chronically.
Hyperosmotic laxative: Onset of effects is 0.5-3 h.		
Lactulose (Chronulac)	Cog S A Motor D Com F 0 0 0 + ++ 0 +	May be used on chronic basis in patients with liver disease. Side effects: Flatulence, intestinal cramps. Chronic use can result in fluid and electrolyte imbalances and dehydration. Drug interactions: Do not use concurrently with antacids, which can change the pH of the bowel and decrease effectiveness.
Polyethylene glycol (Golytely, Colyte, Miralax)	Cog S A Motor D Com F 0 0 0 + ++ 0 +	Golytely or Colyte not for chronic use. Side effects: Flatulence, intestinal cramps. May cause fluid and electrolyte disorders.
Saline osmotic laxatives: Contain electrolytes (e.g., sodium, phosphorus, or magnesium) that draw water into the bowel's lumen, increasing bowel motility and stool transit time. Onset of effects is 0.5-6 h.		
Citrate of magnesia Milk of magnesia Fleet's phospho soda	Cog S A Motor D Com F 0 0 0 + ++ 0 +	For short-term use only. Side effects: Chronic use can result in fluid and electrolyte imbalances and dehydration. Contraindications: Patients with kidney or heart disease.

> *continued*

Table 24.4 › *continued*

Medication	Side effects affecting rehab							Other side effects and considerations
Stimulant laxatives: Used on as-needed basis in most patients; may be used routinely to prevent constipation in patients taking chronic opioids. Directly stimulates enteric neurons and muscle to promote inflammation and accumulation of water and electrolytes to promote gastrointestinal motility. Onset of effects is 6-8 h for bisacodyl and 6-12 h for products containing senna.								
Bisacodyl (Dulcolax, Modane, Correctol) Senna (Senokot)	Cog 0	S 0	A 0	Motor +	D ++	Com 0	F +	Side effects: Chronic use may result in cathartic colon, fluid and electrolyte imbalances, and dehydration. Precautions: Dulcolax and Correctol are enteric coated to prevent irritation of the stomach mucosa and should not be crushed or chewed.
Stimulant products no longer recommended for routine use								
Cascara Castor oil Phenolphthalein	Stimulant agents with toxic effects on the intestinal epithelium and enteric neurons are no longer recommended for routine use. The phenolphthalein products were discontinued in the United States due to concerns about carcinogenicity.							
Stool softeners (wetting agents): Used on as-needed or chronic basis to prevent constipation. Coat the stool and lower the surface tension of the stool to allow mixing of water and fatty deposits, softening the stool to ease defecation; stimulate secretion of intestinal fluid and electrolytes, altering intestinal wall permeability. Onset of effects is 1-3 days.								
Docusate sodium (Colace) Docusate calcium (Surfak)	Cog 0	S 0	A 0	Motor +	D +	Com 0	F +	Side effects: Flatulence, intestinal cramps.
Emollient: Coats stool to assist with passage. Onset of effects is 1-3 days.								
Mineral oil	Cog 0	S 0	A 0	Motor +	D +	Com 0	F +	No longer recommended; interferes with absorption of fat-soluble vitamins. Can cause rectal leakage and, if aspirated, can cause pneumonitis.
Enemas: Administered fluid stimulates an evacuation reflex, distending the bowels. Onset of effects is 1-3 h.								
Saline Tap water Sodium phosphate (Fleet's enema)	Cog +	S 0	A 0	Motor ++	D +	Com 0	F ++	Saline enemas are associated with the least number of complications. Repeated tap-water enemas can cause hyponatremia, and repeated sodium phosphate (Fleet's) enemas can cause hypocalcemia. Monitor for dehydration, electrolyte disturbances, and abdominal cramps.
Opioid antagonist: Used to treat constipation associated with palliative opioid therapy. Onset of effects is 24 h.								
Methylnaltrexone (Relistor)	Cog +	S 0	A 0	Motor +	D ++	Com +	F ++	Side effects: Abdominal cramps (30%), flatulence (40%), fever, dizziness, diarrhea, nausea.

Cog = cognition; S = sedation; A = agitation or mania; Motor = discoordination; D = dysphagia; Com = communication; F = falls.

The likelihood rating scale for encountering the side effects is as follows: 0 = Almost no probability of encountering side effects. 0/+ = Slightly higher probability of encountering side effects. + = Little likelihood of encountering side effects. +/++ = Low probability of encountering side effects; however, probability increases with increased dosage. ++ = Medium likelihood of encountering side effects. +++ = High likelihood of encountering side effects, particularly with high doses. ++++ = Highest likelihood of encountering side effects; best to avoid in at-risk patients.

symptoms include straining on defecation, urgency of defecation, feeling of incomplete bowel movements, and presence of mucus in the stools. The treatment of IBS includes relieving predominant symptoms and modifying factors that contribute to symptoms (Bernardi, 2007; Peura, 2007).

Incidence

The global incidence of IBS is approximately 11%. Prevalence varies extensively among countries and ranges from a high of 30% in Nigeria to a low of 3.5% in Iran (Hungin et al., 2003). IBS affects about 10% of Americans.

Etiology and Pathophysiology

Although the pathogenesis of IBS is multifactorial and is not completely understood, researchers believe that inflammation and infection are important in the etiology of the disease. The complex interplay between the gut lumen, gut mucosa, enteric nervous system (ENS), and central nervous system (CNS; termed the brain–gut axis) can lead to alterations in gut sensation, gut motility, and immune function. Serotonin, an important neurotransmitter in the enteric nervous system, modulates GI motility. Serotonin deficiency, which can be caused by medications that block serotonin, is associated with constipation. On the other hand, serotonin excess, which can be caused by medications that increase serotonin levels, can lead to diarrhea. Psychosocial disturbances such as anxiety, depression, panic disorder, inability to cope, and sleep disorders are also associated with IBS (Bernardi, 2007; Carl & Johnson, 2006; Wallace & Sharkey, 2011).

Nonpharmacologic Therapy

In addition to medication therapy, symptoms of IBS may be improved with alterations in diet, and by instituting a regular exercise regimen as well as psychological therapies. Therapy should be individualized. Patients with fructose malabsorption may benefit with dietary restriction of fructose. Some patients show a reduction in symptoms with a low carbohydrate diet, where others benefit from following a gluten free diet. Lactose intolerance should always be ruled out in patients with IBS. Avoiding lactose in lactose intolerant patients can improve symptoms. Slow increases in dietary fiber may also improve symptoms. Because symptoms may be triggered by stress or concurrent psychiatric symptoms, initiation of psychological therapy including cognitive behavioral therapy, hypnotic therapy, medication treatment of the psychiatric illness, and relaxation techniques may help (Wallace & Sharkey, 2011).

Medication Therapy

Alosetron (Lotronex) is a serotonin-3 receptor antagonist that slows colonic conduction, increases fluid absorption, and improves left colon compliance. It is available under a U.S. Food and Drug Administration Risk Evaluation Mitigation Strategy (REMS) monitoring program for use in patients with diarrhea-predominant IBS who do not respond to standard therapies. Lubiprostone (Amitiza), part of a new class of agents used in IBS, is a fatty acid that activates the chloride-C2 channels in the GI cell wall membrane. The chloride-C2 channels cause intestinal fluid secretion, thus increasing the contents in the colon and enhancing GI motility. Because most of the colonic fluid is reabsorbed, the use of this agent does not lead to fluid or electrolyte losses. Antispasmodic medications and low-dose tricyclic antidepressants can be used to help relieve pain and psychiatric symptoms in patients with pain-predominant IBS. Table 24.5 summarizes medications used to treat IBS (Wallace & Sharkey, 2011).

Evidence shows that intestinal microflora in patients with IBS differs from that found in healthy individuals and that the use of probiotics can help control symptoms. Probiotics are living microorganisms such as the lactic acid-producing bacteria *Bifidobacterium* or *Lactobacillus* found in the intestines of healthy individuals. *Saccharomyces boulardii,* which is a yeast, is also used in probiotic therapy. Probiotics reduce the pH of the intestine, decrease colonization and invasion by pathogenic organisms, and modify the host immune response. Probiotics, which are recommended for all types of IBS, can be added to dairy products as a culture or can be provided as a supplement in tablet, capsule, or powder formulations. Probiotics have been shown to be helpful in treating several GI

See table 24.5 in the web resource for a full list of therapy-specific indications, dosing, and side effects.

Table 24.5 Medications Used to Treat Irritable Bowel Syndrome

Therapy or medication	Side effects affecting rehab							Other side effects or considerations
Probiotic therapy: Used to treat constipation-predominant IBS, diarrhea-predominant IBS, and pain-predominant IBS.								
Bifidobacterium (Align) *Lactobacillus* (Culturelle, Acidophilus ES) *Saccharomyces* (Florastor)	Cog 0	S 0	A 0	Motor 0	D 0	Com 0	F 0	Precautions: Avoid in septic patients or in patients with compromised gastrointestinal integrity to avoid bacteremia. Drug interactions: Space probiotics at least 1-2 h from any antibiotic to avoid killing the bacteria provided in the probiotic supplement.
Nonpharmacologic interventions: Used to treat constipation-predominant IBS, diarrhea-predominant IBS, or pain-predominant IBS. See the nonpharmacologic treatment section of the text for a brief summary of these interventions.								
Dietary interventions: Used to treat diarrhea-predominant IBS.								
Replace fluids and electrolytes with oral rehydration products Rule out lactose intolerance	Cog 0	S 0	A 0	Motor 0	D 0	Com 0	F 0	Avoid caffeine, alcohol, gas-producing beverages such as carbonated drinks, fructose, glutens, artificial sweeteners, and herbals containing senna.
Serotonin antagonist: Used to treat diarrhea-predominant IBS.								
Alosetron (Lotronex)	Cog ++	S ++	A +	Motor ++	D ++	Com +	F ++	Side effects: Ischemic colitis, severe constipation, arrhythmia, fluid and electrolyte disturbances, cognitive disorders, tremors, confusion, sedation, malaise, fatigue, cramps. Prescription and use regulated by a Food and Drug Administration Risk Evaluation and Mitigation Strategy program (REMS).
Opioid agonists: Used to treat diarrhea-predominant IBS.								
Loperamide (Imodium)	Cog ++	S ++	A +	Motor +	D ++	Com +	F ++	Side effects: Blurred vision, constipation, decreased sweating, insomnia, dizziness, somnolence, headache, loss of taste, loss of appetite, xerostomia, nausea. Precautions: Limit to 8 tablets/day to prevent tolerance.
Diphenoxylate with atropine (Lomotil)	Cog ++	S ++	A +	Motor +	D ++	Com +	F ++	Side effects: Blurred vision, constipation, decreased sweating, insomnia, dizziness, somnolence, headache, loss of taste, loss of appetite, xerostomia, nausea. Precautions: Usual dose is 2 tablets, then 1 tablet every 4 h for no more than 48 h to prevent tolerance.

Therapy or medication	Side effects affecting rehab							Other side effects or considerations			
Laxatives: Used to treat constipation-predominant IBS.											
Dietary bran	Cog	S	A	Motor	D	Com	F	Side effects: Flatulence, intestinal cramps.			
Psyllium (Metamucil)	0	0	0	+	++	0	+	Chronic use of osmotic laxatives can result in fluid and electrolyte imbalances and dehydration.			
Osmotic laxatives such as milk of magnesia, lactulose, or polyethylene glycol								Precautions: Avoid lactulose due to bloating and cramping associated with its use which can worsen IBS symptoms.			
Calcium channel activator: Increases fluid secretion by the intestine; used to treat constipation-predominant IBS.											
Lubiprostone (Amitiza)	Cog	S	A	Motor	D	Com	F	Side effects: Nausea (up to 31%), diarrhea (up to 13%), headache (up to 13%).			
	0	0	0	+	++	0	+				
Antispasmodics: Used to treat pain-predominant IBS.											
Dicyclomine (Bentyl)	Cog	S	A	Motor	D	Com	F	Side effects: Strong sedative and anticholinergic effects, dry mouth and throat, increased heart rate, pupil dilation, urinary retention, constipation.			
	+++	+++	++	+++	+	+++	+++				
Hyoscyamine (Levsin)	Cog	S	A	Motor	D	Com	F	At high doses: Hallucinations or delirium, motor impairment (ataxia), flushed skin, blurred vision, abnormal sensitivity to bright light (photophobia), difficulty concentrating, short-term memory loss, visual disturbances, irregular breathing, dizziness, irritability, itchy skin, confusion, decreased body temperature (generally in the hands or feet), erectile dysfunction, excitability.			
	+++	+++	++	+++	+	+++	+++				
								Drug interactions: Additive sedation when used with other central nervous system depressants.			
								Antagonizes dopamine-enhancer therapy used in treatment of Parkinson's disease.			
Tricyclic antidepressants: Used to treat pain-predominant IBS.											
Amitriptyline (Elavil)	Cog	S	A	Motor	D	Com	F	Weight gain	Seizure	Cardiac	Sexual
	++++	++++	0	++	++++	++++	++++	+++	+++	++++	++
Desipramine (Norpramin)	Cog	S	A	Motor	D	Com	F	Weight gain	Seizure	Cardiac	Sexual
	++	++	+	++	++	++	++	+	++	++	++
								Can prolong QT interval and cause arrhythmia.			
Imipramine (Tofranil)	Cog	S	A	Motor	D	Com	F	Weight gain	Seizure	Cardiac	Sexual
	+++	+++	+	++	+++	+++	++++	+++	+++	+++	++
Nortriptyline (Pamelor, Aventyl)	Cog	S	A	Motor	D	Com	F	Weight gain	Seizure	Cardiac	Sexual
	++	++	0	++	++	++	+	+	++	++	++

Cog = cognition; S = sedation; A = agitation or mania; Motor = discoordination; D = dysphagia; Com = communication; F = falls; IBS = irritable bowel syndrome.

Sexual is associated with sexual dysfunction.

The likelihood rating scale for encountering the side effects is as follows: 0 = Almost no probability of encountering side effects. 0/+ = Slightly higher probability of encountering side effects. + = Little likelihood of encountering side effects. +/++ = Low probability of encountering side effects; however, probability increases with increased dosage. ++ = Medium likelihood of encountering side effects. +++ = High likelihood of encountering side effects, particularly with high doses. ++++ = Highest likelihood of encountering side effects; best to avoid in at-risk patients.

disorders, including acute diarrhea, antibiotic-associated diarrhea, *Clostridium difficile* infection, traveler's diarrhea, IBS, and inflammatory bowel disease. Probiotics are also helpful in the treatment of vaginal candidiasis. Side effects of probiotics include bloating and flatulence. Probiotic therapy should be used cautiously in patients who are critically ill or severely immunocompromised, in patients with severe acute pancreatitis, or in patients with central venous catheters because they may cause serious systemic infections in these patients. If a patient is taking an oral antibiotic, probiotics that produce lactic acid should be administered at least 2 h apart from the antibiotic to maintain the efficacy of the probiotic. If the patient is taking an oral antifungal, probiotics containing *Saccharomyces* should be administered at least 2 h apart from the antifungal to maintain the efficacy of the probiotic (Bernardi, 2007; Williams, 2010).

Inflammatory Bowel Disease

Inflammatory bowel disease (IBD) is associated with chronic inflammation of the lining of the GI tract. IBD can affect food intake and can be associated with malabsorption of nutrients, weight loss, malnutrition, weakness, and loss of muscle mass. IBD can reduce appetite and energy, thus interfering with physical, social, and psychological function. Psychosocial disturbances such as anxiety, depression, panic disorder, inability to cope, and sleep disorders are also associated with IBD. Symptoms of IBD can interfere with the patient's ability to complete activities of daily living, maintain an income, and participate in rehabilitation sessions.

IBD comes in two forms: ulcerative colitis (UC) and Crohn's disease (CD). UC is characterized by diffuse inflammation of the superficial mucosa of the rectum and large intestine. In UC, 95% of the cases involve the rectum. Patients with UC are at increased risk of developing colorectal cancer. CD can involve any area of the GI tract but most often involves the colon and small intestine. CD is transmural, meaning that it inflicts damage through each mucosal layer of the GI tract, and is characterized by periods of remission and periods of exacerbation. Immune activation is mediated by the cytokines interferon-gamma and tumor necrosis factor (TNF)-alpha. Increased mucosal levels of TNF-alpha increase production of acute phase reactants, and TNF-alpha promotes the formation of granulomas, the histological hallmark of CD. These granulomas comprise T-cells monocytes, and macrophages. Cytokines such as interferon-gamma regulate the recruitment of these cells to the inflamed tissue (Chan, 2007; Meek, 2002; Schlesselman, 2008).

Incidence

The incidence of CD is 29 to 199/100,000 people. CD affects about 630,000 individuals in the United States and Canada. CD, which is most often diagnosed in early adolescence or early adulthood, affects both sexes equally. Crohn's disease is more common in those individuals that have family members with the disease. It occurs more often in Caucasians and African Americans than in Asians or Hispanics. Identified risk factors include smoking, consumption of lactose or fructose, use of oral contraceptives, and receipt of measles vaccine (Chan, 2007; Schlesselman, 2008). UC most often occurs in persons living in the United Kingdom, Northern Europe, and the United States. UC affects 250,000 to 500,000 people in the United Kingdom and the United States. The economic burden associated with UC in the United States is estimated to be $8.1 billion to $14.9 billion/yr. Onset most frequently occurs between age 15 and 40 yr or between age 50 and 80 yr. The disease affects both sexes equally (Dike et al., 2010).

Etiology and Pathophysiology

Symptoms of CD include abdominal cramping, abdominal pain, anorexia, **cachexia**, diarrhea, **epigastric pain**, fatigue, fever, flu-like symptoms, joint pain, pallor, nausea, vomiting, rectal bleeding, and weight loss. Patients may also experience ocular, dermatologic, hepatic, and rheumatologic symptoms. Rare complications of the disease include toxic megacolon, perianal fistulas, intestinal obstruction, and hypercoagulopathy. Malabsorption of nutrients due to this disease may result in **osteomala-**

cia, osteoporosis, hypocalcemia, and pernicious anemia. The primary goal of treatment is to induce and maintain remission by reducing inflammation, correcting nutritional deficiencies, and managing symptoms.

Symptoms of UC include persistent bloody diarrhea, rectal urgency, and tenesmus. Diagnosis is made via colonoscopy or proctosigmoidoscopy along with biopsy. Biopsy confirms loss of vascular pattern, granularity, friability, and ulceration. Laboratory test results that support the diagnosis include elevated C-reactive protein and erythrocyte sedimentation rates, both of which indicate inflammation. Testing a stool sample is also recommended to rule out infectious causes of the symptoms. UC can be classified as mild, moderate, severe, or fulminant using the UC Activity Index. Patients with mild disease have fewer than 4 stools/day, which may or may not contain blood, no systemic symptoms, and a normal erythrocyte sedimentation rate. Patients with moderate disease have more than 4 stools/day without systemic symptoms. Patients with

severe disease have more than 6 bloody stools/day along with fever, tachycardia, anemia, and an elevated erythrocyte sedimentation rate (ESR). Fulminant disease is associated with more than 10 bloody stools/day, continuous bleeding that necessitates blood transfusions, abdominal distention with tenderness, and colonic distention on X-ray (Dike et al., 2010).

Medication Therapy

Medications used to treat CD or UC are chosen based on the location of the disease and the severity of symptoms. Traditional initial therapy includes aminosalicylates, immunosuppressants, and corticosteroids. Antidiarrheal medications such as loperamide and diphenoxylate–atropine and narcotics are often used to control symptoms and manage pain, and anti-inflammatory agents are used to reduce inflammation. Patients with IBS should receive vitamin and calcium supplements. Table 24.6 summarizes medications used to treat CD and UC (Chan, 2007; Schlesselman, 2008).

 See table 24.6 in the web resource for a full list of medication-specific indications, dosing recommendations, side effects, and other considerations.

Table 24.6 Medications Used to Treat Inflammatory Bowel Disease (Ulcerative Colitis and Crohn's Disease)

Medication	Side effects affecting rehab							Other side effects or considerations
Corticosteroids: Used to induce remission in ulcerative colitis or moderate to severe Crohn's disease.								
Rectal: Hydrocortisone (Cortenema)	Cog +	S 0	A +	Motor +	D +	Com 0	F +	40%-50% of patients become steroid dependent. Supplement daily with calcium (1000 mg/day; 1500 mg/day if >50 yr of age) and vitamin D (400-800 international units).
Rectal: Hydrocortisone (Cortifoam)								Bisphosphonates should be added for patients on steroids >3 mo.
Oral: Prednisone	Cog +	S 0	A +	Motor +	D +	Com 0	F +	Side effects (short-term): Acne, adrenal axis suppression, edema, increased appetite, weight gain, hypertension, mood changes.
Oral: Budesonide (Entocort)								Side effects (long-term): Cataracts, diabetes, muscle atrophy, bone demineralization.
Injectable: Methylprednisolone (Solu-Medrol)	Cog ++	S 0	A ++	Motor +	D +	Com 0	F +	

› continued

Table 24.6 › *continued*

Medication	Side effects affecting rehab							Other side effects or considerations
5-Aminosalicylic acid agents: Used as maintenance therapy in mild to moderate ulcerative colitis or Crohn's disease.								
Oral: Mesalamine (Asacol, Pentasa) Rectal: Mesalamine (Canasa, Rowasa)	Cog 0	S 0	A 0	Motor 0	D +++	Com 0	F 0	Onset is 6 wk-3 mo. Side effects: Asthenia, flu symptoms, abdominal pain, flatulence, arthralgias, lupus-like syndrome, hepatotoxicity, pancreatitis, gastrointestinal upset, bone marrow suppression, interstitial nephritis, interstitial pneumonitis. Monitor with baseline CBC, then repeat weekly for 1 mo, then recheck every 1-2 mo. Contraindications: G6PD deficiency.
Sulfasalazine (Azulfidine)	Cog 0	S 0	A 0	Motor 0	D +++	Com 0	F 0	Onset is 6 wk-3 mo. Side effects: Leukopenia, alopecia, stomatitis, elevated liver enzymes, yellow–orange skin discoloration, photosensitivity, nausea, vomiting, anorexia, rash, hypersensitivity reactions. Minimize nausea, vomiting, diarrhea, and anorexia with low-dose initiation and slow titration. Treat rash, urticaria, serum sickness-like reactions with antihistamines or steroids. Hypersensitivity reactions require discontinuance. Monitor with baseline CBC, then repeat weekly for 1 mo, then recheck every 1-2 mo.
Balsalazide (Colazal) Olsalazine (Dipentum)	Cog 0	S 0	A 0	Motor 0	D +++	Com 0	F 0	Onset is 6 wk-3 mo. Side effects: Asthenia, flu-like symptoms, abdominal pain, flatulence, arthralgias, lupus-like syndrome, hepatotoxicity, pancreatitis, gastrointestinal upset, bone marrow suppression, interstitial nephritis, interstitial pneumonitis. Monitor with baseline CBC, then repeat weekly for 1 mo, then recheck every 1-2 mo.
Immunomodulators: Used to maintain remission in Crohn's disease or ulcerative colitis.								
Azathioprine (Imuran)	Cog 0	S 0	A 0	Motor 0	D +++	Com 0	F 0	Onset is 3-6 mo. Side effects: Reversible dose-related bone marrow suppression (leukopenia, macrocytic anemia, pancytopenia, thrombocytopenia), gastrointestinal intolerance, stomatitis, infection, drug fever, hepatotoxicity, malignancies. Monitor with baseline CBC and AST; repeat every 2 wk for first 2 mo, then every 1-2 mo. Eliminated by kidneys; adjust dose for renal insufficiency. Reduce dose to 25% of original dose if given with allopurinol.

Medication	Side effects affecting rehab							Other side effects or considerations
6-mercaptopurine (Purinethol)	Cog	S	A	Motor	D	Com	F	Onset is 3-6 mo.
	0	0	0	0	++	0	0	Side effects: Bone marrow toxicity, hepato-toxicity, hyperuricemia, nausea, vomiting, anorexia, intestinal ulceration, pancreatitis, skin rash.
								Monitor with baseline CBC and AST; repeat every 2 wk for first 2 mo, then every 1-2 mo.
Methotrexate (Rheumatrex, Trexall)	Cog	S	A	Motor	D	Com	F	Supplement with folic acid.
	0	0	0	0	++	0	0	Onset is 6-8 wk.
								Considered the disease-modifying antirheumatic drug of choice for initiation. Benefits 25%-50% of patients who fail azathioprine or 6-mercaptopurine for maintenance of remission in Crohn's or ulcerative colitis.
								Side effects: Stomatitis (3%-10%), diarrhea, nausea, vomiting (up to 10%), thrombocytopenia (1%-3%), elevated liver function tests (up to 15%; require discontinuance if sustained at more than 2 times normal for > 1 mo), leukopenia (rare), pulmonary fibrosis (rare), pneumonitis (rare).
								Teratogenic.
								Monitor by baseline UA, CBC, and liver function tests (AST/ALT, bilirubin, albumin), and hepatitis B and C testing; repeat CBC, AST, and albumin every 1-2 mo.
Cyclosporine (Neoral, Sandimmune)	Cog	S	A	Motor	D	Com	F	Onset is 1-3 mo.
	0	0	0	+	+++	0	0	Reserved for use in inducing remission in patients with Crohn's disease or UC who fail more conventional therapies.
								Side effects: Hypertension (reversed on discontinuance), increased risk of infection, hyperglycemia, nephrotoxicity (reversed on discontinuance), tremor, gastrointestinal intolerances, hirsutism, gingival hyperplasia.
								Monitor serum creatinine and blood pressure at baseline and monthly.
								Metabolized by the liver (active metabolites) and excreted in the bile.
								Drug interactions: Anticonvulsants, ketoconazole, fluconazole, trimethoprim, erythromycin, verapamil, diltiazem, nonsteroidal anti-inflammatory drugs, or cyclophosphamide.

› continued

Table 24.6 › *continued*

Medication	Side effects affecting rehab							Other side effects or considerations

Antibiotics: Used to treat continued symptoms in combination with immunotherapy in mild to severe ulcerative colitis or Crohn's disease.

Medication	Cog	S	A	Motor	D	Com	F	Other side effects or considerations
Ciprofloxacin (Cipro)	++	0	++	++	++	+	++	Side effects: Drug fever, rash, headache, abdominal pain, pain in the feet and extremities, dizziness, insomnia, malaise, seizures, Achilles tendon rupture or tendinitis, increased risk of arrhythmia and cardiac arrest, taste perversion, abnormal dreams, changes in vision, confusion, behavior changes, hallucinations, speech disorders, arthralgias, myalgias, bone marrow suppression, dysphagia, glossitis, gastritis, nausea, vomiting, stomatitis, *Clostridium difficile* colitis, altered coordination and gait, exacerbation of myasthenia gravis, allergic reactions, liver dysfunction, tendon rupture, renal dysfunction, Stevens-Johnson reaction. Drug interactions: Avoid fluvoxamine (Luvox) and duloxetine (Cymbalta); increases antidepressant levels and can cause hypertensive crisis, hypotension, syncope, and serotonin syndrome. Increases effects of warfarin (Coumadin). Decreased absorption when taken with aluminum, magnesium, calcium-containing antacids, or iron or zinc supplements. Increases caffeine, theophylline, and cyclosporine levels. Cimetidine (Tagamet) and probenecid (Benemid) increase levels of ciprofloxacin. Increased seizure risk when used with foscarnet and nonsteroidal anti-inflammatory drugs. Contraindications: Avoid use in children and pregnant women; causes tooth discoloration and cartilage abnormalities.
Metronidazole (Flagyl)	+	+	0	+	++	+	+	Side effects: Nausea, vomiting, gastrointestinal upset, metallic taste, aseptic meningitis, encephalitis, seizures, brown discoloration of urine. Drug interactions: Disulfiram reaction occurs when used with alcohol. Increases INR when used with warfarin (Coumadin). Phenobarbital and phenytoin increase metabolism and decrease levels and effects.

Medication	Side effects affecting rehab							Other side effects or considerations
Rifaximin (Xifaxan)	Cog	S	A	Motor	D	Com	F	Side effects: Peripheral edema, nausea, dizziness, fatigue, muscle spasm, abdominal pain, vertigo, dry mouth, arthralgias, confusion.
	+	+	0	+	++	+	+	

Tumor necrosis factor-blocking agents: Used in patients with severe ulcerative colitis or Crohn's disease not responsive to standard therapies.

Medication	Side effects affecting rehab							Other side effects or considerations
Infliximab (Remicade)	Cog	S	A	Motor	D	Com	F	Use in combination with methotrexate.
	0	0	0	++	++	0	0	Onset is days to weeks.
								Side effects: Infusion reaction with fever, chills, body aches, and headache; reduce symptoms by slowing the infusion rate and administering diphenhydramine (Benadryl), acetaminophen, and sometimes corticosteroids before infusion.
								Anti-infliximab antibodies occur in 10%-30% of patients, clinical SLE-like syndromes.
								Precautions: Can reactivate latent infections such as tuberculosis or hepatitis B.
								Contraindications: Not recommended for patients with concurrent demyelinating disease or congestive heart failure.
Adalimumab (Humira)	Cog	S	A	Motor	D	Com	F	Usual time to effect is 1-4 wk.
	0	0	0	+	++	0	0	Half-life is approximately 2 wk (range: 10-20 days) after a standard 40 mg dose.
								Side effects: Reactions at injection site, increased upper-respiratory tract infections, bronchitis, urinary tract infection.
								Positive ANA titers with lupus-like disease.
								Precautions: Can reactivate latent infections such as tuberculosis or hepatitis B.
								Contraindications: Patients with concurrent demyelinating disease or congestive heart failure.
Certolizumab (Cimzia)	Cog	S	A	Motor	D	Com	F	Side effects: Headache, rash, cough, abdominal pain, nasopharyngitis, urinary tract infection, upper-respiratory tract infections.
	0	0	0	++	++	0	0	Precautions: Can reactivate latent infections such as tuberculosis or hepatitis B.
								Contraindications: Patients with concurrent demyelinating disease or congestive heart failure.

Cog = cognition; S = sedation; A = agitation or mania; Motor = discoordination; D = dysphagia; Com = communication; F = falls; CBC = complete blood count; AST = aspartate aminotransferase; ALT = alanine transaminase; UA = urinalysis; INR = international normalized ratio; SLE = systemic lupus erythematosus; ANA = antinuclear antibody; G6PD = glucose-6-phosphate dehydrogenase; UC = ulcerative colitis.

The likelihood rating scale for encountering the side effects is as follows: 0 = Almost no probability of encountering side effects. + = Little likelihood of encountering side effects. +/++ = Low probability of encountering side effects; however, probability increases with increased dosage. ++ = Medium likelihood of encountering side effects. +++ = High likelihood of encountering side effects, particularly with high doses. ++++ = Highest likelihood of encountering side effects; best to avoid in at-risk patients.

Corticosteroids

Corticosteroids are the main agents used to induce remission and stop disease progression in patients with moderate to severe CD or UC. Topical use of budesonide (suppositories, foams, or enemas) may be considered in order to minimize side effects associated with steroid use (Chan, 2007; Dike et al., 2010).

Aminosalicylates

Aminosalicylates are the main agents used to induce and maintain remission in patients with mild to moderate UC. These agents are also used off label to maintain remission in patients with mild to moderate CD. Sulfasalazine is a combination of sulfapyridine and 5-aminosalicylic acid (5-ASA) and mesalamine. The product divides into active components once ingested and absorbed. Side effects are associated with the sulfa component and include headache, nausea, vomiting, anorexia, and dyspepsia. Patients should take the sulfasalazine with food to minimize GI side effects. Because the product inhibits folate absorption, patients should receive folate supplementation to prevent anemia. To avoid associated hemolytic anemia, the product should not be administered in patients with glucose-6-phosphate dehydrogenase (G6PD) deficiency (Chan, 2007; Dike et al., 2010).

Immunomodulators

Azathioprine and its metabolite 6-mercaptopurine are effective in maintaining remission, but effects may take 3 to 6 mo. About 25% to 50% of patients who do not tolerate azathioprine or 6-mercaptopurine benefit from the use of methotrexate. Cyclosporine, which is reserved for use in patients who fail other therapies, is effective in inducing remission. However, relapse frequently occurs upon discontinuance (Chan, 2007; Dike et al., 2010).

Antibiotics

Metronidazole and ciprofloxacin are used in the treatment of CD. However, use of these agents is controversial because they improve symptoms but do not induce remission. Rifaximin in doses of 200 mg 3 times/day for 16 wk induced remission in 59% of patients in some small studies (Chan, 2007).

TNF-Blocking Agents

Infliximab (Remicade) is a human chimeric monoclonal antibody product that binds to TNF-alpha and neutralizes its inflammatory effect on the GI mucosa. It is approved for use in patients with CD or UC who do not adequately respond to therapy with an aminosalicylate, corticosteroid, or immunosuppressant agent. Clinical response to this therapy occurs in 81% of patients. Human antichimeric antibodies can develop in patients treated with infliximab and can cause delayed hypersensitivity reactions and a decrease in therapeutic response. Patients who develop these antibodies can be treated with the alternant monoclonal antibody products. Researchers are currently investigating several new monoclonal antibody products for use in patients with IBD (Chan, 2007; Dike et al., 2010; Schlesselman, 2008).

Dyspepsia and Disorders Associated With Delayed Gastric Emptying

All people have experienced heartburn or dyspepsia. Gastroesophageal reflux usually occurs after a meal when the lower esophageal sphincter (LES) fails to contain gastric acid in the stomach and the acid refluxes into the esophagus, causing symptoms of heartburn. Recurrent heartburn or dyspepsia may indicate a more serious condition such as peptic ulcer disease (PUD) or gastroesophageal reflux disease (GERD). The rehabilitation therapist, who will care for patients with chronic dyspepsia or delayed gastric emptying, should be aware of methods of minimizing symptoms during the rehabilitation session and the effect of medication use on the patient. Altering positioning during exercise to minimize reflux of gastric contents and associated discomfort can help the patient participate in rehabilitation sessions. When assessing the patient, the rehabilitation therapist should ask the patient if positioning is associated with these GI symptoms. Scheduling the sessions for times that allow meals to be digested before exercise can contribute to successful rehabilitation (Peters et al., 2010).

Delayed gastric emptying can be associated with the disorders gastroparesis and **achalasia**. Gastroparesis, a disorder of slowed gastric emptying, is a common cause of nausea, vomiting, and postprandial abdominal fullness. Complications associated with gastroparesis can include weight loss along with malnutrition, blood glucose fluctuations, and **bezoar** formation that could be life threatening. Phytobezoars comprise undigested plant material such as seeds, fruit pith, or pits and are frequently reported in patients with impaired digestion and decreased gastric motility. Medication bezoars comprise mostly tablets or semiliquid masses of drugs.

Esophageal achalasia, a motility disorder, involves an absence of esophageal peristalsis and incomplete relaxation of the lower esophageal sphincter (LES). Subsequent retention of undigested foods in the esophagus leads to nocturnal regurgitation and pulmonary aspiration of the esophageal contents. Achalasia is associated with dysphagia, chest pain, weight loss, and, in severe cases, megaesophagus (dilation of the esophagus) (Hermes & Huang, 2007).

Peptic ulcer disease (PUD) presents with epigastric pain that is relieved by eating and is associated with more invasive involvement of the gastric muscularis mucosa than is seen with the superficial damage to the mucosa that occurs with **gastritis**. PUD is classified as peptic, gastric, or esophageal based on the location and is caused by damage to the mucosa by excessive gastric acid (hydrochloric acid and pepsin) when the mucosa loses its natural protective barriers to gastric acid as a result of *Helicobacter pylori* infection, the use of nonsteroidal anti-inflammatory drugs (NSAIDs) or steroids, or stress-related mucosal damage seen with critical illness (Hoogerwerf & Pasricha, 2001; Peters et al., 2010).

Gastroesophageal reflux disease (GERD) is associated with frequent, persistent reflux that may be associated with damage to the esophageal mucosa. Symptoms of GERD include heartburn, regurgitation, dysphagia, coughing, bronchoconstriction, hoarseness, and atypical chest pain that can be mistaken for acute myocardial infarction. Complications associated with GERD can include esophageal ulcer, **stricture**, and **Barrett's esophagus**, a precancerous condition that can result from repeated irritation of the esophageal mucosa. Another frequent complication of GERD is aspiration of the gastric contents into the lungs, which can result in damage to the bronchioles and worsen asthma symptoms or cause aspiration pneumonia (Chan, 2007; Peters et al., 2010; Williams, 2002).

Incidence

Twenty percent of Americans have functional dyspepsia. Delayed gastric emptying is seen in 25% to 40% of these patients. Ten percent of Americans have experienced PUD. Patients with Parkinson's disease and diabetes frequently have gastroparesis (delayed gastric emptying) and complications associated with gastroparesis. Gastroparesis occurs in 20% to 40% of patients with diabetes. GERD is commonly seen in adult patients. Obese patients are at increased risk for GERD. Factors such as diet and medication use can also contribute to symptoms of GERD (Chan, 2007; Peters et al., 2010; Williams, 2002).

GERD is also a common problem in children. GERD starts in infancy in about 18% of children with GERD. Symptoms of GERD are frequently managed by repositioning the child with the head elevated to allow gravity to help minimize symptoms of reflux. Prematurity and neurologic impairment (e.g., cerebral palsy) are common causes of dysphagia in pediatric patients. Children with cerebral palsy typically manage solid boluses more easily than liquid boluses and manage small liquid boluses more easily than large liquid boluses. Childhood achalasia appears to be more common in boys than in girls. Cognitive, developmental, and behavioral issues can affect treatment options in cases of pediatric dysphagia (Paik, 2010; Wallace & Sharkey, 2011).

Etiology and Pathophysiology

The mucosa is normally protected by mucus, secreted bicarbonate, mucosal blood flow, and epithelial defense. Histamine is released when gastric acid invades a weakened area of the GI tract; this stimulates secretion of more gastric acid. Endogenous prostaglandins control the production of mucus and mucosal blood flow. The use of agents that interfere with prostaglandin production, such as NSAIDs and steroids, is a common cause of dyspepsia and PUD. PUD can also occur as a result of gastric *Helicobacter pylori* infection with associated inflammation, increased production of cytotoxins and ammonia by the bacteria, and increased production of gastric acid triggered by the presence of the bacteria (Peters et al., 2010).

GERD occurs when the sphincter between the esophagus and stomach, designed to keep stomach contents in the stomach, becomes less efficient. This can result in regurgitation of gastric (stomach) contents. GERD can result in damage to the esophagus such as stricture or Barrett's esophagus or can result in aspiration pneumonia. Asthmatic symptoms can also be exacerbated due to aspiration of gastric acids into the lungs.

Primary achalasia is caused by a general failure of distal esophageal inhibitory neurons and results in reduced LES relaxation, increased LES tone, and lack of peristalsis of the esophagus. Secondary achalasia is associated with another disease and occurs in patients with Chagas disease, Parkinson's disease, and malignancy. Primary treatment of gastroparesis and achalasia includes dietary manipulations and pharmacotherapy with antiemetics and prokinetic agents (medications that promote gastric motility). Refractory symptoms may require placement of a jejunostomy tube, implantation of a gastric electric stimulator, or botulinum toxin injections. Invasive therapies such as pneumatic balloon dilation and cardiomyotomy are the most effective but can be associated with esophageal stricture or perforation (Bernardi, 2002; Pasricha, 2001; Short & Thomas, 1992).

Medication Therapy

Dyspepsia or indigestion is commonly treated with over-the-counter antacids agents that neutralize or decrease production of stomach acid. Antacids such as calcium carbonate or aluminum and magnesium hydroxides (Tums, Maalox, Mylanta) may also be used. These products have a rapid onset of action (usually 30 min-1 h) and reduce stomach acidity and relieve discomfort associated with refluxed acidic contents. Histamine-2 blockers, which include famotidine (Pepcid), cimetidine (Tagamet), ranitidine (Zantac), and nizatidine (Axid), are routinely used to treat PUD, a disease associated with an imbalance between mucosal defense factors that prevent injury of the GI tract (bicarbonate, mucin, prostaglandins, nitrous oxide) and products that can promote injury to the mucosal lining of GI tract by increasing its vulnerability to gastric acid and pepsin. Patients with peptic ulcers associated with the bacteria *Helicobacter pylori* require a 6 wk drug regimen that includes a proton pump inhibitor (PPI), which is a more potent reducer of gastric acid production, along with two antibiotics, clarithromycin (Biaxin) plus either metronidazole (Flagyl) or amoxicillin (Pasricha, 2001; Wallace & Sharkey, 2011).

Proton pump inhibitors (PPIs) are the mainstay of therapy in the management of GERD. PPIs include omeprazole (Prilosec), esomeprazole (Nexium), lansoprazole (Prevacid), rabeprazole (Aciphex), and pantoprazole (Protonix). These agents have a delayed onset of action; maximal effects are seen after 3 to 5 days of continuous therapy. Table 24.7 includes additional information on these medications. Standard antacids such as calcium carbonate or aluminum and magnesium hydroxides (Tums, Maalox, Mylanta) and the histamine-2 blockers are generally ineffective in managing GERD (Wallace & Sharkey, 2011). Baclofen (Lioresal) has also been shown to improve duodenal reflux that is not controlled by PPI therapy alone (Koek et al., 2003).

LES relaxation is triggered at the level of the medullary brainstem in response to stomach distention. The inhibitory neurotransmitter gamma amino butyric acid (GABA) influences respiration, esophageal motility, and swallowing control. The GABA receptor agonist baclofen (Lioresal) reduces the rate of transient LES relaxations. Baclofen (Lioresal) can increase basal LES pressure, reduce LES relaxation rate, and reduce the number of episodes of reflux in healthy individuals by 40% to 60% (Lidums et al., 2000).

See table 24.7 in the web resource for a full list of medication-specific indications, dosing recommendations, side effects, and drug interactions and precautions.

Table 24.7 Medications Used to Treat Gastric-Emptying Disorders

Medication	Side effects affecting rehab							Other side effects or considerations
Agents that affect LES function								
Nifedipine (Procardia XL) Calcium channel blocker that relaxes LES in treatment of achalasia or gastroparesis	Cog +	S 0	A +	Motor +	D ++	Com +	F ++	Side effects: Dizziness, flushing, headache, gingival hyperplasia, peripheral edema, mood changes, gastrointestinal side effects. Food and drug interactions: Grapefruit juice (>200 ml) can increase levels of this medication and should not be consumed within 2 h before or 4 h after administration. Decreases liver metabolism of carbamazepine (Tegretol), simvastatin (Zocor), atorvastatin (Lipitor), and lovastatin (Mevacor). This can lead to toxicity from these drugs.
Baclofen (Lioresal) Muscle relaxant that inhibits LES relaxation and reduces symptoms of reflux mediated by gamma amino butyric acid	Cog ++	S +++	A ++	Motor +++	D ++	Com ++	F +++	Eliminated by the kidneys; reduce dose with renal dysfunction. Side effects: Initial sedation, muscle weakness, ataxia, orthostatic hypotension, fatigue, headache, nausea, dizziness; confusion and hallucinations reported in the elderly or those with history of stroke. Abrupt discontinuance results in rebound increase in spasticity, rhabdomyolysis, disorientation, hallucination, and seizures.
Botulinum toxin (Botox) Inhibits the release of acetylcholine from nerve terminals in the LES; can induce LES	Cog +	S ++	A +	Motor ++	D +++	Com +	F +	Side effects: Anxiety, back pain, dizziness, drowsiness, dry eyes, dry mouth, flu-like symptoms, headache, increased cough, indigestion, nausea, neck pain, runny nose, sensitivity to light, sweating, stomach upset, reactions at injection site (pain, redness, swelling, or tenderness), weakness of the muscles at or near the injection site.
Prokinetic agents								
Metoclopramide (Reglan) Prokinetic, improves LES function in GERD and promotes gastric emptying; antiemetic agent	Cog +++	S +++	A ++	Motor +++	D +	Com +++	F +++	Common side effects: Restlessness, drowsiness, dizziness, lassitude, dystonia. Infrequent side effects: Headache, extrapyramidal effects such as oculogyric crisis, hypotension, hypertension, hyperprolactinemia leading to galactorrhea, constipation, depression. Drug interactions: Additive sedation when used with other CNS depressants. Antagonizes dopamine-enhancer therapy used in treatment of Parkinson's disease.

› continued

Table 24.7 › *continued*

Medication	Side effects affecting rehab							Other side effects or considerations
Cisapride (Propulsid) Promotes gastric emptying and gastrointestinal motility	Cog ++	S ++	A 0	Motor ++	D ++	Com +	F ++	Withdrawn from the U.S. market due to associated serious cardiac arrhythmias and deaths. Now available for compassionate use only for patients that cannot be treated with other agents. Side effects: Diarrhea, abdominal cramping, nausea, flatulence, dry mouth, headache, dizziness, somnolence, fatigue, bone marrow suppression, depression, hepatitis.
Erythromycin Stimulates motilin receptors in the gastrointestinal smooth muscle, promoting peristalsis	Cog +	S 0	A 0	Motor ++	D +	Com +	F ++	Side effects: Allergic reactions, rash, hearing loss when used in renal failure, muscle weakness, hepatotoxicity, QT prolongation, gastrointestinal upset. Drug interactions: Increased risk for arrhythmia when used with other agents that prolong QT prolongation (e.g., antiarrhythmics, antipsychotics, antidepressants, anesthetics).
Proton pump inhibitors: Reduce acid production.								
Omeprazole (Prilosec) Esomeprazole (Nexium) Lansoprazole (Prevacid) Rabeprazole (Aciphex) Pantoprazole (Protonix)	Cog 0	S 0	A 0	Motor +	D +	Com 0	F +	Side effects: Abdominal pain, diarrhea, headache, dizziness, reduced calcium and magnesium absorption, increased bone fracture. Drug interactions: Can reduce effectiveness of clopidogrel (Plavix) therapy.
Antireflux agent: Produces a foam layer on top of stomach contents, reducing reflux of stomach acid.								
Alginic acid (Gaviscon)	Cog +	S 0	A 0	Motor +	D +	Com 0	F +	Side effects: Decreased absorption of phosphate and magnesium, osteomalacia, encephalopathy, seizures, speech disorders, tremor, dysarthria associated with aluminum toxicity when used chronically in renal failure. Drug interactions: May reduce the absorption of products containing aluminum or calcium or of tetracycline antibiotics; avoid in patients with renal failure due to risk of aluminum toxicity.

Cog = cognition; S = sedation; A = agitation or mania; Motor = discoordination; D = dysphagia; Com = communication; F = falls; LES = lower esophageal sphincter; GERD = gastroesophageal reflux disease; CNS = central nervous system.

The likelihood rating scale for encountering the side effects is as follows: 0 = Almost no probability of encountering side effects. + = Little likelihood of encountering side effects. +/++ = Low probability of encountering side effects; however, probability increases with increased dosage. ++ = Medium likelihood of encountering side effects. +++ = High likelihood of encountering side effects, particularly with high doses. ++++ = Highest likelihood of encountering side effects; best to avoid in at-risk patients.

Medications used to treat gastroparesis and achalasia include prokinetic agents, nitrates (used to reduce esophageal spasm), and botulinum toxin injections. Prokinetic agents are useful in augmenting LES contraction and promoting peristalsis, which helps to empty stomach contents. Pharmacologic therapies used to reduce symptoms of LES spasm include calcium channel blockers and long-acting nitrates. Nifedipine (Procardia, Adalat) is a calcium channel antagonist that reduces influx of calcium into the LES, thus inducing LES relaxation. Nitrates such as isosorbide dinitrate (Isordil) have also been used for this indication but with less success due to associated symptoms of hypotension and dizziness.

Botulinum toxin A (Botox) has been used with success to treat refractory gastroparesis and achalasia, and effects can be sustained for several months. Botox may also be injected into the cricopharyngeal muscle to treat other forms of dysphagia associated with cricopharyngeal muscle spasm or hypertonicity. Injections can lead to positive results such as the ability to eat solid foods without aspiration. Botox has also been used to treat diffuse esophageal spasm. Table 24.7 provides additional detail on the medications used to treat GERD, achalasia, and gastroparesis (Cheng et al., 2006a; Cheng et al., 2006b; Hermes & Huang, 2007).

PATIENT CASE 2

K.T. is a 5-yr-old male who is the smallest child in his class and a fussy eater. He avoids meats with his meals, complains that "foods get stuck going down," and prefers fruits and vegetables when he does eat. After eating a good-sized meal, he frequently coughs, gags, and then vomits his meal. His mother is concerned about his small size and is afraid his diet is inadequate. His physician has diagnosed him with GERD and has referred him to the speech–language pathologist for evaluation and recommendations for treating his dysphagia.

Question
Which of K.T.'s symptoms are consistent with GERD?

Answer
K.T.'s symptoms that may point to GERD-associated dysphagia include low weight, being a fussy eater, avoiding certain foods, complaining of food getting stuck, and postprandial coughing, gagging, and vomiting.

Question
K.T.'s mom asks what can be done to improve her son's GERD symptoms. What information can the rehabilitation specialist provide?

Answer
Infants and children can be treated with a prokinetic agent such as metoclopramide (Reglan) to improve GI motility and gastric emptying. The prokinetic medication is combined with an antacid medication to minimize acid damage to the esophagus that can occur with regurgitation. Complications of such regurgitation can include aspiration and aspiration pneumonia, Barrett's esophagus, and strictures (Bernardi, 2002; Mercado-Deane et al., 2001; Paik, 2010; Pasricha, 2001; Williams, 2002).

In addition to medication therapy, changes in diet can help minimize symptoms of GERD. Avoiding large meals and eating smaller, more frequent meals can help reduce symptoms. Avoiding heavy meals before bedtime, minimizing the fat content of meals, providing more protein in meals, and avoiding foods that trigger reflux symptoms can also help. Foods that can worsen symptoms of GERD include chocolate, peppermint, beverages containing caffeine (e.g., coffee, tea, or colas), tomato juice, citrus juices, onions, garlic, and foods that are spicy. Conversely, high-protein meals increase the tone of the LES and decrease GERD symptoms. In addition, raising the head of the bed by 30° helps relieve nighttime reflux symptoms by using gravity to assist with the transit of food. In the case of infants, repositioning them during and after feeding and when sleeping can minimize symptoms of GERD (Carl & Johnson, 2006; Paik, 2010).

The rehabilitation therapist can play a very important role by counseling the patient with GERD about lifestyle changes. Avoiding alcohol, quitting smoking, reducing stress, and reducing weight in patients who are overweight can help improve symptoms of GERD in adults. Patients should avoid exercising or reclining immediately after meals to minimize symptoms associated with reflux. Exercises that involve bending and positioning the head below the stomach should be avoided; the rehabilitation therapist should design sessions with this in mind. Rehabilitation sessions should be scheduled for at least 1 to 2 h after meals (Carl & Johnson, 2006).

Medications can increase symptoms of regurgitation and reflux by decreasing the resting tone of the LES. The following medications should be avoided whenever possible in patients with GERD. When they cannot be avoided, the patient should be treated with the lowest effective dose and should avoid exercising and reclining for at least 3 to 4 h after taking these medications.

- Antiemetics such as promethazine (Phenergan) or prochlorperazine (Compazine)
- Antidepressants with high anticholinergic activity such as amitriptyline (Elavil)
- Barbiturates such as phenobarbital
- Antihistamines such as diphenhydramine (Benadryl)
- Antipsychotics with high anticholinergic effects such as thioridazine (Mellaril)
- Benzodiazepines such as diazepam (Valium) or temazepam (Restoril)
- Beta blockers such as propranolol (Inderal), atenolol (Tenormin), and metoprolol (Lopressor)
- Theophylline (Theo-Dur)
- Calcium channel blockers used to treat hypertension such as nifedipine (Procardia), diltiazem (Cardizem), and verapamil (Isoptin)
- Estrogen products
- Narcotics with high anticholinergic effects such as morphine or meperidine (Demerol)

- Nitrates such as nitroglycerin, isosorbide mononitrate (Imdur)
- Skeletal muscle relaxants such as baclofen (Lioresal)

Eosinophilic Esophagitis

The rehabilitation therapist who cares for patients with GERD should be aware of a newly discovered disease called eosinophilic esophagitis (EE). EE is an allergic inflammatory disorder with symptoms of dysphagia, food impaction, heartburn, regurgitation, abdominal pain, chest pain, and failure to thrive. In the past, patients with EE were misdiagnosed as having GERD. However, EE differs in etiology and requires different medication therapy to control symptoms. It is diagnosed by the clinical symptoms listed earlier, the presence of more than 15 eosinophils per high-power field, and lack of response to PPI therapy. Increased levels of interleukins 4, 5, and 13 and mast cells are present in the esophagus of patients with EE (Wood, 2010).

Incidence and Etiology

EE occurs in adults and children. Of patients with EE, 50% to 80% have concurrent allergic disorders such as atopic dermatitis, allergic rhinitis, asthma, or eczema (Wood, 2010).

Medication Therapy

Medications that have been used to treat EE include steroid therapy such as inhaled fluticasone (metered-dose inhaler administered 2-4 times/day without a spacer to allow the steroid to deposit in the esophagus rather than in the lungs), oral viscous budesonide (doses of 1-2 mg/day), montelukast (Singulair) 20 to 30 mg/day, and oral steroids used to treat acute exacerbations of the disease. Other anti-inflammatory medications currently being studied in clinical trials include anti-interleukin-5 and monoclonal antibody therapies (Wood, 2010).

Dysphagia

The rehabilitation therapist will encounter many patients with dysphagia. Complications of dysphagia can include aspiration pneumonia, malnutrition, dehydration, weight loss, and airway obstruction. Dysphagia can significantly affect the patient's ability to participate in rehabilitation and can reduce appetite and energy, thus interfering with physical, social, and psychological function. The rehabilitation therapist should ask the patient about symptoms of dysphagia and should re-evaluate patients for symptoms of dysphagia with any change in medication therapy or diet. Oral or pharyngeal dysphagia can be associated with the following symptoms: coughing or choking upon swallowing, difficulty initiating a swallow, food sticking in the throat, sialorrhea, unexplained weight loss, change in dietary habits, recurrent pneumonia, change in voice or speech (wet voice), or nasal regurgitation. Esophageal dysphagia can be associated with the following symptoms: sensation of food sticking in the chest or throat, oral or pharyngeal regurgitation, or change in dietary habits (Carl & Johnson, 2006; Paik, 2010).

Incidence

Approximately 6.5 million Americans suffer from dysphagia. The incidence of dysphagia varies among health care environments. For example, studies report that 14% of patients in acute-care facilities, 35% of patients in rehabilitation centers, and 40% to 50% of patients in skilled nursing facilities have dysphagia (Carl & Johnson, 2006; Marik & Kaplan, 2003). Neurologic swallowing disorders are encountered more frequently in rehabilitation medicine than in most other medical specialties. Stroke is the leading cause of neurologic dysphagia. Approximately 51% to 73% of patients with stroke have dysphagia, which is the most significant risk factor for the development of pneumonia (Katzan et al., 2003; Mann et al., 2000; Paciaroni et al., 2004). Other frequent causes of dysphagia in rehabilitation medicine include traumatic brain injury, motor neuron disease (e.g., amyotrophic lateral sclerosis, Parkinson's disease, and other degenerative disorders), poliomyelitis, multiple sclerosis, myasthenia gravis, myopathy, GI surgery, head and neck surgery (oral cavity cancer), cervical or spinal injury, ventilator dependency, cerebral palsy, and other movement disorders

(Hunt & Walker, 1989; Leslie et al., 2003; Lovell et al., 2005; Mayer, 2004; Morgan et al., 2003; Nelson et al., 2002; Sheikh et al., 2001).

Etiology and Pathophysiology

Dysphagia affects approximately 25% of patients admitted to acute-care hospitals, 40% of patients in rehabilitation centers, and 30% to 75% of patients in skilled nursing facilities. Dysphagia introduces many confounding variables and significantly affects the outcome of rehabilitation. The consequences of dysphagia (e.g., aspiration pneumonia, malnutrition, dehydration, weight loss, and airway obstruction) can be serious, particularly in the elderly (Carl & Johnson, 2006; Howden, 2004; Martino et al., 2005; Paik, 2010; Palmer et al., 2000; Wilkins et al., 2007).

PATIENT CASE 3

U.M. is an 87-yr-old female who is referred for assistance with strength exercises and gait training after a prolonged hospitalization for a stroke complicated by pneumonia. U.M. is 5 ft 2 in. (1.57 m) tall, weighs 102 lb (46.3 kg), and has lost 20 lb (9.1 kg) over the past 4 wk. U.M.'s daughter states that U.M. has no appetite and wakes up coughing and choking at night, which has prevented her from sleeping well.

Question
What signs and symptoms indicate that U.M. may have dysphagia?

Answer
Unexplained weight loss, coughing and choking at night, changes in dietary habits, and a history of pneumonia all indicate that U.M. may have dysphagia.

Patients who are elderly and have had a stroke are at particularly high risk for developing eating and swallowing disorders. Patients suspected of having dysphagia should undergo an initial bedside swallow evaluation and if dysphagia is found, should be referred for further evaluation by a speech–language pathologist (SLP). The SLP may perform an instrumental study if pharyngeal dysphagia is suspected. The SLP further defines the type and severity of the dysphagia and develops a plan for treatment. The clinical dietitian should be consulted to provide an appropriate dysphagia diet and diet education based on the type of dysphagia the SLP identifies and the food and fluid restrictions recommended.

Aspiration is the passage of food or liquid through the vocal folds. People who aspirate are at increased risk for pneumonia. People without swallowing abnormalities routinely aspirate microscopic amounts of food and liquid. Gross aspiration, however, is abnormal and may lead to respiratory complications. If cough is impaired, such as after a stroke, aspiration may occur. Aspiration pneumonia accounts for about 34% of all stroke-related deaths and is the third highest cause of death during the first month after a stroke. Note, however, that not all of these cases of pneumonia are attributable to the aspiration of food. Early detection and treatment of dysphagia in patients who have sustained a stroke is critical (Caruso & Passali, 2006; Paik, 2010).

Patients with dysphagia should continue to self-feed if at all possible. Incidence of pneumonia is generally lower in patients who self-feed (Rosenvinge & Starke, 2005). Patients with feeding issues may present a more complex problem for the rehabilitation team. Typically, the SLP works on the patient's swallowing problem and the occupational therapist works on hand-to-mouth activities involved in eating. All disciplines including physical therapy and nursing are concerned with the patient's posture and muscle strength. The physical therapist can instruct the patient and family in postural awareness and prescribe therapeutic exercises that correct forward head posture, forward shoulder posture, and tight anterior neck muscles that can result in contracture of the cervical flexors. Weak neck extensors and tight neck flexors can result in a chin-to-chest posture that does not provide the optimal length tension relationship for force development in the swallowing muscles.

Oral hygiene and dental care are extremely important when working to prevent pneumonia. Dried secretions that accumulate on the tongue and palate reduce oral sensitivity and promote bacterial growth. The elderly have an increased incidence of oropharyngeal colonization with respiratory pathogens, a well-known risk factor for pneumonia. Decreased salivary production and abnormalities in swallowing can change the amount of bacteria retained in the mouth. Lemon glycerin swabs or a damp washcloth can be used to remove the secretions (Carl & Johnson, 2006; Paik, 2010; Siepler, 2002; Spieker, 2000; Terrado et al., 2001; Vogel et al., 2000; Willoughby, 1983).

The SLP can recommend two types of exercise to the patient with dysphagia: compensatory exercises that do not change the physiology of the swallow (such as head positioning) and therapeutic exercises that change the physiology of the swallow (such as oral motor exercises). The patient performs exercises that facilitate oral motor strength, range of motion, and coordination multiple times per day (Carl & Johnson, 2006; Paik, 2010).

Medication-Induced Dysphagia

Some medications can cause or worsen dysphagia. These medications can be categorized as medications that depress CNS function, medications that affect GI tract secretions and lubrication, and medications that affect GI motility mediated by the autonomic and enteric nervous systems. Many medications fall into more than one category. Table 24.8 summarizes medication classes and associated side effects that can contribute to dysphagia in rehabilitation patients (Carl & Johnson, 2006, 2008; Siepler, 2002; Spieker, 2000; Terrado et al., 2001; Voge et al., 2000; Willoughby, 1983).

Medications That Affect Motor Function

Medications that depress neurotransmission or activity in the central nervous system (CNS) are called CNS depressants. CNS depressants include antipsychotics, antidepressants, sedatives, antianxiety agents, muscle relaxants and anticonvulsants. These medications change levels of the neurotransmitters dopamine, histamine, serotonin, and GABA in the CNS. Changes in these neurotransmitters can cause sedation, impaired motor function, and cognitive difficulties. Impaired motor function can affect all phases of the swallow. CNS depres-

Table 24.8   Medication Classes With Associated Side Effects That Contribute to Dysphagia

Medication	Alters taste, smell, and appetite	Alters cognition	Alters motor function	Alters gastrointestinal motility	Causes gastrointestinal injury
Antipsychotics	Yes	Yes	Yes	Yes	
Antidepressants	Yes	Yes	Yes	Yes	
Antianxiety and sleep medications	Yes	Yes	Yes	Yes	
Anticonvulsants	Yes	Yes	Yes		Mucositis and Stevens-Johnson syndrome; Dilantin causes gingival hyperplasia.
Parkinson's medications	Yes	Yes	Yes	Yes	
Lithium	Yes		Yes		
Alzheimer's disease medications	Yes	Yes	Yes	Yes	
Antihistamines	Yes	Yes	Yes	Yes	
Anticholinergics	Yes	Yes	Yes	Yes	
Cardiac medications	Yes			Worsen gastroesophageal reflux disease	
Opiate pain medications	Yes	Yes	Yes	Yes	
Nonsteroidal anti-inflammatory drugs	Yes	Yes, in the elderly			Gastrointestinal bleeding and ulceration.
Steroid medications	Yes	Yes	Yes		Gastrointestinal bleeding and ulceration.
Potassium supplements	Yes			Yes	Potassium tablets can lodge in esophagus.
Iron supplements	Yes			Yes	Iron tablets can lodge in esophagus.
Osteoporosis medications					Boniva, Fosamax, and Actonel can lodge in esophagus.
Antibiotics	Yes			Yes	Clindamycin, tetracycline, and sulfonamides can result in allergic rash which can progress to exfoliative mucosal damage such as with Stevens-Johnson syndrome.

sants can interfere with brainstem swallowing function, oral and pharyngeal sensation, arousal, and voluntary muscle control involved in eating and swallowing (Alvi, 1999; Bloom, 2001; Carl & Johnson, 2006, 2008; Hoffman, 2001; Markowitz & Morton, 2002).

Antipsychotic medications decrease dopamine in the basal ganglia, limbic system, hypothalamus, brainstem, and medulla. Decreasing dopamine can improve behavior and perception in patients with schizophrenia but can also cause extrapyramidal side effects such as pill rolling, cogwheel rigidity, resting and intentional tremors, akathisia, dystonia, and dysarthria that can contribute to dysphagia. The extrapyramidal side effects of dystonia with altered abilities to chew and swallow and impaired GI transit also increase the probability of choking in this population. Tardive dyskinesia (TD) is permanent motor dysfunction associated with long-term use of antipsychotic medications even after medication discontinuance. TD is associated with a high risk of dysphagia and an increased risk of choking and aspiration in the psychiatric patient (Carl & Johnson, 2006; Siepler, 2002; Spieker, 2000; Terrado et al., 2001; Vogel et al., 2000).

PATIENT CASE 4

R.P. is a 45-yr-old male who is 6 ft 2 in. (1.9 m) tall and weighs 350 lb (158.8 kg). R.P. has a 25 yr history of schizophrenia. His medical history includes myocardial infarction, hypertension, type 2 diabetes, and hyperlipidemia. He is admitted for acute psychotic symptoms that include hallucinations, severe agitation, and combative behavior. He is treated with intramuscular Geodon on a stat basis and continued on an as-needed basis to treat further combative behavior. A nicotine patch is also placed. His home medications, including aspirin, Tenormin, Lisinopril, Glucophage, Geodon, and Zyprexa, are restarted. Twenty four h later he is calm and no longer displays combative behavior, but some visual and auditory hallucinations persist. Three days later he has a fever to 102 °F and an elevated white blood cell count. A chest X-ray and cultures are done and R.P. is diagnosed with pneumonia. Antibiotics are started and the SLP is consulted to determine whether the patient is aspirating.

Question
What are some risk factors for dysphagia identified in R.P.?

Answer
Sedation and extrapyramidal side effects from R.P.'s antipsychotic medications and his obesity may contribute to aspiration and dysphagia.

Medications That Affect GI Secretions

Medications that reduce secretion production and lubrication of the GI tract, starting with the nasal passages and oral secretions and ending with rectal mucosa, can also cause eating and swallowing disorders and gastrointestinal motility dysfunction, resulting in reduced food intake and nutrition. Medication-induced decreases in smell and taste can affect the anticipatory phase of swallowing. Impaired lubrication of nasal passages can reduce smell, which can affect appetite and taste. The lack of saliva production can reduce the taste of foods and thus reduce appetite. A lack of bolus formation and lubrication affect the oral preparatory and oral phases of swallowing. Subsequently, the patient has difficulty forming a cohesive bolus, masticating, and moving the bolus through the system. Saliva dilutes the bacteria counts in the mouth and neutralizes acids that enter the mouth. Saliva is also important for maintaining intact dentition and mucosa. The patient with reduced saliva production may also have increasing difficulty with the swallow trigger and moving the bolus through the pharynx and esophagus. Medications that decrease lubrication of the lower GI tract can cause slowed motility and constipation and subsequently reduce appetite and oral intake (Campbell-Taylor, 2001; Carl & Johnson, 2006; Johnson, 2013; Logemann et al., 2003; Pedersen et al., 2002).

Acetylcholine and histamine are neurotransmitters that stimulate secretion production in the GI tract at the cholinergic and muscarinic receptors via the parasympathetic nervous system. Medications that impair the effects of these neurotransmitters are known as anticholinergic medications. Anticholinergic medications reduce GI secretions and can interfere with GI motility. Many medications have anticholinergic effects, resulting in xerostomia and reduced GI function. **Xerostomia** is one of the most prevalent symptoms seen in the elderly population. Many medications prescribed for the elderly have anticholinergic effects, which can worsen dry mouth. Medications known to cause xerostomia include antihistamines, antidepressants, muscle relaxants, sedatives, antiparkinson agents, and antipsychotics. Bowel or urinary incontinence is often treated with anticholinergic agents such as propantheline (Pro-Banthine), tolterodine (Detrol, Detrol LA), oxybutynin (Ditropan, Ditropan LA), and dicyclomine (Bentyl) or tricyclic antidepressants such as imipramine (Tofranil). The anticholinergic agents scopolamine (Transderm Scop) and glycopyrrolate (Robinul), are used to decrease drooling. In addition to reviewing the patient's prescription medications, the rehabilitation therapist should be aware of the patient's nonprescription medications that can cause anticholinergic effects. For instance, many nonprescription medications advertised as sleep aids or for relief of allergy, cough, and cold symptoms contain antihistamines such as diphenhydramine (Benadryl) and doxylamine. The combination of prescription and over-the-counter medications can greatly exacerbate the anticholinergic effects on the patient. Table 24.9 lists recommended treatments for patients with xerostomia or mucositis (Balmer & Valley, 2002; Johnson, 2013).

Medications That Affect GI Motility

Changes in GI motility can result in decreased gastric emptying, peristalsis, and esophageal sphincter functioning. The action of the neurotransmitters acetylcholine, dopamine, serotonin, and norepinephrine in the GI tract mediates GI motility. Acetylcholine is the primary neurotransmitter that affects GI activity.

Numerous medications can reduce the activity of these neurotransmitters, including antipsychotics such as olanzapine (Zyprexa), antihistamines such as hydroxyzine (Atarax), opiate pain medications such as oxycodone, and antidepressants with pronounced anticholinergic effects such as amitriptyline (Elavil). Oral intake can be adversely affected by nausea and vomiting associated with agents such as opiate pain medications and chemotherapy medications used to treat cancer (Gutstein & Akil, 2001; Max & American Pain Society, 1999). Benzodiazepines such as diazepam (Valium), calcium channel blockers such as nifedipine (Procardia), antipsychotics such as haloperidol (Haldol), barbiturates such as phenobarbital, antihistamines such as diphenhydramine (Benadryl), nitroglycerin, baclofen (Lioresal), and estrogen-replacement medications such as conjugated estrogens (Premarin) can affect LES tone and worsen symptoms of GERD (Campbell-Taylor, 1996; Carl & Johnson, 2006, 2008; Jaspersen, 2000; Markowitz & Morton, 2002; Rooney & Johnson, 2000; Williams, 2002).

PATIENT CASE 5

W.P. is a 69-yr-old male who underwent a resection of oral cancer 6 mo ago followed by 3 cycles of chemotherapy and radiation. He is referred to therapy for problems with

Table 24.9   Interventions That Minimize Dysphagia With Xerostomia or Mucositis

Use over-the-counter saliva substitutes (e.g., Biotene, Oralube, Xero-Lube, Plax, Oral Balance gel) to improve mouth lubrication and enhance swallowing.

Use prescription Salagen (contains pilocarpine) or cevimeline (Evoxac) to enhance saliva production in patients with dry mouth.

Maintain hydration by drinking water or sucking ice.

Chew sugarless gum or suck on sugarless hard candy.

Change the medications or dose of medications causing xerostomia.

Minimize with **cryotherapy** or administer amifostine with chemotherapy doses.

Treat with frequent saline rinses, topical anesthetics, and magic mouthwash.

Avoid irritating mouth products that contain alcohol.

Provide meticulous oral care with use of toothettes when tooth brush cannot be used, mouth swabs, and antibacterial rinses such as chlorhexidine mouthwash (Peridex) at least 3-4 times/day to reduce bacterial counts in the mouth and reduce aspiration pneumonia.

eating and swallowing that have resulted in a 30 lb (13.6 kg) weight loss in the past 3 mo. W.P.'s medication list includes the following: nicotine 21 mg patch/day for smoking cessation, fentanyl (Duragesic) 100 µg patch every 72 h for pain, oxycodone (Oxy IR) 20 mg by mouth every 3 h as needed for breakthrough pain, promethazine (Phenergan) 25 mg by mouth every 6 h as needed for nausea and vomiting, aspirin 81 mg/day, metoprolol (Toprol XL) 50 mg/day for blood pressure, lisinopril (Prinivil) 20 mg/day for blood pressure, and atorvastatin (Lipitor) 10 mg/day for cholesterol.

Question

What risk factors for dysphagia does W.P. have?

Answer

Surgery of the mouth, chemotherapy, and radiation of the mouth can all contribute to eating and swallowing disorders. Misalignment of dentition, inflammatory reactions, and stomatitis associated with chemotherapy and radiation therapy can contribute to difficulty chewing and swallowing. Radiation damage to the salivary glands may contribute to significant xerostomia as well. Medication therapy can add to the risk of dysphagia. Opiate pain medications can contribute to xerostomia, sedation, impaired motor function, and slowed GI transit. W.P. can experience severe constipation if a scheduled bowel regimen that includes adequate fluid and fiber intake, exercise, and an adequately dosed laxative such as Senokot-S is not incorporated into his plan of care. The promethazine prescribed for nausea has anticholinergic side effects and can contribute to dysphagia by potentiating dry mouth and sedation. Promethazine is a phenothiazine derivative that can be associated with extrapyramidal side effects such as dystonia and tremor, which can further contribute to dysphagia. Finally, anticholinergic medications frequently cause confusion and orthostasis in the older patient. The rehabilitation therapist should incorporate fall risk precautions into W.P.'s sessions.

Medication-Induced GI Injury

A number of medications can damage the GI tract. For example, stomatitis and **mucositis** are associated with medications used to treat cancer. Stomatitis is also associated with medications used to treat rheumatoid arthritis. Other medications that can damage the GI tract include NSAIDs such as ibuprofen (Motrin) or naproxen (Naprosyn), aspirin, antiviral medications, and tetracycline antibiotics. A rare but severe allergic reaction called Stevens-Johnson syndrome can result in sloughing of the skin and mucosal tissue and can occur with the use of anticonvulsants such as carbamazepine (Tegretol) and phenytoin (Dilantin) and the antibiotic sulfamethoxazole–trimethoprim (Septra, Bactrim) (Balmer & Valley, 2002; Boyce, 1998; Carl & Johnson, 2006; Chabner et al., 2001).

Medications that are not completely swallowed and that become embedded in the esophagus have been associated with direct esophageal injury. The following medications increase the risk of esophageal injury (Carl & Johnson, 2006; O'Neill, 2003; Ravich, 1997).

- Potassium supplements (Slow-K, K-Dur)
- Theophylline (Theo-dur)
- Quinidine (Quinidex, Quinaglute)
- Iron supplements
- Bisphosphonate medications used to treat osteoporosis: alendronate (Fosamax), risedronate (Actonel), and ibandronate (Boniva)
- Tetracycline antibiotics or clindamycin
- Corticosteroids such as prednisone, methylprednisolone, and dexamethasone (Decadron)
- Aspirin and NSAIDs

Taking medications with little or no fluid immediately before bedtime can increase the risk of medication-induced esophageal injury, particularly in patients with extended GI transit time. To avoid medication-induced esophageal injury patients should take all medications with at least 3 oz (88.7 ml) of fluid. If the patient has difficulty swallowing a pill, the patient should take a sip of fluid first, swallow the pill, and then drink the rest of the fluid. Patients should take bedtime medications in an upright position at least 10 min before reclining. Patients who are bedridden or who have delayed esophageal transit times or esophageal compression should take liquid medications whenever possible. Medications that have delayed dissolution rate or come in large dosage forms that are not easily swallowed have been associated with becoming lodged in the esophageal passageway. Medications dosed once/day and the high-risk medications, such as the bisphosphonates listed previously, should be taken early in the day unless side effects such as sedation make bedtime dosing more desirable (Carl & Johnson, 2006; Gallagher, 2010).

Rehabilitation Considerations in Medication Review and Patient Education

With admission of a new patient to rehabilitation service, the rehabilitation specialist should take a careful medication history to identify any medication issues that may affect rehabilitation progress. In addition, the patient should also be questioned each session regarding any newly initiated medications or changes in dosage and asked about any new symptoms associated with these changes (Carl & Johnson, 2006).

The rehabilitation therapist should educate the patient and family about safe use of medications and encourage healthy lifestyle changes (e.g., smoking cessation, reduction of alcohol intake, exercise, cognitive and behavioral therapy, stress-management techniques, and weight loss) that will reduce many of the symptoms involved in GI disorders. The rehabilitation therapist should also counsel patients about the foods, nonpharmacologic interventions, and over-the-counter medications that exacerbate GERD and GI disorders and instruct the patient and family to monitor

for any changes in dietary intake or weight loss with the addition of any new medication (Carl & Johnson, 2006).

Medications should always be started at a low dose and slowly titrated up based on the patient's tolerance. The "start low and go slow" principle particularly applies to the elderly population. If new symptoms appear, the rehabilitation therapist may contact the prescriber, who may reduce the patient's dose, and contact the patient's pharmacist, who may review the patient's entire medication regimen to identify any drug interactions that may be causing the new symptoms. Reducing the dose and simplifying the medication regimen whenever possible is always preferred over adding another medication to control a new side effect (Carl & Johnson, 2006).

The interdisciplinary team should periodically review the patient's drug regimen to see whether any medications are no longer necessary. The more medications a patient takes, the higher the likelihood a drug interaction, side effect, or medication error will occur and the higher the likelihood that the patient will not adhere to the regimen. Patients should avoid combining over-the-counter medications with prescription medications unless approved by their physician. Patients should be encouraged to use the pharmacist as a resource for selecting over-the-counter and prescription medications and for reviewing and simplifying the patient's medication regimen (Carl & Johnson, 2006).

Summary

This chapter reviews commonly encountered GI disorders that may affect rehabilitation patients, including nausea and vomiting, constipation, dyspepsia, achalasia, gastroparesis, GERD, irritable bowel syndrome (IBS), inflammatory bowel disease (Crohn's disease and ulcerative colitis), dysphagia, and medication-induced GI injury. This chapter also discusses guidelines for safe use of these medications and important points regarding these medications to include in patient education.

APPENDIX

Medications Delivered by Iontophoresis and Phonophoresis

Joseph Murphy and Joseph Gallo

The rehabilitation specialist will encounter patients receiving medication therapies via special delivery methods known as iontophoresis and phonophoresis. This appendix introduces the use of these methods for delivering medications.

Iontophoresis

Iontophoresis is a commonly used electrophysical agent in the field of rehabilitation. It is a noninvasive method of transcutaneous drug delivery that uses low intensities of direct current to deliver medication. Iontophoresis facilitates or enhances the transport of ions transdermally into the subcutaneous tissue. The movement of **ions** into living tissue depends on the principle of electrostatic repulsion of like charges; this is the driving force of iontophoresis. Iontophoresis has gained popularity as a noninvasive alternative to needle injections in the treatment of various musculoskeletal conditions. The use of iontophoresis to deliver medications has several advantages, including avoidance of gastric upset, elimination of the need for syringe injections, and the ability to drive many different ions (drugs).

The iontophoresis device is a portable, battery-powered electrotherapy device that uses a type of electrical current called direct current (figure A.1). Three types of currents are used in electrotherapy: pulsed current, alternating current, and direct current. Iontophoresis cannot be delivered using pulsed current. Some limited research has focused on attempting to use alternating current to drive

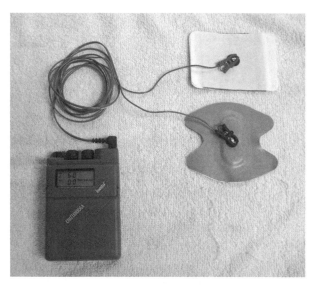

Figure A.1 Empi Dupel iontophoressor.
Courtesy of Joe Gallo.

medication; however, it has yet to be perfected and limited peer-reviewed research supports its use. For these reasons, alternating-current iontophoressors are not yet commercially available. Research has shown that direct current is effective in transporting medications through the skin and into the subcutaneous tissue. The rehabilitation specialist must take care to properly dose the direct current to avoid skin burns. Direct current is more concentrated than are pulsed or alternating current and therefore can be more caustic to the skin, especially in fair-skinned individuals.

Iontophoressors have two poles: the negative pole, which is termed the cathode, and the positive pole, which is termed the anode. Most manufacturers denote the cathode with black or with a negative (−) sign and the anode with red or with a positive (+) sign. The drug used in an iontophoresis treatment has either positive or negative polarity. Because iontophoresis is based on the principle of electrostatic repulsion (like charges repelling), the clinician must use the same polarity of current as the polarity of the medication being delivered. For example, the drug dexamethasone is negatively charged. Therefore, it must be driven by the cathode (negative pole). The like charges repel the drug through the **avascula**r outer portion of the skin (stratum corneum) into the more vascular subcutaneous tissue. Two electrodes are used to complete the electrical circuit.

The drug solution is placed under the active electrode (delivery electrode). The dispersive or return electrode, which is used to complete the electrical circuit, should be placed at least 4 in. (10.1 cm) from the delivery electrode to prevent current from bridging superficially over skin (figure A.2). The clinician must understand the tissue being targeted. Iontophoresis is generally limited to tissues that are within 2 cm of the surface of the skin (Starkey, 2004). The exact depth of penetration is not clear and likely depends on a host of variables related to the medication being delivered, the iontophoresis parameters used, and the physiology of the individual receiving the treatment (e.g., level of hydration of the skin, vascularity

of tissue, and so on). The reported depth of penetration of medications delivered iontophoretically varies by study and ranges from 3 to 20 mm (Glass et al., 1980). Because its depth of penetration is relatively superficial, iontophoresis cannot reach some deeper structures.

Direct current has certain physiologic effects even without the use of medications. The physiologic effects depend on whether the cathode or the anode is selected as the active electrode. Table A.1 lists the physiologic effects of direct current.

Table A.1   Physiologic Effects of Direct Current

Cathode (−)*	Anode (+)
Attracts positive ions	Attracts negative ions
Alkaline reaction occurs under electrode.	Acid (HCl) forms under electrode.
(NaOH is formed).	Increases density of protein (sclerotic effect).
Decreases density of protein (sclerotic effect).	Decreased nerve excitability via hyperpolarization.
Increases nerve excitability via depolarization.	Coagulation of microcirculation (capillary coagulation occurs).

*The cathode can be more caustic than the anode, resulting in an increased risk for skin burn due to alkaline reaction.

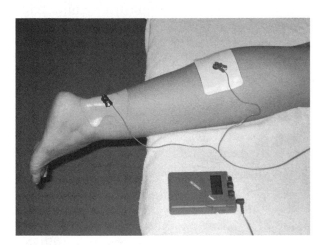

Figure A.2 Delivery of medication to the Achilles tendon through the drug-saturated active electrode. The dispersive electrode (larger square electrode) is placed over the lower calf.

Courtesy of Joe Gallo.

Current intensities used in iontophoresis range from 1.0 to 4.0 mA. Intensities between 2.5 and 3.0 mA are commonly used. Amplitude is dictated by patient tolerance, the pole driving the drug (e.g., the negative electrode is more caustic to the skin), the size of the electrode, and the duration of treatment.

Dosing Iontophoresis

The dosage of iontophoresis is measured in milliamperes per minute. The number of milliamps selected multiplied by the number of minutes determines the dosage. For example, 3 mA for a duration of 20 min equals a dose of 60 mA/min. Dosages used in iontophoresis range from 40 to 80 mA/min. Studies that report successful outcomes with iontophoresis commonly use doses in the range of 60 to 80 mA/min. These ranges have been suggested for clinical use, especially in instances when the patient is unresponsive to lower doses (Ciccone, 2008). The duration of treatment varies depending on the intensity selected. For example, if the clinician choses 3 mA as the treatment intensity, a dose of 60 mA/min will be administered for a total of 20 min (table A.2). Some patients cannot tolerate the higher current intensities and therefore require a lower intensity and, hence, a longer treatment time.

Table A.2   Current Intensity and Treatment Duration for Iontophoresis

Current intensity (mA)	Treatment duration (min)	Dose (mA/min)
1	60	60
2	30	60
3	20	60
4	15	60

A study by Panus and colleagues (1999) demonstrated that the delivery of ketoprofen (–) into pig skin was twice as much when 4 mA was used for 40 min (160 mA/min) compared with when 2 mA was used for 80 min (160 mA/min). The results of this study support using more milliamperes (if tolerated) over a shorter period of time to maximize drug delivery. Conversely, another study reports achieving effective drug delivery with low-intensity (0.05-0.16 mA), battery-powered 12 h iontophoresis patches (figure A.3) (Anderson et al., 2003). The traditional higher-intensity, shorter-duration iontophoresis treatments delivered from a portable iontophoressor continue to be widely used in the rehabilitation field. Additional research is necessary to determine optimal intensities and durations of iontophoresis treatment. Clinically, the iontophoresis patch systems (figure A.3) provide a low-dose, long-duration treatment option for individuals who are unable to tolerate traditional higher-intensity iontophoresis due to discomfort or adverse skin responses.

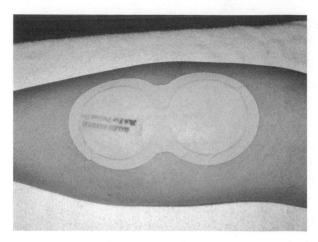

Figure A.3   Wireless iontopatch.
Courtesy of Joe Gallo.

Other Considerations

The rehabilitation specialist must keep in mind several additional considerations before using iontophoresis.

- Iontophoresis can either save costs or be an unnecessary expense. This depends largely on the clinician's ability to select patient cases that will likely respond to the medication used as well as the clinician's ability to monitor the patient's response to treatment closely so that treatment can be discontinued when the patient has achieved maximum benefit or when it becomes clear that the patient is nonresponsive. The single-use commercial electrodes and medication cost approximately $10/treatment.

- Buffers are built into the active electrode of commercially available iontophoresis electrodes to moderate alkaline and acidic pH values under the electrode. It is advisable to use only commercially available iontophoresis electrodes to minimize the chances of adverse skin responses.

- Driving two different ions (positive and negative) at the same time is not recommended. In the past, some clinicians have done this by changing the active pole halfway through treatment. It is advisable to choose only one drug to ensure maximum treatment effect. The medication must be prescribed by a licensed prescriber.

• Heating agents should not be used in conjunction with iontophoresis. The increased blood flow created by the heating agent may wash the drug out of the local area.

• Iontophoresis typically works more effectively in conditions involving superficial muscle, tendon, or bursa. However, treatment is not usually effective when the target tissue is deeper than 2 cm. For example, the patient with a supraspinatus tendinopathy and a large, well-developed deltoid may not be a good candidate for this treatment because it is unlikely that the medication will penetrate through the deltoid to the underlying **supraspinatus** muscle.

Contraindications to Iontophoresis

The rehabilitation specialist should keep in mind the following contraindications when using iontophoresis:

• Iontophoresis should not be used if any contraindications to the use of electrotherapy are present.

• Iontophoresis should not be used if the patient has a known drug allergy to the ion being used.

• Iontophoresis should not be used if there is a lack of sensation in the area to be treated.

• Iontophoresis should not be used if skin breakdown is present in the area to be treated.

• Iontophoresis should not be used if there is sensitivity to direct current (excessive skin irritation).

• Iodine (sclerolytic agent used to break down scar tissue) should not be used in patients with allergies to seafood.

• Zinc, copper, and magnesium-based medications should not be used in patients with sensitivities to metals.

• Salicylates should not be used in patients with known allergies to aspirin.

• Medications that would not normally be prescribed during pregnancy should not be delivered iontophoretically during pregnancy.

• Iontophoresis should not be delivered to the regions of the abdomen, low back, or pelvis during pregnancy.

• Iontophoresis should not be delivered over the temporal region or eyes.

• Iontophoresis should not be administered in the presence of any electrical devices implanted in the patient's body (e.g., pacemaker).

Application Technique

Because ions penetrate mainly through skin pores, hair follicles, and sebaceous glands, skin preparation is important. Before treatment, the rehabilitation specialist should test the patient's skin for sensation and inspect for any broken or damaged skin. Some clinicians advocate trimming or shaving excessive hair that is directly in the treatment area to improve conductivity and drug delivery. Areas that have been shaved should not be treated with iontophoresis until 24 h after shaving. The treatment area should be cleaned with an isopropyl alcohol swab to remove impurities that can decrease the conductance of electricity and potentially lead to skin irritation.

The drug solution is applied to the reservoir in the active electrode. Each size of electrode is designed to hold a manufacturer-suggested number of milliliters of medication. Once the active electrode is ready to be positioned over the target tissue, the clinician must be certain that the active electrode is in full contact with the skin. This will ensure that current density is uniform throughout the electrode and minimize the likelihood of discomfort or skin irritation.

The dispersive electrode should be placed at least 4 in. (10.1 cm) from the active electrode to prevent the current from bridging superficially over the skin. The rehabilitation specialist first selects a total dosage in milliamperes per minute and then sets the intensity. Intensities between 2.0 and 3.0 mA are commonly used. Higher intensities can be used in subsequent treatments based on the patient's response. Current intensity must be based on patient tolerance. The patient should feel a "pins and needles" sensation (some patients describe it as a prickly sensation) but should not feel any burning. Once the dosage and current intensity are set, the iontophoresis device automatically adjusts the treatment time to deliver the specified dosage. After treatment, the rehabilitation specialist should inspect the skin for any unusual irritation. Some skin redness in the area where the treatment was delivered is not reason for concern unless the redness does not resolve within 1 to 3 h after treatment. If the redness persists or any adverse skin response is present, iontophoresis should be discontinued. Some clinicians advocate treating mild skin irritation with aloe after the treatment session (Ciccone, 2008).

Medications Commonly Delivered Using Iontophoresis

The following section describes the polarity, indications, and physiologic effects of medications that the rehabilitation specialist commonly delivers iontophoretically. Additionally, table A.3 lists commonly used iontophoresis

Table A.3   Ions (Drugs) Delivered With Iontophoresis

Drug	Polarity	Indication	Concentration
Acetic acid	Negative (-)	Calcium deposits Myositic ossificans Calcific tendinopathy Bone spurs	2%-5% solution
Dexamethasone phosphate	Negative (-)	Acute inflammation	4% solution (4 mg/ml in aqueous solution)
Calcium chloride	Positive (+)	Skeletal muscle spasms	2% aqueous solution
Copper	Positive (+)	Fungal infection	2%
Hyaluronidase	Positive (+)	Subacute and chronic local edema	Reconstitute with 0.9% sodium chloride to provide 150 µg/ml solution
Iodine	Negative (-)	Scar tissue Adhesions Adhesive capsulitis (sclerolytic effect)	5% solution
Ketoprofen	Negative (-)	Chronic inflammation	2%-10% solution
Lidocaine	Positive (+)	Pain reliever (local anesthetic)	4%-5% solution
Magnesium Sulfate	Positive (+)	Muscle spasm or hyperexcitability (muscle relaxant), vasodilator	2% aqueous solution
Salicylates	Negative (-)	Inflammation and pain (aspirin-based medication with analgesic and anti-inflammatory effects)	2%-3% solution
Sodium salicylate	Negative (-)	Plantar wart	2% solution
Tap water	Negative/positive (-/+ depending on local water source)	Hyperhidrosis	

medications, as well as the polarity, concentration, and indication(s) for each of the ions.

Acetic Acid

Acetic acid is a negatively charged medication that is used to break down calcific deposits such as **myositis** ossificans and bone spurs. Gulick (2000) reported favorable results of acetic acid iontophoresis on reabsorption of heel spurs. Acetic acid has also been used to treat chronic tissue degeneration associated with **plantar fasciosis**. Researchers have theorized that chronically inflamed tissue develops a higher concentration of insoluble calcium carbonate that contributes to pain and scar tissue. Researchers further theorize that the acetic acid combines with the calcium carbonate to form a more soluble calcium acetate, which can be dissolved in the local blood circulation and removed from the injury site (Costa & Dyson, 2007). Japour and colleagues (1999) treated 35 patients experiencing chronic heel pain with acetic acid iontophoresis. In 94% of these patients, heel pain was completely or substantially relieved after an average of 5.7 sessions of acetic acid iontophoresis over an average period of 2.8 wk. The results of this study are consistent with more recent understanding of this condition. Based on histological studies, chronic heel pain and chronic tendinopathies are less likely to be related to inflammation and more likely to be related to degenerative changes in the plantar fascia or tendon. This helps explain why patients with acute plantar fasciitis or tendonitis often respond to anti-inflammatory medications but those with chronic plantar fascia or tendon conditions do not.

Treatment of Acute and Chronic Inflammation

Glucocorticoids are anti-inflammatory steroid medications. The glucocorticoid dexamethasone phosphate (−) is the medication most commonly delivered via iontophoresis (Gurney & Wascher, 2008). It is typically used in a 0.4% solution (4 mg/ml in aqueous solution). Because it is negatively charged, it should be put under the cathode so that it

can be driven into the subcutaneous tissue via electrostatic repulsion. A recent human-tissue biopsy study found that iontophoresis (40 mA/min dose) significantly enhanced the absorption of dexamethasone into the semitendinosus tendon compared with passive diffusion (Gurney & Wascher, 2008). The iontophoresis treatment was administered to the skin overlying the semitendinosus tendon before the tendon was harvested for use as a surgical graft for reconstruction of the anterior cruciate ligament. The tissue was extracted and analyzed for dexamethasone levels within 4 h of treatment. It would be of great interest in future studies to determine whether higher doses of iontophoresis (e.g., 60 mA/min dose) would yield a greater concentration of dexamethasone in the tissue compared with the 40 mA/min dose used in the present study.

Dexamethasone inhibits prostaglandin synthesis and inhibits the migration of scavenger white blood cells at the injury site. It is indicated in acute inflammatory conditions. A prescription for the medication must be obtained from a licensed prescriber, and a pharmacist or compound chemist prepares the solution. The unwanted potential side effects of dexamethasone include breakdown of tendon, muscle, bone, or other collagenous tissue and hormonal imbalances due to suppression of the adrenal gland. These side effects are typically not seen with judicious delivery of dexamethasone via iontophoresis. To minimize unwanted side effects, a minimum of one recovery day between iontophoresis treatments is recommended. It is advisable to avoid excessive iontophoresis treatments with dexamethasone. Generally, a course of six to eight treatments should provide desirable results. After three to four treatments, the clinician should know whether the patient is responding positively to the modality or medication. A study by Nirschl and colleagues (2003) showed decreased pain and tenderness in patients with lateral epicondylitis. This study and others show that dexamethasone iontophoresis provides short-term relief in acute inflammatory conditions such as lateral epicondylitis. In instances where no relief is achieved, the tissue may no longer be in an active inflammatory state but instead may be in a more chronic degenerative state, called tendinosis. The clinician must realize that a patient may not be responding to anti-inflammatory treatment because they do not have an acute inflammatory condition.

Ketoprofen

The nonsteroidal anti-inflammatory ketoprofen (2%-10%) has been gaining popularity as an alternative to dexamethasone. Ketoprofen is thought to be effective for the treatment of chronic inflammation. Iontophoretic delivery of ketoprofen has been demonstrated in rats, pig skin models, and human cadaver skin (Banga, 2011). Although human studies are limited, Panus and colleagues (1997) reported transdermal iontophoretic delivery of ketoprofen into the wrist of human subjects. Ketoprofen was detected in blood samples from the veins of the ipsilateral arm 40 min after treatment and in urine samples taken 16 h postiontophoresis.

Iodine

Use of iodine iontophoresis has been advocated for the treatment of scar tissue and adhesions (Tannenbaum, 1980). Because iodine is negatively charged, it should be driven from the cathode (negative pole). Iodine is believed to have a sclerolytic effect. It is possible to achieve positive results in breaking down scar tissue using iodine iontophoresis; however, the clinician must verify that sensation is intact over the scar tissue to avoid burning the patient's skin.

Table A.3 outlines medications that are commonly delivered iontophoretically. Additional research is necessary to further identify best practices of iontophoresis and drug selection for different conditions. Research is evolving in using iontophoresis to deliver a wide range of other molecules, including insulin, leuprolide, calcitonin analogs, cyclosporine, and beta blockers (Cameron, 2009).

Phonophoresis

Phonophoresis (figure A.4) is the use of therapeutic ultrasound to deliver medication into human tissue. The application of ultrasound in conjunction with a topical drug preparation as part of the conduction medium was first introduced in the 1950s and largely focused on using hydrocortisone-based creams, which were later found to be an ineffective transmission medium for ultrasound. Today a variety of analgesics and anti-inflammatory medications are commonly used as phonophoresis agents. The properties of ultrasound energy enhance drug delivery by facilitating increased permeability of the skin, enhancing diffusion into the subcutaneous tissue, and allowing the medication to be picked up into microcirculation. Ultrasound gel is considered the gold standard for transmitting ultrasound energy; it transmits up to 96% of the ultrasound energy (Cameron & Monroe, 1992). The prescriber must select a medication that transmits ultrasound energy effectively (see table A.4). If the ultrasound waves cannot transmit through the coupling agent that is below the ultrasound transducer head, the ultrasound energy will not be able to reach the skin interface to enhance the delivery of the medication. Properly selected and prepared phonophoresis medications are often mixed with ultrasound gel to enhance medication delivery. Other medications have adequate properties and can transmit ultrasound without being mixed into ultrasound gel. Cameron and Monroe (1992) evaluated the transmission of commonly used coupling media and medications. The results are presented in table A.5 (see

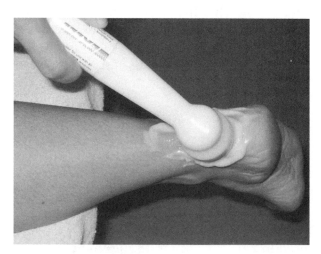

Figure A.4   Phonophoresis.
Courtesy of Joe Gallo.

Table A.4 Commonly Used Phonophoresis Medications

Medication	Concentration (%)	Indication
Corticosteroids		
Dexamethasone in ultrasound gel	0.4	Inflammation
Fluocinonide (Lidex gel)	0.05	Inflammation
Betamethasone 0.05% in ultrasound gel	0.05	Inflammation
Nonsteroidal anti-inflammatory drugs		
Ketoprofen	2-10	Inflammation
Ibuprofen	2-5	Inflammation
Trolamine salicylate	10	Inflammation
Sodium salicylate	3	Inflammation
Methyl salicylate (Thera-Gesic cream)	15	Inflammation
Diclofenac (Voltaren)	1	Inflammation
Analgesics		
Lidocaine	5	Pain, trigger points
Biofreeze (topical analgesic) mixed 1:1 with ultrasound gel	Menthol 3.5 and camphor 0.2	Pain, superficial counterirritant

later in this appendix). The data is important because it allows clinicians to choose coupling agents that effectively transmit ultrasound and avoid those that are poor transmitters of ultrasound.

Application Technique

The standard and most widely used application technique for phonophoresis is performed the same as when using standard gel as a coupling media. The medication is applied liberally on the surface of the skin over the target tissue, and the ultrasound transducer head is slowly moved over the local area at a rate of 2 to 6 cm/s (figure A.4). The total treatment area should not exceed approximately two times the size of the ultrasound transducer head. Treating areas larger than this is likely to minimize the effectiveness of the treatment. A recent study by Saliba and colleagues (2007) advocated for an alternative application technique. The authors delivered a 2 g dose of 0.33% dexamethasone cream by applying it to the skin over the forearm and covering it with a Tegaderm occlusive dressing for 30 min before beginning the phonophoresis treatment. The occlusive dressing remained in place for the duration of the treatment. Standard ultrasound gel was applied over the top of the occlusive dressing and the ultrasound treatment was completed (3 MHz, 1.0 W/cm^2, 5 min). The occlusive dressing was removed immediately after treatment. The total concentration of dexamethasone in the serum was higher in subjects receiving dexamethasone phonophoresis than in those receiving passive diffusion (sham ultrasound, 0.0 W/cm^2). The drug concentration increased over time after treatment was completed and was still elevated at 10 h posttreatment.

A third application technique that has been used clinically involves gently rubbing the cream or ointment-based medication into the skin and then applying ultrasound gel over it before administering the ultrasound. Little data is available to support this application method. The use of this method is more likely related to the past widespread use of hydrocortisone creams that did not transmit ultrasound; this method was advocated in an attempt to mitigate the poor transmission properties of the medication. Further research is necessary to determine the application technique that best optimizes phonophoretic delivery of medications.

Ultrasound Parameters for Phonophoresis

In the past, the transdermal delivery of medication with ultrasound was believed to be mostly related to the thermal effects of ultrasound. This formed the basis for the practice of using continuous-mode ultrasound (thermal ultrasound) to deliver medications. More recent research indicates that the nonthermal effects of ultrasound, including stable cavitation, microstreaming, and enhanced permeability of the skin membrane, are the more likely mechanisms for transdermal drug delivery via phonophoresis (Cagnie et al., 2003). Researchers now believe that the transmission of medication occurs largely through increased permeability of the skin and by subcutaneous microcirculation. The use of either 1 or 3 MHz pulsed ultrasound (20% duty cycle), 0.5 to 0.75 W/cm^2, for 5 to 10 min has been advocated for phonophoresis applications (Cameron, 2009). Researchers believe that these parameters maximize skin permeability to help get the drug into microcirculation. Furthermore, because this application is commonly used to treat acute and subacute inflammatory conditions, these parameters are prudent in that they minimize unwanted increases in tissue temperature associated with thermal ultrasound. Increased tissue temperature and blood flow could aggravate acute conditions and theoretically may wash the drug out of the local area. Gallo and colleagues (2004) found that 3 MHz continuous ultrasound (100% duty cycle) at 0.5 W/cm^2 produced the same temperature increase at 2 cm depth in the human gastrocnemius muscle as 3 MHz pulsed ultrasound with a duty cycle of 50% and an intensity of 1.0 W/cm^2; both treatments were delivered for 10 min. The authors concluded that clinicians should take caution to select a sufficiently low duty cycle (e.g., 20% duty cycle) and intensity (e.g., ≤0.5 W/cm^2) to prevent inadvertent heating and increased blood flow to acute inflammatory conditions. It is plausible that if too much heating were to occur during phonophoresis, the increased blood flow and increases in local metabolism may wash the drug out of the intended area of delivery. Further research is needed to determine optimal parameters for delivering phonophoresis.

Phonophoresis Medications and Coupling Media

A pharmacist specializing in compound chemistry should prepare phonophoresis coupling media. In many instances the drug is mixed into standard ultrasound gel in the correct formulation. In other instances the medication is already in a medium that effectively transmits ultrasound. The prescribing physician or other licensed prescriber and the rehabilitation professional must screen the patient for drug allergies and negative drug interactions that may occur with other medications the patient is taking.

The clinician should choose only phonophoresis coupling agents that transmit ultrasound waves (see table A.5). Not all phonophoresis agents meet this criterion. For example, hydrocortisone has a poor transmission rate of between 0% and 36% (Cameron & Monroe, 1992).

Research in the area of phonophoresis agents has been conflicting. Many of the early studies explored the use of hydrocortisone as a phonophoresis medication. Based on the work of Cameron and Monroe (1992), it is now clear that hydrocortisone is not an effective coupling agent for use in phonophoresis. As a result, dexamethasone (corticosteroid) became a popular phonophoresis medication for treating inflammatory conditions. Dexamethasone mixed with ultrasound transmission gel was found to have ultrasound transmission quality of 95% to 98% (Byl et al., 1993). Concern exists about excessive use of dexamethasone as a phonophoresis agent. Six or fewer treatments of dexamethasone has not been shown to cause adrenal suppression and has been deemed a safe number of treatments (Franklin et al., 1995). In the past, clinicians tended to overuse dexamethasone in treating inflammatory conditions. Currently, ketoprofen has gained popularity as a nonsteroidal anti-inflammatory for treating chronic inflammatory musculoskeletal conditions.

Table A.5 Ultrasound Transmission by Phonophoresis Media

Product	Transmission relative to water (%)
Good transmission	
Fluocinonide 0.05% (Lidex gel)[a]	97
Methyl salicylate 15% (Thera-Gesic cream)[b]	97
Mineral oil[c]	97
Ultrasound gel[d]	96
Ultrasound lotion[e]	90
Betamethasone 0.05%[f] in ultrasound gel[d]	88
Poor transmission	
Betamethasone 0.5% (Diprolene ointment)[g]	36
Hydrocortisone powder 1%[b] in ultrasound gel[d]	29
Hydrocortisone powder 10%[b] in ultrasound gel[d]	7
Hydrocortisone 1% (Cortril ointment)[i]	0
Eucerin cream[j]	0
Hydrocortisone cream 10%[k]	0
Hydrocortisone cream 10%[k] mixed with equal weight ultrasound gel[d]	0
Trolamine salicylate 10% (Myoflex cream)[l]	0
Triamcinolone acetonide cream 0.1%[k]	0
Velva hydrocortisone cream 10%[h]	0
Velva hydrocortisone cream 10%[h] mixed with equal weight ultrasound gel[d]	0
White petrolatum[m]	0
Other	
Chempad-L[n]	68
Polyethylene wrap[o]	98

[a]Syntex Laboratories Inc., 3401 Hillview Ave., P.O. Box 10850, Palo Alto, CA 94303.

[b]Mission Pharmacal Co., 1325 E. Durango, San Antonio, TX 78210.

[c]Pennex Corp., Eastern Avenue at Pennex Drive, Verona, PA 15147.

[d]Ultraphonic, Pharmaceutical Innovations Inc., 897 Frelinghuysen Dr., Newark, NJ 07114.

[e]Polysonic, Parker Laboratories Inc., 307 Washington St., Orange, NJ 07114.

[f]Pharmfair Inc., 110 Kennedy Dr., Haupauge, NY 11788.

[g]Schering Corp., 2000 Galloping Hill Rd., Kenilworth, NJ 07033.

[h]Purepace Pharmaceutical Co., 200 Elmora Ave., Elizabeth, NJ 07207.

[i]Pfizer Labs Division, Pfizer Inc., 235 E. 42nd St., New York, NY 10017.

[j]Beiersdorf Inc., P.O. Box 5529, Norwalk, CT 06856-5529.

[k]E. Fougera & Co., 60 Baylis Rd., Melville, NY 11747.

[l]Rorer Consumer Pharmaceuticals, Division of Rhone-Poulenc Rorer Pharmaceuticals Inc., 500 Virginia Dr., Fort Washington, PA 19034.

[m]Universal Cooperatives Inc., 7801 Metro Pkway., Minneapolis, MN 55425.

[n]Henley International, 104 Industrial Blvd., Sugar Land, TX 77478.

[o]Saran Wrap, Dow Brands Inc., 9550 Zionsville Rd., Indianapolis, IN 46268.

Reprinted from Cameron, M.H. and Monroe, L.G., "Relative transmission of ultrasound by media customarily used for phonophoresis," *Physical Therapy* 72(2): 142-148, with permission of the American Physical Therapy Association. This material is copyrighted, and any further reproduction or distribution required written permission from APTA.

Compared with oral intake, phonophoresis delivers a higher concentration of medication to the local target tissue and eliminates gastric upset associated with oral intake of certain medications. Phonophoresis can also be a good alternative to painful injections. It is less costly than iontophoresis because costly electrodes are unnecessary. The pulsed ultrasound makes the skin more permeable, and the medication is transported through the skin as a result. The clinician must be aware that the drug will travel systemically once it enters through the skin. Therefore, the patient must be screened for drug allergies and sensitivities. Also, medications that would not be prescribed during pregnancy should also not be delivered via phonophoresis. In addition, if a patient is already taking a medication, the same medication should not be delivered phonophoretically due to the risk of compounding the adverse effects of the medication. For example, a patient who is taking corticosteroids to treat asthma should not be administered additional dexamethasone via phonophoresis to treat a musculoskeletal condition (Cameron, 2009). Because therapeutic ultrasound is used to deliver medication, the patient should also be screened for all contraindications to therapeutic ultrasound.

Some have been skeptical about whether phonophoresis could effectively deliver medications to the subcutaneous tissue. Darrow and colleagues (1999) found no detectable level of dexamethasone in the blood at 15 and 30 min after phonophoretic delivery of dexamethasone. Cagnie and colleagues (2003) performed a study that shed light on one reason why previous studies were not able to isolate significant amounts of phonophoretically driven medications in the blood or urine. They administered 2.5% ketoprofen (Fastum gel) to the knee via phonophoresis 1 h before arthroscopic knee surgery. At the time of surgery, a tissue biopsy was taken of the synovium of the knee. Significant concentrations of ketoprofen were found in the synovium whereas negligible amounts were found in the blood (measured 2 h posttreatment), indicating that the drug does transmit into the subcutaneous tissue and that it initially stays local. According to the work of Ballerini and colleagues (1986), ketoprofen concentration in plasma does not reach a peak until the 6th h after topical application and remains constant until the 12th h after treatment. Cagnie and colleagues (2003) further identified that pulsed ultrasound produced consistently higher drug concentrations (1 MHz, 20% duty cycle, 1.5 W/cm², 5 min) compared with continuous ultrasound (1 MHz, 100% duty cycle, 1.5 W/cm², 5 min). Based on this research, it is not surprising that ketoprofen has gained popularity as a nonsteroidal anti-inflammatory agent for treating subacute and chronic inflammation.

Analgesics

Although not all topical analgesics are effective ultrasound coupling agents, some research has been carried out on several over-the-counter topical analgesics. Myrer and colleagues (2001) compared Biofreeze (menthol 3.5%) mixed 1:1 with ultrasound gel with Nature's Chemist (menthol 16%) mixed 1:1 with ultrasound gel. It is believed that topical analgesics such as these modulate pain largely by stimulating the cutaneous receptors and thus creating a counterirritant effect. The researchers concluded that both preparations were effective coupling agents with good transmission of ultrasound similar to the ultrasound gel. No data were collected to determine whether any of the active ingredient(s) of either topical analgesic made it into the subcutaneous tissue. For this reason, these agents likely are better classified as topical analgesics that transmit ultrasound effectively rather than as phonophoresis agents. Although both of these topical analgesics transmit ultrasound effectively, no compelling evidence to date suggests that using them as a coupling agent adds any benefit over simply applying the topical after the ultrasound treatment. Thera-Gesic (methyl salicylate 15%) is an over-the-counter preparation that has been shown to transmit therapeutic ultrasound effectively (97% transmission). Because this product is salicylate based, it should not be used as coupling media or a phonophoresis agent in individuals with aspirin allergies. If the medication does cross through the skin into the subcutaneous tissue, the drug can become systemic.

Clinicians commonly ask which mode of drug delivery—iontophoresis or phonophoresis—is more effective. The research available to date makes a case that each is a promising method of drug delivery. Additional studies comparing the two methods are necessary to better determine best practices for each modality. Future iontophoresis and phonophoresis studies should focus on identifying the optimal dosages of electricity and ultra-sound to effectively deliver medications to the subcutaneous tissue for specific clinical conditions. Additional research is also necessary to determine which medications and concentrations are most effective in creating clinically meaningful physiologic changes that enhance or accelerate recovery from specific musculoskeletal conditions. Finally, continued research focusing on the efficacy of these systems for delivering medications in the treatment of nonmusculoskeletal conditions is necessary.

GLOSSARY

ablation—Removal of a body part or the destruction of its function by a surgical procedure, morbid process, or presence or application of a noxious substance.

acetaminophen—A medicine used to relieve pain and reduce fevers.

acetylcholine—A derivative of choline that is released at the ends of nerve fibers in the somatic and parasympathetic nervous systems and is involved in the transmission of nerve impulses in the body.

achalasia—Failure of a range of muscle fibers to relax; refers especially to visceral openings (e.g., the pylorus, cardia, or other sphincter muscles).

actin—One of the protein components in muscle into which actinomyocin can be split; acts with myosin in muscle contraction.

action tremors—Tremors associated with a voluntary muscle contraction.

acute coronary syndrome—A general term for clinical syndromes caused by reduced blood flow in coronary arteries (e.g., unstable angina, acute myocardial infarction).

adenoma—A benign epithelial neoplasm of epithelial tissue in which the tumor cells form glands or glandlike structures in the stroma.

adipose—Of, relating to, or comprising animal fat.

adynamic ileus—Nonmechanical bowel obstruction.

agonist—A substance that can combine with a cell receptor to produce a reaction typical of that substance.

agoraphobia—Fear of open spaces.

agranulocytosis—An acute condition characterized by pronounced leukopenia and a great reduction in the number of polymorphonuclear leukocytes (frequently less than 500 granulocytes/cm^3). Infected ulcers are likely to develop in the throat, intestinal tract, and other mucous membranes as well as the skin.

akathisia—Muscular restlessness characterized by the inability to sit still, often subsequent to administration of neuroleptic drugs.

akinesia—Slowness or loss of normal motor function that results in impaired muscle movement.

aldosterone—The steroid hormone secreted by the adrenal cortex that regulates the salt and water balance in the body.

aldosteronism—A disorder marked by excessive secretion of the hormone aldosterone, which can cause weakness, cardiac irregularities, and abnormally high blood pressure.

allodynia—Pain that results from a noninjurious stimulus to the skin.

amino acid—Any of various organic acids that contain both an amino group and a carboxyl group, especially any of the 20 or more compounds that link together to form proteins.

amphetamine—A colorless, volatile liquid used primarily as a central nervous system stimulant.

amygdala—An almond-shaped mass of gray matter in the front part of the temporal lobe of the cerebrum.

amyloid—Starch-like deposit resulting from tissue degeneration.

anaerobic—Living without oxygen.

analgesic—A medication capable of reducing or eliminating pain.

anaphylactic shock—A severe, sometimes fatal allergic reaction characterized by a severe decrease in blood pressure and difficulty breathing.

anastomosis—An opening created between two or more normally separate spaces or organs by surgery, trauma, or disease.

anemia—Any condition in which the number of red blood cells per cubic millimeter, the amount of hemoglobin in 100 ml of blood, or the volume of packed red blood cells per 100 ml of blood are less than normal.

aneurysm—Circumscribed dilation of an artery or cardiac chamber in direct communication with the lumen, usually resulting from an acquired or congenital weakness of the wall of the artery or chamber.

angina—A severe, often constricting pain or sensation of pressure; usually refers to angina pectoris.

angiotensin—Any of a group of peptides with vasoconstrictive activity that functions physiologically in controlling arterial pressure.

anhedonia—Absence of pleasure from the performance of acts that would normally be pleasurable.

ankylosing spondylitis—Arthritis of the spine that may progress to bony ankylosis and ossification of the anterior and posterior longitudinal ligaments; resembles rheumatoid arthritis.

anomia—Difficulty finding words.

anorexia nervosa—A psychophysiological disorder characterized by fear of becoming obese, a distorted self-image, a persistent aversion to food, and severe weight loss; often marked by hyperactivity, self-induced vomiting, and other physiological changes.

antacid—Medication used to counteract acidity, particularly in the stomach.

antagonist—Something (e.g., a muscle, disease, or physiological process) that neutralizes or impedes the action or effect of another.

anterograde amnesia—A condition in which the patient cannot recall events that occurred after the onset of amnesia.

antianxiety agent—Any of several drugs used to treat anxiety without causing excessive sedation.

antibacterial—Any of several drugs used to destroy or inhibit the growth of bacteria.

antibiotic—A substance that can destroy or inhibit the growth of other microorganisms.

anticholinergic—An agent that is antagonistic to the action of parasympathetic or other cholinergic nerve fibers.

anticoagulant—A substance that delays or prevents the clotting of blood.

anticonvulsant—A drug that prevents or relieves convulsions.

antidepressant—A drug used to prevent or relieve mental depression.

antidiarrheal—A medication used to prevent or treat diarrhea.

antidiuretic hormone—A nonapeptide neurohypophyseal hormone obtained from the posterior lobe of the pituitary that causes water retention and contraction of smooth muscle, notably that of all blood vessels; also called vasopressin and pitressin.

antiemetic—A medication that prevents vomiting.

antifungal—A medication that destroys or inhibits the growth of fungi.

antigen—A toxin or other foreign substance that induces an immune response in the body, especially the production of antibodies.

antihistamine—Any of several drugs used to counteract the physiological effects of histamine; usually used to treat allergic reactions.

antimetabolite—A substance that closely resembles an essential metabolite and competes with, interferes with, or replaces the metabolite in physiological reactions.

antipsychotic—Any of several drugs used to diminish the symptoms of a psychotic disorder (e.g., schizophrenia, paranoia, or manic–depressive psychosis).

antipyretic—An agent that reduces or prevents fever.

antispasmodic—A drug used to prevent or relieve convulsions or spasms.

anxiolytic—An agent that relieves anxiety.

arrhythmia—Loss or abnormality of rhythm; especially denotes an irregularity of the heartbeat.

arteriosclerosis—A group of diseases characterized by a thickening and loss of elasticity of the arterial walls.

articular—Of or relating to a joint or joints.

aspiration—The drawing of a foreign substance, such as the gastric contents, into the respiratory tract during inhalation.

asthenia—Loss or lack of bodily strength.

asthma—An inflammatory disease of the lungs characterized by (in most cases) reversible airway obstruction.

ataxia—Loss of the ability to coordinate muscle movement.

atherosclerosis—Arteriosclerosis characterized by irregularly distributed lipid deposits in the intima of large and medium arteries; causes narrowing of arterial lumens and eventually proceeds to fibrosis and calcification.

atonic—Relating to, caused by, or exhibiting lack of muscle tone.

atrial fibrillation—Fibrillation in which the normal rhythmical contractions of the cardiac atria are replaced by rapid irregular twitching of the muscular wall that causes the ventricles to respond irregularly.

autolysis—The destruction of tissues or cells of an organism by the action of substances such as enzymes that are produced within the organism.

autonomic nervous system—Part of the nervous system that regulates involuntary movement (e.g., the smooth muscles, heart, and intestines). This system is divided into two parts: the sympathetic nervous system and the parasympathetic nervous system.

avascular—Not associated with or supplied by blood vessels.

axon—The usually long process of a nerve fiber that generally conducts impulses away from the body of the nerve cell.

bacteria—A unicellular prokaryotic microorganism that usually multiplies by cell division and has a cell wall that provides a constancy of form. Bacteria may be aerobic or anaerobic, motile or nonmotile, and free living, saprophytic, commensal, parasitic, or pathogenic.

barbiturate—Barbituric acid derivative that acts as a central nervous system depressant.

Barrett's esophagus—Metaplasia of the lower esophagus that is characterized by replacement of squamous epithelium with columnar epithelium.

B-cell—An immunologically important lymphocyte that is not thymus dependent, is short lived, and is responsible for the production of immunoglobulins. It is the precursor of the plasma cell and expresses, but does not release, surface immunoglobulins. It does not play a direct role in cell-mediated immunity.

benzodiazepine—Any of a group of psychotropic agents used as antianxiety agents, muscle relaxants, sedatives, and hypnotics.

bezoar—A hard, indigestible mass of material formed in the alimentary canal.

bisphosphonate—Class of drugs that prevent the loss of bone mass.

blood–brain barrier—A protective network of blood vessels and cells that filters blood flowing to the brain.

bradycardia—A slowing of the heart rate.

bradykinesia—Extreme slowness in movement.

bradykinin—A biologically active polypeptide that forms from a blood plasma globulin and mediates the inflammatory response, increases vasodilation, and causes contraction of the smooth muscle.

bronchiole—Smaller, tubular extensions of the bronchus.

bronchospasm—A contraction of smooth muscle in the walls of the bronchi and bronchioles that causes narrowing of the lumen.

cachexia—Weight loss, wasting of muscle, loss of appetite, and general debility that can occur with a chronic disease.

calcitonin—A peptide hormone produced by the parathyroid, thyroid, and thymus glands; its action is opposite to that of parathyroid hormone in that calcitonin increases deposition of calcium and phosphate in bone and lowers the level of calcium in blood.

calorimetry—Measurement of the amount of heat produced or absorbed in a chemical reaction, change of state, or formation of a solution; used to determine nutritional needs.

cancer—General term frequently used to indicate any of various types of malignant neoplasms, most of which invade surrounding tissues, may metastasize to several sites, and are likely to recur after attempted removal and to kill the patient unless adequately treated.

cannabinoid—Organic substance present in cannabis (marijuana).

carbuncle—An abscess larger than a boil.

cardiac arrhythmia—Abnormality in cardiac activation.

cardiomegaly—Cardiac enlargement.

catabolism—The breakdown of complex substances such as muscle tissue into simpler substances.

catatonia—An abnormal condition associated with schizophrenia; characterized by stupor, mania, and rigidity.

catecholamines—Neurotransmitters that are chemically related; include epinephrine, norepinephrine, and dopamine.

chelate—To remove a heavy metal (e.g., lead or mercury) from the bloodstream by means of another substance that binds the metal.

chemoreceptor—A site of action that reacts to chemical stimuli such as a neurotransmitter or medication.

cholinergic—Relating to nerve cells or fibers that employ acetylcholine as the neurotransmitter.

choreoathetoid movements—Abnormal choreic (irregular migrating contraction) or atheroid (twisting and writhing) movements.

chronic bronchitis—A condition of the bronchial tree characterized by cough, hypersecretion of mucus, and expectoration of sputum over a long period of time; associated with frequent bronchial infections. Usually caused by inhalation, over a prolonged period, of air contaminated by dust or noxious gases of combustion.

chronic obstructive pulmonary disease—General term used for diseases that cause permanent or temporary narrowing of small bronchi in which forced expiratory flow is slowed. Term is especially used when no etiologic or more specific term can be applied.

chronotropic—Affecting the rate of rhythmic movements (e.g., the heartbeat).

claudication—Severe, cramp-like pain that occurs in the legs or arms during exercise.

clonus—A form of movement marked by contractions and relaxations of a muscle, occurring in rapid succession, after forcible extension or flexion of a body part.

cognition—A group of mental processes that includes attention, memory, producing and understanding language, learning, reasoning, problem solving, and decision making.

cogwheel rigidity—Rigidity in which the muscles respond with cogwheel-like jerks, as in Parkinson's disease.

conditioned responses—A new or modified response elicited by a stimulus after conditioning.

congestive heart failure—Inadequacy of the heart to maintain the circulation of blood. Congestion and edema develop in the tissues as a result.

conjugation—The temporary union of two bacterial cells.

coronary artery disease—Narrowing of the lumen of one or more of the coronary arteries, usually due to atherosclerosis or myocardial ischemia. Can cause congestive heart failure, angina pectoris, or myocardial infarction.

coronary heart disease—A narrowing of the small blood vessels that supply blood and oxygen to the heart.

corticosteroid—Any of the steroid hormones produced by the adrenal cortex or their synthetic equivalents.

creatinine—A nitrogenous organic acid found in muscle tissue that is used as a measurement of renal function.

cryotherapy—The local or general reduction of temperature in medical therapy by applying cold to reduce inflammation or slow metabolic processes.

Cushing's syndrome—A syndrome caused by increased production of adrenocorticotropic hormone (ACTH) from a tumor in the adrenal cortex or of the anterior lobe of the pituitary gland.

cyanosis—A dark-bluish or purplish discoloration of the skin and mucous membrane due to deficient oxygenation of the blood. Evident when reduced hemoglobin in the blood exceeds 5 g/100 ml.

cystitis—Inflammation of the urinary bladder.

cytokines—Any of numerous hormone-like, low-molecular-weight proteins, secreted by various cell types, that regulate the intensity and duration of immune response and mediate cell-to-cell communication.

cytotoxic—Relating to, or producing, a toxic effect on cells.

declarative memory—Recall of episodic, semantic, and lexical memories.

decongestant—A medication or treatment that reduces swelling and congestion, usually of the sinuses.

deglutition—The act of swallowing.

dehiscence—A bursting open or splitting along natural or sutured lines.

demyelination—The destruction or removal of the outside protective myelin sheath of a nerve fiber.

dendrite—Any of the various branched extensions of a nerve cell that conduct impulses from adjacent cells in toward the body of the nerve cell.

depolarization—The initiation of an electrical impulse by elimination or neutralization of polarity in nerve cells.

diabetes mellitus—A chronic metabolic disorder in which the use of carbohydrate is impaired and the use of lipid and protein is enhanced. It is caused by an absolute or relative deficiency of insulin and is characterized, in more severe cases, by chronic hyperglycemia, glycosuria, water and electrolyte loss, ketoacidosis, and coma. Long-term complications include neuropathy, retinopathy, nephropathy, generalized degenerative changes in large and small blood vessels, and increased susceptibility to infection.

diabetic ketoacidosis—Buildup of ketones in blood due to breakdown of stored fats for energy; a complication of diabetes mellitus. Untreated, it can lead to coma and death.

diaphoresis—Acute and profuse perspiration.

diplopia—Double vision.

diuresis—Promotion of increased production of urine.

diuretic—Any substance that increases diuresis.

dopamine—A monoamine (catecholamine) neurotransmitter, formed in the brain, that is essential to the normal functioning of the central nervous system.

drug compartment—Where a medication eventually collects in the body after the bloodstream delivers it to the tissues.

drug receptor—Any part of a cell, usually a large protein molecule, on the cell surface or in the cytoplasm with which a drug molecule interacts to trigger a response or effect.

dysarthria—Difficulty articulating words due to emotional stress or to paralysis, incoordination, or spasticity of the muscles used in speaking.

dysesthesias—Impairment of sensation, especially that of touch.

dyskinesia—Impairment of the ability to control movements; characterized by spasmodic or repetitive motions or lack of coordination.

dyslipidemia—An abnormal amount of lipids in the blood.

dysmetria—Inability to control the range of motion of movement in muscular activity.

dyspepsia—Indigestion.

dysphagia—Difficulty in swallowing.

dysphoria—An emotional state characterized by anxiety and depression.

dyspnea—Shortness of breath or difficulty breathing.

dysprosody—Speech disorder characterized by alterations in the intensity, timing and rhythm, cadence, or intonation of words.

dystonia—Abnormal increase in tonicity of tissue.

dysuria—Difficult or painful urination.

echolalia—The immediate and involuntary repetition of words and phrases just spoken by others; often a symptom of autism or some types of schizophrenia.

ectopic focus—An irritable zone of myocardium capable of initiating ectopic beats or assuming the function of a pacemaker.

edema—Accumulation of serous fluid in tissue spaces or a body cavity.

ejection fraction—The blood present in the ventricle at the end of diastole and expelled during the contraction of the heart.

embolus—A mass that travels in the bloodstream and lodges in a blood vessel, thus obstructing or occluding the vessel.

emesis—The act of vomiting.

emollient—Substance used to soften and sooth the skin.

emphysema—A condition of the lung characterized by increased size of the air spaces distal to the terminal bronchiole, with destructive changes in their walls and reduction in their number.

encoding—The first of three stages in the memory process, involving processes associated with receiving or registering stimuli through one or more of the senses and modifying that information.

endogenous—Originating in the body.

enteral—Administered via the gastrointestinal tract.

enteric—Relating to the intestinal tract.

enuresis—Involuntary discharge or leakage of urine.

epididymitis—Inflammation of the epididymis.

epigastric pain—Pain in the upper-middle region of the abdomen near the stomach.

epinephrine—A hormone of the adrenal medulla that is the most potent stimulant of the sympathetic nervous system. Causes increased heart rate increased force of contraction, and vasoconstriction.

episodic memory—A form of memory based on personal experience.

erythema—Redness of the skin caused by dilatation and congestion of the capillaries; most often a sign of inflammation and infection.

erythropoietin—A protein containing sialic acid that enhances erythropoiesis by stimulating the formation of proerythroblasts and release of reticulocytes from bone marrow. It is formed by the kidney and liver, and possibly by other tissues, and can be detected in human plasma and urine.

esophagitis—Inflammation of the esophagus.

ethanol—Ethyl alcohol or grain alcohol.

euphoria—A feeling of great happiness or well-being, commonly exaggerated and not necessarily well founded.

euvolemia—Presence of the normal amounts of fluids in the body.

exacerbation—Increased and usually acute symptoms or severity of a disease.

extrapyramidal—Relating to or involving neural pathways situated outside or independent of the pyramidal tracts of the brain.

extrapyramidal disease—A degenerative disease, such as parkinsonism or chorea, that affects the corpus striatum of the brain or other part of the extrapyramidal motor system and is characterized by tremor, muscular rigidity or weakness, and involuntary movements.

extrapyramidal motor system—Any of the various brain structures affecting bodily movement, excluding the motor neurons, the motor cortex, and the pyramidal tract and including the corpus striatum, its substantia nigra and subthalamic nucleus, and its connections with the midbrain.

exudate—A fluid that is exuded out of tissue or its capillaries due to injury, infection, or inflammation.

fasciculation—Involuntary contractions or twitching of groups of muscle fibers; a coarser form of muscular contraction than fibrillation.

fasciitis—Reactive proliferation of fibroblasts in fascia.

febrile—Of, relating to, or characterized by fever.

ferritin—An iron-containing protein complex found principally in the intestinal mucosa, liver, and spleen that functions as the primary form of iron storage for the body.

FEV1—The maximal volume that can be expired in a specific time interval when starting from maximal inspiration. A subscript annotation normally indicates the duration (in seconds) of expiration.

fibrillation—A small, local, involuntary, muscular contraction, due to spontaneous activation of single muscle cells or muscle fibers whose nerve supply has been damaged or cut off.

fibromyalgia—Fibromyalgia is a neurosensory disorder characterized by widespread muscle pain, joint stiffness, and fatigue.

first-pass effect—The metabolism of orally administered drugs by gastrointestinal and hepatic enzymes, resulting in a significant reduction of the amount of unmetabolized drug reaching the systemic circulation.

flank—The side of the body between the pelvis or hip and the last rib.

folliculitis—Inflammation of a follicle, especially a hair follicle.

frontal lobe—The largest portion of each cerebral hemisphere; anterior to the central sulcus.

fungus—A general term that encompasses the diverse morphologic forms of yeasts and molds. Fungi share with bacteria the important ability to break down complex organic substances of almost every type (cellulose) and are essential to the recycling of carbon and other elements in the cycle of life.

furuncles—Boils.

gamma amino butyric acid—An amino acid found in the central nervous system that is associated with transmission of inhibitory nerve impulses.

gangrene—Necrosis due to obstruction, loss, or diminution of blood supply. It may be localized to a small area or involve an entire extremity or organ (e.g., bowel), and may be wet or dry.

gastritis—Chronic or acute inflammation of the stomach, especially of the mucous membrane of the stomach.

gastroparesis—Mild paralysis of the muscular coat of the stomach.

gingival hyperplasia—An increase in the tissue elements and bulk of the gum tissue.

glomerulus—Olfactory nerve ending comprising a cluster of axon terminals and dendrites and the initial sites for olfactory processing. The renal glomerulus, which is surrounded by the Bowman's capsule in the kidney, is a capillary tuft that performs the first step in filtering blood for formation of urine.

glucagon—A hormone secreted by alpha cells in the liver that initiates an increase in blood sugar levels by stimulating the breakdown of glycogen by the liver.

glucocorticoids—Any steroid-like compound capable of promoting hepatic glycogen deposition and of exerting a clinically useful anti-inflammatory effect.

gluconeogenesis—Formation of glycogen from noncarbohydrates, such as protein or fat.

glucosuria—Excretion of glucose in the urine.

glutamate—An amino acid that functions as a neurotransmitter and promotes excitation of nerve function in the central nervous system.

glycogenolysis—The hydrolysis of glycogen to glucose.

goiter—A chronic enlargement of the thyroid gland, not due to a neoplasm, occurring endemically in certain localities (especially regions where glaciation occurred and the soil is low in iodine) and sporadically elsewhere.

gout—A disorder of purine metabolism, occurring especially in men, characterized by a raised but variable blood uric acid level and severe, recurrent acute arthritis resulting from deposition of sodium urate crystals in connective tissues and articular cartilage.

Graves' disease—Toxic goiter characterized by diffuse hyperplasia of the thyroid gland; a form of hyperthyroidism. Exophthalmos is a common, but not invariable, concomitant finding.

gynecomastia—Excessive development of the male mammary glands; sometimes causes the glands to secrete milk.

half-life—Time required for the level of a substance to decline to half its initial level.

hallucination—Perception in a conscious and awake state in the absence of external stimuli that has qualities of real perception in that it is vivid, substantial, and located in external objective space. Hallucinations may be visual, auditory, or olfactory.

Hashimoto's disease—An autoimmune disease of the thyroid gland resulting in diffuse goiter, infiltration of the thyroid gland, and hypothyroidism.

hematoma—A bruise or localized swelling filled with blood due to a break in a blood vessel.

hematuria—The abnormal presence of blood in the urine.

hepatolenticular degeneration—An inherited disorder of copper metabolism characterized by cirrhosis, generation of the basal ganglia, and deposition of green pigment in the periphery of the cornea.

hepatotoxic—Having the potential to cause, or causing, damage to the liver.

hirsutism—Excessive growth of facial or body hair in women.

histamine—A neurotransmitter that is a powerful stimulant of gastric secretion, constrictor of bronchial smooth muscle, and mediator of inflammatory changes associated with allergic reactions.

hydrolysis—Decomposition of a clinical compound by a chemical reaction upon exposure to water.

hyperalgesia—Extreme sensitivity to pain.

hypercapnia—An increased concentration of carbon dioxide in the blood; usually associated with a decline in respirations.

hyperglycemia—An abnormally high concentration of glucose in the circulating blood; seen especially in patients with diabetes mellitus.

hyperkalemia—An abnormally high concentration of potassium in the blood.

hyperlipidemia—Elevated levels of lipids in the blood plasma.

hyperplasia—Abnormal increase in tissue or organ cell size or mass.

hypertension—High blood pressure; transitory or sustained elevation of systemic arterial blood pressure to a level that is likely to induce cardiovascular damage or other adverse consequences. Hypertension has been arbitrarily defined as systolic blood pressure above 140 mm Hg or diastolic blood pressure above 90 mm Hg.

hypertensive crisis—Dangerously high blood pressure of acute onset.

hyperthyroidism—An abnormality of the thyroid gland in which secretion of thyroid hormone is usually increased and no longer under the regulatory control of hypothalamic–pituitary centers. Characterized by a hypermetabolic state, usually accompanied by weight loss, tremulousness, elevated plasma levels of thyroxine or tri-iodothyronine, and sometimes exophthalmos. May progress to severe weakness, wasting, hyperpyrexia, and other manifestations of thyroid storm. Often associated with Graves' disease.

hypertonia—Abnormal increase in muscle tension accompanied by the reduced ability of a muscle to stretch.

hypnotic—A medication or substance that induces sleep.

hypocalcemia—Lower-than-normal levels of calcium in the blood.

hypoglycemia—Symptoms resulting from low blood glucose (normal glucose range is 60-100 mg/dl or 3.3-5.6 mmol/L) that are either autonomic (include sweating, trembling, feelings of warmth, anxiety, and nausea) or neuroglycopenic (include feelings of dizziness, confusion, tiredness, difficulty speaking, headache, and inability to concentrate).

hyponatremia—Abnormally low concentration of sodium ions in the blood.

hypophonia—Soft speech due to discoordination of the vocal muscles.

hypothyroidism—Diminished production of thyroid hormone that leads to clinical manifestations of thyroid insufficiency, including low metabolic rate, tendency to gain weight, somnolence, and sometimes myxedema.

hypovolemic—Abnormally low levels of fluid in the body.

hypoxia—Insufficient oxygen in the blood; usually associated with difficulty breathing.

iatrogenic—Induced in a patient by a physician's activity, manner, or therapy.

idiopathic—A symptom or disease that has no known cause.

ileum—The third and terminal portion of the small intestine.

immunosuppressant—A substance or medication that suppresses the body's immune response.

inanition—Exhaustion or disease resulting from a lack of nourishment.

inotropic—A medication or substance that increases the contraction of cardiac muscle.

interleukin—The name given to a group of multifunctional cytokines after their amino acid structure is known. Interleukins are synthesized by lymphocytes, monocytes, macrophages, and certain other cells.

interstitial—Relating to or situated in the small, narrow spaces between tissues or parts of an organ.

intra-articular—Within the cavity of a joint.

intrathecal—Introduced into the space under the arachnoid membrane in the spinal cord.

ion—An atom or a group of atoms that has acquired a net electric charge by gaining (positive charge) or losing (negative charge) one or more electrons.

ionize—To dissociate noncharged atoms or molecules into positively or negatively electrically charged atoms or molecules, usually when exposed to water.

iontophoresis—The use of an electric current to introduce the ions of a medication into bodily tissues.

ischemia—Local loss of blood supply due to mechanical obstruction (mainly arterial narrowing or disruption) of the blood vessel.

ketoacidosis—Acidosis caused by the increased production of ketone bodies, as in diabetics with extremely high levels of glucose.

lacrimation—Excessive secretion of tears.

lassitude—A sense of weariness, lack of energy, or listlessness.

laxative—Having the action of loosening the bowels.

Lennox-Gastaut syndrome—A generalized myoclonic astatic epilepsy that occurs in children as a result of various cerebral afflictions such as perinatal hypoxia, hemorrhage, encephalitis, and maldevelopment of the brain.

leukocytosis—An abnormally large increase in the number of white blood cells in the blood that often occurs as a response to an acute infection.

leukopenia—An abnormally low number of white blood cells in the blood.

levodopa—The levorotatory form of dopa. Dopa is converted to the catecholamines norepinephrine, epinephrine, and dopamine. Levodopa is a medication used to treat Parkinson's disease.

Lewy bodies—Spherical, eosinophilic, intracellular structures found in the substantia nigra in patients with Parkinson's disease.

Lewy body dementia—Type of dementia closely allied to both Alzheimer's and Parkinson's diseases. It is characterized anatomically by the presence of Lewy bodies, clumps of alpha-synuclein, and ubiquitin protein in neurons, detectable in post-mortem brain biopsies.

lexical memory—Recall of words, organized by sound and meaning (e.g., able to judge a string of letters is a word).

lipophilic—Tending to collect and dissolve in fatty tissue (lipids).

lockout time—Setting on an infusion device that limits the frequency of doses delivered.

locus coeruleus—A blue area of the brain stem with many norepinephrine-containing neurons.

long-term memory—Recall of items considered to be permanently stored in memory.

lumen—An inner cavity of a tubular organ (e.g., a blood vessel).

Lyme disease—An inflammatory disease transmitted by ticks and characterized initially by symptoms including fever, joint pain, and headache. If untreated, it can result in chronic arthritis dysfunction of the nerves and heart.

lysis—The rupture or destruction of cells.

maceration—Destruction of the skin associated with the skin being consistently wet. The skin softens, turns white, and can be easily infected.

macronutrient—A nutrient required in large amounts for the normal growth and development of an organism (e.g., carbohydrates, proteins, fats).

maculopapular rash—A rash characterized by raised, spotted lesions.

malignant hyperthermia—Life-threatening adverse reaction to the use of anesthetics and antipsychotic medications that includes rapid onset of extremely high fever and muscle rigidity.

masked facies—Lacking in facial expression as typically seen with Parkinson's disease.

megarectum—Abnormal dilation of rectum that interferes with normal rectal function and bowel movements.

metabolic autoinduction—Ability of a drug to induce enzymes that enhance its own metabolism.

metabolism—Refers to all the physical and chemical processes in the body that convert or use energy.

metabolite—A substance produced by metabolism by the body's enzyme systems or the liver.

metacognition—Ability to know one's cognitive status. Some degree of metacognition must be present for there to be improvement in cognitive deficits.

metastasis—The spread of a disease process from one part of the body to another, as in the appearance of neoplasms in parts of the body remote from the site of the primary tumor. Results from dissemination of tumor cells by the lymphatics or blood vessels or by direct extension through serous cavities or subarachnoid or other spaces.

microbe—A microorganism, especially a bacterium that causes disease.

miosis—Constriction of the pupil of the eye resulting from a normal response to an increase in light or caused by certain drugs or pathological conditions.

monoamine—An amine compound containing one amino (nitrogen-containing) group; especially a compound that functions as a neurotransmitter (e.g., the catecholamines).

monoamine oxidase—An enzyme in the cells of most tissues that catalyzes the oxidative metabolism of monoamines such as norepinephrine, epinephrine, and dopamine.

monoamine oxidase inhibitor—Class of antidepressant medications that block the action of monoamine oxidase in the brain, thus increasing levels of monoamines.

morphology—The science concerned with the configuration or the structure of animals and plants.

MRSA—Methicillin-resistant *Staphylococcus aureus*.

mucocutaneous—Relating to skin and mucous membrane.

mucolytic agents—Substances capable of dissolving, digesting, or liquefying mucus.

mucositis—Inflammation and ulceration of mucous membranes.

muscarinic—A type of acetylcholine receptor that responds to the neurotransmitter muscarine.

mutism—A rare childhood condition characterized by a consistent failure to speak in situations where talking is expected. The child has the ability to converse normally and does so, for example, in the home, but consistently fails to speak in specific situations such as at school or with strangers.

myalgia—Muscle pain or tenderness.

mydriasis—Abnormal pupil dilation caused by medication.

myelinated—A nerve covered with a myelin sheath.

myelosuppression—A reduction in the ability of the bone marrow to produce platelets, red blood cells, and white blood cells. Typically caused by cancer chemotherapy and radiation therapy. During the period of myelosuppression, patients may be at an increased risk of infection or bleeding or may experience symptoms of anemia.

myenteric plexus—A ganglionated plexus of unmyelinated fibers lying in the muscular coat of the stomach, intestines, and esophagus.

myocardium—The middle layer of the heart consisting of cardiac muscle.

myoclonus—Muscle twitching; seizures.

myoglobin—The oxygen-transporting protein of muscle that resembles blood hemoglobin in function but has only one heme as part of the molecule and is one fourth of the molecular weight.

myopathy—Dysfunction of the muscle, including weakness and soreness.

myosin—The most common protein in muscle cells; a globulin responsible for the elastic and contractile rhapsodies of muscle; combines with actin to form actomyosin.

myositis—Inflammation of a muscle.

myxedema—Hypothyroidism characterized by a relatively hard edema of subcutaneous tissue along with increased content of mucins (proteoglycans) in the interstitial fluid, somnolence, slow mentation, dryness and loss of hair, increased fluid in body cavities such as the pericardial sac, subnormal temperature, hoarseness, muscle weakness, and slow return of a muscle to the neutral position after a tendon jerk; usually caused by removal or loss of functioning thyroid tissue.

nadir—The lowest value of blood counts after chemotherapy.

necrolysis—Loosening and death of tissue.

necrosis—Death of tissue due to injury or disease.

necrotizing—That which causes the death of tissues or organisms.

neoadjuvant—The administration of an agent before a main treatment.

neologisms—Nonsensical word produced in error as seen in persons with aphasia.

neostriatum—The caudate nucleus and putamen considered as one and distinguished from the globus pallidus.

nephropathy—Impairment of function or disease involving the kidney.

nephrotoxicity—Toxicity to the kidneys.

neuralgia—Severe pain extending along a nerve or groups of nerves. Severe, throbbing, or stabbing pain in the course or distribution of a nerve.

neuritis—Inflammation of nerves characterized by pain, loss of reflex, and muscle atrophy.

neuroleptic—A tranquilizing drug, especially one used to treat mental disorders.

neuroleptic malignant syndrome—Hyperthermia in reaction to the use of neuroleptic drugs; accompanied by extrapyramidal and autonomic disturbances (e.g., fever and muscle rigidity) that may be fatal.

neurolysis—Breaking down or destruction of nerve tissue.

neuron—Any of the impulse-conducting cells that constitute the brain, spinal column, and nervous system. The neuron consists of a nucleated cell body with one or more dendrites and a single axon.

neuropathic pain—Pain that results from a disturbance of function or pathologic change in a nerve. Pain in one nerve is termed mononeuropathy, pain in several nerves is termed mononeuropathy multiplex, and pain that is diffuse and bilateral is termed polyneuropathy.

neuropathy—Dysfunction or disease associated with nerve function.

neurotransmitter—Any of the various chemical substances (e.g., acetylcholine) that transmit nerve impulses across a synapse.

neutropenia—The presence of an abnormally small number of neutrophils (white blood cells) in the circulating blood.

nociceptive—The perception of external injurious stimuli.

nocturia—Purposeful urination at night after waking from sleep. Typically caused by nocturnal urine volume in excess of bladder capacity or incomplete emptying of the bladder because of lower urinary tract obstruction or detrusor instability.

nondeclarative memory—Recall of habits, procedural memory (motor skills and cognitive operations), priming, and conditioned responses.

norepinephrine—A substance, both a hormone and neurotransmitter, secreted by the adrenal medulla and the nerve endings of the sympathetic nervous system to cause fight or flight response such as vasoconstriction and increased heart rate, blood pressure, and blood glucose levels.

nosocomial—A new disorder (not the patient's original condition) associated with being treated in a hospital, such as a hospital-acquired infection.

nystagmus—A rapid, involuntary oscillatory motion of the eyeball.

oculogyric—Describing the circular rotation of the eyes.

oliguria—Infrequent urination or decreased amounts of urine production, such as is seen in renal failure.

onset of action—The time required after administration of a drug for a response to be observed.

opiate—A drug, hormone, or other chemical substance that has sedative or narcotic effects similar to those of opium or its derivatives.

orthopnea—Discomfort in breathing; especially associated with a reclining position.

orthostasis—Referred to as "standing upright," often used interchangeably with "orthostatic hypotension," a condition in which people develop low blood pressure within three minutes of standing. Although this is technically incorrect, this usage is very common.

orthostatic hypotension—Low blood pressure associated with a change in position; most often caused by moving from a lying or sitting position to a standing position.

osteoarthritis—Arthritis characterized by erosion of articular cartilage (either primary or secondary to trauma or other conditions) that becomes soft, frayed, and thinned and is accompanied by eburnation of subchondral bone and outgrowths of marginal osteophytes.

osteomalacia—A disease occurring primarily in adults that results from a deficiency in vitamin D or calcium and is characterized by a softening of the bones and accompanying pain and weakness.

osteoporosis—Reduction in the quantity of bone or atrophy of skeletal tissue; an age-related disorder characterized by decreased bone mass and loss of normal skeletal microarchitecture that leads to increased susceptibility to fractures.

ototoxicity—Toxicity resulting in loss or impairment of hearing.

oxidation—A metabolic process involving the breakdown of a substance when combined with oxygen.

oxidative stress—Increased oxidation associated with the release of free radicals and tissue damage.

Paget's disease—A disease usually in which the bones become enlarged, often resulting in fracture or deformation.

pain—Suffering, either physical or mental; a stimuli on the sensory nerves that causes distress or extreme agony.

pannus—A membrane of granulation tissue covering the normal surface of the articular cartilages in rheumatoid arthritis.

paraphasia—Aphasia in which one loses the power of speaking correctly, substitutes one word for another, and jumbles words and sentences in such a way that makes speech unintelligible.

parasite—An organism that lives on or in another and draws its nourishment therefrom.

parasympathetic nervous system—A part of the autonomic nervous system that facilitates digestive, sleep, and restorative functions.

parathyroid gland—One of two small paired endocrine glands, superior and inferior, usually found embedded in the connective tissue capsule on the posterior surface of the thyroid gland. They secrete parathyroid hormone that regulates metabolism of calcium and phosphorus.

parathyroid hormone—A hormone produced by the parathyroid glands that regulates the amount of calcium and phosphorus in the body.

parenteral—Delivered by intravenous, intramuscular, or subcutaneous injection.

paresthesias—Skin sensation such as burning, itching, or tingling.

parietal lobe—The middle portion of each cerebral hemisphere; separated from the frontal lobe by the central sulcus, from the temporal lobe by the lateral sulcus, and from the occipital lobe only partially by the parieto-occipital sulcus on its medial aspect.

Parkinson's disease—A progressive nervous disease occurring most often after the age of 50 that is associated with the destruction of brain cells that produce dopamine and is characterized by muscular tremor, slowing of movement, partial facial paralysis, peculiarity of gait and posture, and weakness.

perineurally—Situated around a nerve.

peripheral artery disease—Any disorder that involves the arteries outside of, or peripheral to, the heart.

perseveration—Uncontrollable repetition of a particular response, such as a word, phrase, or gesture, despite the absence or cessation of a stimulus, usually caused by brain injury or other organic disorder.

phagocytosis—The process of ingestion and digestion by cells of solid substances (e.g., other cells, bacteria, bits of necrotic tissue, foreign particles).

pharmacokinetics—The study of how medications are absorbed, distributed, metabolized, and eliminated in the body; tracks the travel of medication throughout the body.

pharmacotherapy—The study of the use of medications to prevent, diagnose, and cure disease.

pharyngitis—Inflammation of the mucous membrane and underlying parts of the pharynx.

phenothiazine—Any of a group of drugs chemically related to the antipsychotic chlorpromazine, including several antipsychotic, antiemetic, and antihistamine medications.

phlebitis—Inflammation of a vein.

photic—Relating to light.

plantar fasciosis—Chronic heel pain at the origin of the plantar fascia.

polyarthralgia—Simultaneous inflammation of several joints.

polydipsia—Excessive thirst.

polyuria—Frequent and excessive excretion of urine.

popliteal—Relating to the poples (back part of the knee).

postherpetic neuralgia—Nerve pain originating in an area formerly infected with herpes virus.

postictal—Occurring after a seizure.

postprandial—Occurring after a meal.

potentiate—To enhance or increase the effects.

prednisone—A synthetic steroid used to treat cancer or inflammation.

priming—The implicit memory effect in which exposure to a stimulus influences response to a later stimulus.

prion—An infectious proteinaceous particle of nonnucleic acid composition; the causative agent, either on a sporadic, genetic,

or infectious basis, of neurodegenerative diseases in animals and humans.

procedural memory—Memory for how to do things. Procedural memory guides the processes individuals perform and most frequently resides below the level of conscious awareness.

progressive supranuclear palsy—A heterogeneous degeneration involving the brainstem, basal ganglia, and cerebellum accompanied by nuchal dystonia and dementia.

prokinetic—A drug that works to speed up the emptying of the stomach and the motility of the intestines.

prophylaxis—Prevention of disease or of a process that can lead to a disease.

prosody—The varying rhythm, intensity, and frequency of speech that are interpreted as stress or intonation that aid meaning transmission.

prostaglandin—Hormone-like substance produced in the tissues. Prostaglandin is derived from amino acids and mediates a range of functions, including inflammation, metabolism, and nerve transmission.

prostatitis—Inflammation of the prostate gland.

pruritus—Severe itching.

psoriatic arthritis—The concurrence of psoriasis and polyarthritis. Resembles rheumatoid arthritis but thought to be a specific disease entity. Seronegative for rheumatoid factor and often involves the digits.

psychosis—Symptom or feature of mental illness typically characterized by radical changes in personality, impaired functioning, and a distorted or nonexistent sense of objective reality.

psychotropic—Having an altering effect on perception or behavior.

purulent—Containing, discharging, or associated with the production of pus.

pyridoxine—Vitamin B_6; a pyridine derivative that occurs especially in cereals, yeast, liver, and fish; serves as a coenzyme in amino acid synthesis.

pyruvate—A ketone made from glucose through glycolysis.

quinidine—An alkaloid medication used to treat cardiac arrhythmias.

Raynaud's disease—A circulatory disorder that affects the hands and feet. Caused by insufficient blood supply to these parts and results in cyanosis, numbness, pain, and, in extreme cases, gangrene.

receptor—A molecular structure or site on the surface or interior of a cell that binds with substances such as hormones, antigens, drugs, or neurotransmitters.

reduction—The amount by which something is lessened.

refractory—Resistant to treatment.

resistance—The natural or acquired ability of an organism to maintain its immunity to or to oppose the effects of an antagonistic agent (e.g., a toxin, drug, or pathogenic microorganism).

resting tremors—Tremor occurring in a relaxed and supported limb or other bodily part; it is sometimes abnormal, as in parkinsonism.

retch—To attempt to vomit.

reticulospinal tract—Any of several fiber tracts descending to the spinal cord from the reticular formation of the pons and medulla oblongata.

retrieval—The process of getting information out of memory.

reuptake—The reabsorption of a substance by a cell.

Reye syndrome—An acute encephalopathy characterized by fever, vomiting, fatty infiltration of the liver, disorientation, and coma. Occurs mainly in children and usually follows a viral infection such as chicken pox or influenza.

rhabdomyolysis—Rapid breakdown of skeletal muscle due to injury to muscle tissue. The muscle damage may be caused by physical (e.g., crush injury), chemical, or biological factors. The destruction of the muscle leads to the release of the breakdown products of damaged muscle cells into the bloodstream; some of these, such as myoglobin (a protein), are harmful to the kidney and may lead to acute kidney failure.

rheumatoid arthritis—A generalized disease, occurring more often in women, that primarily affects connective tissue. Arthritis is the dominant clinical manifestation and involves many joints, especially those of the hands and feet. It is accompanied by thickening of articular soft tissue and extension of synovial tissue over articular cartilages, which become eroded. The course is variable but often is chronic and progressive, leading to deformities and disability.

rhinorrhea—Discharge of a thin watery nasal fluid. Can also be used to describe the flow of cerebrospinal fluid from the nose after an injury to the head.

sarcoma—A malignant tumor arising from connective tissues.

sarcoplasmic reticulum—The endoplasmic reticulum found in the striated muscle fibers.

scleroderma—An autoimmune disease characterized by the swelling and thickening of skin or fibrous tissue.

seizures—Abnormal electrical conduction in the brain, resulting in the abrupt onset of transient neurologic symptoms such as involuntary muscle movements, sensory disturbances, and altered consciousness. Also called *convulsion*.

semantic memory—The knowledge of facts learned over time, such as multiplication tables, vocabulary, and spelling.

sensory memory—The lowest form of memory, responsible for attention to encode and store information.

seroma—A mass or swelling caused by the localized accumulation of serum in a tissue or organ.

serotonin—A neurotransmitter found in animal and human tissue (especially the brain, blood serum, and gastric mucous membranes) that promotes vasoconstriction, stimulation of the smooth muscles, transmission of impulses between nerve cells, and regulation of cyclic body processes.

serotonin receptor antagonists—Drugs that bind to but do not activate serotonin receptors, thereby blocking the actions of serotonin.

serotonin syndrome—A potentially life-threatening syndrome that results from excessive levels of serotonin. Symptoms can include agitation, hallucinations, loss of coordination, overactive reflexes, elevated heart rate and blood pressure, nausea, and vomiting.

sialorrhea—Excessive production and flow of saliva.

side effect—An undesired effect associated with medication use.

slough—A layer of dead tissue separated from surrounding living tissue.

somatic—Relating to the wall of a body cavity.

somatic nervous system—The portion of the nervous system that regulates voluntary movement.

somatosensory—Perception of sensory stimuli from the skin and internal organs.

somnolence—Sleepiness or drowsiness.

staphylococcus—Gram-positive bacteria that are potential pathogens, causing local lesions and serious opportunistic infections which can result in serious infection and systemic disease.

status epilepticus—A form of seizure in which one major tonic–clonic seizure succeeds another with little or no intermission.

steady-state—A stable condition that does not change over time or in which change in one direction is continually balanced by change in another.

Stevens-Johnson syndrome—Severe inflammatory skin or mucous eruption that may be accompanied by sloughing; usually a result of a sensitivity reaction to a medication.

stomatitis—Inflammation of the mucous membrane of the mouth.

storage—The second of three stages in the memory process, involving mental processes associated with retention of stimuli that have been registered and modified by encoding.

streptococcus—A bacterium often found in the throat and on the skin.

striatum—A collective term for the caudate nucleus, the putamen, and the globus pallidus, which form the corpus striatum.

stricture—Narrowing of a hollow structure, such as the esophagus.

stridor—Abnormal, high-pitched, musical breathing sound caused by a blockage in the throat or voice box (larynx). It is usually heard when taking in a breath.

stroke—Any acute clinical event related to impairment of cerebral circulation that lasts longer than 24 h.

substance P—A peptide neurotransmitter comprising 11 amino acyl residues normally present in minute quantities in the nervous system and intestines of humans and various animals and in inflamed tissue. Primarily involved in pain transmission; one of the most potent compounds affecting smooth muscle (dilation of blood vessels and contraction of intestine) and thus presumed to play a role in inflammation.

substantia nigra—A layer of large, pigmented nerve cells in the mesencephalon that produce dopamine. Destruction of dopamine neurons in the substantia nigra is associated with Parkinson's disease.

supraspinatus—One of four rotator cuff muscles that abducts the arm at the shoulder.

sympathetic nervous system—The part of the autonomic nervous system originating in the thoracic and lumbar regions of the spinal cord that mediates the fight or flight response, which includes increased heart rate and blood pressure.

sympathomimetic—Producing physiological effects resembling those caused by the action of the sympathetic nervous system.

synapse—The junction across which a nerve impulse passes from an axon terminal to a neuron, muscle cell, or gland cell; the space between one neuron and another where a nerve impulse is transmitted.

synovial membrane—Soft tissue that lines the noncartilaginous surfaces in joints with cavities (e.g., the knee).

synovitis—Inflammation of a synovial membrane.

systemic lupus erythematosus—An autoimmune inflammatory disease of the connective tissues occurring mainly among middle-aged women, chiefly characterized by skin eruptions, joint pain, recurrent pleurisy, and kidney disease.

tachypnea—Rapid breathing.

tardive dyskinesia—A chronic disorder of the nervous system characterized by involuntary, jerky movements of the face, tongue, jaws, trunk, and limbs. Usually develops as a late side effect of prolonged treatment with antipsychotic drugs.

T-cell—A lymphocyte formed in the bone marrow. It migrates from the bone marrow to the thymic cortex to become an immunologically competent cell. T lymphocytes have long lifespans (months to years) and are responsible for cell-mediated immunity.

temporal lobe—The lowest of the major subdivisions of the cortical mantle of the brain; contains the sensory center for hearing and forms the rear two thirds of the ventral surface of the cerebral hemisphere.

teratogenesis—Development of malformation of the fetus.

tetany—A condition characterized by painful, prolonged muscle contraction; usually associated with abnormal calcium levels.

tetracyclines—A class of antibiotics that includes minocycline, tetracycline, oxytetracycline, and doxycycline.

therapeutic index—The ratio between the toxic dose and the therapeutic dose of a drug, used as a measure of the relative safety of the drug for a particular treatment.

thrombocytopenia—A condition in which an abnormally low number of platelets circulate in the blood.

thrombosis—Formation or presence of a fibrinous clot; most often formed in a blood vessel or heart chamber.

thyroid gland—An endocrine (ductless) gland consisting of irregularly spheroid follicles. Lies in front and to the sides of the upper part of the trachea and lower part of the larynx and is of horseshoe shape; has two lateral lobes connected by a narrow central portion (the isthmus) and occasionally an elongated off-shoot (the pyramidal lobe) that passes upward from the isthmus in front of the larynx. It secretes thyroid hormone and calcitonin.

thyrotoxicosis—A toxic condition that results from excessive amounts of thyroid hormones in the body.

thyrotropin—A glycoprotein hormone produced by the anterior lobe of the hypophysis that stimulates the growth and function of the thyroid gland; also used as a diagnostic test to differentiate primary and secondary hypothyroidism.

thyroxine—The l-isomer is the active iodine compound existing normally in the thyroid gland and extracted therefrom in crystalline form for therapeutic use; also prepared synthetically. Used to relieve hypothyroidism and myxedema.

tinnitus—A sound, such as buzzing or ringing, in one or both ears.

tonic—Condition characterized by continuous tension or contraction of muscles.

torsades de pointes—A type of ventricular tachycardia with a spiral-like appearance ("twisting of the points") and complexes that at first look positive and then negative on an electrocardiogram. It is precipitated by a long QT interval, which is often induced by drugs (quinidine, procainamide, or disopyramide), but which may be the result of hypokalemia, hypomagnesemia, or profound bradycardia. The first line of treatment is IV magnesium sulfate, as well as defibrillation if the patient is unstable.

transient ischemic attack—A sudden focal loss of neurologic function; complete recovery usually occurs within 24 h. Caused by a brief period of inadequate perfusion in a portion of the territory of the carotid or vertebral basilar arteries.

tremors—Unintentional trembling or shaking movements in one or more parts of the body. Most tremors occur in the hands.

tricyclic antidepressants—A class of antidepressants whose chemical structures contain three rings of atoms.

trigeminal neuralgia—Facial neuralgia associated with the trigeminal nerve.

tri-iodothyronine—Used in the treatment of thyroid deficiency syndromes.

tumor lysis syndrome—Hyperphosphatemia, hypocalcemia, hyperkalemia, and hyperuricemia after induction chemotherapy of malignant neoplasms. Believed to be caused by the release of intracellular products by cell lysis.

tumor necrosis factor alpha—A pleiotropic cytokine synthesized widely throughout the female reproductive tract.

tyramine—An amino acid, found in certain cheeses and other foods, that is a precursor of the catecholamines and that can cause adverse effects in patients using monoamine oxidase inhibitors.

urea—The main nitrogen-containing substance found in urine; formed in the metabolic processes of protein.

urethritis—Inflammation of the urethra.

valproic acid—An anticonvulsive drug used to treat seizures.

vascular dementia—General term describing problems with reasoning, planning, judgment, memory, and other thought processes caused by brain damage from impaired blood flow to the brain.

vasculitis—Inflammation of a blood or lymph vessel.

vasoconstriction—Constriction of a blood vessel.

vasoconstrictor—Medication that causes constriction of the blood vessels, resulting in an increase in blood pressure.

vasodilation—Dilation of a blood vessel.

vasopressor—Medication that causes constriction of the blood vessels, usually resulting in an increase in blood pressure.

vermicular movement—Wavelike muscular contractions.

vestibulospinal tract—Descending spinal tracts of the ventromedial pathway that originate in the medulla. Motion of fluid in the vestibular labyrinth activates hair cells that signal the vestibular nuclei via cranial nerve VIII.

virus—A term for a group of infectious agents that, with few exceptions, are capable of passing through fine filters that retain most bacteria, are usually not visible through the light of a microscope, lack independent metabolism, and are incapable of growth or reproduction apart from living cells. The complete particle usually contains either deoxynucleic acid or ribonucleic acid, not both, and is usually covered by a protein shell or capsid that protects the nucleic acid.

Wernicke's encephalopathy—A disease of the nervous system caused by a thiamine deficiency and characterized by abnormal eye movements, loss of muscle coordination, tremors, confusion, and amnesia.

xerostomia—Dryness of the mouth resulting from diminished or arrested salivary secretion.

REFERENCES

Chapter 1

Bauer, L.A. (2002). Clinical pharmacokinetics and pharmacodynamics. In J.T. DiPiro, R.L. Talbert, G.C. Yee, G.R. Matske, B.G. Wells, et al. (Eds.), *Pharmacotherapy: A pathophysiologic approach* (5th ed., pp. 33-55). Stamford, CT: Appleton & Lange.

Blumenthal, D.K., & Garrison, J.C. (2011). Pharmacodynamics: Molecular mechanisms of drug action. In L.L. Brunton, B.A. Chabner, & B.C. Knollman (Eds.), *Goodman and Gillman's the pharmacological basis of therapeutics* (12th ed., pp. 41-72). New York: McGraw-Hill.

Buxton, I.L., & Benet, L.Z. (2011). Pharmacokinetics: The dynamics of drug absorption, distribution, metabolism, and elimination. In L.L. Brunton, B.A. Chabner, & B.C. Knollman (Eds.), *Goodman and Gillman's the pharmacological basis of therapeutics* (12th ed., pp. 17-39). New York: McGraw-Hill.

Campbell-Taylor, I. (2001). *Medications and dysphagia* (pp. 1-32). Stow, OH: Interactive Therapeutics.

Carl, L.C, & Johnson, P.R. (2006). *Drugs and dysphagia: How medications can affect eating and swallowing* (pp. 3-30). Austin, TX: Pro-Ed.

Ciccone, C.D. (2002). *Pharmacology in rehabilitation* (3rd ed., pp. 3-58). Philadelphia: Davis.

Gadson, B. (2006). *Pharmacology for physical therapists*. Philadelphia: Elsevier.

Institute for Safe Medication Practices. (2011). www.ismp.org/

Malone, T. (1989). *Physical and occupational therapy: Drug implications for practice* (pp. 1-35). Philadelphia: Lippincott.

Niles, A.S. (2001). Principles of therapeutics. In J.G. Hardman, L.E. Limbird, & A.G. Gillman (Eds.), *Goodman and Gillman's the pharmacological basis of therapeutics* (10th ed., pp. 45-66). New York: McGraw-Hill.

Rivera, S.M., & Gilman, A.G. (2011). Drug invention and the pharmaceutical industry. In L.L. Brunton, B.A. Chabner, & B.C. Knollman (Eds.), *Goodman and Gillman's the pharmacological basis of therapeutics* (12th ed., pp. 1-16). New York: McGraw-Hill.

Ross, E.M., & Kenakin, T.P. (2001). Pharmodynamics: Mechanisms of drug action and relationship between drug concentration and effect. In J. G. Hardman, L.E. Limbird, & A.G. Gillman (Eds.), *Goodman and Gillman's the pharmacological basis of therapeutics* (10th ed., pp. 31-44). New York: McGraw-Hill.

Vogel, D., Carter, J.E., & Carter, P.B. (2000). *The effects of drugs on communication disorders* (pp. 1-60). San Diego: Singular.

Wilkinson, G.R. (2001). Pharmacokinetics: The dynamics of drug absorption, distribution, and elimination. In J.G. Hardman, L.E. Limbird, & A.G. Gillman (Eds.), *Goodman and Gillman's the pharmacological basis of therapeutics* (10th ed., pp. 31-66). New York: McGraw-Hill.

Chapter 2

Bayles, K., & Tomoeda, C. (2007). *Cognitive communication disorders in dementia*. San Diego: Plural.

Berube, M. (2002). *The American Heritage Stedman's medical dictionary*. Boston: Houghton Mifflin.

Brown, J.W. (1972). *Aphasia, apraxia and agnosia: Clinical and theoretical aspects*. Springfield, IL: Charles C. Thomas.

Carl, L.C., & Johnson, P.R. (2006). *Drugs and dysphagia*. Austin, TX: Pro-Ed.

Casper, M. (2007, February). *Addressing the needs of patients with dementia across the healthcare continuum: Comprehensive assessment and treatment planning for communication, cognition and swallowing*. Paper presented at Northern Speech Services Professional Seminar, San Diego.

Cone, W. (2005). *Stop memory loss*. Pacific Palisades, CA: Matteson Books.

Cone, W. (2008, July). *Aging and cognition*. Paper presented at Health Education Seminars, Tampa.

Drewe, E. (1975). Go–no-go learning after frontal lobe lesion in humans. *Cortex*, 11(1):8-16.

Emilien, G., Durlach, C., Minaker, K., Winblad, B., Gauthier, S., and Maloteaux, J. (2004). *Alzheimer disease: neuropsychology and pharmacology*. Basel: Birkhäuser Verlag.

Gardiner, J.M. (2001). Episodic memory and autonoetic consciousness: A first-person approach. *Philosophical Transactions of the Royal Society Biological Sciences*, 356(1413):1351-1361.

Grimsley, S.R. (1998). Mood disorders. In *Pharmacotherapy self-assessment program—Book 4: Neurology & psychiatry* (3rd ed.) (pp. 119-163). Kansas City, MO: American College of Clinical Pharmacy.

Grimsley, S.R., Huang, V., & Gortney, J.S. (2006). Risk for serotonin syndrome with concomitant administration of linezolid and serotonin agonists. *Pharmacotherapy*, 26(12):1784-1793.

Iversen, L.L., Iversen, S.D., Bloom, F.E., & Roth, R.H. (2009). *Introduction to neuropsychopharmacology*. New York: Oxford University Press.

Kolb, B., & Milner, B. (1981). Performance of complex arm and facial movements after focal brain lesions. *Neuropsychologia*, 19(4):505-514.

Kuypers, H. (1981). Anatomy of the descending pathways. In V. Brooks (Ed.), *The nervous system, handbook of physiology* (Vol. 2). Baltimore: Williams & Wilkins.

Leonard, G., Jones, L., & Milner, B. (1988). Residual impairment in handgrip strength after unilateral frontal-lobe lesions. *Neuropsychologia*, 26(4):555-564.

Levin, H.S. (1990). Memory deficit after closed head injury. *Journal of Clinical and Experimental Neuropsychology*, 12(1):129-153.

Mahendra, N., & Apple, A. (2007). Human memory systems: A framework for understanding. *ASHA Leader*, 12(16):8-11.

Mendez, M.F., & Cummings, J. (2003). *Dementia: A clinical approach*. Oxford: Butterworth-Heinemann Medical.

Miller, L. (1985). Cognitive risk taking after frontal or temporal lobectomy: The synthesis of fragmented visual information. *Neuropsychologia*, 23(3):359-369.

Milner, B. (1964). Some effects of frontal lobectomy in man. In J. Warren & K. Akert (Eds.), *The frontal granular cortex and behavior (pp. 313-331)*. New York: McGraw-Hill.

Parente, R., & Herrmann, D. (2003). *Retraining cognition: Techniques and applications*. Austin, TX: Pro-Ed.

Sander, A.M., Nakase, R., Constantinidou, F., Wertheimer, J., & Paul, D.R. (2007). Memory assessment on an interdisciplinary rehabilitation team: A theoretically based framework. *American Journal of Speech Language Pathology*, 16(4):316-330.

Semmes, J., Weinstein, S., Ghent, L., & Teuber, H. (1963). Impaired orientation in personal and extrapersonal space. *Brain*, 86(4):747-772.

Vogel, D., Carter, J., & Carter, P.B. (2000). *The effects of drugs on communication disorders* (2nd ed.). San Diego: Singular.

Wiig, E., Zureich, P., Radford, N., & Ross-Swain, D. (2008, November). *Cognitive speed, frontal/temporal parietal executive functions across the lifespan.* Paper presented at American Speech Language Hearing Association Annual Convention, Chicago.

Zemlin, W.R. (1998). *Speech and hearing: Anatomy and physiology* (4th ed.). Boston: Allyn & Bacon.

Chapter 3

Alvi, A. (1999). Iatrogenic swallowing disorders: Medications. In R.L. Carrau & T. Murry (Eds.), *Comprehensive management of swallowing disorders* (pp. 119-124). San Diego: Singular.

Awdishu, L., & Mehta, R.L. (2007). Drug issues in renal replacement therapies. In T. Dunsworth & J. Cheng (Eds.), *Pharmacotherapy self-assessment program* (6th ed.) (pp. 91-105). Lenexa, KS: American College of Clinical Pharmacology.

Barber, J.R., & Teasley, K.M. (1984). Nutrition support of patients with severe hepatic failure. *Clinical Pharmacology*, 3(3):245-253.

Beck, F.K., & Rosenthal, T.C. (2002). Prealbumin: A marker for nutritional evaluation. *American Family Physician*, 65(8):1575-1578.

Brooks, M.J., & Melnik, G. (1995). The refeeding syndrome: An approach to understanding its complications and preventing its occurrence. *Pharmacotherapy*, 15(6):713-726.

Btaiche, I.F., & Khalidi, N. (2004a). Metabolic complications of parenteral nutrition in adults: Part 1. *American Journal of Health-System Pharmacy*, 61(18):1938-1949.

Btaiche, I.F., & Khalidi, N. (2004b). Metabolic complications of parenteral nutrition in adults: Part 2. *American Journal of Health-System Pharmacy*, 61(24):2050-2059.

Buchman, A.L. (2006). Total parenteral nutrition: Challenges and practice in the cirrhotic patient. *Transplantation Proceedings*, 38(6):1659-1663.

Campbell-Taylor, I. (1996). Drugs, dysphagia, and nutrition. In C. Van Riper (Ed.), *Dietetics in development and psychiatric disorders* (pp. 24-29). Chicago: American Dietetic Association.

Campbell-Taylor, I. (2001). *Medications and dysphagia* (pp. 1-32). Stow, OH: Interactive Therapeutics.

Carey, C.F., Lee, H.H., & Woeltje, K.F. (Eds.). (1998). *The Washington manual of medical therapeutics* (29th ed.). Philadelphia: Lipincott Williams & Wilkins.

Carl, L.L., & Johnson, P.J. (2006). *Drugs and dysphagia*. Austin, TX: Pro-Ed.

Carl, L.L., & Johnson, P.J. (2010). Drugs and dysphagia. In A.M. Furkim (Ed.), *Disfagias orofaringia* (Vol. 3). Barueri, Sao Paulo, Brazil: Pro-Fono.

Carson, J.S., & Gormican, A. (1976). Disease mediation relationships in altered taste sensitivity. *Journal of the American Dietetic Association*, 68(6):550-553.

Charney, P.J. (1995). Nutritional assessment in the 1990s: Where are we now? *Nutrition in Clinical Practice*, 10(4):131-139.

Chima, C.S., Meyer, L., Hummell, C., Heyja, R., Paganinin, E.P., & Weynski, A. (1993). Protein catabolic rate in patients with acute renal failure on CAVH and TPN. *Journal of the American Society of Nephrology*, 3(8):1516-1521.

Cochran, E.R., Kamper, C.A., Phelps, S.J., & Brown, R.O. (1989). Parenteral nutrition in the critically ill patient. *Clinical Pharmacy*, 8(11):783-799.

DeHart, R.M., & Worthington, M.A. (2005). Nutritional considerations in major organ failure. In J.T. Dipiro, R.T. Talbert, G.C. Yee, G.R. Matske, B.G. Wells, et al. (Eds.), *Pharmacotherapy: A pathophysiologic approach* (5th ed.) (pp. 2519-2530). New York: McGraw-Hill.

Delich, P.C., Siepler, J.K., & Parker, P. (2007). Liver disease. In Gottschlich, M.M., DeLegge, M.H., Mattox, T., Mueller, C., & Worthingon. P. (Eds.), *A case based approach: The adult patient*(pp 540-557). Silver Spring, MD: American Society for Parenteral and Enteral Nutrition.

Dombrowski, S.R., & Mirtallo, J.M. (1984). Drug therapy and nutritional management of patients with gastrointestinal fistulas. *Clinical Pharmacy*, 3(3):264-272.

Douglass, H.O. (1984). Nutritional support of the cancer patient. *Hospital Formulary*, 19:220-234.

Farthing, M.G. (1983). Gastrointestinal dysfunction and IBS. *Clinical Nutrition* 2(4):5-17.

Feinstein, E.I. (1988). TPN support of patients with acute renal failure. *Nutrition in Clinical Practice*, 3(1):9-13.

Finley, R.S., & LaCivitia, C.L. (1992). Neoplastic diseases. In M.A. Koda-Kimball & L.Y. Young (Eds.), *Applied therapeutics: The clinical use of drugs* (5th ed.) (sections 52-7 & 52-31). Vancouver, WA: Applied Therapeutics.

Fischbach, F. (2002). *Common laboratory and diagnostic tests* (3rd ed.). New York: Lippincott Williams & Wilkins.

Frankenfield, D., Roth-Yousey, L., & Compher, C.C. (2005). Comparison of predictive equations for resting metabolic rate in healthy nonobese and obese adults: A systematic review. *Journal of the American Dietetic Association*, 105(5):775-789.

Gardner, T.B., & Berk, B.S. (2010). Acute pancreatitis. Available: www.emedicine.com/med/topic1720.htm

Gossum, A.V., Lemoyne, M., Geig, P.D., & Jeejebhoy, K.N. (1988). Lipid associated total parenteral nutrition in patients with severe acute pancreatitis. *Journal of Parenteral and Enteral Nutrition*, 12(3):250-255.

Gottschlich, M.M. (2007). *Nutrition support core curriculum: A case based approach—The adult patient*. Silver Spring, MD: ASPEN.

Griffin, J.P. (1992). Drug induced disorders of taste. *Adverse Drug Reactions*, 11(4):229-239.

Grunwald, P.E. (2003). Supportive care II. In Mueller, B.A., Dunsworth, T.S., Fagan, S.C., Hayner, M.S., O'Connel, M.B., Schumock, G.T., Thompson, D.F., Tisdale, J.E., Witt, D.M., and Zaharowitz, B.J. *Pharmacotherapy self-assessment program—Book 10: Hematology and oncology* (4th ed.) (pp. 113-135). Kansas City, MO: American College of Clinical Pharmacy.

Hamaoui, E. (1986). Nutritional support in hepatic disease. *Endoscopic Review*, November:35-38.

Harm, P. (1990). Indications for intradialytic parenteral nutrition. *Nephrology News and Issues*, July:19-22.

Harohalli, R., Shashidhar, H.R., & Grigsby, D.G. (2010). Malnutrition. Available: http://emedicine.medscape.com/article/985140-overview

Henkin, R.L. (1994). Drug induced taste and smell disorders: Incidence, mechanism, and management related to treatment of sensory receptor dysfunction. *Drug Safety*, 11(5):318-337.

Hoffer, L.J. (2003). Protein and energy provision in critical illness. *American Journal of Clinical Nutrition*, 78:906-911.

Horton, M.W., & Godley, P.J. (1988). Continuous ateriovenous hemofiltration: An alternative to hemodialysis. *American Journal of Hospital Pharmacy*, 45(6):1361-1368.

Huckabee, M.L., & Pelletier, C.A. (1999). *Management of adult neurogenic dysphagia*. San Diego: Singular.

Ignoffo, R.J. (1992). Parenteral nutrition support in patients with cancer. *Pharmacotherapy*, 12(4):353-357.

Ireton-Jones, C.S., Borman, K.R., & Turner, W.W. (1993). Nutrition considerations in the management of ventilator-dependent patients. *Nutrition in Clinical Practice*, 8(2):60-64.

Kayser-Jones, J. (2000). Improving the nutritional care of nursing home residents. *Nursing Homes Long Term Care Management*, 49(10):56-59.

Kayser-Jones, J., Schell, E.S., Porter, C., Barbaccia, J.C., & Shaw, H. (1999). Factors contributing to dehydration in nursing homes: Inadequate staffing and lack of professional supervision. *Journal of the American Geriatrics Society*, 47(10):1187-1194.

Krenitsky J. (2004). Nutrition in renal failure: Myths and management. *Practical Gastroenterology*, 4:40-59.

Krishnan, K. (2012). Tumor lysis syndrome. Available: http://emedicine.medscape.com/article/282171

Kumpf, V.J., & Gervasi, J. (2007). Complications of parenteral mutrition. In Gottschlich, M.M., DeLegge, M.H., Mattox, T., Mueller, C., & Worthingon. P. (Eds.) *A case based approach: The adult patient* (pp. 323-339). Silver Spring, MD: American Society for Parenteral and Enteral Nutrition.

Lamb, W.H. (2010). Diabetes mellitus, type 1. Available: http://emedicine.medscape.com/article/919999-overview

Langley, G. (2007). Fluid, electrolytes, and acid–base disorders. In Gottschlich, M.M., DeLegge, M.H., Mattox, T., Mueller, C., & Worthingon. P. (Eds.) *A case based approach: The adult patient* (pp104-129). Silver Spring, MD: American Society for Parenteral and Enteral Nutrition.

Lemoyne, M., & Jeejeebhoy, K.N. (1986). Total parenteral nutrition in the critically ill patient. *Chest*, 89(4):568-575.

Mayo Clinic. (2010). Diabetes diet: Create your own healthy eating plan. Available: www.mayoclinic.com/health/diabetes-diet/DA00027

McClave, S.A., Marindale, R.G., Vanek, V.W., McCarthy, M., Roberts, P., Taylor, B., & Cresci, G. (2009). Guidelines for the provision and assessment of nutrition support therapy in the adult critically ill patient: Society of Critical Care Medicine (SCCM) and American Society for Parenteral and Enteral Nutrition (ASPEN). *Journal of Parenteral and Enteral Nutrition*, 33(3):277-316.

McDonald, G.A., & Dubose, T.D. (1993). Hyponatremia in the cancer patient. *Oncology*, 7(9):55-62.

McDonnell, M.E., & Aprovian, C.M. (2007). Diabetes mellitus. In Gottschlich, M.M., DeLegge, M.H., Mattox, T., Mueller, C., & Worthingon. P. (Eds.) *A case based approach: The adult patient* (pp 676-694). Silver Spring, MD: American Society for Parenteral and Enteral Nutrition.

McMahon, M., Manji, N., Driscoll, D.F., & Bistraian, B.R. (1989). Parenteral nutrition in patients with diabetes mellitus: Theoretical and practical considerations. *Journal of Parenteral and Enteral Nutrition*, 13(5):545-553.

Mifflin, M.D., St. Jeor, S.T., Hill, L.A., Scott, B.J., Daugherty, S.A., & Koh, Y.O. (1990). A new predictive equation for resting energy expenditure in healthy individuals. *American Journal of Clinical Nutrition*, 51(2):241-247.

Mirtallo, J.M. (2007) Overview of parenteral nutrition. In Gottschlich, M.M., DeLegge, M.H., Mattox, T., Mueller, C., & Worthingon. P. *The A.S.P.E.N. Nutrition Support Core Curriculum A case-based approach—The adult patient* (pp. 264-322). Silver Spring, MD: American Society for Parenteral and Enteral Nutrition.

Mirtallo, J.M., Kudsk, K.A., & Ebbert, M.L. (1984). Nutritional support of patients with renal disease. *Clinical Pharmacy*, 3(3):253-263.

Morley, J.E., & Kraenzle, D. (1994). Causes of weight loss in a community nursing home. *Journal of the American Geriatrics Society*, 42(6):583-585.

Moses, S. (2010). Dysphagia diet. Available: www.fpnotebook.com/pharm/neuro/dysphgDt.htm

Parrish, C.R., Krenitsky, J., Willcutts, K., & Radigan, A.E. (2007). Gastrointestinal disease. In Gottschlich, M.M., DeLegge, M.H., Mattox, T., Mueller, C., & Worthingon. P. (Eds.) *A case based approach: The adult patient* (pp 508-539). Silver Spring, MD: American Society for Parenteral and Enteral Nutrition.

Pisters, P.W., & Ranson, J.H. (1992). Nutritional support for acute pancreatitis. *Surgery, Gynecolology, and Obstetrics*, 175(3):275-284.

Rabinowitz, S.S., Katturupalli, M., & Rogers, G. (2010). Failure to thrive: Treatment medication. Available: http://emedicine.medscape.com/articl/

Roberts, S., & Mattox, T. (2007). Cancer. In Gottschlich, M.M., DeLegge, M.H., Mattox, T., Mueller, C., & Worthingon. P. (Eds.) *A case based approach: The adult patient* (pp. 649-675). Silver Spring, MD: American Society for Parenteral and Enteral Nutrition.

Scheinfeld, N.S., & Mokashi, A. (2010). Protein-energy malnutrition. Available: http://emedicine.medscape.com/article/1104623-overview

Sherman, A.L., & Echeverry, D. (2010). Diabetic neuropathy: Treatment and medication. Available: http://emedicine.medscape.com/article/315434-treatment.Sitzmann

Sitzmann, J.V., Steinborn, P.A., Zinner, M.J., & Cameron, J.L. (1989). Total parenteral nutrition and alternate energy substrates in treatment of severe acute pancreatitis. *Surg Gynecol Obstet*, 168(4):311-317.

Sundaram, A., Koutkia, P., & Apovian, C.M. (2002). Nutritional management of short bowel syndrome in adults. *Journal of Clinical Gastroenterology*, 34(3):207-220.

Tiu, A., & McClave, S. (2007). Pancreatitis. In Gottschlich, M.M., DeLegge, M.H., Mattox, T., Mueller, C., & Worthingon. P. (Eds.) *A case based approach: The adult patient* (pp. 558-574) Silver Spring, MD: American Society for Parenteral and Enteral Nutrition.

Votey, S.R., & Peters, A.L. (2010). Diabetes mellitus, type 2—A review: Treatment and medication. Available: http://emedicine.medscape.com/article/766143-treatment

Willoughby, J.T. (1983). Drug induced abnormalities of taste sensation. *Adverse Drug Reaction Bulletin*, 2:368-371.

Winchester, C., Pelletier, C., & Johnson, P.R. (2001). Feeding dependency issues in the long term care environment. *Swallowing and Swallowing Disorders (Dysphagia)*. 10:19-24.

Wolk, R., Moore, E., & Foulks, C. (2007). Renal disease. In Gottschlich, M.M., DeLegge, M.H., Mattox, T., Mueller, C., & Worthingon. P., (Eds.) *A case based approach: The adult patient* (pp. 575-598). Silver Spring, MD: American Society for Parenteral and Enteral Nutrition.

Chapter 4

Alpert, M. (2001). Reflections of depression in acoustic measures in the patient's speech. *Journal of Affective Disorders*, 66(1):59-69.

Alvi, A. (1999). Iatrogenic swallowing disorders: Medications. In R.L. Carrau & T. Murry (Eds.), *Comprehensive management of swallowing disorders* (pp. 119-124). San Diego: Singular.

Baldessarini, R.J. (2001). Drugs and the treatment of psychiatric disorders: Depression and anxiety disorders. In J.G. Hardman, L.E. Limbird, & A.G. Gillman (Eds.), *Goodman and Gillman's the pharmacological basis of therapeutics* (10th ed.) (pp. 447-483). New York: McGraw-Hill.

Basso, M., & Bornstein, R. (1999). Relative memory deficits in recurrent versus first episode depression on a word list learning task. *Neuropsychology*, 13(4):557-563.

Bate, G., Wright, M., Rozenbilds, U., & Geffen, L. (1993). A comparison of cognitive impairments in dementia of the Alzheimer type and depression in the elderly. *Dementia*, 4(5):294-300.

Baylor, S.D., & Patterson, B.Y. (2009). Psychotropic medication during pregnancy. *U.S. Pharmacist*, 34(9):58-68.

Bloom, F.E. (2001). Neurotransmission and the central nervous system. In J.G. Hardman, L.E. Limbird, & A.G. Gillman (Eds.), *Goodman and Gillman's the pharmacological basis of therapeutics* (10th ed.) (pp. 293-320). New York: McGraw-Hill.

Blumenthal, J.A., Babyak, M.A., Moore, K.A., Craighead, W.E., Herman, S., Khatri, P., et al. (1999). Effects of exercise training on older patients with major depression. *Archives of Internal Medicine*, 159(19):2349-2356.

Bostick, J.R., & Diez, H.L. (2008). Optimizing care for patients with depression in the community pharmacy setting. *U.S. Pharmacist*, 33(11):24-38.

Brooks, M. (2011). Problem solving therapy curbs disability in depressed, cognitively impaired elderly. *Archives of General Psychiatry*, 68(1):33-41.

Brown, C.H. (2008). Overview of drug-drug interactions with SSRIs. *U.S. Pharmacist-Health Systems Edition*, January:3-19.

Burt, T., Prudic, J., Peyser, S., Clark, J., & Sackeim, H. (2000). Learning and memory in bipolar and unipolar major depression: Effects of aging. *Cognitive and Behavioral Neurology*, 13(4):246-253.

Butters, M., Becker, J., Nebes, R., Zmuda, M., Mulsant, B., Pollock, B., & Reynolds, C. (2000). Changes in cognitive functioning following treatment of late life depression. *American Journal of Psychiatry*, 157(12):1912-1914.

Campbell-Taylor, I. (1996). Drugs, dysphagia and nutrition. In C. Van Riper (Ed.), *Dietetics in development and psychiatric disorders* (pp. 24-29). Chicago: American Dietetic Association.

Campbell-Taylor, I. (2001). *Medications and dysphagia*. Stow, OH: Interactive Therapeutics.

Carl, L., & Johnson, P. (2006). *Drugs and dysphagia*. Austin, TX: Pro-Ed.

Chapman, A.L., St. Dennis, C., & Cohen, L.J. (2003). Escitalopram: Clinical implications of stereochemistry in an expanding drug class. *Advances in Pharmacy*, 1(3):253-265.

Ciccone, C.D. (2002). *Pharmacology in rehabilitation* (3rd ed.). Philadelphia: Davis.

Clark, L., Iversen, S.D., & Goodwin, G.M. (2001). A neuropsychological investigation of prefrontal cortex involvement in acute mania. *The American Journal of Psychiatry*, 158(10):1605-1611.

Darby, J., Simmons, N., & Berger, P. (1984). Speech and voice parameters of depression: A pilot study. *Journal of Communication Disorders*, 17(2):75-85.

DeSimone, E.M., Lindley, T.J., & Wilcox, S.M. (2006). Antidepressants and suicide in children. *U.S. Pharmacist*, 31(2):40-47.

Dopheide, J.A. (2006). Recognizing and treating depression in children and adolescents. *American Journal of Health-System Pharmacy*, 63(February):233-243.

Drayton, S.J. (2011). Bipolar disorder. In J.T. DiPiro, R.L. Talbert, G.C. Yee, G.R. Matske, B.G. Wells, & L.M. Posey (Eds.), *Pharmacotherapy: A pathophysiologic approach* (8th ed.) (pp. 1191-1208). Stamford, CT: Appleton & Lange.

Dunlay, M., Strutt, A., Levin, H., Jankovic, J., Lai, E., Grossman, R., & York, M. (2008). Depressed mood and memory impairment before and after unilateral posterventral pallidotomy in Parkin-son's disease. *Journal of Neuropsychiatry and Clinical Neurosciences*, 20(3):357-363.

Eligring, H. (1989). *Non-verbal communication in depression*. New York: Cambridge University Press.

Emery, O., & Breslau, L. (1989). Language deficits in depression: Comparisons with SDAT and normal aging. *The Erotological Society of America*, 44(3):M85-M92.

Endicott, J., Rajagopalan, K., Minkwitx, M., & Macfadden, W. (2007). A randomized double blind placebo controlled study of quetiapine in the treatment of bipolar I and II depression: Improvements in quality of life. *International Clinical Psychopharmacology*, 22(1):29-37.

Fahlander, K., Berger, A., Wahlin, A., & Backman, L. (1999). Depression does not aggravate the episodic memory deficits associated with Alzheimer's disease. *Neuropsychology*, 13(4):532-538.

Feinberg, M. (1997). The effect of medications on swallowing. In B.C. Sones (Ed.), *Dysphagia: A continuum of care* (pp. 107-118). Gaithersburg, MD: Aspen.

Fitz, A., & Teri, L. (1994). Depression, cognition, and functional ability in patients with Alzheimer's disease. *Journal of American Geriatric Society*, 42(2):186-191.

Flint, A.J., Black, S.E., & Campbell-Taylor, I. (1993). Abnormal speech articulation, psychomotor retardation, and subcortical dysfunction in major depression. *Journal of Psychiatric Research*, 27(3):309-319.

Fossati, P. (2002). Influence of age and executive functioning on verbal memory of inpatients with depression. *Journal of Affective Disorders*, 68(2):261-271.

Fossati, P., Harvey, P., LeBastard, G., Ergis, A., Jouvent, R., & Alliaire, J. (2004). Verbal memory performance of patients with a first depressive episode and patients with unipolar and bipolar recurrent depression. *Journal of Psychiatric Research*, 38(2):137-144.

Gibbons, R.D., Hur, K., Bhaumik, D.H., & Mann, J.J. (2005). The relationship between antidepressant medication use and the rate of suicide. *Archives of General Psychiatry*, 62(2), 165-172.

Glassman, A.H., Roose, S.P., & Bigger, J.T. (1993). The safety of tricyclic antidepressants in cardiac patients: Risk-benefit reconsidered. *Journal of the American Medical Association*, 269(20):2673-2675.

Goodman, C.C., Boissonnault, W.G., & Fuller, K.S. (2003). *Pathology: Implications for the physical therapist* (2nd ed.). Philadelphia: Saunders.

Greden, J., & Carroll, B. (1980). Decrease in speech pause times with treatment of endogenous depression. *Biological Psychology*, 15(4):575-587.

Guthrie, E.W. (2007). Discontinuing antidepressants requires special care. *Pharmacy Today*, November:24.

Hart, R., Kwentus, J., Hamer, R., & Taylor, J. (1987). Selective reminding procedure in depression and dementia. *Psychological Aging*, 2(2):111-1153.

Harvey, P., LeBastard, G., Pochon, J., Levy, R., Alliaire, J., Dubois, B., & Fossati, P. (2004). Executive functions and updating of the contents of working memory in unipolar depression. *Journal of Psychiatric Research*, 38(6):567-576.

Hazif, T., Billion, T., Peix, R., Faugeron, P., & Clement, J. (2009). Depression and frontal dysfunction: Risks for the elderly? *L'Encephale*, 35(4):361-369.

Hill, C., Stoudemire, A., Morris, R., Martino-Saltzman, D., & Markwalter, H. (1993). Similarities and differences in memory deficits in patients with primary dementia and depression related cognitive dysfunction. *Journal of Neuropsychiatry and Clinical Neurosciences*, 5(3):277-282.

Jackson, C.W. (2002). Mood disorders. In Mueller, B.A., Bertch, K.E., Dunsworth, T.S., Fagan, S.C., Hayney, M.S., O'Connell, M.B., Schumock, G.T., Thompson, D.F., Tisdale, J.E., Witt. D.M., & Zaharowitz, B.J. (Eds.) *Pharmacotherapy self-assessment program. Book 7: Neurology and psychiatry* (4th ed.) (pp. 203-250). Kansas City, MO: American College of Clinical Pharmacy.

Jacobson, S.A., Pies, R.W., & Katz, I.R. (2007). *Clinical manual of geriatric psychopharmacology*. Washington, DC: American Psychiatric.

Jann, M.W., & Slade, J.H. (2007). Antidepressant agents for the treatment of chronic pain and depression. *Pharmacotherapy*, 27(11):1571-1587.

Kando, J.C., Wells, B.G., & Hayes, P.E. (2002). Depressive disorders. In J.T. DiPiro, R.L. Talbert, G.C. Yee, G.R. Matske, B.G. Wells, & L.M. Posey (Eds.), *Pharmacotherapy: A pathophysiologic approach* (5th ed.) (pp. 1243-1264). Stamford, CT: Appleton & Lange.

Kemrak, W.R., & Kenna, G.A. (2008). Association of antipsychotic and antidepressant drugs with Q-T prolongation. *American Journal of Health System Pharmacy*, 65(1):29-38.

Kindermann, S., Kalayam, B., Brown, G., Burdick, K., & Alexopoulos, G. (2000). Executive functions and P300 latency in elderly depressed patients and control subjects. *American Journal of Geriatric Psychiatry*, 8(1):57-65.

Kirkwood, C.A., Phipps, L.B., & Wells, B.G. (2011). Anxiety disorders II: Posttraumatic stress disorder and obsessive compulsive disorder. In J.T. DiPiro, R.L. Talbert, G.C. Yee, G.R. Matske, B.G. Wells, & L.M. Posey (Eds.), *Pharmacotherapy: A pathophysiologic approach* (8th ed.) (pp. 1229-1241). Stamford, CT: Appleton & Lange.

Kizibash, A., Vanderploeg, R., & Curtiss, G. (2002). The effects of depression and anxiety on memory performance. *Archives of Clinical Neuropsychology*, 17(1):57-67.

Lichtman, J.H., Bigger, J.T., Blumenthal, J.A., Frasure-Smith, N., Kaufmann, P.G., Lesperance, F., et al. (2008). Depression and coronary heart disease: Recommendations for screening, referral, and treatment. *Circulation*, 118(17):1768-1775.

Martinez-Aran, A., Vieta, E., Colom, F., Torrent, C., Sanchez-Marino, J., Reinares, M., et al. (2004). Cognitive impairment in euthymic bipolar patients: Implications for clinical and functional outcomes. *Bipolar Disorders*, 6(3):224-232.

Mascarenas, C.A. (2012). Major depressive disorder. In Richardson, M.M., Chessman, K.H., Chants, C., Finks, S.W., Hemstreet, B.A., Hume, A.L., Hutchison, L.C., Jaoyuj, E.I., NcCullum, M., Segarra-Newham, M., & Shere, J.T. (Eds.) *Pharmacotherapy self-assessment program. Book 10: Neurology and psychiatry* (7th ed.) (pp. 7-26). Kansas City, MO: American College of Clinical Pharmacy.

McCain, J.A. (2009). Antidepressants and suicide in adolescents and adults: A public heath experiment with unintended consequences. *Pharmacy and Therapeutics*, 34(7):355-367.

Merikangas, K.R., Jin, R., He, J.P., Kessler, R.C., Lee, S., Sampson, N.A., et al. (2011). Prevalence and correlates of bipolar spectrum disorder in the world mental health survey initiative. *Archives of General Psychiatry*, 68(3):241.

Meyer, J.M. (2011). Pharmacotherapy of psychosis and mania. In L. Brunton, B. Chabner, & B. Knollman (Eds.), *Goodman and Gillman's the pharmacological basis of therapeutics* (12th ed.) (pp. 517-455). New York: McGraw-Hill.

Miller, J.R., & Miller, C.W. (2012). Bipolar disorder. In Richardson, M.M., Chessman, K.H., Chants, C., Finks, S.W., Hemstreet, B.A., Hume, A.L., Hutchison, L.C., Jaoyuj, E.I., NcCullum, M., Segarra-Newham, M., & Shere, J.T. (Eds.) *Pharmacotherapy self-*

assessment program. Book 10: Neurology and psychiatry (7th ed.) (pp. 27-44). Kansas City, MO: American College of Clinical Pharmacy.

Nebes, R., Mulsant, B., Pollock, B., Zmuda, M., Houck, P., & Reynolds, C. (2000). Decreased working memory and processing speed mediate cognitive impairment in geriatric depression. *Psychological Medicine*, 30(3):679-691.

O'Donnell, J.M., & Shelton, R.C. (2011). Drug therapy of depression and anxiety disorders. In L. Brunton, B. Chabner, & B. Knollman (Eds.), *Goodman and Gillman's the pharmacological basis of therapeutics* (12th ed.) (pp. 397-415). New York: McGraw-Hill.

Rooney, J., & Johnson, P. (2000). Potentiation of the dysphagia process through psychotropic use in the long term care facility. *ASHA Special Interest Division 13 Dysphagia Newsletter*, 9(3):4-6.

Rubinsztein, J.S., Fletcher, P.C., Rogers, R.D., Ho, L.W., Aigbirhio, F.I., Paykel, E.S., Robbins, T.W., & Sahakian, B.J. (2001). Decision-making in mania: A PET study. *Brain*, 124(12):2550-2563.

Rude, S., Gortner, E., & Pennebaker, J. (2004). Language use of depressed and depression—Vulnerable college students. *Cognition and Emotion*, 18(8):1121-1133.

Sapolsky, R. (2001). Depression, antidepressants and the shrinking hippocampus. *Proceedings of the National Academy of Sciences*, 98(22):12320-12322.

Schuck, R., Dubois, B., Lepine, J., Gallarda, T., Olie, J., Goni, S., & Troy, S. (2003). Validation of the short cognitive battery (B2C): Value in screening for Alzheimer's disease and depressive disorders in psychiatric practice. Encephale, 29(3):266-272.

Sigfried, N., Schouws, S.N., Stek, M.L., Comijs, H.C., & Beekman, A.T. (2010). Risk factors for cognitive impairment in elderly bipolar patients. *Journal of Affective Disorders*, 125(1-3):330-335.

Suslow, T. (2009). Estimating verbal intelligence in unipolar depression: Comparison of word definition and word recognition. *Nordic Journal of Psychiatry*, 63(2):120-123.

Svarstad, B.L., Bultman, D.C., & Mount, J.K. (2004). Patient counseling provided in community pharmacies: Effects of state regulation, pharmacist age, and busyness. *Journal of American Pharmacy Association*, 44(1):22-29.

Teasdale, J., Fogarty, S., & Williams, M. (1980). Speech rate as a measure of short-term variation in depression. *British Journal of Social and Clinical Psychology*, 19(3):271-278.

Teter, C.J., Kando, J.C., & Wells, B.G. (2011). Major depressive disorder. In J.T. DiPiro, R.L. Talbert, G.C. Yee, G.R. Matske, B.G. Wells, & L.M. Posey (Eds.), *Pharmacotherapy: A pathophysiologic approach* (8th ed.) (pp. 1173-1190). Stamford, CT: Appleton & Lange.

Thase, M.E., Macfadden, W., Weisler, R.H., Chang, W., Paulsson, B., Khan, A., et al. (2006). Efficacy of quetiapine monotherapy in bipolar I and II depression: A double-blind randomized placebo-controlled study. *Journal of Clinical Psychopharmacolology*, 26(6):600-609.

Tomporowski, P.D. (2003). Effects of acute bouts of exercise on cognition. *Acta Psychologica*.References and further reading may be available for this article. To view references and further reading you must 112(3):297-324.

Tom-Revson, C., & Lee, B. (2006). Use of psychotropics in children and adolescents. *U.S. Pharmacist*, November:30-37.

Uston, T.B., Ayuso-Mateos, J.L., Chatterjii, S., Mathers, C., & Murray, C.L. (2004). Global burden of depressive disorders in the year 2000. *British Journal of Psychiatry*, 184:386-392.

Vogel, D., Carter, J., & Carter, P. (2000). *The effects of drugs on communication disorders* (2nd ed.). San Diego: Singular.

Watanabe, M.D. (2007). Pharmacotherapy for bipolar disorder: An updated review. *U.S. Pharmacist*, November:26-32.

Zemrak, W., & Kenna, G.A. (2008). Association of antipsychotic and antidepressant drugs with QT interval prolongation. *American Journal Health System Pharmacology*, 65(11):1029-1038.

Chapter 5

Baldessarini, R.J. (2001). Drugs and the treatment of psychiatric disorders: Psychosis and mania. In J.G. Hardman, L.E. Limbird, & A.G. Gillman (Eds.), *Goodman and Gillman's the pharmacological basis of therapeutics* (10th ed.) (pp. 285-540). New York: McGraw-Hill.

Barch, D. (1997). The effect of language production manipulations on negative thought disorder and discourse coherence disturbances in schizophrenia. *Psychiatry Research*, 71(2):115-127.

Baylor, S.D., & Patterson, B.Y. (2009). Psychotropic medications during pregnancy. *U.S. Pharmacist*, September:58-68.

Bellnier, T.J. (2002). Continuum of care: Stabilizing the acutely agitated patient. *American Journal of Health-System Pharmacy*, 59(Suppl. 5):12-18.

Benjamin, S., & Munetz, M.R. (1994). CMHC practices related to tardive dyskinesia screening and informed consent for neuroleptic drugs. *Hospital Community Psychiatry*, 45(4):343-346.

Cameron, M.H., & Monroe, L.G. (2007). *Physical rehabilitation: Evidenced based examination, evaluation, and intervention.* St. Louis: Saunders.

Campbell-Taylor, I. (1996). Drugs, dysphagia and nutrition. In C. Van Riper (Ed.), *Dietetics in development and psychiatric disorders* (pp. 24-29). Chicago: American Dietetic Association.

Campbell-Taylor, I. (2001). *Medications and dysphagia* (pp. 1-32). Stow, OH: Interactive Therapeutics.

Carl, L., & Johnson, P. (2006). *Drugs and dysphagia.* Austin, TX: Pro-Ed.

Chang, J.T., Morton, S.C., Rubenstein, L.Z., Mojica, W.A., Maglione, M., Suttorp, M.J., et al. (2004). Interventions for the prevention of falls in older adults: A systematic review and meta-analysis of randomized clinical trials. *British Medical Journal*, 328(7441):680-686.

Cohen, A.S., & Docherty, N.M. (2004). Affective reactivity of speech and emotional experience in patients with schizophrenia. *Schizophrenia Research*, 69(1):7-14.

Crismon, M.L., Argo, T.R., & Buckley, P.F. (2011). Schizophrenia. In J.T. DiPiro, R.L. Talbert, G.C. Yee, G.R. Matzke, B.G. Wells, & L.M. Posey (Eds.), *Pharmacotherapy: A pathophysiologic approach* (8th ed.) (pp. 1147-1172). Stamford, CT: Appleton & Lange.

Crismon, M.L., & Dornson, P.G. (2002). Schizophrenia. In J.T. DiPiro, R.L. Talbert, G.C. Yee, G.R. Matzke, B.G. Wells, & L.M. Posey (Eds.), *Pharmacotherapy: A pathophysiologic approach* (5th ed.) (pp. 1219-1242). Stamford, CT: Appleton & Lange.

Dolder, C., Nelson, M., & Deyo, Z. (2008). Paliperidone for schizophrenia. *American Journal of Health-System Pharmacy*, 65(5):403-413.

Eon, S., & Durham, J. (2009). Schizophrenia: A review of pharmacologic and nonpharmacologic treatments. *U.S. Pharmacist*, November:2-20.

Feinberg, M. (1997). The effect of medications on swallowing. In B.C. Sones (Ed.), *Dysphagia: A continuum of care* (pp. 107-118). Gaithersburg, MD: Aspen.

Gawel, M.J. (1981). The effects of drugs on speech. *International Journal of Language and Communication Disorders*, 16(1):51-57.

Gerratt, B.R., Goetz, C.G., & Fisher, H.B. (1984). Speech abnormalities in tardive dyskinesia. *Arch Neurol*, 41(3):273-276.

Goldberg, T.E., Dodge, M., Aloia, M., Egan, M.F., & Weinberger, D.R. (2000). Effects of neuroleptic medications on speech disorganization in schizophrenia: Biasing associative networks toward meaning. *Psychological Medicine*, 30(5):1123-1130.

Goldberg, T.E., & Weinberger, D.R. (1995). Thought disorder, working memory and attention: Interrelationships and the effects of neuroleptic medications. *International Clinical Psychopharmacology*, 10(3):99-104.

Green, M.F. (2002). Recent studies on the neurocognitive effects of second-generation antipsychotic medications. *Schizophrenia*, 15(1):25-29.

Guthrie, S.K. (2002a). Managing psychiatric drug therapy across the continuum of care: Focus on the schizophrenic patient. *American Journal of Health-System Pharmacy*, 59(Suppl. 5):3-4.

Guthrie, S.K. (2002b). Clinical issues associated with maintenance treatment of patients with schizophrenia. *American Journal of Health-System Pharmacy*, 59(Suppl. 5):19-24.

Hall, K.D. (2001). *Pediatric dysphagia resource guide.* San Diego: Singular/Thompson Learning.

Harvey, P.D., & Serper, M.R. (1990). Linguistic and cognitive failures in schizophrenia: A multi-variant analysis. *The Journal of Nervous and Mental Disease*, 178(8):487-494.

Iversen, L.L., Iversen, S.D., Bloom, F.E., & Roth, R.H. (2009). *Introduction to neuropsychopharmacology.* New York: Oxford University Press.

Jacobson, S.A., Pies, R.W., & Katz, I.R. (2007). *Clinical manual of geriatric psychopharmacology.* Washington, DC: American Psychiatric.

Johnson, P. (2001). Drug interactions with antipsychotic medications in the population with dementia. *ASHA Special Interest Division 13 Dysphagia Newsletter*, 10(3):25-27.

Laporta, M., Archambault, D., Ross-Chouinard, A., & Chouinard, G. (1990). Articulatory impairment associated with tardive dyskinesia. *The Journal of Nervous and Mental Disease*, 78(10):660-662.

Lee, P.E., Gill, S.S., Freedman, M., Bronskill, S.E., Hillmer, M.P., & Rochon, P.A. (2004). Atypical antipsychotic drugs in the treatment of behavioral and psychological symptoms of dementia: Systemic review. *British Medical Journal*, 329(7457):75.

Leger, J.M., Moulias, R., Vellas, B., Monfort, J.C., Chapuy, P., Robert, P., Knellesen, S., & Gerard, D. (2000). Causes and consequences of elderly's agitated and aggressive behavior. *Encephale*, 26(1): 32–43.

Lindenmayer, J.P. (2000). The pathophysiology of agitation. *J Clin Psychiatry*, 61(Suppl 14):5-10.

Maguire, G.A. (2002). Comprehensive understanding of schizophrenia and its treatment. *American Journal of Health-System Pharmacy*, 59(Suppl. 5):4-11.

Markowitz, J.S., & Morton, W.A. (2002). Psychoses. In Mueller, B.A., Bertch, K.E., Dunsworth, T.S., Fagan, S.C., Hayney, M.S., O'Connell, M.B., Schumock, G.T., Thompson, D.F., Tisdale, J.E., Witt. D.M., & Zaharowitz, B.J. (Eds.) *Pharmacotherapy self-assessment program. Book 7: Neurology and psychiatry* (4th ed.) (pp. 99-139). Kansas City, MO: American College of Clinical Pharmacy.

Masand, P.S. (2007). Differential pharmacology of atypical antipsychotics: Clinical implications. *American Journal of Health-System Pharmacy*, 64(Suppl. 1):3-8.

Melinder, M., & Barch, D. (2003). The influence of a working memory load manipulation on language production in schizophrenia. *Schizophrenia Bulletin*, 29(3):473-485.

Meyer, J.M. (2011). Pharmacotherapy of psychosis and mania. In L.L. Brunton, B.A. Chabner, & B.C. Knollman (Eds.), *Goodman and Gillman's the pharmacological basis of therapeutics* (12th ed.) (pp. 417-455). New York: McGraw-Hill.

Miller, K.M., & Holliday, K.L. (2012). Schizophrenia and other psychosis. In Richardson, M.M., Chessman, K.H., Chants, C., Finks, S.W., Hemstreet, B.A., Hume, A.L., Hutchison, L.C., Jaoyuj, E.I., NcCullum, M., Segarra-Newham, M., & Shere, J.T. (Eds.) *Pharmacotherapy self-assessment program. Book 10: Neurology and psychiatry* (7th ed.) (pp. 45-64). Kansas City, MO: American College of Clinical Pharmacy.

Munetz, M.R., & Benjamin, S. (1988). How to examine patients using the abnormal involuntary movement scale. *Hospital Community Psychiatry*, 39(11):1172-1177.

Nasrallah, H.A., & Newcomer, J.W. (2004). Atypical antipsychotics and metabolic dysregulation: Evaluating the risk/benefit equation and improving the standard of care. *Journal of Clinical Psychopharmacology*, 24:S7-S14.

O'Keefe, C., & Noordsy, D. (2002). Prevention and reversal of weight gain associated with antipsychotic treatment. *Journal of Clinical Outcomes Management*, 9(10):575-582.

Patel, K.H., & Hlavinka, P.F. (2007). Schizophrenia: Optimal therapy with second-generation antipsychotic agents. *Pharmacy Today*, 13(11):71-84.

Petersen, L., Jeppesen, P., Thorup, A., Abel, M.B., Ohlenschlager, J., Chistensen, T.O., et al. (2005). A randomized multicenter trial of integrated versus standard treatment for patients with a first episode of psychotic illness. *British Medical Journal*, 331(7517):602-608.

Pierce, J.D., O'Neill, J.H., & Talaga, M.C. (2008). *Handbook of clinical psychopharmacology for therapists* (5th ed.). Oakland: New Harbinger.

Preston, J., & Johnson, J. (2009). *Clinical psychopharmacology*. Miami, FL: MedMaster.

Rooney, J., & Johnson, P. (2000). Potentiation of the dysphagia process through psychotropic use in the long term care facility. *ASHA Special Interest Division 13 Dysphagia Newsletter*, 9(3):4-6.

Rose, D.J. (2003). *Fall proof: A comprehensive balance and mobility training program*. Champaign, IL: Human Kinetics.

Salome, F., Boyer, P., & Fayol, M. (2000). The effects of psychoactive drugs and neuroleptics on language in normal subjects and schizophrenic subjects: A review. *European Psychiatry*, 15(8):461-469.

Schatzberg, A.F., Cole, J.O., & DeBattista, C. (2007). Manual of clinical psychopharmacology (6th ed.). Washington, DC: American Psychiatric.

Seale, C., Chaplin, R., Lelliott, P., & Quirk, A. (2007). Antipsychotic medication, sedation, and mental clouding: An observational study of psychiatric consultations. *Social Science and Medicine*, 65(4):698-711.

Siegel, L.K., & Hansten, P. (1993). *Consumers guide to drug interactions*. New York: McMillan.

Singer, B.A., Levien, T.L., & Baker, D.E. (2003). Aripiprazole: A new atypical antipsychotic that stabilizes the dopamine-serotonin system. *Advances in Pharmacy*, 1(3):198-210.

Sommer, I.E., Diederen, K.M., Dirk-Blom, J., Willems, A., Kushan, L., Slotema, K., et al. (2008). Auditory verbal hallucinations predominately activate the right inferior frontal area. *Brain*, 131(12):3169-3177.

Sumiyoshi, C. (2001). Semantic structure in schizophrenia as assessed by the category fluency test: Effect of verbal intelligence and age of onset. *Psychiatry Research*, 105(3):187-199.

Sumiyoshi, C., Sumiyoshi, T., Nohara, I., Yamashita, M., Matsui, M., Kurachi, M., & Niwa, S. (2005). Disorganization of semantic memory underlies alogia in schizophrenia: An analysis of verbal fluency performance in Japanese subjects. *Schizophrenia Research*, 74(1):91-100.

Sumiyoshi, C., Sumiyoshi, T., Roy, A., Jayathilake, K., & Meltzer, H.Y. (2006). Atypical antipsychotic drugs and organization of long-term semantic memory. *The International Journal of Neuropsychopharmacology*, 9(6):677-683.

Tahir, R. (2007). Metabolic effects of atypical antipsychotics. *U.S. Pharmacist*, November:3-14.

Tanzi, M.G. (2009). Iloperidone: An atypical antipsychotic. *Pharmacy Today*, July:29.

Terri, Y.C. (2008). Adherence key to effective management of schizophrenia. *Pharmacy Times*, March:46-49.

Tom-Revzon, C, & Lee, B. (2006). Use of psychotropics in children and adolescents. *U.S. Pharmacist*, November:30-37.

Vogel, D., Carter, J.E., & Carter, P.B. (2000). *The effects of drugs on communication disorders* (2nd ed.). San Diego: Thomson Learning.

Wang, P.S., Schneeweiss, S., Avorn, J., Fischer, M.A., Mogun, H., Solomon, D.H., & Brookhart, M.A. (2005). Risk of death in elderly users of conventional vs. atypical antipsychotic medications. *New England Journal of Medicine*, 353(22):2335-2341.

Weiden, P.J., & Miller, A.L. (2001). Which side effects really matter? Screening for common and distressing side effects of antipsychotic medications. *Journal of Psychiatric Practice*, 7(1):41-47.

Whall, A.L., Engle, A., Bobel, L., & Haberland, L. (1983). Development of a screening program for tardive dyskinesia: Feasility issues. *Nursing Research*, 32(3):151-156.

Wick, J.Y., & Zanni, G.R. (2006). Drug-induced weight gain: Schizophrenia and atypicals. Available: www.pharmacytimes.com/publications/issue/2006/2006-07/2006-07-5677

Woodruff, P.R., Wright, I.C., Bullmore, E.T., Brammer, M., Howard, R.J., Williams, S.C., et al. (1997). Auditory hallucinations and the temporal cortical response to speech in schizophrenia: A functional magnetic resonance imaging study. *American Journal of Psychiatry*, 154(12):1676-1682.

Zagaria, M.E. (2008). Antipsychotics in seniors: Misuse warning update. *U.S. Pharmacist*, 33(11):20-22.

Zasler, N., Katz, D., & Zafonte, R. (2006). Brain injury medicine: Principles and practice. New York: Demos Publishing.

Zemrak W.R., & Kenna, G.A. (2008). Association of antipsychotic and antidepressant drugs with QT interval prolongation. *American Journal of Health-System Pharmacy*, 65(11):1029-1038.

Chapter 6

Allen, C. Blue, T. Earhart, C. (1995). *Understanding cognitive performance modes*. Ormond Beach, Florida: Allen Conferences.

Barna, M.M., & Hughes, F.I. (2009). Alzheimer's disease: Slowing down the course. *Pharmacy Times*, 20(March):28-32.

Barrett-Connor, E., & Kritz-Silverstein, D. (1993). Estrogen replacement therapy and cognitive function in older women. *Journal of the American Medical Association*, 269(20):2637-2641.

Bayles, K. & Tomoeda, C. (2007). *Cognitive-communication disorders of dementia*. San Diego: Plural Publishing.

Beier, M.T. (2007). Pharmacotherapy for behavioral and psychological symptoms of dementia in the elderly. *American Journal of Health-System Pharmacy*, 64(Suppl. 1):S9-S17.

Belden, H. (2007). Try to remember: More targeted treatment and better disease identification aim to get at the root of Alzheimer's disease. *Drug Topics*, January:28-33.

Berman, K, & Brodaty, H. (2004). Tocopherol (vitamin E) in Alzheimer's disease and other neurodegenerative disorders. *CNS Drugs*, 18(12):807-825.

Berumen, J. (2003). Incidence of delirium, risk factors, and long-term survival of elderly patients hospitalized in a medical specialty teaching hospital in Mexico City. *International Psychogeriatrics*, 15 (4):325-336.

Boothby, L.A., & Doering, P.L. (2004). New drug update 2003. *Drug Topics*, March:84-85.

Brinton, R.D. (2004). Impact of estrogen therapy on Alzheimer's disease. *CNS Drugs*, 18(7):405-422.

Brush, J., Sanford, J., Fleder, H., Bruce, C., & Calkins, M. (2011). Evaluating and modifying the communication environment for people with dementia. *American Speech-Language-Hearing Association Perspectives on Gerontology*, 16(2):32-40.

Brush, J.A., & Camp, C.J. (1998, July). *A therapy technique for improving memory: Spaced retrieval*. Presentation at Menorah Park Center for Senior Living, Beachwood, OH.

Burns, A., Rossor, M., Hecker, J., Gauthier, S., Petit, H., Moller, et al. (1999). The effects of donepezil in Alzheimer's disease: Results from a multinational trial. *Dementia and Geriatric Cognitive Disorders*, 10(3):237-244.

Camp, C.J. (1999). *Montessori-based activities for persons with dementia*. Presentation at Menorah Park Center for Senior Living, Beachwood, OH.

Caufield, J.S. (2007). Inappropriate prescribing in geriatric patients: Dementia and falls prevention. *Drug Topics*, January:42-50.

Cummings, J.L. (2004). Alzheimer's disease. *New England Journal of Medicine*, 351(1):56-67.

Cummings, J.L., & Benson, D.F. (1983). *Dementia: A clinical approach*. Stoneham, MA: Butterworth.

Defilippi, J.L., Crismon, M.L., & Clark, W.R. (2002). Alzheimer's disease. In J.T. DiPiro, R.L. Talbert, G.C. Yee, G.R. Matske, B.G. Wells, & L.M. Posey (Eds.), *Pharmacotherapy: A pathophysiologic approach* (5th ed.) (pp. 1165-1182). Stamford, CT: Appleton & Lange.

Eisner, E. (2001). *Can do activities for adults with Alzheimer's disease*. Austin, TX: Pro-Ed.

Elias, M.F., Beiser, A., Wolf, P.A., Au, R., White, R.F., & D'Agostino, R.B. (2000). The pre-clinical phase of Alzheimer's disease. A 22 year prospective study of the Framingham cohort. *Archives of Neurology*, 57(6):808-813.

Emilien, G., Durlach, C., Minaker, K.L., Winblad, B., Gauthier, S., & Maloteaux, J. (2004). *Alzheimer disease: Neuropsychology and pharmacology*. Berlin: Birkhauser Verlag.

Farlow, M.R., Tariot, P.N., Grossberg, G.T., Gergel, I., Graham, S., & Jin, J. (2003). Memantine/donepezil dual therapy is superior to placebo/donepezil therapy for treatment of moderate to severe Alzheimer's disease. *Neurology*, 60(Suppl. 1):A412.

Feldman, H., Gauthier, S., Hecker, J., Vellas, B., Subbiah, P., & Whalen, E. (2001). Donepezil improved the clinical state and quality of life in moderate to severe Alzheimer's disease. *Neurology*, 57(4):613-620.

Fleischmann, D.A., & Gabrieli, J.E. (1998). Repetition priming in normal aging and Alzheimer's disease: A review of findings and theories. *Psychology and Aging*, 13(1):88-119.

Gogia, P.P., & Rastogi, N. (2009). *Clinical Alzheimer rehabilitation*. New York: Springer.

Higuera, D., Harmon, A., Honeywell, M., & Emmanuel, F. (2008). At home test for Alzheimer's disease. *U.S. Pharmacist*, 33(6):49-50.

Hilas, O., & Ezzo, D.C. (2012). Dementias and related neuropsychiatric issues. In Richardson, M.M., Chessman, K.H., Chants, C., Finks, S.W., Hemstreet, B.A., Hume, A.L., Hutchison, L.C.,

Jaoyuj, E.I., NcCullum, M., Segarra-Newham, M., & Shere, J.T. (Eds.) *Pharmacotherapy self-assessment program. Book 10: Neurology and psychiatry* (7th ed.) (pp. 91-110). Kansas City, MO: American College of Clinical Pharmacy.

Ho, Y., & Chagan, L. (2004). Memantine: A new treatment option for patients with moderate to severe Alzheimer's disease. *Pharmacy and Therapeutics*, 29(3):162-165.

Hopper, T., Mahendra, N., Kim, E., Azuma, T., Bayles, K., Cleary, S., et al. (2005). Evidenced-based practice recommendations for working with individuals with dementia: Spaced-retrieval training. *Journal of Medical Speech-Language Pathology*, 13(4):xxvii-xxxiv.

Iversen, L.L., Iversen, S.D., Bloom, F.E., & Roth, R.H. (2009). *Introduction to neuropsychopharmacology*. New York: Oxford University Press.

Jacobson, S.A., Pies, R.W., & Katz, R.I. (2007). *Clinical manual of geriatric psychopharmacology*. Washington, DC: American Psychiatric.

Jick, H., Zolbeg, G.L., Jick, S.S., Seshadri, S., & Drachman, D.A. (2000). Statins and the risk of dementia. *Lancet*, 356(11):1627-1631.

Johnson, P. (2013). The effects of medication on cognition in long-term care. *Seminars in Speech and Language* 34(01):018-028.

Kayrak, M., Yazici, M., Ayhan, S.S., Koc, F., & Ulgen, M.S. (2008). Complete atrioventricular block associated with rivastigmine therapy. *American Journal of Health-System Pharmacy*, 65(11):1051-1053.

Knudsen, D.S. (2007). Complexities of AD require extensive counseling. *Pharmacy Times*, November:64-67.

Langmore, S.E., Terpenning, M.S., Schork, A., Chen, Y., Murray, J.T., Lopatin, D., et al. (1998). Predictors of aspiration pneumonia: How important is dysphagia? *Dysphagia*, 13(2):69-81.

Le Bars, P.L., Katz, M.M., Berman, N., Itil, T.M., Freedman, A.M., & Schatzberg, A.F. (1997). A placebo-controlled double-blind randomized trial of an extract of ginkgo biloba for dementia. *Journal of the American Medical Association*, 278(16):1327-1332.

Lukatela, K., Malloy, P., Jenkins, P., & Cohen, R. (1998). The naming deficit in early Alzheimer's and vascular disease. *Neuropsychologylogy*, 22(6):565-572.

Mahendra, N., Kim, E., Bayles, K., Hopper, T., & Azuma, T. (2005). Evidence-based practice recommendations for working with dementia: Computer assisted cognitive interventions (CACIs). *Journal of Medical Speech-Language Pathology*, 13(3):xxxv-xliv.

Mancano, M.A. (2004). New drugs of 2003. *Pharmacy Times*, March:96.

Mendez, M.F., & Cummings, J.L. (2003). *Dementia: A clinical approach* (3rd ed.). Philadelphia: Butterworth Heinemann.

Mergenhagen, K.A., & Arif, S. (2008). Delirium in the elderly: Medications, causes and treatments. *U.S. Pharmacist*, 33(6):59-68.

Milman, L., Holland, A., Kaszniak, A.W., D'Agostino, J., Garret, M., & Rapcsak, S. (2008). Initial validity and reliability of the SCCAN: Using tailored testing to assess adult cognition and communication. *Journal of Speech, Language, and Hearing Research*, 51(February):49-69.

Mulnard, R.A., Cotman, C.W., Kawas, C., Van Dyck, C.H., Sano, M., Doody, R., et al. (2000). Estrogen replacement therapy for the treatment of mild to moderate Alzheimer's disease. *Journal of the American Medical Association*, 283(8):1007-1015.

Nasreddine, Z., Phillips, N., Bedirian, V., Charbonneau, S., Whitehead, V., & Collin, I. (2005). The Montréal cognitive assessment,

MoCA: A brief screening tool for mild cognitive impairment. *American Geriatrics Society*, 53(4):695-699.

Nickerson, J.L., & Sherman, J. (2007). Memory screening and diagnosis of Alzheimer's disease. *Pharmacy Times*, March supplement:7.

Orgogozo, J.M., Rigaud, A.S., Stoffler, A., Mobius, H.J., & Forette, F. (2002). Efficacy and safety of Memantine in patients with mild to moderate vascular dementia: A randomized, placebo-controlled trial. *Stroke*, 33(7):1834-1839.

Ousset, P.J., Viallard, G., Puel, M., Celsis, P., Demonet, J.F., & Cardebat, D. (2002). Lexical therapy and episodic word learning in dementia of the Alzheimer type. *Brain and Language*, 80(1):14-20.

Parashos, S.A., Johnson, M.L., Erickson-Davis, C., & Wielinski, C.L. (2009). Assessing cognition in Parkinson disease. The use of the cognitive linguistic quick test. *Journal of Geriatric Psychiatry and Neurology*, 22(4):228-234.

Pavlis, C.J., Kutscher, E.C., Carnahan, R.M., Kennedy, W.K., Gerpen, S.V., & Schlenker, E. (2007). Rivastigmine induced dystonia. *American Journal of Health-System Pharmacy*, H64(23):2468-2470.

Perry, R.J., Watson, P., & Hodges, J.R. (2000). The nature and staging of attention dysfunction in the early (minimal and mild) Alzheimer's disease: Relationship to episodic and semantic memory impairment. *Neuropsychology*, 38(3):252-271.

Pirmohamed, J.S., Meakin, S., Green, S., Scott, A.K., Walley, T.J., Farrar, K., et al. (2004). Adverse drug reactions as cause of admission to hospital: Prospective analysis of 18,820 patients. *British Medical Journal*, 329(7456):15-19.

Pomerantz, J.M. (2008). Exercise and cognition: What's the connection? *Drug Benefit Trends*, 20(1):35-36.

Reisberg, B., Doody, R., Stoffler, A., Schmitt, F., Ferris, S., & Mobius, H.J. (2003). Memantine in moderate to severe Alzheimer's disease. *New England Journal of Medicine*, 348(14):1333-1341.

Reisberg, B., Ferris, S.H., Leon, M.J., & Crook, T. (1982). The global deterioration scale for assessment of primary degenerative dementia. *American Journal of Psychiatry*, 139(9):1136-1139.

Robishaw, S., & Beadle, M. (2010). Vascular dementia. *U.S. Pharmacist*, 35(1):46-48.

Rush Alzheimer's Disease Center. (2004). *The Rush manual for caregivers* (6th ed.). Chicago: Rush University Medical Center.

Sano, M., Ernesto, C., Thomas, R.G., Klauber, M.R., Schafer, K., Grundman, et al. (1997). A controlled trial of selegiline, alpha-tocopherol, or both as treatment for Alzheimer's disease. *New England Journal of Medicine*, 336(17):1216-1222.

Shankle, W.R., Romney, A.K., Hara, J., Fortier, D., Dick, M.B., Chen, J.M., et al. (2005). Methods to improve the detection of mild cognitive impairment. *Proceedings of National Academy of Science*, 102(13):4919-4924.

Shirley, K.L. (2002). Dementia. In In Mueller, B.A., Bertch, K.E., Dunsworth, T.S., Fagan, S.C., Hayney, M.S., O'Connell, M.B., Schumock, G.T., Thompson, D.F., Tisdale, J.E., Witt. D.M., & Zaharowitz, B.J. (Eds). *Pharmacotherapy self-assessment program. Book 7: Neurology and psychiatry* (4th ed.) (pp. 167-202). Kansas City, MO: American College of Clinical Pharmacy.

Sikdar, K.C., Dowden, J., Alaghehbandan, R., MacDonald, D., Peter, P., & Gadag, V. (2012). Adverse drug reactions in elderly hospitalized patients: A 12-year population-based retrospective cohort study. *Annals of Pharmacotherapy*, 44(7-8):641-649.

Sohlberg, M.M. & Mateer, C. (2001). Cognitive rehabilitation: An integrated neuropsychological approach, New York: The Guilford Press.

Sohlberg, M.M., Ehlardt, L., & Kennedy, M. (2005). Instructional techniques in cognitive rehabilitation: A preliminary report. *Seminars in Speech and Language*, 26(4):268-279.

Sohlberg, M.M. & Turkstra, L. (2011). Optimizing cognitive rehabilitation. New York: The Guilford Press.

Sonnett, T., Setter, S.M., & Greeley, D.R. (2006). Dementia with Lewy bodies. *U.S. Pharmacist*, April:12-28.

Standaert, D.G., & Young, A.B. (2001). Treatment of central nervous system degenerative disorders. In J.G. Hardman, L.E. Limbird, & A.G. Gillman (Eds.), *Goodman and Gillman's the pharmacological basis of therapeutics* (10th ed.) (pp. 547-568). New York: McGraw-Hill.

Stewart, W.F., Kawas, C., Corrada, M., & Metter, E.J. (1997). Risk of Alzheimer's disease and duration of NSAID use. *Neurology*, 48(3):627-632.

Sucher, B.J., & Mehlhorn, A.J. (2007). Alzheimer's disease: Practical management of cognitive symptoms. *U.S. Pharmacist Health Systems Edition*, 32(June):45-53.

Swanson, M.T. (2009). Homotaurine: A failed drug for Alzheimer's disease and now a nutraceutical for memory protection. *American Journal of Health-System Pharmacy*, 66(November):1950-1953.

Taylor, P. (2011). Anticholinesterase agents. In J.T. DiPiro, R.L. Talbert, G.C. Yee, G.R. Matske, B.G. Wells, & L.M. Posey (Eds.), *Pharmacotherapy: A pathophysiologic approach* (8th ed.) (pp. 239-254). Stamford, CT: Appleton & Lange.

Van Dongen, M.C., Van Rossum, E., Kessels, A.G., Sielhorst, H.J., & Knipschild, P.G. (2000). The efficacy of ginko for elderly people with dementia and age related memory impairment: New results of a randomized clinical trial. *Journal of American Geriatrics Society*, 48(10):1183-1194.

Wick, J.Y. (2008). Dementia: Many facets, no cure. *Pharmacy Times*, February:8.

Wilcock, G., Mobius, H.J., & Stoffler, A. (2002). A double blind, placebo controlled multi-centre study of memantine in mild to moderate vascular dementia. *International Clinical Psychopharmacology*, 17(6):297-305.

Zagaria, M.A. (2006). Agitation and aggression in the elderly. *U. S. Pharmacist*, November:20-28.

Chapter 7

Alvi, A. (1999). Iatrogenic swallowing disorders: Medications. In R.L. Carrau & T. Murry (Eds.), *Comprehensive management of swallowing disorders* (pp. 119-124). San Diego: Singular.

Asperheim, M.K. (2002). *Pharmacology: an introductory text*. Philadelphia: W.B. Saunders.

Ayers, C.R., Thorp, S.R., & Wetherell, J.L. (2009). Anxiety disorders and hoarding in older adults. In M.M. Antony & M.B. Stein (Eds.), *Oxford handbook of anxiety and related disorders* (pp. 625-635). New York: Oxford University Press.

Baldessarini, R.J. (2001). Drugs and the treatment of psychiatric disorders: Depression and anxiety disorders. In J.G. Hardman, L.E. Limbird, & A.G. Gillman (Eds.), *Goodman and Gillman's the pharmacological basis of therapeutics* (10th ed.) (pp. 447-483). New York: McGraw-Hill.

Cameron, L.D., & Leventhal, H. (2003). *The self-regulation of health and illness behavior*. New York: Routledge Taylor Francis.

Campbell-Taylor, I. (1996). Drugs, dysphagia and nutrition. In C. Van Riper (Ed.), *Dietetics in development and psychiatric disorders* (pp. 24-29). Chicago: American Dietetic Association.

Campbell-Taylor, I. (2001). *Medications and dysphagia* (pp. 1-32). Stow, OH: Interactive Therapeutics.

Carl, L., & Johnson, P. (2006). *Drugs and dysphagia*. Austin, TX: Pro-Ed.

Charney, D.S. (2001). Hypnotics and sedatives. In J.G. Hardman, L.E. Limbird, & A.G. Gillman (Eds.), *Goodman and Gillman's the pharmacological basis of therapeutics* (10th ed.) (pp. 399-427). New York: McGraw-Hill.

Chavez, B. (2006). A review of pharmacotherapy for PTSD. *U.S. Pharmacist*, 31(11):31-38.

Ciccone, C.D. (2007). *Pharmacology in rehabilitation*. Philadelphia, PA: F.A. Davis Company.

Cumming, R.G., & Le Couteur, D.G. (2003). Benzodiazepines and risk of hip fractures in older people: A review of the evidence. *CNS Drugs*, 17(11):825-837.

Curtis, J.L., & Jermain, D.M. (2002). Sleep disorders. In J.T. DiPiro, R.L. Talbert, G.C. Yee, G.R. Matske, B.G. Wells, & L.M. Posey (Eds.), *Pharmacotherapy: A pathophysiologic approach* (5th ed.) (pp. 1323-1333). Stamford, CT: Appleton & Lange.

Dopheide, J.A., & Kushida, C.A. (2005). Newer options in the management of insomnia. *U.S. Pharmacist*, October:102-112.

Eaton-Maxwell, A., Ndefo, U.A., Ebeid, A., Ramirez, R., Patel, K., & Begnaud, D. (2010). The use of psychotherapeutic medications in war veterans. *U.S. Pharmacist*, 35(11):94-102.

Garuti, G., Cilione, C., Dell'Orso, D., Gorini, P., Lorenzi, M.C., Totaro, et al. (2003). Impact of comprehensive pulmonary rehabilitation on anxiety and depression in hospitalized COPD patients. *Monaldi Archives for Chest Disease*, 59(1):56-61.

Goodman, C.C., Boissonnault, W.G., & Fuller, K.S. (2003). Pathology: Implications for the physical therapist (2nd ed.). Philadelphia: Saunders.

Halas, C.J. (2006). Eszopiclone. *American Journal of Health-System Pharmacy*, 63(1):41-48.

Hulisz, D., & Duff, C. (2009). Assisting seniors with insomnia: A comprehensive approach. *U.S. Pharmacist*, 34(6):38-47.

Iverson, L.L., Iverson, S.D., Bloom, F.E. & Roth, R.H. (2009). *Introduction to neuropsychopharmacology*. Oxford: Oxford University Press, Inc.

Jacobson, S.A., Pies, R.W., & Katz, I.R. (2007). *Clinical manual of geriatric psychopharmacology*. Washington, DC: American Psychiatric.

Jarvis, C.I., Morin, A.K., & Lynch, A.M. (2008). Pharmacotherapeutic options for chronic insomnia. *U.S. Pharmacist*, 34(6):60-69.

Kirkwood, C.K., & Melton, S.T. (2002). Anxiety disorders. In J.T. DiPiro, R.L. Talbert, G.C. Yee, G.R. Matske, B.G. Wells, & L.M. Posey (Eds.), *Pharmacotherapy: A pathophysiologic approach* (5th ed.) (pp. 1289-1310). Stamford, CT: Appleton & Lange.

Knudsen, D. (2008). Sleep disorders: Treatment options for a tiring problem. *Pharmacy Times*, March:24-26.

Mai, E., & Buysse, D. (2008). Insomnia: Prevalence, impact, pathogenesis, differential diagnosis, and evaluation. *Sleep Medicine Clinics*, 3(2):167-174.

Matthew, S.J., & Hoffman, E.J. (2009). Pharmacotherapy for generalized anxiety disorder. In M.M. Antony & M.B. Stein (Eds.), *Oxford handbook of anxiety and related disorders* (pp. 350-363). New York: Oxford University Press.

Passarella, S., & Duong, M.T. (2008). Diagnosis and treatment of insomnia. *American Journal of Health-System Pharmacy*, 65(10):927-934.

Peel, C., & Mossberg, K.A. (1995). Effects of cardiovascular medications on exercise responses. *Physical Therapy*, 75(5):387-396.

Preston, J.D., O'Neill, J.H., & Talaga, M.C. (2008). *Handbook of clinical psychopharmacology for therapists* (5th ed.). Oakland: New Harbinger.

Saljoughian, M. (2006). Anxiety disorders. *U.S. Pharmacist-Health System*, November:HS3-HS13.

Sherwood, D.A., & Rey, J.A. (2007). Stop losing sleep over insomnia. *Drug Topics*, July:31-40.

Taylor, H.R., & Cates, M.E. (2008). Prazosin for treatment of nightmares related to posttraumatic stress disorder. *American Journal of Health-System Pharmacy*, 65(April):716-722.

Chapter 8

Alvi, A. (1999). Iatrogenic swallowing disorders: Medications. In R.L. Carrau & T. Murry (Eds.), *Comprehensive management of swallowing disorders* (pp. 119-124). San Diego: Singular.

Bohan, K.H., Masuri, T.F., & Wilson, N.M. (2007). Anticonvulsant hypersensitivity syndrome: Implications for pharmaceutical care. *Pharmacotherapy*, 27(10):1425-1439.

Campbell-Taylor, I. (1996). Drugs, dysphagia and nutrition. In C. Van Riper (Ed.), *Dietetics in development and psychiatric disorders* (pp. 24-29). Chicago: American Dietetic Association.

Campbell-Taylor, I. (2001). *Medications and dysphagia* (pp. 1-32). Stow, OH: Interactive Therapeutics.

Carl, L., & Johnson, P. (2006). *Drugs and dysphagia*. Austin, TX: Pro-Ed.

Ciccone, C.D. (2007). *Pharmacology in rehabilitation* (4th ed.). Philadelphia: Davis.

Farooq, M.U., Bhatt, A., Mahd, A., Gupta, T., Khasnis, A., & Kasab, M.Y. (2009). Levetiracetam for managing neurologic and psychiatric disorders. *American Journal of Health-System Pharmacy*, 66(6):541-561.

Feinberg, M. (1997). The effect of medications on swallowing. In B.C. Sones (Ed.), *Dysphagia: A continuum of care* (pp. 107-118). Gaithersburg, MD: Aspen.

French, J.A., Kanner, A.M., Bautista, J., Abou-Khalil, B., Browne, T., Harden, C.L., et al. (2004). Efficacy and tolerability of the new antiepileptic drugs. *Neurology*, 62(8):1261-1273.

Garnett, W.R. (2005). Evaluation of the use of antiepileptic drugs for epilepsy and non-epilepsy indications. *U.S. Pharmacist*, October:88-100.

Gidal, B.E., Garnett, W.R., & Graves, N.M. (2002). Epilepsy. In J.T. DiPiro, R.L. Talbert, G.C. Yee, G.R. Matske, B.G. Wells, & L.M. Posey (Eds.), *Pharmacotherapy: A pathophysiologic approach* (5th ed.) (pp. 1031-1059). Stamford, CT: Appleton & Lange.

Goodman, C.C., Boissonnault, W.G., & Fuller, K.S. (2003). *Pathology: Implications for the physical therapist* (2nd ed.). Philadelphia: Saunders.

Guthrie, E.W. (2006). Epilepsy in children. *U.S. Pharmacist-Health System Edition*, November:17-28.

Hauser, W.A., & Beghi, E. (2008). First seizure definitions and worldwide incidence and mortality. *Epilepsia*, 49(Suppl. 1):8-12.

Iversen, L.L., Iverson, S.D., Bloom, F.E., & Roth, R.H. (2009). *Introduction to neuropsychopharmacology*. New York: Oxford University Press.

Magill-Lewis, J. (2006). Taking control of epilepsy. *Drug Topics*, March:30-34.

McNamara, J.O. (2001). Drugs effective in the therapy of the epilepsies. In J.G. Hardman, L.E. Limbird, & A.G. Gillman (Eds.), *Goodman and Gillman's the pharmacological basis of therapeutics* (10th ed.) (pp. 521-547). New York: McGraw-Hill.

Motamedi, G.K., & Meader, K.J. (2008). Cognition. In S.C. Schachter, G.L. Holmes, & D.G. Kasteleijn-Nolst Trenite (Eds.), *Behavioral aspects of epilepsy: Principles and practice* (pp. 281-287). New York: Demos Medical.

Pesaturo, K.A., Spooner, L.M., & Belliveau, P. (2011). Vigabatrin for infantile spasms. *Pharmacotherapy*, 31(3):298-311.

Rogers, S.J., & Cavezos, J.E. (2011). Epilepsy. In J.T. DiPiro, R.L. Talbert, G.C. Yee, G.R. Matske, B.G. Wells, & L.M. Posey (Eds.), *Pharmacotherapy: A pathophysiologic approach* (8th ed.) (pp. 979-1003). Stamford, CT: Appleton & Lange.

Schachter, S.C., Holmes, G.L., & Kasteleijn-Nolst Trenite, D.G. (2008). *Behavioral aspects of epilepsy: Principles and practice*. New York: Demos Medical.

Talati, R., White, C.M., & Coleman, C.I. (2009). Eslicarbazepine: A novel antiepileptic agent designed for improved efficacy and safety. *Formulary*, 44:357-361.

Vingerhoets, G. (2008). Cognition. In S.C. Schachter, G.L. Holmes, & D.G. Kasteleijn-Nolst Trenite (Eds.), *Behavioral aspects of epilepsy: Principles and practice* (pp. 155-161). New York: Demos Medical.

Weinberg, M.E. (2008). Treatment of seizures in a hospital care setting. *U.S. Pharmacist-Health System Edition*, November:5-15.

Welty, T.E. (2002). The pharmacotherapy of epilepsy. In *Pharmacotherapy self-assessment program. Book 7: Neurology and psychiatry* (4th ed.) (pp. 43-66). Kansas City, MO: American College of Clinical Pharmacy.

Wolff, D.L., & Graves, N.M. (2006). Epilepsy. In *Pharmacotherapy self-assessment program. Book 4: Neurology and psychiatry* (3rd ed.) (pp. 1-26). Kansas City, MO: American College of Clinical Pharmacy.

Zagaria, M.E. (2008). Causes of seizures in the elderly. *U.S. Pharmacist*, 33(1):27-31.

Chapter 9

Ahsan, S.F., Meleca, R.J., & Dworkin, J.P. (2000). Botulinum toxin injection of the cricopharyngeus muscle for the treatment of dysphagia. *Otolaryngology*, 122(5):691-695.

Albright, A.L., Barron, W.B., Fasick, M.P., Polinko, P., & Janosky, J. (2003). Continuous intrathecal baclofen infusion for spasticity of cerebral origin. *Journal of American Medical Association*, 270(20):2475-2477.

Biltzer, A. (1997). Cricopharyngeal muscle spasms and dysphagia. *Operative Techniques in Otolaryngology*, 8(4):191-192.

Bjornson, K., McLaughlin, J., Loeser, J., Nowak-Cooperman, K., Russel, M., Bader, K., & Desmond, S. (2003). Oral motor, communication, and nutritional status of children during intrathecal baclofen therapy. *Archives of Physical Medicine and Rehabilitation*, 84(4):500-506.

Boone, D.R,. & McFarlane, S.C. (2000). *The voice and voice therapy* (6th ed.). Boston: Allyn & Bacon.

Brin, M.F. (1997). Botulinum toxin: Chemistry, pharmacology, toxicity, and immunology. *Muscle Nerve*, 6(Suppl.):S146-S168.

Cameron, M.H., & Monroe, L.G. (2007). Pediatric nonprogressive central nervous system disorders. In M.H. Cameron & L.G. Monroe (Eds.), *Physical rehabilitation*. St. Louis: Saunders.

Carl, L., & Johnson, P. (2006). *Drugs and dysphagia*. Austin, TX: Pro-Ed.

Chou, R., Peterson, K., & Helfand, M. (2004). Comparative efficacy and safety of skeletal muscle relaxants for spasticity and musculoskeletal conditions: A systematic review. *Journal of Pain and Symptom Management*, 28(2):140-175.

Ciccone, C.D. (2007). *Pharmacology in rehabilitation* (4th ed.). Philadelphia: Davis.

Cunningham, S.J., & Teller, D. (2004, October). *Botox therapy in the laryngopharynx*. Lecture at University of Texas Medical Branch, Galveston, TX.

Dario, A., & Tomei, G. (2004). A benefit–risk assessment of baclofen in severe spinal spasticity. *Drug Safety*, 27(11):799-818.

Dillon, C., Paulose-Ram, R., Hirsch, R., & Gu, Q. (2004). Skeletal muscle relaxant use in the United States: Data from the third national health and nutrition examination survey. *Spine*, 29(8):892-896.

Gallichio, J.E. (2004). Pharmacologic management of spasticity following stroke. *Physical Therapy*, 84(10):973-981.

Houglum, J.E., Haarrelson, G.L., & Leaver-Dunn, D. (2005). *Principles of pharmacology for athletic trainers*. Thorofare, NJ: Slack.

Hudson, J. (2008). Spasticity. Retrieved from http://neurosurgery.med.sc.edu/patientcare/spasticity.asp

Hunter, O.K., & Freeman, M. (2008). Cervical sprain and strain. Available: http://emedicine.medscape.com/article/306176-overview

Koek, G.H., Sifrim, D., Lerut, T., Janssens, J., & Tack, J. (2003). Effect of the GABA agonist baclofen in patients with symptoms and duodeno-gastro-oesophageal reflux refractory to proton pump inhibitors. *Gut*, 52(10):1397-1402.

Kopec, K. (2008). Cerebral palsy: Pharmacologic treatment of spasticity. *U.S. Pharmacist*, 33(1):22-26.

Leary, S.M., Gilpin, P., & Lockley, L. (2006). Intrathecal baclofen therapy improves functional intelligibility of speech in cerebral palsy. *Clinical Rehabilitation*, 20(3):228-231.

Lidums, I., Lehmann, A., Checklin, H., Dent, J., & Holloway, R. (2000). Control of transient lower esophageal sphincter relaxations and reflux by the GABA agonist baclofen in normal subjects. *Gastroenterology*, 118(1):7-13.

Magee, D.J. (2007). Principles and concepts. In D.J. Magee (Ed.), *Orthopedic physical assessment* (p. 37). St. Louis: Saunders.

Merello, M., Garcia, H., Nogues, M., & Leiguarda, R. (1994). Mastication muscle spasm in a non-Japanese patient with Satoyoshi syndrome successfully treated with botulinum toxin. *Movement Disorders*, 9(1):104-105.

Milanov, I., & Georgiev, D. (1994). Mechanisms of tizanidine action on spasticity. *Acta Neurologica Scandinavica*, 89(4):274-279.

Mullarkey, T. (2009). Considerations in the treatment of spasticity with intrathecal baclofen. *American Journal of Health-System Pharmacy*, 66(Suppl. 5):S14-S22.

Murry, T., & Woodsen, G.E. (1995). Combined-modality treatment of adductor spasmodic dystonia with botulinum toxin and voice therapy. *Journal of Voice*, 9(4):460-465.

National Institute of Neurological Diseases and Stroke. (2011). *Stroke*. Bethesda, MD: National Institutes of Health.

O'Brien, G.F., Seeberger, L.G., & Smith, D.B. (1996). Spasticity after stroke: Epidemiology and optimal treatment. *Drugs and Aging*, 9(5):332-340.

Omari, T., Benninga, M., Sansom, L., Butler, R., Dent, J., & Davidson, G. (2006). Effect of baclofen on esophagogastric utility and gastroesophageal reflux in children with gastroesophageal reflux disease: A randomized controlled trial. *The Journal of Pediatrics*, 149(4):468-474.

Ozcakir, S., & Sivrioglu, K. (2007). Botulinum toxin in poststroke spasticity. *Clinical Medicine Research*, 5(2):132-138.

Peng, C.T., Ger, J., Yang, C.C., Tsai, W.J., Deng, J.F., & Bullard, M.J. (1998). Prolonged severe withdrawal symptoms after acute or chronic baclofen overdose. *Clinical Toxicology*, 36(4):359-363.

Purves, D., Augustine, G.J., Fitzpatrick, D., Katz, L.C., LaManita, A.S., McNamara, J.O., & Williams, M. (2001). Lower motor neuron circuits and motor control. *Neuroscience* (2nd ed.). Sunderland, MA: Sinauer Associates.

Rietman, J.S., & Geertzen, J.B. (2007). Efficacy of intrathecal baclofen delivery in the management of severe spasticity in upper motor neuron syndrome. *ACTA Neurochirurgica*, 97(Suppl. Part 1):205-211.

Rubin, D.I. (2007). Epidemiology and risk factors for spine pain. *Neurologic Clinics*, 25(2):353-371.

Satkunam, L.E. (2003). Rehabilitation medicine: Management of adult spasticity. *Canadian Medical Association*, 169(11):1173-1179.

Sullivan, J.E., & Hedman, L.D. (2004). A home program of sensory and neuromuscular electrical stimulation with upper-limb task practice in a patient 5 years after a stroke. *Physical Therapy*, 84(11):1045-1054.

Tsering D., Kissinger P., & Hoadley D. (1998). Knowledge and attitudes about HIV/AIDS among health care professionals serving Tibetan refugees in northern India. *International Journal of STD & AIDS*, 9(1):58-9.

VanDenburgh, A., Eisele, O., Varon, S.F., & Horak, H. (2010). Spasticity: Characterization and treatment considerations. *Allergan Neurosciences*, (March) pp. 1-16.

Vittal, H., & Pasricha, P.J. (2006). Botulinum toxin for gastrointestinal disorders: Therapy and mechanisms. *Neurotoxicity Research*, 9(2):149-159.

Walker, R.H., Danisi, F.O., Swope, D.M., Goodman, R.R., Germano, I.M., & Brin, M.F. (2000). Intrathecal baclofen for dystonia: Benefits and complications during six years of experience. *Movement Disorders*, 15(6):1242-1247.

Wilson-Howle, J. (1999). Cerebral palsy. In S. Campbell (Ed.), *Decision making in pediatric neurologic physical therapy*. New York: Churchill Livingstone.

Wise, J., & Conklin, J.L. (2004). Gastroesophageal reflux disease and baclofen: Is there a light at the end of the tunnel? *Current Gastroenterology Reports*, 6(3):213-219.

Zhang, Q., Lehmann, A., Rigda, R., Dent, J., & Holloway, R.H. (2002). Control of transient lower oesophageal sphincter relaxations and reflux by the GABA agonist baclofen in patients with gastroesophageal reflux disease. *Gut*, 50(1):19-24.

Chapter 10

Alvi, A. (1999). Iatrogenic swallowing disorders: Medications. In R.L. Carrau & T. Murry (Eds.), *Comprehensive management of swallowing disorders* (pp. 119-124). San Diego: Singular.

Antonopoulos, M.S., & Kim, K.S. (2007). Selegiline orally disintegrating tablets (Zelapar)—A new formulation of an old drug for Parkinson's disease. *Pharmacy and Therapeutics Journal*, 32(12):653-659.

Behrman A.L., Teitelbaum, P., & Cauraugh, J. (1998). Verbal instructional sets to normalize the temporal and spatial variables in Parkinson's disease. *Journal of Neurology, Neurosurgery, and Psychiatry*, 65(4):580-582.

Brunt, D., Protas, E., & Bishop, M. (2008). Gait characteristics and intervention strategies in patients with Parkinson's disease. In M. Trail, E.J. Protas, & E.C. Lai (Eds.), *Neurorehabilitation in Parkinson's disease* (pp. 153-174). Thorofare, NJ: Slack.

Campbell-Taylor, I. (1996). Drugs, dysphagia and nutrition. In C. Van Riper (Ed.), *Dietetics in development and psychiatric disorders* (pp. 24-29). Chicago: American Dietetic Association.

Campbell-Taylor, I. (2001). *Medications and dysphagia* (p.1-32). Stow, OH: Interactive Therapeutics.

Carl, L.C., & Johnson, P.R. (2006). *Drugs and dysphagia: How medications can affect eating and swallowing*. Austin, TX: Pro-Ed.

Chen, J.J. (2002). Movement disorders: Parkinson's disease and essential tremor. In Mueller, B.A., Bertch, K.E., Dunsworth,

T.S., Fagan, S.C., Hayney, M.S., O'Connell, M.B., Schumock, G.T., Thompson, D.F., Tisdale, J.E., Witt, D.M., & Zaharowitz, B.J. *Pharmacotherapy self-assessment program. Book 7: Neurology and psychiatry* (4th ed.) (pp. 1-42). Kansas City, MO: American College of Clinical Pharmacy.

Chen, J.J. (2012). Parkinson disease. In Richardson, M.M., Chessman, K.H., Chant,C., Finks, S.W., Hemstreet, B.A., Hume, A.L., Hutchison, L.C., Karpiuk, E.L., MCCollum, M., Segarra-Newnham, M., & Sherer, J.T. *Pharmacotherapy self-assessment program. Book 10: Neurology and psychiatry*. (7th ed.) (pp. 111-132). Kansas City, MO: American College of Clinical Pharmacy.

Chen, J.J., Lew, M.F., & Siderowf, A. (2009). Treatment strategies and quality of care indicators for patients with Parkinson's disease. *Journal of Managed Care Pharmacy*, 15(3):S1-S21.

Chen, J.J., & Swope, D.M. (2007). Pharmacotherapy for Parkinson's disease. *Pharmacotherapy*, 27(12 Part 2):161S-173S.

Chen, J.J., Swope, D.M., Dashtipour, K., & Lyons, K.E. (2009). Transdermal rotigotine: A clinically innovative dopamine-receptor agonist for the management of Parkinson's disease. *Pharmacotherapy*, 29(12):1452-1467.

Ciccone, C.D. (2007). *Pharmacology in rehabilitation* (4th ed.). Philadelphia: Davis.

DeLetter, M., Santens, P., & Van Borsel, J. (2005). The effects of levodopa on word intelligibility in Parkinson's disease. *Journal Community Disorders*, 38(3):187-196.

Factor, S.A., & Weiner, W.J. (2008). *Parkinson's disease: Diagnosis and clinical management*. New York: Demos Medical.

Faulkner, M.A. (2006). The role of the pharmacist in the management of Parkinson's disease. *U.S. Pharmacist*, 31(9):105-116.

Feinberg, M. (1997). The effect of medications on swallowing. In B.C. Sones (Ed.), *Dysphagia: A continuum of care* (pp. 107-118). Gaithersburg, MD: Aspen.

Fernandez, H.H., & Chen, J.J. (2007). Monoamine oxidase-b inhibition in the treatment of Parkinson's disease. *Pharmacotherapy*, 27(12 Part 2):174S-185S.

Fox, C.M., Ramig, L., Sapir, S., Halpern, A., Cable, J., Mahler, L.A., & Farley, B.G. (2008). Voice and speech disorders in Parkinson's disease and their treatment. In M. Trail, E.J. Protas, & E.C. Lai (Eds.), *Neurorehabilitation in Parkinson's disease* (pp. 240-276). Thorofare, NJ: Slack.

Fuh, J.L., Lee, R.C., Wang, S.J., Chiang, J.H., & Liu, H.C. (1997). Swallowing difficulty in Parkinson's disease. *Clinical Neurological Neurosurgery*, 99(2):106-112.

Gallena, S., Smith, P.J., Zeffirp, T., & Ludlow, C.L. (2001). Effects of levodopa on laryngeal muscle activity for voice onset and offset in Parkinson's disease. *Journal of Speech Language Hearing Research*, 44(6):1284-1299.

Hopfer-Deglin, J., & Hazard Vallerand, A. (2010). *Med notes* (3rd ed.). Philadelphia: Davis.

Hou, J.G., & Lai, E.C. (2008). Overview of Parkinson's disease: Clinical features, diagnosis and management. In M. Trail, E.J. Protas, & E.C. Lai (Eds.), *Neurorehabilitation in Parkinson's disease* (pp. 1-39). Thorofare, NJ: Slack.

Hunter, P.C., Crameri, J., & Austin, S. (1997). Response of parkinsonian swallowing dysfunction to dopaminergic stimulation. *Journal of Neurology, Neurosurgery, and Psychiatry*, 63(5):579-583.

Iversen, L.L., Iversen, S.D., Bloom, F.E., & Roth, R.H. (2009). *Introduction to neuropsychopharmacology*. Oxford, NY: Oxford University Press.

Jacobson, S.A., Pies, R.W., & Katz, I.R. (2007). *Clinical manual of geriatric psychopharmacology*. Washington, DC: American Psychiatric.

Kyle, J.A., & Kyle, L.R. (2007). A Parkinson's disease primer. *Drug Topics*, October:26-34.

Langston, J.W., Waters, C., & Watts, R.L. (2007). Lifelong management of Parkinson's disease: Diagnosis, treatment and emerging therapies. Proceedings from a Live Meeting Series. AAF-MED/Schwarz Pharma Program.

Lertxundi, U., Peral, J.M., Mora, U., Domingo-Echaburu, S., Martinez-Bengoechea, M.J., & Garcia-Monco, J.C. (2008). Anti-dopaminergic therapy for managing comorbidities in patients with Parkinson's disease. *American Journal of Health-System Pharmacy*, 65(5):414-419.

Lew, M. (2007). Overview of Parkinson's disease. *Pharmacotherapy*, 27(12 Part 2):153S-160S.

Lo, K., Leung, K., & Shek, A. (2007). Management of Parkinson disease: Current treatments, recent advances, and future development. *Formulary*, 42(September):529-544.

Marder, K.S., & Jacobs, D.M. (2008). Dementia. In S.A. Factor & W.J. Weiner (Eds.), *Parkinson's disease: Diagnosis and clinical management* (pp. 147-158). New York: Demos Medical.

Morris, M.E., Grad, D., Huxham, F., Menz, H.B., Dobson, F., Piry-aprasarth, P., et al. (2008). Optimizing movement and preventing falls in Parkinson's disease: Strategies for patients and caregivers. In M. Trail, E.J. Protas, & E.C. Lai (Eds.), *Neurorehabilitation in Parkinson's disease* (pp. 177-185). Thorofare, NJ: Slack.

Nelson, M.V., Berchou, R.C., & LeWitt, P.A. (2002). Parkinson's disease. In J.T. DiPiro, R.L. Talbert, G.C. Yee, G.R. Matske, B.G. Wells, & L.M. Posey (Eds.), *Pharmacotherapy: A pathophysiologic approach* (5th ed.) (pp. 1089-1102). Stamford, CT: Appleton & Lange.

Pagni, C.A., Zeme, S., & Zemga, F. (2003). Further experience with extradural motor cortex stimulation for treatment of advanced Parkinson's disease. *Journal of Neurosurgical Science*, 47(4):189-193.

Parkinson Study Group. (2004). A controlled, randomized delayed-start study of rasagiline in early Parkinson disease. *Archives of Neurology*, 61(4):561-566.

Protas, E.J., Stanley, R.K., & Jankovic, P.T. (1996). Cardiovascular and metabolic responses to upper and lower extremity training in men with idiopathic Parkinson's disease. *Physical Therapy*, 76(1):34-40.

Quigley, E.M. (2008). Gastrointestinal features. In S.A. Factor & W.J. Weiner (Eds.), *Parkinson's disease: Diagnosis and clinical management* (pp. 99-105). New York: Demos Medical.

Rascol, O., Payoux, P., Ory, F., Ferreira, J.J., Brefel-Courbon, C., & Montastruc, J.L. (2003). Limitations of current Parkinson's disease therapy. *Annals of Neurology*, 53(Suppl. 3):3-15.

Sapir, S., Ramig, L.O., & Fox, C.M. (2008). Voice, speech, and swallowing disorders. In S.A. Factor & W.J. Weiner (Eds.), *Parkinson's disease: Diagnosis and clinical management* (pp. 77-97). New York: Demos Medical.

Schwartz, J. (2003). Rationale for dopamine agonist use as monotherapy in Parkinson's disease. *Current Opinion in Neurology*, 16(Suppl. 1):S27-S33.

Standaert, D.G., & Young, A.B. (2001). Treatment of central nervous system degenerative disorders. In J.G. Hardman, L.E. Limbird, & A.G. Gillman (Eds.), *Goodman and Gillman's the pharmacological basis of therapeutics* (10th ed.) (pp. 547-568). New York: McGraw-Hill.

Talati, R., White, C.M., & Coleman, C.I. (2007). Rotigotine: The first transdermal nonergot-derived dopamine agonist for the treatment of Parkinson disease. *Formulary*, 42(November):633-646.

Tanzi, M.G. (2007). Rotigotine: Transdermal dopamine agonist for Parkinson's disease. *Pharmacy Today*, August:28-30.

Trail, M., Protas, E.J., & Lai, E.C. (2008). *Neurorehabilitation in Parkinson's disease*. Thorofare, NJ: Slack.

Twelves, D., Perkins, K., & Counsell, C. (2002). Systematic review of incidence studies of Parkinson's disease. *Movement Disorders*, 18(1):19-31.

Weintraub, D., Comella, C.L., & Horn, S. (2008a). Parkinson's disease—Part 1: Pathophysiology, symptoms, burden, diagnosis, and assessment. *American Journal of Managed Care*, 14(2 Suppl.):S40-S48.

Weintraub, D., Comella, C.L., & Horn, S. (2008b). Parkinson's disease—Part 2: Treatment of motor symptoms. *American Journal of Managed Care*, 14(2 Suppl.):S49-S58.

Weintraub, D., Comella, C.L., & Horn, S. (2008c). Parkinson's disease—Part 3: Neuropsychiatric symptoms. *American Journal of Managed Care*, 14(2 Suppl.):S59-S69.

Wood, B. (2010). Eosinophilic esophagitis: A new disease. *U.S. Pharmacist*, 35(12):44-50.

Wood, B. (2011). *Parkinson's disease*. Available: http://toolkit.parkinson.org/content/orthostatic-hypotension.

York, M.K., & Alvarez, J.A. (2008). Cognitive impairments associated with Parkinson's disease. In M. Trail, E.J. Protas, & E.C. Lai (Eds.), *Neurorehabilitation in Parkinson's disease*. Thorofare, NJ: Slack.

Yorkston, K.M., Miller, R.M., & Strand, E.A. (2004). *Management of speech and swallowing disorders in degenerative diseases* (2nd ed.). Austin, TX: Pro-Ed.

Zweig, R.M., & Elliott, D. (2008). Sensory symptoms. In S.A. Factor & W.J. Weiner (Eds.), *Parkinson's disease: Diagnosis and clinical management* (2nd ed.) (pp. 65-76). New York: Demos Medical.

Chapter 11

Armon, C. (2010). Amyotrophic lateral sclerosis. Available: http://emedicine.medscape.com/article/1170097-overview

Awwad, S., & Mal'uf, R. (2010). Myasthenia gravis: Treatment and medication. Available: http://emedicine.medscape.com/article/1216417-treatment

Bainbridge, J.L. (2007). Mastering multiple sclerosis: Challenges and opportunities for managed care pharmacists. *University of Tennessee Advanced Studies in Pharmacy*, 4(11):311-313.

Bennett, J.L. (2007). Treating relapsing–remitting multiple sclerosis II: Strategies for patients not responding to primary treatments. *University of Tennessee Advanced Studies in Pharmacy*, 4(11):324-329.

Carr, A., Cardwell, C., McCarron, P., & McConville, J. (2010). A systematic review of population based epidemiological studies in myasthenia gravis. *BMC Neurology*, 10(46):10-46.

Chitsaz, A., Janghorbani, M., Shaygannejad, V., Ashtari, F., Heshmatipour, M., & Freeman, J. (2009). Sensory complaints of the upper extremities in multiple sclerosis: Relative efficacy of nortriptyline and transcutaneous electrical nerve stimulation. *Clinical Journal of Pain*, 25(4):281-285.

Ciccone, C.D. (2007). *Pharmacology in rehabilitation* (4th ed.). Philadelphia: Davis.

Cohen, J.A., Goodman, A.D., Kooijmans, M.F., Rudick, R.A., Simonian, N.A., & Tsao E.C. et al. (2002). Benefit of interferon beta-1a on MSFC progression in secondary progressive MS. *Neurology*, 59(5):679-687.

Cree, B. (2006). Emerging monoclonal antibody therapies for multiple sclerosis. *Neurologist*, 12(4):171-178.

Cronin, S., Hardiman, O., & Traynor, B.J. (2007). Ethnic variation in the incidence of ALS. *Neurology*, 68(13):1002-1007.

DeLuca, J. (1999). Speed of information processing as a key deficit in multiple sclerosis: Implications for rehabilitation. *Journal of Neurology, Neurosurgery, and Psychiatry*, 67(5):661-663.

Drory, V.E., Goltsman, E., Reznik, J.G., Mosek, A., & Korczyn, A.D. (2001). The value of muscle exercise in patients with amyotrophic lateral sclerosis. *Journal of Neurological Sciences*, 191(1-2):133-137.

Feret, B. (2009). Fampridine-SR: A potassium-channel blocker for the improvement of walking ability in patients with MS. *Formulary*, 44(10):293-299.

Gawronski, K.M., Rainka, M.M., Patel, M.J., & Gengo, F.M. (2010). Treatment options for multiple sclerosis: Current and emerging therapies. *Pharmacotherapy*, 30(9):916-917.

Gehlsen, G.M., Grigsby, S.A., & Winant, D.M. (1984). Effects of an aquatic fitness program on the muscular strength and endurance of patients with multiple sclerosis. *Physical Therapy*, 64(5):653-657.

Grasso, M.G., Troisi, E., Rizzi, F., Morelli, D., & Paolucci, S. (2005). Prognostic factors in multidisciplinary rehabilitation treatment in multiple sclerosis: An outcome study. *Multiple Sclerosis*, 11(6):719-724.

Guthrie, E.W. (2005). Overview of multiple sclerosis. *U.S. Pharmacist*, September:73-80.

Guthrie, E.W. (2007a). Multiple sclerosis. In Dunsworth, T.S., Richardson, M.M., Schwartz, W.B., Cheng, J.W.M., Chessman, K.H., Hume, A.L., Hutchison, L.C., Jackson, A.B., Karpiuk, E.L., Martin. L.G., Semla, T.P., & Wittbrodt, E.T. *Pharmacotherapy self-assessment program. Book 3: Neurology and psychiatry* (6th ed.) (pp. 1-17). Kansas City, MO: American College of Clinical Pharmacy.

Guthrie, E.W. (2007b). Multiple sclerosis: A primer and update. *University of Tennessee Advanced Studies in Pharmacy*, 4(11):313-317.

Havercamp, L.J., Appel, V., & Appel, S.H. (1995). Natural history of amyotrophic lateral sclerosis in database population—Validation of a scoring system and a model for survival prediction. *Brain*, 118(Part 3):707-719.

Iversen, L.L., Iversen, S.D., Bloom, F.E., & Roth, R.H. (2009). *Introduction to neuropsychopharmacology*. New York: Oxford University Press.

Jacobson, S.A., Pies, R.W., & Katz, I.R. (2007). *Clinical manual of geriatric psychopharmacology*. Washington, DC: American Psychiatric.

Khan, F., Pallant, J.F., Brand, C., & Kilpatrick, T.J. (2008). Effectiveness of rehabilitation intervention in persons with multiple sclerosis: A randomized controlled study. *Journal of Neurology, Neurosurgery, and Psychiatry*, 79(11):1230-1235.

Kurtzke, J.F., & Wallin, M.T. (2000). Epidemiology. In J.S. Burks & K.P. Johnson (Eds.), *Multiple sclerosis: Diagnosis, medical management, and rehabilitation*. New York: Demos.

Litzinger, M.J., & Litzinger, M. (2009). Multiple sclerosis: A therapeutic overview. *U.S. Pharmacy-Health Systems Edition*, 34(1):3-9.

Lo, A.C., & Triche, E.W. (2008). Improving gait in multiple sclerosis using robot assisted, body weight supported treadmill training. *Neurorehabilitation and Neural Repair*, 22(6):661-671.

Lohi, E., Lindberg, C., & Anderson, O. (1993). Physical training in myasthenia gravis. *Archives of Physical Medicine and Rehabilitation*, 74(11):1178-1189.

Mendez, M.F., & Cummings, J.L. (2003). *Dementia: A clinical approach*. Philadelphia: Butterworth Heinemann.

Perez, B. (2009). Fampridine-SR: A potassium channel blocker for the improvement of walking ability in patients with MS. *Formulary*, October:293-300.

Rosati, G. (2001). The prevalence of multiple sclerosis in the world: An update. *Neurological Science*, 22(2):117-139.

Rosenzweig, T.M., Hartman, S., & MacKenzie, E. (2010). Disease modifying therapy in adult relapsing–remitting multiple sclerosis. *Formulary*, 45:252-262.

Ryan, M. (2007). Treating relapsing–remitting multiple sclerosis I: The primary disease-modifying drugs. *University of Tennessee Advanced Studies in Pharmacy*, 4(11):318-322.

Shah, A. (2011). Myasthenia gravis. Available: http://emedicine.medscape.com/article/1171206-overview

Sobieraj, D.M. (2010). Fingolimod: A potential first-in-class oral therapy for the treatment of relapsing–remitting multiple sclerosis. *Formulary*, 45(August):245-251.

Tanzi, M.G. (2010). Fingolimod provides oral option for relapsing MS. *Pharmacy Today*, November:29-30.

Vogel, D., Carter, J.E., & Carter, P.B. (2000). *The effects of drugs on communication disorders* (2nd ed.). San Diego: Singular.

Yorkston, K.M., Miller, R.M., & Strand, E.A. (2004). *Management of speech and swallowing disorders in degenerative diseases* (2nd ed.). Austin, TX: Pro-Ed.

Chapter 12

Brown, C.H. (2010). Drug induced serotonin syndrome. *U.S. Pharmacist-Health System Edition*, November:16-21.

Carl, L., & Johnson, P. (2006). *Drugs and dysphagia*. Austin, TX: Pro-Ed.

Chen, J.J. (2002). Movement disorders: Parkinson's disease and essential tremor. In Mueller, B.A., Bertch, K.E., Dunsworth, T.S., Fagan, S.C., Hayney, M.S., O'Connell, M.B., Schumock, G.T., Thompson, D.F., Tisdale, J.E., Witt, D.M., & Zaharowitz, B.J. *Pharmacotherapy self-assessment program. Book 4: Neurology and psychiatry* (3rd ed.) (pp. 1-42). Kansas City, MO: American College of Clinical Pharmacy.

Cheng, C.M., Chen, J.S., & Patel, R.P. (2006). Unlabeled uses of botulinum toxins: A review— Part 1. *American Journal of Health-System Pharmacy*, 63(2):145-152.

Ciccone, C.D. (2007). *Pharmacology in rehabilitation* (4th ed.). Philadelphia: Davis.

Crystal, H.A. (2010). Dementia with Lewy bodies treatment and management. Available: http://emedicine.medscape.com/article/1135041-treatment

DeRuiter, J., & Holston, P.L. (2009). Review of selected NMEs for 2009. *U.S. Pharmacist-Health System Edition*, October:3-13.

DeSimone, E.M., & Petrov, K. (2009). Restless legs syndrome: A common, underdiagnosed disorder. *U.S. Pharmacist*, 34(1):24-29.

Eggenberger, E.R., & Vanek, Z.F. (2010). Progressive supranuclear palsy: Treatment and medications. Available: http://emedicine.medscape.com/article/1151430-treatment

Emilien, G., Durlach, C., Minaker, K.L., Winblad, B., Gauthier, S., & Maloteaux, J. (2004). *Alzheimer disease: Neuropsychology and pharmacology*. Berlin: Birkhauser Verlag.

Grimsley, S.R. (1998). Mood disorders. In Carter, B.L., Lake, K.D., Raebel, M.A., Bertch, K.E., Israel, M.K., Jermain, D.M., Kelly, H.W., Lam, N.P., Mueller, B.A., & Thompson, D.F. *Pharmacotherapy self-assessment program. Book 4: Neurology and psychiatry* (3rd ed.) (pp. 119-163). Kansas City, MO: American College of Clinical Pharmacy.

Heidebrink, J. (2002). Is dementia with Lewy bodies the second most common cause of dementia? *Journal of Geriatric Psychiatry and Neurology*, 15(4):182-187.

Huang, V., & Gortney, J.S. (2006). Risk of serotonin syndrome with concomitant administration of linezolid and serotonin agonists. *Pharmacotherapy*, 26(12):1784-1793.

Iversen, L.L., Iversen, S.D., Bloom, F.E., & Roth, R.H. (2009). *Introduction to neuropsychopharmacology*. New York: Oxford University Press.

Jacobson, S.A., Pies, R.W., & Katz, I.R. (2007). *Clinical manual of geriatric psychopharmacology*. Washington, DC: American Psychiatric.

Kishel, J.J., & Palkovic, L. (2006). Serotonin syndrome associated with linezolid administration. *U.S. Pharmacist–Health System Edition*, November:41-42.

Lorenz, D., Frederiksen, H., Moises, H., Kopper, F., Deuschl, G., & Christensen, K. (2004). High concordance for essential tremor in monozygotic twins of old age. *Neurology*, 62(2):208-211.

Mendez, M.F., & Cummings, J.L. (2003). *Dementia: A clinical approach*. Philadelphia: Butterworth Heinemann.

Narita, M., Tsuji, B.T., & Yu, V.L. (2007). Linezolid-associated peripheral and optic neuropathy, lactic acidosis, and serotonin syndrome. *Pharmacotherapy*, 27(8):1189-1197.

Neumiller, J.J., Wood, L., Dobbins, E., Setter, S.M., & Greeley, D.R. (2009). Tetrabenazine for the treatment of Huntington's chorea. *U.S. Pharmacist*, 34(1):47-55.

Preston, J.D., O'Neill, J.H., & Talaga, M.C. (2008). *Handbook of clinical psychopharmacology for therapists*. Oakland: New Harbinger.

Robishaw, S., & Beadle, M. (2010). Vascular dementia. *U.S. Pharmacist*, 35(1):46-48.

Ryan, M., & Slevin, J.T. (2006). Restless legs syndrome. *American Journal of Health-System Pharmacy*, 63(17):1599-1612.

Smeltzer, S., & Bare, B. (2000). *Brunner and Suddarth's textbook of medical-surgical nursing* (9th ed.). Philadelphia: Lippincott.

Sohlberg, M., & Turkstra, L. (2011). *Optimizing cognitive rehabilitation*. New York: Guilford Press.

Sonnett, T., Setter, S.M., & Greeley, D.R. (2006). Dementia with Lewy bodies. *U.S. Pharmacist-Health System Edition*, April:12-28.

Spillantini, M.G., Bird, T., & Bernardino, G. (2006). Frontotemporal dementia and parkinsonism linked to chromosome 17: A new group of tauopathies. *Brain Pathology*, 8(2):387-402.

Tison, F., Crochard, A., Leger, D., Bouee, S., Lainey, E., & Hasnaoui, A. (2005). Epidemiology of restless legs syndrome in French adults. A nationwide survey. *Neurology*, 65(2):239-246.

Vogel, D., Carter, J., & Carter, P. (2000). *The effects of drugs on communication disorders*. San Diego: Singular.

Walshe, J., & Cox, D. (1998). Effect of treatment of Wilson's disease on natural history of haemochromatosis. *Lancet*, 352(9122):112-113.

Yorkston, K.M., Miller, R.M., & Strand, E.A. (2004). *Management of speech and swallowing disorders in degenerative diseases* (2nd ed.). Austin, TX: Pro-Ed.

Chapter 13

Acute Pain Management Guidelines Panel. (1992). *Acute pain management: Operative or medical procedures and trauma—Clinical practice guideline*. U.S. Department of Health and Human Services Public Health Service Agency for Healthcare Policy and Research: Rockville, Maryland.

Aegis Therapies (2010). *Pain management workbook*. Aegis Therapies: Plano, Texas.

Blommel, M. L. and Blommel, A. L. (2007). Pregabalin: An antiepileptic agent useful for neuropathic pain. *American Journal of Health-System Pharmacy*, 64(14):1475-1482.

Bone, M., Critchley, P., & Buggy, D.J. (2002) Gabapentin use in post amputation phantom limb pain: A randomized, double-blind, placebo-controlled, cross-over study. *Regional Anesthesia and Pain Medicine*, 27(5):481-486.

Brenton-Wood, B. (2009). Understanding the pharmacologic therapy for patients afflicted with complex regional pain syndrome. *U.S. Pharmacist-Health System Edition*, May:3-7.

Cameron, M.H., & Monroe, L.G. (2007). *Physical rehabilitation: Evidence-based examination, evaluation, and intervention*. St. Louis: Saunders Elsevier.

Campbell-Taylor, I. (1996). Drugs, dysphagia and nutrition. In C. Van Riper (Ed.), *Dietetics in development and psychiatric disorders* (pp. 24-29). Chicago: American Dietetic Association.

Campbell-Taylor, I. (2001). *Medications and dysphagia* (pp. 1-32). Stow, OH: Interactive Therapeutics.

Carl, L., & Johnson, P.R. (2006). *Drugs and dysphagia*. Austin, TX: Pro-Ed.

Caufield, J.S. (2006). Management of chronic non-malignant pain. *Drug Topics*, March:39-48.

Ciccone, C.D. (2007). *Pharmacology in rehabilitation* (4th ed.). Philadelphia: Davis.

Dubinsky, R.M., Kabbani, H., El-Chami, Z., Boutwell, C., & Ali, H. (2004). Practice parameter: Treatment of post herpetic neuralgia: An evidenced based report of the American Academy of Neurology. *Neurology*, 63(6):959-965.

Dworkin, R.H., Corbin, A.E., Young, J.P., Sharma, U., LaMoreaux, L., Bockbrader, H., et al. (2007). Resource use associated with topiramate in migraine prophylaxis. *American Journal of Health-System Pharmacy*, 64(14):1483-1491.

Eidelman, A., White, T., & Swarm, R.A. (2007). Interventional therapies for cancer pain management: Important adjuvants to systemic analgesics. *Journal of the National Comprehensive Cancer Network*, 5(8):753-760.

Finnerup, N.B., Otto, M., McQuay, H.J., Jensen, T.S., & Sindrup, S.H. (2005). Algorithm for neuropathic pain treatment: An evidence-based proposal. *Pain*, 118(3):289-305.

Ghafoor, V.L., Epshteyn, M., Carlson, G.H., Terhaar, D.M., Charry, O., & Phelps, P.K. (2007). Intrathecal drug therapy for long term pain management. *American Journal of Health-System Pharmacy*, 64(23):2447-2461.

Gutstein, H.B., & Akil, H. (2001). Opioid analgesics. In J.G. Hardman & L.E. Limbird (Eds.), *Goodman and Gillman's the pharmacological basis of therapeutics* (10th ed.) (pp. 569-619). New York: McGraw-Hill.

Hartrick, C., Van Hove, I., Stegmann, J.U., Oh, C., & Upmalis, D. (2009). Efficacy and tolerability of tapentadol immediate release and oxycodone HCl immediate release in patients awaiting primary joint replacement surgery for end-stage joint disease: A 10-day, phase III, randomized, double-blind, active- and placebo-controlled study. *Clinical Therapeutics*, 31(2):260-271.

Hulisz, D., & Moore, N. (2007). Chronic pain management: Role of newer antidepressants and anticonvulsants. *U.S. Pharmacist*, 32(5):55-61.

Hutchinson, R.W. (2007). Challenges in acute post-operative pain management. *American Journal of Health-System Pharmacy*, 64(Suppl. 4):S2-S5.

Iversen, L.L., Iversen, S.D., Bloom, F.E., & Roth, R.H. (2009). *Introduction to neuropsychopharmacology*. New York: Oxford University Press.

Jacobson, S.A., Pies, R.W., & Katz, I.R. (2007). *Clinical manual of geriatric psychopharmacology*. Washington, DC: American Psychiatric.

Jacox, A., Carr, D.B., & Payne, R. (1994). *Management of cancer pain: Clinical practice guidelines*. Agency for Health Care Policy and Research publication no. 94-0592 (pp. 39-74). Rockville, MD:, U.S. Department of Health and Human Services.

Jann, M.W., & Slade, J.H. (2007). Antidepressant agents for the treatment of chronic pain and depression. *Pharmacotherapy*, 27(11):1571-1587.

Max, M.B., Payne, R., & Edwards, W.T. (1999). *Principles of analgesic use in the treatment of acute pain and cancer pain* (4th ed.) (pp. 1-64). Glenview, IL: American Pain Society.

Metzger, S.E. (2009). New products bulletin: Nucynta (tapentadol). *Pharmacy Today*, September(Suppl.):3-16.

Montfort, E.G., Witte, A.P., & Ward, K. (2010). Neuropathic pain: A review of diabetic neuropathy. *U.S. Pharmacist-Health System Edition*, May:8-15.

Moultry, A.M., & Poon, I.O. (2009). The use of antidepressants for chronic pain. *U.S. Pharmacist*, 34(5):26-34.

Nucynta (Tapentadol). (2009). Product information available at www.nucynta.com

Phillips, S.E. (2007). Pain assessment in the elderly. *U.S. Pharmacist*, May:37-52.

Preston, J. D., O'Neill, J.H., & Talaga, M.C. (2008). *Handbook of clinical psychopharmacology for therapists* (5th ed.). Oakland: New Harbinger.

Puig, M., Montes, A., & Marrugat, J. (2001). Management of postoperative pain in Spain. *Acta Anaesthesiologica Scandinavica*, 45(4):465-470.

Roberts, L.J., & Morrow, J.D. (2001). Analgesic, antipyretic and antiinflammatory agents and drugs employed in the treatment of gout. In J.G. Hardman & L.E. Limbird (Eds.), *Goodman and Gillman's the pharmacological basis of therapeutics* (10th ed.) (pp. 687-731). New York: McGraw-Hill.

Rosenstock, J., Tuchman, M., LaMoreaux, L., & Sharma, U. (2004). Pregabalin for the treatment of painful diabetic peripheral neuropathy: A double blind placebo controlled trial. *Pain*, 110(3):628-638.

Sluka, K.A. (2001). Basic science mechanisms of TENS and clinical implications. *American Pain Society*, 11(2):12-25.

Strassels, S.A., McNicol, E., & Suleman, R. (2007). Acute pain pharmacotherapy. *U.S. Pharmacist-Health System Edition*, May:5-19.

Swarm, R., Benedetti, C., Cleeland, C., deLeon-Casasola, O.A., Eiler, J.G., Grossman, S.A., et al. (2007). Adult cancer pain: Clinical practice guidelines in oncology. *Journal of National Comprehensive Cancer Network*, 5(8):726-760.

Tanzi, M.G. (2009). Tapentadol: An opioid with a dual mode of action. *Pharmacy Today*, Septermber:20.

Teague, A. (2007). Neuropathic pain calls for a range of treatment options. *Pharmacy Times*, September:32-33.

Toth, J.A. (2009). Concepts in cancer pain management. *U.S. Pharmacist*, 34(11):3-12.

Viscusi, E.R. (2007). Emerging treatment modalities: Balancing efficacy and safety. *American Journal of Health-System Pharmacy*, 64(Suppl. 4):S6-S11.

Westanmo, A.D., Gayken, G., & Haight, R. (2005). Duloxetine: a balanced *and* selective norepinephrine- *and* serotonin-reuptake inhibitor *American Journal of Health-System Pharmacy*, 62(23):2481-2490.

Wiffen, P.J., McQuay, H.J., Edwards, J.E., & Moore, R.A. (2005). Gabapentin for acute and chronic pain. Available: www.ncbi.nlm.gov/pubmed/16034978

Zagaria, M.E. (2009). Assessing pain in the cognitively impaired. *U.S. Pharmacist*, 34(5):21-34.

Zichterman, A. (2007). Opioid pharmacology and considerations in pain management. *U.S. Pharmacist-Health System Edition*, May:77-87.

Chapter 14

Adams, P.F., Hendershot, G.E., & Marano, M.A. (1999). Current estimates from the national health interview survey, 1996. *Vital and Health Statistics*, 200(October):1-203.

Black, L.M., Persons, R.K., & Jamieson, M.S. (2009). What is the best way to manage phantom limb pain? *The Journal of Family Practice*, 58(3):155-158.

Bomburg, N. (2012). Epidemiology: trigeminal neuralgia—the disease is not as rare as previously thought. Retrieved from: www.prnewswire.com/news-releases/epidemiology-trigeminal-neuralgia----the-disease-is-not-as-rare-as-previously-thought-158892165.html

Bone, M., Critchley, P., & Buggy, D.J. (2002) Gabapentin in post amputation phantom limb pain: A randomized, double-blind, placebo-controlled, cross-over study. *Regional Anesthesia and Pain Medicine*, 27(5):481-486.

Brenton-Wood, B. (2009). Understanding the pharmacologic therapy for patients afflicted with complex regional pain syndrome. *U.S. Pharmacist-Health System Edition*, 34(5):3-7.

Cameron, M.H., & Monroe, L.G. (2007). *Physical rehabilitation: Evidence-based examination, evaluation, and intervention*. St. Louis: Saunders Elsevier.

Chabal, C., Fishbain, D., Weaver, M., Heine, L., & Wipperman, M. (1998). Long-term transcutaneous electrical nerve stimulation (TENS) use: Impact on medication utilization and physical therapy costs. *Clinical Journal of Pain*, 14(1):66-73.

Chan, B.L., Witt, R., Charrow, A.P., Magee, A., Howard, R., Pasquina, P.F., et al. (2007). Mirror therapy for phantom limb pain. *New England Journal of Medicine*, 357(21):2206-2207.

Cheng, C.M., Chen, J.S., & Patel, R.P. (2006a). Unlabeled uses of botulinum toxins: A review—Part 1. *American Journal of Health-System Pharmacy*, 63(2):145-152.

Cheng, C.M., Chen, J.S., & Patel, R.P. (2006b). Unlabeled uses of botulinum toxins: A review—Part 2. *American Journal of Health-System Pharmacy*, 63(3):225-232.

Demaagd, G. (2008a). The pharmacological management of migraine—Part 1: Overview and abortive therapy. *Pharmacy and Therapeutics*, 33(3):404-418.

Demaagd, G. (2008b). The pharmacological management of migraine—Part 2: Preventative therapy. *Pharmacy and Therapeutics*, 33(8):480-490.

de Mos, M., de Bruin, A.J., Dieleman, J.P., Stricker, B.H., & Sturkenboom, M.M. (2006). The incidence of complex regional pain syndrome: A population-based study. *Pain*, 129(1-2):12-20.

Eidelman, A., White, T., & Swarm, R.A. (2007). Interventional therapies for cancer pain management: Important adjuvants to systemic analgesics. *Journal of the National Comprehensive Cancer Network*, 5(8):753-760.

English, C., Rey, J.A., & Rufin, C. (2010). Milnacipran (Savella): A treatment option for fibromyalgia. *Pharmacy and Therapeutics*, 35(5):261-288.

Feliu, A.L., Rupnow, M.T., Blount, A., Boccuzzi, S.J., & Vermilyea, J. (2007). Resource use associated with topiramate in migraine prophylaxis. *American Journal of Health-System Pharmacy*, 64(14):1483-1491.

Finnerup, N.B., Otto, M., McQuay, H.J., Jensen, T.S., & Sindrup, S.H. (2005). Algorithm for neuropathic pain treatment: An evidence-based proposal. *Pain*, 118(3):289-305.

Flor, H., Nikolajsen, L., & Jensen, S.T. (2006). Phantom limb pain: A case of maladaptive CNS plasticity? *Nature Reviews Neuroscience*, 7(November):873-881.

Ghafoor, V.L., Epshteyn, M., Carlson, G.H., Terhaar, D.M., Charry, O., & Phelps, P.K. (2007). Intrathecal drug therapy for long term pain management. *American Journal of Health-System Pharmacy*, 64(23):2447-2461.

Gibson, J.L. (2010). Over the counter use of neuroactive peptides for the treatment of chronic pain. *U.S. Pharmacist*, 35(12):106-115.

Gutstein, H.B., & Akil, H. (2001). Opioid analgesics. In J.G. Hardman, L.E. Limbird, & A.G. Gilman (Eds.), *Goodman and Gillman's the pharmacological basis of therapeutics* (10th ed.) (pp. 569-619). New York: McGraw-Hill.

Harden R.N., & Cole P.A. (1998). New developments in rehabilitation of neuropathic pain syndromes. *Neurologic Clinics*, 16(4):937-50.

Hartrick, C., Van Hove, I., Stegman, J.U., Oh, C., & Upmalis, D. (2009). Efficacy and tolerability of tapentadol immediate release and oxycodone HCl immediate release in patients awaiting primary joint replacement surgery for end-stage joint disease: A 10-day, phase III, randomized, double-blind, active- and placebo-controlled study. *Clinical Therapeutics*, 31(2):260-271.

Jensen, T.S., Krebs, B., Nielsen, J., & Rasmussen, P. (1985). Immediate and long-term phantom limb pain in amputees: incidence, clinical characteristics and relationship to pre-amputation limb pain. *Pain*, 21(3):267-278.

Leonardi, M., Steiner, T., Scher, A., & Lipton, R. (2005). The global burden of migraine: Measuring disability in headache disorders with WHO's Classification of Functioning, Disability and Health (ICF). *The Journal of Headache and Pain*, 6(6):429-440.

Levy, M. (1996). Pharmacologic treatment of cancer pain. *New England Journal of Medicine* 335(15):1124-1132.

Marlowe, K. (2007). A multidisciplinary approach to complex regional pain syndrome. *U.S. Pharmacist-Health System Edition*, May:44-50.

Matthews, M., & Horton, E. (2007). Managing central pain syndromes. *U.S. Pharmacist-Health System Edition*, 32(5):20-32.

Morin, A.K. (2009). Fibromyalgia: A review of management options. *Formulary*, 44(December): 362-373.

Moultry, A.M., & Poon, I.O. (2009). The use of antidepressants for chronic pain. *U.S. Pharmacist*, 34(5):26-34.

Neumann, L., & Busklia, D. (2003). Epidemiology of fibromyalgia. *Current Pain and Headache Reports*, 7(5):362-368.

Nickerson, B. (2009). Recent advances in the treatment of pain associated with fibromyalgia. *U.S. Pharmacist*, 34(9):49-85.

Parillo, S.J., & O'Conner, R.E. (2011). Complex regional pain syndrome in emergency medicine Available: http://emedicine.medscape.com/article/793370-overview

Parkes, M. (1973). Factors determining the persistence of phantom pain in the amputee. *Journal of Psychosomatic Research*, 17(2):97-108.

Ramachandran, V.S., & Altschuler, E.L. (2009). The use of visual feedback, in particular mirror visual feedback, in restoring brain function. *Brain*, 132(7):1693-1710.

Robinson, L.R., Czemiecki, J.M., Ehde, D.M., Edwards, W.T., Judish, D.A., Goldberg, M.L., et al. (2004). Trial of amitriptyline for relief of pain in amputees: Results of a randomized controlled study. *Archives of Physical Medicine and Rehabilitation*, 85(1):1-6.

Siddall P.J., McClelland J.M., Rutkowski S.B., Cousins M.J. (2003). A longitudinal study of the prevalence and characteristics of pain in the first 5 years following spinal cord injury. *Pain.*, Jun;103(3):249-57.

Sluka, K.A. (2001). Basic science mechanisms of TENS and clinical implications. *American Pain Society Bulletin*, 11(2):10-13.

Swarm, R., Benedetti, C., Cleeland, C., deLeon-Casasola, O.A., Eiler, J.G., Grossman, S.A., et al. (2007). Adult cancer pain: Clinical practice guidelines in oncology. *Journal of the National Comprehensive Cancer Network*, 5(8):726-760.

Teague, A. (2007). Neuropathic pain calls for a range of treatment options. *Pharmacy Times*, September:32-33.

Toth, J.A. (2009). Concepts in cancer pain management. *U.S. Pharmacist*, 34(11):3-12.

Ziegler-Graham, K., MacKenzie, E.J., Ephraim, P.L., Travison, T.G., & Brookmeyer, R. (2008). Estimating the prevalence of limb loss in the United States: 2005 to 2050. *Archives of Physical Medicine and Rehabilitation*, 89(3):422-442.

Chapter 15

Calvanio, R., Burke, D.T., Kim, H.J., Cheng, J., Lepak, P., Leonard, J., et al. (2000). Naltrexone: Effects on motor function, speech, and activities of daily living in a patient with traumatic brain injury. *Brain Injury*, 14(10):933-942.

Carl, L., & Johnson, P. (2006). *Drugs and dysphagia: How medications affect eating and swallowing*. Austin, TX: Pro-Ed.

Centers for Disease Control and Prevention. (2012). Alcohol use and health. Available: http://www.cdc.gov/alcohol/

Ciccone, C.D. (2007). *Pharmacology in rehabilitation* (4th ed.). Philadelphia: Davis.

Davis, P.E., Liddiard, H., & McMillan, T.E. (2002). Neuropsychological deficits and opiate abuse. *Drug and Alcohol Dependence*, 67(1):105-108.

Epstein, E.E., Ginsburg, B.E., Hesselbrock, V.M., & Schwartz, J.C. (1994). Alcohol and drug abusers subtyped by antisocial personality and primary or secondary depressive disorder. *Annals of the New York Academy of Sciences*, 708(February):187-201.

Hanley, M.J., & Kenna, G.A. (2008). Quetiapine: Treatment for substance abuse and drug of abuse. *American Journal of Health-System Pharmacy*, 65(7):611-618.

Herring, M.P., O'Connor, P.J., & Dishman, R.K. (2010). The effect of exercise training on anxiety symptoms among patients: A systematic review. *Archives of Internal Medicine*, 170(4):321-331.

Jacobson, S.A., Pies, R.W., & Katz, I.R. (2007). *Clinical manual of geriatric psychopharmacology*. Washington, DC: American Psychiatric.

Johnson, R.E., Strain, E.C., & Amass, L. (2003). Buprenorphine: How to use it right. *Drug and Alcohol Dependence*, 70(Suppl. 2):S59-S77.

Kenna, G.A. (2007a). Substance use disorders. In Dunsworth, T.S., Rchardson, M.M., Schwartz, W.B., Cheng, J.W.M., Chessman, K.H., Hume, A.L., Hutchison, L.C., Jackson, A.B., Karpiuk, E.L., Martin, L.G., Semla, T.P., & Wittbrodt, E.T. *Pharmacotherapy self-assessment program. Book 3: Neurology and psychiatry* (6th ed.) (pp. 135-156). Kansas City, MO: American College of Clinical Pharmacy.

Kenna, G.A. (2007b). Substance use disorders: Therapeutic approaches for more complex diagnoses. In Dunsworth, T.S., Rchardson, M.M., Schwartz, W.B., Cheng, J.W.M., Chessman, K.H., Hume, A.L., Hutchison, L.C., Jackson, A.B., Karpiuk, E.L.,

Martin, L.G., Semla, T.P., & Wittbrodt, E.T. *Pharmacotherapy self-assessment program. Book 3: Neurology and psychiatry* (6th ed.) (pp. 157-175). Kansas City, MO: American College of Clinical Pharmacy.

Lintzeris, N., Bammer, G., Jolley, D.J., & Whelan, G. (2003). Buprenorphine dosing regime for inpatient heroin withdrawal: A symptom-triggered dose titration study. *Drug and Alcohol Dependence*, 70(3):287-294.

Poldrugo, F. (2006). Acamprosate treatment in a long-term community based alcohol rehabilitation program. *Addiction*, 92(11):1537-1546.

Preston, J.D., O'Neal, J.H., & Talaga, M.C. (2008). *Handbook of clinical psychopharmacology for therapists*. Oakland: New Harbinger.

Preston, K.L., Umbricht, A., & Epstein, D.H. (2000). Methadone dose increase and abstinence reinforcement for treatment of continued heroin use during methadone maintenance. *Archives of General Psychiatry*, 57(4):395-404.

Sproule, B.A. (2002). Substance abuse. In Mueller, B.A., Bertch, K.E., Dunsworth, T.S., Fagan, S.C., Hayney, M.S., O'Connell, M.B., Schumock, G.T., Thompson, D.F., Tisdale, J.E., Witt, D.M., & Zarowitz, B.J. *Pharmacotherapy self-assessment program. Book 7: Neurology and psychiatry* (4th ed.) (pp. 133-166). Kansas City, MO: American College of Clinical Pharmacy.

Chapter 16

Alzen, E., Ljubuncic, Z., Ljubuncic, P., Alzen, I., & Potasman, I. (2007). Risk factors for methicillin-resistant *Staphylococcus aureus* colonization in a geriatric rehabilitation hospital. *Journal of Gerontology Series A: Biological Sciences and Medical Sciences*, 62(10):1152-1156.

American Thoracic Society and Infectious Diseases Society of America. (2005). Guidelines for the management of adults with hospital acquired, ventilator-associated and healthcare-associated pneumonia. *American Journal of Respiratory Critical Care Medicine*, 171:388-416.

Bennett, N.T., & Schultz, G.S. (1993). Growth factors and wound healing—Part 1: Role in normal and chronic wound healing. *American Journal of Surgery*, 166:74-81.

Bratzler, D.W., Houck, P.M., Richards, C., Steele, L., Dellinger, E.P., Fry, D.E., et al. (2005). Use of antimicrobial prophylaxis for major surgery: Baseline results from the national surgical infection prevention project. *Archives of Surgery*, 140(2):174-182.

Brill, L.R., Cavanagh, P.R., Doucette, M.M., & Ulbrecht, J.S. (1994). Prevention, protection and recurrence reduction of diabetic neuropathic foot ulcers. In Boulton, A.J.M., Cavanagh, P.R., & Rayman, G. Curative Technologies Inc.

Bryant, R.A. (2003). *Acute and chronic wounds: Nursing management*. Philadelphia: Mosby Yearbook.

Cameron, M.H. (2003). *Physical agents in rehabilitation* (2nd ed.). St. Louis: Saunders.

Centers for Medicare and Medicaid Services. (2011). Immunizations http://www.cms.gov/Medicare/Prevention/Immunizations/Downloads/2012-2013_Flu_Guide.pdf

Chambers, H.F. (2004). Beta-lactam antibiotics and other inhibitors of cell wall synthesis. In B.G. Katzung (Ed.), *Basic and clinical pharmacology* (9th ed.). New York: Lange Medical Books/McGraw-Hill.

Ciccone, C.D. (2007). *Pharmacology in rehabilitation* (4th ed.). Philadelphia: Davis.

Cleveland Clinic. (2009). Chronic venous insufficiency. Available: http://my.clevelandclinic.org/disorders/venous_insufficiency/hvi_chronic_venous_insufficiency.aspx

Cleveland Clinic. (2010). Antibiotic-associated diarrhea. Available: www.clevelandclinicmed.com/medicalpubs/diseasemanagement/gastroenterolgy/antibiotic-associated-diarrhea/

Cohen, S.H., Gerding, D.N., Johnson, S., Kelly, C.P., Loo, V.G., McDonald, L.C., et al. (2010). Clinical practice guidelines for *Clostridium difficile* infection in adults: 2010 update by the Society of Healthcare Epidemiology of America (SHEA) and the Infectious Disease Society of America (ISDA). *Infection Control and Hospital Epidemiology*, 31(5):431-455.

Cotter, M., Donlon, S., Roche, F., Byrne, H., & Fitzpatrick, F. (2012). Healthcare-associated infection in Irish long-term care facilities: Results from the first national prevalence study. *Journal of Hospital Infection*, 80(3):212-216.

Cuna, B.A. (2007). *Antibiotic essentials* (6th ed.). Royal Oak, MI: Physician's Press.

Danziger, L.H., Fish, D.N., & Pendland, S.L. (2002). Skin and soft tissue infections. In J.T. DiPiro, R.L. Talbert, G.C. Yee, G.R. Matzke, B.G. Wells, & L.M. Posey (Eds.), *Pharmacotherapy: A pathophysiologic approach* (5th ed.) (pp. 1885-1898). Stamford, CT: Appleton & Lange.

Dosick, S.M. (1996). *Management of ulcers on the ischemic limb*. New York: Curative Health Services.

Driscoll, P. (2009). Incidence and prevalence of wounds by etiology. Available: http://mediligence.com/blog/2009/12/13/incidence-and-prevalence-of-wounds-by-etioogy/

Duerden, M.C., Bergeron, J., Baker, R.L., & Braddom, R.L. (1997). Controlling the spread of vancomycin-resistant enterocci with the rehabilitation cohort unit. *Archives of Physical Medicine and Rehabilitation*, 78(5):553-555.

Eaglstein, W.H. (1990). *Wound care manual: New directions in wound healing*. Princeton, NJ: Squibb & Sons.

Estrada, C.A., Young, J.A., Nifong, L.W., & Chitwood, W.R. (2003). Outcomes and perioperative hyperglycemia in patients with or without diabetes mellitus undergoing coronary artery bypass grafting. *Annals of Thoracic Surgery*, 75(5):1392-1399.

Fine, M.J., Auble, T.E., Yealy, D.M., Hanusa, B.H., Weissfeld, L.A., Singer, D.E., et al. (1997). A prediction rule to identify low-risk patients with community-acquired pneumonia. *New England Journal of Medicine*, 336(4):243-250.

Flaherty, P.J., Liljestrand, J.S., & O'Brien, T.F. (1984). Infection control surveillance in a rehabilitation hospital. *Archives of Physical Medicine and Rehabilitation*, 65(6):313-315.

Friedman, C., & Petersen, K.H. (2004). *Infection control in ambulatory care*. Sudbury, MA: Jones & Bartlett.

Gabriel, A., Camp, M.C., & Paletta, C. (2010). Vascular ulcers. Available: http://emedicine.medscape.com/article/1298345-overview

Gerberdin, J.L. (2002). Hospital-onset infections: A patient safety issue. *Annals of Internal Medicine*, 137(8):665-670.

Gupta, K., Hooton, T.M., Naber, K.G., Wolit, B., Colgan, R., Miller, L.G., et al. (2011). International clinical practice guidelines for the treatment of acute and uncomplicated cystitis and pyelonephritis in women: A 2010 update by the Infectious Disease Society of America and the European Society for Microbiology and Infectious Diseases. *Clinical Infectious Diseases*, 52(5):103-120.

Hain, D., & Hain, T. (2012). Situation of the worldwide incidence of MRSA. Available: http://www.hain-lifescience.de.en/products/microbiology/mrsa/situation-of-the-worldwide-incidence-of-mrsa.html

Haley, R.W., Culver, D.H., White, J.W., Morgan, W.N., & Emori, T.G. (1985). The nationwide nosocomial infection rate. *American Journal of Epidemiology*, 121(2):159-167.

Halsey, J. (2008). Current and future treatment modalities for *Clostridium difficile* associated disease. *American Journal of Health-System Pharmacy*, 65(April):705-715.

Hernandez, K., Ramos, E., Seas, C., & Henostroza, G. (2005). Incidence of and risk factors for surgical-site infections in a Peruvian hospital. *Infection Control and Hospital Epidemiology*, 26(5):473-477.

Hershkovitz, A., Beloosesky, Y., Pomp, N., & Brill, S. (2002). Is routine screening for urinary tract infection in rehabilitation day hospital elderly patients that necessary? *Archives of Gerontology and Geriatrics*, 34(1):29-36.

Holloway, G.A. (1996). Arterial ulcers: assessment and diagnosis. *Ostomy Wound Manage*, Apr;42(3):46-8, 50-1.

Hooton, T.M., Bradley, S.F., Cardenas, D.D., Colgan, R., Geerlings, S.E., Rice, J.C., et al. (2010). Diagnosis, prevention and treatment of catheter associated urinary tract infection in adults: 2009 clinical practice guidelines from the Infectious Diseases Society of America. *Clinical Infectious Disease*, 50(5):625-663.

Houck, P.M., Bratzler, D.W., Nsa, W., Ma, A., & Bartlett, J.G. (2004). Timing of antibiotic administration and outcomes for Medicare patients hospitalized with pneumonia. *Archives of Internal Medicine*, 164(6):637-644.

Howes, D.S. (2010). Urinary tract infection, female: Treatment and medication. Available: http://emedicine.medscape.com/article/778670-treatment

Inge, L.D. (2010). Management of catheter associated urinary tract infections. *U.S. Pharmacist-Health System Edition*, August:6-10.

Katzung, B.G. (2004). *Basic and clinical pharmacology* (9th ed.). New York: Lange Medical Books/McGraw-Hill.

Kingsley, A. (2001). A proactive approach to wound infection. *Nursing Standard*, 15(30):50-54, 56, 58.

Kjonniksen, I., Andersen, B.M., Sondenaa, V.G., & Segadal, L. (2002). Preoperative hair removal—A systematic literature review. *AORN Journal*, 75(5):928-938, 940.

Knox, M. (2009). Superbugs and healthcare infection control. *Rainbow Visions Magazine*, 6(3):1-4.

Krasner, D., Margolis, D.J., Ordona, R.U., & Rodeheaver, G.T. (1996). *Treatment of chronic wounds: Prevention and management of pressure ulcers*. Hauppauge, NY: Curative Health Services.

Latham, R., Lancaster, A.D., Covington, J.F., Pirolo, J.S., & Thomas, C.S. (2001). The association of diabetes and glucose control with surgical-site infections among cardiothoracic surgery patients. *Infection Control and Hospital Epidemiology*, 22(10):607-612.

Lipsky, B.A., Berendt, A.R., Deery, H.G., Embil, J.M., Joseph, W.S., Karchmer, A.W., et al. (2004). ISDA guideline for the diagnosis and treatment of diabetic foot infections. *Clinical Infectious Disease*, 39(7):885-910.

Liu, C. (2011). *New clinical guidelines for MRSA treatment*. Atlanta: Centers for Disease Control and Prevention.

Lutfiyya, M.N., Henley, E., Chang, L.F., & Wessel Reyburn, S. (2006). Diagnosis and treatment of community-acquired pneumonia. *American Academy of Family Physicians*, 73(3):442-450.

Mandell, L.A., Wunderink, R.G., Anzueto, A., Bartlett, J.G., Campbell, C.D., Dean, N.C., et al. (2007). Infectious Disease Society of America/American Thoracic Society consensus guidelines on the management of community-acquired pneumonia in adults. *Clinical Infectious Diseases*, 44(Suppl. 2):27-72.

McGuickin, M., Taylor, A., Martin, V., Porten, L., & Salcido, R. (2004). Evaluation of a patient education model for increasing hand hygiene compliance in an inpatient rehabilitation unit. *American Journal of Infection Control*, 32(4):235-238.

Mulder, G.D., Jeter, J.F., & Haberer, P.A. (1992). *Clinician's pocket guide to chronic wound repair* (2nd ed.). Ambler, PA: Springhouse.

Mylotte, J.M., Graham, R., Kahler, L., Young, L., & Goodnough, S. (2001). Impact of nosocomial infection on length of stay and functional improvement among patients admitted to an acute rehabilitation unit. *Infection Control and Hospital Epidemiology*, 22(2):83-87.

Mylotte, J.M., Graham, R., Kahler, L., Young, L., & Goodnough, S. (2000a). Epidemiology of nosocomial infection and resistant organisms in patients admitted for the first time to an acute rehabilitation unit. *Clinical Infectious Diseases*, 30(3):425-432.

Mylotte, J.M., Kahler, L., Graham, R., Young, L., & Goodnough, S. (2000b). Perspective surveillance for antibiotic resistant organisms in patients with spinal cord injury admitted to an acute rehabilitation unit. *American Journal of Infection Control*, 28(4):291-297.

National Institute of Allergy and Infectious Disease. (2000). *Antimicrobial resistance: NIAID fact sheet*. Bethesda, MD: National Institutes of Health.

Nicolle, L.E., Bradley, S., Colgan, R., Rice, J.C., Schaeffer, A., & Hooten, T.M. (2005). Infectious Diseases Society of America guidelines for diagnosis and treatment of asymptomatic bacteriuria in adults. *Clinical Infectious Diseases*, 40(5):643-654.

O'Connor, K.A., Kingston, M., O'Donovan, M., Cryan, B., Twomey, C., & O'Mahony, D. (2004). Antibiotic prescribing policy and *Clostridium difficile* diarrhea. *Quarterly Journal of Medicine*, 97(7):423-429.

Pailaud, E., Herbaud, S., Callet, P., Lejonc, J., Campillo, B., & Bories, P. (2005). Relations between undernutrition and nosocomial infections in elderly patients. *Age and Aging*, 34(6):619-625.

Papanas, N., & Maltezos, E. (2009). The diabetic foot. *Hippokratia*, 13(4):199-204.

Petri, W.A. (2011). Sulfonamides, trimethoprim-sulfamethoxazole, quinolones and agents for urinary tract infections. In L.L. Brunton, B.A. Chabner, & B.C. Knolimann (Eds.), *Goodman and Gillman's the pharmacological basis of therapeutics* (12th ed.) (pp. 1463-1476). New York: McGraw-Hill.

Raad, I., & Maki, D. (2007). Intravascular catheter-related infections: Advances in diagnosis, prevention, and management. *The Lancet Infectious Diseases*, 7(10):645-657.

Safrin, S. (2004). Antiviral agents. In B.G. Katzung (Ed.), *Basic and clinical pharmacology* (9th ed.). New York: Lange Medical Books/McGraw-Hill.

Schmitt, S.K. (2005). Community acquired pneumonia. Available: http://www.clevelandclinicmeded.com/medicalpubs/diseasemanagement/infectious-disease/community-acquired-pneumonia

Select Medical Corporation. (2010). *Outpatient division clinical operations policy and procedures manual: Version 2.6*. Mechanicsburg, PA: Select Medical Corporation.

Sherman, J.J. (2010). Diabetic foot ulcer assessment and treatment: A pharmacist's guide. *U.S. Pharmacist*, 35(6):38-44.

Shammash, J.B., Trost, J.C., Gold, J.M., Berlin, J.A., Golden, M.A., & Kimmel, S.E. (2001). Perioperative beta-blocker withdrawal and mortality in vascular surgical patients. *American Heart Journal*, 141(1):148-153.

Shuman, M., Lee, D.T., Trigoboff, E., & Opler, L.A. (2012). Hematologic impact of antibiotic administration on patients taking clozapine. *Innov Clin Neurosci*. Nov;9(11-12):18-30.

Singhal, H. (2006). Wound infections. Available: www.emedicine.com/MED/topic2422.htm

Stevens, D.L., Bisno, A.L., Chambers, H.F., Evans, E.D., Dellinger, P., Goldstein, E.C., et al. (2005). IDSA practice guidelines for the diagnosis and management of skin and soft tissue infections. *Clinical Infectious Disease*, 41(10):1373-1406.

Stotts, N., Deosaransingh, K., Roll, J., & Newman, J. (1998). Underutilization of pressure ulcer risk assessment in hip fracture patients. *Advances in Wound Care*, 11(1):32-38.

Vaishnavi, C. (2009). Established and potential risk factors for *Clostridium difficile* infection. *Indian Journal of Medicine and Microbiology*, 27(4):289-300.

Welte, T., & Kohnlein, T. (2009). Global and local epidemiology of community acquired pneumonia. *Seminars in Respiratory and Critical Care*, 30(2):127-135.

Wound Source. (2011). Arterial ulcers. Available: www.woundsource.com/article/arterial-ulcers-and-wound-care-symptoms-causes-treatments-and-risks

Wu, J., & Baguley, I.J. (2005). Urinary retention in a general rehabilitation unit: Prevalence, clinical outcome and the role of screening. *Archives of Physical Medicine and Rehabilitation*, 86(9):1772-1777.

Chapter 17

Altman, R.D., Hochberg, M.C., Moskowitcz, R.W., & Schnitzer, T.J. (2000). Recommendations for the medical management of osteoarthritis of the hip and knee: 2000 update—American College of Rheumatology subcommittee on osteoarthritis guidelines. *Arthritis Rheumatism*, 43(9):1905-1915.

Arnett, F.C., Edworthy, S.M., Bloch, D.A., McShane, D.J., Fries, J.F., Cooper, N.S., et al. (1988). The American Rheumatism Association 1987 revised criteria for the classification of rheumatoid arthritis. *Arthritis and Rheumatism*, 31(3):315-324.

Arrich, J., Piribauer, F., Mad, P., Schmid, D., Klaushofer, K., & Mullner, M. (2005). Intra-articular hyaluronic acid for the treatment of osteoarthritis of the knee: Systematic review and meta-analysis. *Canadian Medical Association Journal*, 172(8):1039-1043.

Arroll, B., & Goodyear-Smith, F. (2004). Corticosteroid injections for osteoarthritis of the knee: Meta-analysis. *British Medical Journal*, 328(7444):869-870.

Bellamy, N., Campbell, J., Robinson, V., Gee, T., Bourne, R., & Wells, G. (2006). Viscosupplementation for the treatment of osteoarthritis of the knee. *Cochrane Database Systematic Reviews*, 19(2):CD005321.

Boh, L.E., & Elliott, M.E. (2002). Osteoarthritis. In J.T. DiPiro, R.L. Talbert, G.C. Yee, G.R. Matzke, B.G. Wells, & L.M. Posey (Eds.), *Pharmacotherapy: A pathophysiologic approach* (5th ed.) (pp. 1639-1658). Stamford, CT: Appleton & Lange.

Brooks, P. (2003). Inflammation as an important feature of osteoarthritis. *Bulletin of the World Health Organization*, 81(9):689-690.

Brosseau, L., Welch, V., Wells, G.A., Tugwell, P., de Bie, R., Gam, A., et al. (2000). Low level laser therapy for osteoarthritis and rheumatoid arthritis: A meta-analysis. *Journal of Rheumatology*, 27(8):1961-1969.

Carl, L., & Johnson, P. (2006). *Drugs and dysphagia*. Austin, TX: Pro-Ed.

Carmona, L., Villaverde, V., Hernandez-Gargia, C., Ballina, J., Gabriel, R., & Laffon, A. (2002). The prevalence of rheumatoid arthritis in the general population of Spain. *Rheumatology*, 41(1):88-95.

Centers for Disease Control and Prevention. (1990). Arthritis prevalence and activity limitations—United States. *Morbidity and Mortality Weekly Report*, 43(24):433-438.

Centers for Disease Control and Prevention. (2001). Prevalence of disabilities and associated health conditions among adults—United States, 1999. *Morbidity and Mortality Weekly Report*, 50(7):120-125.

Cooper, C., Snow, S., McAlindon, T.E., Kellingray, S., Stuart, B., Coggon, D., et al. (2000). Risk factors for the incidence and progression of radiographic knee osteoarthritis. *Arthritis and Rheumatism*, 43(5):995-1000.

Cooper, N.J. (2000). Economic burden of rheumatoid arthritis: A systematic review. *Rheumatology*, 39:28-33.

Emery, P., Breedveld, F.C., Dougados, M., Kalden, J.R., Schiff, M.H., & Smolen, J.S. (2002). Early referral recommendations for newly diagnosed rheumatoid arthritis: Evidence based development of a clinical guide. *Annals Rheumatic Diseases*, 61(4):290-297.

European Conference Against Rheumatism. (2010). Rheumatism classification criteria for rheumatoid arthritis. Available: www.eular.org

Feibel, A., & Fast, A. (1976). Deep heating of joints: A reconsideration. *Archives of Physical Medicine and Rehabilitation*, 57(11):513-514.

Firestein, G.S., & Corr, M. (2005). Common mechanisms in immune-mediated inflammatory disease. *Journal of Rheumatology*, 73(Suppl.):8-13.

Fuchs, H.A., Kaye, J.J., Callahan, L.F., Nance, E.P., & Pincus, T. (1989). Evidence of significant radiographic damage in rheumatoid arthritis within the first 2 years of disease. *Journal of Rheumatology*, 16(5):585-591.

Gottlieb, A., Korman, N.J., Gordon, K.B., Feldman, S.R., Lebwohl, M., Koo, J.Y., et al. (2008). Guidelines of care for the management of psoriasis and psoriatic arthritis: Section 2. Psoriatic arthritis: Overview and guidelines of care for treatment with an emphasis on the biologics. *Journal of American Academy of Dermatology*, 58(5):851-864.

Groher, M. (1997). *Dysphagia: Diagnosis and management*. Boston: Butterworth-Heinemann.

Grosser, T., Smyth, E., & FitzGerald, G.A. (2011). Anti-inflammatory, antipyretic, and analgesic agents; Pharmacotherapy of gout. In L.L. Brunton, B.A. Chabner, & B.C. Knollmann (Eds.), *Goodman and Gillman's the pharmacological basis of therapeutics* (12th ed.) (pp. 959-1004). New York: McGraw-Hill.

Harris, E.D. (1990). Rheumatoid arthritis: Pathophysiology and implications for therapy. *New England Journal of Medicine*, 322(18):1277-1289.

Hawkins, D.W., & Rahn, D.W. (2002). Gout and hyperuricemia. In J.T. DiPiro, R.L. Talbert, G.C. Yee, G.R. Matzke, B.G. Wells, & L.M. Posey (Eds.), *Pharmacotherapy: A pathophysiologic approach* (5th ed.) (pp. 1659-1664). Stamford, CT: Appleton & Lange.

Helms, S., & Darbishire, P.L. (2010). An overview of systemic lupus erythematosis. *U.S. Pharmacist*, September:14-25.

Hochberg, M.C. (1981). Adult and juvenile rheumatoid arthritis: Current epidemiologic concepts. *Epidemiology Review*, 3:27-44.

Hummer, L., & Wigley, L, (2010). John Hopkins Scleroderma Center. Available: www.hopkins.org/patients/scleroderma-treatment-options/

Issa, S.N., & Ruderman, E.M. (2004). Damage control in rheumatoid arthritis: Hard-hitting, early treatment is crucial to curbing joint destruction. *Postgraduate Medicine*, 116:14-24.

Jackson, D.W., Scheer, M.J., & Simon, T.M. (2001). Cartilage substitutes: Overview of basic science and treatment options. *Journal of American Academy of Orthopaedic Surgery*, 9(1):37-52.

Johnson, H.J., & Heim-Duthey, K.L. (2002). Renal transplantation. In J.T. DiPiro, R.L. Talbert, G.C. Yee, G.R. Matzke, B.G. Wells, & L.M. Posey (Eds.), *Pharmacotherapy: A pathophysiologic approach* (5th ed.) (pp. 843-866). Stamford, CT: Appleton & Lange.

Kagilaski, J. (1981). "Baggietherapy": Simple pain relief for arthritic knees. *Journal of the American Medical Association*, 246(4):317-318.

Khan, M.A. (1998). Spondyloarthropathies: Ankylosing spondylitis. In J.H. Klippel & P.A. Dieppe (Eds.), *Rheumatology* (Vol. 2, 2nd ed.) (pp.70-76). Philadelphia: Mosby.

Klippel, J. (Ed.). (2008). *Primer on the rheumatic diseases* (13th ed.). New York: Springer.

Krenty, A.M., Bennett, W.A., & Vincenti, F. (2011). Immunosuppressants, tolerogens and immunostimulants. In L.L. Brunton, B.A. Chabner, & B.C. Knollmann (Eds.), *Goodman and Gillman's the pharmacological basis of therapeutics* (12th ed.) (pp. 1005-1029). New York: McGraw-Hill.

Kwoh, C.K., Roemer, F.W., Hannon, M.J., Guermazi, A., Green, S.M., & Boudreau, R.M. (2009). *The joints on glucosamine (JOG) study: A randomized, double-blind, placebo-controlled trial to assess the structural benefit of glucosamine in knee osteoarthritis based on 3T MRI.* Presentation no. 1942. Presented at ACR/ARHP Annual Scientific Meeting, Philadelphia.

Lawrence, R.C., Felson, D.T., Helmick, C.G., Arnold, L.M., Choi, H., Deyo, R.A., et al. (2008). Estimates of the prevalence of arthritis and other rheumatic conditions in the United States—Part II. *Arthritis and Rheumatism*, 58(1):26-35.

Lawrence, R.C., Hochberg, M.C., Kelsey, J.L., McDuffie, F.C., Medsger, T.A., Felts, W.R., et al. (1989). Estimates of the prevalence of selected arthritic and musculoskeletal diseases in the United States. *Journal of Rheumatology*, 16(4):427-444.

Lorig, K.R., Mazonson, P.D., & Holman, H.R. (1993). Evidence suggesting that health education for self-management in patients with chronic arthritis has sustained health benefits while reducing health care costs. *Arthritis and Rheumatism*, 36(4):439-446.

Matsumoto, A.K., Bathon, J., & Bingham, C.O. (2010). The John Hopkins Arthritis Center. Available: www.hopkins-arthritis.org/arthritis-info/rheumatoid/rheum_treat.html#cytotoxic

Mattje, G.D., & Turato, E.R. (2006). Life experiences with systemic lupus erythematosus as reported in outpatients' perspective: A clinical-qualitative study in Brazil. *Rev Latino-am Enfermagem Julho-Agosto*, 14(4):475-482.

Mayers, M.D. (2005). *The scleroderma book: A guide for patients and families.* New York: Oxford University Press.

Medical Disability Advisor. (2010). Gout: M.D. guidelines. Available: www.mdguidelines.com/gou

Miller, S.A., & Bartels, C.L. (2009). Dietary supplements. In Richardson, M.M., Chant, C., Cheng, J.W.M., Chessman, K.H., Hume, A.L., Hutchison, L.C., Jackson, A.B., Karpiuk, E.L., Martin, L.G., & Semla, T.P. *Pharmacotherapy self-assessment program. Book 9: Gastroenterology and nutrition* (6th ed.) (pp. 167-184). Kansas City, MO: American College of Clinical Pharmacy.

National Psoriasis Foundation. (2010). Statistics. Available: www.psoiriasis.org/netcommunity/learn_statistics

Osteoarthritis Research Society International. (2010). Treatment guidelines for hips and knees. Accessed: www.oarsi.org/index2.cfm?section=Publications_and_Newsroom&content=OAGuidelines

Phillips, C.R., & Brasington, R.D. (2010). Osteoarthritis treatment update: Are NSAIDs still in the picture? *The Journal of Musculoskeletal Medicine*, 27(2):65-71.

Porter, R.S., & Kaplan, J.L. (2006). *The Merck manual.* Rathway, NJ: Merck.

Rabinovich, C.E. (2010). Juvenile rheumatoid arthritis: Treatment and medication. Available: http://emedicine.medscape.com/article/1007276-treatmen

Roth, S.H., & Shainhouse, J.Z. (2004). Efficacy and safety of a topical diclofenac solution (Pennsaid) in the treatment of primary osteoarthritis of the knee: A randomized, double-blind, vehicle-controlled clinical trial. *Archives of Internal Medicine*, 164(18):2017-2023.

Roubenoff, R., Klag, M.J., Mead, L.A., Kung-Yee, L., Seidler, A.J., & Hochberg, M.C. (1991). Incidence and risk factors for gout in white men. *Journal of the American Medical Association*, 1266(21):3004-3007.

Schur, P. (1993). Clinical features of SLE. In W.N. Kelly, C.B. Sledge, & E.D. Harris (Eds.), *Textbook of rheumatology* (4th ed.). Philadelphia: Saunders.

Statsny, P. (1978). Association of the B-cell alloantigen DRw4 with rheumatoid arthritis. *New England Journal of Medicine*, 298(16):869-871.

Stevens, M.B. (1983). Musculoskeletal manifestations. In P.H. Schur (Ed.), *The clinical management of systemic lupus erythematosus.* Orlando, FL: Grune & Stratton.

Sturmer, T., Brenner, H., Koenig, W., & Gunther, K.P. (2004). Severity and extent of osteoarthritis and low grade systemic inflammation as assessed by high sensitivity C reactive protein. *Annals of Rheumatic Diseases*, 63(2):200-205.

Tan, E.M., Cohen, A.S., Fries, J.F., Masi, A.T., McShane, D.J., Rothfield, N.F., et al. (1982). The 1982 criteria for classification of systemic lupus erytematosus. *Arthritis and Rheumatism*, 25(11):1271-1277.

Towheed, T.E., Maxwell, L., Judd, M.G., Catton, M., Hochberg, M.C., & Wells, G. (2006). Acetaminophen for osteoarthritis. *Cochrane Database Systematic Reviews*, 1:CD00425.

Veale, D., Rogers, S., & Fitzgerald, O. (1994). Classification of clinical subjects in psoriatic arthritis. *British Journal of Rheumatology*, 33(2):133-138.

Vlad, S.C., LaValley, M.P., McAlindon, T.E., & Felson, D.T. (2007). Glucosamine for pain in osteoarthritis: Why do trial results differ? *Arthritis and Rheumatism*, 56(7):2267-2277.

Walker, J.M. (1998). Pathomechanics and classification of cartilage lesions, facilitation or repair. *Journal of Orthopedic and Sports Physical Therapy*, 28(4):216-231.

Wong, R., Davis, A., Badley, E., Grewal, R., & Mohammed, M. (2010). *Prevalence of arthritis and rheumatic diseases around the world.* Toronto: Canada Arthritis Community Research and Evaluation Unit, Toronto Western Research Institute.

Zaka, R., & Williams, C.J. (2006). New developments in the epidemiology and genetics of gout. *Current Rheumatology Reports*, 8(3):215-223.

Zhang, W., Moskowitz, R.W., Nuki, G., Abramson, S., Altman, R.D., Arden, N., et al. (2008). OARSI recommendations for the management of hip and knee osteoarthritis, Part II: OARSI evidence-based, expert consensus guidelines. *Osteoarthritis and Cartilage*, 16(2):137-162.

Chapter 18

American Cancer Society. (2011). Cancer research. Retrieved from http://www.cancer.org/research.index

Balmer, C.M., & Valley, A.W. (2002). Basic principles of cancer treatment and cancer chemotherapy. In J.T. DiPiro, R.L. Talbert, G.C. Yee, G.R. Matzke, B.G. Wells, & L.M. Posey (Eds.), *Pharmacotherapy: A pathophysiologic approach* (5th ed.) (pp. 2175-2222). Stamford, CT: Appleton & Lange.

Berger, A.M., & Kilroy, T.J. (1997). Oral complications. In V.T. DeVita, S. Hellman, & S.A. Rosenburg (Eds.), *Cancer principles and practice of oncology* (5th ed.) (pp. 2714-2725). Philadelphia: Lippincott Williams & Wilkins.

Bishop, M.A. (2010). Monoclonal antibodies. Available: www.meds.com/immunotherapy/monoclonal_antibodies.html

Bubalo, J.S. (2009). Supportive care. In M. Richardson, C. Chant, J.W. Cheng, K.H. Chessman, A.L. Hume, & L.C. Hutchison (Eds.), *Pharmacotherapy self-assessment program: Oncology* (6th ed.) (pp. 89-100). Lenexa, KS: American College of Clinical Pharmacy.

Carl, L., & Johnson, P. (2006). *Drugs and dysphagia.* Austin, TX: Pro-Ed.

Center, M., & Siegel, R. Jemal, A. (2011). *Global cancer facts and figures.* Atlanta: American Cancer Society.

Chabner, B.A., Ryan, D.P., Paz-Ares, L., Garcia-Carbonera, R., & Calabresi, P. (2001). Antineoplastic agents. In J.G. Hardman, L.E. Limbird, & A.G. Gillman (Eds.), *Goodman and Gillman's the pharmacological basis of therapeutics* (10th ed.). New York: McGraw-Hill.

Chu, E., & DeVita, V.T. (2010). *Physician's cancer chemotherapy drug manual.* Sudbury, MA: Jones & Bartlett.

Douglass, H.O. (1984). Nutritional support of the cancer patient. *Hospital Formulary,* 19:220-234.

FDA. (2012). Approved risk evaluation and mitigation strategies (REMS). Available: www.fda.gov/Drugs/default.htm

Finley, R.S., & LaCivitia, C.L. (1992). Neoplastic diseases. In M.A. Koda-Kimball & L.Y. Young (Eds.), *Applied therapeutics: The clinical use of drugs* (5th ed.). Vancouver, WA: Applied Therapeutics.

Grunwald, P.E. (2003). Supportive care II. In Dunsworth, T. & Cheng, J. (Eds.), *Pharmacotherapy self-assessment program. Book 10: Hematology and oncology* (4th ed.) (pp. 113-135). Kansas City, MO: American College of Clinical Pharmacy.

Kaplan, R.J., & Zandt, J.E. (2010). Cancer and rehabilitation. Available: http://emedicine.medscape.com/article/320261-overview

Krishnan, K., & Hammad, A. (2009). Tumor lysis syndrome: Treatment and medication. Available: http://emedicine.medscape.com/article/283171-treatment

Weber, J. (2010). Cytokines and cancer therapy. Available: www.meds.com/immunotherapy/cytokines.html

Chapter 19

Almeida, O.P., & Flicker, L. (2001). The mind of a failing heart: A systematic review of the association between congestive heart failure and cognitive functioning. *Internal Medicine Journal,* 31(5):290-295.

Almeida, O.P., & Tamai, S. (2001a). Clinical treatment reverses attentional deficits in congestive heart failure. *BMC Geriatrics,* 1(2):1-2.

Almeida, O.P., & Tamai, S. (2001b). Congestive heart failure and cognitive functioning amongst older adults. *Arquivos de Neuropsiquiatria,* 59(2): 10-20.

American College of Cardiology and American Heart Association. (2005). Guideline update for the diagnosis and management of chronic heart failure in the adult. *Journal of American College of Cardiology,* 46:1116-1143.

American Heart Association. (2006). Heart disease and stroke statistics: 2006 update. *Circulation,* 113(6):e85-e151.

American Heart Association. (2012). What is cardiovascular disease (heart disease)? Available: www.heart.org/HEARTORG/Caregiver/Resources/WhatisCardiovascularDisease/What-is-Cardiovascular-Disease_UCM_301852_Article.jsp

Bauman, J.L., & Scoen, M.D. (2002). Arrhythmias. In J.T. DiPiro, R.L. Talbert, G.C. Yee, G.R. Matzke, B.G. Wells, & L.M. Posey (Eds.), *Pharmacotherapy: A pathophysiologic approach* (5th ed.) (pp. 272-303). Stamford, CT: Appleton & Lange.

Bennett, S.J., & Sauve, M.J. (2003). Cognitive deficits in patients with heart failure: A review of the literature. *Journal of Cardiovascular Nursing,* 18(3):219-242.

Berrios-Colon, E., & Cha, A. (2010). The treatment and management of atrial fibrillation. *U.S. Pharmacist,* 35(2):46-53.

Brawner, C.A. (2010). Prescribing exercise in cardiac rehabilitation without an exercise test. *American Academy of Sports Medicine Certified News,* 20(January-March):1.

Brawner, C.A., Ehrman, J.K., Schairer, J.R., Cao, J.J., & Keteyian, S.J. (2004). Predicting maximum heart rate among patients with coronary heart disease receiving beta-adrenergic blockade therapy. *American Heart Journal,* 148(5):910-914.

Carter, B.L., & Saseen, J.J. (2002). Hypertension. In J.T. DiPiro, R.L. Talbert, G.C. Yee, G.R. Matzke, B.G. Wells, & L.M. Posey (Eds.), *Pharmacotherapy: A pathophysiologic approach* (5th ed.) (pp. 157-183). Stamford, CT: Appleton & Lange.

Ciccone, C.D. (2007). *Pharmacology in rehabilitation* (4th ed.). Philadelphia: Davis.

Coe, D.P., & Fiatarone-Singh, M.A. (2010). Exercise prescription in special populations. In J.K. Ehrman (Ed.), *American College of Sports Medicine resource manual for guidelines for exercise testing and prescription* (6th ed.) (pp. 559-571). Philadelphia: Lippincott Williams & Wilkins.

Colbert, B.J., & Mason, B.J. (2002). *Integrated cardiopulmonary pharmacology.* Upper Saddle River, NJ: Prentice Hall.

Cuccurullo, S. (2004). *Physical medicine and rehabilitation board review.* New York: Demos Medical.

Dobesch, P.P., & Stacy, Z.A. (2011). Management of chronic stable angina. In Richardson , M., Chant, C., Cheng, J.W.M., Chessman, K.H., Hume, A.L., Hutchison, L.C., et.al. *Pharmacotherapy self-assessment program. Book 1: Cardiology* (7th ed.) (pp. 43-64). Kansas City, MO: American College of Clinical Pharmacy.

Draskovich, C.D., & O'Dell, K.M. (2010). Dronedarone for atrial fibrillation: An update of clinical evidence. *Formulary,* 45:275-283.

Elkayam, U., Bitar, F., Kiramijyian, S., Hatamizadeh, P., Binkley, P.F., & Leier, C. (2007). Vasodilators. In J.D. Hosenpud & B.H. Greenberg (Eds.), *Congestive heart failure* (3rd ed.). Philadelphia: Lippincott Williams & Wilkins.

Evans, L., Probert, H., & Shuldham, C. (2009). Cardiac rehabilitation—Past to present. *Journal of Research in Nursing,* 14(3):223-240.

Jennings, H.R, Cook, T.S. (2010). Hypertension: clinical practice updates. In Richardson, M., Chant, C., Cheng, J.W.M., et al., (Eds). Pharmacotherapy self-assessment program, 7th ed. *Cardiology.* Lenexa, KS: American College of Clinical Pharmacy.

Johnson, J.A., Parker, R.B., & Patterson, J.H. (2002). Heart failure. In J.T. DiPiro, R.L. Talbert, G.C. Yee, G.R. Matzke, B.G. Wells, & L.M. Posey (Eds.), *Pharmacotherapy: A pathophysiologic approach* (5th ed.) (pp. 185-218). Stamford, CT: Appleton & Lange.

Jones, D.L., Adams, R.J., Brown, T.M., Camethon, M., Dai, S., DeSimone, G., et al. (2010). Heart disease and stroke statistics—2010 update: A report from the American Heart Association. *Circulation,* 121(7):e46-e215.

Marcy, T.R., & Ripley, T.L. (2006). Aldosterone antagonists in the treatment of heart failure. *American Journal of Health-System Pharmacy,* 63(1):49-58.

Maron, B.A., & Rocco, T.P. (2011). Pharmacotherapy of congestive heart failure. In J.G. Hardman, L.E. Limbird, & A.G. Gillman (Eds.), *Goodman and Gillman's the pharmacological basis of therapeutics* (12th ed.) (pp. 789-813). New York: McGraw-Hill.

Mayo Clinic. (2010). Complications of hypertension. Available: www.mayoclinic.com/health/high-blood-pressure/DS00100/DSECTION=complications

McKhann, G., Goldsbough, M., Borowisz, L.M., Seines, O., Melilis, E., Enger, C., et al. (1997). Cognitive outcome after coronary artery bypass. *The Annals of Thoracic Surgery*, 63(2):510-515.

Michel, T., & Hoffman, B.B. (2011). Treatment of ischemia and hypertension. In J.G. Hardman, L.E. Limbird, & A.G. Gillman (Eds.), *Goodman and Gillman's the pharmacological basis of therapeutics* (12th ed.) (pp. 745-813). New York: McGraw-Hill.

Moller, J., Cluitmans, P., Rasmussen, L., Houx, P., Rasmussen, H., Canet, J., et al. (1998). Long-term postoperative cognitive dysfunction in the elderly. *Lancet*, 351(9106):857-861.

Murray, L. (2006). Cardiovascular disease: Effects upon cognition and communication. *ASHA Leader*, 11(May):10-23.

Newman, M.F., Croughwell, N.D., Blumenthal, J.A., White, W.D., Lewis, J.B., Smith, L.R., et al. (1994). Effect of aging on cerebral autoregulation during cardiopulmonary bypass: Association with postoperative cognitive dysfunction. *Circulation*, 90(5 Part 2):243-249.

Quinn, C. (2006). *100 questions and answers about congestive heart failure*. Sudbury, MA: Jones & Bartlett.

Sampson, K.J., & Kass, R.S. (2011). Anti-arrhythmic drugs. In J.G. Hardman, L.E. Limbird, & A.G. Gillman (Eds.), *Goodman and Gillman's the pharmacological basis of therapeutics* (12th ed.) (pp. 815-848). New York: McGraw-Hill.

Sanoski, C.A. (2011). Atrial and ventricular arrhythmias: Evolving practices. In Richardson, M., Chant, C., Cheng, J.W.M., Chessman, K.H., Hume, A.L., Hutchison, L.C., et.al. (Eds.). *Pharmacotherapy self-assessment program. Book 1: Cardiology* (7th ed.) (pp. 125-151). Kansas City, MO: American College of Clinical Pharmacy.

Schairer, J.R., Jarvis, R.A., Ehrman, J.K., & Keteyian, S.J. (2010). *American College of Sports Medicine resource manual for guidelines for exercise testing and prescription* (6th ed.) (pp. 559-571). Philadelphia: Lippincott Williams & Wilkins.

Seines, O.A., & McKhann, G.M. (2005). Neurocognitive complications after coronary artery bypass surgery. *Annals of Neurology*, 57(5):615-621.

Selnes, O.A., Grega, M.A., Borowicz, L.M., Royall, R.M., McKhann, G.M., & Baumgarter, W.A. (2003). Cognitive changes with coronary heart disease: A prospective study of coronary artery bypass graft patients and nonsurgical controls. *Annals of Thoracic Surgery*, 75(5):1377-1384.

Singh, V.D., Schocken, D.D., & Williams, K. (2008). Cardiac rehabilitation. Available: http://emedicine.com/article/319683-overview

Taylor, A., Bell, J., & Lough, F. (2001). Cardiac rehabilitation. In J.A. Pryor & S.A. Prasad (Eds.), *Physiotherapy for respiratory and cardiac problems* (3rd ed.). Edinburgh: Churchill Livingstone.

Trojano, L., Raffaele, A.I., Acanfora, D., Picone, C., Mecocci, P., & Rengo, F. (2003). Cognitive impairment: A key feature of congestive heart failure in the elderly. *Journal of Neurology*, 250(12):1456-1463.

World Health Organization. (2012). World life expectancy—Coronary heart disease. Available: www.worldlifeeexpectancy.com/world-health-rankings

Young, J.B., & Mills, R.M. (2004). *Management of heart failure* (2nd ed.). West Islip, NY: Professional Communications.

Youse, K.M. (2008). Medications that exacerbate or induce cognitive communication deficits. *Perspectives on Neurophysiology and Neurogenic Speech and Language Disorders*, 18:137-143.

Zheng, Z.J., Croft, J.B., & Giles, W.H. (2002). State specific mortality from sudden cardiac death—United States, 1999. *Morbidity and Mortality Weekly Report*, 51:123-126.

Zuccala, G., Cattel, C., Manes-Gravina, E., Di Niro, M.G., Cocchi, A., & Bernabei, R. (1997). Left ventricular dysfunction: Clue to cognitive impairment in older patients with heart failure. *Journal Neurological Neurosurgical Psychiatry*, 63(4):509-512.

Chapter 20

Adams, R.J., Zoppo, G.D., Alberts, M.J., Bhatt, D.L., Brass, L., Furlan, A., et al. (2007). Guidelines for the early management of adults with ischemic stroke. *Stroke*, 38(5):1655-1711.

American Heart Association. (2010). Heart disease and stroke statistics. *Circulation*, 121:e46-e215.

American Heart Association. (2012a). Coronary artery disease—The ABCs of CAD. Available: www.heart.org/HEARTORG/Conditions/More/MyHeartandStrokeNews/Coronary-Artery-Disease---The-ABCs-of-CAD_UCM_436416_Article.jsp

American Heart Association. (2012b). Heart disease and stroke statistics. *Circulation*, 125:188-197.

ATP III pocket guideline. (2004). Circulation. Available: www.nhlbi.nih.gov/guidelines/cholesterol/index.htm

Bath, P., Boysen, G., Donnan, G., Kaste, M., Lees, K.R., Olsen, T., et al. (2001). Hypertension in acute stroke: What to do? *Stroke*, 32(7):1697-1698.

Beers, M.H., & Porter, R.S. (2006). *The Merck manual of diagnosis and therapy* (18th ed.). Whitehouse Station, NJ: Merck Research Laboratories.

Bersot, T.P. (2011). Drug therapy for hypercholesterolemia and dyslipidemia. In J.G. Hardman, L.E. Limbird, & A.G. Gillman (Eds.), *Goodman and Gillman's the pharmacological basis of therapeutics* (12th ed.) (pp. 877-908). New York: McGraw-Hill.

Carter, B.L. & Saseen J.J. (2002). Hypertension. In DiPiro, J.T., Talbert, R.L., Yee, G.C., Matzke, G.R., Wells, B.G., & Posey, L.M. (Eds.), *Pharmacotherapy: a pathophysiologic approach.* (5th ed.) (pp.157-183). Stamford, CT: Appleton and Lange.

Cerebral Embolism Study Group. (1989). Cardiogenic brain embolism: The second report of the Cerebral Embolism Task Force. *Archives of Neurology*, 46(7):727-743.

Ciccone, C.D. (2007). *Pharmacology in rehabilitation* (4th ed.). Philadelphia: Davis.

Clarify. (2009). The burden of coronary artery disease. Available: www.clarify-registry.com/healthcare-professionals/about-coronary-artery-disease/1-the-burden-of-cad

Colbert, B.J., & Mason, B.J. (2002). *Integrated cardiopulmonary pharmacology.* Upper Saddle River, NJ: Prentice Hall.

Collins, R., Armitage, J., Parish, S., Sleight, P., & Peto, R. (2004). Effects of cholesterol lowering with simvastatin on stroke and other major vascular events in 20536 people with cerebrovascular disease or other high-risk conditions. *Lancet*, 363(9411):757-767.

Del Zoppo, G.J., Saver, J.L., Jauch, E.C., & Adams, H.P. (2009). Expansion of the time window for treatment of acute ischemic stroke with intravenous tissue plasminogen activator. A scientific advisory from the AHA/ASA. *Stroke*, 40(8):1-4.

Dobesch, P.P., Stacy, Z.A. (2011). Management of chronic stable angina, In Richardson, M., Chant, C., Cheng, J.W.M., Chessman, K.H., Hume, A.L., Hutchison, L.C., et.al (Eds.) *Pharmacotherapy self-assessment program*. Book 1: Cardiology (7th Edition, p. 43-64). Kansas City: American College of Clinical Pharmacy.

Dromerick, A. (2003). Evidence-based rehabilitation: The case for and against constraint-induced movement therapy. *Journal of Rehabilitation Research and Development*, 40(1):vii-ix.

Easton, J.D., Saver, J.L., Albers, G.W., Chaturvedi, S., Feldnab, E., Hatsukami, R.T., et al. (2009). AHA/ASA scientific statement: Definition and evaluation of transient ischemic attack. Available: http://stroke.ahajournals.org/content/40/6/2276.full

Fonarow, G.C., Gregory, T., Driskill, M., Stewart, M.D., Beam, C., Butler, J., et al. (2010). Hospital certification for optimizing cardiovascular disease and stroke quality of care and outcomes. *Circulation*, 122(23):2459-2469.

Friedman, G.D., Loveland, D.B., & Ehrlich, P.S. (1968). Relationship of stroke to other cardiovascular disease. *Circulation*, 38(3):533-541.

Furie, K.L., Kasner, S.E., Adams, R.J., Albers, G.W., Fagan, S.C., Halperin, J.L., et al. (2011). Guidelines for the prevention of stroke in patients with stroke or transient ischemic attack: A guideline for healthcare professionals from the American Heart Association/American Stroke Association. *Stroke*, 42(1):227-276.

Goldstein, L.B., Bushnell, C.D., Adams, R.J., Appal, L.J., Braun, L.T., Chaturvdi, S., et al. (2011). Guidelines for the primary prevention of stroke: A guideline for healthcare. *Stroke*, 42:517-584.

Goldstein, L.B., & Simel, D.L. (2005). "Is this patient having a stroke?" *Journal of the American Medical Association*, 293(19):2391-2402.

Goodman, C.C., Boissonnault, W.G., & Fuller, K.S. (2008). *Pathology: Implications for the physical therapist* (3rd ed.). Philadelphia: Saunders.

Grundy, S. (2001). National cholesterol education program expert panel on detection, evaluation and treatment of high blood cholesterol in adults. *Journal of the American Medical Association*, 285(19):2486-2497.

Harrington, C. (2003). Managing hypertension in patients with stroke. *Critical Care Nurse*, 23(3):30-38.

Harris, K. (2008). *The worldwide burden of peripheral artery disease*. London: Inter-Society Consensus for the Management of PAD.

Hart, R.G., Coull, B.M., & Hart, D. (1983). Early recurrent embolism associated with nonvalvular atrial fibrillation: A retrospective study. *Stroke*, 14(5):688-693.

Hart, R.G., & Halperin, J.L. (2001). Atrial fibrillation and stroke: Concepts and controversies. *Stroke*, 32(3):803-808.

Heart Protection Study Collaborative Group. (2002). MRC/BHF heart protection study of cholesterol lowering with simvastatin in 20,536 high-risk individuals: A randomized placebo-controlled trial. *Lancet*, 360(9326):7-22.

Hiatt, W.R., Wolfel, E.E., & Regensteiner, J.G. (1991). Exercise in the treatment of intermittent claudication due to peripheral arterial disease. *Vascular Medicine*, 2(1):61-70.

Knopp, R. (1999). Drug treatment of lipid disorders. *New England Journal of Medicine*, 321(7):498-511.

Liu-DeRyke, X., & Baldwin, K.A. (2012). Management of acute ischemic stroke and transient ischemic attack. In Richardson, M., Chant, C., Cheng, J.W.M., Chessman, K.H., Hume, A.L., Hutchison, L.C., et.al (Eds.) *Pharmacotherapy self-assessment program. Book 10: Cardiology* (7th ed.) (pp. 71-90). Kansas City, MO: American College of Clinical Pharmacy.

Mehler, P.S., Coll, J.R., Estacio, R., Esler, A., Schrier, R.W., & Hiatt, W.R. (2003). Intensive blood pressure control reduces the risk of cardiovascular events in patients with peripheral arterial disease and type 2 diabetes. *Circulation*, 107(5):753-756.

Michel, T., & Hoffman, B.B. (2011). Treatment of ischemia and hypertension. In J.G. Hardman, L.E. Limbird, & A.G. Gillman (Eds.), *Goodman and Gillman's the pharmacological basis of therapeutics* (12th ed.) (pp. 745-813). New York: McGraw-Hill.

Muls, E., Klanowski, J., Scheen, A., & Van Gaal, L. (2001). The effects of orlistat on weight and on serum lipids in obese patients with hypercholesterolemia: A randomized double-blind, placebo-controlled, multicentre study. *International Journal of Obesity and Related Metabolic Disorders*, 25(11):1714-1721.

Murabito, J.M., Evans, J.C., D'Agostino, R.B., Wilson, P.W., & Kannel, W.B. (2005). Temporal trends in the incidence of intermittent claudication from 1950 to 1999. *American Journal of Epidemiology*, 162(5):430-437.

National Stroke Association. (2010). Prevention. Available: http://www.stroke.org/site/PageServer?pagename=SS_Mag_fall2010_prevention

O'Donnell, M.E., Badger, S.A., Sharif, M.A., Young, I.S., Lee, B., & Soong, C.V. (2009). The vascular and biochemical effects of cilostazol in patients with peripheral arterial disease. *Journal of Vascular Surgery*, 49(5):1226-1234.

Peel, C., & Mossberg, K.A. (1995). Effects of cardiovascular medications on exercise responses. *Physical Therapy*, 75(5):387-396.

Pradaxa. (2012). Product information. Available: www.pradaxa.com/index.jsp

Rodgers, H., Atkinson, C., Bond, S., Suddes, M., Dobson, R., & Curless, R. (1999). Randomized controlled trial of a comprehensive stroke education program for patients and caregivers. *Stroke*, 30(12):2585-2591.

Rowe, V.L. (2009). Peripheral arterial occlusive disease: Treatment and medication. Available: http://emedicine.medscape.com/article/460178-treatment

Sacco, R.L., Adams, R., Albers, G., Alberts, M.J., Benavente, O., Furie, K., et al. (2006). Guidelines for the prevention of stroke in patients with ischemic stroke or transient ischemic attack. *Stroke*, 37(2):577-617.

Sanoski, C.A. (2011). Atrial and ventricular arrhythmias: Evolving practices. In Richardson, M., Chant, C., Cheng, J.W.M., Chessman, K.H., Hume, A.L., Hutchison, L.C., et.al. (Eds.) *Pharmacotherapy self-assessment program. Book 1: Cardiology* (7th ed.) (pp. 125-151). Kansas City, MO: American College of Clinical Pharmacy.

Schell Frazier, M., & Wist Drzymkowski, J. (2004). *Essentials of human diseases and conditions* (3rd ed.). St. Louis: Elsevier.

Semplicini, A., Maresca, A., Boscolo, G., Sartori, M., Rocchi, R., Giantin, V., et al. (2003). Hypertension in acute ischemic stroke: A compensatory mechanism or an additional damaging factor? *Archives of Internal Medicine*, 163(2):211-216.

Sisson, E., & Van Tassell, B.W. (2011). Dyslipidemias: Updates and new controversies In Richardson, M., Chant, C., Cheng, J.W.M., Chessman, K.H., Hume, A.L., Hutchison, L.C., et.al. (Eds). *Pharmacotherapy self-assessment program. Book 1: Cardiology* (7th ed.) (pp. 25-42). Kansas City, MO: American College of Clinical Pharmacy.

SPARCL Investigators. (2006). The stroke prevention by aggressive reduction in cholesterol levels (SPARCL) study. *Cerebrovascular Disease*, 21(Suppl. 4):1.

Summers, D., Leonard, A., Wentworth, D., Saver, J.L., Simpson, J., Spilker, J.A., et al. (2009). Comprehensive overview of nursing and interdisciplinary care of the acute ischemic stroke patient: A scientific statement from the American Heart Association. *Stroke*, 40(8):2911-2944.

Talbert, R. (2005). *Hyperlipidemia*. In J.T. DiPiro, R.L. Talbert, & G.C. Yee (Eds.), *Pharmacotherapy: A pathophysiologic approach* (6th ed.) (pp. 429-452). New York: McGraw-Hill.

Tamparo, C.D., & Lewis, M.A. (2000). *Diseases of the human body* (3rd ed.). Philadelphia: Davis.

Wall, H.K., Beagan, B.M., & O'Neill, J.H. (2008). Addressing stroke signs and symptoms through public education: The stroke heroes act fAST campaign. *Prevention of Chronic Disease*, 5(2):A49.

Weitz, J.I. (2011). Blood coagulation and anticoagulant, fibronolyic, and antiplatelet drugs. In J.G. Hardman, L.E. Limbird, & A.G. Gillman (Eds.), *Goodman and Gillman's the pharmacological basis of therapeutics* (12th ed.) (pp. 849-876). New York: McGraw-Hill.

World Health Organization. (2012). The atlas of heart disease and stroke: The global burden of stroke. Available: www.who.int/cardiovascular_diseases/en/cvd_atlas_15_burden_stroke.pdf

Chapter 21

Brock, C.M. (2010). DDP-4 inhibitors: What is their place in therapy, diabetes and pharmaceutical care? *U.S. Pharmacist*, May(Suppl.):8-13.

DeHart, R.M., & Worthington, M.A. (2005). Nutritional considerations in major organ failure. In J.T. Dipiro, R.T. Talbert, G.C. Yee, G.R. Matzke, B.G. Wells, & M.L. Posey (Eds.), *Pharmacotherapy: A pathophysiologic approach* (5th ed.) (p. 2519-2530). New York: McGraw-Hill.

Drabb, S.R. (2009a). Liraglutide: A new option for the treatment of type 2 diabetes mellitus. *Pharmacotherapy*, 29(12 Part 2):23S-25S.

Drabb, S.R. (2009b). Clinical studies of liraglutide, a novel, once daily human glucagon-like peptide-1 analog for improved management of type 2 diabetes mellitus. *Pharmacotherapy*, 29(12 Part 2):43S-55S.

Grossman, S. (2009). Differentiating incretin therapies based on structure, activity, and metabolism: Focus on liraglutide. *Pharmacotherapy*, 29(12 Part 2):25S-33S.

Inarcchi, S.E., Bergenstal, R.M., Buse, J.B., Diamant, M., Ferrannu, E., Nauck, M., Peteres, A.L., Tsapas, A., Wender, R. & Matthews, D.R. (2012). Management of hyperglycemia in type 2 diabetes: a patient-centered approach position statement of the American Diabetes Association (ADA) and the European Association for the Study of Diabetes. (EASD). *Diabetes Care*, 35(6):1364-1379.

Joffe, D.L., Leahy, J.L., & Marquess, J.G. (2010). New options for glycemic control in type 2 diabetes. Available: www.uspharmacist.com/about_usp/

Lamb, W.H. (2011). Diabetes mellitus: Type 1. Available: http://emedicine.medscape.com/article/919999-overview

Leahy, J.L., & Marquess, J.G. (2010). New options for glycemic control in type 2 diabetes: What pharmacists need to know about GLP-1 agonists. *U.S. Pharmacist-Diabetes and Pharmaceutical Care*, 35(5 Suppl.):19-24.

Marquess, J.G. (2010). Maximizing the benefits of GLP-1 agonists in type 2 diabetes: Successful patient strategies, diabetes and pharmaceutical care. *U.S. Pharmacist*, (May Suppl.):29-33.

Montfort, E.G., Witte, A.P., & Ward, K. (2010). Neuropathic pain: A review of diabetic neuropathy. *U.S. Pharmacist-Health System Edition*, May:8-15.

Quinn, J.A., Snyder, S.L., Berghoff, J.L., Colombo, C.S., Jacobi, J. (2006). A practical approach to hyperglycemia management in the intensive care unit: Evaluation of an intensive insulin infusion protocol. *Pharmacotherapy*, 26(10), 1410-1420.

Rochester, C.D., Leon, N., Domrowskiv, R., & Haines, S.T. (2010). Collaborative drug therapy management for initiating and adjusting insulin therapy in patients with type 2 diabetes mellitus. *American Journal of Health System Pharmacists*, 67(1):42-48.

Sherman, J.J. (2010). Diabetic foot ulcer assessment and treatment: A pharmacist's guide. *U.S. Pharmacist*, 35(6):38-44.

Votey, S.R., & Peters, A.L. (2010). Diabetes mellitus: Type 2—A review: Treatment and medication. Available: http://emedicine.com/article/766143-treatment

White, J.R. (2010). Insulin analogues: What are the clinical implications of structural differences? *U.S. Pharmacist*, May(Suppl.):3-7.

World Health Organization. (2012). Diabetes global incidence (No.326) (Fact sheet). Retrieved from www.who.int/diabetes/facts/world_figures/en/

Zaharowitz, B.J., & Conner, C. (2009). The intersection of safety and adherence: New incretin-based therapies in patients with type 2 diabetes mellitus. *Pharmacotherapy*, 29(12):55S-67S.

Chapter 22

Adams, P.F., Barnes, P.M., & Vickerie, J.L. (2008) Summary health statistics for the U.S. population: National Health Interview Survey, 2007. *Vital Health Stat 10*(238):1-104.

Beers, M.H., & Porter, R.S. (2006). *The Merck manual of diagnosis and therapy* (18th ed.). Whitehouse Station, NJ: Merck Research Laboratories.

Boueri, F.M., Bucher-Bartelson, B.L., Glenn, K.A., & Make, B.J. (2001). Quality of life measured with a generic instrument (short form-36) improves following pulmonary rehabilitation in patients with COPD. *Chest*, 119(1):77-84.

Bourbeau, J., Julien, M., Maltais, F., Rouleau, M., Beaupré, A., Bégin, R., et al. (2003). Reduction of hospital utilization in patients with chronic obstructive pulmonary disease: A disease-specific self-management intervention. *Archives of Internal Medicine*, 163(5):585.

Braman, S. (2006). The global burden of asthma. *Chest*, 130(1 Suppl.):4S-12S.

Brenes, G.A. (2003). Anxiety and chronic obstructive pulmonary disease: Prevalence, impact, and treatment. *Psychosomatic Medicine*, 65(6):963-970.

Brenner, B.E. (2010). Asthma. Available: http://emedicine.medscape.com/article/806890-overview

Brown, J.B., Votto, J.J., Trailers, R.S., Haggerty, M.C., Woolley, R.C., Banmdyopadhyay, T., et al. (2000). Functional status and survival following pulmonary rehabilitation *Chest*, 118(3):697-703.

Buist, A.S., McBurnie, M.A., Vollmer, W.M., Gillespie, S., Burney P., Mannino, D.M., & Nizakowska-Mogilnicka, E. (2007). International variation in prevalence of COPD (the BOLD Study): A population-based prevalence study. *Lancet*, 370(9589):741-750.

Carl, L., & Johnson, P. (2006). *Drugs and dysphagia*. Austin, TX: Pro-Ed.

Cerveri, I., Accordini, S., Veriato, G., Zoia, M.C., Casali, L., Burney, P., et al. (2001). Variations in the prevalence across countries of chronic bronchitis and smoking habits in young adults. *European Respiratory Journal*, 18(1):85-92.

Ciccone, C.D. (2007). *Pharmacology in rehabilitation* (4th ed.). Philadelphia: Davis.

DeHart, R.M., & Worthington, M.A. (2005). Nutritional considerations in major organ failure. In J.T. Dipiro, R.T. Talbert, G.C. Yee, G.R. Matske, B.G. Wells, & L.M. Posey (Eds.), *Pharmacotherapy: A pathophysiologic approach* (5th ed.) (pp. 2519-2530). New York: McGraw-Hill.

Derkacz, M., Mosiewicz, J., & Myslinski, W. (2007). Cognitive dysfunction in patients with chronic obstructive pulmonary disease. *Wiadomosci Lekarskie*, 60(3-4):143-147.

Devine, E.C., & Pearcy, J. (1996). Meta-analyses of the effects of psychoeducational care in adults with chronic obstructive pulmonary disease. *Patient Education and Counseling*, 29(2):167-178.

DiMeo, F., Pedone, C., Lubich, S., Pizzoli, C., Traballesi, M., & Incalzi, R.A. (2008). Age does not hamper the response to pulmonary rehabilitation of COPD patients. *Age and Aging*, 37(5):530-535.

Drive, A.G., McAlevy, M.T., & Smith, J.L. (1982). Nutritional assessment of patients with COPD and acute respiratory failure. *Chest*, 82(5):568-571.

Emory, K.E., Kaplan, R.M., Wamboklt, F.S., Zhang, L., & Make, B.J. (2008). Cognitive and psychological issues in emphysema. *Proceedings of the American Thoracic Society*, 1(5):556-560.

Finnerty, J.P., Keeping, D.M., Bullough, I., & Jones, J. (2001). The effectiveness of outpatient pulmonary rehabilitation in chronic lung disease. *Chest*, 119(6):1705-1710.

Fischer, M., Scharloo, M., Weinman, J., & Kaptein, A. (2007). Respiratory rehabilitation. In P. Kennedy (Ed.), *Psychological management of physical disabilities* (pp. 124-148). London: Routledge Taylor & Francis.

Gardenhire, D.S. (2008a). Cough and cold agents. In D.S. Gardenhire (Ed.), *Rau's respiratory care pharmacology* (7th ed.) (pp. 305-315). St. Louis: Mosby Elsevier.

Gardenhire, D.S. (2008b). Adrenergic (sympathomimetic) bronchodilators. In D.S. Gardenhire (Ed.), *Rau's respiratory care pharmacology* (7th ed.) (pp. 103-131). St. Louis: Mosby Elsevier.

Gardenhire, D.S. (2008c). Corticosteroids in respiratory care. In D.S. Gardenhire (Ed.), *Rau's respiratory care pharmacology* (7th ed.) (pp. 204-225). St. Louis: Mosby Elsevier.

Gardenhire, D.S. (2008d). Xanthines. In D.S. Gardenhire (Ed.), *Rau's respiratory care pharmacology* (7th ed.) (pp. 150-161). St. Louis: Mosby Elsevier.

Garrod, R., Parl, E.A., & Wedzicha, J.A. (2000). Supplemental oxygen during pulmonary rehabilitation in patients with COPD with exercise hypoxemia. *Thorax*, 55(7):539-543.

GOLD. (2013). The global initiative for chronic obstructive lung disease. Available: www.goldcopd.org/Guidelines/guidelines-resources.html.

Gross, R.D., Atwood, C.W., Ross, S.B., Olszewski, J.W., & Eichhorn, K.A. (2009). The coordination of breathing and swallowing in chronic obstructive pulmonary disease. *American Journal of Respiratory and Critical Care Medicine*, 179(7):559-565.

Harding, S.M. (2002). Oropharyngeal dysfunction in COPD patients. *Chest*, 121(2):315-317.

Hill, N.S. (2006). Pulmonary rehabilitation. *Proceedings of the American Thoraxic Society*, 3(1):66-74.

Hitner, H., & Nagle, B. (2001a). Bronchodilator drugs and the treatment of asthma. In S.R. Levine & A.J. McLaughlin (Eds.), *Pharmacology in respiratory care* (pp.253-270). New York: McGraw-Hill.

Hitner, H., & Nagle, B. (2001b). Drugs affecting the sympathetic nervous system. In S.R. Levine & A.J. McLaughlin (Eds.), *Pharmacology in respiratory care* (pp. 77-94). New York: McGraw-Hill.

Hitner, H., & Nagle, B. (2001c). Adrenal steroids. In S.R. Levine & A.J. McLaughlin (Eds.), *Pharmacology in respiratory care* (pp. 271-288). New York: McGraw-Hill.

Incalzi, R.A., Fuso, I., DeRosa, M., Forastiiere, F., Rapiti, E., Nardecchia, B., et al. (1997). Comorbidity contributes to predict mortality of patients with chronic obstructive pulmonary disease. *European Respiratory Journal*, 10(12):2794-2800.

Incalzi, R.A., Marra, C., Giordano, A., Calcagni, M.L., Cappa, A., Basso, S., et al. (2003). Cognitive impairment in chronic obstructive pulmonary disease. *Journal of Neurology*, 250(3):325-332.

Kamanger, N., & Nikhani, N.S. (2010). Chronic obstructive pulmonary disease. Available: http://emedicine.medscape.com/article/297664-overview

Kim, H.F., Kunik, M.E., Molinari, V.A., Hillman, S.L., Lalani, S., Orengo, C.A., et al. (2000). Functional impairment in COPD patients: The impact of anxiety and depression. *Psychosomatics*, 41(6):465-471.

Koppers, R.J., Vos, P.J., Boot, C.R., & Folgering, H.T. (2006). Exercise performance improves in patients with COPD due to respiratory muscle endurance training. *Chest*, 129(4):886-892.

Kozora, E., Emery, C., Kaplan, R.M., Wamboldt, F.S., Zhang, L., & Make, B.J. (2008). Cognitive and psychological issues in emphysema. *Proceedings of the American Thoracic Society*, 5(4):556-560.

MacIntyre, N.R., Cook, D.J., Ely, E.W., Epstein, S.K., Fink, J.B., Heffner, J.E., et al. (2001). Evidence based guidelines for weaning and discontinuing ventilatory support. *Chest*, 120(6 Suppl.):375-396.

McKinstry, A., Tranter, M., & Sweeney, J. (2010). Outcomes of dysphagia intervention in a pulmonary rehabilitation program. *Dysphagia*, 25(2):104-111.

Mokhlesi, B. (2003). Clinical impressions gastroesophageal reflux disease and swallowing dysfunction in COPD. *American Journal of Respiratory Medicine*, 2(2):117-121.

Mokhlesi, B., Logemann, J.A., Rademaker, A.E., Stangel, C.E., & Corbridge, T.C. (2002). Oropharyngeal deglutition in stable COPD. *Chest*, 121(2):361-369.

Mokhlesi, B., Morris, A.L., Cheng-Fang, H., Barrett, T.A., & Kamp, D.W. (2001). Increased prevalence of gastroesophageal reflux symptoms in patients with COPD. *Chest*, 119(4):1043-1048.

Mueller, R.E., Petty, T.L., & Filley, G.F. (1970). Ventilation and arterial blood gas changes induced by pursed lips breathing. *Journal of Applied Physiology*, 28(6):784-789.

Prosser, T.R., & Bollmeier, S.G. (2008). Chronic obstructive pulmonary disease. In Hume, A.L., Khachikian, D., & Kucera, M. (Eds.), *Pharmacotherapy self-assessment program. Clinical pharmacy book 6: Cardiology* (6th ed.) (pp. 1-20). Kansas City, MO: American College of Clinical Pharmacy.

Puhan, M.A., Frey, M., Büchi, S., & Schunemann, H.J. (2008). The minimal important difference of the hospital anxiety and depression scale in patients with chronic obstructive pulmonary disease. *Health Quality Life Outcomes*, 6:46.

Raissy, H.H., & Kelly, H.W. (2008). Update on guidelines and controversies in the treatment of asthma. In J. Cheng (Ed.), *Pharmacotherapy self-assessment program. Book 6: Cardiology* (6th ed.) (pp. 21-42). Kansas City, MO: American College of Clinical Pharmacy.

Reardon, J.E., Awad, E., Normandin, E.F., Vale, F.B., Clark, B., & Zu Wallack, R. (1994). The effect of comprehensive outpatient pulmonary rehabilitation on dyspnea. *Chest*, 105(4):1046-1052.

Sergysels, R., Decoster, A., Degre, S., & Denolin, H. (1979). Functional evaluation of a physical rehabilitation program including breathing exercises and bicycle training in chronic obstructive pulmonary disease. *Respiration*, 38(2):105-111.

Sharma, S., & Arneja, A. (2010). Pulmonary rehabilitation. Available: http://emedicine.medscape.com/article/319885-overview

Springhouse. (2009). *Clinical pharmacology made incredibly easy* (3rd ed.). Philadelphia: Wolters Kluwer/Lippincott Williams & Wilkins.

Troosters, T., Gosselink, R., & Decramer, M. (2000). Short-and long-term effects of outpatient rehabilitation in patients with chronic obstructive pulmonary disease: A randomized trial. *American Journal of Medicine*, 109(3):207-212.

U.S. Preventative Services Task Force. (2009). Counseling and interventions to prevent tobacco use and tobacco-caused disease in adults and pregnant women: U.S. Preventative Services Task Force reaffirmation recommendation statement. *Annals of Internal Medicine*, 150(8):551-555.

van Durme, Y., Verhamme, K., Stijnen, T., van Rooij, F., Van Pottelberge, G., Hofman, A., et al. (2009). Prevalence, incidence, and lifetime risk for the development of COPD in the elderly: The Rotterdam study. *Chest*, 135(2):368-377.

World Health Organization. (2004). World health report 2004. Available: http://www.who.int/whr/2004/annex/topic/en/annex_2_pdf

Chapter 23

American Association of Orthopedic Surgeons. (2009). Position statement 1113: Osteoporosis/bone health in adults as a national public health priority. Available: http://www.aaos.org/about/papers/position/1113.asp

Beers, M.H., & Porter, R.S. (2006). *The Merck manual of diagnosis and therapy* (18th ed.) (pp. 1252-1253). Whitehouse Station, NJ: Merck Research Laboratories.

Bharaktiya, S., Griffing, G., Orlander, P., Woodhouse, W., & Davis, A. (2012). Hypothyroidism. Available: http://emedicine.medscape.com/article/122393-overview

Bilezikian, J.P., Potts, J.T., & Fuleihan, G.E. (2002). Summary statement from a workshop on asymptomatic primary hyperparathyroidism: A perspective for the 21st century. *Journal of Bone and Mineral Research*, 17(Suppl. 2):2-11.

Blackwell, J. (2004). Evaluation and treatment of hyperthyroidism and hypothyroidism. *Journal of American Academy of Nurse Practitioners*, 16(10):422-425.

Boissonnault, W.G. (1995). *Examination in physical therapy practice: Screening for medical disease* (2nd ed.). Philadelphia: Churchill Livingstone.

Brent, G.A., & Koenig, R.J. (2011). Thyroid and anti-thyroid drugs. In L.L. Brunton, B.A. Chabner, & B.C. Knollmann (Eds.), *Goodman and Gillman's the pharmacological basis of therapeutics* (12th ed.) (pp. 1129-1161). New York: McGraw Hill.

Bringhurst, F.R., Demay, M.B., & Kronenberg, H.M. (2008). Disorders of mineral metabolism. In H.M. Kronenberg, M. Schlomo, K.S. Polansky, & P.R. Larsen (Eds.). *Williams textbook of endocrinology* (11th ed.) (pp 1203-1268). St. Louis: Saunders.

Chen, H., Parkerson, S., & Udelsman, R. (1998). Parathyroidectomy in the elderly: Do the benefits outweigh the risks? *World Journal of Surgery*, 22(6):531-535.

Chow, D. (2011). Rehabilitation for Paget's disease. Available: http://emedicine.medscape.com/article/311688-overview#a30.

Clarke, B.L. (2008). Parathyroid adenomas and hyperplasia. In Hay, I.D. & Wass, J.A. (Eds.) *Clinical Endocrine Oncology* (pp 172-179). Malden, MA: Blackwell Publishing.

Cleveland Clinic. (2009). Paget's disease. Available: http://my.clevelandclinic.org/disorders/pagets_disease/hic_pagets_disease.aspx

Cohen, J. (2008). Paget's disease: Definition, causes, symptoms and treatment. Available: http://acontreacourant.com/?p=627

Delange, F. (1998). Screening for congenital hypothyroidism used as an indicator of the degree of iodine deficiency and of its control. *Thyroid*, 8(12):1185-1192.

Franklyn, J.A. (1994). The management of hyperthyroidism. *New England Journal of Medicine*, 330(24):1731-1738.

Frazier, M., & Drzymkowski, J. (2004). *Essentials of human diseases and conditions* (3rd ed.). St. Louis: Elsevier.

Friedman, P.A. (2011). *Agents affecting mineral ion homeostasis and bone turnover.* In L.L. Brunton, B.A. Chabner, & B.C. Knollmann (Eds.), Goodman and Gillman's the pharmacological basis of therapeutics (12th ed.) (pp. 1275-1306). New York: McGraw-Hill.

Goodman, C.C., Boissonnault, W.G., & Fuller, K.S. (2003). *Pathology: Implications for the physical therapist* (2nd ed.). Philadelphia: Saunders.

Guildiken, B., Guildiken, S., Turgut, N., Yuce, M., Arikan, E., & Tugrul, A. (2006). Dysphagia as a primary manifestation of hyperthyroidism: A case report. *Acta Clinica Belgica*, 61(1):35- 37.

Guyton, A.C., & Hall, J.E. (2010). *Textbook of medical physiology* (12th ed.). Philadelphia: Saunders.

Howard, A. (2009). Change lifestyle and rebalance an underactive thyroid. Available: www.naturalnews.com/027241_thyroid_food_body.html

Kennedy, J.W., & Carlo, J.F. (1996). The ABCs of managing hyperthyroidism in the older patient. *Geriatrics*, 51(5):22-32.

Klein, I., & Ojamaa, K. (1996). The cardiovascular system in hypothyroidism. In L. Braverman & R. Utiger (Eds.), Werner and Ingbar's the thyroid (7th ed.) (p. 799). Philadelphia: Lippincott-Raven.

Kocabas, H., Yazicioglu, G., & Karaman, N.S. (2009). Isokinetic evaluation of muscle strength in patients with thyroid dysfunction. *Isokinetics and Exercise Science*, 17:69-72.

Konstantitinos, P., Ramona, D., Sheikh, H., & Argento, V. (2011). Thyrotoxic dysphagia in an 82-year-old male. *Case Reports in Medicine*, 2011(929523):1-3.

McConnell, R. (2007). Toward optimal health: Improved thyroid disease management in women. *Journal of Women's Health*, 16(4):458-462.

McGrogan, A., Seaman, H.E., & Wright, J.W. (2008). The incidence of autoimmune thyroid disease: A systematic review of the literature. *Clinical Endocrinology*, 69(5):687-696.

Medical Disability Advisor. (2010). Hypoparathyroidism. Available: www.mdguidelines.com/hypoparathyroidism

Mehta, A., Voight, J., Pahuja, D., & Devi, S.S. (2010). Hyperthyroidism: Exploring treatment strategies. *U.S. Pharmacist*, 35(6):45-54.

Norman, J. (2010). Hyperthyroidism: Overactivity of the thyroid gland. Available: www.endocrineweb.com/conditions/hyperthyroidism/hypterthyroidism-overactivity-thyroid-gland-0

O'Connell, M.B., & Elliott, M.E. (2002). Osteoporosis and osteomalacia. In J.T. DiPiro, R.L. Talbert, G.C. Yee, G.R. Matske, B.G. Wells, & L.M. Posey (Eds.), *Pharmacotherapy: A pathophysiologic approach* (5th ed.) (pp. 1599-1621). Stamford, CT: Appleton & Lange.

Pederson, B., Laurberg, P., Knudsen, N., Jorgensen, T., Perrild, H., Ovesen, L., et al. (2006). Increase in incidence of hyperthyroidism predominantly occurs in young people after iodine fortification of salt in Denmark. *Journal of Clinical Endocrinology and Metabolism*, 91(10):3830-3834.

Reasner, C.A., & Talbert, R.L. (2011). Thyroid disorders. In J.T. DiPiro, R.L. Talbert, G.C. Yee, G.R. Matske, B.G. Wells, & L.M. Posey (Eds.), *Pharmacotherapy: A pathophysiologic approach* (5th ed.) (pp. 1359-1378). Stamford, CT: Appleton & Lange.

Regina-Cammon, S.A., Knauff, C.A., & McNeely, E.D. (2002). *Atlas of pathophysiology*. Springhouse, PA: Springhouse.

Reid, J.R., & Wheeler, S.F. (2005). Hyperthyroidism: Diagnosis and treatment. *American Family Physician*, 72(4):623-630.

Schapira, A.H., & Griggs, R.C. (2000). Endocrine myopathies. In Schapira, A.H. & Griggs, R.C. (Eds.), *Muscle disease* (Vol. 6.) (pp. 181-192). Burlington, MA: Butterworth-Heinemann.

Shomon, M. (2010). Thyroid awareness month. Available: www.thyroidawarenessmonth.com/thyroid-gland.htm

Springhouse. (2008). *Professional guide to diseases* (9th ed.). Philadelphia: Lippincott Williams & Wilkins.

Tamparo, C.D., & Lewis, M.A. (2000). *Diseases of the human body* (3rd ed.). Philadelphia: Davis.

Tfelt-Hansen, J., & Brown, E.M. (2005). The calcium-sensing receptor in normal physiology and pathophysiology: A review. *Critical Reviews in Clinical Laboratory Sciences*, 42(1):35-70.

Vestergaard, P., Mollerup, C.L., & Frokjær, V.G. (2000). Cohort study of risk of fracture before and after surgery for primary hyperparathyroidism. *British Medical Journal*, 321(7261):598-602.

Vestergaard, P., & Mosekilde, L. (2003). Cohort study on effects of parathyroid surgery on multiple outcomes in primary hyperparathyroidism. *British Medical Journal*, 327(7414):530-534.

Wysolmerski, J.J., & Insogna, K.L. (2008). The parathyroid glands, hypercalcemia, and hypocalcemia. In H.M. Kronenberg, M. Schlomo, K.S. Polansky, & P.R. Larsen (Eds.), *Williams textbook of endocrinology* (11th ed.). St. Louis: Saunders.

Chapter 24

Alvi, A. (1999). Iatrogenic swallowing disorders: Medications. In R.L. Carrau & T. Murry (Eds.), *Comprehensive management of swallowing disorders* (pp. 119-124). San Diego: Singular.

Balmer, C.M., & Valley, A.W. (2002). Basic principles of cancer treatment and cancer chemotherapy. In J.T. DiPiro, R.L. Talbert, G.C. Yee, G.R. Matske, B.G. Wells, & L.M. Posey (Eds.), *Pharmacotherapy: A pathophysiologic approach* (5th ed.) (pp. 2175-2222). Stamford, CT: Appleton & Lange.

Bernardi, R.R. (2002). Peptic ulcer disease. In J.T. DiPiro, R.L. Talbert, G.C. Yee, G.R. Matske, B.G. Wells, & L.M. Posey (Eds.), *Pharmacotherapy: A pathophysiologic approach* (5th ed.) (pp. 603-624). Stamford, CT: Appleton & Lange.

Bernardi, R.R. (2007). Irritable bowel syndrome: Update on medical management and the use of probioitcs. *U.S. Pharmacist*, October:77-88.

Bloom, F.E. (2001). Neurotransmission and the central nervous system. In J.G. Hardman, L.E. Limbird, & A.G. Gillman (Eds.), *Goodman and Gillman's the pharmacological basis of therapeutics* (10th ed.) (pp. 293-320). New York: McGraw-Hill.

Boyce, H.W. (1998). Drug induced esophageal damage: Diseases of medical progress. *Gastrointestinal Endoscopy*, 47(6):547-550.

Bubalo, J.S. (2009). Supportive care: Oncology. In M. Richardson, C. Chant, J.W. Cheng, K.H. Chessman, A.L. Hume, L.C. Hutchison, et al. (Eds.), *Pharmacotherapy self-assessment program* (6th ed.) (pp. 89-100). Lenexa, KS: American College of Clinical Pharmacy.

Campbell-Taylor, I. (1996). Drugs, dysphagia and nutrition. In C. Van Riper (Ed.), *Dietetics in development and psychiatric disorders* (pp. 24-29). Chicago: American Dietetic Association.

Campbell-Taylor, I. (2001). *Medications and dysphagia* (pp. 1-32). Stow, OH: Interactive Therapeutics.

Carl, L.C., & Johnson, P.R. (2006). *Drugs and dysphagia: How medications can affect eating and swallowing.* Austin, TX: Pro-Ed.

Carl, L.C. & Johnson, P.R. (2008). Drugs and dysphagia: Perspectives on swallowing and swallowing disorders. *Dysphagia* 17: 4 143-4148.

Johnson, P.R. (2013). The effects of medication on cognition in long-term care. *Semin Speech Lang*, 34(1): 18-27.

Caruso, G., & Passali, F.M. (2006). ENT manifestations of gastroesophageal reflux in children. *Acta Otorhinolaryngolica Italica*, 26(5):252-255.

Cash, B.D. (2007). Novel mechanisms: Paving the way to relief in chronic constipation. *U.S. Pharmacist*, December:3-11.

Cassagnol, M., Saad, M., Ahmed, E., & Ezzo, D. (2010). Review of current chronic constipation guidelines. *U.S. Pharmacist*, December:74-81.

Chabner, B.A., Ryan, D.P., Paz-Ares, L., Garcia-Carbonero, R., & Calabresi, P. (2001). Antineoplastic agents. In J.G. Hardman, L.E. Limbird, & A.G. Gillman (Eds.), *Goodman and Gillman's the pharmacological basis of therapeutics* (10th ed.) (pp. 1389-1461). New York: McGraw-Hill.

Chan, J. (2007). A review on the management of Crohn's disease. *U.S. Pharmacist*, January:HS18-HS33.

Cheng, C.M., Chen, J.S., & Patel, R.P. (2006a). Unlabeled uses of botulinum toxins: A review— Part 1. *American Journal of Health-System Pharmacy*, 63(2):145-152.

Cheng, C.M., Chen, J.S., & Patel, R.P. (2006b). Unlabeled uses of botulinum toxins: A review—Part 2. *American Journal of Health-System Pharmacy*, 63(3):225-232.

Dike, U.A., Honeywell, M.S., Welch, T.M., Soto, C., & Michel, D. (2010). Ulcerative colitis: Therapeutic management update. *U.S. Pharmacist*, December:HS21-HS26.

Eng, M., & White, P. (2007). Postoperative nausea and vomiting: An update on its prevention and treatment. *Pharmacology and Physiology in Anesthetic Practice Updates*, 1(1):7-19.

Gallagher, L. (2010). The impact of prescribed medication on swallowing: An overview. *ASHA Perspectives on Swallowing and Swallowing Disorders (Dysphagia)*, 19:98-102.

Gutstein, H.B., & Akil, H. (2001). Opioid analgesics. In J.G. Hardman, L.E. Limbird, & A.G. Gillman (Eds.), *Goodman and Gillman's the pharmacological basis of therapeutics* (10th ed.) (pp. 569-619). New York: McGraw-Hill.

Hermes, E.R., & Huang, S. (2007). Botulinum toxin type A for treatment of refractory gastroparesis. *American Journal of Heath-System Pharmacy*, 64(21):2237-2240.

Hoffman, B.B. (2001). Neurotransmission: The autonomic and somatic motor nervous systems. In J.G. Hardman, L.E. Limbird, & A.G. Gillman (Eds.), *Goodman and Gillman's the pharmacological basis of therapeutics* (10th ed.) (pp. 115-154). New York: McGraw-Hill.

Hoogerwerf, W.A., & Pasricha, P. (2001). Agents used for control of gastric acidity and treatment of peptic ulcers and gastroesophageal reflux disease. In J.G. Hardman, L.E. Limbird, & A.G. Gillman (Eds.), *Goodman and Gillman's the pharmacological basis of therapeutics* (10th ed.) (pp. 1005-1020). New York: McGraw-Hill.

Howden, C.W. (2004). Management of acid-related disorders in patients with dysphagia. *American Journal of Medicine*, 117(5A):44S-48S.

Hungin, A.S., Whorwell, P.J., Tack, J., & Mearins, F. (2003). The prevalence, patterns and impact of irritable bowel syndrome: An international survey of 40,000 subjects. *Aliment Pharmacology and Therapeutics*, 17(5):643-650.

Hunt, V.P., & Walker, F.O. (1989). Dysphagia in Huntington's disease. *Journal of Neuroscience Nursing*, 21(2):92-95.

Jaspersen, D. (2000). Drug induced esophageal disorders. *Drug Safety*, 22(3):237-249.

Katzan, I.L., Cebul, R.D., Husak, S.H., Dawson, N.V., & Baker, D.W. (2003). The effect of pneumonia on mortality among patients hospitalized for acute stroke. *Neurology*, 60(4):620-625.

Kloth, D.D. (2009). New pharmacologic findings for the treatment of PONV and PDNV. *American Journal of Health-System Pharmacy*, 66(Suppl. 1):S11-S8.

Koek, G.H., Sifrim D., Lerut T., Janssens J., & Tack, J. (2003). Effect of the GABAβ agonist baclofen in patients with symptoms and duodeno-gastro-oesophageal reflux refactory to proton pump inhibitors. *Gut*, 52(10):1397-1402.

Kraft, M.D. (2007). Emerging pharmacologic options for treating postoperative ileus. *American Journal of Health-System Pharmacy*, 64(Suppl. 12):S13-S20.

Leslie, P., Carding, P.N., & Wilson, J.A. (2003). Investigation and management of chronic dysphagia. *British Medical Journal*, 326(7386):433-436.

Lidums I., Lehmann A., Checklin H., Dent J., & Holloway R.H. (2000). Control of transient lower esophageal sphincter relaxations and reflux by GABA$_B$ baclofen in normal subjects. *Gastroenterology*. 118(1):7-13.

Logemann, J.A., Pauloski, B.R., Rademaker, A.W., Lazarus, C.L., Mittal, B., Gaziano, J., et al. (2003). Xerostomia: 12 month changes in saliva production and its relationship to perception and performance of swallow intake, and diet after chemo radiation. *Head and Neck*, 25(6):432-437.

Lovell, S.J., Wong, H.B., Loh, K.S., Ngo, R.Y., & Wilson, J.A. (2005). Impact of dysphagia on quality of life in nasopharyngeal carcinoma. *Head and Neck*, 27(10):864-872.

Mann, G., Hankey, G.J., & Cameron, D. (2000). Swallowing disorders following acute stroke: Prevalence and diagnostic accuracy. *Cerebrovascular Disease*, 10(5):380-386.

Marik, P.E., & Kaplan, D. (2003). Aspiration pneumonia and dysphagia in the elderly. *Chest*, 124(1):328-336.

Markowitz, J.S., & Morton, W.A. (2002). Psychoses. In M.M. Richardson & C.C. Chant (Eds.), *Pharmacotherapy self-assessment program. Book 7: Neurology and psychiatry* (4th ed.) (pp. 99-139). Kansas City, MO: American College of Clinical Pharmacy.

Martino, R., Foley, N., Bhogal, S., Diamant, N., Speechley, M., & Teasell, R. (2005). Dysphagia after stroke: Incidence, diagnosis, and pulmonary complications. *Stroke*, 36(12):2756-2763.

Max, M.B., & American Pain Society. (1999). *Principles of analgesic use in the treatment of acute pain and cancer pain* (4th ed.). Glenview, IL: American Pain Society.

Mayer, V. (2004). The challenges of managing dysphagia in brain-injured patients. *British Journal of Community Nursing*, 9(2):67-73.

Meek, P.D. (2002). Recent concepts in the treatment of irritable bowel syndrome. In M.M. Richardson & C.C. Chant (Eds.), *Pharmacotherapy self-assessment program. Book 8: Gastroenterology and nutrition* (4th ed.) (pp. 69-95). Kansas City, MO: American College of Clinical Pharmacy.

Mercado-Deane, M.G., Burton, E.M., Harlow, S.A., Glover, A.S., Deane, D.A., Guill, M.F., et al. (2001). Swallowing dysfunction in infants less than 1 year of age. *Pediatric Radiology*, 31(6):423-428.

Morgan, A., Ward, E., Murdoch, B., Kennedy, B., & Murison, R. (2003). Incidence, characteristics, and predictive factors for dysphagia after pediatric traumatic brain injury. *Journal of Head Trauma and Rehabilitation*, 18(3):239-251.

Nelson, M.V., Berchou, R.C., & LeWitt, P.A. (2002). Parkinson's disease. In J.T. DiPiro, R L. Talbert, G.C. Yee, G.R. Matske, B.G. Wells, & L.M. Posey (Eds.), *Pharmacotherapy: A pathophysi-ologic approach* (5th ed.) (pp. 1289-1102). Stamford, CT: Appleton & Lange.

O'Neill, J.L. (2003). Drug-induced esophageal injuries and dysphagia. *Annals of Pharmacotherapy*, 37(11):1675-1684.

Paciaroni, M., Mazzotta, G., Corea, F., Caso, V., Venti, M., Milia, P., et al. (2004). Dysphagia following stroke. *European Neurology*, 51(3):162-167.

Paik, N.J. (2010). Dysphagia. Available: http://emedicine.com/article/324096-overview

Palmer, J.B., Drennan, J.C., & Baba, M. (2000). Evaluation and treatment of swallowing impairments. *American Family Physician*, 61(8):2453-2462.

Pasricha, P.J. (2001). Prokinetic agents, antiemetics and agents used in irritable bowel syndrome. In J.G. Hardman, L.E. Limbird, & A.G. Gillman (Eds.), *Goodman and Gillman's the pharmacological basis of therapeutics* (10th ed.) (pp. 1021-1035). New York: McGraw-Hill.

Pedersen, A.M., Bardow, A., Beir Jensen, S., & Nauntofte, B. (2002). Saliva and gastrointestinal functions of taste, mastication, swallowing and digestion. *Oral Diseases*, 8(3):117-129.

Peters, G.L., Rosselli, J.L., & Kerr, J.L. (2010). Overview of peptic ulcer disease. *U.S. Pharmacist*, December:29-43.

Peura, D.A. (2007). The constipation conundrum: What now in chronic constipation and IBS-C. *U.S. Pharmacist-Self Study Supplement*, September:3-12.

Ravich, W. (1997). Esophageal dysphagia. In M.E. Groher (Ed.), *Dysphagia, diagnoses and management* (3rd ed.) (pp. 107-129). Boston: Butterworth-Heinemann.

Rooney, J., & Johnson, P. (2000). Potentiation of the dysphagia process through psychotropic use in the long term care facility. *ASHA Special Interest Division 13 Dysphagia Newsletter*, 9(3):4-6.

Rosenvinge, S.K., & Starke, I.D. (2005). Improving care for patients with dysphagia. *Age and Aging*, 34(6):587-593.

Schlesselman, L.S. (2008). Certolizumab pegol: A pegolated anti-TNF-alpha antibody fragment for the treatment of Crohn's disease. *Formulary*, 43:22-28.

Sharley, K.A., & Wallace, J.L. (2011). Treatment of disorders of bowel motility and water flux: Antiemetics agents used in biliary and pancreatic disease. In J.G. Hardman, L.E. Limbird, & A.G. Gillman (Eds.), *Goodman and Gillman's the pharmacological basis of therapeutics* (12th ed.) (pp. 1323-1349). New York: McGraw-Hill.

Sheikh, S., Allen, E., Shell, R., Hruschak, J., Iram, D., Castile, R., et al. (2001). Chronic aspiration without gastroesophageal reflux as a cause of chronic respiratory symptoms in neurologically normal infants. *Chest*, 120(4):1190-1195.

Short, T.P., & Thomas, E. (1992). An overview of the role of calcium antagonists in the treatment of achalasia and diffuse esophageal spasm. *Drugs*, 43(2):177-184.

Siepler, J.K. (2002). Gastroesophageal reflux disease. In M.M. Richardson & C.C. Chant (Eds.), *Pharmacotherapy self-assessment program. Book 8: Gastroenterology and nutrition* (4th ed.) (pp. 1-28). Kansas City, MO: American College of Clinical Pharmacy.

Spieker, M.R. (2000). Evaluating dysphagia. *American Family Physician*, 61(12):3639-3648.

Terrado, M., Russell, C., & Bowman, J.B. (2001). Dysphagia: An overview. *MedSurg Nursing*, 10(5):233-248.

Vogel, D., Carter, J.E., & Carter, P.B. (2000). *The effects of drugs on communication disorders*. San Diego; Singular.

Wald, A., Kamm, M.A., Muller-Lissner, S.A., Scarpignato, C., Marx, W., & Schuijt, C. (2006). The BI Omnibus study:

An international survey of community prevalence of constipation and laxative use in adults. *Digestive Disorders Week*, May:368-371.

Wallace, J.L., & Sharkey, K.A. (2011). Pharmacotherapy of gastric acidity, peptic ulcers, and gastroesophageal reflux disease. In J.G. Hardman, L.E. Limbird, & A.G. Gillman (Eds.), *Goodman and Gillman's the pharmacological basis of therapeutics* (12th ed.) (pp. 1309-1322). New York: McGraw-Hill.

Wender, R. (2009). Do current antiemetic practices result in positive patient outcomes? Results of a new study. *American Journal of Health-System Pharmacy*, 66(Suppl.):S3-S10.

Wilkins, T., Gillies, R.A., Thomas, A.M., & Wagner, P.J. (2007). The prevalence of dysphagia in primary care patients: A Hamesnet Research Network study. *Journal of the American Board of Family Medicine*, 20(2):144-150.

Williams, D.B. (2002). Gastroesophageal reflux disease. In J.T. DiPiro, R.L. Talbert, G.C. Yee, G.R. Matske, B.G. Wells, & L.M. Posey (Eds.), *Pharmacotherapy: A pathophysiologic approach* (5th ed.) (pp. 585-602). Stamford, CT: Appleton & Lange.

Williams, N.T. (2010). Probiotics. *American Journal of Health-System Pharmacy*, 67(6):449-458.

Willoughby, J.T. (1983). Drug induced abnormalities of taste sensation. *Adverse Drug Reaction Bulletin*, 2:368-371.

Wood, B. (2010). Eosinophilic esophagitis: A new disease. *U.S. Pharmacist*, December:44-50.

Appendix

Anderson, C.R., Morris, R.L., Boch, S.D., Panus, P.C., & Sembrowich, W.I. (2003). Effects of iontophoresis current magnitude and duration on dexamethasone deposition and localized drug retention. *Physical Therapy*, 83(2):161-170.

Ballerini, R., Casini, A., Chinol, M., Mannucci, C., Giaccai, L., & Salvi, M. (1986). Study on the absorption of ketoprofen topically administered in man: Comparison between tissue and plasma levels. *International Journal of Clinical Pharmacology Research*, 6(1):69-72.

Banga, A.K. (2011). *Transdermal and intradermal delivery of therapeutic agents: Application of physical technologies* (pp. 171-193). Boca Raton, FL: CRC Press.

Byl, N.N., McKenzie, A., Halliday, B., Wong, T., & O'Connell, J. (1993). The effects of phonophoresis with corticosteroids: A controlled pilot study. *Journal of Orthopaedic Sports Physical Therapy*, 18(5):590-600.

Cagnie, B., Vinck, E., Rimbaut, S., & Vanderstraeten, G. (2003). Phonophoresis versus topical application of ketoprofen: Comparison between tissue and plasma levels. *Physical Therapy*, 83(8):701-712.

Cameron, M.H. (2009). *Physical agents in rehabilitation* (3rd ed.). St. Louis: Saunders.

Cameron, M.H., & Monroe, L.G. (1992). Relative transmission of ultrasound by media customarily used for phonophoresis. *Physical Therapy*, 72(2):142-148.

Ciccone, C.D. (2008). Electrical stimulation for the delivery of medications: Iontophoresis. In A.J. Robinson & L. Snyder-Mackler (Eds.), *Clinical electrophysiology* (3rd ed.) (pp. 351-388). Philadelphia, PA: Lippincott Williams & Wilkins.

Costa, I.A., & Dyson, A. (2007). The integration of acetic acid iontophoresis, orthotic therapy and physical rehabilitation for chronic plantar fasciitis: A case study. *Journal of Canadian Chiropractic Association*, 51(3):166-174.

Darrow, H., Schulties, S., Draper, D., Ricard, M., & Measom, G.J. (1999). Serum dexamethasone levels after decadron phonophoresis. *Journal of Athletic Training*, 34(4):338-341.

Franklin, M.E., Smith, S.T., Chenier, T.C., & Franklin, R.C. (1995). Effects of phonophoresis with dexamethasone on adrenal function. *Journal of Orthopaedic Sports Physical Therapy*, 22(3):103-107.

Gallo, J.A., Draper, D.O., Brody, L.T., & Fellingham, G.W. (2004). A comparison of human muscle temperature increases during 3-MHz continuous and pulsed ultrasound with equivalent temporal average intensities. *Journal of Orthopaedic Sports Physical Therapy*, 34(7):395-401.

Glass, J.M., Stephen, R.L., & Jacobsen, S.C. (1980). The quality and distribution of radio labeled dexamethasone delivered to tissue by iontophoresis. *International Journal of Dermatology*, 19(9):519-525.

Gulick, D.T. (2000). Effects of acetic acid iontophoresis on heel spur reabsorption. *Physical Therapy Case Reports*, 3(2):64-70.

Gurney, B., & Wascher, D.C. (2008). Absorption of dexamethasone sodium phosphate in human connective tissue using iontophoresis. *American Journal of Sports Medicine*, 36(4):753-759.

Japour, C.L., Vohra, R., Vohra, P.K., Garfunkle, L., & Chin, N. (1999). Management of heel pain syndrome with acetic acid iontophoresis. *Journal of American Podiatric Medical Association*, 89(5):251-257.

Myrer, W.J., Measom, G.J., & Fellingham, G.W. (2001) Intramuscular temperature rises with topical analgesics used as coupling agents during therapeutic ultrasound. *Journal of Athletic Training*, 36(1):20-26.

Nirschl, R.P., Rodin, D.M., & Ochiai, D.H. (2003). Iontophoretic administration of dexamethasone sodium phosphate for acute epicondylitis: A randomized double blinded, placebo controlled study. *American Journal of Sports Medicine*, 31(2):189-195.

Panus, P.C., Campbell J., Kulkami, S.B., Herrick, R.T., Ravis, W.R., & Banga A.K. (1997). Transdermal iontophoretic delivery of ketoprofen through human cadaver skin and in humans. *Journal of Controlled Release*, 44(2-3):113-121.

Panus, P.C., Ferslew, K.E., Tober-Meyer, B., & Kao, R.L. (1999). Ketoprofen tissue permeation in swine following cathodic iontophoresis. *Physical Therapy*, 79(1):40-49.

Saliba, S., Mistry, D.J., Perrin, D.H., Giek, J., & Weltman, A. (2007). Phonophoresis and absorption of dexamethasone in the presence of an occlusive dressing. *Journal of Athletic Training*, 42(3):349-354.

Starkey, C. (2004). *Therapeutic modalities* (3rd ed.). Philadelphia: Davis.

Tannenbaum, M. (1980). Iodine iontophoresis in reduction of scar tissue. *Physical Therapy*, 60(6):792.

INDEX

Subject Index
Page numbers followed by a *t* indicate a
table.

ABOUT THE AUTHORS

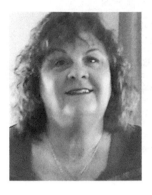

Lynette L. Carl, BS, PharmD, BCPS, CP, is an assistant professor of clinical practice at the University of Florida College of Pharmacy and an adjunct faculty member teaching pharmacotherapeutics at South University in Tampa, Florida.

Carl has more than 25 years of experience as a clinical pharmacist and consultant pharmacist. In 1997, Carl became a board-certified pharmacotherapy specialist, the highest accomplishment for a clinical pharmacist.

Carl has many years of experience in pharmacy management and in providing patient care as a clinical pharmacy specialist. She has significant experience in developing clinical pharmacy programs to improve clinical pharmacy practice and patient care. She is a frequent presenter on medication use to professionals and students of many disciplines in health care. Carl coauthored a text on drugs and dysphagia and is working on a second text covering medication-induced dysphagia in pediatrics.

Carl is a member of the American College of Clinical Pharmacy, American Society of Health-System Pharmacists, Florida Society of Health-System Pharmacists, Southwest Society of Health-System Pharmacists, American Society for Parenteral and Enteral Nutrition, and the Florida Society for Parenteral and Enteral Nutrition.

In her spare time, Carl enjoys traveling, snorkeling, fishing, and playing with her dogs. She and her husband, Randel Sturgeon, reside in Indian Rocks Beach, Florida.

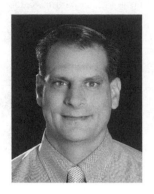

Joseph A. Gallo, DSc, ATC, PT, earned his doctorate degree in sport physical therapy, his master's degree in physical therapy, and his bachelor of science degree in physical education and athletic training. He serves as director and associate professor of the athletic training program in the sport and movement science department at Salem State University in Salem, Massachusetts. Dr. Gallo has served as an adjunct faculty member in the Notre Dame College physical therapy program and Franklin Pierce University doctor of physical therapy program. He was an instructor and director of rehabilitation for the Keene State College athletic training program in Keene, New Hampshire, and professor and director of the Hesser College physical therapist assistant program. Gallo also worked as a high school and college athletic trainer and delivered rehabilitation services in outpatient clinics, subacute settings, and in-home settings. Gallo has published his research in the *Journal of Orthopaedic & Sports Physical Therapy* and the *Chinese Journal of Sports Medicine*. He is a nationally recognized speaker who has presented over 300 courses to rehabilitation professionals throughout the United States. Gallo is currently a certified instructor for the VitalStim certification course teaching NMES for the treatment of dysphagia. He is also a United States Professional Tennis Association teaching professional, the founder and director of Summer's Edge Tennis School, and the men's tennis coach for Salem State University. Joe enjoys running, playing tennis, hiking, and camping with his wife, Gina. They live in Salem, Massachusetts.

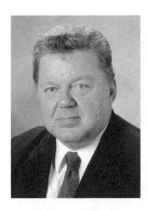

Peter R. Johnson, PhD, CCC-SLP, earned his MS and PhD in speech-language pathology from the University of Pittsburgh and an executive graduate degree in health care financial management from Ohio State University. He has worked in acute-care hospitals, home care, outpatient clinics, and long-term care and has written numerous articles on rehabilitation. Johnson served as a column editor for the American Speech-Language-Hearing Association Special Interest Division (ASHA SID) 13 Dysphagia newsletter and for the ASHA SID 11 newsletter. He was on the executive board of the Florida Association of Speech-Language Pathologists and Audiologists. He is a three-time recipient of the President's Award and the Outstanding Service Award.

Johnson has coauthored two books, *Business Matters: A Guide for Speech–Language Pathologists* and *Drugs and Dysphagia: How Medications Can Affect Eating and Swallowing*. He is currently working on another book on cognition and dementia.

Johnson has lectured at various hospitals and universities on the subject of cognition, dysphagia, and polypharmacy. He is currently the speech mentor for Select Medical Rehabilitation Services, where he develops continuing education programs as well as one-to-one mentoring. He is also the vice chair of the Florida Department of Health licensing board for speech-language pathologists and audiologists. Johnson is an adjunct faculty and dissertation chair for Nova Southeastern University.

Johnson enjoys sailing, reading, and teaching. He and his wife, Joanne, live in Port Richey, Florida.

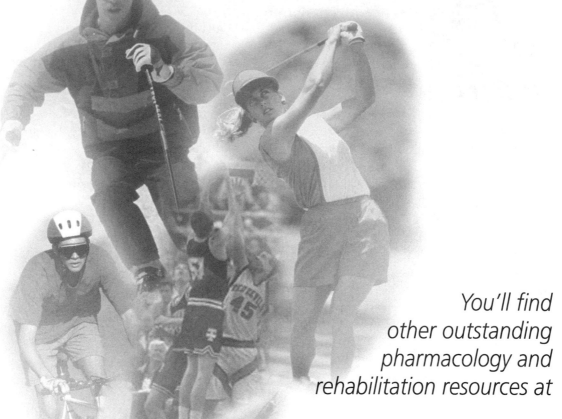